Clinical Naturopathy:
an evidence-based guide to practice

Clinical Naturopathy:
an evidence-based guide to practice

Jerome Sarris • Jon Wardle

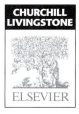

Sydney   Edinburgh   London   New York   Philadelphia   St Louis   Toronto

Disclaimer

Complementary medicine and pharmacology are ever-changing fields. Standard safety precautions must be followed but, as new research and clinical experience broaden our knowledge, changes in treatment become necessary or appropriate. The authors and publisher have, in so far as it is possible, taken every care to ensure that the information contained within the text is as accurate and as up-to-date as possible. Readers are, however, advised to always check available product information with the herb, supplement or drug manufacturer to verify the recommended dose, the method and duration of administration, and contraindications. It is the responsibility of the treating person to determine dosages and the best treatment for the patient. Neither the publisher nor the editors assume any responsibility for any injury and/or damage to persons or property.

Churchill Livingstone
is an imprint of Elsevier

Elsevier Australia. ACN 001 002 357
(a division of Reed International Books Australia Pty Ltd)
Tower 1, 475 Victoria Avenue, Chatswood, NSW 2067

National Library of Australia Cataloguing-in-Publication Data

Sarris, Jerome.

Clinical naturopathy: an evidence-based guide to practice/
        Jerome Sarris, Jon Wardle.

ISBN: 978 0 7295 3926 5 (pbk.)

Includes index.
Bibliography.

Naturopathy.

Wardle, Jon.

615.535

Publisher: Sophie Kaliniecki
Developmental Editor: Sabrina Chew
Publishing Services Manager: Helena Klijn
Editorial Coordinator: Eleanor Cant
Edited by Joy Window
Proofread by Tim Learner
Design by Lisa Petroff
Index by Master Indexing
Typeset by TNQ Books and Journals
Printed by 1010 Printing International

CONTENTS

FOREWORD

Naturopathy, the subject of this book, is an eclectic healthcare practice, the scope of which differs somewhat in different parts of the world. In Australia, the two core modalities of naturopathy are herbal medicine (phytotherapy) and nutritional medicine. A key feature of naturopathy is the holistic approach to the patient, who is not simply seen as a biological organism but also as an emotional and social being, whose health is affected by many external factors. Accordingly, treatments are highly individualised to meet the specific needs of each individual patient.

Naturopathy, and complementary and alternative medicine (CAM) in general, has come a long way in the last couple of decades. When I first developed an interest in natural and complementary medicine, some 30 years ago, it was undeniably fringe in the Western industrialised world. It was a kind of underground, alternative health movement, the followers of which were mostly people who led rather alternative lifestyles or at least had a somewhat alternative outlook on life in general. Natural and complementary medicine, or alternative medicine as it was mostly known then, had little and mostly acrimonious interaction with mainstream healthcare, and medical practitioners in particular were mostly scathing about the ineffectiveness and dangers of these 'unproven' therapies and medicines. There were exceptions, of course. In some European countries, homoeopathy was embraced by many medical practitioners, and in Germany general practitioners were prescribing large amounts of herbal medicines, as had always been the norm. But this kind of practice was considered to be neither alternative, complementary, natural nor fringe, because it was perpetrated by medical doctors.

Globally, the situation back then was very different, and indeed this remains the case. Many therapies that in the West are considered part of CAM are in other parts of the world traditional medical systems. It is estimated that more than 80% of the world's population still depends on traditional medicine for their primary healthcare. The traditional medical system that serves the largest number of people in this way today is undoubtedly traditional Chinese medicine.

It is somewhat ironic that herbal medicine is considered to be part of CAM in most Western countries, because pharmacy and the pharmaceutical industry both have their roots in herbal medicine and a large proportion of modern pharmaceutical drugs are still directly or indirectly derived from plant compounds.

In Australia, the developments in naturopathy and other CAM practices over the past two decades have been consumer driven. Despite these modalities being excluded from the public health insurance scheme, Australian healthcare consumers have clearly demonstrated that they want CAM to be part of the available health services, even if they have to bear the entire cost. Survey data show that two-thirds of Australian adults use some form of CAM, that the total number of visits to CAM practitioners and medical practitioners are equal, and that Australians spend in excess of $4 billion on CAM annually.[1]

Naturopathy is not only one of the largest CAM professions in Australia, but also among the fastest growing, with the number of naturopathic practitioners increasing by 56% between 1996 and 2006.[2]

In response to the consumer demand for CAM, Southern Cross University in 1995 started its Bachelor of Naturopathy program, the first of its kind in a publicly funded university in the Western world. Today, an increasing number of qualified naturopaths attain postgraduate qualifications including doctorates, a fact well illustrated by the editors and many of the contributors to this work. Naturopathic practitioners now interact extensively with other health professionals, and most private health funds offer rebates for naturopathic consultations. Consumers increasingly want the best of both worlds: integrated healthcare that optimises outcomes.

The publication of this text is another indication that the naturopathic profession is coming of age. There are still precious few books on naturopathy that are written as scholarly texts. Documenting and consolidating the body of knowledge of a discipline in scholarly texts is an important step in the process of professionalisation, and this text makes a significant contribution in this regard.

The reference to evidence-based practice in the title is particularly noteworthy. Being an eclectic discipline, naturopathy draws upon both traditional knowledge and scientific data, including findings from clinical research. Some may find the suggestion that the practice of naturopathy can be evidence-based a contradiction in terms. On the other hand, some naturopaths may approach the notion of evidence-based naturopathic practice with great caution and scepticism, concerned that the potent paradigm of evidence-based healthcare will destroy the very core of naturopathic practice, with its emphasis on holism and individualised treatment.

This concern is understandable, because the face of evidence-based medicine to a large extent is the systematic review of randomised controlled trials. Naturopathy is not well supported by this type of evidence, because the randomised controlled trial as a research method is not readily applied to a practice characterised by highly individualised treatments. However, naturopaths would be well advised to familiarise themselves with the full definition of evidence-based medicine. It not only calls for clinical decision making to be based on the best available research evidence, but also for the integration of this information with the clinical expertise of the practitioner and the values and circumstances of the patient. If the term 'evidence' is taken to include traditional knowledge from a history of use in a traditional medical system (the approach adopted by the Therapeutic Goods Administration in the regulation of complementary medicines in Australia), then the concept of evidence-based naturopathic practice should become widely acceptable to practitioners.

Practising in an evidence-based paradigm also means having the ability to critically evaluate information and the willingness to re-evaluate treatments as new evidence becomes available. There is no doubt that some practices that are widespread today will be modified or abandoned in the future, because new evidence will demonstrate that they are ineffective or unsafe. In this respect naturopathy is no different from conventional medicine. The shared goal must be to provide patients with effective and safe treatments.

This text will greatly assist practitioners and students in developing their naturopathic practice in an evidence-based framework. It takes a systems-based approach and features unique key treatment protocols outlining the naturopathic approaches to each condition. This is supported by treatment decision trees and evidence tables that summarise major treatments in an easily accessible format.

I congratulate the editors and contributors on what is an important milestone in the continuing development of naturopathic medicine.

Hans Wohlmuth, PhD
School of Health and Human Sciences
Southern Cross University
Lismore, New South Wales

References

1. Australian Bureau of Statistics (2008). Australian social trends: complementary therapies. Available from: http://www.abs.gov.au/AUSSTATS/abs@.nsf/DetailsPage/4102.02008?OpenDocument

2. Xue CCL, et al. Complementary and alternative medicine use in Australia: a national population-based survey. *Journal of Alternative and Complementary Medicine* 2007;13:643–650.

PREFACE

The practice of naturopathy is developing from a traditional healing art into an evidence-based science. While the clinical application of naturopathy is becoming more homogenised with medical science, this need not be at the expense of its intrinsic core principles—'treating the causes, and the whole person', or 'supporting the body/mind to heal itself via the least harmful methods'. Indeed, naturopathy takes its very name from one of these principles—'nature cure'.

While books exist detailing the evidence of individual complementary or alternative medicines (CAM) such as herbal medicines or nutrients, currently few books exist that explore in any great depth the principles and processes involving the clinical practice of naturopathy. Naturopathic practice is defined far more by the principles it adopts in the treatment process, rather than the specific interventions used. It was our intention to publish a book that not only detailed the evidence of common CAM interventions, but also explored the key protocols and integrative methods used by naturopaths in treating disease and illness.

The differences between orthodox and holistic medicine is evident even beyond the interventions used. As practitioners and users of CAM services would attest to, while conventional medicine concentrates on a reductive process in diagnosis and treatment (with often a symptomatic focus), naturopaths perceive causes of ill health as being multifactorial; bodily systems are regarded as interrelated, and it is accepted that psychological, social, environmental and spiritual aspects strongly influence health. With respect to the intricacies of naturopathic practice, the diagnostic art is often complex. For example, a conventional medical practitioner may treat a patient's headache symptomatically with an analgesic; in contrast a CAM practitioner may take a detailed case study involving an analysis of signs and symptoms from various bodily systems (in addition to transpersonal elements). In this example, they may conclude that the cause of the headache may involve many factors such as poor sleep posture, a dietary intolerance, dehydration and anxiety from an external stressor. An individualised treatment would then be subsequently formulated to address the underlying causes and the symptoms.

The purpose of this text was to articulate 'evidence-based' clinical practice (principles, treatment protocols and interventions) in a reader-friendly format for the practitioner, academic and student. To this end, naturopathic leaders in their fields were chosen to facilitate the dissemination of broad clinical expertise in conjunction with evidence-based guidelines. While universal structure and formatting were broadly standardised, each contributor was granted a degree of autonomy to allow them to manifest their expertise. This may be observed, for example, in subtle differences in the decision tree or evidence box styles in the various chapters. At times throughout the development of the manuscript there were difficult decisions about what constitutes 'core naturopathic practice'. Given the international scope of this text we thought it appropriate to focus on those core therapeutic modalities that are most likely to be universally engaged by naturopaths. Thereby, this text focuses on nutritional, dietary, herbal and lifestyle treatments, making mention of other therapeutic options where appropriate. While it is acknowledged that other therapies such as homoeopathy, physical manipulation and traditional Chinese medicine are practised by naturopaths in various jurisdictions, we considered these as distinct and separate modalities, often acknowledging them as 'integrative treatments' in the chapters.

The introductory section on 'case taking' and 'naturopathic diagnostic techniques' provides a platform to understand the practice of naturopathy. The body of the book is structured around body systems such as the digestive system, with two or three important health conditions within that system treated. The use of a case study is employed to give a clinical context to the condition covered in the chapter (rather than focusing on the treatment of a specialised case). The next section focuses on specialised conditions such as cancer and autommunity—conditions that are generally not constrained by systematic categorisation. A subsequent section is about special considerations for patients at various stages of the life cycle (paediatrics, fertility and ageing), highlighting the varying foundational requirements for growth, development and optimal function at these different life stages. The final section explores the interwoven tapestry of naturopathic and orthodox medical practice used in an integrative manner to treat serious diseases such as HIV and cancer. As readers will note, the book contains many sections on material that has rarely or never before been published, such as pain management, in-depth case-taking protocols, practical assessment of drug-CAM interactions and integrative treatment of psychiatric disorders. This innovation extends to the appendices, which include clinically relevant information such as diagnostic ranges for standard pathology tests and nutrient status, a CAM–chemotherapeutic interaction chart, a drug–CAM interaction chart and traditional Chinese medicine diagnostic figures.

A strength of this book is that it explores the key principles and philosophies utilised in modern naturopathy for the treatment of a range of conditions. The essence of this is detailed in the 'Key treatment protocols' section in each chapter. An additional strength is the critical evaluation of the current evidence of both the naturopathic diagnostic and practice methods, and CAM interventions. This differentiates *Clinical Naturopathy: an evidence-based guide to practice* from some other publications that, while informative, often do not provide an evidence-based, referenced critique of the treatment protocols or CAM interventions.

To provide a balanced and truly academic discussion, the limitations of the book must be outlined. First, it is recognised that it is not possible to detail all possible diseases and illnesses that are encountered in clinical practice. However, as all naturopaths know, 'people' are treated, not 'diseases', and each person manifests a unique combination of variations of signs and symptoms rather than a solitary diagnosed disease. Regardless, categorisation by major diseases and illnesses is a necessity to provide a framework with which to discuss naturopathic treatment protocols and interventions. The protocols and principles discussed in each chapter will in many cases be clinically relevant to the treatment of various other conditions.

With respect to the evidence reviewed, it should be noted that we focus primarily on the major evidence from clinical trials over that of in vivo or in vitro studies. Traditional evidence is discussed when relevant. It will be apparent to the reader that not every method, diagnostic technique or intervention included in this book has solid clinical evidence. Some methods such as iridology have only emerging evidence, and some herbal medicines or nutrients have only traditional evidence. This is recognised by us. Where scientific evidence is deficient, this is highlighted. To ignore those treatments and practices that form core parts of modern naturopathic practice based purely on their foundation of traditional over modern scientific evidence would be remiss. For example, discussing naturopathic treatment of many gastrointestinal disorders without referencing *Ulmus fulva* (slippery elm), or talking about female reproductive disorders without referencing the role of 'anti-spasmodics' or 'uterine tonics', would be unrepresentative of contemporary naturopathic practice. Research is undoubtedly the best way to uncover 'new knowledge' and test 'old knowledge'. One of the developments we hope to see arise from this text (which catalogues many contemporary naturopathic treatments) is a further interest in conducting research that accurately reflects and tests naturopathic clinical practice.

A significant challenge in the construction of the manuscript was to find the balance between traditional practice and modern practice. Some practitioners of naturopathy prefer an intuitive approach using their self-evolved diagnostics and treatment protocols, and folkloric prescriptions; others may be more biomedically trained, strictly using interventions that have clinically validated evidence. We have done our best to balance these sometimes competing perspectives of naturopathic practice by maintaining the principles of holistic practice in concert with modern clinical evidence. Of course the argument over what constitutes 'evidence' is a book of its own, and a Pandora's box that for now we will leave sealed ...

We aimed to make this an easy-to-read clinical text, and because of this the use of p values and effect sizes were omitted from the narrative and limited to the evidence tables. In light of this, the term 'significant' was used when an intervention was revealed to have a p value of < 0.05 (likely to occur less than 5% due to chance). As this is meant to be a clinical reference, rather than a purely academic tome, detailed analysis of each and every trial was not entered into. However, all treatments have been duly referenced and readers are encouraged to explore these further. A selection of relevant further reading has been listed by individual contributors for those who wish to investigate chapter content even further. With over 4500 references we believe this to be a positive direction—albeit a small foundational one—towards the development of evidence-based naturopathic practice.

The future direction of naturopathy and CAM appears positive, with mainstream acceptance evolving in countries such Australia, USA, UK, Germany, Canada and South Africa. To maintain the evolution of the profession and to enable more effective healers, education is paramount. *Clinical Naturopathy: an evidence-based guide to practice* was developed to be at the forefront of naturopathic education in the 21st century. This book is designed for the naturopath, the allied health or orthodox medical practitioner, the researcher and anyone with an interest in principles, practices and treatments of natural medicine. Enjoy!

Jerome Sarris and Jon Wardle

ACKNOWLEDGEMENTS

For my father Mark – This dragon is slain for you
For Kath – My muse who inspires me in ways she does not even realise

We would like to thank the contributors who helped to shape *Clinical Naturopathy* into a unique contribution to the field. We would also like to thank the countless peers that assisted us in the creative process, through kind words, scholarly advice or simply putting up with our many personalities that the project unearthed. Thanks are also extended to the talented and supportive Elsevier staff: Eleanor Cant, Sophie Kaliniecki, Sunalie Silva, Joy Window and particularly Sabrina Chew for their tireless efforts throughout the development of the manuscript. Finally, we would like to acknowledge all of the students, practitioners and academics who strive to evolve and enhance their knowledge of the art and science of naturopathy for the easing of human suffering and the betterment of humanity.

ABOUT THE EDITORS

Jerome Sarris ND (ACNM), PhD (UQ), MHSc HMed (UNE), Adv Dip Acu (ACNM), MNHAA
NHMRC Research Fellow, Faculty of Medicine, Department of Psychiatry, The University of Melbourne and Brain Sciences Institute, Swinburne University of Technology, Victoria
Formerly Researcher, Lecturer, School of Medicine, Department of Psychiatry, The University of Queensland, Australia

Jerome has practised as a clinical naturopath and acupuncturist, and currently researches, publishes and lectures internationally in the area of CAM and integrative medicine in mental health, in particular depression and anxiety. He has coordinated and conducted a number of clinical trials involving herbal medicines, and holds a prestigious NHMRC Australian Clinical Research Fellowship.

Jon Wardle ND (ACNM), MPH (UQ)
NHMRC Public Health Research Scholar, School of Population Health, University of Queensland
Director, Research Capacity Building Stream, Network of Researchers in the Public Health of Complementary and Alternative Medicine (NORPHCAM)
Trans-Pacific Fellow, School of Medicine, University of Washington
Naturopathic Practitioner, Herbs on the Hill, Brisbane, Queensland

Jon practises as a naturopath in Brisbane and is a National Health and Medical Research Council Public Health Scholar at the School of Population Health, University of Queensland. He is a founding Director of the Network of Researchers in the Public Health of Complementary and Alternative Medicine (NORPHCAM) and is on the editorial board of several journals, including the International Journal of Naturopathic Medicine. Jon lectures internationally on CAM and writes several popular Australian health columns, in addition to his academic publishing endeavours.

CONTRIBUTORS

Michael Alexander ND, BPharm, MNHAA , MACNEM, MAIPM
Adjunct Lecturer, Faculty of Pharmacy, Latrobe University
Pharmacist, Naturopathic practitioner, Victoria, Australia

Leslie Axelrod ND, LAc
Professor of Clinical Sciences, Southwest College of Naturopathic Medicine
Private practitioner, Arizona, USA

Michelle Boyd ND (ACNM), GCert HEd (UQ), MNHAA
Lecturer, Endeavour College of Natural Health
Private practitioner, Queensland, Australia

Joanne Bradbury ND (CSU), BA (UNSW), BNat(Hons) (SCU)
University of Queensland, Department of Pharmacy and Southern Cross University, New South Wales, Australia

David Casteleijn ND (ACNM), MHSc HMed (UNE)
Lecturer, Faculty of Naturopathy, Endeavour College of Natural Health
Private practitioner, Queensland, Australia

Greg Connolly ND, BA, FANTA
Lecturer and Clinic Supervisor, Southern School of Natural Therapies
Private practitioner, Victoria, Australia

Kieran Cooley ND (CCNM), BSc (UoS)
Associate Director of Research, Assistant Professor, Department of Research and Clinical Epidemiology, Canadian College of Naturopathic Medicine, Toronto, Ontario, Canada

Jane Daley ND (CSU), DBM (NCC), GradCertAppSc (SUT), MNHAA
Lecturer, Faculty of Naturopathy, Southern School of Natural Therapies
Private practitioner, Victoria, Australia

Gary Deed MBBS (UQ), Dip Herb Med, FACNEM
Integrative medical practitioner, Queensland, Australia
Senior Adjunct Lecturer, School of Health Sciences, RMIT University, Victoria

Tessa Finney-Brown ND (ECNH)
Private practitioner, Queensland, Australia

Tini Gruner ND MSc, DipPsychTher, DipTeach, PhD, MANPA, MNSA
Adjunct Professor, Lecturer, Clinic Supervisor, Course Coordinator, School of Health & Human Sciences, Southern Cross University
Private practitioner, New South Wales, Australia

Jason A. Hawrelak ND (SCU), BNat(Hons), PhD (SCU), MNHAA
Private practitioner, Goulds Naturopathica, Tasmania, Australia

Jennifer Hillier BHSc (QUK), ND (CCNM)
Clinic Faculty and Assistant Professor, Canadian College of Naturopathic Medicine, Toronto, Ontario, Canada
Private practitioner, Canada

Christina Kure ND (SSNT), BAppSci (SUT)
National Institute of Complementary Medicine (NICM) Collaborative Centre for the Study of Natural Medicines and Neurocognition in Health and Disease, Swinburne University of Technology, Victoria, Australia

James Lake MD
Adjunct Clinical Assistant Professor, Department of Psychiatry and Behavioral Sciences, Stanford
Clinical Assistant Professor, Department of Medicine, Arizona Center for Integrative Medicine
Chair, American Psychiatric Association Caucus on Complementary, Alternative and Integrative Medicine, California, USA

Matthew J. Leach ND, RN, BN(Hons), Dip Clin Nutr, PhD, MATMS
Registered Nurse, Naturopath
Research Fellow, School of Nursing and Midwifery University of South Australia, South Australia, Australia

Vicki Mortimer ND (NCC, CSU), RN, RM (Sydney, Edinburgh)
Head of Program and Lecturer in naturopathy, University of Western Sydney
Naturopathy Clinical Manager, University of Western Sydney, New South Wales, Australia

Paul J. Orrock ND (NSWCNT), DBM, MAppSc (VU), GCert HEd (SCU)
Senior Lecturer, School of Health and Human Sciences—Natural and Complementary Medicine, Southern Cross University
Private practitioner, New South Wales, Australia

Jerome Sarris ND (ACNM), PhD (UQ), MHSc HMed (UNE), Adv Dip Acu (ACNM), MNHAA
NHMRC Research Fellow, Faculty of Medicine, Department of Psychiatry, The University of Melbourne, and Brain Sciences Institute, Swinburne University of Technology, Victoria, Australia
Formerly Researcher, Lecturer, School of Medicine, Department of Psychiatry, The University of Queensland

Janet Schloss ND (ACNM), Dip Nut (ACNM), PGrad Cert Nut (RMIT), BARM (GU)
Lecturer, Endeavour College of Natural Health
Private practitioner, Queensland, Australia

Niikee Schoendorfer ND (CSU), MHSc NMed (UNE), GCert HEd (UQ), Nutr Dip (ACNM)
Children's Nutrition Research Centre, School of Medicine, University of Queensland
Lecturer, Endeavour College of Natural Health, Queensland, Australia

Justin Sinclair ND, MHerbMed (USyd), BHSc (UNE), DBM, DRM, Dip Nut, Dip Hom (ACNT), MNHAA, MATMS
Senior Lecturer, Faculty of Naturopathy, School of Holistic Medicine, Endeavour College of Natural Health, Queensland, Australia

Amie Steel ND (ACNM), MPH (UQ), MANTA
Sessional Lecturer, Faculty of Holistic Medicine, Endeavour College of Natural Health, Queensland
Private practitioner, Queensland, Australia

Jon Wardle ND (ACNM), MPH (UQ)
NHMRC Public Health Research Scholar, School of Population Health, University of Queensland
Director, Research Capacity Building Stream, Network of Researchers in the Public Health of Complementary and Alternative Medicine (NORPHCAM)
Trans-Pacific Fellow, School of Medicine, University of Washington
Naturopathic practitioner, Herbs on the Hill, Queensland, Australia

REVIEWERS

Sandy Davidson ND, Grad Dip Pub Health, Adv Dip Naturopathy
Naturopathic practitioner and lecturer at Australasian College of Natural Therapies and Nature Care College, NSW, Australia

Jane Hills ND (ACNT), BHSc (UNE), MATMS
Lecturer, Faculty of Natural Therapies, Australasian College of Natural Therapies, NSW, Australia
Private Practitioner, NSW, Australia

Rebecca Hughes ND (SCU), MNHAA
Teacher, Advanced Diploma of Naturopathy, Canberra Institute of Technology, ACT
Private practitioner, ACT, Australia

Siobhan Jordan ND (NCC), BHSc (CSU), Dip Nut (NCC), Grad Cert PHC (Flinders University), MATMS
Private practitioner and health writer, NSW, Australia

Steve Lawson MEd, BSc(CompMed), AdvDipNat, GradDipMFR, GradDipCST, DTS, DRM
Director of Education, Nature Care College, Australia

Phil Rasmussen MPharm, MNIMH, MPS, Dip Herb Med, MNHAA, MNZAMH
Medical herbalist and pharmacist, Auckland
Honorary Lecturer, Faculty of Health Sciences, University of Auckland, Auckland

Ses Salmond ND (NCC), Dip Bot Med (NCC), Dip Nutri (NCC), BA (MU), FNHAA
Senior Lecturer, Western Herbal Medicine Department, Nature Care College, NSW
Herbalist, naturopath and homoeopath, Leichhardt Women's Community Health Centre, NSW
Private practitioner, NSW, Australia

Alicia Tan BNat (SCU), MANTA
Teacher, Centre for Health, Community and Wellbeing, Canberra Institute of Technology, ACT, Australia
Private practitioner, natural medicine Consultant, ACT and internationally

P. Spero Tsindos ND (NSWCNM) GCert Health Promotion (Deakin), GCert Education (UQ), MPH (Deakin), MANPA
Program leader, Department of Occidental Medicine, Endeavour College of Natural Health, Melbourne
Private practitioner, Victoria, Australia

Samantha Warner ND (PANT), MANTA
Lecturer, Paramount College and Australian Institute of Holistic Medicine, WA
Private practitioner, Western Australia

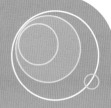

PART A
Naturopathic clinical skills

The practice of any therapeutic modality is as much art as it is science. Previously, the practice of traditional natural medicine took little time to learn, but a lifetime to master. Young apprentices would sit at the feet of practitioners with a broad mastery of clinical experience and learn this art firsthand. Modern graduates can now 'learn' naturopathic practice in an intensive manner (and the content is increasing all the time), but this should not be viewed as a replacement of an art that takes years to master. While the balance of naturopathic education has shifted in modern times to a broader scientific and evidence-based paradigm, the profession must remain diligent that this does not come at the expense of the underpinning traditional principles.

Case taking has been included in this section as it forms the core foundation of naturopathic practice; most of the information required for treatment can be elicited through the interview and patient observation. Comprehensive case taking has long been one of the strengths of naturopathic practice and is the reason traditionally a naturopathic consultation takes considerably longer than a conventional one. The naturopathic consultation allows the practitioner to 'release their inner detective', narrowing down health suspects until an underlying cause or causes can be found. The consultation process itself can also be therapeutic—and 'non-specific' effects from the therapeutic relationship can provide up to one-third of the outcome in every consultation. This can be a powerful tool for the practitioner if mastered properly.

One of the key challenges to any emerging and rapidly growing profession is reconciling traditional and emerging knowledge. Contemporary naturopathic practice makes use of new scientific diagnostic techniques while also paying homage to traditional knowledge. With respect to diagnostic techniques, practitioners must weigh up factors such as the evidence level of the intervention and the potential discomfort and cost of the process, before deciding on the diagnostic tool. Medical diagnostic procedures (which can sometimes be expensive and invasive) are generally used only when required or when pertinent information cannot be attained via simpler and cheaper means. Contemporary naturopaths are as comfortable using modern and laboratory diagnostic techniques like blood tests or bioimpedance analysis as they are with traditional arts such as tongue diagnosis or iridology. Each of these has a place in contemporary naturopathic practice. However, the art lies in using these tools judiciously—many criticisms of traditional naturopathic diagnostic techniques come not from the use of the techniques themselves, but rather their use in inappropriate circumstances. This part of the book recognises that many of these older and more traditional techniques lack a conventional evidence base, but given their use in contemporary naturopathic medicine it would be remiss to not include them. While their efficacy may be difficult to prove by quantitative studies, these traditional techniques often provide qualitative information on the patient's health and vitality, which when used in combination with scientific-based tools provides a rich diagnostic picture.

By highlighting the way in which naturopathic practitioners can use the case taking method and the appropriate use of diagnostic techniques, this part aims to provide a sound basis for modern clinical naturopathic practice, combining the best of traditional and contemporary techniques in an attempt to marry the art and science of naturopathic practice.

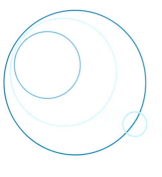

1

Naturopathic case taking

Greg Connolly
BA, ND

NATUROPATHIC PHILOSOPHY AND PRINCIPLES

For naturopaths, the patient-centred approach to case taking with its emphasis on rapport, empathy and authenticity is a vital part of the healing process. It is based not just on current accepted health practices but on the philosophy and principles that have underpinned naturopathy since its beginnings. This chapter examines how to establish and maintain a therapeutic relationship with patients through the process of a holistic consultation in the light of these values and practices. This chapter also presents a model of the structure and process of holistic case taking that will facilitate this consultation and provide both patient and naturopath with the knowledge and insight needed for healing and wellness.

Historical precursors

Having a philosophy by which to practice gives a clearer understanding of what constitutes good health, how illness is caused, what the role of the practitioner should be, and the type of treatments that should be given.[1] Naturopathy has a loosely defined set of principles that have arisen from three interrelated philosophical sources. The first main source is the *historical precursors* of eclectic health-care practices that formed naturopathy in the 19th and 20th centuries.[2] Allied to this are two other essential philosophical concepts intertwined with the historical development of naturopathy: *vitalism*[3,4] and *holism*[5].

The tenets of naturopathic philosophy have developed from its chequered historical background, which includes the traditions of Hippocratic health, herbal medicine, homoeopathy, nature cure, hydrotherapy, dietetics and manipulative therapies.[6] In modern times naturopathic philosophy has borrowed from the social movements of the 1960s and 1970s that fostered independence from authoritative structures and challenged the dependency upon technology and drugs for health care. These social movements emphasised a holistic approach to the environment and ecology with a yearning for health care that was natural and promoted self-reliance harking back to late 19th-century principles of nature care philosophy.[7] Naturopathy also borrowed from other counterculture movements and began to be suffused with New Age themes of transpersonal and humanistic psychology, spirituality, metaphysics and new science paradigms.[8] Since the 1980s naturopathy has increasingly used scientific research to increase understanding of body systems and validate treatments.[9,10]

From this variety of sources, naturopathy has consolidated a number of core principles. These principles have had many diverse adherents and an eclectic variety of blended philosophies. Notwithstanding this, there are key concepts within naturopathy that are agreed upon and are flexible enough to accommodate a broad range of styles in naturopathic practice.[11]

The historical precursors of naturopathy emphasise the responsibility of the patient in following a healthy lifestyle with a balance of work, recreation, exercise, meditation and rest; eating healthily, and having fresh air, water and sunshine; regular detoxification and cleansing; healthy emotions within healthy relationships; an ethical life; and a healthy environment. These views highlight the fact that each patient is unique and, in light of this, naturopathic treatments for each patient are tailored to addressing the individual factors that cause their ill health. An essential part of a holistic consultation is the education of the patient to promote healthy living, self-care, preventive medicine and the unique factors affecting their vitality.[12]

Vitalism

A fundamental belief of naturopathy is that ill health begins with a loss of vitality. Health is positive vitality and not just an absence of medical findings of disease. Health is restored by raising the vitality of the patient, initiating the regenerative capacity for self-healing. The vital force is diminished by a range of physical, mental, emotional, spiritual and environmental factors.[13]

Vitalism is the belief that living things depend on the action of a special energy or force that guides the processes of metabolism, growth, reproduction, adaptation and interaction.[14] This vital force is capable of interactions with material matter, such as a person's biochemistry, and these interactions of the vital force are necessary for life to exist. The vital force is non-material and occurs only in living things. It is the guiding force that accounts not only for the maintenance of life, but for the development and activities of living organisms such as the progression from seed to plant, or the development of an embryo to a living being.[15]

The vital force is seen to be different from all the other forces recognised by physics and chemistry. And, most importantly, living organisms are more than just the effects of physics and chemistry. Vitalists agree with the value of biochemistry and physics in physiology but claim that such sciences will never fully comprehend the nature of life. Conversely, vitalism is not the same as a traditional religious view of life. Vitalists do not necessarily attribute the vital force to a creator, a god or a supernatural being, although vitalism can be compatible with such views. This is considered a 'strong' interpretation of vitalism. Naturopaths use a 'moderate' form of vitalism: *vis medicatrix naturae,* or the healing power of nature.[1]

Vis medicatrix naturae defines health as good vitality where the vital force flows energetically through a person's being, sustaining and replenishing us, whereas ill health is a disturbance of vital energy.[3] While naturopaths agree with modern pathology about the concepts of disease (cellular dysfunction, genetics, accidents, toxins and microbes), naturopathic philosophy further believes that a person's vital force determines their susceptibility to illness, the amount of treatment necessary, the vigour of treatment and the speed of recovery.[16] Those with poor vitality will succumb more quickly, require more treatment, need gentler treatments and take longer to recover.[17]

Vis medicatrix naturae sees the role of the practitioner as finding the cause (*tolle causum*) of the disturbance of vital force. The practitioner must then use treatments that are gentle, safe, non-invasive techniques from nature to restore the vital force; and to use preventative medicine by teaching (*docere*—doctor as teacher) the principles of good health.[18]

Vitality and disease

Vitalistic theory merges with naturopathy in the understanding of how disease progresses (see Table 1.1). The *acute* stages of disease have active, heightened responses to challenges within the body systems. When the vital force is strong it reacts to an acute crisis by mobilising forces within the body to 'throw off' the disease.[17] The effect on vitality is usually only temporary as the body reacts with pain, redness, heat and swelling. If this stage is not dealt with appropriately where suppressive medicines are used the vital force is weakened and acute illnesses begin to become *subacute*. This is where there are less activity, less pain and less reaction within the body, accompanied by a lingering loss of vitality, mild toxicity and sluggishness. The patient begins to feel more persistently 'not quite right' but nothing will show up on medical tests and, in the absence of disease, the patient will be declared 'healthy' in biomedical terms. If the patient continues without addressing their health and lifestyle in a holistic way they can begin to

EFFECTS ON HEALTH AND VITALITY

- Constitutional strength—familial, genetic, congenital
- Diet—excess and deficiency
- Fresh air, water, sunlight, nature
- Lifestyle—work, education, exercise, rest, recreation
- Disease
- Injury
- Toxaemia—external (such as pollution, pesticides and drugs) and internal (such as metabolic byproducts and cell waste)
- Organs of detoxification—liver, kidney and lymph
- Organs of elimination—bowel, gallbladder, bladder, respiratory, skin
- Emotions and relationships
- Culture, creativity, arts
- Philosophy, religion and an ethical life
- Community, environment and ecology
- Social, economic and political factors

Table 1.1 Stages of disease

STAGE	ACUTE	SUBACUTE	CHRONIC	DEGENERATIVE
Symptoms	Pain, heat, redness, swelling, high activity, discharges, sensitivities	Lowered activity, relapsing symptoms	Persistent symptoms, constant discomfort, accumulation of cellular debris	Overwhelmed with toxicity, cellular destruction, mental and spiritual decay
Toxicity	Toxic discharges	Toxic absorption	Toxic encumbrance	Toxic necrosis
Vitality	Temporarily weak vitality	Variable vitality, ill at ease, not quite right, sluggish	Poor vitality, malaise, susceptible to other physical, mental or spiritual distress	Very low vitality, pernicious disruption of life processes at all levels

experience *chronic* diseases where there are long-term, persistent health problems. This is highlighted by weakened vitality, poor immune responses, toxicity, metabolic sluggishness, and the relationships between systems both within and outside the patient becomes dysfunctional. The final stage of disease is *destructive* where there are tissue breakdown, cellular dysfunction, low vitality and high toxicity.[19]

In traditional naturopathic theory the above concepts emphasise the connections between lowered vitality and ill health. Traditional naturopathic philosophy also emphasises that the return of vitality through naturopathic treatment will bring about healing. The stages of this healing are succinctly summarised by Dr Constantine Hering, a 19th-century physician, and these principles of healing are known as Hering's Law of Cure.[19,20]

HERING'S LAW OF CURE

- Healing begins on the inside in the vital organs first, from the most important organs to the least important organs. The outer surfaces are healed last.
- Healing begins from the middle of the body out to the extremities.
- Healing begins from the top and goes down the body.
- Retracing—healing begins on the most recent problems back to the original problems.
- Healing crisis—as retracing and healing take place the body will re-experience any prior illness where the vital force was inappropriately treated. In re-experiencing the symptoms the patient will awaken their vitality and have an inner sense that the cleansing 'is doing them good'. A healing crisis is usually of a brief duration.

Holism

Another essential principle of naturopathy developed from its eclectic history is the importance of a holistic perspective to explore, understand and treat the patient. Holism comes from the Greek word *holos*, meaning whole.[21,22] The concept of holism has a more formal description in general philosophy and has three main beliefs.[23] First, it is important to consider an organism as a whole. The best way to study the behaviour of a complex system is to treat it as a whole and not merely to analyse the structure and behaviour of its component parts. It is the principles governing the behaviour of the whole system rather than its parts that best elucidate an understanding of the system.

Secondly, every system within the organism loses some of its characteristics when any of its components undergo change. The component parts of a system will lose their nature, function, significance and even their existence when removed from their interconnection with the rest of the systems that support them. An organism is said to differ from a mere mechanism by reason of its interdependence with nature and its parts in the whole. For instance, any changes that occur in the nervous system can cause changes in other systems such as musculoskeletal, cognition and mood, and digestion. Or, more widely, any changes that occur in social relationships have an effect on the nervous system and vice versa.

Thirdly, the important characteristics of an organism do not occur at the physical and chemical levels but at a higher level where there is a holistic integration of systems within the whole being. There are important interrelations that define the systems and these may be completely missed in a 'parts-only perspective'. These interrelations are completely independent of the parts. For instance, the digestive tract is functional only when its blood supply, nerve supply, enzymes and hormones are integrated and unified by complex interrelationships.

In naturopathic health care, holism is the understanding that a person's health functions as a whole, unified, complex system in balance. When any one part of their human experience suffers, a person's entire sense of being may suffer.

PATIENT-CENTRED APPROACH TO HOLISTIC CONSULTATION

One of the most difficult duties as a human being is to listen to the voices of those who suffer … listening is hard but fundamentally a moral act.[24]

The holistic consultation and treatment of the whole person includes emotional, mental, spiritual, physical and environmental factors, and it aims to promote wellbeing through the whole person rather than just the symptomatic relief of a disease. To best enhance this holistic consultative process a 'patient-centred' approach is used. This is where the emphasis is on patient autonomy; the patient and practitioner are in an equal relationship that values and respects the wants and needs of the patient.[25] The role of the practitioner is to develop a therapeutic relationship of rapport, empathy and authenticity to serve the patient's choices and engender the healing process.

An essential component of developing a therapeutic relationship with the patient is the ability to listen.[26] Naturopaths must never forget that each patient is an individual with their own unique story of illness and treatment. The patient needs to be allowed to tell that story and in turn the naturopathic practitioner needs to listen with sensitive, authentic attention and empathy. This disciplined type of therapeutic listening bonds the patient and practitioner and enhances the effectiveness of treatment.[27]

When patients feel listened to, they open up and declare hidden information that can be clinically significant to the type of treatment given and to how well that treatment works. A clinical example is where a stressed final year secondary student wanted 'something natural' to help her sleep. As she spoke about her situation, another deeper narrative slowly unfolded in which she divulged that she had been sexually assaulted by an ex-boyfriend and her current anxiety centred upon thoughts of self-harm. The act of listening not only deepened rapport and established trust and empathy but also led to better clinical support for her with a referral to a psychologist.

If a naturopath does not holistically enquire into the causes of a patient's presenting complaint and merely follows a protocol—in this case, an insomnia prescription—they may be, at the very least, clinically ineffective in treating insomnia or, worse, prolonging the patient's suffering and increasing her risk of self-harm.

A practitioner needs to be aware that a holistic consultation is not a routine event for the patient. It is dense with meaning and can represent a turning point for them.[28] Fully listening to a patient's concerns in a patient-centred holistic consultation helps the naturopath to explore and understand what is at stake and why it matters so much.[29] With this knowledge it is then possible to provide appropriate and effective treatment. Establishing rapport, empathy and authenticity in a patient-centred holistic consultation also enhances the practitioner's ongoing ability to assess recovery and to achieve the patient-centred aim of independent self-care.[30]

This therapeutic relationship depends upon the practitioner being proficient in consulting skills, communication skills and counselling skills. This chapter now focuses on consulting skills and the reader is recommended to the 'Further reading' section at the end of this chapter for texts discussing communication skills and counselling skills.

It should also be noted that some patients present to clinic with little or no prior understanding of what the naturopathic consultation involves. Some preliminary steps can be taken to facilitate a better understanding for the patient. Initially, a practitioner's website can provide explanatory details of naturopathic philosophy, treatment modalities and the consulting process. This can be reinforced with clinic brochures in the reception area of the clinic. As the holistic consultation begins the practitioner can sensitively enquire as to the patient's level of understanding of naturopathy and what their expectations about the consultation are.

Phases of the holistic consultation

Adapting the Nelson-Jones[31] model, there are five phases to the holistic patient centred consultation. These are to:

1. *explore* the range of problems
2. *understand* each problem
3. determine the *goals*
4. provide *treatments*, and
5. consolidate the patient's *independence.*

In a brief acute case of a minor condition, such as a minor head cold, these five phases can be completed over a single session. In a complex case with multiple pathologies and a myriad of personal issues, the phases discussed below can occur and recur over a long period of time and completion may entail many sessions.

Explore

The task here is to establish rapport with the patient and to help the patient reveal, identify and describe their problems. The naturopath can facilitate this by providing a structure for the interview and fostering an ambience where the patient's views are valued and important. The naturopath's empathy with the patient will sensitise the practitioner to the tone, pace, depth and breadth of their enquiry into the patient's health issues. The enquiry should be patient-centred, where the patient sets the parameters of what they feel comfortable discussing while the naturopath maintains a heightened awareness of the clinical significance of what they are saying—or indeed not saying. The patient in this process has an opportunity to share their thoughts and feelings and for the naturopath to join with them in identifying the problem areas in their health from a holistic perspective.

Understand

Understanding the problems involves a focused attempt to gather more specific details of the problems experienced by the patient. The naturopath's facilitation skills will help the patient accurately focus on symptoms while also using the naturopath's clinical skills in physical examination, body sign observations, reviewing medical reports and completing a systems history to gain and impart a holistic overview. The knowledge gained from this helps the patient to acknowledge areas of strength and weakness in their health and to develop new insights and perceptions that will help them to relate to their health issues holistically. It is also appropriate in this phase to seek referrals for further diagnosis where necessary from biomedical or allied health professionals.

Set goals

The next step is to work with the patient to negotiate goals and strategies to achieve positive outcomes for their health. The naturopath needs to discuss with the patient the types of modalities that can be used and which treatments are expected to be efficacious. It is appropriate at this juncture to give a prognosis of what can be reasonably achieved within a specified time. The patient has now an opportunity to ask questions, discuss costs and be in an active position to make an informed choice in setting goals and deciding on the best treatment options. The patient should be encouraged to acknowledge their active participation in their health improvement. They can also discuss with the naturopath their preferences for various modalities, and the naturopath can highlight what they can expect as their health improves.

Treatment

The task now is to assist the patient in gaining better vitality, building health resources and skills, and lessening health deficits. The patient's role is to acquire self-help skills. Active encouragement is crucial in developing and maintaining the patient's self-motivation. Encourage the patient to acquire books, internet resources and community resources and to undertake courses to further self-support the recovery. The issues of compliance, or how well the patient can follow a treatment plan, can be discussed with the patient in a supportive way by identifying any possible difficulties. The treatment plan may need to be modified or strategies developed to ensure the patient gains the full benefit of their treatment program.

Potential barriers to treatment need to be anticipated, assessed and discussed, with contingencies put in place within the treatment plan to account for these. For example, if the treatment goal is weight loss and exercise is suggested as a primary treatment strategy, then the attitude of the patient towards exercise needs to be assessed. If those potential barriers are anticipated, plans can be suggested that overcome them and improve compliance, for example by exercising with a friend rather than alone.

Also in this phase the need for 'follow-up' is assessed. The patient may require further appointments to refine the processes of exploring, understanding, goal setting and treatment of their health issues. At this point, referrals to other practitioners for treatment may also be necessary where it can be seen that this would be beneficial.

Independence

The final step in the patient-centred therapeutic process is to consolidate the patient's independence. The task is to ensure the patients have the necessary self-help skills and are prepared for the naturopath's helping role to end. At this stage, both the naturopath and the patient review the progress and goal achievements. The naturopath can assist the patient plan independent control of their health. The patient should be encouraged to share their thoughts on their own progress, as well as any exit issues, such as their readiness for self-management. The patient now can consolidate all their learning and is ready to implement self-help skills in daily life.

STRUCTURE AND TECHNIQUE OF CASE TAKING

Basic case-taking skills take 1 or 2 years to develop and a diligent naturopath over the years will be constantly improving and refining techniques.[32] It may be overwhelming in the first few cases for novice practitioners, especially if the case (or the patient!) is complex. At times a patient may be difficult, angry or demanding and a practitioner

FROM NOVICE TO EXPERIENCED NATUROPATH

Novice naturopaths: tend to use learned protocols that give treatment programs for a disease or syndrome.

Advanced beginners: soon find that the 'one-size-fits-all' approach, besides being counter to naturopathic philosophy, is problematic and begin to adapt and vary the protocols to each patient.

Competent naturopaths: begin to develop their own independent strategies for patients.

Professional naturopaths: develop treatments based on traditional learning, evidenced-based practice and their intuition in selecting treatments that best align with the patient's individual holistic causes of ill health.

Experienced naturopaths: are immersed in an intuitive proficiency where they understand tradition and evidence; can listen carefully and sensitively to the patient's issues; adapt readily and easily to the patient's personality; motivate and educate the patient; are aware of the nuances in patient rapport, red flags and need for referrals; and are calm, gentle and understanding in the face of uncertainty and suffering.

Source: Adapted from Boon et al. 2006.[33]

needs to have insight and strategies for dealing with this (see 'Further reading' at the end of this chapter, which highlights useful texts discussing these issues).

Novice practitioners may wish to begin any case, no matter how chronic or complex, by starting with a good case history of one key ailment that bothers the patient. This is designated as the 'presenting complaint'.[34] For example if the patient has five health issues to discuss, negotiate with the patient what is most important to them to work on first.

The presenting complaint

• *Location*: Ask about the nature of the problem. Get an idea of the physical, emotional, spiritual and environmental dimensions of the problem. Note if it affects a certain location of the anatomy or a physiological system. Be aware that certain conditions have multiple locations, such as arthritis or systemic lupus erythematosus (SLE).

• *Onset*: Ask about the factors that seemed to initiate or trigger the problem. In a holistic manner, enquire as to what was occurring for the patient before and at the start of the problems. When did the problems first start?

• *Course*: Ask whether the problem seems to be constant (there all the time with minimal variation) or fluctuating (there all the time but varies in presentation and intensity) or intermittent (it stops and starts or happens occasionally). The treatment of headaches, for example, could be quite different if they are constant or fluctuating or happen twice a week or twice a year.

• *Duration*: Ask when the problem first started if it has been constant or fluctuating, and also how long an episode of the problem endures if it is intermittent.

• *Sensation/quality*: Ask the patient to describe in their own words how the patient experiences their symptoms via the five senses of feeling (such as ache, burn, numb, pinch, stab, throb, hot, cold, itch, anxious, sad, dizzy, nauseous, twisting, wrenching or tingling); sight (such as colour, consistency, texture or shape); sound (such as crepitation, rattling, gasping, rumbling or buzzing), odour (such as fetid, ketosis, fishy, yeasty or sharp) and taste (such as bitter, salty, rancid, bloody or metallic). Note that a loss of any sensation is also clinically significant.

- *Intensity*: Ask about how mild, moderate or severe the problem is. Be aware that different personalities may under-report or over-report the severity. You can get the patient to give it a score out of 10 to make a useful comparison on follow-up visits.
- *Modalities*: What makes it better or worse? Time of day, week, season, or year; situation, such as in bed, at work, in hot weather; or certain activities may trigger it; or certain emotional or spiritual crises may trigger the problem.
- *Radiates*: Does the problem shift, extend or move around one location or between other locations?
- *Concomitants*: When the problem occurs is there any other part of the person that seems to be affected? Examples are irritability with hot flushes; loss of appetite with depression; and headaches with existential crises.
- *Past history*: In an acute case this can be a previous history of this presenting complaint. It can also include a general past history of all health issues.
- *Family history*: As above, this can be a family history of the presenting complaint as well as a general history of all health issues in the family.
- *Medications*: Include all medical, naturopathic, Chinese medicine and other health modalities, including self-prescribed supplements. It often occurs that the presenting complaint is directly linked to a side effect or interaction of medications.
- *Diet*: Discuss a typical day's diet. For a more comprehensive approach the naturopath can give the patient a diet diary to record their diet and symptoms over a 1- or 2-week period and review this in a follow-up appointment.
- *Observation of body signs and relevant physical examinations* (refer to Chapter 2 on diagnosis).
- *Timeline:* The information gathered can also be represented in the format of a timeline that illustrates the sequence of events.

This single issue case-taking process can take 20–45 minutes for novice practitioners in the early days of training or practice. It is always important not to spend an overly long time in getting the case details. There has to be sufficient time also for explaining the holistic diagnosis and naturopathic understanding of why this problem is occurring; treatment goals; prognosis; remedy preparation and label instructions; doing the account; and booking the patient for the next appointment. Bear in mind that the patient is likely to be unwell, tired, in pain or have restless children in tow and it is a strain on the patient to have them there for 1 or 2 hours while trying to pack too much into the first session. It is more appropriate to use the second and third appointments to gather further information. Psychologists, for example, may spend at least the first five to 10 sessions getting a general background and then may spend the next year or more listening to the patient's life narrative on a once-a-week basis.

Holistic review

As part of a holistic consultation it is essential to enquire into a broad range of factors. This is where the consultation moves beyond the presenting complaint.[35] It encompasses a review of the patient's:

- past history
- family history
- lifestyle history
- mind/emotion/spirit history, and
- body systems.

This can be done in any order that seems most comfortable between practitioner and patient. A holistic assessment is made of the patient's vitality and symptoms by exploring the physical, mental, social and spiritual factors that affect them. A simple model of holistic assessment is first to explore the factors affecting the patient's constitutional strength, which are the physical and mental attributes they are born with. This includes genetics, temperament and the inherent strengths and weaknesses of different physiological systems. Secondly, factors that occur over time are considered. These include the family and culture that the patient grew up with and the socioeconomic status and environment that they live in. They also include the types of diseases or traumas the patient has had, the diets and lifestyle they have followed and the patterns of adaptive behaviour that they have adopted. Thirdly, a holistic assessment needs to consider important, dramatic events that have overwhelmed an otherwise healthy person, such as severe stress, trauma or toxicity. Fourthly, the factors that trigger disturbances to vitality such as stress, injury, infection, toxicity, allergens and drugs need to be considered. Finally, a holistic assessment of the factors that sustain ongoing health issues, such as psychological, social, economic, environmental and ecological factors, is made.[36]

Galland[37] cautions that care must be taken in holistic assessments. Careful listening to the patient is required, as the range of possibilities is extensive. The assessment needs to be comprehensive as there can be multiple factors that reinforce each other and the practitioner needs to constantly reassess the patient who has complex symptoms to avoid misdiagnosis. The practitioner also needs to be flexible as the same symptom in two different people, for example joint pain, may have different triggers; conversely, the same trigger, for example hot weather, may induce headache in one person and asthma in another.

Past history
- General level of vitality and health in infancy, childhood, teens, twenties and subsequent decades; the effect on vitality of life stages such as puberty, education, relationships, marriage, pregnancy, parenting, work, menopause/andropause, retiring
- Immunisations, vaccinations, reactions
- Allergies, intolerances
- Childhood illnesses; either minor but persistent, or major, episodes requiring medical supervision, hospitalisation, surgery, medication
- Major illnesses, accidents, genetic issues, hospitalisations, disabilities
- Past use of medications

Family history
- Major diseases, syndromes and level of vitality that affect family members
- Causes of mortality in family
- Familial, hereditary, genetic issues

Lifestyle history
- Exercise, fitness, coordination, mobility, flexibility, strength, stamina, aerobic capacity
- Recreation, entertainment, rest, holidays
- Alcohol consumption, coffee/tea consumption, smoking, recreational drug use
- Daily exposure to toxins, pollutants, chemicals
- Education
- Work conditions (exposure to toxins; stress, injury)
- Home conditions

- Social, economic, financial and political conditions
- Health issues with class, race, religion or gender
- Travel
- Military service

Mind/emotion/spirit

- Life satisfaction; relationships; connectedness to friends, family, colleagues, community, society
- Reactions to stress, grief, trauma; coping mechanisms; resilience, vulnerability
- Moods, perceptions, sensitivities, motivation, will, intensity, personal characteristics, attachments, obsessions
- Attitudes, optimism
- Mental capacities, performance, confidence, procrastinations, decision making ability
- Speech, gesture, posture, thinking, feeling, behaviour
- Creativity, arts, music, dance, theatre, sculpture, hobbies, collecting
- Religion, spirituality, philosophy, self-discovery, ethics, purpose of existence, world view, meditation, revelation, prayer, metaphysics
- Spiritual and cultural issues in health care

Body systems

In each of these sections, if there are relevant symptoms to discuss then follow the format as given regarding the presenting complaint, such as location, duration, onset, course, sensation and so forth:

- *general*: fatigue, pallor, fever, chills, sweats; proneness to infection; allergies, intolerances; weight, posture, build; age, stage of life; gender
- *gastrointestinal*: problems with mouth, gums, tongue, oesophagus, swallowing, reflux, eructation, stomach pain, gastritis, ulcers, bloating, fullness, appetite, nausea, vomiting, cramping, flatulence, stool (frequency, consistency, colour, odour, blood), haemorrhoids, fissures; infections (viral, bacterial, fungal, protozoal); polyps, tumours
- *hepatic-biliary:* jaundice, cirrhosis, gallstones, abnormal liver function tests, bile duct inflammation or obstruction, right shoulder or flank pain, ascites
- *respiratory*: pain; difficulty or obstruction in breathing; wheezing, shortness of breath; cough; sputum; smoking; asthma
- *head/neurologic*: headaches, migraines, dizziness, fainting, epilepsy, head trauma, confusion, memory loss; eyes (vision, discharge, pain, redness, change in appearance of eye such as unequal pupils, cataracts, glaucoma)
- *ear, nose, throat*: pain, hearing problems, sense of smell, sense of taste, sinus, rhinitis, allergens, discharges, change in voice, gums, teeth, lips, tongue, tonsils, adenoids, mouth ulcers
- *cardiovascular*: chest pain; palpitations, arrhythmias; oedema; dyspnoea; blood pressure; cholesterol; anaemia; blood disorders; claudication; varicosities; circulation—cold hands/feet; bruising; bleeding
- *lymph nodes*: sore, swollen, infected
- *endocrine*: pituitary/hypothalamus; thyroid (hyper and hypo symptoms); thymus; pancreas (pancreatitis, diabetes, hypoglycaemia); adrenal (Addison's, fatigue, immune, oedema); ovary/testes
- *female*: breast—pain, tender, lumps, change in appearance, galactorrhea; menses, menarche, hormonal contraceptives, frequency, duration, volume, colour, consistency, pain, PMT; libido, sexual function, pain, itch, discharge, infections, Pap smears,

surgery, investigations, uterine, ovarian, fallopian, cervical, vaginal; polycystic ovarian syndrome, endometriosis; fertility, pregnancies, births; menopause, hot flushes, headaches, mood, vaginal dryness, weight gain

- *males*: infection, discharge, lesions, sexual dysfunction (libido, erection, ejaculation), pain, infertility, testes, prostate (benign prostate hyperplasia, prostatitis, cancer), varicocele, phimosis, balanitis
- *genitourinary*: frequency, volume, colour, odour, infections, blood, urgency, incontinence, pain (flank, suprapubic, urethral), rigors; dribbling, hesitancy; calculi; kidneys, ureters, bladder, urethra; abnormal urinary test results; renal effects on sodium, blood pressure, acid/base balance, fluid retention
- *peripheral neurologic*: weakness, abnormal sensation, numbness, coordination, loco motor, paralysis, tremor
- *musculoskeletal*: bone deformities, ligament, tendon, muscle, joints, discs, inflammation, pain, swelling, redness, hot, cold, stiffness, crepitation, range of motion, functional loss
- *Skin, hair, nails*: rash, itch, eruption, discharge, flaking, erosive, pitting, peeling, lumps, cysts, change in colour, texture, shape; hair loss, dandruff.

In chronic, complex cases with multiple symptoms and pathologies it may take two or three sessions to get a complete and accurate history. As a novice practitioner gains more experience, all the details of complex cases can be gained in one to two sessions.

POSOLOGY

Posology is the determination of the appropriate dosage of remedies for the patient. In general terms if a patient has good vitality they can handle the rigour of more remedies at higher doses and more aggressive treatment regimens of exercise and detoxification if required. For those patients with moderate vitality their treatment is modified with milder doses of tonics and supplements in an effort to strengthen vitality and prevent relapses occurring. Patients with weakened vitality are best administered treatments that offer gentle relief of symptoms and the mildest of programs to support the affected systems. This is done through toning, building and adaptogenic remedies.

These general guidelines for dosages and range of remedies are modified by the *pace*, *intensity*, *location* and *natural history* of the illness. First, vary the treatment according to the pace of the symptoms. The dosage and range of remedies will vary according to the symptoms being slow and sluggish as compared to symptoms that are rapid in onset. Secondly, the intensity of the symptoms dictates that a higher dose is required for symptoms of a florid, aggressive nature with a potential for pathological sequelae. The naturopath may also have to factor in that some patients are particularly stressed by the symptoms and demand more urgent treatment programs than is necessarily required. Thirdly, the location of the illness may change the posology as symptoms in the eye, for example, are more sensitive than in the heel of the foot. Fourthly, treatments will vary according to the natural history of an illness where dosages change between the onset, middle and resolution of an illness.

SIGNPOSTS FOR RECOVERY

Patients always ask 'When will I get better?' Prognosis is the forecast of the course of a disease. With illnesses that are familiar, such as a head cold, it is relatively predictable how long it takes for symptoms to resolve with treatment. As a novice practitioner progresses through their career and experiences a wider range of patients, the ability to give an accurate prognosis of a variety of health problems improves. However, there are always instances when it is very difficult to predict how a patient's illness will respond to treatment and over what period of time. In instances of difficulty with predicting how long a patient will take to recover it is better to approach the issue from another angle. That is, rather than trying to give the patient a definitive time frame of amelioration of the illness it is better to give estimations of what signposts or stages the patient is expected to experience and leave the issue of duration open-ended. This prevents the frustration a patient may experience when told they should be better by a certain date but they are not.

The first signpost for recovery is that the condition has stabilised and is no longer deteriorating. Secondly, the intensity of symptoms begins reducing. Thirdly, the symptoms are no longer constant. Fourthly, the symptoms no longer fluctuate. Fifthly, there are longer periods of intermittence and, if they do return, the symptoms are milder and of shorter duration. And finally there is remission or cure. The patient is asked to watch for these stages as signs of improvement. Discuss with the patient the fact that it is often too difficult to give an exact time estimation as to how long each stage of recovery will take.

To assist in prognostic skills the following practice tips will be useful. For a known disease or syndrome there is excellent information in pathology texts and medical journals that indicates the natural history of a disease—that is, how a disease behaves and over what period of time. Secondly, check the naturopathic information from academic notes, texts, journals and seminars on the action of naturopathic remedies and how long these remedies take to reduce symptoms. Also enquire further from senior naturopathic colleagues, mentors and academic staff who can give information of how this disease normally behaves and how it responds to the proposed treatments. Thirdly, having established a good knowledge of how the disease behaves and the efficacy of the treatments, make an assessment of the patient's capabilities and compliance with following the treatment plan. This is where a holistic understanding of the patient's vitality, preferences for modalities and personal circumstances will help in judging when the patient will improve.

CASE TAKING—THE RETURN VISIT

Novice practitioners can sometimes feel confusion as to what they are supposed to say or do in the return visit. For 'follow-up' of acute, minor cases, use the guidelines below. For 'follow-up' of complex, chronic cases see the following section, 'Case taking–advanced'.

At the end of the first session

The return visit is made easier for novice practitioners if they get into the habit of making notes at the end of the initial visit as a reminder of what needs to be done at the next session. At the end of the first visit history form, make a box with the heading 'Follow-up'. In this box write down any items the practitioner promised the patient to look into. Also in this box write down the patient's symptoms to review in follow-up; for example, check temperature, mucus (colour, consistency), sneezing and fatigue to compare with the first session to gauge treatment response. Also write in this box any other issues that the practitioner or the patient wanted to explore for the second session but did not get time for in the first session.

What to do in the second session

Before the patient arrives the practitioner needs to re-familiarise themselves with the patient's case. This can include the patient's personal and social anecdotes of things that they were going to be doing during the week, such as family functions, outings with friends, work issues or relationship issues. To quickly re-establish rapport the practitioner can remind themselves of how the patient was feeling in the first session.

An important feature of the follow-up session is to review the patient's symptoms. This enables the practitioner to make comparisons of the patient's progress and to gauge the effectiveness of the treatment program. Make new notes on what changes have occurred in signs and symptoms since the previous visit. It may be necessary to repeat any physical examinations that were done in the first session, such as vitals. The practitioner needs to enquire how the patient managed with the remedies and lifestyle advice and check whether the patient was taking the remedies in the manner prescribed.

If acute symptoms have resolved, then reiterate to the patient holistic, preventive measures to maintain good health and to avoid the symptoms reoccurring. If acute symptoms have not resolved, then explore the reasons for this. Confirm that the original diagnosis and naturopathic understanding were correct. This may require referrals to other health professionals for further diagnostic assessment and testing. Check antecedents, triggers and mediators as discussed earlier. For example, the patient may still be under the same stresses at work, or their diet may need further support. Check materia medica selection and posology and that the patient knows how to take the remedies properly; check patient compliance or any difficulties with taking the remedies, managing the diet or following exercise programs. Check information on the expected prognosis and natural history of the condition. That is, how long does a particular condition normally take to clear up? For example, some sinus conditions take a few weeks to heal and there may be little change in the first week. Often the reason for lack of improvement is obvious and it is easy to make adjustments to the treatment program or support the patient with ways to achieve their health goals. At other times, there are cases that, even with the best intentions of the practitioner and the patient, are not responding very well. It is appropriate here to seek the patient's permission to discuss their case with colleagues or a mentor with experience in similar cases. It can happen that the practitioner needs to refer the patient to another modality that might have more success with that particular condition. For example with persistent back pain the patient can be referred to remedial massage, chiropractic, physiotherapy or osteopathy.

The second visit also allows the opportunity to discuss if there are any other different issues or symptoms not mentioned in the first visit. First, ask the patient if there are other concerns they have that they wish to talk about. This needs to be done every session. It may take some patients many repeated sessions to gain the trust to discuss sensitive issues like a past history of bulimia, sexual abuse or a worrisome ailment they feel embarrassed about. The practitioner can also initiate discussion on any issues that are apparent, for example if the patient looks pale or jaundiced or their thyroid looks swollen, or has signs of body systems under stress that were not part of the initial discussions.

The second session allows completion of any further history that may have not been obtained in the first session or going into issues in more depth if that seems appropriate. At the end of the second session the practitioner always has to remember to draw up a 'Follow-up' box on the end of the history forms so they know what needs to be done in the third session. This needs to be done for every subsequent session.

CASE TAKING—ADVANCED

Getting the details of chronic complex cases requires careful attention. As previously stated getting these details could take a number of sessions for novice practitioners. The written data obtained need to be accurate, comprehensive and easily recoverable. The practitioner should be able to quickly find any data on any question from any session because all the data are put into specific locations in the history form.

The case history requires the patient's words verbatim if possible. However, this does not mean that every word is written in the order that the patient has said it. Patients tend to talk by random association where one thing reminds them of something else and will jump from topic to topic and back again. The skill is allowing this to occur to obtain rich information but also to do three other things simultaneously. The first is to write or type fluently key words or phrases while maintaining eye contact and rapport. The second is to write in such a way that the practitioner does not end up with line after line of the patient's words on a blank sheet in a disorganised fashion. After six or seven sessions there will be 10 or 20 pages of notes and it is very embarrassing when it takes 5 minutes to check some detail the patient has asked about! Instead, the history forms should have predefined sections where the patient's verbatim data can go. If the answers and details about, say, body systems are put in predefined sections on the history form under the heading 'Body systems', the information can be located in a matter of seconds. For example, information on coughing goes under 'Respiratory'; information on depression goes under 'Mind'. In later sessions when the practitioner wants to compare coughs or depressive symptoms the information is easy to find. Also, by following a format for history taking the practitioner can see the gaps in the history form. This then is a reminder to get the relevant information for those sections that have been missed. For example there may be a blank space on the history form under 'Circulation' and this will prompt the practitioner to complete this part of the history.

Thirdly, the art of patient interviews is to gauge when to gently direct or turn the patient's conversation towards information that the practitioner wishes to gain. If the practitioner is too directive the patient will learn only to briefly answer in a perfunctory way and to wait for the next question. This static style is quite mechanical and only emphasises to the patient that the practitioner's questions are more important than the patient's needs. This could stifle much rich information about the patient's personal thoughts, symptoms and motivations that can be discovered by a spontaneous, free-flowing conversation. On the other hand, if the practitioner is too non-directive the patient may digress into sessions of repetitive minutiae on one symptom; or random generalisations that do not articulate context or specificity; or the conversation is extended into blander areas to avoid enquiry into sensitive issues.

Complex cases: an example of how to summarise complex data

Case Study

'John' is an 84-year-old male. He is a very friendly and cheerful fellow of slim build and, considering the range of health issues he has, he is mobile and independent and pursues hobbies in music and literature. He has health issues with diabetes, asthma, insomnia, stress, headaches, elevated cholesterol, palpitations, skin rash, sciatica, sinusitis, depression, reflux and diarrhoea. Other issues can come and go, and these are recorded in a similar fashion, as in the box below, by adding more bottom rows. All symptoms are chronic, some are constant, some fluctuate and some are intermittent.

Table 1.2 Case history summary table

SYMPTOMS	FEBRUARY	MARCH	APRIL
Diabetes	Stable (6–7 on rising)	Same	
Asthma	Stable (same)	Same	
Insomnia	> 8/10; herbs good	> 9/10	
Stress	> 8/10; herbs good	Same	
Headache	> 4/10; occurs 2/7–mild	> 8/10	
Cholesterol	No data this month	Total 5.8; LDL 2.6; Tryg 2.6	
Palpitation	> 8/10 for magnesium	Same	
Skin rash	> 4/10–shrunk 1 cm	< 2/10; increased 2 cm; hot weather	
Sinusitis	> generally; but worse in last 2 days	Clear	
Depression	> 8/10 with herbs	All good	
Reflux	Same—still occurs after meals	Same	
Diarrhoea	Variable—no incontinence this month	Same	

Note: > means 'better'. Improvement or deterioration is given a score out of 10. For example > 8/10 means that symptoms have improved and are now 80% of normal.

After taking a couple of sessions to get full details of his complete case history the practitioner's subsequent sessions now involve tracking and reviewing his symptoms and response to treatment. This can be done on a simple spreadsheet by asking specific questions in each category and recording it in a summary table (such as Table 1.2). Every month the practitioner checks these symptoms and adds or subtracts other symptoms that come and go.

This simple method keeps track of the patient's 12 or more symptoms and pathologies. Within each session the treatment program can be reviewed and adjusted to address the patient's changing circumstances. If clarification or comparison of the past history of the patient's symptoms is required it can be readily accessed in the written history form in good detail. Discussion can then be directed to what symptoms bother the patient the most and to jointly decide whether or not to treat particular symptoms, given that the patient is already on multiple medications. Thus the patient's wishes and values are respected and the patient feels secure in the knowledge that all his issues are being addressed in a holistic way.

Further reading

The following texts provide more specific strategies to enhance communication skills and counselling skills to add to your consulting skills as outlined in this chapter.

Active listening. Australian Family Physician, 2005. Online. Available: http://www.racgp.org.au/afp/200512/200512robinson.pdf

Cava R. Dealing with difficult people. Sydney: Pan Macmillan, 2000.

Egan G. The skilled helper: a problem management approach to healing. 6th edn. Pacific Grove: Brooks Cole Publishing, 1998.

Geldard D, Geldard K. Basic personal counselling: a training manual for counsellors. 5th edn. Frenchs Forest: Pearson Prentice Hall, 2005.

Interpersonal counselling in general practice. Australian Family Physician, 2004. Online. Available: http://www.racgp.org.au/afp/200405/20040510judd.pdf

Ivey AE, Ivey MB. Intentional interviewing and counselling: facilitating client development in a multicultural society. Pacific Grove: Thomson Brooks Cole, 2003.

Murtagh JE. General practice. 3rd edn. North Ryde: McGraw-Hill Australia, 2006. Chapter 4 Communication skills. Chapter 5 Counselling skills. Chapter 6 Difficult, demanding and trying patients.

Navigating through the swampy lowlands. Dealing with the patient when the diagnosis is unclear. Australian Family Physician, 2006. Online. Available: http://www.racgp.org.au/afp/200612/20061205 stone.pdf

Nelson-Jones R. Human relating skills. 3rd edn. Marrickville: Harcourt Brace, 1996.

Surviving the 'heartsink' experience. Family Practice, 1995. Online. Available: http://fampra.oxfordjournals.org/cgi/content/abstract/12/2/176

References

1. Coulter ID, Willis, M. The rise and rise of complementary and alternative medicine: a sociological perspective. Med J Aust 2004;180:587.
2. Pizzorno JE, Snider P. Naturopathic medicine. In: Micozzi M, ed. Fundamentals of complementary and integrative medicine. 3rd edn. St Louis: Saunders Elsevier, 2006:221–255.
3. Kaptchuck TJ. Vitalism. In: Micozzi M, ed. Fundamentals of complementary and integrative medicine. 3rd edn. St Louis: Saunders Elsevier, 2006:53–63.
4. Bradley R. Philosophy of natural medicine. In: Pizzorno JE, Murray MT, eds. Textbook of natural medicine. 2nd edn. Edinburgh: Churchill Livingstone, 1999:42–44.
5. Di Stefano V. Holism and complementary medicine: origin and principles. Sydney: Allen & Unwin, 2006:Chapter 4.
6. Cody G. History of naturopathic medicine. In: Pizzorno JE, Murray MT, eds. Textbook of natural medicine. 2nd edn. Edinburgh: Churchill Livingstone, 1999:41–49.
7. Schneirov M, Geczik J. Alternative health care and the challenges of institutionalization. Health 2002;6(2):201–220.
8. Baer HA, Coulter ID. Introduction – taking stock of integrative medicine; broadening biomedicine or co-option of complementary and alternative medicine? Health Sociology Review 2008;17(4):332.
9. Braun L, Cohen M. Herbs and natural supplements: an evidence based guide. 2nd edn. Sydney: Churchill Livingstone, 2007:71–73.
10. Ernst E. The clinical researcher. Journal of Complementary Medicine 2004;3(1):44–45.
11. Bradley R. Philosophy of natural medicine. In: Pizzorno JE, Murray MT, eds. Textbook of natural medicine. 2nd edn. Edinburgh: Churchill Livingstone, 1999:41.
12. Hoffman D. The herbal handbook: a user's guide to medical herbalism. Rochester: Healing Arts Press, 1988:18–19.
13. Di Stefano V. Holism and complementary medicine: origin and principles. Sydney: Allen & Unwin, 2006:107–108.
14. Kirschner M, et al. Molecular vitalism. Cell 2000;100(1):87.
15. Bechtel W, et al. Vitalism. In: Concise Routledge Encyclopedia of Philosophy. London: Routledge, 2000:919.
16. Turner RN. The foundations of health. In: Naturopathic medicine. England: Thorsons Publishing Group, 1990:17–27.
17. Jacka J. A philosophy of healing. Melbourne: Inkata Press, 1997:36–38.
18. Pizzorno JE, Snider P. Naturopathic medicine. In: Micozzi M, ed. Fundamentals of complementary and integrative medicine. 3rd edn. St Louis: Saunders Elsevier, 2006:236–238.
19. Jensen B, ed. Iridology: the science and practice in the healing arts. Volume 2. Escondido: Bernard Jensen Publisher, 1982:181–183.
20. Models for the study of whole systems. In: Bell IR, Koithan M, eds. Integrative Cancer Therapies 2006:5(4):295.
21. Dunne R, Watkins J. Complementary medicine–some definitions. Journal of the Royal Society of Health 1997;117(5):287–291.
22. Moore B, ed. The Australian Oxford Dictionary. 2nd edn. South Melbourne: Oxford University Press, 2004:598.
23. Wentzel J. Holism. In: Van Huyssteen W, et al, eds. Encyclopedia of Science and Religion. 2nd edn. New York: Thomson Gale Macmillan Reference, 2003:412–414.
24. Frank A. The wounded story teller: body, illness and ethics. Chicago: University of Chicago Press, 1995:25.
25. Emmanuel E, Emmanuel K. Four models of the physician–patient relationship. JAMA 1992;267(16): 2225–2226.
26. Connelly J. Narrative possibilities: using mindfulness in clinical practice. Perspectives in Biology and Medicine 2005;48(1):84.
27. Charon R. The ethicality of narrative medicine. In: Hurwitz B, Greenhalgh T, Skultans V, eds. Narrative research in health and illness. Massachusetts: Blackwell Publishing, 2004:30.
28. Mattingly C. Performance Narratives in the clinical world. In: Hurwitz B, Greenhalgh T, Skultans V, eds. Narrative research in health and illness. Massachusetts: Blackwell Publishing, 2004:73.
29. Berlinger N. After harm: medical harm and the ethics of forgiveness. Baltimore: Johns Hopkins University Press, 2005:3.
30. Kumar P, Clarke M, eds. Kumar & Clark Clinical Medicine. Edinburgh, New York: WB Saunders, 2005:8.
31. Nelson-Jones R. Practical counselling and helping skills. 2nd edn. Marrickville: Holt Rhinehart Wilson/Harcourt Brace Jovanovich Group (Australia), 1988:92.
32. Murtagh JE. General practice. 3rd edn. North Ryde: McGraw-Hill Australia, 2006:chapters 4–5.
33. Boon NA, et al, eds. Davidson's principles and practice of medicine. 20th edn. Philadelphia: Churchill Livingstone Elsevier, 2006:6.
34. Bates B, et al. A guide to physical examination and history taking. Philadelphia: J.B. Lippincott Company, 1995.
35. Seidel H, et al. Mosby's guide to physical examination. St Louis: Mosby Elsevier, 2006:9, 22.
36. Galland L. Power healing: use the new integrated medicine to cure yourself. New York: Random House, 1997:52–84.
37. Galland L. Power healing: use the new integrated medicine to cure yourself. New York: Random House, 1997:64.

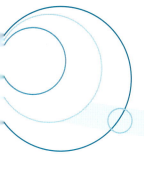

2

Naturopathic diagnostic techniques

Niikee Schoendorfer
ND, MHSc

INTRODUCTION

An important aspect of naturopathic clinical practice is the use of diagnostic techniques to ascertain the patient's state of health or disease. Naturopathy makes use of orthodox medical diagnostic techniques involving pathology testing and clinical examination, but also uses a combination of several other modalities such as a broader physical examination to incorporate traditional theories, dietary assessment and other pathology testing techniques not currently endorsed by mainstream medicine.

The diagnostic process should flow from an extensive case history and physical examination to a differential diagnosis that lists possible alternatives for the presentations within the patient. An awareness of different types of pathology that may lead to particular signs and symptoms will assist the naturopath to narrow down the list of possibilities and select the most likely hypothesis.[1]

Further investigations, including pertinent biochemical evaluations, should then be performed to point to a more definitive diagnosis. This diagnosis, along with any other health issues that may have presented during the investigation, should all be used to address a patient from a holistic perspective and develop an adequate management plan. Clinical methods of diagnosis are best used in combination, and when interpreted alone possess definite disadvantages. Physical signs in conjunction with dietary and biochemical methods may provide a clearer picture of the physiology or pathophysiology at play in each individual. This chapter provides an overview of a variety of physical examination techniques such as anthropometric data, body signs and symptoms, gastrointestinal palpation and iridology, as well as an outline of dietary assessment methods and biochemical evaluations via a variety of pathology testing methods. Some of these types of assays have robust scientific bases, while others that have not been so extensively studied have

NATUROPATHIC DIAGNOSTIC TECHNIQUES

Evidence-based
- Physical examination:
  - anthropometric data
  - body signs and symptoms
  - gastrointestinal palpation
- Dietary assessment
- Pathology testing—blood, urine, stool, saliva, hair
- Factors affecting nutritional status

Traditional or emerging evidence-based
- Iridology
- Dark field microscopy
- Bioelectrical impedance
- Humoral theory
- Adapted traditional Chinese medicine diagnostic techniques

been included as an overview of available techniques. The chapter then concludes with some useful traditional Chinese medicine analytical methods that have been adapted for naturopathic diagnostic purposes. A section on factors that affect nutritional status has also been included as a tool to assist with identifying potential confounding variables that should also be taken into consideration.

EVIDENCE-BASED CLINICAL DIAGNOSTIC TECHNIQUES

Physical examination

Naturopathic physical examination should be systematic and precisely recorded, while relating particular signs to standardised definitions. Assessment of a patient begins as soon as the consultation starts. A person's disposition, facial complexion and expression, body size and shape, mobility, gait and posture, as well as the way they conduct or hold themselves, may provide important clues in relation to their mental and physical states.[1] A general inspection of the whole body may reveal external evidence of a disease, for example obesity, wasting, arthritis, abnormal stature or development, presence of pain, jaundice, pallor or cyanosis.[2]

Warm, sweaty palms on the initial handshake may indicate an overactive thyroid due to increased circulation with blood vessel dilation. In contrast, an underactive thyroid may cause the hands to be cool and dry in texture.[3] Persons with alcohol dependence may attempt to conceal their addiction; however, certain signs may provide indicators such as plethoric faces, rhinophymic noses and alcoholic aroma. Smokers may also be revealed by their scent or nicotine-stained fingers. A person's facial expression may portray psychiatric illness such as depression, while conversation may alert to an anxiety disorder. In developing countries, malnutrition with subsequent wasting and loss of weight is a relatively common occurrence; however, when these signs appear in more developed populations, naturopaths should be alerted to potential underlying pathological conditions such as diabetes, thyrotoxicosis, malabsorption syndromes or chronic infections.[4]

Anthropometric data

To begin a regular physical examination, a person's anthropometric data—including height, weight, waist and hip measures, as well as skin fold or bioelectrical impedance analysis (BIA) to give an estimation of body fat percentages and lean mass—can be collected. Next, a methodical inspection of the hands and nails, skin colour and texture, hair, face and mouth including the tongue, eyes, irises and sclera, concluding with gastrointestinal palpation.

Height and weight should be determined to assess if a person is over- or underweight. Waist to hip ratio (WHR) is the most useful predictor of cardiovascular disease mortality while body mass index (BMI = weight (kg)/height (m²)) may be a better predictor of increased mortality from raised blood pressure (see Table 2.1).[5]

Some form of body composition analysis, whether via skin fold or BIA, should also be performed to determine lean mass or protein sufficiency. Protein insufficiency may have widespread ramifications. Hypoproteinaemia can cause deviations in circulating levels of certain micronutrients, such as iron,[6] zinc, copper[7] and potentially selenium.[8]

Body signs and symptoms

Physical signs may be important aids in identifying nutritional dysfunction, though care should also be taken during case taking as particular signs may not be specific and may relate to non-biological factors (such as injury or excessive sun exposure). Signs may also differ between populations and may also vary over time periods within a population.[9] Any findings suggesting an abnormality should be considered a clue rather than a diagnosis. Table 2.2 outlines a variety of signs and symptoms as documented in research literature.

Bioelectrical impedance analysis

Bioelectrical impedance analysis measures the impedance or opposition to the flow of an electric current (usually 50 kHz) through the body fluids contained mainly in the lean and fat tissue. This is generally low in lean tissue, where intracellular fluid and electrolytes are primarily contained, but high in fat tissue. In practice, a small constant current is passed between electrodes spanning the body and the voltage drop between electrodes provides a measure of impedance. The resulting impedance reading is proportional to the total body water volume. Prediction equations are used to convert impedance to a corresponding estimate of total body water.[127] Lean body mass is then calculated from this estimate using an assumed hydration fraction for lean tissue. Fat mass may then be calculated by subtracting lean mass from total body weight. Although commonly accepted as a measure of these markers many naturopathic practitioners adopt novel conclusions from this technique that are yet to build an evidentiary base.

Table 2.1 Data that predict increased mortality from cardiovascular disease and raised blood pressure[5]

FEMALES	MALES
WHR > 0.8	WHR > 0.9
Waist circumference of > 88	Waist circumference of > 102
BMI > 25	BMI > 30

Table 2.2 Body signs and symptoms in nutritional deficiency

SYSTEM	SIGN	POSSIBLE NUTRIENT DEFICIENCIES
Biliary	Fatty liver deposits	Omega-6 EFA[10]
Cardiovascular	Cardiac arrhythmias, atherosclerosis Hypertension Tachycardia Palpitations	Mg[11] Mg,[11] Ca[12] Fe[13] Vitamin B12,[14] Fe[13]
Eyes	Bitot's spots—current or may be artefact of past deficiency Dry eyes Night blindness Amblyopia Corneal vascularisation Retinal haemorrhage Photophobia Blurred vision Pallor of conjunctiva Blue sclera	Vitamin A[15] Vitamin A,[16] EFA[17] Vitamin A,[16] Zn[13] Vitamin B1[13] Vitamin B2[18] Fe[13] Vitamin B2, B3, Zn[17] Omega-3 EFA[19,10] Fe[20] Fe[21]
Face	Nasolabial dermatitis Red, scaly, greasy, painful rashes on external ears and eyelids Seborrheic dermatitis of the mouth, nose and ears with cheilosis Smell dysfunction Symmetrical dry scaly dermatitis of the nose, mouth and eyes progressing to pustular and erosive Hyperpigmentation around mouth, eye and malar areas	Vitamin B2[17] Vitamin B2[13] Vitamin B6[17] Zn[22] Mg[17] Protein[17]
Endocrine	Abnormal glucose tolerance Reduced pancreatic insulin Goitre	Mg,[23] chromium[24] Mg[23] Iodine[25]
Gastrointestinal	Abdominal pain Digestive disturbances, indigestion Loss of appetite Flatulence and constipation Diarrhoea Weight loss, anorexia Nausea, vomiting Colon cancer Malabsorption Pica	Vitamin B3[17] Vitamin B3,[17] B12,[13] Se[26] Vitamin B12,[14] Zn[22] Vitamin B12[14] Vitamin B3,[17] Zn[27] Vitamin B1,[28] B3,[26] B12,[13] folate,[26] biotin,[29] Mg[30] Biotin,[29] Mg[30] Ca[30] Zn[27] Fe[31]
Genitourinary	Lesions of the scrotum and vulva Perirectal ulcerations Perineal seborrheic dermatitis Reproductive failure Male infertility Sexual immaturity Menstrual irregularity Urinary frequency and loss of libido	Vitamin B2[17] Folate[17] Folate[17] Omega-6 EFA[10] Se[32] Zn[22] Fe[13] Fe[13]

(Continued)

Table 2.2 Body signs and symptoms in nutritional deficiency *(Continued)*

SYSTEM	SIGN	POSSIBLE NUTRIENT DEFICIENCIES
Hair	Premature greying of hair	Vitamin B12,[17] protein,[17] biotin[33]
	Hair loss	EFA,[33] Fe,[33] Se,[26] protein[17]
	Hair thinning with loss of colour	Biotin[17]
	Sparse growth	Omega-6 EFA,[34] protein[20]
	Alopecia with loss of eyelashes in some cases	Zn[17]
	Depigmentation	Cu,[17] Se,[17] protein[20]
	Lack of eyelashes and eyebrows	Cu[17]
	Brittle, dry, split, lustreless	Fe,[21] protein[17]
Haematological	Impaired synthesis of red blood cells	Vitamin A[35]
	Depressed immunity with increased infections	Vitamin A,[16] folate,[36] omega-6 EFA,[34] Zn[17,37]
	Hypochromic, microcytic anaemia	Vitamin B6,[7] Fe[31]
	Megaloblastic anaemia	Vitamin B12[14]
	Markedly increased serum lactate dehydrogenase	Vitamin B12[38]
	Haemolytic anaemia	Vitamin E,[39,40] EFA,[41] Se[31]
	Excessive bleeding	Vitamin K[13]
	Capillary fragility	Vitamin C,[26] EFA[17]
	Distended blood vessels	Cu[17]
Mouth	Impaired taste	Vitamin A,[13] Zn[22]
	Red painful tongue	Vitamin B1,[17] B12, folate[13]
	Mouth pain and tenderness	Vitamin B2[42]
	Glossydinia (tongue pain)	Fe[21]
	Glossitis (tongue inflammation)	Vitamin B3,[17] B6,[43] B12,[44] B12,[17] Zn,[13] Fe[17]
	Magenta coloured glossitis	Vitamin B2[18]
	Aphthous stomatitis	Vitamin B1,[17] folate,[26] Fe[21]
	Angular stomatitis/ angular cheilosis	Vitamin B2,[18] B3,[20] folate[26]
	Stomatitis (mouth inflammation)	Vitamin B6,[43] B12[44]
	Cheilosis/cheilitis (lip cracking and inflammation)	Vitamin B2,[18] B3,[20] folate[17]
	Bright red painful 'raw beef' tongue with fissures	Vitamin B3[17]
	Smooth shiny tongue	Vitamin B12, folate,[13] biotin,[33] Fe[17]
	Greyish mucous membranes	Biotin[17]
	Pallor mucous membranes	Folate,[26] Fe[20]
	Mucosal ulceration	Folate[17]
	Haemorrhagic gingivitis	Vitamin C[45]
	Dry	EFA[17]
	Garlic breath	Se[26]
	Metallic taste	Se[26]

(Continued)

Gastrointestinal palpation

Gastrointestinal palpation should be performed only by practitioners trained in this skill and when deemed appropriate through the case-taking process. In addition to its more generalised conventional application, it may also be a beneficial technique to alert a practitioner to an underlying digestive dysfunction in a naturopathic consult.

Palpitation of the abdominal area may reveal various underlying organ pathologies such as liver disease or gall bladder insufficiencies (see Figure 2.1a):

- Muscle guarding may indicate pain—voluntary guarding may occur in people who are cold, tense or ticklish, and relaxation techniques may reduce this type.
- Tenderness or rigidity may also be indicative of underlying pathology in the palpated area,[64] such as rectal sheath sensitivity, which may indicate dysbiosis.

Table 2.2 Body signs and symptoms in nutritional deficiency *(Continued)*

SYSTEM	SIGN	POSSIBLE NUTRIENT DEFICIENCIES
Musculoskeletal	Growth retardation	Vitamin A,[16] EFA,[34,41] Mg,[30] Zn[22]
	Malaise	Vitamin B1[28]
	Flabby muscles	Fe[46]
	Fatigue, weakness	Vitamin B1,[28] B2,[42] B3, B5,[17] B12,[26] C,[45] Fe[46]
	Muscle pain and weakness	Se[46]
	Proximal muscle weakness	Vitamin D[47]
	Leg pains and weakness	Omega-3 EFA[19]
	Leg cramps	Vitamin B5[17]
	Tenderness of hands and feet 'burning foot syndrome'	Vitamin B5[17]
	Joint pains	Vitamin C[26]
	Bone disorders	Vitamin C,[26] D[47]
	Connective tissue disorders	Vitamin C[26]
	Bowing of the arms, knock-knees or outward bowing	Vitamin D[48]
	Muscle fasciculation, muscle spasms	Mg,[23] Ca[49]
	Osteopenia, osteoporosis	Ca[50]
Nails	Eggshell nails	Vitamin A[51]
	Variable brown–black pigmentation	Vitamin B12[52]
	Splinter haemorrhages near the distal ends of nails	Vitamin C[13]
	Brittle	EFA,[17] Fe[53]
	Variable white pigmentation of the nails	Ca[52]
	Spoon shaped nails (koilonychias)	Fe[17]
	Fragile, thin, longitudinally ridged	Fe[21]
	White nail beds	Se[17]
	Poor growth	Protein[20]
Nervous	Peripheral neuropathy	Vitamin E,[26] chromium,[24] Se[26]
	Peripheral neuropathy presenting mainly with symmetric foot drop	Vitamin B1[13]
	Tingling and numb extremities	Vitamin B12[54]
	Anxiety	Vitamin B3[26]
	Irritability	Vitamin B1,[28] B3,[26] B6,[43] C,[45] E,[14] Se[26]
	Nervousness	Mg[11]
	Tremor	Mg[13]
	Convolutions	Ca[49]
Neurological	Balance disturbances	Vitamin A,[13] B12,[54] E[55]
	Ataxia with loss of position and vibratory sense	Vitamin B1[13]
	Paresthesia	Omega-3 EFA[19]
	Burning paresthesia in the feet	Vitamin B1[13]
	Sleeplessness	Vitamin B1,[28] folate[26]
	Personality changes	Vitamin B2[42]
	Depression	Vitamin B1,[28] B3,[17] Mg[11]
	Depression with confusion	Vitamin B6,[43] B12,[56] folate[26]
	Confusion	Zn[27]
	Headaches with fatigue	Vitamin B6,[26] Fe[13]
	Memory loss	Vitamin B12[54]
	Learning deficits	Omega-3 EFA,[10] iodine[57]
	Apathy	Mg,[11] Zn[27]
	Delirium, hallucinations	Mg[11]
	Behaviour disorders	Zn[27]
	Tinnitus and vertigo	Fe[13]

(Continued)

Table 2.2 Body signs and symptoms in nutritional deficiency *(Continued)*

SYSTEM	SIGN	POSSIBLE NUTRIENT DEFICIENCIES
Other nutrients	Impaired iron mobilisation with increased stores and decrease in plasma iron	Vitamin A[58]
	Calcium/potassium abnormalities	Mg[59,60]
	Impaired vitamin A metabolism	Zn[61]
Respiratory	Impaired lung function and wheezing	Mg[62]
	Dyspnoea on exertion	Vitamin B12,[14] Fe[20]
Skin	Perifollicular hyperkeratosis on the lateral aspects of the upper arms and the thighs	Vitamin A, B complex, EFAs,[13] C[17]
	Xerotic, wrinkled skin covered with fine scales 'toad skin'	Vitamin A[17]
	Seborrheic dermatitis	Vitamin B2[18]
	Symmetrical dermatitis on dorsal surface of hands with erythema, slight oedema, pruritus and burning	Vitamin B3[17]
	Symmetric hyperpigmentation on distal extremities involving the palms	Vitamin B12[17]
	Petechiae	Folate,[31] C[14]
	Pallor	Vitamin B12, folate,[26] biotin,[29,26] protein[17]
	Diffuse hyperpigmentation	Folate[17]
	Depigmentation	Cu,[17] Se[17]
	Dry scaly dermatitis first appearing around the eyes, nose and mouth	Biotin[29]
	Dry flaky skin progressing to scaling dermatitis starting on the nasolabial folds and eyebrows and spreading across the face and neck	Omega-6 EFA[63]
	Poor wound healing	Vitamin C,[14] EFA,[34,17] Zn,[17,13]
	Peripheral oedema	Protein[20]
	Oedema	Vitamin E[14]
	Dryness and depigmentation in premature infants	Vitamin E[17]
	Atopic eczema and dermatitis	EFA[33]
	Dry	EFA[17]
	Inelastic	Cu[17]
	Pruritus	Fe[21]
	Thin, dull, greyish	Protein[20]
	Cyanosis in cold weather	Protein[17]

- The liver may be enlarged; this may indicate toxicity or dysfunctions causing hepato-megaly.
- The spleen may be enlarged, signifying immune system upregulation or trauma.

Palpation may also locate a mass. If so, it must be distinguished from a normally palpable structure or enlarged organ and note must be taken of its location, size, shape, tenderness, consistency, surface, mobility, pulsatility and tenderness. Gastrointestinal palpation may also be used in conjunction with other abdominal physical examinations, such as auscultation and percussion, to elicit required information. An example of this is that a fluid wave indicates ascites, which may occur with heart failure, portal hypertension, cirrhosis of the liver, hepatitis, pancreatitis and cancer.[64]

Prior to commencing palpation, the abdomen should be viewed for any intestinal bloating or asymmetry, prior to palpating each organ individually. On palpation look for any tenderness or muscular guarding, which may indicate potential issues in that region. When palpating, keep one hand flat; this will be in contact with the abdomen

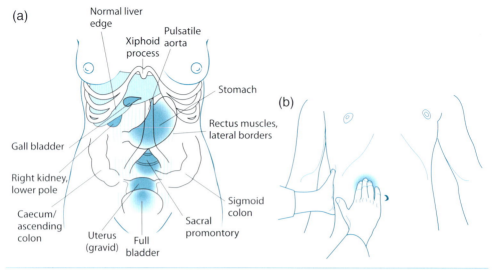

Figure 2.1 (a) Normally palpable abdominal structures (b) Palpating the liver
Source: Adapted from Jarvis 2007[64]

and the other on top to apply pressure for palpation. Initially, gentle pressure should be applied, then pressure more deeply.

Palpation should begin in the upper middle region below the ribcage where the stomach is located. To the right along the line of the ribs is the gallbladder and further to the right is the liver. Across on the far left of the stomach, the spleen is located somewhat deeper than the previous organs. If you roll the person onto their right side the pancreas may be felt if deep pressure is placed from near the side moving toward the midline and slightly upward. Next the area around the umbilicus is the small intestines, while slightly above and toward the right is the duodenum. Distal to the small intestine is the ascending colon with the appendix situated below the latter. The jejunum is located to the left of the small intestine; continuing in this direction the descending colon with the sigmoid is found below. From this position moving medially, above the pubic bone, is the rectal sheath (see Figure 2.1).

Nutritional assessment

Clinical signs due to insufficient nutrition may occur primarily due to underlying changes in metabolic processes.[65] Optimal nutrition is indispensible for proper physiological functioning, where adequate intakes need to be considered with factors such as impaired digestion and absorption. Excessive losses may result from chronic haemorrhage or catabolic states, as well as from the use of certain medications such as diuretics or corticosteroids.[66] At any time a need is elevated, the risk of developing a deficiency is increased. Adequate macro- and micronutrients are crucial for growth and maintenance of tissues, preventing cell damage and mutation,[67] as well as immune system function[68] and may decrease the likelihood of chronic disease development. It is considered by some investigators that an underlying condition linked to nutritional status may cause undefined or subsyndromal symptoms such as irritability, insomnia, lethargy and difficulty in concentrating.[69] If tissue stores become depleted, various clinical manifestations may become apparent and, if left untreated, progress to deficiency disease states.

For example, protein deficiency can affect the status of many other nutrients, namely type II nutrients such as phosphorus, potassium, sodium, chlorine, water, nitrogen, sulfur, zinc and magnesium, as well as the essential amino acids. Deficiency of any one of these nutrients may result in cessation of growth, increased catabolism and, eventually, loss of all tissue components.[70] These nutrients are required to be absorbed in approximately the same ratios as occur in the body. Secondary deficiencies may manifest if supplements that do not contain all of the necessary nutrients for tissue synthesis are given. It is possible to unbalance the diet and cause a greater level of malnutrition via the dilution of any potentially existing marginal levels of these nutrients.[71] The *Oxford Textbook of Medicine* states:

> *These types of deficiency states have always posed problems for clinicians because of the difficulty in making a diagnosis, the non-specificity of weight loss and the lack of confirmatory tests. This has led these nutrients to be largely ignored and their importance to be grossly underestimated. As a group, their deficiency is responsible for malnutrition in half the world's children and to the unrecognised problems of ill health in many others.*[70]

These interactions may be bidirectional. For example, protein deficiency can significantly affect vitamin A metabolism, and in turn its deficiency can influence protein metabolism. Protein insufficiency principally affects vitamin A status via mechanisms such as impeding intestinal absorption, release from the liver and blood transport. In light of this, protein deficiency can lead to a secondary deficiency of this vitamin, despite an adequate intake. Vitamin A deficiency, on the other hand, can also influence the metabolism of proteins by lowering the plasma levels of retinol-binding protein, impairing nitrogen balance and decreasing the synthesis of other specific proteins such as enzymes and hormones.[35]

Dietary assessment

In naturopathic practice, dietary assessment forms an integral part of the diagnostic process. While signs and symptoms (discussed previously) and blood tests (to follow) may reveal nutritional deficiencies, dietary assessment may reveal patterns of macro- or micronutrient intake. In general, dietary analysis involves the naturopath recording the patient's dietary habits and making an assessment of which nutrients are in excess or deficiency. In addition, recording the patient's dietary habits can allow the naturopath to observe the preferred eating patterns of the patient and allow them to individually tailor a dietary prescription that can improve compliance. In brief, the typical Western diet can be high in refined carbohydrates and saturated fats, while low in lean protein, complex carbohydrates and fibre as well as micronutrients (such as B vitamins, vitamin C, zinc, magnesium and calcium), essential fatty acids and other beneficial phytochemicals. After an assessment is made, general dietary advice or a more complex nutritional program can be instituted by the naturopath.

Dietary assessment methods may be controversial as they require a patient's recall of either their usual or their actual diet and may be influenced by the patient not consuming a representative diet during the assessment period, along with variations in perceived quantities also having the potential to occur. Retrospective methods such as 24-hour recall, semi-quantitative food frequency questionnaires and diet histories all have the disadvantage of assessing memory, which may limit the quality of information presented. Factors that have been documented to affect recall accuracy include food consumption patterns, gender, age, weight status and even mood.[72]

Other methods such as 3–7-day food diaries and weighed food records may be better alternatives. This information is documented at the actual time the food is consumed. The information gained from such exercises may be analysed by various software programs to provide a more detailed assessments of actual nutrient intakes.[73] Various commercial programs are available. Alternatively, food table information databases are accessible on the internet for various nations including Australia,[74] the USA,[75] Canada[76] and Europe.[77] These methods may also be subject to the bias of variations in a patient's change of dietary choices during the assessment period, as well as deviations in perceived quantities for the former method. Although weighed records may be the most accurate, this process is extremely labour intensive and may have issues with compliance. Digestion and absorption may also affect the accuracy of intake estimates on body status.[14]

Prior to undertaking such an investigation, people should be assured that they will not be judged on their food diaries and the more accurate the information they provide, the better they can be assisted to improve their overall health. Again, these types of methods should be used as another piece to the complex physiological puzzle.

Pathology testing

Blood analysis

The analysis of blood cells may be a useful tool to confirm a suspected dysfunction or deficiency. These may also play an important role in monitoring the efficacy of a treatment program and to highlight improvements in a patient's condition. Particular reference ranges for specific assays may be laboratory, age and gender specific; therefore it is best to consult national standards for their appropriate values. A list of Australian reference ranges can be found in Appendix 4.

For example, glucose tolerance testing may be a useful tool to assess blood sugar regulation (see Figures 2.2 and 2.3). The test is performed immediately following a fast of at least 8 hours, but no more than 16 hours. A fasting blood glucose test is performed immediately prior to the glucose tolerance testing. If the level is ≥ 7.0 mmol/L, the glucose tolerance testing is usually not performed, as this level is diagnostic of diabetes mellitus. Gestational diabetes mellitus or suspected diabetes may be indicated when the fasting glucose is 5.5–6.9 mmol/L or a random glucose level is 7.8–11.0 mmol/L. A dose of oral glucose is then administered at 75 g for an adult and 1.75 g/kg body weight (75 g maximum) for children, after an overnight fast in subjects consuming at least 150 g of carbohydrate daily for 3 days prior to the test.[78] Medications that impair glucose tolerance, such as diuretics, glucocorticoids, nicotinic acid and phenytoin, may invalidate results.[79]

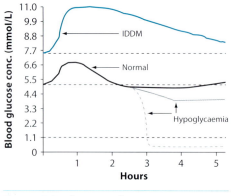

Figure 2.2 Glucose tolerance test interpretation

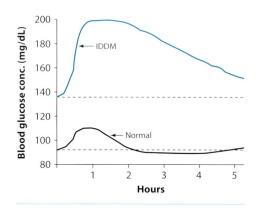

Figure 2.3 Blood glucose reference levels

Blood glucose reference intervals
Normal: fasting < 5.5 mmol/L
    2 hour < 7.8 mmol/L
Impaired glucose tolerance: fasting < 5.5 mmol/L
    2 hour 7.8–11.0 mmol/L
Impaired fasting glycaemia: fasting 5.5–6.9 mmol/L
    2 hour < 7.8 mmol/L
Diabetes mellitus: fasting ≥ 7.0 mmol/L
    2 hour ≥ 11.1 mmol/L[78]
Reactive hypoglycaemia: fasting < 5.5 mmol/L
    2 hour < 7.8 mmol/L
    after 3 hours decrease ≥ 1.1 mmol/L below fasting.[79]

A selection of more commonly used blood pathology tests, along with potential indicators, is outlined in the appendices.

Validity of direct micronutrient analyses

Assessment of mineral status has traditionally included body signs and symptoms, although in recent times it has relied on the quantification of mineral element concentrations in a variety of components and cells in the blood. This strategy is based on the assumption that circulating mineral concentrations reflect organ and tissue mineral contents. Although methods such as these have been used, it has not been a sensitive approach for the evaluation of the total body nutritional status of mineral elements.[80]

The term 'acute phase response' is used to describe a short-term metabolic change, encompassing increased plasma levels of particular proteins and decreased levels of others. These responses occur not only in tissue injury such as infection, surgical or other trauma, burns, tissue infarction and a variety of idiopathic inflammatory states, but have also been documented in pregnancy, during the first few days in a neonate's life and in neoplastic states.[81] Several frequently used indicators of micronutrient status are affected by the acute phase response and may not effectively reflect micronutrient status. During an acute phase response, there can be a redistribution of micronutrients without actual alterations in the total body content of the micronutrient, resulting in commonly used serum indicators producing inaccurate measurements. On the other hand, requirements or losses may be amplified during this time and also occasionally in combination with impaired assimilation, inevitably resulting in an alteration in body stores.[82]

Micronutrients are also disseminated among circulating, storage and tissue pools, depending on the chemical nature of their environment. Physiological stress, intercompartmental fluid shifts, acid–base balance and recent dietary intake can all influence a nutrient's existence within a particular pool. Hypoproteinaemia during malnutrition alters the circulating levels of certain nutrients such as iron,[6] zinc, copper[7] and potentially selenium,[8] regardless of tissue store adequacy, due to them circulating in plasma bound to protein carriers.[67] Plasma levels of vitamins A, C, E and B6 have also been shown to be altered during an acute phase response.[83] In these instances a measure of an acute phase protein such as C-reactive protein, would be useful in identifying the presence of an acute phase response.[6]

Furthermore, levels of micronutrients may also be modified during the haemodilution at certain stages of pregnancy or surgery and have been shown to be influenced by exercise, with the most evident changes occurring throughout the inflammatory processes of infection[84] or trauma. Nutrient levels in both plasma and serum may also appear to be sufficient, even when there is verification of functional impairment due to the serum concentrations of some nutrients, such as calcium, vitamin A and zinc, being strongly homeostatically regulated,[85,86] therefore providing little information on total body status. In cases such as these, alternative biochemical indicators may be needed, such as the assay of intracellular enzymes or other metabolites known to be dependent upon an adequate supply of a micronutrient.[87]

Functional laboratory tests assess the extent of functional impairments during a specific nutrient deficiency and as such have greater biological implication than commonly used static laboratory tests. Functional biochemical tests may involve the measurement of an abnormal metabolic product in blood or urine samples, which is caused by the overflow of an intermediary by-product, due to a lack of a nutrient-dependent enzyme. For some nutrients, reduction in the activity of enzymes that require a nutrient as a coenzyme or prosthetic group can also be assayed.[26] Here the underlying assumption is that loss of such functions is biologically more important than the levels of a mineral element in circulation or in a tissue or organ. In light of this concept, various functional parameters may serve as diagnostic tests to verify the adequacy of a variety of vitamins and minerals to permit cells, tissues, organs, anatomical systems and the individual to optimally carry out nutrient-dependent biological functions.[80]

Table 2.3 outlines specific nutrients and the best readily available assessment methods to determine status, as well as factors that may affect results.

Urine testing
Nutrient status assessment
Assessment of the majority of vitamins and trace elements in urine is of limited value as most are not under homeostatic regulation. Excretion may be a direct measure of intake as opposed to active retention even in cases of whole body deficiency. Large dosages of supplements at any given time can lead to high levels of excretion.[14] Urine specimens may be used for the assessment of recent dietary intake of some trace elements such as chromium, iodine and selenium, as well as protein and the water-soluble B and C vitamins, if renal function is normal. This type of assessment is invalid in cases where metabolites are not excreted in proportion to amounts consumed, absorbed and metabolised, such as vitamins A, D, E and K.[26]

In relation to the minerals for which the kidneys are not involved in maintaining homeostasis, measurement of urinary excretion rates does not provide useful information on dietary intake or mineral status. In contrast, excretion rates of iodine for which the kidneys have a prominent role in homeostasis provide a useful biomarker of dietary intake of this mineral.[97] In circumstances such as infections, after trauma, with the use of antibiotics or other medications, as well as in conditions that produce negative balance, increases in urinary excretion may occur regardless of depletion of body nutrient stores.[26]

Urinary organic acid assays
These tests may be a useful tool for the detection of organic acids or heavy metals. Organic acids derived from the metabolic conversion of dietary proteins, fats and carbohydrates provide a unique chemical profile of cellular health. Key intermediate metabolic markers of cellular physiology are quantified to assess compromised energy production, detoxification, intestinal microbial activity, neurotransmitter metabolism and nutrient deficiencies. Clinically, these markers offer valuable information into possible causative factors of dysfunctional cellular physiology physical and mental performance, as well as overall health status.[98]

Table 2.3 Assessment methods for nutrients

NUTRIENT	ASSAY	CONFOUNDING VARIABLES
Vitamin A	Retinol binding protein: transthyretin (prealbumin)	Vitamin A is strongly homeostatically regulated.[88] Acute phase response will decrease levels irrespective of tissue status.[14] Protein energy malnutrition may affect the binding of retinol.[89] Ratio < 0.36 → marginal deficiency.[89]
B1	Red cell thiamine pyrophosphate	
B2	Erythrocyte glutathione reductase activity coefficient	Severe tissue deficiency may reduce apo-enzyme activity → falsely elevated activity coefficient.[14] Decreased values may exist with a negative nitrogen balance.[26]
B6	Urinary kynurenate or xanthure-nate + PLP coenzyme	Interferences in the tryptophan pathway → increased metabolic flux by corticoids and oestrogens. Bacterial endotoxins, viral infections, protein intake, exercise, lean body mass and pregnancy → increased metabolite excretion.[88] No single marker adequately reflects status; a combination may be the best approach.[14]
B12	Methylmalonic acid in serum	
Folic acid	Red cell folate	
Vitamin C	Leukocyte vitamin C	Complex methodology → issues with accuracy and precision.[90] Acute disease → increased uptake by leukocytes.[87]
Vitamin D	25-hydroxy vitamin D	Initial chromatographic sample clean-up is essential for accurate results.[91] Oral contraceptive use → increased levels due to oestrogen increasing levels of vitamin D-binding protein.[26]
Vitamin E	Plasma α-tocopherol:cholesterol ratio	Acute phase inflammatory response decreases circulating levels.[92] Ratio < 2.2 µmol α-tocopherol/mmol cholesterol is associated with deficiency.
Magnesium	Red cell magnesium	
Calcium	Osteocalcin	Serum calcium is strongly homeostatically regulated. Alcohol intake and vitamin D status.[26]
Zinc	Plasma zinc	Acute phase response lowers circulating levels irrespective of body status.[6]
Selenium	Red cell glutathione peroxidase	Deficiencies of iron, vitamin B12 or essential fatty acids, exposure to pro-oxidants, toxins or heavy metals.[93]

(Continued)

Table 2.3 Assessment methods for nutrients *(Continued)*

NUTRIENT	ASSAY	CONFOUNDING VARIABLES
Iodine	Thyroglobulin	High variability between methods and laboratories.[94] Administration of thyroid hormone decreases levels.[95] Values increased in thyroid cancer, pregnancy, thyroiditis, thyrotoxicosis.[95]
Iron	Soluble transferrin receptor:ferritin ratio	Any change in erythropoiesis such as folate or B12 deficiency increases transferrin receptor, while inflammation increases ferritin, therefore a ratio may be more ideal. Receptor values > 8.5 mg/L and ferritin < 12 mg/L is indicative of deficiency.[96]

Urinalysis

Dipstick urinalysis is a method of urine analysis involving dipping a plastic strip with a series of pads that change colour according to specific chemical reactions into a sample of urine. Results are then read off this strip by comparing it to a chart that shows levels of substances in the urine, depending on the colour change that occurred. A variety of substances, including protein, glucose, bilirubin, blood and pH, may be investigated at one time. Despite being simple, fast and easy to use, many dipsticks may not be completely accurate and therefore may provide false positive results.[99]

Urinary indicans

The production of indicans such as indoxyl potassium sulfate and indoxyl glucoronate is thought to reflect bacterial activity in the small and large intestines. As such it has been used as an indicator of intestinal toxaemia and overgrowth of anaerobic bacteria, although research on this method has been quite limited. A positive test may indicate hypochlorhydria, bacterial overgrowth in the small intestine,[100] malabsorption of protein or a high protein diet.[101]

Stool/digestive tests

Stool analysis can be used to provide an overview or the components of digestion, absorption, intestinal function and microbial flora, as well as identifying the presence of any pathogenic bacteria, yeasts or parasites. These types of tests can be extremely useful as dysfunctions of any of these elements may play a crucial role in the underlying cause of many health conditions (refer further to the section on the gastrointestinal system).

Breath testing

Breath testing is a useful method of distinguishing small intestine bacterial overgrowth from other digestive disorders. The hydrogen and methane breath test uses a challenge dose of lactulose or glucose after an overnight fast in order to identify bacterial overgrowth in the small intestine. If dysbiosis exists in the small intestine, the bacteria will ferment the challenge substance and produce increased methane and hydrogen in the breath. Testing for both hydrogen and methane is more sensitive than testing for hydrogen alone, as fasting breath hydrogen levels can be suppressed by methanogenic bacteria.[102]

Alternatively, a challenge dose of lactose may be used to identify lactose intolerance.

Saliva

Salivary testing to measure levels of hormones such as cortisol and the sex steroid hormones has many advantages, both scientific and practical, over serum testing. The non-protein bound or unbound fractions of these hormones are measured, as opposed to the total levels, which are quantitated in serum measures. As these steroid hormones are predominantly bound to specific protein carriers, it is the free hormones that are considered to best reflect a person's hormonally related symptoms.[103] On the other hand, saliva levels of DHEA, thyroxine and cortisone may be of little value due to changes in their concentrations dependent upon salivary flow rate, enzymatic production or degradation by the salivary glands themselves, as well as contamination by plasma exudates, respectively.[104]

Hair

Hair analysis is one of the most meaningful and representative methods to detect and monitor heavy metal toxicity[105] or the ingestion of drugs, although its usefulness in identifying nutrient status remains controversial. Despite its many advantages such as its non-invasive manner, a number of pitfalls exist in using hair in nutritional assessment, including the wide variability in levels reported in healthy people; this may be due to methods of sampling and sample preparation, as well as alterations caused by shampoos, hair treatments and other forms of environmental contamination that may make mineral content inconsistent throughout the length of the hair strand.[106] Furthermore, results of measuring metal concentrations in hair, even under ideal circumstances, may not correlate with those obtained in blood pathology.[107]

FACTORS AFFECTING NUTRITIONAL STATUS

A variety of factors may influence nutritional status other than dietary insufficiency and therefore should be taken into account if a particular deficiency is suspected or a specific condition is present. Some conditions may increase the need for a particular nutrient, while others may interfere with its absorption or excretion.

Examples of these include omega-3 essential fatty acid status being affected by excessive omega-6 due to their competition for the enzyme delta-6-desaturase, or the antagonism between zinc and copper.[30] A variety of genetic polymorphisms that may affect the absorption of a nutrient or its bioavailability on a number of different levels depending on the position of the amino acid replacement on the nucleotide base within the DNA strand also exist.[108–110] A comprehensive examination of this issue is placed in Appendix 5.

IMPORTANT!

Traditional diagnostic techniques although widely used by naturopaths, are still building an evidentiary base. The next section is descriptive only and represents how these are is currently used in clinical practice, rather than promoting it as an evidence-based tool.

TRADITIONAL OR EMERGING DIAGNOSTIC TECHNIQUES

Iridology

Iridology is the study and analysis of the neuro-optic reflex, which is thought to have the potential to reveal disharmonies in the body ranging from pathological, structural and functional to psychological and emotional. Its roots stem as far back as the advanced ancient cultures of the Egyptians, Chinese and Greeks, and in more recent times the development of the German and American schools of iridology has seen numerous scientists and doctors accumulating knowledge of this area through their own personal research. Iris analysis as a tool of diagnosis has been officially accepted in the former Soviet Union (1984), South Korea (1996–97) and Belarus (2002).[111] It should be noted that much of the information discussed in this section has been derived from this empirical knowledge and currently lacks firm evidentiary support. While orthodox medical practice uses certain diagnostic signs of the iris (the arcus senilis or calcium ring), many other signs have not been adopted into conventional practice. A key point regarding the practice of iridology is that signs are considered to be reflective of a 'constitutional health pattern', rather than an indication of a specific disease, surgery or medications.

Iridology has the potential to reveal inherent strengths and weaknesses of organs, glands and tissues of the body, as well as the quality of assimilation of nutrients, inflammation and toxicity, circulatory and lymphatic congestion. It is not meant to nor does it reveal specific disease processes. Of the published evidence, negative studies exist for iridology to detect cancer,[112] gall bladder disease[113] and kidney disease,[114] concluding that this practice was no better than chance at detecting these conditions. Positive studies do exist for broader constitutional correlations, for example hypertension, TNF alpha gene and iris constitution.[115,116] As the skilled iridologist may be able to identify inherited or acquired health dispositions, as well as potential strengths and weaknesses within a system, the endpoint of final disease may not always manifest in these people and therefore the practitioner will be unable to place a definitive diagnosis. Here is the importance of using this science as an adjunct to the overall health assessment, giving possible clues to assist in piecing together the complex biological system of each patient.

A variety of positive articles have also been published, although many of these have been uncontrolled and unmasked investigations.[117,118] Much of the literature on iridology is published in non-English (predominantly Portuguese and Russian) literature and is therefore either difficult to source or not included in many systematic reviews.[119] A methodologically rigorous longitudinal study on the ability of both iridology and sclerology to detect or predict predisposed vulnerability to type 2 diabetes is currently being currently undertaken.[120] However, in general the evidence base for iridology remains poor to date, and even by naturopathic standards current approaches to iridology remain a relatively recent diagnostic invention.

In an iris evaluation the most outstanding iris signs and impressions should first be documented. Overall integrity of the fibres will give an indication of the ability of a patient to resist negative influences to their health. Next, constitutional types and subtypes, overall pigmentation patterns, then specific structural and pigmentation signs according to appearance and location on the iris chart should be noted (see Table 2.4). The area from the pupil and extending out concentrically through the digestive and nervous zones to the outer circulatory zone should also be examined sequentially.

Table 2.4 Subtypes according to structure

IRIS	IRIS CONSTITUTION	POTENTIAL PREDISPOSITIONS
	Neurogenic Iris is mainly blue and have tight, delicately arranged, thin, stretched iris fibres that appear to look like fine silk.	• Headaches and vascular spasms, especially in cerebral vessels • Weakness in the nervous system • Ulcers • Skin eruptions due to nervous dysfunction such as herpes or shingles • Weakened endocrine glands may also manifest particularly of the thyroid and adrenals
	Neuro-lymphatic Constitution is generally blue and often with large pupils and looser, wavy, brightened fibres.	• Anxiety conditions • The nervous system can affect circulation very strongly with corresponding fainting spells and dizziness, hypothermia and migraines due to vaso-motor disturbances. • Lymphatic congestion and inflammation • Diseases involving the mucous membranes and nervous system, including neurodermatitis, stress-related asthma, irritable bowel syndrome, nausea and burping
	Connective tissue Iris may be blue, blue-grey or occasionally brown, character-ised by very loose, widened iris fibres with many spaces in the iris fabric, separated fibres with a 'torn up' appearance.	• Connective and elastic tissue weakness, leading to condi-tions of prolapse, especially of the abdominal organs, varicosities and circulation issues due to weakened venous structure, haemor-rhoids, spinal anomalies and hernias. • General stagnation, low vital energy and weak stamina along with adrenal dysfunction
	Anxiety tetanic This is seen in any colour iris and consist of circular rings or half rings, spread concentri-cally throughout the iris. These are generally caused by a buckling of the fibres due to prolonged, excessive stress and neuromuscular tension of psychosomatic aetiology.	• Muscle tension and headaches • Gastrointestinal disorders such as ulcers, colitis and ner-vous stomach with intestinal spasms • Tachycardia, angina and circulatory disorders • Blood sugar dysregulation • Hyperthyroidism • Dark, deeper rings may be indicative of potassium deficiency. • Lighter shallow rings may indicate increased magne-sium requirement.

(Continued)

Table 2.4 Subtypes according to structure *(Continued)*

IRIS	IRIS CONSTITUTION	POTENTIAL PREDISPOSITIONS
	Hormonal Present in blue or brown iris, with spaces in the iris fabric positioned in a geometric pattern around the autonomic nerve wreath. These holes may be open or closed, small or large with fibres presenting underneath. A study found lacunae on a hypertonic autonomic nerve wreath a common finding in women with polycystic ovarian syndrome. This was frequently accompanied with dilated pupils (73%),[122] which is also commonly associated with fatigue and adrenal weakness.	• Weakness in the endocrine system, mainly thyroid, adrenal, pituitary and pancreas • Weakness in the endodermal lining of the gastrointestinal system, causing problems with glandular secretions and irregularity of the bowels • Smaller holes are evidence of more functional disturbances of the glands. • Larger holes indicate greater organic and congenital degeneration of the glands. • Issues with the central nervous system can lead to fluid retention, blood pressure and body weight fluctuations, basal metabolism disturbances, low motivation and drive with a need for extra sleep.

Source: Bernard Jensen International

The constitutional framework of German iridology is based on inherent iris signs that have been clinically researched and verified for pathology that may potentially occur if preventive measures are not taken (see Table 2.5). The iris may be categorised by basic colour, along with structures and colours: blue eyes being 'lymphatic', light brown 'biliary' and true brown eyes 'haematogenic'. These categories have been further subdivided into subtypes according to structure and overlying colours. Overall pigmentation patterns and structural signs can also be observed in relation to their location on the iris chart. Classical American-style iridology also focuses on structure and colours in specific regions of the iris, related to the various organ reflex positions. Here the depth of the openings of iris tissue are assessed; the deeper the lesion, the more chronic and degenerative condition. This theory also incorporates the idea of concentric circle zones radiating from the pupil to the periphery, with the pupil reflecting the central nervous system and the areas surrounding indicating in sequence, the digestive zone, blood and primary lymph nodes, endocrine glands, skeletal and muscular systems, secondary lymphatic system, skin and the blood capillaries that feed it. A study has demonstrated that almost half of the 87 hypertensive subjects displayed connective tissue weakness in the cardiac and renal positions in the iris.[121]

Figure 2.4 outlines the American chart and has been reproduced with permission from Bernard Jensen International.

To optimise the diagnostic benefits of iridology, a thorough assessment of the iris and surrounding sclera should be performed. It is paramount for naturopaths to be aware that, due to a lack of rigorous evidence at present, iridology should be considered more of an 'art' than a science. Clinical diagnoses should not be made via iridology alone, and the tool should be incorporated into an array of diagnostic techniques in order to provide a balanced, comprehensive and holistic framework.

Table 2.5 Basic iris signs

IRIS SIGN	REASON
Small pupil (miosis)	• 'Hypertension' of the nervous system and related structures • Orthodox medical texts suggest that pupil constriction may be due to diabetes or neurosyphilis, as well as possibly by Horner's syndrome in which lesions are found anywhere along the sympathetic nerve pathway.[4]
Large pupil (mydriasis)	• 'Hypotension' (and possible 'exhaustion') of the nervous system • Weakened adrenal glands • Predisposing to hypoglycaemia • Absent tendon-jerks in the limbs[4] • Sympathetic overactivity such as hyperthyroidism and anxiety,[2] which can lead to adrenal insufficiency
Pupil border and surrounding area	• Brightly coloured red or orange ring encircling the pupil—digestive insufficiency • Marked white ring—increased stomach acidity • Grey ring—under-acidity in the stomach and sluggish digestion • 'Toxic' colon—variety of dark brown or black deposits in zone 2 of the iris or dark elongated lines branching out from that region like spokes of a wheel • Cogwheel teeth border—spinal weakness • Thickened border—circulatory problems • Partial atrophy of inner border—endocrine dysfunction (in one study 78% of PCOS cases and 80% of subjects with endometriosis)[111]
Autonomic nerve wreath /collarette	• White inflamed fibres—nerve irritations • Constricted—bowel contraction and structure • Distended wreath—under-functioning intestines with poor peristalsis and slow motility • Thick or raised—excessive energy in the gastrointestinal tract and may predispose to diarrhoea, colic and spasms • Thin, delicate or intermittent wreath—poor absorption of minerals along with poor assimilation of vitamins • Jagged or star-shaped—spastic colon with irritability, strictures and potential inflammation
Outer edge of the iris periphery	• Dark ring—under-active, sluggishly eliminating skin with metabolic wastes accumulating • Blue ring—congestion or restriction in the venous blood supply causing reduced circulation, lowered oxygen and cold extremities • Translucent to opaque coating over the top portion of the iris—reduced oxygen transport to the brain leading to mental fatigue, poor memory and concentration (a study on 150 Alzheimer's patients documented the presence of a frontal arcus in many of the subjects)[123] • White or cream deposit in the cornea—high cholesterol or calcium build-up in the joints and tissues (according to orthodox medicine, infiltration of lipids and associated with hypercholesterolaemia and diabetes)[124]
Hyperpigmentation spots	• Potential dysfunctions, depending on colours and their location • Black—liver • Yellow—kidney • Orange—pancreas

Source: Bernard Jensen International

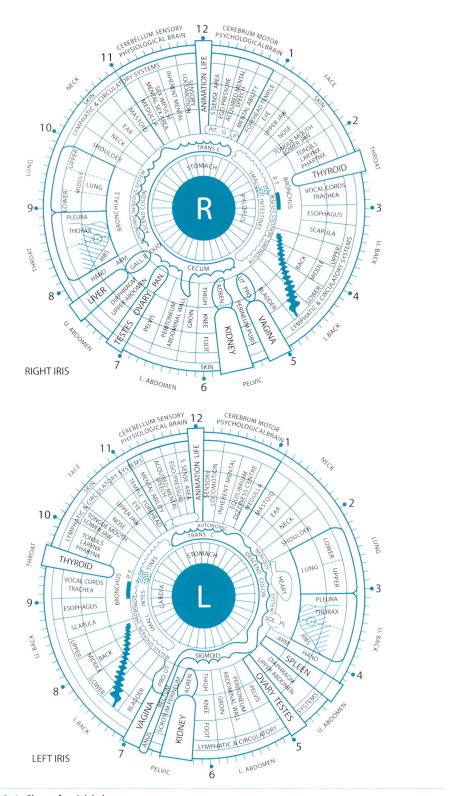

Figure 2.4 Chart for iridology
Source: Bernard Jensen International with permission

IRIDOLOGY AND PERSONALITY: ANY LINK?

Some systems of iridology advocate a connection between people's personality traits and their iris colour or iris structural features.

Aside from anecdotal reports, there have been several studies conducted (varying in methodological standard) over the past 30 years exploring the relationship.

Current evidence indicates the following:

- There may be a link with iris colour to personality in children.
- Hypotheses suggest that various encoding genes may express in different iris colours and features. These may be influenced by hormones and neurochemicals.
- When people age (> 9 years old), the association of personality to irises has been noted to disappear.
- Although a recent study found a connection between crypts and furrows and changes on the Neuroticism–Extroversion–Openness Inventory personality scale, these were not significant when conservative statistical methods were employed.[125]
- There is currently no solid evidence that consistently supports the link between iris colours or architectural features and personality traits in adults.

Dark field microscopy

Dark field microscopy or live blood-cell examination is a method of screening patients for abnormal cell morphology and for the detection of uncharacteristic substances within blood. This type of assessment may be clinically useful for identifying bacterial forms, blood cell morphology and the effects of cell-mediated immune responses. However, as stated in a position statement by the Council on Diagnosis and Internal Disorders, 'There is no direct correlation that can be ascertained with certainty regarding any defined nutritional component and the particular morphology that might be seen under the microscope'.[126] This council does, however, believe live blood analysis to be a beneficial diagnostic laboratory technique when used as a method of screening patients for abnormal cell morphology and for the identification of abnormal biological contents in blood plasma.[126]

CAUTION REGARDING CHOICE OF TECHNIQUES

Many 'new' diagnostic techniques are often commercial or proprietary in nature, incurring significant costs to both patient and naturopath. Although some may be based on a sound theory, practice or evidence base, others may often exaggerate or over-extrapolate diagnostic ability or have no diagnostic usefulness. Naturopathic practitioners need to apply critical analysis to their choice of diagnostic tools.

Humoral theory

Humoral medicine was the predominant type of medicine practised in England by orthodox naturopaths from the 1200s to 1800s.[128] The theory was based on early Greek manuscripts, believed to be written by Hippocrates in the 5th century BC. The four

Table 2.6 The interrelationships between humours, the mind and the body[128]

HUMOURS	QUANTITIES	TEMPERAMENT	ORGANS
Blood	Hot and wet	Sanguine	Heart
Phlegm	Cold and wet	Phlegmatic	Brain
Yellow bile	Hot and dry	Choleric	Liver
Black bile	Cold and dry	Melancholic	Spleen

humours doctrine states that the body consists of blood, phlegm, yellow and black bile. When the body is healthy, each is proportional in strength and quantity; however, if an imbalance has occurred, illness results.[128] As this balance is different in every person, it is necessary to determine the patient's normal humoral condition before an assessment can be made of the changes that caused the illness.[129] Extensive case taking from patients included pulse, urine inspection and symptoms of humoral changes such as heightened colour, quickening of pulse, swollen veins or headaches indicative of excess blood. Excessive phlegm may manifest as catarrh, slow pulse, indigestion or poor appetite, too much yellow bile as jaundice, and surplus black bile as mental disturbances such as nightmares or depression. A variety of treatments may have been employed and include medicines, dietary measures, bloodletting, purging and counter-irritation.[128]

The use of humoral diagnostic techniques, while outdated, may still provide a diagnostic framework for the modern naturopath to use in combination with validated scientific methods. Scientific inquiry has not validated humoralism, and in fact the emergence of post-1800s medical science has in a sense discredited the paradigm, so the humoral model does not fit into a classic scientific model. Like traditional Chinese medicine, it can be seen as a model unto itself.

Naturopaths are advised to base diagnostic assessment on case taking and evidence-based techniques, but the humoral diagnostic technique may provide a supplementary approach to fine-tune analysis or the patient's health state, and afford a richer understanding of the person beyond quantitative assessment. As revealed in Table 2.6 and Figure 2.5, the four humours describe energetic qualities that may be found in somatic or psychological presentations in people. Example of various conditions and tongue and pulse signs are:

- **cold-dry (melancholic)**
  Condition: for example, osteoarthritis, dandruff, poor circulation, dysmenorrhoea
  Tongue: cracked body, dry white coat
  Pulse: slow, deep, possibly tight
  Treatment: warming, moistening interventions
- **cold-damp (phlegmatic)**
  Condition: for example, certain tumours/cysts, asthma, common cold, oedema, depression
  Tongue: greasy thick white coat
  Pulse: slow, slippery
  Treatment: warming, drying interventions
- **hot-dry (choleric)**
  Condition: for example, menopausal symptoms, psoriasis, anxiety, ulcers
  Tongue: red cracked body/yellow dry/no coat

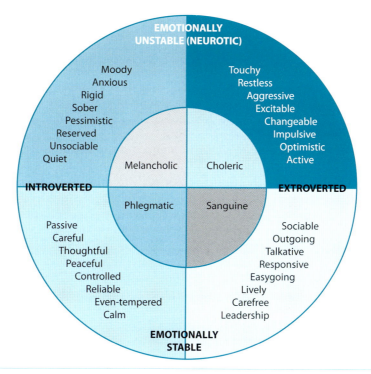

Figure 2.5 The four humours and their attributes
Source: Eysenck HJ, Eysenck MW. Personality and individual differences. Plenum Publishing, 1958

Pulse: rapid, thin
Treatment: cooling, moistening interventions

- **hot-damp (sanguine)**
  Condition: for example, rheumatoid osteoarthritis, weepy eczema, fatty liver
  Tongue: red beefy body/greasy yellow coat
  Pulse: rapid, slippery
  Treatment: cooling, drying interventions.

The philosophy of treating a humoral presentation is to use its 'energetic opposite'. For example to treat a classically melancholic condition such as osteoarthritis, the use of warming circulatory stimulants may be of assistance. Or in the case of a choleric condition such as psoriasis or dry eczema, the use of cooling moistening treatments may help. Below is a brief list of herbal energetic examples that may be used to treat the opposite humoral presentation:[130]

- *heating*: stimulating and warming—sulfur-containing or volatile-oil rich phytomedicines
  for example, garlic, ginger, cayenne, valerian, thyme, rosemary
- *cooling*: cleansing and draining—bitter principles, cooling volatile oils or phenols
  for example, gentian, globe artichoke, goldenseal, willow bark
- *moistening*: demulcent and soothing—mucilaginous or viscous agents
  for example, marshmallow root, slippery elm, liquorice, rehmannia
- *drying*: astringing and diuretic tannin-rich or pungent herbs
  for example, cranesbill, sage, mandarin peel, dandelion leaf.

Adapted traditional Chinese medicine diagnostic techniques

Although traditional Chinese medicine diagnosis does not have a developed evidence base in terms of Western scientific method, it does have a history of development by empirical observation and testing spanning thousands of years. There is also evidence of concordance of diagnosis by different traditional Chinese medicine practitioners for a number of conditions.[131]

Traditional Chinese medicine is similar to humoralism in regard to its view of health and disease.[132] The traditional Chinese medicine energetic model can be adapted for use in the naturopathic context, with the Western theory of 'vital force' being analogous with the traditional Chinese medicine theory of Qi. The concept of Qi is fundamental to Chinese medical thinking. Its five major functions are responsible for a person's physical integrity and for any changes they may experience.[133] Qi is said to be the source of all movement and harmonious transformation in the body; it protects and warms the body, as well as governs retention of the body's substances and organs. There are three major patterns of disharmony associated with Qi: deficient or empty, excessive or stagnant, and unregulated or disharmonious.[131] Qi and the principles of the six pernicious influences can add insight into a patient's condition and assist with selection of the right prescription.

Traditional Chinese medicine has a unique diagnostic framework, which can be adapted for naturopathic practice. Conditions can be divided into three patterns of disharmony: deficient, excessive or unregulated. General signs and symptoms may provide diagnostic detail of which state the body/mind is in, and prescriptive recommendations. Table 2.7 details basic traditional Chinese medicine diagnostic patterns and clinical recommendations for application in naturopathic practice. It should be noted that this table is only theoretical (for further reference to traditional Chinese medicine diagnostic techniques, see Appendices 7, 8 and 9).

Table 2.7 Adapted traditional Chinese medicine diagnostic patterns[134,135]

PATTERN OF DISHARMONY	SYMPTOMS	PATIENT SIGNS	PATIENT RECOMMENDATIONS
Deficient May arise due to lack of quality sleep, high work or emotional demands, chronic illness, poor nutrition, genetic weakness, surgery or childbirth	• Poor digestive function and appetite • Muscle weakness or fatigue which improves with rest • Insufficient circulation • Pallor • Inability of an organ to perform its function (e.g. kidney in fluid regulation, pancreas in digestion)	*Tongue* may have a pale body *Pulse* may feel weak and fine	• *Herbs*: tonifying, building, warming or sweet types of herbs or nutritionals including adaptogens, nervines, immunostimulants or tissue-trophorestoratives should be selected.[135] • *Foods*: High protein foods, complex carbohydrates and warm meals. • A patient with this type of presentation should avoid depurative herbal formulas and fasting diets that may further deplete remaining 'vital force'.

(Continued)

Table 2.7 Adapted traditional Chinese medicine diagnostic patterns *(Continued)*

PATTERN OF DISHARMONY	SYMPTOMS	PATIENT SIGNS	PATIENT RECOMMENDATIONS
Excessive (or stagnant) Any condition that is said to be a somatic or energetic overabundance	• Fevers • High blood pressure • Constipation • Obesity or fluid retention • Skin formations or exudates • Autoimmune conditions • Aches and pains	*Tongue* may present with a thick coat *Pulse* may feel full, strong and hard	• *Herbs*: Herbs such as those which drain, expel or sedate, or strong tasting herbs such as bitter or pungent can be chosen. • *Foods*: Cleansing diets with fruits and vegetables, pungent spices and water.
Unregulated Unbalanced and disharmonious 'vital force'	• Gastrointestinal irregularities • Hormonal fluctuations • Emotional lability • Muscle spasms or cramping	*Tongue*: Difficult to apply diagnostically *Pulse* may feel erratic and changeable	• *Herb*: Botanicals which benefit these types of conditions are harmonisers such as carminatives, antispasmodics, hormonal modulators or mood regulators.[135] • *Foods*: Diets should be comprised of a balance of building and cleansing foods, while avoiding an excess of either.

CHOOSING DIAGNOSTIC METHODS

There is a vast array of diagnostic tools and techniques available to naturopaths; these are best used in combination.

When interpreted alone many have explicit shortcomings due to the lack of available evidence of efficacy. Each person's needs should be evaluated and investigations adjusted accordingly, always keeping in mind what level of evidence is available, as well as the relative strengths and weaknesses of each (see Table 2.8).

It is essential for the naturopath to always be mindful of the costs associated with pathology testing and only make use of these if necessary to investigate a particular condition or dysfunction, if the results will determine the mode of treatment. If a particular test will have no bearing on the management plan, it is unnecessary to have these

CONSIDER COST

- While modern technology may provide added diagnostic techniques that may be valuable, they also may be expensive.
- Naturopaths should be judicious regarding which tests they advise their patients to undertake to avoid overburdening their patients financially.
- Naturopathic diagnosis should always be founded on solid case-taking skills. In many cases a thorough case history and physical examination will elicit the same information as many diagnostic tests.

Table 2.8 Review of the major evidence

TECHNIQUE	EVIDENCE	COMMENT	EVIDENCE RATING
Anthropometric data	Established public health application	Has a valuable place in clinical assessment	4–5
Body signs and symptoms	Semi-established public health applications	Some controlled studies with mixed results	3–4
Palpation	Established traditional use in the orthodox medicine	Semi-established public health applications	3–4
Iridology	Established traditional use in naturopathy	Many open studies	2
Dietary assessment	Controlled studies with mixed results	Strength varies depending on method	3–4
Pathology testing	Several robust controlled studies, established public health application	Strength depending on method and adequacy for particular investigation	4–5
Bioelectrical Impedance (novel calcuations) or dark field microscopy	Lacking in controlled studies	Based on theoretical concepts More evidence is required	1–2
Traditional Chinese medicine diagnosis	Established traditional use in traditional Chinese medicine	Many open studies	3

Evidence rating: 1 = poor (no clinical studies, mainly anecdotal), 2 = average (open studies, some traditional evidence), 3 = moderate (some controlled studies with mixed results, established traditional use), 4 = good (controlled studies with mainly positive results, semi-established public health applications), 5 = strong (several robust controlled studies, established public health application)

carried out. It is likely that patients have already had a test, if not a number of them, performed by their general practitioners and in these cases it is beneficial to seek the results.

Most important is to always consider biological individuality, where diagnostic tools and treatments should be tailored to suit individual needs and not have individuals fit into specific predetermined treatment protocols. The naturopath should also always be clear to patients as to whether diagnostic techniques are in the 'orthodox' or 'naturopathic' tradition.

KEY POINTS

- Naturopathic practice often uses a variety of 'evidence-based clinical' and 'traditional' techniques.
- Consider the levels of evidence and limitations to methods.
- Only use extra, costly diagnostic tools if it is likely the technique will positively benefit the diagnosis and treatment of the patient.
- Individualise the use of diagnostic techniques for different patients and health conditions.
- Use diagnostic techniques holistically, professionally and sensitively.

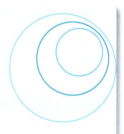

Acknowledgment

The author would like to acknowledge Milo Milosevic for his assistance in the iridology section and Jerome Sarris for his assistance with naturopathic interpretations of traditional Chinese and humoral medical theory.

Further reading

Gibson R. Principles of nutritional assessment. 2nd edn. USA: Oxford University Press, 2005.

Olgilvie C, Evans CC. Symptoms and signs in clinical medicine: an introduction to medical diagnostics. 12th edn. Oxford: Butterworth–Heinemann, 1997.

Heimburger D, et al. Clinical manifestations of nutrient deficiencies and toxicities: a resume. In: Heimburger D, Shils M, McLaren D. Modern nutrition in health and disease. USA: Lippincott Williams & Wilkins, 2006.

Maciocia G. The foundations of Chinese medicine. New York: Churchill Livingstone, 1996.

References

1. Model D. Making sense of clinical examination of the adult patient. New York: Oxford University Press, 2006.
2. Olgilvie C, Evans CC. Symptoms and signs in clinical medicine: an introduction to medical diagnostics. 12th edn. Oxford: Butterworth–Heinemann, 1997.
3. Welsby PD. Clinical history taking and examination. New York: Churchill Livingstone, 1995.
4. Toghill P. First impressions. In: Toghill PJ, ed. Examining patients: an introduction to clinical medicine. London: Edward Arnold, 1995.
5. Welborn T, et al. Waist–hip ratio is the dominant risk factor predicting cardiovascular death in Australia. Med J Aust 2003;179(11):580–585.
6. Shenkin A. Trace elements and inflammatory response: implications for nutritional support. Nutrition 1995;11 (1 Suppl):100–105.
7. Sauberlich HE. Laboratory tests for the assessment of nutritional status. 2nd edn. USA: CRC Press, 1999.
8. Maehira F, et al. Selenium regulates transcription factor NF-[kappa]B activation during the acute phase reaction. Clin Chim Acta 2003;334(1–2):163–171.
9. WHO. Clinical assessment of nutritional status. AJPH 1973;63 Suppl:18–27.
10. Anderson GJ, Connor WE. On the demonstration of omega-3 essential-fatty-acid deficiency in humans. Am J Clin Nutr 1989;49(4):585–587.
11. Rude RK. Magnesium deficiency: a cause of heterogenous disease in humans. J Bone Miner Res 1998;13(4):749–758.
12. Allender PS, et al. Dietary calcium and blood pressure: a meta-analysis of randomized clinical trials. Ann Intern Med 1996;124(9):825–831.
13. Heimburger D, et al. Clinical manifestations of nutrient deficiencies and toxicities: a resume in Modern Nutrition in Health and disease. USA: Lippincott Williams & Wilkins, 2006.
14. Shenkin A, et al. Vitamins and trace elements. In: Burtis C, et al., eds. Tietz textbook of clinical chemistry and molecular diagnostics. Missouri: Elsevier Saunders, 2006.
15. Olson J. Vitamin A. In: Ziegler EE, Filer Jr LJ, eds. Present knowledge in nutrition. Washington: ILSI Press, 1996:109–117.
16. Sommer A, Davidson FR. Assessment and control of vitamin A deficiency: the Annecy accords. J Nutr 2002;132(9):2845S–2850S.
17. Ryan AS, Goldsmith LA. Nutrition and the skin. Clin Dermatol 1996;14(4):389–406.
18. Thurnham DI. Red cell enzyme tests of vitamin status: do marginal deficiencies have any physiological significance? Proc Nutr Soc 1981;40(2):155–163.
19. Holman RT, et al. A case of human linolenic acid deficiency involving neurological abnormalities. Am J Clin Nutr 1982;35(3):617–623.
20. Pencharz PB. Making a nutritional assessment. Can Med Assoc J 1982;127(9):823–835.
21. Sato S. Iron deficiency: structural and microchemical changes in hair, nails and skin. Semin Dermatol 1991;10:313–319.
22. Shankar AH, Prasad AS. Zinc and immune function: the biological basis of altered resistance to infection. Am J Clin Nutr 1998;68(2 Suppl):447S–463S.
23. Kubena KS, Durlach J. Historical review of the effects of marginal intake of magnesium in chronic experimental magnesium deficiency. Magnes Res 1990;3(3):219–226.
24. Jeejeebhoy KN, et al. Chromium deficiency, glucose intolerance, and neuropathy reversed by chromium supplementation, in a patient receiving long-term total parenteral nutrition. Am J Clin Nutr 1977;30(4):531–538.
25. Delange F. Physiopathology of iodine nutrition. In: Chandra RK, ed. Trace elements in nutrition of children. New York: Raven Press, 1985:291–296.
26. Gibson R. Principles of nutritional assessment. 2nd edn. USA: Oxford University Press, 2005.
27. Hopper N. Zinc metalloproteases in health and disease. London: Taylor & Francis Ltd, 1996:1–22.
28. Smidt L, et al. Influence of thiamin supplementation on the health and general well-being of an elderly Irish population with marginal thiamin deficiency. J Gerontol 1991;46:M16–M22.
29. Carlson GL, et al. Biotin deficiency complicating long-term total parenteral nutrition in an adult patient. Clin Nutr 1995;14(3):186–190.
30. Groff J, Gropper S. Advanced nutrition and human metabolism. 3rd edn. USA: Wadsworth/Thompson Learning, 2000.
31. Smith H. Diagnosis in paediatric haematology.. New York: Churchill Livingstone, 1996:6–40.
32. Rayman MP. The importance of selenium to human health. Lancet 2000;356(9225):233–241.
33. Rushton DH. Nutritional factors and hair loss. Clin Exp Dermatol 2002;27(5):400–408.
34. Paulsrud JR, et al. Essential fatty acid deficiency in infants induced by fat-free intravenous feeding. Am J Clin Nutr 1972;25(9):897–904.
35. Mejia L. Vitamin A–nutrient interrelationships. In: Bauernfeind J, ed. Vitamin A deficiency and its control. Orlando: Academic Press, 1986.

36. Chandra RK, Newberne PM. Nutrition, immunity and infection. New York: Plenum Press, 1977:37–86.
37. Prasad AS. Effects of zinc deficiency on immune functions. Journal of Trace Elements in Experimental Medicine 2000;13(1):1–20.
38. Stabler SP, et al. Clinical spectrum and diagnosis of cobalamin deficiency. Blood 1990;76(5):871–881.
39. Wilfond BS, et al. Severe hemolytic anemia associated with vitamin E deficiency in infants with cystic fibrosis: implications for neonatal screening. Clin Pediatr 1994;33(1):2–7.
40. Johnson L, et al. Boggs Jnr, TR. The premature infant, vitamin E deficiency and retrolental fibroplasia. Am J Clin Nutr 1974;27(10):1158–1173.
41. Mead JF. The non-eicosanoid functions of the essential fatty acids. J Lipid Res 1984;25(13):1517–1521.
42. Rivlin R. Riboflavin. In: Ziegler EE, Filer LJ Jr, eds. Present knowledge in nutrition. Washington: ILSI Press, 1996:167–173.
43. Leklem J. Vitamin B6. In: Ziegler EE, Filer LJ Jr, eds. Present knowledge in nutrition. Washington: ILSI Press, 1996:175–183.
44. Field EA, et al. Oral signs and symptoms in patients with undiagnosed vitamin B_{12} deficiency. J Oral Pathol Med 1995;24(10):468–470.
45. Leggott PJ. The effect of controlled ascorbic acid depletion and supplementation on periodontal health. J Periodontol 1986;57:480–485.
46. Hambidge K. Clinical deficiencies: when to suspect there is a problem. In: Chandra RK, ed. Trace elements in nutrition of children. New York: Raven Press, 1985.
47. Haddad JG, Stamp TCB. Circulating 25-hydroxyvitamin D in man. Am J Med 1974;57(1):57–62.
48. Welch TR, et al. Vitamin D-deficient rickets: the reemergence of a once-conquered disease. J Pediatr 2000;137(2):143–145.
49. Arnaud C. Calcium and phosphorus. In: Ziegler EE, Filer LJ Jr, eds. Present knowledge in nutrition. Washington: ILSI Press, 1996:245–255.
50. Cumming RG. Calcium intake and bone mass: a quantitative review of the evidence. Calcif Tissue Int 1990;47(4):194–201.
51. Daniel R, et al. Nails in systemic disease. Dermatol Clin 1985;3(3):465–483.
52. Daniel R. Nail pigmentation abnormalities. Dermatol Clin 1985;3(3):431–443.
53. Kechijian P. Brittle fingernails. Dermatol Clin 1985;3(3):421–429.
54. Goodman K, Salt W. Vitamin B12 deficiency: important concepts in recognition. Postgrad Med 1990;88:147–158.
55. Kalra V, et al. Vitamin E deficiency and associated neurological deficits in children with protein-energy malnutrition. J Trop Pediatr 1998;44(5):291–295.
56. Healton EBMD, et al. Neurologic aspects of cobalamin deficiency. Medicine 1991;70(4):229–245.
57. Hetzel BS. Iodine and neuropsychological development. J Nutr 2000;130(2):489S–491S.
58. Mohanram M, Reddy V. Utilisation of radioactive iron in vitamin A deficient children. Proceedings of the International Congress of Nutrition, 1981.
59. Maclean AR, Renwick C. Audit of pre-operative starvation. Anaesthesia 1993;48(2):164–166.
60. Whang R, et al. Magnesium homeostasis and clinical disorders of magnesium deficiency. Ann Pharmacother 1994;28(2):220–226.
61. Baly DL, et al. Studies of marginal zinc deprivation in rhesus monkeys. III. Effects on vitamin A metabolism. Am J Clin Nutr 1984;40(2):199–207.
62. Britton J, et al. Dietary magnesium, lung function, wheezing, and airway hyper-reactivity in a random adult population sample. Lancet 1994;344(8919):357–362.
63. Fleming CR, et al. Essential fatty acid deficiency in adults receiving total parenteral nutrition. Am J Clin Nutr 1976;29(9):976–983.
64. Jarvis C. Physical examination and health assessment. St Louis: Elsevier Saunders, 2007.
65. Mertz W. Metabolism and metabolic effects of trace elements. In: Chandra RK, ed. Trace elements in nutrition of children. New York: Raven Press, 1985:107–117.
66. Salmenpera L. Detecting subclinical deficiency of essential trace elements in children with special reference to zinc and selenium. Clin Biochem 1997;30(2):115–120.
67. Prelack K, Sheridan RL. Micronutrient supplementation in the critically ill patient: strategies for clinical practice. J Trauma 2001;51(3):601–620.
68. Chandra RK, Sarchielli P. Immunocompetence methodology. In: Fidanza F, ed. Nutritional status assessment – a manual for population studies. London: Chapman & Hall, 1991:425–441.
69. Holmes S. Undernutrition in hospital patients. Nurs Stand 2003;17(19):45–52:quiz 54–55.
70. Golden M. Severe malnutrition. In: Weatherall D, et al., eds. Oxford textbook of medicine. 3rd edn. Oxford: Oxford University Press, 1995:1279–1280.
71. Golden MH. Malnutrition. In: Guandalini S, ed. Textbook of pediatric gastroenterology and nutrition. London: Taylor & Francis, 2004:489–525.
72. Krall EA, et al. Factors influencing accuracy of dietary recall. Nutr Res 1988;8(7):829–841.
73. Nelson M. Methods and validity of dietary assessment. In: Garrow JS, et al., eds. Human nutrition and dietetics. Edinburgh: Churchill Livingstone, 2000:311–331.
74. Food Standards Australia New Zealand, NUTTAB database. Online. Available: http://www.foodstandards.gov.au/monitoringandsurveillance/nuttab2006/.
75. Agricultural Research Service, USDA, USDA Nutrient database. Online. Available: http://www.nal.usda.gov/fnic/foodcomp/search/.
76. Health Canada, Canada. Online. Available: http://www.hc-sc.gc.ca/fn-an/nutrition/fiche-nutri-data/index-eng.php.
77. European Food Information Resource Network, EuroFIR, Food Composition Databases. Online. Available: http://www.eurofir.net/public.asp?id=8778 2009.
78. Royal College of Pathologists of Australasia, RCPA Manual. 2004. Online. Available: http://www.rcpamanual.edu.au/sections/pathologytestindex.asp?s=33
79. Pizzorno J, Murray M. Textbook of natural medicine. London: Churchill Livingstone, 1999.
80. Lukaski HC, Penland JG. Functional changes appropriate for determining mineral element requirements. J Nutr 1996;126(9S):2354S.
81. Kushner I. The phenomenon of the acute phase response. Ann N Y Acad Sci 1982:39–48.
82. Wieringa FT, et al. Estimation of the effect of the acute phase response on indicators of micronutrient status in Indonesian infants. J Nutr 2002;132(10):3061–3066.
83. Louw JAMF, et al. Blood vitamin concentrations during the acute-phase response. Crit Care Med 1992;20(7):934–941.
84. Tomkins A. Assessing micronutrient status in the presence of inflammation. J Nutr 2003;133(5 Suppl 2):1649S–1655S.
85. Ruz M, et al. Development of a dietary model for the study of mild zinc deficiency in humans and evaluation of some biochemical and functional indices of zinc status. Am J Clin Nutr 1991;53(5):1295–1303.
86. Hambidge M. Biomarkers of trace mineral intake and status. J Nutr 2003;133(Suppl 3):948S–955S.
87. Fell G, Talwar D. Assessment of status [review article]. Curr Opin Clin Nutr Metab Care 1998;1(6):491–497.
88. Bates C. Vitamin analysis. Ann Clin Biochem 1997;34:599–626.

89. Rosales FJ, et al. Determination of a cut-off value for the molar ratio of retinol-binding protein to transthyretin (RBP: TTR) in Bangladeshi patients with low hepatic vitamin A stores. J Nutr 2002;132(12):3687–3692.

90. Bates C, et al. Vitamin C. In: Fidanza F, ed. Nutritional status assessment – a manual for population studies. London: Chapman & Hall, 1991:309–319.

91. Maiani G, et al. Vitamin A. Int J Vitam Nutr Res 1993;63(4):252–257.

92. Talwar D, et al. Effect of inflammation on measures of antioxidant status in patients with non-small cell lung cancer. Am J Clin Nutr 1997;66(5):1283–1285.

93. Ganther HE. Selenium and glutathione peroxidase in health and disease: a review. In: Prasad AS, Oberleas D, eds. Trace elements in human health and disease. New York: Academic Press, 1976.

94. Spencer CA, Wang CC. Thyroglobulin measurement. Techniques, clinical benefits, and pitfalls. Endocrinol Metab Clin North Am 1995;24(4):841–863.

95. Van Leeuwen A, et al. Davis's comprehensive handbook of laboratory and diagnostic tests with nursing implications. 2nd edn. Philadelphia: FA Davis Company, 2006.

96. Skikne BS, et al. Serum transferrin receptor: a quantitative measure of tissue iron deficiency. Blood 1990;75(9):1870–1876.

97. Sweetman L. Qualitative and quantitative analysis of organic acids in physiologic fluids for diagnosis of the organic acidurias. In: Nyhan W, ed. Abnormalities in amino acid metabolism in clinical medicine. Norwalk: Appleton-Century-Crofts, 1984:419–453.

98. Newman M, et al. Urinary organic acid analysis: a powerful clinical tool, potentially muddled by poor testing methods. US BioTek Laboratories, 2004. Online. Available: http://www.usbiotek.com/Downloads/information/MarkOATLArticle-V6.pdf

99. Talley NJ, O'Connor S. Clinical examination: a systematic guide to physical diagnosis. 4th edn. Sydney: MacLennan & Petty, 2001.

100. Neale G, Tabaqchali S. The British society of gastroenterology. Gut 1966;7(6):708–718.

101. Greenberger N, et al. Urine indican excretion in malabsorption disorders. Gastroenterology 1968;55:204–211.

102. Hamilton LH. Breath testing and gastroenterology. Menomonee Falls, Wisconsin: Quintron Division, The EF Brewer Company, 1992.

103. Lac G. Saliva assays in clinical and research biology. Pathol Biol 2001;49(8):660–667.

104. Vining RF, McGinley RA. The measurement of hormones in saliva: possibilities and pitfalls. J Steroid Biochem 1987;27(1–3):81–94.

105. Jenkins DW. Toxic trace metals in mammalian hair and nails. US Environmental Protection Agency. Number 600/4-79-049, 1979.

106. Haddy T, et al. Minerals in hair, serum and urine of healthy and anemic black children. Public Health Rep 1991;106(5):557–563.

107. Rivlin RS. Misuse of hair analysis for nutritional assessment. Am J Med 1983;75(3):489–493.

108. Zeisel SH. Genetic polymorphisms in methyl-group metabolism and epigenetics: lessons from humans and mouse models. Brain Res 2008;1237:5–11.

109. Yates Z, Lucock M. Interaction between common folate polymorphisms and B-vitamin nutritional status modulates homocysteine and risk for a thrombotic event. Mol Genet Metab 2003;79(3):201–213.

110. Whitehead VM. Acquired and inherited disorders of cobalamin and folate in children. Br J Haematol 2006;134(2):125–136.

111. Andrews J. Endocrinology and iridology. Corona: John Andrews Iridology, 2006.

112. Munstedt K, et al. Can iridology detect susceptibility to cancer? A prospective case-controlled study. J Altern Complementary Med 2005;11(3):515–519.

113. Knipschild P. Looking for gall bladder disease in the patient's iris. Br Med J 1988;297:1578–1581.

114. Simon A, et al. An evaluation of iridology. JAMA 1979;242(13):1385–1389.

115. Yoo C, et al. Relationship between iris constitution analysis and TNF-alpha gene polymorphism in hypertensives. Am J Chin Med 2007;35(4):621–629.

116. Cho J, et al. Angiotensinogen gene polymorphism predicts hypertension, and iridological constitutional classification enhances the risk for hypertension in Koreans. Int J Neurosci 2008;118(5):635–645.

117. Pokanevych V. Iridology in Ukraine. Lik Sprava 1998;3:152–156.

118. Zubareva TV, Gadakchian KA. The use of iridoscopy in prophylactic examinations. Oftalmologicheskii Zhumal 1989;4:233–235.

119. Salles L, Silva M. [Iridology: a systematic review]. Rev Esc Enferm USP 2008;42(3):596–600.

120. Personal communication, L. Mehlmauer.

121. Jae-Young U, et al. Novel approach of molecular genetic understanding of iridology: relationship between iris constitution and angiotensin converting enzyme gene polymorphism. Am J Chin Med 2005;33(3):501–505.

122. Andrews J. Polycystic ovary syndrome research and iridology profiles. Advanced Iridology Research Journal 2006;6:16–20.

123. Dailakis M. New research in Alzheimer's disease and iridology. Advanced Iridology Research Journal 2006;6:9–10.

124. Mir MA. Atlas of clinical diagnosis. 2nd edn. London: Elsevier, 2003.

125. Larsson M, et al. Associations between iris characteristics and personality in adulthood. Biol Psychol 2007;75:165–175.

126. American Chiropractic Association. The internist. In: Position statement of the Council on Diagnosis and Internal Disorders of the American Chiropractic Association, 1996.

127. Sun SS, et al. Development of bioelectrical impedance analysis prediction equations for body composition with the use of a multicomponent model for use in epidemiologic surveys [see comment]. Am J Clin Nutr 2003;77(2):331–340.

128. Jackson WA. A short guide to humoral medicine. Trends Pharmacol Sci 2001;22(9):487–489.

129. Earles MP. Hall's prescriptions. In: Lane J, ed. John Hall and his patients. Stratford-upon-Avon: The Shakespeare Birthplace Trust, 1996:xxxi–xl.

130. Holmes P. The energetics of western herbs. Berkeley: NatTrop Publishing, 1993.

131. O'Brien K, Birch S. A review of the reliability of traditional East Asian medicine diagnoses. J Altern Complement Med 2009;15(4):353–366.

132. Zhang D. Humoralism and its influence on western medicine. Zhonghua Yi Shi Za Zhi 2001;31(3):141–147.

133. Chen B-L, ed. Classic of difficulties with explanation in vernacular language. Beijing: People's Health Press, 1963.

134. Kaptchuk TJ. Chinese medicine: the web that has no weaver. London: Rider Books, 1983.

135. Ross J. Combining western herbs and Chinese medicine: principles, practice and materia medica. Seattle: Greenfields Press, 2006.

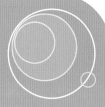

PART B
Common clinical conditions

The practice of naturopathy is evolving from a traditional art into an evidence-based science; however while more evidence is accumulating in respect to individual interventions, the protocols and processes used by naturopaths to treat people are only now beginning to be explored by researchers. As discussed in the Preface, the concept of what constitutes 'evidence' is a contentious issue in the field. The focus of the following sections is on revealing both traditional and scientific evidence in naturopathic medicine.

This part is divided into sections based on systems, and outlines major health conditions that are commonly encountered in clinical practice by naturopaths. The structure used in the chapters details the fundamentals of the condition such as aetiology, risk factors, conventional treatments and the evidence-based CAM interventions commonly used in treatment. Most importantly, however, is the emphasis on the exploration of the principles and protocols used in naturopathic practice. Due to practical constraints, not all diseases are covered. The aim is to cover the key principles and protocols used to treat major conditions, and this knowledge can be extrapolated to treat similar conditions requiring comparable principles and protocols. A caveat is that the chapters focus on a specific disease whereas in naturopathy individuals, rather than diseases, are treated. Naturopaths commonly employ a complex variety of treatment principles and hold a regard for the intimate dynamics of intersystem relationships. The condition-based structure used can, however, be used as an ideal cataloguing technique to explore the major principles and practices used in naturopathy, even if it does not broadly represent the way disease is categorised in naturopathic practice.

Tables, figures, charts and a 'review of the evidence' table provide a format in which the contributors can detail their expertise in a reader-friendly style. The 'naturopathic treatment decision tree' elegantly manifests the clinical process of treatment. The contributors were chosen as experts in their fields and were given individual licence as to the format of the decision trees to allow for a personalised expression of their clinical knowledge. Case studies detailed at the end of each chapter are designed to provide a clinical example of the condition covered. All cases are theoretical examples, and are designed to give details of the common signs and symptoms of the condition covered. The case study is included to put theoretical information from the chapter in a context that clearly relates to clinical practice. It is recognised that the condition outlined is a simplistic example and does not necessarily truly reflect a normal, complex case.

Section 1 Gastrointestinal system

The gastrointestinal system is traditionally thought to be the root of naturopathic treatment, with many diseases being considered colloquially to 'all come down to the gut'. The functions of the gastrointestinal tract are systemically important, with control over ingestion, digestion, absorption and elimination of food by-products. Conditions of the gastrointestinal tract form a major part of primary care practice – it is estimated that 10% of all primary care practitioner visits are for indigestion alone, and a further 5% for diarrhoea. The gastrointestinal system can be broadly broken down into the upper and lower tract (although the system is more complex).

Conditions commonly encountered in naturopathic practice of the upper gastrointestinal tract include functional disorders such as dyspepsia and gastro-oesophageal reflux, inflammatory conditions such as mouth ulcers, oesophagitis and gastritis. Dental hygiene is also an important consideration in treatment of alimentary canal diseases. Common conditions of the lower gastrointestinal tract include functional disorders such as irritable bowel syndrome, gastrointestinal infections and dysbiosis, constipation and inflammatory diseases such as ulcerative colitis.

So central is the role of the gastrointestinal system to good health that the correction of gastrointestinal complaints offers a valuable strategic therapy in most systemic disorders (particularly those of an inflammatory nature, or where a deficiency of 'vital force' is apparent). Gut-associated lymphatic tissue (GALT) represents nearly 70% of the body's total immune system. Years before 'increased intestinal permeability' and 'probiotics' became catchphrases in modern gastroenterology, naturopaths commonly treated suspected 'leaky gut' and intestinal dysbiosis. Furthermore, removal of allergenic foods and regulating the immune reaction in gut tissue has long been a core naturopathic tenet.

Optimal gastrointestinal function is also essential to ensure appropriate absorption of nutrients. Dietary modification and supplementation can be rendered ineffective if the body does not possess the capacity to adequately absorb these treatments. Chronic malabsorption (even at a subclinical level) is detrimental to the promotion of good health and vitality. Therefore supporting good digestion is an integral adjuvant treatment principle in naturopathic practice.

The elimination aspect of the gastrointestinal tract is also clinically significant. While promoting liver function for elimination is important, the crude imperativeness of promoting elimination through the faeces should also not be underestimated. Metabolic by-products from the liver are removed via the faeces, and if transit time is long, they will be reabsorbed by the enterohepatic circulatory system. The success of any program aimed at eliminating toxins is utterly reliant on improving the gastrointestinal system's multiple elimination pathways.

Common naturopathic prescriptions used to treat GS disorders involve dietary modification, lifestyle advice, herbal medicines and nutraceuticals. Evidently, dietary changes are the most fundamental treatment for most GS conditions, and commonly involve elimination and challenge diets, and specific dietary advice to address intolerances, deficiencies and special needs. Herbal medicine actions often include anti-inflammatory, antimicrobial or astringent activity, which are particularly effective as the botanical will come into direct contact with intestinal tissue. Nutrients are commonly supplemented in cases of deficiency, although some may provide a specific activity such as reducing inflammation or repairing intestinal tissue. The role of microflora is a vital component of intestinal and systemic health (and is discussed in depth in the section).

In many cases traditional naturopathic treatments for improving digestion will have a role in improving hepatic and biliary function as well (and vice versa), as these systems are considered to be inextricably linked. This chapter however focuses mainly on common GS disorders, rather than the hepatobiliary system, which is also covered in other chapters (see Chapters 19 and 24).

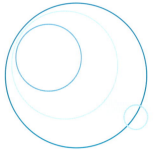

3
Irritable bowel syndrome: constipation-predominant (C-IBS)

Jason Hawrelak
ND, BNat (Hons), PhD

AETIOLOGY

Irritable bowel syndrome (IBS) is a functional gastrointestinal disorder characterised by altered bowel habit and abdominal pain.[1] It is a chronic disorder of unclear aetiology.[2] Recent research, however, has brought to light a number of possible aetiological factors:

- *enhanced visceral perception*. Patients with IBS have been found to have increased visceral sensation and visceral hyperalgesia compared to healthy controls.[3,4]
- *low-grade inflammation*. Irritable bowel syndrome patients show no identifiable inflammation on routine colonic biopsies. However, some do show increased expression of inflammatory markers (increased enterochromaffin and mast cell numbers, increased intraepithelial T-lymphocytes and increased mucosal interleukin-1β messenger RNA), suggesting low-grade inflammation is present. This mild mucosal inflammation is theorised to cause local disruptions to neuromuscular function.[4,5]
- *altered gastrointestinal tract (GIT) motility*. Subjects suffering from C-IBS have been found to have significant delays in overall colonic transit time and decreased numbers of fast and propagated colonic contractions compared to healthy controls.[6] There also appears to be impaired transit of intestinal gas.[7]
- *altered GIT microflora (dysbiosis)*. Colonic fermentation studies have found patients with IBS produce significantly more colonic hydrogen than healthy controls,[8] as well as having altered faecal short-chain fatty acid profiles.[9] Additional studies have found the GIT microflora of IBS patients to differ from that of healthy controls, most notably lower faecal concentrations of bifidobacteria and lactobacilli and higher concentrations of Enterobacteriaceae.[10–12]

RISK FACTORS

Several factors that appear to play a role in initiating and maintaining IBS have been identified. These factors include a genetic predisposition, a history of enteric infections, antibiotic use, a history of stressful life events, and concurrent anxiety and/or depressive disorders:

- It is believed that a genetic disposition may contribute to the development of IBS in some patients.[13,14] This predisposition may not be disease-specific, but more related to alterations in the responsiveness of the central nervous system to stimuli.
- Several studies have shown a relationship between acute gastrointestinal infections and the onset of IBS symptoms.[15–17] It has been postulated that long-lasting alterations in mucosal function and structure may be responsible for postinfective IBS. These alterations include increased intestinal permeability, increased expression of inflammatory markers (such as interleukin-1β), and neuromuscular dysfunction.[17,18]
- Two studies have found an association between antibiotic use and increased frequency of IBS symptoms.[19,20] This association is thought to be mediated via antibiotic-induced alterations in the GIT microflora and/or enhanced visceral sensitivity.
- Stressful and traumatic life events are frequently reported to precede the initial onset of IBS symptoms and symptom flare-ups in patients already suffering from IBS.[21,22] Additionally, IBS has consistently been found to have a high degree of psychiatric comorbidities, such as dysthymia, depression, panic disorder and generalised anxiety disorder.[23,24]

CONVENTIONAL TREATMENT

Many agents are currently used for the treatment of IBS and no one agent has proven particularly effective and/or free from side effects.[25–27] Key classes of medications used to treat C-IBS include antispasmodics, antidepressants, laxatives and 5-hydroxytryptamine type 4 receptor agonists (such as tegaserod). Therapeutic gains (the difference in treatment response between placebo and active therapy) have often been minimal with these agents[28] and adverse events severe.[29]

> **NATUROPATHIC TREATMENT AIMS**
> - Optimise GIT microflora.
> - Promote daily, easy-to-pass bowel movements.
> - Manage GIT symptoms.
> - Support the nervous system.
> - Decrease gut inflammation and diminish visceral hypersensitivity.
> - Improve liver function.

KEY TREATMENT PROTOCOLS

GIT microflora: overview

The microflora of the GIT represents an ecosystem of the highest complexity.[30] The microflora is believed to be composed of over 50 genera of bacteria,[31] accounting for over 500 different species.[32] The adult human GIT is estimated to contain 10^{14} viable microorganisms, which is 10 times the number of eukaryotic cells found within the entire human body.[33] Some researchers have called this microbial population the 'microbe' organ – an organ that is similar in size to the liver (1–1.5 kg in weight).[34] Indeed, this 'microbe' organ is now recognised as rivalling the liver in the number of biochemical transformations and reactions in which it participates.[35]

The microflora plays many critical roles in the body; thus, there are many areas of host health that can be compromised when the microflora is altered. The GIT microflora is involved in the stimulation of the immune system, synthesis of vitamins (B group and K), enhancement of GIT motility and function, digestion and nutrient absorption, inhibition of pathogens (colonisation resistance), metabolism of plant compounds (for example, phytoestrogens and glycosides), and production of short-chain fatty acids and polyamines.[30,36,37]

The colon is the most heavily colonised area of the GIT and this microbial ecosystem is believed to play the greatest role in human health. The colonic microflora is composed almost entirely of anaerobic bacteria, with the largest two genera being *Bacteroides* (accounting for up to 30% of all organisms) and *Bifidobacterium* (which can constitute up to 25% of total faecal counts). Other numerically important anaerobes include eubacteria, lactobacilli, clostridia and gram-positive cocci. Existing in smaller proportions are coliforms, methanogens, enterococci and dissimilatory sulfate-reducing bacteria. These important groups of bacteria have been divided into species that exert either beneficial or harmful effects on the host, as outlined in Figure 3.1.[37] When the beneficial species are present in insufficient numbers or when concentrations of

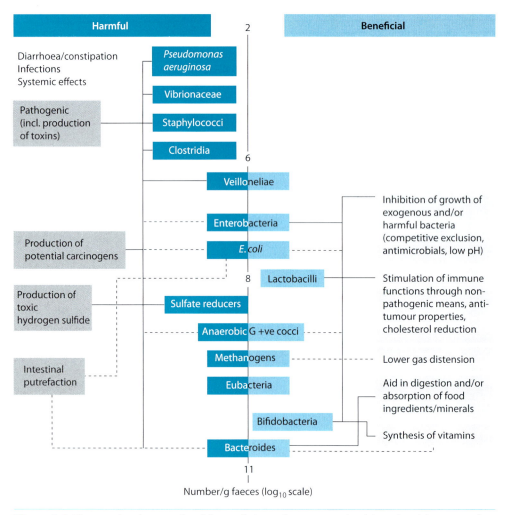

Figure 3.1 The predominant microbiota of the colon categorised into health-promoting and potentially harmful groups.[31]

potentially harmful bacteria are relatively high, then dysbiosis is said to result. Dysbiosis is a state in which the microflora produces harmful effects through one or more of the following factors: (1) qualitative and quantitative changes in the intestinal flora itself; (2) changes in their metabolic activities; and (3) changes in their local distribution.[38]

Optimise the GIT microflora

In the naturopathic treatment of C-IBS, dysbiosis is viewed as one of the most important aetiological factors. Hence, treatments aimed at addressing this imbalance are seen as crucial to the management of this condition. Treatments aimed at improving the GIT ecosystem can be divided into three categories: probiotics, prebiotics and synbiotics.

Probiotics

The term 'probiotic' is derived from the Greek and literally means 'for life'. It was first coined in 1965 by Lilley and Stillwell to describe substances secreted by one microorganism that stimulate the growth of another.[39] In 1974, Parker modified this definition to 'organisms and substances which contribute to intestinal microbial balance'.[40] The current World Health Organization definition of probiotics is 'live microorganisms which when administered in adequate amounts confer a health benefit on the host'.[41] Probiotic organisms can be found in fermented foods (such as yoghurt, sauerkraut and kefir), as well as supplements. The microorganisms found in these products are typically lactobacilli and bifidobacteria.[42]

Probiotics have a long history of successful use in the treatment of IBS. In fact the first case series detailing the efficacy of a **Lactobacillus acidophilus** supplement in IBS was published in 1955.[43] A recent systematic review and meta-analysis of randomised, controlled trials found probiotic use to be associated with improvements in global IBS symptoms compared to placebo and reductions in abdominal pain.[44] It is well-known, however, that efficacy in this condition, as it is in all conditions, is strain dependent. Commercially available probiotic strains that have shown efficacy in the treatment of IBS include **L. fermentum** PCC[45,46] and **L. plantarum** 299V.[47,48] Commercially-available strains found to be ineffective in the management of IBS include *L. acidophilus* NCFM[49] and *L. rhamnosus* GG.[50,51]

To achieve the desired therapeutic results, it is imperative to prescribe the precise probiotic strains that have demonstrated therapeutic and clinical efficacy in the condition in question. Strains that work in one condition will not necessarily be effective in other conditions. For example, *Lactobacillus rhamnosus* GG appears to be effective in the prevention of antibiotic-associated side effects,[65] but not of any demonstrable benefit in urinary tract infections.[66] Tables 3.2 and 3.3 outline the most appropriate probiotic strains and prebiotic to use for specific disease conditions, as determined by human trials.

Delivery of probiotics

Probiotic organisms can be delivered through a variety of mechanisms: fermented foods (such as yoghurt, kim chi and sauerkraut), capsules, tablets and powders. Each method has its advantages and disadvantages, which are listed in Table 3.1.

Prebiotics

A prebiotic is defined as 'a nondigestible food ingredient that beneficially affects the host by selectively stimulating the growth and/or activity of one or a limited number of bacteria in the colon.'[53] For food ingredients to be classified as prebiotics, they must:
- be neither digested nor absorbed in the stomach or small intestine[42]
- act as a selective food source for one or a limited number of potentially beneficial commensal bacteria in the large intestine[42]

Table 3.1 Mechanisms of delivery of probiotics, and their advantages and disadvantages

DELIVERY SYSTEM	ADVANTAGES	DISADVANTAGES
Fermented foods	• Affordable and accessible • Easily incorporated into daily lifestyle • Additional nutritional benefits • Enhanced bacterial survival through upper GIT (100 × less can be given per dose if given in a dairy base)[52] • Effective in upper GIT	• May contain dairy proteins or lactose • Unsuitable when travelling • Unsuitable for vegans (if dairy-based)
Capsules	• Ease of administration • No binders	• Not therapeutic for upper GIT unless opened or chewed • May contain allergenic excipients • Higher cost
Tablets	• Ease of administration • Effective in upper GIT (if chewed)	• May contain allergenic binders and excipients such as gluten • Higher cost
Powders	• Effective in upper GIT • Dosage easily adjusted • May be incorporated into food and drinks • No binders	• May contain allergenic excipients • Higher cost

• change the colonic microflora ecosystem towards a healthier composition,[42] and
• induce luminal or systemic changes that improve the health of the host.[37]

Most emphasis to date has been on finding and trialling food sources that are used by lactic acid-producing bacteria. This is due to the health-promoting properties of these organisms.[42] The best known lactic acid-producing bacteria belong to the genera *Lactobacillus* and *Bifidobacterium*. Commonly used prebiotics include **lactulose**, **fructo-oligosaccharides** (FOS), and **galacto-oligosaccharides** (GOS). The most appropriate prebiotics to use for specific health conditions are highlighted in Table 3.3.

One trial has been performed investigating the efficacy of FOS in IBS with disappointing results.[54] However, the dose of FOS used in the study (20 g/day in a single dose) is known to cause significant gastrointestinal side effects (such as bloating, distension, borborygmi and increased flatulence).[55] Thus it is not surprising that FOS failed

PREBIOTICS VERSUS COLONIC FOODS

There are a number of other substances that are frequently referred to as prebiotics. Many of these, however, fail to meet the criteria outlined above. Slippery elm, psyllium husks, guar gum and pectin would more accurately be described as colonic foods rather than prebiotics as they appear to lack the selectivity of fermentation that is required of prebiotics.[56–58] Other substances, such as polydextrose and larch arabinogalactans, have been shown to increase the growth of beneficial bacteria in human trials.[59–60] However, they have thus far been the subject of inadequate research to determine if they meet all of the prebiotic requirements.

Table 3.2 Most appropriate probiotic strains for specific disease conditions

CONDITION		EVIDENCE LEVEL	MOST APPROPRIATE PROBIOTIC STRAINS	REFERENCE
Irritable bowel syndrome		II	*Lactobacillus fermentum* PCC	67,68
		II	*Lactobacillus plantarum* 299V	69,70
		II	VSL#3	33,34
Ulcerative colitis	Inducing remission	III	VSL#3	71
	Maintaining remission	II	*Lactobacillus rhamnosus* GG	72
		III	VSL#3	73
	Preventing pouchitis	II	VSL#3	74
		III	*Lactobacillus rhamnosus* GG	75
Viral gastroenteritis	Prevention	II	*Lactobacillus rhamnosus* GG	76
		II	*Bifidobacterium lactis* Bb12	77,78
	Treatment	I	*Lactobacillus rhamnosus* GG	79
		II	*Lactobacillus reuteri* MM53	80,81
Helicobacter pylori infection		II	*Lactobacillus reuteri* MM53	82
		III	*Lactobacillus acidophilus* La5 and *Bifidobacterium animalis* subsp. *lactis* Bb12	83
Colic		II	*Lactobacillus reuteri* MM53	84
Collagenous colitis		II	*Lactobacillus acidophilus* La5 and *Bifidobacterium animalis* subsp. *lactis* Bb12	85
Constipation		II	*Lactobacillus casei* Shirota	86
		II	*Bifidobacterium animalis* subsp. *lactis* Bb12	87
Antibiotic use		I	*Lactobacillus rhamnosus* GG	88
		II	*Lactobacillus reuteri* MM53	89
		II	*Lactobacillus acidophilus* La5 and *Bifidobacterium animalis* subsp. *lactis* Bb12	90

Table 3.2 Most appropriate probiotic strains for specific disease conditions *(Continued)*

CONDITION		EVIDENCE LEVEL	MOST APPROPRIATE PROBIOTIC STRAINS	REFERENCE
Bacterial gastro-enteritis	CD[α]	III	*Lactobacillus rhamnosus* GG	91,92
		III	*Lactobacillus plantarum* 299V	93
	VRE[β]	II	*Lactobacillus rhamnosus* GG	94
Radiation-induced diarrhoea		II	VSL#3	95
Prevention of dental caries		II	*Lactobacillus rhamnosus* GG	96
Lowered immunity: decreased rates of infection		II	*Lactobacillus rhamnosus* GG	97
		II	*Lactobacillus reuteri* MM53	98,99
		II	*Lactobacillus acidophilus* NCFM and *Bifidobacterium animalis* subsp. *lactis* Bi-07	100
		II	*Lactobacillus acidophilus* NCFM	100
		II	*Bifidobacterium lactis* HN019	101
Atopic eczema	Prevention	II	*Lactobacillus rhamnosus* GG	102,103
		II	*Lactobacillus rhamnosus* HN001	104
	Treatment	II	*Lactobacillus fermentum* PCC	105
Vaginal candidiasis		III	*Lactobacillus acidophilus* La5	106

* Levels of evidence: I = systematic review or meta-analysis of randomised, controlled trials (RCTs); II = positive finding from one or more double-blind RCT; III = positive results in one or more open-label trial
CD[α] = Clostridium difficile
VRE[β] = vancomycin-resistant enterococci
VSL#3 = a unique multistrain product containing strains of B. longum, B. infantis, B. breve, L. acidophilus, L. casei, L. plantarum, L. delbruekii spp. bulgaricus and Streptococcus thermophilus

to reduce these same GIT symptoms in trial participants. It is possible that administration of lower doses of FOS (for example, 3 g/day) or other prebiotic agents (lactulose or GOS) will result in better clinical outcomes.

Synbiotics

Synbiotics are products that contain both probiotic and prebiotic agents.[61] The combination is theorised to enhance the survival of the probiotic bacteria through the upper GIT, improve implantation of the probiotic in the colon, and have a stimulating effect on the growth and/or activities of both the exogenously provided probiotic strains and the endogenous inhabitants of the bowel.[62] Synbiotics are a promising treatment avenue in C-IBS with two recently published, open-label trials finding a synbiotic preparation

Table 3.3 Prebiotics for disease conditions

DISEASE CONDITIONS	PREBIOTIC
Prevention of UTIs	Lactulose (25 g/day)
Lowered immunity: decreased rates of infection	FOS (2 g/day in infants)
Poor calcium absorption	FOS (8 g/day)
Atopic eczema: prevention in infants	GOS and FOS (0.8 g/100 mL formula)
Constipation	• Lactulose (10–40 g/day) • GOS (9 g/day) • FOS (10 g/day)

(containing a daily dose of 5×10^9 CFU *Bifidobacterium longum* strain W11 and 2.5 g **fructo-oligosaccharides**) to significantly decrease abdominal pain and bloating in patients with C-IBS, as well as increasing stool frequency.[63,64]

Promote daily, easy-to-pass bowel movements

C-IBS is associated with infrequent bowel movements and hard lumpy stools. Interventions aimed at increasing stool frequency and softening the stools are thus well-indicated. The three main tools used to address this issue are fibre, fluid and exercise.

Epidemiological studies have consistently found correlations between dietary fibre intake and improved bowel function.[107,108] As the amount of dietary fibre in the diet is increased, mean gastrointestinal transit time decreases, stool frequency increases and stools become softer and easier to pass.[107] Clinical trials of fibre supplementation have also consistently found increased bowel movement frequency and improved stool consistency.[109]

HOW DOES DIETARY FIBRE WORK?

There appear to be at least five ways by which dietary fibre consumption improves laxation. First, plant cell walls that resist microfloral degradation are able to exert a physical bulking effect by retaining water within their cellular structure. This increased bulk stimulates colonic movement. Secondly, the vast majority of consumed dietary fibre is extensively broken down and metabolised by the colonic microflora. This stimulates microbial growth, leading to an increase in microbial products and microbes themselves in faeces – again leading to an increase in faecal bulk. Thirdly, the increase in faecal bulk speeds up the faeces' rate of passage through the bowel. As transit time decreases, the efficiency with which the bacteria grow improves – further bulking the stools. Shortened transit time also leads to reduced water absorption by the colon and, hence, moister stools. Fourthly, fermentation of dietary fibre by the colonic microflora results in the production of hydrogen, methane and carbon dioxide gas. When trapped within the gut contents they further add to stool bulk.[116] Lastly, other end-products of fermentation (short-chain fatty acids, particularly acetate) enhance muscular contraction in the colon.[117,118]

A recent systematic review and meta-analysis found fibre to significantly improve global IBS symptoms (see Table 3.4, the review of evidence table) and IBS-related constipation. However, fibre supplementation was found to significantly worsen abdominal pain. When soluble fibre was examined in isolation, it was found to induce a greater reduction in global IBS symptoms and to improve constipation in C-IBS subjects. Conversely, insoluble fibre supplementation was found to have no significant effect upon global IBS symptoms, although it did improve constipation. The authors concluded that fibre supplementation appears to be of benefit in improving global IBS symptoms and particularly constipation; it does not, however, improve IBS-related abdominal pain.[110]

The findings from this systematic review suggest that sources of soluble fibre would be more appropriate therapeutic tools than sources of insoluble fibre in the treatment of C-IBS. Good sources of supplemental soluble fibre include ground flaxseeds,[111] slippery elm powder,[112] psyllium husks,[113] oat bran[114] and pectin.[115]

Fluid intake

Ensuring the intake of adequate fluid is also a vital, although under-researched, therapeutic tool. Positive associations have been observed between bowel movement frequency and fluid intake in epidemiological research.[108] Stool frequency and stool weight have also been found to be significantly decreased during enforced periods of low fluid intake in prospective, human research.[119] Adequate fluid intake is usually described as 2100–2600 mL daily, although this would need to be increased in warmer climates.[120]

Exercise

Epidemiological research has found an association between level of physical activity and frequency of bowel habit, with lower levels of physical activity being linked with impaired bowel habit.[121] This link between physical activity levels and bowel health is widely known amongst the general populace, with even Roald Dahl remarking in his *Revolting Rhymes*:[122]

> *An early morning stroll is good for people on the whole.*
> *It makes your appetite improve,*
> *It also helps your bowels to move.*

In support of this connection, prospective human research has found that daily moderate exercise is capable of significantly accelerating gastrointestinal transit time, which should equate to softer, easier-to-pass stools.[123] Additionally, a recently published, randomised, controlled trial found daily exercise to significantly improve constipation-related symptoms in IBS subjects.[124]

Manage GIT symptoms

Although it is a benign disorder, IBS is associated with significant impairments in quality of life.[134] Recent research has found that three gastrointestinal symptoms (straining at stool, abdominal pain and abdominal bloating) have the greatest negative impact upon quality of life in IBS sufferers.[135] Providing relief from these symptoms should thus be at the forefront of naturopathic management of this condition.

Straining at stool is usually addressed with the agents and interventions discussed in the 'Promote daily, easy-to-pass bowel movements' section above. Occasionally, however, laxative herbs are needed at the onset of treatment. Sometimes gentle **laxatives** like *Glycyrrhiza glabra* are adequate. In more severe cases of constipation, the anthraquinone-containing laxatives can be used: *Senna* spp., *Rhamnus purshiana*, *Rumex*

WHAT IS A 'NORMAL' BOWEL PATTERN?

This question should really be broken up into two questions: what is a 'normal' bowel habit and what is a 'healthy' or 'optimal' bowel habit? A 'normal' bowel habit has been defined by conventional medicine as between three bowel movements per day to three bowel movements per week. These frequencies are based on epidemiological studies conducted on Western populations which have found the vast majority of individuals to have a bowel frequency within this range, with the most common frequency being once daily.[125,126] Constipation is thus defined as less than three bowel movements per week.[127]

Naturopaths would generally not consider patients who experience three bowel movements per week to have a 'normal' bowel habit. Naturopath Henry Lindlahr stated in his 1919 classic *Natural Therapeutics* that 'normally a person should have a copious movement of the bowels once in twenty-four hours – twice is better'.[128] Studies looking at non-Western populations eating traditional fibre-rich diets found defecation frequencies to average two or three times daily.[129] Other studies looking at vegans eating high-fibre diets (about 47 g fibre daily) have found a mean bowel movement frequency of $\geq$ 1.5 per day.[107,108] From these data we can gather that individuals consuming a high-fibre, plant-based diet pass stools more frequently than individuals consuming the typical low-fibre, Western diet (about 11–16 g fibre daily).[130] Optimal bowel frequency should be considered to be one, two or three movements daily. Naturopaths generally consider patients as being constipated if they experience less than one bowel movement daily.

Bowel habit: men versus women

Studies have consistently found men to have an increased frequency of daily bowel movements, to produce a greater quantity of faeces daily, to have shorter gastrointestinal transit times and to have softer, less-formed faeces than women.[107,108,125] Stool form and bowel movement frequency also appears to vary in women according to the menstrual cycle. During the luteal phase of the cycle, gastrointestinal transit time significantly slows, resulting in more formed, harder stools.[107]

What is the 'perfect' bowel movement?

In terms of consistency, the most common stool passed by typical Western populations is well-formed (sausage or snake-like) with either cracks on its surface or a smooth and soft surface (types 3 and 4 in Figure 3.2).[125] Populations consuming a predominantly plant-based, high-fibre diet, on the other hand, have softer, bulkier stools that tend to be less formed and more 'mushy' (type 5). These stools are associated with shorter gastrointestinal transit times, whereas harder stools are associated with longer transit times.[107] So, what is the perfect bowel movement? Optimal stool form should vary between well-formed, sausage-like stools with cracks on its surface (type 3) through to softer blobs with clear-cut edges (type 5). In addition, there should be little-to-no straining at stool, little urgency and a feeling of complete evacuation after the event.[131]

What stimulates the bowels to move?

Colonic motility is the key factor determining the whens and whys of bowel movements. The greatest stimulant of colonic contractile activity is morning awakening. Colonic motility is greatly reduced and sometimes even completely abolished during sleep. Upon awakening contractile activity increases briskly.[133] Not surprisingly, population studies have found that the vast majority of bowel

WHAT IS A 'NORMAL' BOWEL PATTERN?—(Continued)

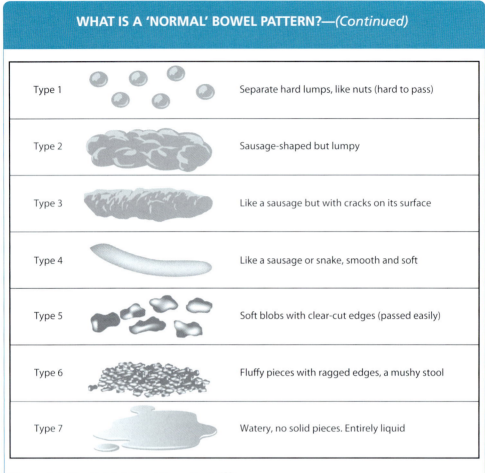

Type 1	Separate hard lumps, like nuts (hard to pass)
Type 2	Sausage-shaped but lumpy
Type 3	Like a sausage but with cracks on its surface
Type 4	Like a sausage or snake, smooth and soft
Type 5	Soft blobs with clear-cut edges (passed easily)
Type 6	Fluffy pieces with ragged edges, a mushy stool
Type 7	Watery, no solid pieces. Entirely liquid

Figure 3.2 The Bristol Stool Form Scale[132]

movements occur between 6 and 9 a.m.[125] The other main stimulus of colonic motility is eating – referred to as the *colonic motor response to eating* or the *gastrocolonic reflex*. Within minutes of consuming the first mouthful of food, colonic contractile activity begins, and lasts for at least 3 hours.[133] In Western populations, a second peak of defecation frequency has been observed at 6–7 p.m., the time at which the largest meal of the day is typically consumed.[125]

crispus or *Juglans cinerea*. The use of these agents can result in griping abdominal pain; concurrent administration of carminatives and antispasmodics is thus highly recommended. If anthraquinone-containing laxatives are used, the aim should be to use them for a short-term period only.

Abdominal pain and bloating can be addressed using a combination of carminatives and antispasmodics. Useful **carminatives** include *Mentha piperita*, *Mentha spicata*, *Carum carvi*, *Foeniculum vulgare*, *Citrus reticulata*, *Coriandrum sativum*, *Elettaria cardamomum*, *Origanum vulgare* and *Anethum graveolens*. Commonly prescribed **GIT antispasmodics** include *Matricaria recutita*, *Viburnum opulus*, *Dioscorea villosa*, *Melissa officinalis* and *Zingiber officinale*.

Support the nervous system

Given that C-IBS is often associated with depression[23,24] and given the link between perceived stress levels and IBS-symptom severity,[21,22] support for the nervous system is also an important component of naturopathic management. Mood has also been shown to affect bowel habit, with depression significantly slowing gastrointestinal transit time and anxiety significantly speeding it.[136]

Both nervines and adaptogens have a role to play in the treatment of C-IBS. Depending upon patient presentation, **thymoleptics** (*Hypericum perforatum*, *Albizzia julibrissin*, *Crocus sativus*, *Sceletium tortuosum* or *Leonurus cardiaca*) or **anxiolytics** (*Passiflora incarnata*, *Valeriana officinalis* or *Lavandula angustifolia*) can be used alongside **trophorestoratives** (for example, *Verbena officinalis* or green seed *Avena sativa*). If patients are currently experiencing conditions of high stress, adaptogens will also play an important role in management. If fatigue is part of the patient presentation, stimulating **adaptogens** such as *Rhodiola rosea*, *Panax ginseng* and *Eleutherococcus senticosus* may be the best choices. If anxiety or overstimulation is present, relaxing adaptogens may be more appropriate (for example, *Withania somnifera*, *Schisandra chinensis* or *Ganoderma lucidum*).

Decrease gut inflammation and diminish visceral hypersensitivity

Patients with IBS have been shown to have increased visceral sensation and may suffer from mild colonic mucosal inflammation.[3,4] Ingestion of **gastrointestinal anti-inflammatories** such as *Curcuma longa*, *Glycyrrhiza glabra* and *Matricaria recutita* may help decrease this inflammation. Recent research has found a combination of peppermint (*Mentha piperita*) and caraway (*Carum carvi*) essential oils effective in decreasing visceral hypersensitivity in an animal model of IBS.[137] A proprietary herbal preparation (**Iberogast**) has also been found to decrease visceral hypersensitivity in an animal model.[138] Iberogast is an ethanolic extract containing *Iberis amara*, *Angelica archangelica*, *Silybum marianum*, *Carum carvi*, *Glycyrrhiza glabra*, *Chelidonium majus*, *Matricaria recutita*, *Melissa officinalis* and *Mentha piperita*.

Improve liver function

Poor liver function is viewed by some practitioners as an important contributing factor in IBS.[139] Liver congestion has also long been seen by naturopaths as a common cause of constipation[128] and bile salts are well-known laxative agents.[140] Accordingly, patients with C-IBS can sometimes receive benefit from the ingestion of **cholagogues** (*Cynara scolymus*, *Curcuma longa*, *Taraxacum officinale radix*, *Chelidonium majus*, *Berberis vulgaris* or *Juglans cinerea*). See Chapter 19 for information on liver function and detoxification.

In support of the use of cholagogues in C-IBS, two clinical trials have been conducted on herbal cholagogues with both trials finding evidence of therapeutic effectiveness. In a post-marketing surveillance study *Cynara scolymus* extract was found to significantly decrease abdominal pain, bloating, flatulence and constipation in subjects with IBS over a 6-week period.[141] In an open-label trial, two different doses of turmeric extract (*Curcuma longa*) were examined to assess their effects on IBS symptoms.[142] Both extracts were found over an 8-week period to significantly reduce abdominal pain/discomfort scores from baseline. Additionally, bowel pattern was found to normalise. There were, however, no significant differences between the high and low dose groups.

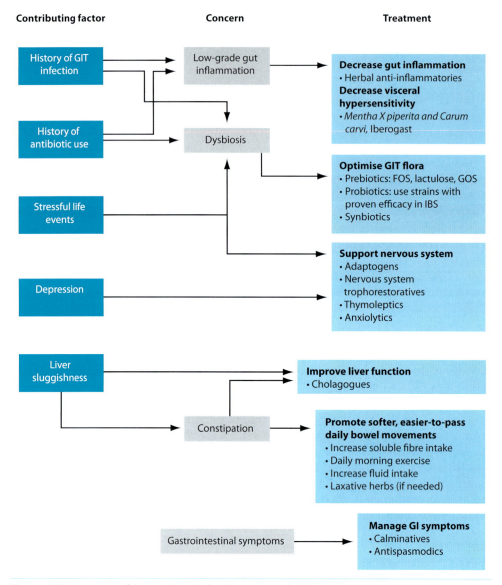

Figure 3.3 Naturopathic treatment decision tree—C-IBS

INTEGRATIVE MEDICAL CONSIDERATIONS
Referral

In many ways, IBS is a clinical diagnosis – a diagnosis is based on the presence of typical signs and symptoms (see the box on the Rome III criteria for current diagnostic criteria). Specificity of using the Rome criteria for the diagnosis of IBS has been found to be about 98% in the absence of 'alarm features'. Hence further investigations are typically not required to confirm the diagnosis and exclude organic disease. If 'alarm features' are present, however, referral for further investigation is recommended. 'Alarm features' include the presence of blood in the stools, weight loss, fever and family history of colon cancer.[4] Any change in bowel pattern in individuals over 45 years of age is also an 'alarm feature' requiring further investigation.[165]

DIARRHOEA-PREDOMINANT IBS

Diarrhoea-predominant IBS (D-IBS) is defined as IBS with loose (mushy) or watery stools ≥ 25% of bowel movements (type 6 or 7 on the Bristol Stool Form Scale) and hard or lumpy stools < 25% of movements (Bristol Stool Form Scale types 1 and 2).[127] Management of D-IBS shares a number of treatment goals with C-IBS, such as optimising the GIT microflora, supporting the nervous system, decreasing gut inflammation, and managing acute symptoms such as abdominal pain and bloating. However, there is a focus on decreasing bowel movement frequency and solidifying the stools. If anxiety plays a pivotal role in bowel symptoms and particularly in increased stool frequency, then supporting the nervous system with anxiolytics, nervous system trophorestoratives, adaptogens and thymoleptics (as discussed above) is well-indicated. Herbal antidiarrhoeal agents will have a more direct effect in the bowel. Herbal antidiarrhoeal agents can be divided into those that are tannin-based and those that are not. Tannin-based agents include *Quercus robor*, *Polygonum bistorta*, *Geranium maculatum*, *Croton lechlerii* and *Agrimonia eupatoria*. In Western herbal medicine, two of the few non-tannin based antidiarrhoeal agents currently in use are nutmeg (*Myristica fragrans*) and black pepper (*Piper nigrum*) – although black pepper can be too 'spicy' for some patients with D-IBS. The benefit of utilising non-tannin antidiarrhoeals is that they can be mixed together with alkaloid-containing herbs without causing precipitation.

REDISCOVERING OUR HERBAL ROOTS

Western herbalists have always been eclectic, using herbs from many different locations and herbal traditions. Western herbalists have also, until recently, been intimately involved with making the medicines they use. In Australia today, industry supplies herbal medicines to the bulk of practitioners, meaning that very few herbalists have a close connection to the plant medicines they currently use in practice. This situation has also indirectly limited the materia medica most practitioners can practise with. Only those herbs that are commercially profitable become available to use; the others become 'lost'. There is, however, a renaissance of sorts occurring in Australia today, with practitioners reconnecting with the herbs they use as medicines, with a growing number of herbalists returning to making their own medicines.

 A number of herbs with specific actions very helpful to GIT disorders have been 'lost' to modern Australian practitioners. Some of these and their actions are discussed below:

• **Nutmeg (*Myristica fragrans*)**: In the Banda Islands of Indonesia where nutmeg is native, nutmeg is used to treat abdominal cramping, excessive flatulence, nausea and vomiting, restlessness and insomnia.[143] Nutmeg was used by the eclectics to alleviate nausea, vomiting, abdominal pain, flatulence and diarrhoea.[144] It is used in traditional Chinese medicine for the treatment of abdominal pain and distension, vomiting and chronic diarrhoea.[145] Similarly

REDISCOVERING OUR HERBAL ROOTS *(Continued)*

in Ayurveda, nutmeg is used for diarrhoea, excessive intestinal gas, nervous disorders and insomnia.[146] Animal studies have found nutmeg to possess antisecretory activity and to slow gastrointestinal transit time.[147] It has also been found to exhibit antidepressant-like activity[148] and anxiolytic activity.[149]

- **Black pepper (*Piper nigrum*)**: The eclectic physicians considered black pepper to be a digestive stimulant, carminative, antiemetic, and circulatory stimulant.[150] In Ayurvedic medicine, it is used for indigestion, colic, diarrhoea and cold extremities, as well as for its adjuvant action.[146] In traditional Chinese medicine, it is used for vomiting, diarrhoea and abdominal pain.[145] Animal research has supported its role as a digestive stimulant, where it has been found to stimulate gastric acid secretion,[151,152] enhance bile flow[153] and improve functioning of digestive enzymes.[154] Black pepper has also been found to slow gastrointestinal transit[155] and to exhibit antisecretory action[156] – both of which support its traditional application in diarrhoea.

- **Caraway (*Carum carvi*)**: While still a commonly used cooking spice, caraway seeds have lost their place in the materia medica of most Australian herbalists. Weiss describes caraway, traditionally viewed as a carminative and gastrointestinal antispasmodic, as 'one of our most reliable and powerful carminatives'.[157] Human trials have found a combination of caraway and peppermint essential oils effective in alleviating the symptoms of functional dyspepsia, such as abdominal pain and the sensation of fullness and heaviness postmeals.[158–160]

- **Saffron (*Crocus sativus*)**: The stigma of saffron has long been revered as both medicine and spice. In the Middle East, where it was originally cultivated, saffron is considered an antispasmodic, thymoleptic, carminative, cognition enhancer, aphrodisiac and emmenagogue.[161] It is used in traditional Chinese medicine primarily for its ability to invigorate the blood, dispel stasis and unblock the menses, and a text from the Mongol dynasty states that 'long-term ingestion causes a person's heart to be happy'.[145] In 1862, an English herbalist Christopher Catton was quoted as remarking that 'saffron hath power to quicken the spirits, and the virtue thereof pierceth by and by to the heart, provoking laughter and merrines'.[162] Recent human research has confirmed this thymoleptic activity, with randomised, controlled trials finding saffron stigma as effective as pharmaceutical antidepressants in the treatment of mild-to-moderate depression.[163,164]

ROME III DIAGNOSTIC CRITERIA FOR C-IBS

1. Recurrent abdominal pain or discomfort at least 3 days per month in the last 3 months, associated with 2 or more of the following:
   - improvement with defecation
   - onset associated with change in stool frequency
   - onset associated with change in stool form.
2. Hard and lumpy stools (Bristol Stool Form Scale types 1 and 2) occur at least 25% of the time and loose (mushy) or watery stools occur less than 25% of the time (Bristol Stool Form Scale types 6 and 7).[127]

Traditional Chinese medicine

Initial research suggested that acupuncture may have a role to play in the management of IBS.[166] Follow-up research using more rigorous designs has not backed this up, however[167,168] and a recent systematic review of randomised, controlled trials failed to find acupuncture more effective than sham acupuncture in the management of IBS symptoms.[169] The results of a recent systematic review of herbal medicines in IBS found Chinese herbal medicine formulas effective in relieving IBS symptoms, while being very well tolerated. Unfortunately many of the trials were of poor quality, preventing firm conclusions about efficacy from being drawn.[170]

STRAIN SELECTIVITY OF ACTION

Within each species of bacteria there is a multitude of strains. Some probiotic strains are resilient and strong, with a demonstrated capacity to survive passage through the upper GIT and inhibit pathogenic bacteria, whereas others are weak and cannot even survive transit through the stomach. It is vital to note that just because one strain of bacteria in a given species has a proven action or characteristic, it does not mean that another strain will too, even if they are closely related. Strains of bacteria within the same species can have significantly different actions, properties and characteristics, as these are all essentially strain-specific qualities.[171]

Case Study

A 43-year-old married woman presented with **cramping abdominal pain**, **distension**, **excessive flatulence and constipation**. Further questioning reveals that **bowel movements occur once every 2 days** and that she can go several days between movements at times. Symptoms have been present over the previous 13-year period. For the past 2 years she has also been suffering from **upper GIT pain.** This pain started soon after she began taking NSAIDs (Celebrex) for bursitis in her left shoulder. Her GP then prescribed her Nexium in an attempt to help with the upper GIT complaint. Concurrent complaints include raised blood pressure and migraine headaches (about two episodes per month). She is currently going through a **highly stressful period** and is feeling very flat with little vital energy; there has also been a flare-up in her IBS symptoms. Previous investigations included FBC, TFT and abdominal ultrasound, which were all NAD. Current medications and supplements were Celebrex, Nexium, Coversyl, B vitamins and a probiotic (*Lactobacillus acidophilus* NCFM strain).

SUGGESTIVE SYMPTOMS

- Abdominal pain or discomfort
  - typically relieved by defecation
  - often associated with changes in stool frequency and/or appearance
- Abdominal bloating and distension
- Infrequent bowel movements (strictly speaking < 3 movements/week)
- Hard, lumpy stools
- Straining at stool passage
- Passage of mucus per rectum

Example treatment

The patient was encouraged to seek counselling to help her through the recent marital upheavals. It was also suggested that she take a brisk walk first thing each morning for 30 minutes along the beach. She was prescribed the liquid herbal formula displayed in the table at a dose of 7.5 mL twice daily. *Albizzia julibrissin* is a Chinese herb used to treat depression, anxiety and insomnia. It is particularly indicated in times of grief and 'heartache' caused by substantial loss. *Schisandra chinensis* and *Eleutherococcus senticosus* were both used for their adaptogenic qualities.

Iberogast was prescribed to address the visceral hypersensitivity seen in IBS and to reduce the main gastrointestinal symptoms of pain, bloating, distension and excessive flatulence. She was advised to cease taking *Lactobacillus acidophilus* NCFM, as this strain has been found to be ineffective in IBS.[49] Instead *L. fermentum* PCC was prescribed – a probiotic strain clinically proven to reduce abdominal pain and bloating, and to decrease flatulence in IBS sufferers (see the box on strain specificity of action).[46] Freshly ground flaxseeds were

Herbal formula	
Schisandra chinensis 1:2	30 mL
Albizzia julibrissin 1:2	40 mL
Eleutherococcus senticosus 1:2	30 mL
100 mL 7.5 mL b.d.	
Iberogast 20 drops t.d.s.	

Nutritional prescription

Lactobacillus fermentum PCC 1 billion CFU daily with meals
Ground flaxseeds (*Linum usitatissimum*) 2 tab/day
Ulmus fulva powder 1 tsp t.d.s.
Curcuma longa extract 1 tablet daily

Continued prescription

B-vitamin complex
Coversyl

used as a source of soluble fibre to promote laxation. Slippery elm powder was prescribed to decrease the gastric irritation caused by the Celebrex. Additionally, she was put on a turmeric extract primarily to reduce the bursitis-related pain and inflammation, but also for its GI anti-inflammatory and cholagogue actions. After 7 days of taking the turmeric extract and slippery elm she was advised to start weaning off the Celebrex and Nexium. She was advised to continue taking the B-complex and the Coversyl.

She was also given dietary advice, as her diet was low in fruit, vegetables and whole grains. She was advised to consume at least two serves of fruit daily, to increase her vegetable intake and to choose wholegrain options over their processed counterparts whenever possible. Her fluid intake was already good (about 2 litres daily) and needed no modification.

Expected outcomes and follow-up protocols

If treated with carminatives and GI antispasmodics (or, in this case, Iberogast), gastrointestinal symptoms such as cramping pain and bloating should improve rapidly over the next few days. In the author's experience, the key to keeping C-IBS symptoms under control is to ensure daily, easy-to-pass bowel movements. If the bowels are kept moving regularly, this tends to prevent the other GI symptoms (for example, bloating and cramping) from occurring – the pain and bloating is actually secondary to the constipation. If patients are able to implement dietary changes that successfully increase their fibre intake, exercise regularly and ingest adequate amounts of fluid, then this is usually adequate to maintain daily bowel movements for most individuals suffering from C-IBS. The addition of a soluble-fibre source, such as ground flaxseeds, is usually needed in the short-term and is obviously healthy to take long-term if need be – the consumption of freshly milled flaxseeds has a number of ancillary health benefits. Initially, the carminative, anti-inflammatory and antispasmodic herbs should be taken throughout the day every day, but after a few weeks their use can be reserved as prophylaxis for situations that are known to cause symptom flare-ups and to treat flare-ups. Nervines and adaptogens provide restoration over the long term, so their use should be continued until both the practitioner and the patient are confident that they are no longer needed. Pro-, pre- and synbiotics can (in IBS) be considered disease-modifying agents that need to be taken long-term for their benefits to be truly felt.

Table 3.4 Review of the major evidence

INTERVENTION	METHODOLOGY	RESULT	COMMENT
Probiotics[44]	Systematic review and meta-analysis of probiotics in IBS; 20 RCTs included in analysis (n = 1404 subjects)	Probiotic use was associated with improvement in global IBS symptoms compared to placebo [pooled relative risk (RRpooled) 0.77, 95% CI = 0.62–0.94]. Probiotic use was also associated with less abdominal pain compared to placebo [RRpooled = 0.78 (0.69–0.88), 95% CI 0.45–0.81].	Probiotics as a whole appear effective in the treatment of IBS, but some probiotic strains were not found to be effective; efficacy is a strain-specific attribute.
Lactobacillus fermentum PCC[46]	6-week, RDBPCCO (n = 19); 6.0 × 10^9 CFU/day of Lactobacillus fermentum strain PCC vs placebo; subjects met Rome II criteria	Significant reduction in abdominal pain (p = 0.041), constipation (p = 0.045), alternating bowel habit (p = 0.021), flatulence (p = 0.001), and bloating scores (p = 0.006) after lactobacilli treatment period, but not after placebo period; patients perceived that L. fermentum PCC relieved their IBS symptoms significantly better than placebo (p = 0.015).	The results from this small study suggest that L. fermentum PCC should be the strain of choice in the treatment of IBS, as it seems to modify a number of symptoms.
Lactobacillus plantarum 299V[48]	4-week, RDBPC (n = 40); 2.0 × 10^{10} CFU/day of Lactobacillus plantarum strain 299V vs placebo; subjects met Manning criteria	All subjects in the probiotic group reported improvements in abdominal pain versus only 58% of controls (p = 0.0012); 95% rated their overall IBS symptoms as improved compared to 15% of controls (p < 0.0001).	L. plantarum appears to be beneficial in reducing IBS symptoms.
Galacto-oligosaccharides (GOS)[172]	12-week, RSBPCCO (n = 44), 3–arm; 3.5 g/day GOS or 7 g/day GOS vs placebo; subjects met Rome II criteria	When subjects taking 3.5 g/day, significant improvements were observed in stool consistency (p < 0.05), flatulence (p < 0.05), bloating (p < 0.05) and overall IBS symptom scores (p < 0.05) compared to placebo. When subjects taking 7.0 g/day, significant improvements observed in subjective assessment of global IBS symptom score (p < 0.05) and anxiety scores (p < 0.05) compared to placebo controls.	The lower dose of GOS (3.5 g/day) appears to be more effective than the higher dose in reducing IBS symptoms. The higher dose was also associated with a significant increase in bloating scores relative to baseline at the end of the 4-week intervention period.

Table 3.4 Review of the major evidence (*Continued*)

INTERVENTION	METHODOLOGY	RESULT	COMMENT
Peppermint (*Mentha piperita*) essential oil[173]	2-week, RDBPC (*n* = 42); 100–200 mg TDS vs placebo; subjects met Rome I or Manning criteria	Significant reduction in severity of abdominal pain ($p < 0.03$) and significant improvement in global IBS symptoms ($p < 0.001$) compared to placebo	Although this trial was positive, others using peppermint oil have been inconclusive.
Padma lax – a tableted combination of herbs, heavy kaolin, sodium bicarbonate and sodium sulfate[174]	12-week, RDBPC (*n* = 80); 482 mg b.d. vs placebo; subjects met Rome I criteria (all suffered from C-IBS)	Significant increase in stool frequency ($p = 0.002$) and a significant improvement in gastroenterologist-rated constipation severity ($p = 0.0001$) compared to placebo; significant reduction in presence of moderate to severe pain ($p = 0.05$) and effect of pain on daily activities ($p = 0.002$) compared to placebo	Despite the fact that some herbal authorities do not recommend the prescription of anthraquinone-containing herbs in IBS, these results clearly demonstrate that they can be efficacious in increasing stool frequency and reducing abdominal pain.
Carmint™ – an aqueous-ethanolic extract of *Melissa officinalis*, *Mentha spicata* and *Coriandrum sativum*[175]	8-week, RDBPC (*n* = 32); Carmint™ (30 drops t.d.s. after each meal) vs placebo; Carmint™ or placebo was combined with loperamide in D-IBS and psyllium husk (1 spoonful daily) in C-IBS or alternating-IBS; subjects met Rome II criteria	Significantly decreased the severity ($p = 0.016$) and frequency ($p = 0.001$) of abdominal pain/discomfort and the severity ($p = 0.02$) and frequency of bloating ($p = 0.002$) compared to placebo	Significant differences in abdominal pain and bloating severity in favour of Carmint™ were noted from the beginning of the second week of treatment.

Note: R = randomised, CT = controlled trial, DB = double-blind, PC= placebo-controlled, CO = crossover, SB = single-blind

KEY POINTS

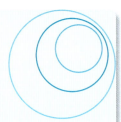

- IBS is a commonly encountered condition in naturopathic practice, typically diagnosed on clinical findings (the presence of typical signs and symptoms). Be aware of alarm features, which indicate the need for referral and/or further investigation.
- Dysbiosis appears to be a key aetiological factor in IBS and treatments aimed at addressing this imbalance (probiotics, prebiotics and synbiotics) have shown great promise in its treatment.
- In C-IBS, one of the main treatment aims should be to promote daily, easy-to-pass bowel movements.
- In some patients, stress will be *the* key contributing factor to their IBS symptoms. Avoid the temptation to focus solely on the gastrointestinal tract to the neglect of the nervous system.
- Remember that, although addressing aetiological factors is important in the long-term, providing relief of gastrointestinal symptoms (such as abdominal pain and bloating) needs to be done in the short-term to ensure the patient will come back.

Further reading

Azpiroz F, et al. Mechanisms of hypersensitivity in IBS and functional disorders. Neurogastroenterol Motil 2007;19(Suppl. 1):62–88.

Hawrelak JA, Myers SP. The causes of intestinal dysbiosis: a review. Altern Med Rev 2004;9(2):180–197.

Spiller R. Review article: probiotics and prebiotics in irritable bowel syndrome. Aliment Pharmacol Ther 2008;28:385–396.

Ohman L, Simren M. New insights into the pathogenesis and pathophysiology of irritable bowel syndrome. Dig Liver Dis 2007;39(3):201–215.

References

1. American Gastroenterology Association. Irritable bowel syndrome: a technical review for practice guideline development. Gastroenterology 2002;112:2120–2137.
2. Mayer EA. Emerging disease model for functional gastrointestinal disorders. Am J Med 1999;107(5A):12S–19S.
3. Delvaux M. Role of visceral sensitivity in the pathophysiology of irritable bowel syndrome. Gut 2002;51(Suppl. 1):i67–i71.
4. Camilleri M, et al. Consensus report: clinical perspectives, mechanisms, diagnosis and management of irritable bowel syndrome. Aliment Pharmacol Ther 2002;16:1407–1430.
5. Bercik P, et al. Is irritable bowel syndrome a low-grade inflammatory bowel disease? Gastroenterol Clin North Am 2005;34:235–245.
6. Coulie B. Role of GI motor abnormalities in irritable bowel syndrome. Acta Gastroenterol Belg 2001;64:276–280.
7. Serra J, et al. Impaired transit and tolerance of intestinal gas in irritable bowel syndrome. Gut 2001;48:14–19.
8. King TS, et al. Abnormal colonic fermentation in irritable bowel syndrome. Lancet 1998;352:1187–1189.
9. Treem WR, et al. Fecal short-chain fatty acids in patients with diarrhea-predominant irritable bowel syndrome: in vitro studies of carbohydrate fermentation. J Pediatr Gastroenterol Nutr 1996;23:280–286.
10. Si JM, et al. Intestinal microecology and quality of life in irritable bowel syndrome patients. World J Gastroenterol 2005;10:1802–1805.
11. Malinen E, et al. Analysis of the fecal microbiota of irritable bowel syndrome patients and healthy controls with real-time PCR. Am J Gastroenterol 2005;100:373–382.
12. Balsari A, et al. The fecal microbial population in the irritable bowel syndrome. Microbiologica 1982;5:185–194.
13. Morris-Yates AD, et al. Evidence of a genetic contribution to self reported symptoms of irritable bowel syndrome. Gastroenterol 1995;108:A652.
14. Locke III GR, et al. The irritable bowel syndrome and functional dyspepsia: familial disorders? Gastroenterol 1996;110:A26.
15. Rodriguez LAG, Ruigomez A. Increased risk of irritable bowel syndrome after bacterial gastroenteritis: cohort study. BMJ 1999;318:565–566.
16. McKendrick W, Read NW. Irritable bowel syndrome – post salmonella infection. J Infect 1994;29:1–3.
17. Gwee KA, et al. The role of psychological and biological factors in postinfective gut dysfunction. Gut 1999;44:400–406.
18. Mayer EA. Emerging disease model for functional gastrointestinal disorders. Am J Med 1999;107(5A):12S–19S.
19. Mendall MA, Kumar D. Antibiotic use, childhood affluence and irritable bowel syndrome. Eur J Gastroenterol Hepatol 1998;10:59–62.
20. Maxwell PR, et al. Antibiotics increase functional abdominal symptoms. Am J Gastroenterol 2002;97:104–108.
21. Bennett EJ, et al. Level of chronic stress predicts clinical outcome in irritable bowel syndrome. Gut 1998;43:256–261.
22. Whitehead WE, et al. Symptoms of psychological distress associated with irritable bowel syndrome. Gastroenterol 1998;95:709–714.
23. Masand PS, et al. Major depression and irritable bowel syndrome: is there a relationship? J Clin Psychiatry 1995;56:363–367.
24. Hochstrasser B, Angst J. The Zurich study: XXII. Epidemiology of gastroenterol complaints and comorbidity with anxiety and depression. Eur Arch Psychiatry Clin Neurosci 1996;246:261–272.
25. Wysowski DK, et al. Postmarketing reports of QT prolongation and ventricular arrhythmia in association with cisapride and Food and Drug Administration regulatory actions. Am J Gastroenterol 2001;96:1698–1703.
26. Klein KB. Controlled treatment trials in the irritable bowel syndrome: a critique. Gastroenterology 1988;95:232–241.
27. Friedel D, et al. Ischemic colitis during treatment with alosetron. Gastroenterology 2001;120:557–560.
28. Schoenfeld P. Efficacy of current drug therapies in irritable bowel syndrome: what works and does not work. Gastroenterol Clin N Am 2005;34:319–335.
29. DiBaise JK. Tegaserod-associated ischemic colitis. Pharmacotherapy 2005;25:620–625.
30. Holzapfel WH, et al. Overview of gut flora and probiotics. Int J Food Microbiol 1998;41:85–101.
31. Gibson GR. Dietary modulation of the human gut microflora using prebiotics. Br J Nutr 1998;80(Suppl. 2): S209–S212.
32. Moore WEC, Holdeman LV. Human fecal flora: the normal flora of 20 Japanese-Hawaiians. Appl Microbiol 1974;27:961–979.
33. Savage DC. Microbial ecology of the gastrointestinal tract. Annu Rev Microbiol 1997;3:107–133.
34. Bengmark S. Probiotics and prebiotics in prevention and treatment of gastrointestinal diseases. Gastroenterol Int 1998;11(Suppl. 1):4–7.
35. Macfarlane GT, Macfarlane S. Human colonic microbiota: ecology, physiology and metabolic potential of intestinal bacteria. Scand J Gastroenterol 1997;32(Suppl. 222):3–9.
36. Noack J, et al. Dietary guar gum and pectin stimulate intestinal microbial polyamine synthesis in rats. J Nutr 1998;128:1385–1391.
37. Gibson GR, Roberfroid MB. Dietary modulation of the human colonic microbiota: introducing the concept of prebiotics. J Nutr 1995;125:1401–1412.
38. Hawrelak JA, Myers SP. Intestinal dysbiosis: a review of the literature. Altern Med Rev 2004;9:180–197.
39. Lilley DM, Stillwell RH. Probiotics: growth promoting factors produced by microorganisms. Science 1965;147:747–748.
40. Parker RB. Probiotics, the other half of the antibiotic story. Animal Nut Hlth 1974;29:4–8.
41. Food and Agriculture Organization and World Health Organization Expert Consultation. Evaluation of health and nutritional properties of powder milk and live lactic acid bacteria. Food and Agriculture Organization of the United Nations and World Health Organization 2001.

42. Collins MD, Gibson GR. Probiotics, prebiotics, and synbiotics: approaches for modulating the microbial ecology of the gut. Am J Clin Nutr 1999;69(Suppl):1052S–1057S.

43. Winkelstein A. *Lactobacillus acidophilus* tablets in the therapy of various intestinal disorders: a preliminary report. Am Pract Dig Treat 1955;6:1022–1025.

44. McFarland LV, Dublin S. Meta-analysis of probiotics for the treatment of irritable bowel syndrome. World J Gastroenterol 2008;14:2650–2661.

45. Conway PL, et al. Modulation of faecal enteric bacteria and symptoms of irritable bowel syndrome using *Lactobacillus fermentum* and resistant starch. J Diet Suppl 2005:In press.

46. Amansec S, et al. *Lactobacillus fermentum* PCC™ relieves the symptoms of medically diagnosed irritable bowel syndrome. Unpublished 2005.

47. Nobaek S, et al. Alteration of intestinal microflora is associated with reduction in abdominal bloating and pain in patients with irritable bowel syndrome. Am J Gastroenterol 2000;95(5):1231–1238.

48. Niedzielin K, et al. A controlled, double-blind, randomized study on the efficacy of *Lactobacillus plantarum* 299V in patients with irritable bowel syndrome. Eur J Gastroenterol Hepatol 2001;13:1143–1147.

49. Newcomer AD, et al. Response of patients with irritable bowel syndrome and lactase deficiency using unfermented acidophilus milk. Am J Clin Nutr 1983;38:257–263.

50. O'Sullivan MA, O'Morain CA. Bacterial supplementation in the irritable bowel syndrome: a randomised double-blind placebo-controlled crossover study. Dig Liver Dis 2000;32:294–301.

51. Bausserman M, Michail S. The use of *Lactbacillus GG* in irritable bowel syndrome in children: a double-blind randomized control trial. J Pediatr 2005;147:197–201.

52. Saxelin M. Colonization of the human gastrointestinal tract by probiotic bacteria *(Lactobacillus GG)*. Nutrition Today 1996;31:5S–9S.

53. Roberfroid MB. Prebiotics and synbiotics: concepts and nutritional properties. Br J Nutr 1998;80(Suppl. 2):S197–S202.

54. Olesen M, Gudmand-Hoyer E. Efficacy, safety, and tolerability of fructooligosaccharides in the treatment of irritable bowel syndrome. Am J Clin Nutr 2000;72:1570–1575.

55. Bouhnik Y, et al. Short-chain fructo-oligosaccharide administration dose-dependently increases fecal bifidobacteria in healthy humans. J Nutr 1999;129:113–116.

56. Salyers AA, Leedle JAZ. Carbohydrate metabolism in the human colon. In: Hentges DJ, ed. Human intestinal microflora in health and disease. New York: Academic Press, 1983:129–146.

57. Bernalier A, et al. Biochemistry of Fermentation. In: Gibson GR, Roberfroid M, eds. Colonic microbiota, nutrition and health. Dordoecht: Kluwer Academic Publishers, 1999:37–54.

58. Gibson SAW, Conway PL. Recovery of a probiotic organism from human faeces after oral dosing. In: Gibson SAW, ed. Human health: the contribution of microorganisms. London: Springer-Verlag, 1994:119–121.

59. Robinson RR, et al. Effects of dietary arabinogalactan on gastrointestinal and blood parameters in healthy human subjects. J Am Coll Nutr 2001;20:279–285.

60. Jie Z, et al. Studies on the effects of polydextrose intake on physiologic functions in Chinese people. Am J Clin Nutr 2000;72:1503–1509.

61. Schrezenmeir J, de Vrese M. Probiotics, prebiotics, and synbiotics—approaching a definition. Am J Clin Nutr 2001;73:361–364.

62. Casiraghi MC, et al. Effects of a synbiotic milk product on human intestinal ecosystem. J Appl Microbiol 2007;103:499–506.

63. Dughera L, et al. Effects of symbiotic preparations on constipated irritable bowel syndrome symptoms. Acta Biomed 2007;78:111–116.

64. Colecchia A, et al. Effects of a symbiotic preparation on the clinical manifestations of irritable bowel syndrome, constipation-variant. Results of an open, uncontrolled multicenter study. Minerva Gastroenterol Dietolo 2006;52:349–358.

65. Arvola T, et al. Prophylactic *Lactobacillus GG* reduces antibiotic-associated diarrhea in children with respiratory infections: a randomized study. Pediatrics 1999;104(5):1–4.

66. Kontiokari T, et al. Randomised trial of cranberry-lingonberry juice and *Lactobacillus GG* drink for the prevention of urinary tract infections in women. BMJ 2001;322:1571.

67. Conway PL, et al. Modulation of faecal enteric bacteria and symptoms of irritable bowel syndrome using *Lactobacillus fermentum* and resistant starch. Unpublished 2005.

68. Amansec S, et al. *Lactobacillus fermentum* PCC™ relieves the symptoms of medically diagnosed irritable bowel syndrome (IBS). Unpublished 2005.

69. Nobaek S, et al. Alteration of intestinal microflora is associated with reduction in abdominal bloating and pain in patients with irritable bowel syndrome. Am J Gastroenterol 2000;95(5):1231–1238.

70. Niedzielin K, et al. A controlled, double-blind, randomized study on the efficacy of *Lactobacillus plantarum* 299V in patients with irritable bowel syndrome. Eu J Gastroenterol Hepatol 2001;13:1143–1147.

71. Tursi A, et al. Low-dose balsalazide plus a high-potency probiotic preparation is more effective than balsalazide alone or mesalazine in the treatment of acute mild-to-moderate ulcerative colitis. Med Sci Monit 2004;10:126–131.

72. Zocco MA, et al. Efficacy of *Lactobacillus GG* in maintaining remission of ulcerative colitis. Aliment Pharmacol Ther 2006;23:1567–1574.

73. Venturi A, et al. Impact on the composition of the faecal flora by a new probiotic preparation: preliminary data on maintenance treatment of patients with ulcerative colitis. Aliment Pharmacol Ther 1999;13:1103–1108.

74. Mimura T, et al. Once daily high dose probiotic therapy (VSL#3) for maintaining remission in recurrent or refractory pouchitis. Gut 2004;53:108–114.

75. Gosselink MP, et al. Delay of the first onset of pouchitis by oral intake of the probiotic strain *Lactobacillus rhamnosus GG*. Dis Colon Rectum 2005;47:876–884.

76. Szajewska H, et al. Efficacy of *Lactobacillus GG* in prevention of nosocomial diarrhea in infants. J Pediatr 2001;138:361–365.

77. Chouraqui JP, et al. Acidified milk formula supplemented with Bifidobacteria lactis: impact on infant diarrhea in residential care settings. J Pediatr Gastroenterol Nutr 2004;38:288–292.

78. Saavedra JM, et al. Feeding of *Bifidobacterium bifidum* and *Streptococcus thermophilus* to infants in hospital for prevention of diarrhoea and shedding of rotavirus. Lancet 1994;344:1046–1049.

79. Szajewska H, et al. Meta-analysis: *Lactobacillus GG* for treating acute diarrhoea in children. Aliment Pharmacol Ther 2007;25:871–881.

80. Shomikova AV, et al. *Lactobacillus reuteri* as a therapeutic agent in acute diarrhea in young children. J Pediatr Gastroenterol Nutr 1997;24:399–404.

81. Shornikova AV, et al. Bacteriotherapy with *Lactobacillus reuteri* in rotavirus gastroenteritis. Pediatr Infect Dis 1997;16:1103–1107.

82. Saggioro A, et al. *Helicobacter pylori* eradication with *Lactobacillus reuteri*. A double-blind placebo-controlled study. Dig Liv Dis 2005;37:588.

83. Wang KY, et al. Effects of ingesting *Lactobacillus-* and *Bifidobacterium*-containing yogurt in subjects with colonized *Helicobacter pylori*. Am J Clin Nutr 2004;80:737–741.

84. Savino F, et al. *Lactobacillus reuteri* ATCC 55730 versus simeticone in the treatment of infantile colic: a prospective randomised study. Paediatrics 2005;119:124–130.

85. Wildt S, et al. Probiotic treatment of collagenous colitis: a randomized, double-blind, placebo-controlled trial with *Lactobacillus acidophilus* and *Bifidobacterium animalis subsp lactis*. Inflamm Bowel Dis 2006;12:395–401.

86. Koebnick C, et al. Probiotic beverage containing *Lactobacillus casei* Shirota improves gastrointestinal symptoms in patients with chronic constipation. Can J Gastroenterol 2005;17:655–659.

87. Pitkala KH, et al. Fermented cereal with specific bifidobacteria normalizes bowel movements in elderly nursing home residents. A randomized, controlled trial. J Nutr Health Aging 2007;11:305–311.

88. Hawrelak JA, et al. Is *Lactobacillus rhamnosus GG* effective in preventing the onset of antibiotic-associated diarrhea: a systematic review. Digestion 2005;72:51–56.

89. Lionetti E, et al. The effect of oral administration of *Lactobacillus reuteri* on antibiotic-assocaited gastrointestinal side-effects during *Helicobacter pylori* eradication therapy. 12th National Congress of Italian Society of Pediatric Gastroenterology, 22–24 September 2005.

90. Wenus C, et al. Prevention of antibiotic-associated diarrhoea by a fermented probiotic milk drink. Eur J Clin Nutr 2008;62:299–301.

91. Gorbach SL, et al. Successful treatment of relapsing *Clostridium diffcile* colitis with *Lactobacillus GG*. Lancet 1987;2:1519.

92. Bennett RG, et al. Treatment of relapsing *Clostridium difficile* diarrhea with *Lactobacillus GG*. Nutr Today 1996;31:35S–39S.

93. Klarin B, et al. *Lactobacillus plantarum* 299v reduces colonisation of *Clostridium difficile* in critically ill patients treated with antibiotics. Acta Anaesthesiol Scand 2008;52:1096–1102.

94. Manley KJ, et al. Probiotic treatment of vancomycin-resistant enterococci: a randomised controlled trial. Med J Aust 2007;186:454–457.

95. Delia P, et al. Use of probiotics for prevention of radiation-induced diarrhea. World J Gastroenterol 2007;13:912–915.

96. Nase L, et al. Effect of long-term consumption of a probiotic bacterium, *Lactobacillus rhamnosus GG,* in milk on dental caries and caries risk in children. Caries Res 2001;35:412–420.

97. Hatakka K, et al. Effect of long-term consumption of probiotic milk on infections in children attending day care centres: double-blind, randomised trial. BMJ 2001;322:1327.

98. Weizman Z, et al. Effect of a probiotic infant formula on infections in child care centers: comparison of two probiotic agents. Pediatrics 2005;115:5–9.

99. Tubelius P, et al. Increasing work-place healthiness with the probiotic *Lactobacillus reuteri*: a randomised, double-blind placebo-controlled trial. Environ Health 2005;4:25.

100. Leyer GJ, et al. Probiotic effects on cold and influenza-like symptom incidence and duration in children. Pediatrics 2009;124:172–179.

101. Sazawal S, et al. Efficacy of milk fortified with a probiotic *Bifidobacterium lactis (DR-10)* and prebiotic galacto-oligosaccharides in prevention of morbidity and on nutritional status. Asia Pacific J Clin Nutr 2004;13(Suppl):S28.

102. Kalliomaki M, et al. Probiotics in primary prevention of atopic disease: a randomised, placebo-controlled trial. Lancet 2001;357:1076–1079.

103. Kalliomaki M, et al. Probiotics during the first 7 years of life: a cumulative risk reduction of eczema in a randomised, placebo-controlled trial. J Allergy Clin Immunol 2007;119:1019–1021.

104. Wickens K, et al. A differential effect of 2 probiotics in the prevention of eczema and atopy: a double-blind, randomized, placebo-controlled trial. J Allergy Clin Immunol 2008;122:788–794.

105. Weston A, et al. Effects of probiotics on atopic dermatitis: a randomised controlled trial. Arch Dis Child 2005;90:892–897.

106. Hilton E, et al. Ingestion of yogurt containing *Lactobacillus acidophilus* as prophylaxis for candidal vaginitis. Ann Intern Med 1992;116(5):353–357.

107. Davies GJ, et al. Bowel function measurements of individuals with different eating patterns. Gut 1986;27:164–169.

108. Sanjoaquin MA, et al. Nutrition and lifestyle in relation to bowel movement frequency: a cross-sectional study of 20,630 men and women in EPIC-Oxford. Public Health Nutr 2004;7:77–83.

109. Tramonte SM, et al. The treatment of chronic constipation in adults: a systematic review. J Gen Intern Med 1997;12:15–24.

110. Bijkerk CJ, et al. Systematic review: the role of different types of fibre in the treatment of irritable bowel syndrome. Aliment Pharmacol Ther 2004;19:245–251.

111. Cunnane SC, et al. High a-linolenic acid flaxseed *(Linum usitatissimum)*: some nutritional properties in humans. Br J Nutr 1993;69:443–453.

112. van Wyk BE, Wink M. Medicinal plants of the world. Pretoria, South Africa: Briza, 2004.

113. Sierra M, et al. Therapeutic effects of psyllium in type 2 diabetic patients. Eur J Clin Nutr 2002;56:830–842.

114. Knudsen KEB, Johansen HN. Mode of action of oat bran in the gastrointestinal tract. Eur J Clin Nutr 1995;49(Suppl 3):S163–S169.

115. Southgate DA. Dietary fiber parts of food plants and algae. In: Spiller GA, ed. CRC handbook of dietary fibre in human nutrition. Boca Raton: CRC Press, 2001:11–13.

116. Cummings JH. The effect of dietary fiber on fecal weight and composition. In: Spiller GA, ed. CRC handbook of dietary fibre in human nutrition. Boca Raton: CRC Press, 2001:183–252.

117. Cherbut C, et al. Effects of short-chain fatty acids on gastrointestinal motility. Scand J Gastroenterol 1997;32(Suppl. 222):58–61.

118. Topping DL. Short-chain fatty acids produced by intestinal bacteria. Asia Pacific J Clin Nutr 1996;5(Suppl):15–19.

119. Klauser AG, et al. Low fluid intake lowers stool output in healthy male volunteers. Z Gastroenterol 1990;28:606–609.

120. National Health and Medical Research Council. Nutrient reference values for Australia and New Zealand. National Health and Medical Research Council 2006.

121. Everhart JE, et al. A longitudinal survey of self-reported bowel habits in the United States. Dig Dis Sci 1989;34:1153–1162.

122. Dahl R. Revolting rhymes. London: Puffin Books, 1995.

123. Oettle GJ. Effect of moderate exercise on bowel habit. Gut 1991;32:941–944.

124. Daley AJ, et al. The effects of exercise upon symptoms and quality of life in patients diagnosed with irritable bowel syndrome: a randomised controlled trial. Int J Sports Med 2008;29:778–782.

125. Heaton KW, et al. Defecation frequency and timing, and stool form in the general population: a prospective study. Gut 1992;33:818–824.

126. Bassoti G, et al. An extended assessment of bowel habits in a general population. World J Gastroenterol 2004;10:713–716.

127. Longstreth GF, et al. Functional bowel disorders. Gastroenterol 2006;130:1480–1491.

128. Lindlahr H. Natural therapeutics Volume 2: practice. Essex UK: CW Daniel Company Ltd, 1981.

129. Walker ARP. Nutritionally related disorders/diseases in Africans. Highlights of half a century of research with special reference to unexpected phenomena. In: Kritchevsky D, Bonfield C, eds. Dietary fibre in health and disease. New York: Plenum Press, 1997:1–14.

130. Jones JM. Consumption of dietary fibre 1992–2000. In: Spiller GA, ed. CRC handbook of dietary fibre in human nutrition. Boca Raton: CRC Press, 2001:553–566.

131. Heaton KW, et al. How bad are the symptoms and bowel dysfunction of patients with the irritable bowel syndrome? A prospective, controlled study with emphasis on stool form. Gut 1991;32:73–79.

132. Lewis SJ, Heaton KW. Stool form scale as a useful guide to intestinal transit time. Scand J Gastroenterol 1997;32:920–924.

133. Bassoti G, et al. Human colonic motility: physiological aspects. Int J Colorectal Dis 1995;10:173–180.

134. Gralnek IM, et al. The impact of irritable bowel syndrome on health-related quality of life. Gastroenterology 2000;119:654–660.

135. Spiegel B, et al. Predictors of patient-assessed illness severity in irritable bowel syndrome. Am J Gastroenterol 2008;103:2536–2543.

136. Gorard DA, et al. Intestinal transit in anxiety and depression. Gut 1996;39:551–555.

137. Adam B, et al. A combination of peppermint oil and caraway oil attenuates the post-inflammatory visceral hyperalgesia in a rat model. Scan J Gastroenterol 2006;41:155–160.

138. Muller MH, et al. STW 5 (Iberogast) reduces afferent sensitivity in the rat small intestine. Phytomedicine 2006;13:100–106.

139. Bone K. Phytotherapy and irritable bowel syndrome. Br J Phytotherapy 1997;4:190–198.

140. Bretagne JF, et al. Increased cell loss in the human jejunum induced by laxatives (ricinoleic acid, dioctyl sodium sulphosuccinate, magnesium sulphate, bile salts). Gut 1981;22(264):269.

141. Walker AF, et al. Artichoke leaf extract reduces symptoms of irritable bowel syndrome in a post-marketing surveillance study. Phytother Res 2001;15:58–61.

142. Bundy R, et al. Turmeric extract may improve irritable bowel syndrome symptomology in otherwise healthy adults: a pilot study. J Altern Complement Med 2004;10:1015–1018.

143. Gils CV, Cox PA. Ethnobotany of nutmeg in the Spice Islands. J Ethnopharmacol 1994;42:117–124.

144. Felter HW. The eclectic materia medica, pharmacology and therapeutics. Cincinnati: John K Scudder, 1922.

145. Bensky D, et al. Chinese herbal medicine materia medica. Seattle: Eastland Press, 2004.

146. Khare CP. Indian herbal remedies. Rational western therapy, ayurvedic and other traditional usage, botany. Heidelberg: Springer-Verlag, 2004.

147. Bennett A, et al. The biological activity of eugenol, a major constituent of nutmeg (*Myristica fragrans*): studies on prostaglandins, the intestine and other tissues. Phytother Res 1988;2:124–130.

148. Dhingra D, Sharma A. Antidepressant-like activity of n-hexane extract of nutmeg (*Myristica fragrans*) seeds in mice. J Med Food 2006;9:84–89.

149. Sonavane GS, et al. Anxiogenic activity of *Myristica fragrans* seeds. Pharmacol Biochem Behav 2002;71:247–252.

150. Felter HW, Lloyd JU. King's American dispensatory. Cincinnati: Ohio Valley Company, 1898.

151. Ononiwu IM, et al. Effects of piperine on gastric acid secretion in albino rats. Afr J Med Sci 2002;31:293–295.

152. Vasudevan K, et al. Influence of intragastric perfusion of aqueous spice extracts on acid secretion in anesthetized albino rats. Indian J Gastroenterol 2000;19:53–56.

153. Bhat BG, Chandrasekhara N. Effect of black pepper and piperine on bile secretion and composition in rats. Food/Nahrung 1987;31:913–916.

154. Platel K, Srinivassan K. Influence of dietary spices and their active principles on pancreatic digestive enzymes in albino rats. Food/Nahrung 2000;44(42):46.

155. Izzo AA, et al. Effect of vanilloid drugs on gastrointestinal transit in mice. Br J Pharmacol 2001;132:1411–1416.

156. Bajad S, et al. Antidiarrhoeal activity of piperine in mice. Planta Med 2001;67:284–287.

157. Weiss RF. Herbal medicine. Beaconsfield: Ab Arcanum, 1988.

158. May B, et al. Efficacy of a fixed peppermint oil/caraway oil combination in non-ulcer dyspepsia. Arzneimittel-Forschung 1996;46:1149–1153.

159. May B, et al. Efficacy and tolerability of a fixed combination of peppermint oil and caraway oil in patients suffering from functional dyspepsia. Aliment Pharmacol Ther 2000;14:1671–1677.

160. Madisch A, et al. Treatment of functional dyspepsia with a fixed peppermint oil and caraway oil combination preparation as compared to cisapride. A multicenter, reference-controlled double-blind equivalence study 1999;49:925–932.

161. Rios JL, et al. An update review of saffron and its active constituents. Phytother Res 1996;10:189–193.

162. Pierpoint Johnson C. The useful plants of Great Britain: a treatise upon the principal native vegetables capable of application as food, medicine, or in the arts and manufactures. London: R. Hardwicke, 1862.

163. Noorbala AA, et al. Hydro-alcoholic extract of *Crocus sativus* L. versus fluoxetine in the treatment of mild to moderate depression: a double-blind, randomized pilot trial. J Ethnopharmacol 2005;97:281–284.

164. Akhondzadeh S, et al. Comparison of *Crocus sativus* L. and imipramine in the treatment of mild to moderate depression: a pilot double-blind randomized trial. BMC Complement Altern Med 2004;4:12.

165. Jones J, et al. British Society of Gastroenterology guidelines for management of the irritable bowel syndrome. Gut 2000;47(Suppl. 2):ii1–ii19.

166. Chan J, et al. The role of acupuncture in the treatment of irritable bowel syndrome: a pilot study. Hepatogastroenterology 1997;44:1328–1330.

167. Forbes A, et al. Acupuncture for irritable bowel syndrome: a blinded placebo-controlled trial. World J Gastroenterol 2005;11:4040–4044.

168. Schneider A, et al. Acupuncture treatment in irritable bowel syndrome. Gut 2006;55:649–654.

169. Lim B, et al. Acupuncture for treatment of irritable bowel syndrome. Cochrane Database Syst Rev 2006(4):CD005111.

170. Shi J, et al. Effectiveness and safety of herbal medicines in the treatment of irritable bowel syndrome: a systematic review. World J Gastroenterol 2008;14:454–462.

171. Lewis SJ, Freedman AR. The use of biotherapeutic agents in the prevention and treatment of gastrointestinal disease. Aliment Pharmacol Ther 1998;12:807–822.

172. Silk DB, et al. Clinical trial: the effects of a trans-galactooligosaccharide prebiotic on faecal microbiota and symptoms in irritable bowel syndrome. Aliment Pharmacol Ther 2009;29:508–518.

173. Kline RM, et al. Enteric-coated, pH-dependent peppermint oil capsules for the treatment of irritable bowel syndrome in children. J Pediatr 2001;138:125–128.

174. Sallon S, et al. A novel treatment for constipation-predominant irritable bowel syndrome using Padma®Lax, a Tibetan herbal formula. Digestion 2002;65:161–171.

175. Vejdani R, et al. The efficacy of an herbal medicine, Carmint, on the relief of abdominal pain and bloating n patients with irritable bowel syndrome: a pilot study. Dig Dis Sci 2006;51:1501–1507.

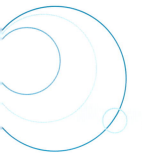

4

Gastro-oesophageal reflux disease

Jason Hawrelak
ND, BNat (Hons), PhD

AETIOLOGY

Gastro-oesophageal reflux disease (GORD) is commonly encountered in clinical practice. Recent research has estimated the prevalence at 10–20% in Western nations.[1] GORD has been defined as 'a condition which develops when the reflux of stomach contents causes troublesome symptoms and/or complications'.[2] Signs and symptoms of GORD result primarily from the recurrent reflux of gastric contents into the oesophagus (Figure 4.1). The pathogenesis of GORD is complex and multifactorial with a number of mechanisms appearing to be involved (Figure 4.2):

- *lower oesophageal sphincter incompetence.* The role of the lower oesophageal sphincter (LOS) is to allow the passage of food into the stomach, while preventing the reflux of gastric contents back into the oesophagus. Patients with GORD have been found to suffer from frequent transient LOS relaxations and decreased LOS resting pressure compared with healthy controls.[3,4]
- *poor oesophageal acid clearance.* Patients with GORD have been found to have less oesophageal peristaltic activity. This results in a reduced capacity to clear reflux contents from the oesophagus.[5] Contact between the refluxed gastric contents and the oesophageal mucosa results in inflammation. This inflammation has been found to further reduce oesophageal peristalsis, further impairing acid clearance, and causing a worsening of reflux symptoms—a vicious circle.[6]
- *slow gastric emptying.* Delayed gastric emptying (particularly of the proximal stomach) has been correlated with increased severity and frequency of reflux episodes in GORD patients.[7] Delayed gastric emptying of ingesta has been postulated to contribute to GORD symptoms via two mechanisms: (1) by increasing the length of time refluxate is available in the stomach; and (2) increasing gastric distension, which has been found to increase the rate of transient LOS relaxations.[8]
- *impaired saliva flow.* Salivary secretion plays an important role in the clearance of regurgitated gastric contents in the oesophagus. GORD patients have been found to suffer from impaired salivary gland function and reduced saliva production.[9]
- *hiatal hernia.* Hiatal hernias have been found to be relatively common in patients suffering from GORD.[10] They appear to promote LOS incompetence via a decrease in

LOS resting pressure,[11,12] and their presence is associated with increased severity of reflux.[13]

- *oxidative stress.* Research has shown that mucosal damage in oesophagitis is mediated, at least in part, by oxygen-derived free radicals.[14] Animal research has also found considerable levels of oxidative stress in the oesophageal mucosa after reflux episodes. This research also noted a significant mucosa protective effect from antioxidant supplementation.[15]
- *food allergy and intolerance.* Gastro-oesophageal reflux in infants and toddlers is frequently linked to a dairy allergy.[16] Patients with gluten intolerance have also been found to have a high prevalence of gastro-oesophageal reflux. Although the exact

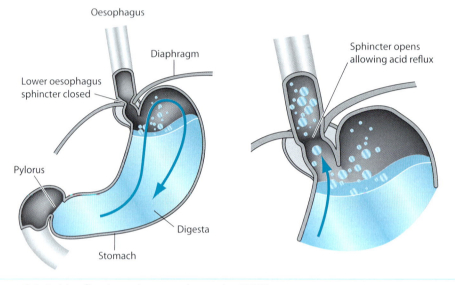

Figure 4.1 Acid reflux into the oesophagus in GORD

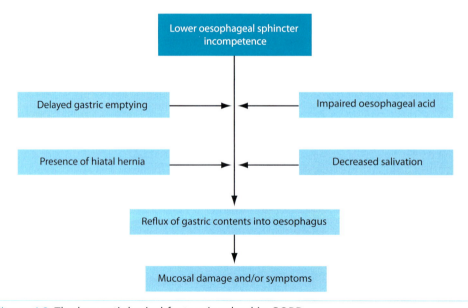

Figure 4.2 The key aetiological factors involved in GORD

mechanism of how gluten exposure leads to gastro-oesophageal reflux is not known, gluten-free diets have been found to significantly reduce GORD symptoms and effectively prevent their recurrence.[17]

RISK FACTORS

A number of risk factors that appear to contribute to the initiation and maintenance of GORD symptoms have been identified. These usually involve lifestyle factors, although genetic influences and medications can also contribute to the disorder:

- *dietary factors*. Dietary factors capable of precipitating reflux episodes include coffee and other caffeinated beverages, alcoholic beverages, chocolate, meals high in fat, and, potentially, peppermint essential oil (for example, peppermint candy).[18] These substances are capable of increasing acid secretion (alcohol, coffee), reducing LOS pressure (alcohol, chocolate, coffee, fatty meals), causing transient LOS relaxations (alcohol, peppermint essential oil), slowing gastric emptying (alcohol, fatty foods) and/or impairing oesophageal motility (alcohol). Agents that can trigger pain by irritating an already inflamed oesophageal mucosa include tomato and citrus juice, soft drinks and spicy foods. From a naturopathic perspective, eating meals too quickly, consuming too large meals, consuming fluids with meals, eating close to bedtime and chewing food inadequately are other potential contributing factors to GORD.
- *high BMI*. Research has found a clear association between reflux symptoms and the presence of overweight or obesity.[19]
- *smoking*. Tobacco smokers report higher rates of reflux symptoms than non-smokers do.[20] This is thought to be caused by smoking-induced decreases in resting LOS pressure. Coughing or even deep inhalation can cause acute increases in intraabdominal pressure capable of overpowering their feeble LOS.[21]
- *psychological stress*. A significant proportion of subjects with GORD have been found to suffer from psychological distress[22] and stress appears to increase sensitivity to heartburn pain in some GORD sufferers.[23]
- *genetic disposition*. A genetic predisposition may contribute to the development of GORD in some patients, with one study estimating that genetic influences comprise almost 30% of attributable risk for GORD.[24]
- *medications*. Nitrates, calcium channel blockers, theophylline, morphine, meperidone, diazepam, barbiturates and sildenafil are all capable of decreasing LOS pressure.[25]

CONVENTIONAL TREATMENT

Conventional treatment aims to reduce the symptoms of GORD and reduce oesophageal damage through the use of antisecretory therapies, such as proton pump inhibitors or histamine type 2 receptor antagonists (H2RAs). Although these agents have been found to be effective in reducing the oesophageal symptoms of GORD and, to a lesser extent, extraoesophageal symptoms,[26] their use is also associated with significant side effects and risks. Common adverse events of antisecretory therapies include diarrhoea, nausea, abdominal pain and headaches.[27] Longer-term use of anti-secretory drugs is associated with increased risk of gastroenteritis,[28] pneumonia,[29] spinal fracture[30] and vitamin and mineral malabsorption.[31,32] More recently, the surgical procedure laparoscopic fundoplication has been advocated in the treatment of GORD.

KEY TREATMENT PROTOCOLS

The naturopathic protocols adopted to treat GORD usually focus on dietary and lifestyle modifications, in addition to botanical treatments. After relieving symptoms, the aim is to initially identify any factors that contribute to GORD and remove these triggers. If inflammation, ulceration or poor motility/sphincter tone is present, herbal or nutritional prescription may be of benefit.

> **NATUROPATHIC TREATMENT AIMS**
> - Relieve symptoms.
> - Treat the cause—eliminate/minimise exacerbating factors:
>   - address dietary factors
>   - address lifestyle factors.
> - Decrease oesophageal inflammation and promote oesophageal healing.
> - Tone the lower oesophageal sphincter.
> - Prevent oesophageal cancer.
> - Promote antioxidant defences.
> - Support the nervous system.

Relieve symptoms

Relief of heartburn is paramount in the management of GORD. Gastrointestinal demulcents are typically very effective in providing prompt relief of heartburn symptoms (usually within minutes of ingestion). Effective **demulcents** include *Althaea officinalis radix*, *Ulmus fulva cortex* and *Glycyrrhiza glabra*.[44] Gastrointestinal demulcents are most effective when administered in powdered form—mixed into a little water or apple juice to form a slurry or gruel. Tablets and capsules will be significantly less effective. Demulcents can be used 'on demand' or taken after meals and/or before bed for a preventative effect.

Eliminate exacerbating factors

Dietary factors

The naturopathic axiom *tolle causum* ('treat the cause') is particularly relevant to the management of GORD. While herbal demulcents can relieve heartburn symptoms effectively and promptly, their use, in some respects, is only palliative if patients continue to indulge in dietary factors known to exacerbate their condition. Avoidance of foods and drinks known to precipitate reflux episodes (for example, chocolate, alcoholic beverages, caffeinated beverages and fatty foods) is an important therapeutic strategy that may produce excellent clinical outcomes (see Chapter 5 on food intolerance/allergy),[33] although it should be noted that an 'evidence-based review' of dietary changes was inconclusive due to insufficient research.[18] The authors did, however, note that there is a definitive link in some sufferers of GORD with food and alcohol, as physiological evidence has demonstrated decreased LOS tone.

Other recommendations, such as taking time when eating, consuming smaller meals and avoiding fluid consumption with meals (both should decrease gastric distension) and chewing food adequately, are traditional naturopathic recommendations.[34] Chewing food as thoroughly as possible is a traditional recommendation which may result in improved salivary gland function over time and, hence, improved oesophageal acid clearance. Changing the evening meal time to earlier in the evening (at least 3–4 hours before bedtime) can also be helpful.[35]

In infants and toddlers with GORD, a dairy-free diet should be implemented. If they are formula-fed, the mother should be encouraged to relactate. The use of an extensively hydrolysed whey formula is the next best option. Soy and goat's milk formulas should be avoided as they share a significant amount of cross-reactivity with cow milk proteins. There have also been a number of studies demonstrating the efficacy of **carob bean**

powder (*Ceratonia siliqua*) as a formula additive.[36,37] Carob powder has been found to significantly decrease the severity and frequency of vomiting in infants with GORD, as well as increasing weight gain.[36] If the infant is exclusively breastfed, then the mother should be placed on a dairy-free diet, as small, but clinically significant, amounts of dairy proteins do appear in the breast milk.

Lifestyle factors

In addition to the dietary factors discussed above, lifestyle factors such as obesity and smoking should be addressed. Weight loss has been shown in some research to result in reduced reflux episodes and should be encouraged in all overweight and obese patients.[38] Cessation of smoking could be recommended for a number of compelling reasons, not the least of which is its effect on oesophageal reflux. Short-term studies (of 24–48 hours duration) have not consistently found a reduction in reflux episodes after smoking cessation.[39,40] However, no longer-term studies have yet been performed and, in light of smoking's well-known adverse effects, GORD patients who smoke should be encouraged to give up. **Herbal thymoleptics**, **anxiolytics** and **adaptogens** could play an important supportive role in this process (see the section on the nervous system).

Raising the head of the bed is another easy-to-implement lifestyle intervention that has demonstrated beneficial effects in GORD.[18] This recommendation is based on the theory that acidic stomach contents will be more likely to reflux when patients are lying flat. Research has, thus far, mostly supported this theory, with intervention trials finding reduced frequency of reflux episodes, shorter reflux episodes and fewer reflux symptoms when bed heads were raised (one trial raised the head by 28 cm).[41]

Decrease oesophageal inflammation and promote oesophageal healing

The reduction of oesophageal inflammation and the promotion of oesophageal healing will help reduce the vicious circle of GORD. As previously discussed, inflammation is a common occurrence in GORD. Demulcents (as discussed above), **anti-inflammatory and vulnerary herbs** may soothe the tissue and enhance healing. Useful anti-inflammatory phytomedicines for the digestive system include *Filipendula ulmaria*, *Glycyrrhiza glabra* and *Matricaria recutita*, while vulnerary herbal medicines traditionally used to help heal the upper gastrointestinal tract include *Althaea officinalis*, *Ulmus fulva*, *Calendula officinalis*, *Symphytum officinale* and *Aloe barbadensis*.[42,43] Given that alcohol is a common reflux exacerbating factor, teas are probably the preferred method of administration.

Given the role of free radicals in reflux-induced oesophageal inflammation,[14] the promotion of antioxidant defences is a worthwhile, but as yet under-researched, therapeutic approach. The incorporation of brightly coloured fruits, vegetables, legumes and whole grains into the diet should be encouraged (see the food nutrient chart in Appendix 4).

PHYTOTHERAPY IN GORD

Aside from the use of carminative herbs in dyspepsia, phytotherapy in most other digestive conditions including GORD is under-researched.

Currently, most evidentiary support is based on traditional use and in vitro studies. This remains a potential area of research.

WHAT ABOUT HYPOCHLORHYDRIA AND DIGESTIVE BITTERS?

A common naturopathic theory is that GORD is actually caused by hypochlorhydria—too little gastric acid.

This theory is based on the idea that sufficient gastric acid in the stomach functions as a signal informing the LOS to remain tightly closed. When there is insufficient gastric acid, the LOS allows the reflux of the gastric contents into the oesophagus where it causes damage and inflammation. Another theory is that insufficient digestion causes fermentation, which creates increased intra-gastric pressure and the subsequent opening of the LOS

At this point in time, however, there is little hard evidence to support either theory.

Given the theoretical causative role of hypochlorhydria in GORD, it is not surprising that bitters have been suggested as potential therapeutic substances.

Bitter herbs tend to be viewed as increasing gastric acid output via taste receptors on the tongue. Independent of this effect on gastric acid output, bitters, such as *Gentiana lutea*, produce a number of effects that are potentially beneficial in GORD.

Bitters increase saliva secretion,[47] speed gastric emptying,[48] and exhibit mucosal protective activity.[49] Caution should be used in their application, however, as any increase in gastric acidity could significantly aggravate GORD symptoms.

Tone the lower oesophageal sphincter

A traditional naturopathic focus of treating GORD is to improve the tone of the smooth muscle of the LOS, thereby enhancing its capacity to hold gastrointestinal contents in the stomach. Poor LOS tone may be potentially improved by the use of **tannin-rich herbs**, which provide astringency and increased tissue tone, in addition to reducing inflammation.[44] Hydrolysable tannin constituents (higher molecule weight tannins) primarily affect astringency.[44] Botanicals that contain these tannins include *Geranium maculatum*, *Achillea millefolium*, *Calendula officinalis*, *Hamamelis virginiana* and *Agrimonia eupatorium*.[45] The naturopath should be aware that long-term use or high doses of tannins may impede digestion. A prudent approach is to co-prescribe a herbal medicine with a bitter principle to stimulant digestion and to provide an adjuvant anti-inflammatory effect. However, to complicate matters, the use of bitters should be monitored carefully as this may worsen some people's GORD.[46]

Prevent oesophageal cancer

One of the more serious complications of GORD is the development of Barrett's oesophagus, a metaplastic change of the lining of the oesophagus that is associated with an increased risk of oesophageal adenocarcinoma.[50] Preventing the development of Barrett's oesophagus and preventing the change of Barrett's oesophagus to adenocarcinoma should be major naturopathic treatment aims. Preventing reflux episodes, reducing oesophageal inflammation and promoting mucosal healing using the strategies discussed above will be part of this approach. Reducing oxidative stress is an additional approach to this issue, as research has found patients with Barrett's oesophagus to have lower plasma concentrations of antioxidants (selenium, vitamin C, β-cryptoxanthine and xanthophyll) than GORD patients without Barrett's oesophagus.[51] This can best

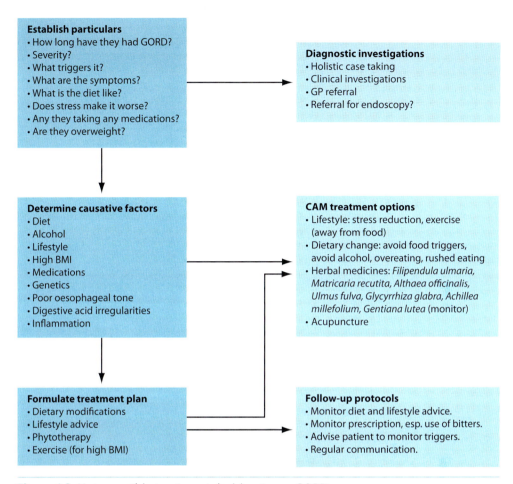

Establish particulars
- How long have they had GORD?
- Severity?
- What triggers it?
- What are the symptoms?
- What is the diet like?
- Does stress make it worse?
- Any they taking any medications?
- Are they overweight?

Diagnostic investigations
- Holistic case taking
- Clinical investigations
- GP referral
- Referral for endoscopy?

Determine causative factors
- Diet
- Alcohol
- Lifestyle
- High BMI
- Medications
- Genetics
- Poor oesophageal tone
- Digestive acid irregularities
- Inflammation

CAM treatment options
- Lifestyle: stress reduction, exercise (away from food)
- Dietary change: avoid food triggers, avoid alcohol, overeating, rushed eating
- Herbal medicines: *Filipendula ulmaria, Matricaria recutita, Althaea officinalis, Ulmus fulva, Glycyrrhiza glabra, Achillea millefolium, Gentiana lutea* (monitor)
- Acupuncture

Formulate treatment plan
- Dietary modifications
- Lifestyle advice
- Phytotherapy
- Exercise (for high BMI)

Follow-up protocols
- Monitor diet and lifestyle advice.
- Monitor prescription, esp. use of bitters.
- Advise patient to monitor triggers.
- Regular communication.

Figure 4.3 Naturopathic treatment decision tree—GORD

be done by encouraging the consumption of antioxidant-rich fruits and vegetables, legumes and whole grain products on a daily basis.

Epidemiological research has found an inverse relationship between dietary intake of zinc and incidence of oesophageal adenocarcinoma[52] and animal models have found zinc deficiency to be a significant contributing factor to the development of Barrett's oesophagus.[53] In light of this research, zinc supplementation may also be warranted in GORD sufferers in an attempt to prevent the development of Barrett's oesophagus (see Chapter 29 on cancer for overarching protocols and interventions).

INTEGRATIVE MEDICAL CONSIDERATIONS
Medical referral
Diagnosis of GORD is typically made clinically, based on the presence of the classic symptoms—a burning feeling rising from the stomach or lower chest up towards the neck (heartburn) and/or the effortless return of stomach contents into the pharynx (regurgitation). The diagnosis is usually confirmed by its good response to therapy. In the conventional medicine, this equates to antacids, proton pump inhibitors or histamine type 2 receptor antagonists. In naturopathic medicine, this could equate to a short

trial of antacids, but more probably a trial of gastrointestinal demulcents. If the patient presents with the classic symptom picture and responds to demulcent therapy, that confirms the diagnosis. If alarm signs and symptoms are present (for example, weight loss, dysphagia, an epigastric mass upon examination, anaemia or signs of internal bleeding), then patients should be referred for further investigation (endoscopy). If the patient presents with the classic symptoms of GORD but does not respond to treatment, then referral is also recommended.[26,54]

Acupuncture

In a recently published clinical trial, the efficacy of acupuncture was compared to doubling the dose of a proton pump inhibitor (PPI) in patients unresponsive to the standard dose of a PPI. Subjects were randomised to receive either 10 acupuncture sessions over a 4-week period in combination with their original PPI or the same PPI at double the daily dose. At the end of a 4-week treatment period, subjects in the acupuncture group

Table 4.1 Digestive complications

CONDITION	SIGNS AND SYMPTOMS[56]	PROTOCOLS[46]	CAM TREATMENTS[42,43,46]
Dyspepsia	GIT discomfort (esp. after meals), bloating and wind, nausea or vomiting	• Regulate GIT motility. • Enhance digestion. • Provide antiemesis. • Soothe tissue. • Reduce intestinal gas.	• Lifestyle: stress reduction • Dietary change: avoid food triggers; reduce greasy foods; avoid alcohol, over-eating, rushed eating • Herbal carminatives, e.g. *Matricaria recutita, Mentha piperita, Melissa officinalis, Cinnamonum zeylanicum, Carum carvi* • Herbal antiemetics, e.g. *Zingiber officinale, Mentha piperita, Citrus reticulata* • Herbal bitters, e.g. *Cynara scolymus, Gentiana lutea, Centaurium erythraea* • Digestive enzymes, e.g. amylase, protases, lipases, HCl • Combination phytotherapy product mainly containing *Iberis amara*
Ulceration	GIT pain relieved by food, worse with hunger signal, relief from antacids/ antiulcer drugs, potential dry blood in stool	• Stop bleeding and pain. • Reduce inflammation. • Heal GIT tissue.	• Lifestyle: stress reduction • Dietary change: avoid food triggers, avoid alcohol, install good eating patterns • Plant demulcents/anti-inflammatories/vulneraries, e.g. *Glycyrrhiza glabra, Althaea officinalis, Ulmus fulva, Achillea* spp., cabbage leaf soup, cabbage juice, sauerkraut • Wound-healing nutrients: zinc, vitamin C, folate, glutamine • Probiotics (see Table 3.2 in Chapter 3 on irritable bowel syndrome)
Gastritis	Similar symptoms to ulceration conditions, may be initiated by alcohol, stress, medications or bacteria overgrowth, e.g. *Helicobacter pylori*.	• Reduce pain. • Reduce inflammation. • Heal GIT tissue. • Eradicate *H. pylori*.	• Lifestyle: stress reduction • Dietary change: avoid food triggers; reduce greasy foods; avoid alcohol, over-eating, rushed eating • Herbal anti-inflammatories, demulcents (see above) • Herbal antimicrobials with demonstrated anti-*H. pylori* activity, e.g., berberine-containing herbs, propolis, *Origanum vulgare, Cinnamonum zeylanicum, Thymus vulgaris*[57–61] • Probiotics (see Table 3.2 in Chapter 3 on irritable bowel syndrome)

(Continued)

Table 4.1 Digestive complications *(Continued)*

CONDITION	SIGNS AND SYMPTOMS[56]	PROTOCOLS[46]	CAM TREATMENTS[42,43,46]
Malabsorption	Bloating and wind, undigested food in the stool, diarrhoea, weight loss over time, nutrient deficiencies	• Enhance digestion. • Supplement nutrients. • Regulate stool. • Reduce symptoms.	• Lifestyle: stress reduction • Dietary change: avoid food triggers; reduce greasy foods; avoid alcohol, over-eating, rushed eating • Herbal digestives (bitters, aromatics—see above) • Nutrients: broad spectrum vitamin/mineral supplement

had significant decreases in daytime heartburn, night-time heartburn, acid regurgitation and dysphagia compared to baseline versus no significant change in the double dose PPI group.[55] In subjects unresponsive to initial naturopathic therapy, referral to a traditional Chinese medicine practitioner may be warranted.

Case Study

A 71-year-old woman presents with **a 15-year history of chronic cough**. The cough is tickly and dry in nature, worse after lying down and extremely disrupting to sleep. She also experiences a **retrosternal burning sensation most mornings after breakfast and most evenings after lying down**. Previous **investigations (barium swallow and endoscopy) revealed signs of gastro-oesophageal reflux** and **slight oesophageal inflammation**. Cardiovascular and respiratory investigations were all negative. She was prescribed Nexium (40 mg once daily) 3 years ago; this has reduced both the heartburn and the cough, but has not eliminated them. Medical history was otherwise unremarkable.

SUGGESTIVE SYMPTOMS

- Sensation of heartburn:
  - A burning feeling rising from the stomach or lower chest up towards the neck
  - Worse postprandially
  - Prompt relief by antacids
- Regurgitation: the effortless return of stomach contents into the pharynx
- Dysphagia
- Extraoesophageal manifestations:
  - chronic cough
  - halitosis
  - dental erosions
  - chronic laryngitis

Example treatment

Upon analysing her diet, it was found to fit the 'standard Australian diet' (SAD)—low in fruits, vegetables and whole grains. In terms of GORD risk factors, she consumed caffeine-containing beverages with each meal, ate lots of fatty foods, consumed chocolate, wine and coffee most evenings after dinner, and ate snacks just before retiring most evenings. To address these GORD risk factors, she was advised not to have any beverages with her meals and to drink fluids only between meals (≥ 1 hr before or ≥ 2 hr after), to switch from full-cream milk to skim, to eliminate all caffeinated and alcoholic beverages, and to avoid other foods known to decrease LOS pressure or worsen GORD symptoms (chocolate, tomatoes and tomato products, and peppermint lollies). She was also advised to eat her evening meals earlier in the evening (prior to 7 p.m.), eat smaller meals in general and advised not to snack after 7 p.m. To help prevent the development of Barrett's oesophagus, she was advised to consume more fruit daily (three to five pieces), vegetables (five serves daily) and whole grains.

Her BMI was within normal range,[21] so there was no need to recommend weight loss. Her incidental exercise levels were quite high—she worked most days each week on her garden acreage—and also walked 3 km at least four times each week.

A herbal tincture was prescribed to acutely relieve her reflux symptoms. *Achillea millefolium* was prescribed in the tincture for its tannic, phenolic and volatile oil compounds that may increase LOS tone and reduce inflammation.[62] *Matricaria recutita* and *Glycyrrhiza glabra* will provide a topical anti-inflammatory activity that should soothe the inflamed

> ### Herbal formula
>
> | | |
> |---|---|
> | *Achillea millfolium* 1:2 | 35 mL |
> | *Matricaria recutita* 1:2 | 35 mL |
> | *Glycyrrhiza glabra* 1:1 | 25 mL |
> | *Gentiana lutea* 1:2 | 5 mL |
> | 5 mL each evening as required | 100 mL |
>
> *Filipendula ulmaria*: 2–3 cups daily between meals using 1 heaped tablespoon per cup
>
> GI demulcent powder: equal parts powdered *Ulmus fulva* bark and *Althaea officinalis* radix—1 heaped teaspoon mixed into a little water after breakfast, after dinner and as needed for relief of reflux symptoms

oesophageal in combination.[42,63,64] *Glycyrrhiza glabra* has the additional benefit of helping to heal the oesophageal mucosa.[46] The use of *Gentiana lutea* as a bitter to enhance digestive activity needs to be monitored as it may potentially cause GORD to be worsened in some individuals.[46,65] As indicated in the case, her digestion seems insufficient (bloating and halitosis); hence the use of a bitter may be warranted. Gastrointestinal demulcents (powdered *Ulmus fulva* and *Althaea officinalis*) were prescribed to relieve the reflux symptoms and to help protect and heal the oesophageal mucosa.[42] Filipendula tea was prescribed to help decrease the oesophageal inflammation and to heal the mucosa. A herbal tincture was prescribed to acutely relieve her symptoms.

As many patients suffering from GORD present with a GORD-related cough (as in this case), it is often advisable to prescribe a herbal mix to provide acute relief of the cough. The herb mix can be taken throughout the day to prevent the cough from

LESSER-KNOWN HERBS FOR GORD-RELATED COUGHS

Sanguinaria canadensis (blood root)
A North American native, blood root is slow growing and rich in alkaloids. It is prescribed only in small doses, as it is emetic in larger doses. Blood root is one of the strongest stimulating expectorants, useful in dry, tickly, unproductive coughs and when the respiratory tract is congested with tenacious, thick, hard-to-expel mucus. Its acrid taste is due to its alkaloid content (principally sanguinarine), which is also responsible for its expectorant activity. After ingestión, blood root alkaloids irrítate the vagus nerve along the GIT, resulting in the secretion of water and thin mucus in the upper GIT and reflexively in the respiratory tract. This can soothe a dry, irritated mucosa or dislodge thick, tenacious mucus from the respiratory tract. This ability to soothe an irritated oesophageal mucosa is what makes it useful in GORD-related coughs.

Ophiopogon japonicus (mondo grass)
Mondo grass is a Chinese herb, traditionally classified as a 'yin' tonic. It is sweet in taste, cooling and moistening in nature and makes a thick, rich, excellent-tasting tincture. In addition to its respiratory demulcent activity, it is also a relaxing nervine, making it a specific for dry, tickly coughs that keep a patient awake at night.

occurring or on an as-needed basis. A typical prescription would contain respiratory demulcents (such as *Glycyrrhiza glabra*, *Althaea officinalis* radix and/or *Ophiopogon japonicus*). This combination effectively soothes the GORD-induced irritation, quickly quelling the tickly cough.

Expected outcomes and follow-up protocols

If the patient successfully implements the dietary recommendations, the GORD symptoms should progressively abate over the course of the following weeks. The signposts of recovery will be seen as a lessening of digestive discomfort, a reduction of regurgitation and other symptoms, such as cough. After cessation of symptoms the patient is advised to continue with the dietary program, the *Filipendula ulmaria* tea and the gastrointestinal-demulcent powder, and to use the tincture as required. After approximately a month of no symptoms the prescription can be used only as required, although the dietary modifications should continue. The practitioner should be aware that patients may most likely occasionally fall back into poor dietary habits (such as drinking excess alcohol or eating known dietary triggers), so understanding and patience is required with the therapeutic relationship.

Table 4.2 Review of the major evidence

INTERVENTION	METHODOLOGY	RESULT	COMMENT
Weight loss[38]	Open-label, prospective trial (n = 34 obese adults with GORD)	Significant correlation between weight loss and oesophageal pH ($p < 0.001$).	Weight loss is a viable treatment option for high BMI patients with GORD.
Carob bean gum added to formula[37]	Randomised, single-blind, placebo-controlled crossover trial (n = 14 infants) Formula with carob gum versus normal formula Carob formula contained 0.4% carob gum Duration 14 days	Regurgitation frequency significantly reduced ($p < 0.0003$). Gastro-oesophageal reflux episodes significantly reduced ($p < 0.02$).	Very positive results—should be considered for paediatric reflux.
Dietary supplement containing melatonin (6 mg), L-tryptophan (200 mg), vitamin B6 (25 mg), folic acid (10 mg), vitamin B12 (50 µg), methionine (100 mg) and betaine (100 mg)[66]	Randomised, single-blind, controlled trial (n = 351 adults with GORD) Dietary supplement versus omeprazole 20 mg/day Duration 40 days	All patients (100%) in the dietary supplement group reported complete relief of GORD symptoms at 40 days versus 65.7% in the omeprazole group ($p < 0.05$) Complete relief was noted after 7 days treatment with the supplement.	These are very promising results, particularly for a formula that does not appear to have a 'gut' focus. More research is needed to tease out how each component contributes to its apparent effectiveness.

Note: Very little research has been done investigating lifestyle interventions, herbal medicines or nutritional interventions in the treatment of GORD. More research is needed.

> **KEY POINTS**
> - GORD is typically diagnosed based on the presence of classic symptoms (heartburn and/or regurgitation), but can also present with extraoesophageal manifestations, such as a chronic cough as the main presenting complaint.
> - Be aware of the alarm features that require immediate referral.
> - Remember the naturopathic axiom *tolle causum* ('treat the cause').
> - In GORD, the cause is often diet- or lifestyle-related; unless these underlying issues are dealt with, treatment is only palliative.
> - GORD symptoms usually respond quickly to gastrointestinal demulcents.
> - Use powders or teas as the preferred methods of application—tablets and capsules will be least effective.

Further reading

American Gastroenterological Association Institute. American Gastroenterological Association Institute technical review on the management of gastroesophageal reflux disease. Gastroenterology 2008;135: 1392–1413.

Baille N. Indigestion: antacids, bitters, digestive enzymes; when to use what? Aust J Med Herbalism 2002;14(4):151–157.

Kaltenbach T, et al. Are lifestyle measures effective in patients with gastroesophageal reflux disease? Arch Intern Med 2006;166:965–971.

References

1. Dent J, et al. Epidemiology of gastro-oesophageal reflux disease: a systematic review. Gut 2005;54:710–717.
2. Vakil N, et al. The Montreal definition and classification of gastroesophageal reflux disease: a global evidence-based consensus. Am J Gastroenterol 2006;101:1900–1920.
3. Cadiot G, et al. Multivariate analysis of pathophysiological factors in reflux oesophagitis. Gut 1997;40:167–174.
4. Dent J, et al. Mechanisms of lower oesophageal sphincter incompetence in patients with symptomatic gastrooesophageal reflux. Gut 1988;29:1020–1028.
5. Anggiansah A, et al. Oesophageal motor responses to gastro-oesophageal reflux in healthy controls and reflux patients. Gut 1997;41:600–605.
6. Stanciu C, Bennett JR. Oesophageal acid clearing: one factor in the production of reflux oesophagitis. Gut 1974;15:852–857.
7. Stacher G, et al. Gastric emptying: a contributory factor in gastro-oesophageal reflux activity? Gut 2000;47:661–666.
8. Holloway RH, et al. Gastric distention: a mechanism for postprandial gastroesophageal reflux. Gastroenterology 1985;89:779–784.
9. Urita Y, et al. Salivary gland scintigraphy in gastro-esophageal reflux disease. Inflammopharmacology 2007;15:141–145.
10. Van Niewenhove YV, et al. Clinical relevance of laparoscopically diagnosed hiatal hernia. Surg Endosc 2009;23:1093–1098.
11. Van Herwaarden MA, et al. Excess gastroesophageal reflux in patients with hiatus hernia is caused by mechanisms other than transient LES relaxations. Gastroenterology 2000;119:1439–1446.
12. Kahrilla PJ, et al. The effect of hiatus hernia on gastro-oesophageal junction pressure. Gut 1999;44:476–482.
13. Jones MP, et al. Hiatal hernia size is the dominant determinant of esophagitis presence and severity in gastro-esophageal reflux disease. Am J Gastroenterol 2001;96:1711–1717.
14. Wetscher GJ, et al. Reflux esophagitis in humans is mediated by oxygen derived free radical. Am J Surg 1995;170:552–557.
15. Oh TY, et al. Oxidative stress is more important than acid in the pathogenesis of reflux oesophagitis in rats. Gut 2001;49:364–371.
16. Salvatore S, Vandenplas Y. Gastroesophageal reflux and cow milk allergy: is there a link? Pediatrics 2002;110:972–984.
17. Usai P, et al. Effect of gluten-free diet on preventing recurrence of gastroesophageal reflux disease-related symptoms in adult celiac patients with nonerosive reflux disease. J Gastroenterol Hepatol 2009;23:1369–1372.
18. Kaltenbach T, et al. Are lifestyle measures effective in patients with gastroesophageal reflux disease? An evidence-based approach. Arch Intern Med 2006;166(8):965–971.
19. Nocon M, et al. Lifestyle factors and symptoms of gastro-oesophageal reflux – a population-based study. Aliment Pharmacol Ther 2006;23:169–174.
20. Watanabe Y, et al. Cigarette smoking and alcohol consumption associated with gastro-oesophageal reflux disease in Japanese men. Scand J Gastroenterol 2003;38:807–811.
21. Kahrilas PJ, Gupta RR. Mechanisms of acid reflux associated with cigarette smoking. Gut 1990;31:4–10.
22. Rey E, et al. Influence of psychological distress on characteristics of symptoms in patients with IBS comorbidity. Dig Dis Sci 2008;54(2):321–327.
23. Bradley LA, et al. The relationship between stress and symptoms of gastroesophageal reflux: the influence of psychological factors. Am J Gastroenterol 1993;88:11–19.
24. Cameron AJ, et al. Gastroesophageal reflux disease in monozygotic and dizygotic twins. Gastroenterology 2002;122:55–59.
25. Castell DO, et al. Review article: the pathophysiology of gastro-oesophageal reflux disease – oesophageal manifestations. Aliment Pharmacol Ther 2004;20(Suppl 9):14–25.
26. American Gastroenterological Association Institute. American Gastroenterological Association Institute technical review on the management of gastroesophageal reflux disease. Gastroenterology 2008;135:1392–1413.

27. Davies M, et al. Safety profile of esomeprazole: results of a prescription monitoring study of 11,595 patients in England. Drug Saf 2008;31:313–323.
28. Canani RB, et al. Therapy with gastric acidity inhibitors increases the risk of acute gastroenteritis and community-acquired pneumonia in children. Pediatrics 2006;117:817–820.
29. Gulmez SE, et al. Use of proton pump inhibitors and the risk of community-acquired pneumonia. Arch Intern Med 2007;167:950–955.
30. Elaine WY, et al. Acid-suppressive medications and risk of bone loss and fracture in older adults. Calcif Tissue Int 2008;83(4):251–259.
31. Ruscin JM, et al. Vitamin B(12) deficiency associated with histamine(2)-receptor antagonists and a proton pump inhibitor. Ann Pharmacother 2002;36:812–816.
32. Kuipers MT, et al. Hypomagnesaemia due to use of proton pump inhibitors – a review. Neth J Med 2009;169:169–172.
33. Semeniuk J, Kaczmarski M. Gastroesophageal reflux (GER) in children and adolescents with regard to food intolerance. Adv Med Sci 2006;51:321–326.
34. Benjamin H. Everybody's guide to nature cure. 2nd edn. London: Health for All Pub. Co., 1961.
35. Duroux P, et al. Early dinner reduces nocturnal gastric acidity. Gut 1989;30:1063–1067.
36. Vivatvakin B, Buachum V. Effect of carob bean on gastric emptying time in Thai infants. Asia Pac J Clin Nutr 2003;12:193–197.
37. Wenzl TG, et al. Effects of thickened feeding on gastro-esophageal reflux in infants: a placebo-controlled crossover study using intraluminal impedance. Pediatrics 2003;111:355–359.
38. Fraser-Moodie CA, et al. Weight loss has an independent beneficial effect on symptoms of gastro-oesophageal reflux in patients who are overweight. Scand J Gastroenterol 1999;34:337–340.
39. Schindlbeck NE, et al. Influence of smoking and esophageal intubation on esophageal pH-metry. Gastroenterology 1987;92:1994–1997.
40. Kadakia SC, et al. Effect of cigarette smoking on gastroesophageal reflux measured by 24-h ambulatory esophageal pH monitoring. Am J Gastroenterol 1995;90:1785–1790.
41. Stanciu C, Bennett JR. Effects of posture on gastro-oesophageal reflux. Digestion 1977;15:104–109.
42. Mills S, Bone K. Principles and practice of phytotherapy. London: Churchill Livingstone, 2000.
43. Blumenthal M, et al. The ABC clinical guide to herbs. Austin: American Botanical Council, 2004.
44. Pengelly A. The constituents of medicinal plants. Vol 2. Glebe, NSW: Fast Books, 1997.
45. Bone K. A clinical guide to blending liquid herbs: herbal formulations for the individual patient. St Louis: Churchill Livingstone, 2003.
46. Baille N. Indigestion: indigestion: antacids, bitters, digestive enzymes: when to use what? Aust J Med Herbalism 2002;14(4):151–157.
47. Borgia M, et al. Pharmaco-logical activity of an herbal extract: controlled clinical study. Curr Ther Res 1981;29:525–536.
48. Metugriachuk Y, et al. Effect of a phyto-compound on delayed gastric emptying in functional dyspepsia: a randomized-controlled study. J Dig Dis 2008;9:204–207.
49. Niiho Y, et al. Gastroprotective effects of bitter principles isolated from gentian root and swertia herb on experimentally-induced gastric lesions in rats. J Nat Med 2006;60:82–88.
50. Shaheen N, Ransohoff DF. Gastroesophageal reflux, Barrett esophagus and esophageal cancer. JAMA 2002;287:1972–1981.
51. Clements DM, et al. A study to determine plasma antioxidant concentrations in patients with Barrett's oesophagus. J Clin Pathol 2005;58:490–492.
52. Chen H, et al. Nutrient intakes and adenocarcinoma of the esophagus and distal stomach. Nutr Cancer 2002;42:33–40.
53. Guy NC, et al. A novel dietary-related model of esophagitis and Barrett's esophagus, a premalignant lesion. Nutr Cancer 2007;59:217–227.
54. DeVault KR, Castell DO. Updated guidelines for the diagnosis and treatment of gastroesophageal reflux disease. Am J Gastroenterol 2005;100:190–200.
55. Dickman R, et al. Clinical trial: acupuncture vs. doubling the proton pump inhibitor dose in refractory heartburn. Aliment Pharmacol Ther 2007;26:1333–1344.
56. Kumar P, Clark M, eds. Clinical medicine. 5th edn. London: W.B. Saunders, 2002.
57. Tabak M, et al. In vitro inhibition of *Helicobacter pylori* by extracts of thyme. J Appl Bacteriol 1996;80:667–672.
58. Tabak M, et al. Cinnamon extracts' inhibitory effect on *Helicobacter pylori*. J Ethnopharmacol 1999;67:269–277.
59. Chung JG, et al. Inhibitory actions of berberine on growth and arylamine N-acetyltransferase activity in strains of *Helicobacter pylori* from peptic ulcer patients. Int J Toxicol 1999;18:35–40.
60. Stamatis G, et al. In vitro anti-*Helicobacter pylori* activity of Greek herbal medicines. J Ethnopharmacol 2003;88:175–179.
61. Nostro A, et al. Effects of combining extracts (from propolis or *Zingiber officinale*) with clarithromycin on *Helicobacter pylori*. Phytother Res 2006;20:187–190.
62. Nemeth E, Bernath J. Biological activities of yarrow species (*Achillea* spp.). Curr Pharm Des 2008;14(29):3151–3167.
63. Aly AM, et al. Licorice: a possible anti-inflammatory and anti-ulcer drug. AAPS PharmSciTech 2005;6(1):E74–E82.
64. Asl MN, Hosseinzadeh H. Review of pharmacological effects of *Glycyrrhiza* sp. and its bioactive compounds. Phytother Res 2008;22(6):709–724.
65. Aktay G, et al. Hepatoprotective effects of Turkish folk remedies on experimental liver injury. J Ethnopharmacol 2000;73(1–2):121–129.
66. Pereira RS. Regression of gastroesophageal reflux disease symptoms using dietary supplementation with melatonin, vitamins and amino acids: comparison with omeprazole. J Pineal Res 2006;41:195–200.

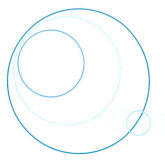

5

Food allergy/ intolerance

Jane Daley
ND

AETIOLOGY

Food reactions can be divided into toxic and non-toxic reactions.[1,2] Toxic food reactions are rare and usually involve food toxins that may be naturally present in food or a consequence of food processing, contaminants or additives, such as aflatoxin found in contaminated grains and peanuts. In the modern world reactions are rare due to diet variety and food-processing standards. They are dose-dependent reactions and have the same effect on everybody. Non-toxic food reactions can be further divided into immune- and non-immune-mediated reactions. Reactions that involve immune activation are mediated by immunoglobulins, especially immunoglobulin E (IgE) but also possibly IgG, IgA and IgM.[2] Non-immune-mediated food hypersensitivity reactions are often termed 'food intolerances' and include fructose and lactose intolerance. There is also another general category called 'undefined'. As the name suggests there is little information about this category, which includes idiosyncratic and psychosomatic food reactions.

Food allergy

Most severe food allergies are IgE-mediated.[3] IgE is associated with receptors on mast cells, fixed cells in the mucosa and skin, and basophils in the blood,[2] and conjugation with an allergen leads to cell granulation and the subsequent release of inflammatory mediators. Vasodilation, exudation, smooth muscle contraction and mucus secretion (largely due to histamine) are common consequences. The greatest concern about an IgE-mediated food allergy is the chance that it will culminate in anaphylaxis. Common food culprits include fish, eggs, cow's milk and peanuts.[4] It is usually a reaction to the protein component of the food such as casein and gluten; if the patient is reacting to another food component, such as lactose, it is more likely to be food intolerance. Other less well-defined food allergies may also occur; these may be IgG-, IgM- or IgA-mediated.

Food intolerance

Food intolerances are much more insidious and often cause delayed symptoms. Food intolerances can be enzymatic, pharmacological or idiosyncratic in nature and are generally thought to be non-immune activated.[2,4,5] Below is an outline of the two most common food intolerances: lactose and fructose.

Lactose intolerance

Lactose intolerance is due to the inability of the body to produce enough lactase to break down the lactose in milk. If lactose is undigested it will pass through to the large colon where it is acted on by colonic flora, causing pain, bloating and osmotic diarrhoea. Lactose is a disaccharide and is metabolised by β-galactosidase (lactase is a subclass of this) to glucose and galactose. Lactose maldigestion effects up to 20% of Caucasians,[6,7] but incidence in some ethnic groups (African, Asian and those from the Baltic states and the Mediterranean) is up to 60%.[6] A recent American study reported the prevalence of lactose intolerance in irritable bowel syndrome to be between 17 and 24%.[8] Lactase deficiency can also be transitory (gastroenteritis) or as a result of mucosal damage (coeliac disease or gastroenteritis).

Fructose intolerance

Fructose is a six-carbon monosaccharide. It is ingested as a monosaccharide, as the disaccharide sucrose (glucose + fructose) or in polymerised forms such as oligosaccharides and polysaccharides.[9] If the degree of polymerisation (DP) is < 10, they are usually referred to as fructo-oligosaccharides and if the DP is ≥ 10 they are usually called inulins.[9] Another form of dietary fructose is the galacto-oligosaccharides (fructose + glucose + galactose), usually present as raffinose. Additional substances also poorly absorbed and readily fermented are:

- sugar alcohols (sorbitol, xylitol, mannitol and maltitol), which occur naturally in some fruits; they are also added as humectants and artificial sweeteners
- polydextrose and isomalt, used as food additives, which behave in a similar way.

Fructose intolerance may be a primary or secondary condition. Hereditary fructose intolerance is a rare autosomal recessive disorder that is due to a deficiency of the liver enzyme fructose-1,6-biphosphate aldolase.[10,11] It is particularly dangerous and can result in vomiting, failure to thrive, hypoglycaemia and liver failure with jaundice and bleeding in children.[10] Secondary fructose intolerance is quite different and much more common. It is usually due to abnormalities in the expression of GLUT5.[12] Recent research suggests that it affects 30% of the population.[13] If fructose is not absorbed in the small intestine it reaches the distal end of the small intestine and the colon where it is fermented by colonic flora to produce hydrogen and carbon dioxide.[9] Fructose is fermented especially quickly, so there is not enough time for gas to be further metabolised or absorbed, increasing intralumen pressure and producing an osmotic effect. Abdominal distension, pain, flatulence and diarrhoea may result. Fructose malabsorption is associated with gastro-oesophageal reflux, small intestinal bacterial overgrowth and depression.[12,14]

RISK FACTORS

Genetics

It appears that genetic predisposition is a strong determining factor in allergic disease. There is an 11–13% risk of developing allergies if there is no parental history, a 20–30% risk if the patient has one allergic parent and 40–60% risk if both parents are allergic.[5]

Twin studies show that environmental factors are important in the development of atopic disease.[15–18]

Gastrointestinal mucosal hyperpermeability

The mucosal barrier in the small intestine is comprised of epithelial cells held together by tight junctions. Various cellular and chemical factors, including extremes of pH, mucus, bile salts, brush border enzymes, together with innate and adaptive immune responses also help to ensnare pathogens or render them harmless.[3] Many factors, including gastrointestinal viral infections and stress, appear to increase intestinal permeability.[17] If this intestinal barrier is compromised proteins, pathogens and antigens may pass through the intestinal wall. A recent study conducted in 20 patients with food allergies and 21 patients with food sensitivities found that they all had increased intestinal permeability as diagnosed by a lactulose/mannitol test.[19] It was also found that the more significant the permeability, the more severe the allergies/intolerances were.

Maternal consumption and early consumption of allergenic foods

Consumption of allergenic foods by the mother during gestation and/or lactation may predispose the child to food allergy.[5] This includes foods the mother is sensitive to or common allergenic foods if the mother has any allergic conditions herself. Similarly, consumption of common allergic foods by the child at an early age may also increase risk. A recent meta-analysis found that a hypoallergenic diet during gestation was useful for the prevention of allergic disease in high risk infants.[20] The authors also found that the best dietary prevention was breastfeeding for at least 4 to 6 months, together with solid food and cow's milk avoidance for 4 months.

Lifestyle factors

Factors such as eating habits, meal frequency, lack of exercise, poor sleep and use of analgesic medication are often thought to increase the likelihood of food sensitivities, or increase the intensity of symptoms in some individuals. A recent Norwegian study, however, found that there was no difference between these factors in a group of adults with abdominal discomfort, self-attributed to food intolerance, and a placebo group.[21] Stress may be an added risk factor for the development of food sensitivities. Stress (physical, biochemical, psychological) induces the central production of corticotrophin-releasing hormone, which in turn suppresses vagal activity.[22]

CONVENTIONAL TREATMENT

There is no particular conventional medical treatment available for IgG-mediated food allergies or food intolerances. Patients with IgE-mediated food allergies are often prescribed epinephrine and antihistamines, and cromoglycate may also be given.[5,23] Strict dietary avoidance is usually recommended for all known food intolerances or allergies and hyposensitisation may be offered.

KEY TREATMENT PROTOCOLS

Case-taking assessment

The first protocol is to assess the particulars of the suspected digestive intolerance/allergy.

A range of questions should first be asked of the patient, such as:

- How long after you eat the suspect foods do you get symptoms? This is called the latency period. If it is immediate or very soon after it is more likely to be an IgE-mediated allergic response.
- How severe are the symptoms? If they are immediate and very severe, it is quite possibly an IgE-mediated allergy. Do the symptoms change in severity and get stronger after repeated exposure? If this is the case it is more likely to be food intolerance.
- How long do the symptoms last? If they last many days after exposure then it is unlikely to be an IgE-mediated allergy.
- Are the symptoms easy and clear to define or more vague?
- Is the symptom present without the offending food?
  A food/symptom diary is often useful in identifying potential allergens or intolerances.

> **NATUROPATHIC TREATMENT AIMS**
> - Identify and remove offending foods and substances.
> - Design an appropriate, healthy diet.
> - Reduce inflammation.
> - Repair intestinal hyperpermeability if required
> - Ensure healthy gastrointestinal function.

Identify and remove offending foods and substances

There are various ways to identify problematic foods and substances, depending on what foods are suspected. A de-challenge re-challenge diet is ideal to assess this (see Figure 5.1). Below is a summary of tests that are useful for the identification of food allergies and intolerances:

- *IgG radioallergosorbent test (RAST)*. This test Measures IgG4 antibodies for specific antigens using the ELISA technique. It is very sensitive and useful for the identification of food intolerances. It tests blood IgG4 reactions to 90 or so different foods.

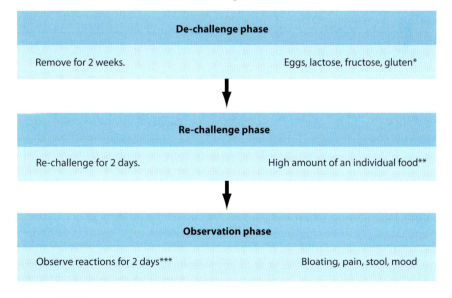

De-challenge phase

Remove for 2 weeks.   Eggs, lactose, fructose, gluten*

Re-challenge phase

Re-challenge for 2 days.   High amount of an individual food**

Observation phase

Observe reactions for 2 days***   Bloating, pain, stool, mood

* Example foods
** Stop eating any foods found to cause reactions
***Have 2 days' break between new challenge foods
Note: After 2-day observation phase, new food can be 're-challenged'.

Figure 5.1 De-challenge re-challenge diet

Various studies have found positive results.[24–28] Some laboratories also offer blood testing for IgE reactions.

- *food avoidance and challenge.* These diets are useful for the identification of food intolerances, but are unsafe for some allergies.
- *hydrogen/methane breath test.* These tests are useful for the identification of lactose and fructose malabsorption.
- *lactulose/mannitol test.* This test is useful for the identification of intestinal permeability.

Once a food has been identified it must be removed from the diet (see Figure 5.1). In the case of IgG-triggered reactions, most of these foods need to be avoided only for a period of time until the reason for their existence is rectified. They can be due to a myriad of causes such as intestinal hyperpermeability, immune dysregulation and poor digestive function. This is also the case for secondary fructose and lactose malabsorption. Foods that provoke an IgE reaction, however, need to be thoroughly avoided.

Design an appropriate healthy diet

Maintenance of a healthy diet is crucial. Many people who have suffered from long-term food allergies or hypersensitivities have self-restricted their diet, in turn leading to various nutrient deficiencies. This is a perilous situation and one that needs addressing immediately if present. Deficiencies of protein, calcium, zinc, iron, vitamin B12 and magnesium are common, and a diet should always be designed with this in mind (see Appendix 4 for nutritional chart). Problematic foods must be avoided and the patient must also be offered as many alternatives as possible as the treatment will often fail if the patient finds compliance difficult.

For patients with lactose intolerance, the severity of symptoms depends on how much lactase is being produced by the small intestine. Many people can tolerate up to 7 g and many up to 12 g.[6] This is important when designing a diet for a lactose-intolerant patient as it is not necessary to take patients off all dairy foods. It is also essential to understand hexose transport in the gastrointestinal tract in order to design a diet for fructose intolerant individuals. GLUT5 is a fructose transporter that is responsible for moving fructose across the brush border; it has a low capacity but is present along the whole length of the small intestine.[12,29] It is this mechanism that is often deficient in fructose intolerance. Glucose enhances the absorption of fructose by its co-presence in the small intestine. GLUT2 (a low-affinity transporter that will carry glucose, fructose and galactose, found on the basolateral membrane) is shunted into the brush border to facilitate the diffusion of glucose.[12,30] This in turn means that higher luminal concentrations of glucose are taken up by the cells via an active process, which in turn activates a system that can more efficiently take up all hexoses including fructose.[12] This becomes very important when designing a diet for fructose intolerance as foods with an amount of glucose equal to or higher than the amount of fructose can be included. Hence it is only foods with higher fructose than glucose that are avoided. See Tables 5.1 and 5.2 for a list of foods to avoid if intolerant to lactose or fructose.

If the patient is avoiding fructose and lactose, or lactose only, it is probably best to avoid fructans, galactans (galacto-oligosaccharides such as raffinose and stacchyose) and polyols (sorbitol, xylitol, mannitol, maltilol) as well.[12] While glucose enhances the absorption of fructose it does not enhance the absorption of fructans, galactans and polyols.

Reduce inflammation

While there is excessive gut inflammation driven by food hypersensitivities, the small intestine does not get a chance to repair.[1] Inflammation causes increased local immune activation, which further damages the gut mucosa and potentially leads to

Table 5.1 Dairy foods to avoid in lactose intolerance

Milk—cow's, sheep's, goat's. More than ½ a cup at any serving.
Yoghurt—more than 100 g a serving (1/2 an average tub).
Ice-cream
Cream cheese

Table 5.2 High fructose foods to avoid (fructose higher than glucose)[9,31]

Fruits—apple, coconut (also coconut milk and cream), grape, guava, honeydew melon, mango, nashi fruit, paw paw/papaya, pear, quince, star fruit, tomato and watermelon. Also all fruit juice, fruit juice concentrate, dried fruit and tinned fruit.
Vegetables—Lebanese cucumber, sweet potatoes
Other—tomato sauce, tomato paste, chutney, relish, plum sauce, sweet and sour sauce, BBQ sauce, high fructose corn syrup, fructose, honey and fortified wines. Inulin and fructo-oligosaccharides should also be avoided.
Fructan-containing foods—vegetables such as artichokes, asparagus, garlic, green beans, leek, onions, spring onion and shallots, and wheat (many breakfast cereals, bread, biscuits, crackers, cakes, pies, pastas, pizzas, and some noodles).

Note: Spring onion, garlic and leek contain longer chains of fructans and may therefore be easier to tolerate for some. Rye, barley, banana and lettuce all contain fructans; however, they appear to be tolerated by most patients.[9]

more sensitivities. Inflammation also increases gut permeability, therefore increasing the amount of food antigens that can cross the bowel wall and provoke an immune response.[19]

There are several nutrients and herbal medicines that may reduce inflammation in the gastrointestinal tract. These include *glutamine, fish oils, Chamomilla recutita, Urtica dioica* and *Curcuma longa*.

Glutamine appears to down-regulate inflammatory mediators in the gastrointestinal system by stimulating the protective stress response in gut cells.[32] The anti-inflammatory effects of **fish oil** have been touted for some time now and these also appear to be relevant to the gut. Although no clinical trials have investigated the effects of fish oil in food intolerance/allergy, randomised clinical trials have demonstrated anti-inflammatory effects in other gastrointestinal disorders such as ulcerative colitis.[33]

Many constituents of **C. recutita** have been found to be anti-inflammatory, including the flavonoids apigenin, apigetrin, rutin and quercetin. *C. recutita* is also antispasmodic, choleretic and antioxidant;[34] however, clinical trials need to be conducted to confirm *C. recutita's* role as an anti-inflammatory in the gut. **U. dioica** is a traditional treatment for inflammation and allergy. The leaf extract IDS 30 was shown to reduce nuclear factor kappa B (NFkB), leading to reductions in cyclooxygenase (COX) and lipooxygenase (LOX) reactions in vitro.[35] The extract may also reduce tumour necrosis factor alpha (TNF-alpha).[36] **Curcuma longa** and in particular its chief constituent, curcumin, inhibit multiple inflammatory mediators such as NFkB, cyclooxygenase-2 (COX-2), LOX and inducible nitric oxide synthase (iNOS).[37] Clinical trials of *C. longa's* anti-inflammatory effects in allergy are lacking; however, these effects are biologically plausible due to the plant's demonstrated efficacy in inflammatory bowel disease.[38,39]

Recent research has shown that inflammation in the small bowel is frequently caused by an immunological cytokine TNF-alpha.[40] It is this cytokine that causes an increase in gastrointestinal permeability, leading to leaky gut syndrome. Both fish oil and *C. longa* have been shown to inhibit TNF-alpha.[41–44]

Repair mucosal hyperpermeability

This is an essential part of the process as a damaged gut wall leads to further inflammation. Limit alcohol, antibiotics, aspirin and other non-steroidal anti-inflammatory drugs if possible as they all damage the gut wall.[45–47] Additionally, encourage reduced exposure to xenobiotics such as pesticides and insecticides as early in vitro evidence suggests they may increase intestinal permeability.[48,49] Support liver function and increase antioxidant status by increased consumption of fruit and vegetables. Encourage the consumption of cruciferous vegetables such as broccoli, cabbage, Brussels sprouts and cauliflower as they all support healthy liver function.[50]

Glutamine, *zinc*, *slippery elm* and *probiotics* may help to heal a damaged gut wall. Glutamine has also been shown to decrease intestinal permeability in animal models[51,52] and two recent randomised clinical trials have demonstrated promising results.[53,54] **Zinc sulfate** (110 mg three times a day, for 8 weeks) decreased intestinal hyperpermeability in Crohn's disease patients in remission;[55] however, zinc supplementation for intestinal permeability in food intolerance/allergy patients has not been studied to date. The dose in this study is extremely high and should only be used for short periods of time. **Slippery elm** is also a prebiotic, which will encourage the growth of healthy bacteria. **Probiotics** including *Lactobacillus* spp. and *Bifidobacterium* spp. will also help to heal the gut wall and may also help to prevent bacterial translocation. Probiotics have been shown to improve immunity, decrease allergies and food intolerances, normalise bowel function, reduce intestinal inflammation and decrease intestinal permeability.[56–58]

Reduce flatulence and abdominal spasm

Herbs such as *Mentha piperita*, *Zingiber officinale*, *Foeniculum vulgare* and *Melissa officinalis* are useful to decrease abdominal spasm and flatulence.[59]

M. piperita is used mainly as a whole plant extract, either as a tea, tincture or fluid extract. It is antispasmodic, antiemetic, antimicrobial, cholagogue, carminative and bitter.[34] Peppermint oil contains on average between 35 and 55% menthol,[34] which is thought to be largely responsible for the plant's spasmolytic activity.[60] *M. piperita* appears to relax the sphincter of Oddi and inhibits the movement of calcium across the cell membrane.[60,61] Nine human studies (n = 269) found that *M. piperita* (0.1–0.24 mL) significantly reduced spasm of the smooth muscle of the gastrointestinal tract.[62] *M. piperita* has also been shown to reduce histamine release in vitro.[63] **Z. officinale** has a spasmolytic effect on the gastrointestinal tract also via a calcium antagonist mechanism.[64] *Z. officinale* is also antiemetic and anti-inflammatory.[59] A combination of ***Foeniculum vulgare*** and ***C. recutita*** has been shown to significantly reduce infantile colic in 93 breastfed infants in a randomised clinical trial after 1 week.[65] Clinical studies are needed to assess the spasmolytic and carminative effects of these herbs in adults.

Ensure healthy gastrointestinal function

Although no research is currently available to support the following protocols, they describe a very traditional way of treating the digestive system. Bitters, cholagogues and choleretics are employed to facilitate and enhance digestion.[66] **Bitter digestives** may be useful to ensure healthy stomach function. These include *Gentiana lutea*, *Taraxacum*

Table 5.3 'Digestive' herbal medicines: summary of main actions[59]

HERB	ACTIONS
Berberis vulgaris	Bitter, choleretic, cholagogue
Chamomilla recutita	Anti-inflammatory, bitter, carminative, spasmolytic
Curcuma longa	Anti-inflammatory
Cynara scolymus	Antiemetic, bitter, choleretic, cholagogue, hepatoprotective, hepatic-trophorestorative
Foeniculum vulgare	Appetite stimulating, carminative, digestive, spasmolytic
Gentiana lutea	Antiemetic, bitter, cholagogue
Hydrastis canadensis	Anti-inflammatory, bitter, choleretic
Iris versicolor	Cholagogue
Melissa officinalis	Carminative, spasmolytic
Mentha piperita	Antiemetic, bitter, carminative, cholagogue, spasmolytic
Rumex crispus	Cholagogue, laxative
Silybum marianum	Antioxidant, choleretic, hepatoprotective, hepatic-trophorestorative
Taraxacum officinale radix	Bitter, choleretic, laxative
Urtica dioica	Antiallergic, anti-inflammatory
Zingiber officinale	Antiemetic, anti-inflammatory, carminative, digestive stimulant, spasmolytic

officinale radix and *Hydrastis canadensis*.[59] **Choleretics** are substances that improve the production of bile by the liver. These could be useful if bile production is compromised; consider *Berberis vulgaris*, *Taraxacum officinale* radix, *Cynara scolymus*, *Silybum marianum*, *Curcuma longa* and *Hydrastis canadensis*.[59,66] A cholagogue may also be helpful. **Cholagogues** are substances that facilitate the release of bile from the gallbladder. They include *Gentiana lutea*, *Berberis vulgaris*, *Cynara scolymus*, *Rumex crispus* and *Iris versicolor*.[59,66] See Table 5.3, summarising the actions for relevant herbs.

INTEGRATIVE MEDICAL CONSIDERATIONS

There are very few integrative medical therapies that can be considered at this present time. Therapies such as homoeopathy and kinesiology are often utilised by patients with food allergies or intolerances; however, there is no current research to support this use. There is a small amount of research to support the use of traditional Chinese medicine in the treatment of asthma and food allergy and two double-blind clinical trials are currently underway in the United States of America to assess the benefit of two different traditional Chinese medicine herbal products.[67]

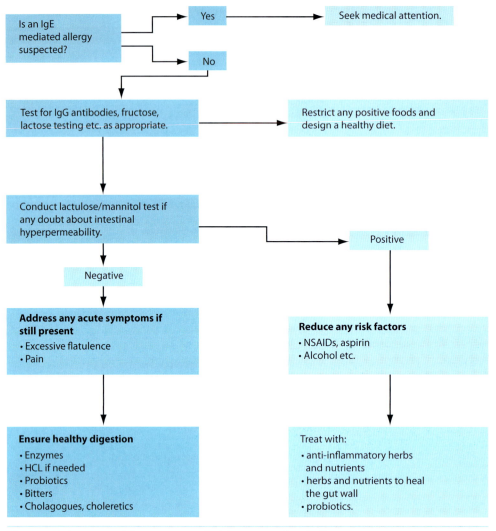

Figure 5.2 Naturopathic treatment decision tree—food allergy

 Case Study

A 26-year-old woman presents with **diarrhoea, abdominal pain** and **flatulence after eating**. She explains that her **stool is always very loose** with occasional bouts of watery diarrhoea. The pain (described as cramping) is under the umbilicus and worse in the lower left quadrant. Her **flatulence** appears to be excessive and foul smelling. She has a **history of a sensitive gut**. She has had various past investigations such as a colonoscopy (bowel mucosa normal), stool test (-ve) and gliadin antibodies (-ve). Past medications have included antibiotics occasionally for sinusitis and over-the-counter antihistamines for hay fever as needed for 5 years.

SUGGESTIVE SYMPTOMS
- Abdominal bloating
- Abdominal distension
- Abdominal pain
- Excessive flatulence
- Onset of symptoms after eating
- Loose stool and/or diarrhoea

Example treatment
Herbal and nutritional prescription

The patient was given a herbal formula containing *Mentha piperita* (carminative, bitter), *Chamomilla recutita* (carminative bitter), *Melissa officinalis* (carminative, bitter) and *Foeniculum vulgare* (carminative) and advised to take 5 mL three times a day to relieve the abdominal symptoms of distension, bloating and flatulence. The patient was assumed to have intestinal hyperpermeability due to the amount of time she had suffered from these gastrointestinal problems. She was prescribed glutamine (1000 mg/day), zinc (20 mg/day) and slippery elm (1 tsp three times a day) to rectify this.

Herbal prescription

Mentha piperita 1:2	20 mL
Chamomilla recutita 1:2	30 mL
Melissa officinalis 1:2	25 mL
Foeniculum vulgare 1:2	25 mL
	100 mL

Dose 5 mL, three times a day.

Nutritional prescription

Glutamine 1000 mg/day
Zinc 20 mg/day
Slippery elm 1 tsp t.d.s.

Dietary and lifestyle modification
Dietary modification

Test results revealed fructose and lactose malabsorption along with IgG antibodies to wheat, rye, dairy, soy and egg white. The patient was advised to avoid these foods and a personal diet was designed for her. The patient was asked to keep a food/symptom diary and to duly record all foods eaten and symptoms including bowel motions.

The low fructose and lactose diet could be prescribed, advising her to avoid foods that contain fructose in higher or equal amounts to glucose, including apple, coconut (also coconut milk and cream), grape, guava, honeydew melon, mango, nashi fruit, paw paw/papaya, pear, quince, star fruit, tomato, and watermelon. She should also avoid fruit juice, fruit juice concentrate, dried fruit and tinned fruit.[9,31] Vegetables such as Lebanese cucumber and sweet potatoes need to be avoided, along with condiments and miscellaneous objects such as tomato sauce, tomato paste, chutney, relish, plum sauce, sweet and sour sauce, BBQ sauce, high fructose corn syrup, fructose, honey and fortified wines. Stone fruits such as peaches, plums and apricots contain sorbitol, which can have similar effects on the gastrointestinal system as free fructose, so effects should be observed.

Avoidance of fructan (chains of fructose units) containing foods such as artichokes, asparagus, garlic, green beans, leek, onions, spring onion, shallots and wheat (many breakfast cereals, bread, biscuits, crackers, cakes, pies, pastas, pizzas, and some noodles) is advised. Inulin and fructo-oligosaccharides should also be avoided. These commonly occur in health food products and prebiotic formulas. Foods such as rye, barley, banana and lettuce all contain fructans, but many people appear to tolerate moderate levels of these foods. Avoid initially, then re-introduce and observe.

Avoidance of foods that contain over 7 g of lactose per serve, which include cow's milk, sheep's milk and goat's milk (more than 1/3 of a cup on average), yoghurt (more than 100 g), ice-cream, cream cheese (more than 100 g) and cream cheese-based dips is also recommended.[31] Exercise caution with low-fat milk and cheddar cheese as some contain high amounts of lactose.

Expected outcomes and follow-up protocols

It is expected that abdominal symptoms such as distension and flatulence would be alleviated within 2 or 3 weeks of adhering to a fructose- and lactose-free diet. The herbal mix should also help to reduce these symptoms, while the causes are rectified.

After 3 or 4 months it is expected that the patient will be able to tolerate small portions of foods that produced a 1+ or 2+ response on the IgG antibody test (eggs and rye in this case). These foods should be re-introduced slowly every 3 to 4 days. If worrying symptoms such as diarrhoea are still present the patient needs to be referred for further testing.

Table 5.4 Review of the major evidence—IBS-based studies

KEY LITERATURE	SUBJECTS	INTERVENTION	OUTCOME MEASURES	RESULTS
Atkinson et al. 2004[24]	RCT in 150 patients with IBS for 12 weeks	Randomised to receive either a diet excluding all foods to which they had raised IgG antibodies or a diet excluding the same number of foods, but not those to which they had antibodies	Changes in IBS symptom severity and global rating scores	26% greater reduction in symptom score ($p < 0.001$). Global scores also significantly improved overall ($p = 0.048$).
Drisko et al. 2006[25]	Open label pilot study in 20 patients with IBS	Food elimination diets based on the results of IgG, IgE, mould tests and hydrogen breath tests. Comprehensive stool testing was also conducted. 100% of patients were found to have dysbiosis and probiotics were given.	Improvements in symptoms and quality of life.	Significant improvements in stool frequency ($p < 0.05$), pain ($p < 0.05$), and IBS-QOL scores ($p < 0.0001$).
Zar et al. 2005[26]	108 patients with IBS and 43 control subjects	IgG, IgE and skin prick for 16 common allergens including milk, eggs, cheese, wheat, rice, potato, chicken, beef, pork, lamb, fish, shrimp, soy, yeast, tomato and peanuts	Antibody levels in IBS patients as compared to non-IBS patients	Serum IgG4 antibodies to wheat, beef, pork, and lamb ware elevated in IBS patients
Zar et al. 2005[28]	25 patients with IBS for 6 months	Exclusion diets based on IgG results	IBS symptoms and quality of life	Significant improvement in the severity of pain ($p < 0.001$), pain frequency ($p = 0.034$) and bloating ($p = 0.001$) at 3 months. Patients were also more satisfied with bowel habits ($p = 0.004$). Follow-up at 6 months showed symptom improvement was maintained.

(Continued)

Table 5.4 Review of the major evidence—IBS-based studies *(Continued)*

KEY LITERATURE	SUBJECTS	INTERVENTION	OUTCOME MEASURES	RESULTS
Shepherd & Gibson 2006[9]	62 patients with IBS and fructose mal-absorption as identified on breath testing	Fructose avoidance	Adherence to diet and symptom improvement	77% adhered to the diet always or frequently. 74% of all patients responded positively in all abdominal symptoms. 85% of patients who adhered to the diet had a significant response as compared to 36% who did not ($p < 0.01$).

Note: RCT = randomised controlled trial, IBS = irritable bowel syndrome

KEY POINTS

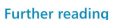

- It is essential to differentiate between different types of allergy and/or intolerance.
- Testing is frequently required and is a valuable clinical tool.
- Diets need to be designed to take into account potential nutrient deficiencies.
- It is essential to identify underlying causes such as inflammation or intestinal hyperpermeability.
- It should be the goal of practitioners to re-introduce foods if possible.

Further reading

David TJ. Adverse reactions and intolerance to foods. Br Med Bull 2000:56(1):34–50.

Gibson PR, et al. Review article: fructose malabsorption and the bigger picture. Aliment Pharmacol Ther 2007;25(4):349 363.

Ortolani C, Pastorello EA. Food allergies and food intolerances. Best Pract Res Clin Gastroenterol 2006;20(3):467–483.

References

1. Montalto M, et al. Adverse reactions to food: allergies and intolerances. Dig Dis 2008;26(2):96–103.
2. Ortolani C, Pastorello EA. Food allergies and food intolerances. Best Pract Res Clin Gastroenterol 2006;20(3):467–483.
3. Sampson HA. Update on food allergy. J Allergy Clin Immunol 2004;113(5):805–819: quiz 820.
4. David TJ. Adverse reactions and intolerance to foods. Br Med Bull 2000;56(1):34–50.
5. Samartín S, et al. Food hypersensitivity. Nutrition Research 2001;21(3):473–497.
6. Savaiano D, et al. Nutrient considerations in lactose intolerance in nutrition in the prevention and treatment of disease. San Diego: Academic Press, 2001:563–575.
7. Suarez F, et al. Lactose intolerance. In: Encyclopedia of food sciences and nutrition. Oxford: Academic Press, 2003:2634–2642.
8. Pimentel M, et al. Breath testing to evaluate lactose intolerance in irritable bowel syndrome correlates with lactulose testing and may not reflect true lactose malabsorption. Am J Gastroenterol 2003;98(12):2700–2704.
9. Shepherd SJ, Gibson PR. Fructose malabsorption and symptoms of irritable bowel syndrome: guidelines for effective dietary management. J Am Diet Assoc 2006;106(10):1631–1639.
10. Wong D. Hereditary fructose intolerance. Mol Genet Metab 2005;85(3):165–167.
11. Yasawy MI, et al. Adult hereditary fructose intolerance. World J Gastroenterol 2009;15(19):2412–2413.

12. Gibson PR, et al. Review article: fructose malabsorption and the bigger picture. Aliment Pharmacol Ther 2007;25(4):349–363.

13. Gibson PR, Shepherd SJ. Personal view: food for thought – western lifestyle and susceptibility to Crohn's disease. The FODMAP hypothesis. Aliment Pharmacol Ther 2005;21(12):1399–1409.

14. Varea V, et al. Malabsorption of carbohydrates and depression in children and adolescents. J Pediatr Gastroenterol Nutr 2005;40(5):561–565.

15. Thomsen SF, et al. Importance of genetic factors in the etiology of atopic dermatitis: a twin study. Allergy Asthma Proc 2007;28(5):535–539.

16. Thomsen SF, et al. Multivariate genetic analysis of atopy phenotypes in a selected sample of twins. Clin Exp Allergy 2006;36(11):1382–1390.

17. Lichtenstein P, Svartengren M. Genes environments and sex: factors of importance in atopic diseases in 7–9-year-old Swedish twins. Allergy 1997;52(11):1079–1086.

18. Wuthrich B, et al. Total and specific IgE (RAST) in atopic twins. Clin Allergy 1981;11(2):147–154.

19. Ventura MT, et al. Intestinal permeability in patients with adverse reactions to food. Dig Liver Dis 2006;38(10):732–736.

20. Host A, et al. Dietary prevention of allergic diseases in infants and small children. Pediatr Allergy Immunol 2008;19(1):1–4.

21. Lind R, et al. Lifestyle of patients with self-reported food hypersensitivity differ little from controls. Gastroenterol Nurs 2008;31(6):401–410.

22. Berstad A, et al. Food hypersensitivity – immunologic (peripheral) or cognitive (central) sensitisation? Psycho-neuroendocrinology 2005;30(10):983–989.

23. Pastar Z, Lipozencic J. Adverse reactions to food and clinical expressions of food allergy. Skinmed 2006;5(3):119–125:quiz 126–127.

24. Atkinson W, et al. Food elimination based on IgG antibodies in irritable bowel syndrome: a randomised controlled trial. Gut 2004;53(10):1459–1464.

25. Drisko J, et al. Treating irritable bowel syndrome with a food elimination diet followed by food challenge and probiotics. J Am Coll Nutr 2006;25(6):514–522.

26. Zar S, et al. Food-specific serum IgG4 and IgE titers to common food antigens in irritable bowel syndrome. Am J Gastroenterol 2005;100(7):1550–1557.

27. Zar S, et al. Food hypersensitivity and irritable bowel syndrome. Aliment Pharmacol Ther 2001;15(4):439–449.

28. Zar S, et al. Food-specific IgG4 antibody-guided exclusion diet improves symptoms and rectal compliance in irritable bowel syndrome. Scand J Gastroenterol 2005;40(7):800–807.

29. Wright EM, et al. Intestinal absorption in health and disease–sugars. Best Pract Res Clin Gastroenterol 2003;17(6):943–956.

30. Sibley E. Carbohydrate intolerance. Curr Opin Gastroenterol 2004;20(2):162–167.

31. FSANZ. Online. Available: http://www.foodstandards.gov.au/2006 May 2009.

32. Wischmeyer PE. Glutamine: role in gut protection in critical illness. Curr Opin Clin Nutr Metab Care 2006;9(5):607–612.

33. De Ley M, et al. Fish oil for induction of remission in ulcerative colitis. Cochrane Database Syst Rev 2007;(4):CD005986.

34. Braun L, Cohen M. Herbs and natural supplements: an evidence-based guide. 2nd edition. Sydney: Elsevier, 2007.

35. Broer J, Behnke B. Immunosuppressant effect of IDS 30, a stinging nettle leaf extract on myeloid dendritic cells in vitro. J Rheumatol 2002;29(4):659–666.

36. Konrad A, et al. Ameliorative effect of IDS 30, a stinging nettle leaf extract, on chronic colitis. Int J Colorectal Dis 2005;20(1):9–17.

37. Bengmark S. Curcumin, an atoxic antioxidant and natural NFkappaB, cyclooxygenase-2, lipooxygenase, and inducible nitric oxide synthase inhibitor: a shield against acute and chronic diseases. J Parenter Enteral Nutr 2006;30(1):45–51.

38. Hanai H, et al. Curcumin maintenance therapy for ulcerative colitis: randomized, multicenter, double-blind, placebo-controlled trial. Clinical Gastroenterology and Hepatology 2006;4(12):1502–1506.

39. Holt PR, et al. Curcumin therapy in inflammatory bowel disease: a pilot study. Dig Dis Sci 2005;50(11):2191–2193.

40. Ye D, et al. Molecular mechanism of tumor necrosis factor-alpha modulation of intestinal epithelial tight junction barrier. Am J Physiol Gastrointest Liver Physiol 2006;290(3):G496–G504.

41. Jagetia GC, Aggarwal BB. 'Spicing up' of the immune system by curcumin. J Clin Immunol 2007;27(1):19–35.

42. Kim YS, et al. Curcumin attenuates inflammatory responses of TNF-alpha-stimulated human endothelial cells. J Cardiovasc Pharmacol 2007;50(1):41–49.

43. Mehra MR, et al. Fish oils produce anti-inflammatory effects and improve body weight in severe heart failure. J Heart Lung Transplant 2006;25(7):834–838.

44. Zhao Y, et al. Eicosapentaenoic acid prevents LPS-induced TNF-alpha expression by preventing NF-kappaB activation. J Am Coll Nutr 2004;23(1):71–78.

45. DeMeo MT, et al. Intestinal permeation and gastrointestinal disease. J Clin Gastroenterol 2002;34(4):385–396.

46. Bode C, Bode JC. Effect of alcohol consumption on the gut. Best Pract Res Clin Gastroenterol 2003;17(4):575–592.

47. Viljoen M, et al. Gastro intestinal hyperpermeability: a review. East Afr Med J 2003;80(6):324–330.

48. Isoda H, et al. Effects of organophosphorous pesticides used in China on various mammalian cells. Environ Sci 2005;12(1):9–19.

49. Singer MM, Tjeerdema RS. Fate and effects of the surfactant sodium dodecyl sulfate. Rev Environ Contam Toxicol 1993;133:95–149.

50. Tanii H, et al. Effects of cruciferous allyl nitrile on phase 2 antioxidant and detoxification enzymes. Med Sci Monit 2008;14(10):BR189–92.

51. Basivireddy J, et al. Oral glutamine attenuates indomethacin-induced small intestinal damage. Clin Sci (Lond) 2004;107(3):281–289.

52. Salman B, et al. Effect of timing of glutamine-enriched enteral nutrition on intestinal damage caused by irradiation. Adv Ther 2007;24(3):648–661.

53. Peng X, et al. Effects of enteral supplementation with glutamine granules on intestinal mucosal barrier function in severe burned patients. Burns 2004;30(2):135–139.

54. Zhou YP, et al. The effect of supplemental enteral glutamine on plasma levels gut function and outcome in severe burns: a randomized, double-blind, controlled clinical trial. JPEN J Parenter Enteral Nutr 2003;27(4):241–245.

55. Sturniolo GC, et al. Zinc supplementation tightens 'leaky gut' in Crohn's disease. Inflamm Bowel Dis 2001;7(2):94–98.

56. Forsyth CB, et al. Lactobacillus GG treatment ameliorates alcohol-induced intestinal oxidative stress, gut leakiness, and liver injury in a rat model of alcoholic steatohepatitis. Alcohol 2009;43(2):163–172.

57. White JS, et al. The probiotic bacterium *Lactobacillus plantarum* species 299 reduces intestinal permeability in experimental biliary obstruction. Lett Appl Microbiol 2006;42(1):19–23.

58. Limdi JK, et al. Do probiotics have a therapeutic role in gastroenterology? World J Gastroenterol 2006;12(34):5447–5457.

59. Bone K. A clinical guide to blending liquid herbs. St Louis: Elsevier, 2003.

60. Grigoleit HG, Grigoleit P. Pharmacology and preclinical pharmacokinetics of peppermint oil. Phytomedicine 2005;12(8):612–616.
61. Giachetti D, et al. Pharmacological activity of *Mentha piperita, Salvia officinalis* and *Rosmarinus officinalis* essences on Oddi's sphincter. Planta Med 1986;52(6):543–544.
62. Grigoleit HG, Grigoleit P. Gastrointestinal clinical pharmacology of peppermint oil. Phytomedicine 2005;12(8):607–611.
63. Inoue T, et al. Antiallergic effect of flavonoid glycosides obtained from *Mentha piperita* L. Biol Pharm Bull 2002;25(2):256–259.
64. Ghayur MN, Gilani AH. Pharmacological basis for the medicinal use of ginger in gastrointestinal disorders. Dig Dis Sci 2005;50(10):1889–1897.
65. Savino F, et al. A randomized double-blind placebo-controlled trial of a standardized extract of *Matricariae recutita, Foeniculum vulgare* and *Melissa officinalis* (ColiMil) in the treatment of breastfed colicky infants. Phytother Res 2005;19(4):335–340.
66. Mills S, Bone K. Principles and practice of phytotherapy. St Louis: Churchill Livingstone, 2000.
67. Li XM. Complementary and alternative medicine in pediatric allergic disorders. Curr Opin Allergy Clin Immunol 2009;9(2):161–167.

Section 2 Respiratory system

The respiratory system is vital for life, providing essential gas exchange of oxygen and carbon dioxide. The lungs, with their combined alveolar surface area of around 140 m^2, are indirectly open to potential airborne pathogens. The extensive, thin and vulnerable alveolar surface is connected to the external environment via the conducting airways from nose to alveoli, and air is filtered, warmed and moistened before reaching the membranes of the lung. Environmental, occupational, psychosocial factors can directly bring about structural, functional and microbiological changes within the upper airways and the lungs. Hence while the treatment of many respiratory disorders may seem to involve basic protocols (for example, antimicrobial, expectorant and bronchodilatory effects), the clinician still needs to view even the most basic respiratory condition within a holistic treatment model.

Common respiratory conditions treated by naturopaths include acute upper and lower respiratory infections (URTIs and LRTIs), encompassing the common cold and seasonal influenzas; acute rhinitis; chronic sinusitis; inflammatory and obstructive conditions such as asthma and chronic obstructive airways disease; and congestive conditions such as bronchitis.

As with all naturopathic treatment, while the specific respiratory condition and its direct symptoms may be the focus of initial treatments (commonly to reduce inflammation and infection), there exists the understanding that the acute presentation is usually due to an underlying imbalance predisposing the person to the condition. With respect to the pathogenesis of acute respiratory infections, the general naturopathic principle centres on the concept of 'vitality'. When a person's vitality and immune competence are low they are more vulnerable to pathogenic invasion. Due to this, prevention via a balanced and healthy lifestyle, a diet rich in nutrients (especially zinc and vitamins A, B, C and E) and low in refined sugars, saturated fats and chemicals, and the use of herbal tonics, may have a protective effect for U/LRTIs. With respect to chronic respiratory conditions such as asthma or emphysema, there is often an inflammatory component that needs to be treated; these conditions require continual treatment, often via an integrative medical approach.

Respiratory conditions are treated by naturopaths via a range of biological interventions. Common nutrients involved in improving respiratory function include omega-3 fatty acids, zinc, magnesium and vitamins A, C and E. Herbal medicine has a long history of use in respiratory disorders, with actions ranging from immune modulation (for example, *Echinacea* spp., *Andrographis paniculata* and *Astragalus membranaceus*); direct antimicrobial activity (for example, *Thymus vulgaris* and *Hydrastis canadensis*); bronchodilatory effects (*Lobelia inflata* and *Adhatoda vasica*) and expectorant activity (*Thymus vulgaris*, *Inula helenium* and *Polygala senega*). However, even simple interventions can have significant therapeutic effects. For example, breathing techniques and exercises are simple, free, require no specific equipment, can be implemented by anyone at any time and can also proffer improvement in patients' lives.

While it is known that the immune and respiratory systems are inextricably connected, a key component of treating respiratory disorders is to search for underlying interactions with other bodily systems, particularly the digestive and nervous systems. The link between these systems is evident, as research in the field of psychoneuroimmunology details. This section outlines these connections and the underlying principles of treating the major respiratory conditions, in addition to providing insights on general immunity-enhancing protocols.

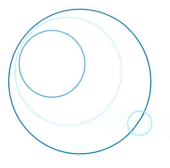

6

Respiratory infections and immune insufficiency

David Casteleijn
ND, RN, MHSc
Tessa Finney-Brown
ND

OVERVIEW

Respiratory infections are caused by pathogenic invasion and colonisation.[1] Upper respiratory tract infections (URTI) involve the nose, sinuses, pharynx or larynx, while lower respiratory tract infections (LRTI) involve the lungs and bronchi, and include pneumonia, lung abscess, acute bronchitis and bronchiectasis.

The term 'coryza' (the common cold) encompasses for a number of viral URTIs with heterogeneous presentation.[1] They may in turn lead to secondary LRTI, or predispose to bacterial URTI. The common cold is most frequently experienced with nasal congestion and drainage, sneezing, sore or scratchy throat, cough and general malaise.[1,2] Influenza is regarded as a separate disease entity, although the two often

> ### GENERAL CLINICAL FEATURES— URTI
> - Nasal congestion and discharge
> - Sneezing
> - Sore or scratchy throat
> - Cough
> - General malaise
> - Fever (sometimes)
> - Headache (sometimes)
> - Myalgia (sometimes)
>
> ### GENERAL CLINICAL FEATURES— LRTI
> - Cough
> - Dyspnoea
> - Weakness
> - High fever
> - Fatigue

overlap.[1] Manifestations of influenza commonly include fever, myalgia, fatigue, malaise, headache, pain behind the eyes, dry cough, runny nose and sore throat (see Table 6.1).[3,4]

Respiratory tract infections (RTIs) are among the most commonly experienced illnesses, and place large economic costs on the community in terms of absences from work and school, and also in visits to medical professionals.[1,2] While most are self-limiting and resolve within time, they can be quite serious. Influenza kills approximately 36,000 in the United States of America every year,[3] with higher mortality rates in the elderly, who have weaker immune systems.[6] Many more Americans (exceeding 200,000) experience complications that require hospital admission.[3]

URTIs are more commonly experienced in the cooler months of the year, and in the rainy periods of tropical areas.[1] Children contract a greater number of infections throughout the year than adults, possible due to their close socialisation in day care and at school.[3,7]

Transmission occurs by one of three main methods:[1–3,7]

1. hand contact with virus-containing secretions, from either the environment or an infected person
2. inhalation of small-particle aerosols
3. direct exposure to large-particle aerosols from an infected person (e.g. via a sneeze or cough).

Most acute respiratory illnesses are viral in origin.[8] There are several viruses which cause the common cold, with rhinoviruses (HRV) playing a prominent aetiological role.[1,2,9] In autumn, the peak time for colds, the HRV accounts for up to 80% of URTIs.[10] Other predominant viral agents include respiratory syncytial virus (RSV), influenza virus (INF) and parainfluenza viruses (PIV).[1,3,8]

Genetics play a large role in immune function, and innate resistance to infection is principally inherited rather than acquired.[11] The set of host genes controlling this is termed the 'resistome', and this varies from person to person.[11] Defective genes in the

Table 6.1 The symptoms of influenza and cold

SYMPTOM	COMMON COLD	INFLUENZA
Onset	Gradual: 1–3 days	Sudden: within a few hours
Site of infection	Upper respiratory tract	Entire respiratory tract
Nasal congestion	Frequent	Occasionally
Rhinorrhea	Frequent	Occasionally
Sneezing	Frequent	Occasionally
Sore throat	Frequent	Occasionally
Cough	Less common	Can be quite severe
Chest discomfort	Mild	Pronounced
Fever	Rare	High
Myalgia	Occasional or insignificant	Severe
Fatigue/malaise	Mild	Long lasting
Headache	Rare, more mild	Prominent and severe
Exhaustion	Rare	Early and prominent

Source: Adapted from Meissner 2005[3] and Roxas & Jurenka 2007[5]

resistome present most strikingly in congenital immunodeficiency syndromes, but variance in the genetic set may also lead to variability in the individual capacity of resistance to infections.[12,13]

Epidemiological data and the evidence from viral-challenge studies suggest that psychological stress is a risk factor for the development of URTI.[14]

Diet also has a key role in immune capacity. Malnourished children in developing countries, particularly those with vitamin A deficiency, are at far higher risk of contracting respiratory infection and also experience more severe morbidity.[15] Many nutrients play a role in responding to microbial and viral challenge, and deficiencies in zinc, vitamin A, C, B6, iron, copper, selenium, protein intake and omega 3 fatty acids have all been shown to negatively affect immune capacity.[6,16–21]

Environmental chemicals are known to be immunotoxic and children exposed to these chemicals at an early age (pre- and postnatally) experience higher rates of respiratory infection than comparative populations with low levels of exposure.[15,22]

An inverse relationship has been demonstrated between the level of physical activity and the number of URTIs experienced by adult males.[23] However, while moderate exercise enhances immune function and lowers the risk of URTI, intensive exertion actually produces a temporary suppressive effect on both the adaptive and the innate systems.[24]

Traditional knowledge links the development of URTI with a drop in body temperature due to cold exposure. This connection was examined in healthy subjects, who each received a 20-minute foot chill at 10°C. Approximately 29% of those receiving a foot chill were diagnosed with a cold 4 days after the chill experience, compared to 9% of control subjects (a significant difference).[25] In another study, a clear connection was demonstrated between the incidence of URTI and LRTI and decreases in average ambient temperature.[26]

PATHOPHYSIOLOGY

The pathogenesis of URTI differs depending on the organism, but generally involves interaction between viral replication and the host immune inflammatory response.[1] Viral infection stimulates a local inflammatory response, which causes the classic symptoms of the common cold—rhinorrhea and nasal obstruction.[1,9] Sneezing and excess mucus production are precipitated by increased cholinergic stimulation in the area.[1] Inflammatory mediators interleukin (IL) 6 and IL-8 appear to be particularly involved, with some studies correlating their concentration in nasal secretions directly with the severity of cold symptoms.[27,28]

Contrastingly, influenza viruses inhabit and replicate in the epithelium of the tracheobronchial area.[4] Here they generate a similar inflammatory response, but also cause overt epithelial toxicity, which contributes to the severity of symptoms.[4,9]

CONVENTIONAL TREATMENT

As the common cold is caused by a multitude of different virus types with varying pathogenic mechanisms, a universal medical treatment remains elusive. Until more effective antiviral treatments are available, the treatment of choice for URTIs remains rest, increased fluids and symptomatic relief (usually with over-the-counter medications).[29]

Nasal congestion and rhinorrhea are the two most vexing symptoms of URTI, and are often addressed with intranasal or oral decongestants (see Table 6.2).[30] Sneezing and rhinorrhoea may be treated with first-generation (but not second-generation) antihistamines though these drugs have no role in shortening the duration of the virus.[30,31] Non-steroidal anti-inflammatory drugs are effective at reducing soreness of the throat, cough and systemic effects of URTI such as fever and malaise.[32] Cough medications, both antitussives and mucolytic agents, are also frequently used, although their efficacy seems variable and limited.[33]

Antibiotic use is contentious in the treatment of URTI. The general consensus is that there is no benefit in treating the common cold with antibiotics.[34] Most studies show no difference in symptom improvement between those treated with antibiotics immediately and those with delayed prescriptions.[35] However, in patients who are more predisposed to complications, such as those with underlying lung disease, evidence does exist to support the use of these drugs in the treatment of URTIs.[34,36]

At present, specific antiviral treatments for respiratory viruses are commercially available only for influenza viruses.[37] Because of the leading role of rhinoviruses in the common cold, effective antivirals against these viruses could be expected to have the greatest effect in the treatment of this disease. Although these agents exist, they are still in the developmental stages, and often are not as clinically efficacious as in vitro studies would suggest; they must be taken early and frequently in order to have an effect, and it is often too late by the time a patient presents to their general practitioner.[2]

KEY TREATMENT PROTOCOLS

From a clinical perspective, it is important to address the acute presentation first. Amelioration of symptoms, limitation of causative pathogens, and strengthening immune defences and clearance will address the patient's immediate concerns and help them to feel better. Once this is resolved, the practitioner should endeavour to restore the health and

Table 6.2 Conventional symptomatic treatment of URTI

URTI SYMPTOM	TREATMENT GOAL	PHARMACOLOGICAL TREATMENT
Nasal congestion	Reduce inflammation and size of nasal turbinates	Decongestants
Rhinorrhoea	Reduce seromucous gland secretion	Anticholinergic Antihistamine (1st generation)
	Reduce goblet cell exocytosis	Antihistamines (?)
Sneezing	Suppress the sneeze reflex	Antihistamine (1st generation)
Sore throat	Reduce pain sensation and diminish pain-invoking cytokines	Analgesic NSAIDs
Cough	Suppress cough reflex	Opiates (antitussive)
	Reduce cytokines (prostaglandins)?	NSAIDs
Malaise, fatigue and other systemic symptoms	Reduce responsible mediators	NSAIDs

Source: Adapted from Gwaltney 2002[32]

wellbeing of the patient, and address causes of immune insufficiency that may predispose to future infections.

Addressing the symptoms

While it is important to take a holistic view of the disease process and underlying causes, symptomatic treatment of URTI is also essential (see Table 6.3). Clearing the infection and ameliorating the symptoms can be accomplished concurrently. Overall, many symptoms are the result of an inflammatory response, and thus reducing this will address the symptom cluster as a whole.

> ## NATUROPATHIC TREATMENT AIMS
> - Treat symptoms (e.g. catarrh/phlegm, cough, fever).
> - Address pathogens (e.g. bacteria, viruses).
> - Support and modulate the immune system.
>
> After cessation of acute infection:
>
> - tonify and restore vitality
> - modulate cortisol response and HPA axis activity (if required)
> - address gastrointestinal dysregulation (if required):
>   - correct poor digestion and malabsorption
>   - reduce intestinal permeability
>   - rebalance intestinal microflora.

Quercetin demonstrates a potent ability to inhibit inflammatory cytokine and chemokine production in acute and chronic inflammation, including the cytokines IL-6 and IL-8, which are both implicated in the aetiology of cold symptoms.[38,39] *Echinacea* **spp.** may also be of use in this regard, as it is known to modulate levels of these two cytokines.[40] (See 'Immune modulation— humoral and cellular immune system' below.)

For the protocols for addressing symptoms such as phlegm, cough and nasal congestion, please refer to Chapter 8 on congestive respiratory illness.

Fever management

Overview

Fever is a state of elevated core temperature, which is part of the defensive response to the invasion of live or inanimate matter recognised as pathogenic or alien.[46] This response is a complex physiological reaction involving a cytokine-mediated rise in core temperature, generation of acute phase reactants, and activation of numerous physiological, endocrinological and immunological systems (see Figure 6.1).[46]

Accompanying the development in antipyretic therapies such as external cooling and specific pharmacological antipyretic agents has come a change in medical philosophy: from fever as a beneficial host defence mechanism to fever as a symptom indicating the need for aggressive therapy.[47]

Treating fever presentation with antipyretic medication is commonly considered by the medical community to do no harm, nor to slow the resolution of common viral and bacterial infections.[48] However, other data suggest a beneficial effect from fever and, correspondingly, adverse effects from antipyretics on infection outcomes. A positive correlation was found between maximum temperature on the day of bacteraemia and survival in a retrospective analysis of 218 patients with bacteraemia.[49] In an examination of factors influencing the prognosis of spontaneous bacterial peritonitis, a positive correlation was identified between a temperature greater than 38°C and likelihood of survival.[50] Paracetamol may potentially prolong chicken pox, as treated subjects experience a longer time to total crusting of lesions than placebo-treated controls,[51] possibly allowing for a longer period of viral spread. Adults infected with rhinovirus exhibit more nasal viral shedding when they receive aspirin than when administered placebo.[52] A trend towards longer duration of rhinoviral shedding was found in association with antipyretic therapy, showing that the use of aspirin or paracetamol is associated with

Table 6.3 Suggested actions and agents for symptomatic relief[41,42–45]

SYMPTOM	ACTION REQUIRED	HERBAL AND NUTRITIONAL REMEDIES
Nasal congestion/ sinusitis	Mucolytic	*Foeniculum vulgare* (fennel), *Trigonella foenum-graecum* (fenugreek), *Armoracia rusticana* (horseradish), *Pimpinella anisum* (anise), N-acetylcysteine, onion, garlic, mustard seeds, papain, bromelain, amylase, sodium chloride, sodium bicarbonate
	Anticatarrhal (upper respiratory tract)	*Glycyrrhiza glabra* (liquorice), *Euphrasia officinalis* (eyebright), *Hydrastis canadensis* (goldenseal), *Plantago lanceolata* (ribwort), *Sambucus nigra* (elder), bromelain, papain
	Mucous membrane trophorestorative	*Euphrasia officinalis* (eyebright), *Hydrastis canadensis* (goldenseal), vitamin A, zinc, glutamine, vitamin C
Phlegm and cough	Mucolytic	*Foeniculum vulgare* (fennel), *Trigonella foenum-graecum* (fenugreek), *Armoracia rusticana* (horseradish), *Pimpinella anisum* (anise), N-acetylcysteine, onion, garlic, mustard seeds, papain, bromelain, amylase, sodium chloride, sodium bicarbonate
	Anticatarrhal (lower respiratory tract)	*Verbascum thapsus* (mullein), *Plantago lanceolata* (ribwort), *Salvia officinalis* (sage), bromelain, papain
	Expectorant	*Glycyrrhiza glabra* (liquorice), *Verbascum thapsus* (mullein), *Inula helenium* (elecampane), *Marrubium vulgare* (white horehound), *Adhatoda vasica* (Malabar nut), *Allium sativum* (garlic)
	Antitussive	*Prunus serotina* (wild cherry), *Althaea officinalis* (marshmallow), *Glycyrrhiza glabra* (liquorice)
Fever	Diaphoretic	*Achillea millefolium* (yarrow), *Sambucus nigra* (elder), *Bupleurum falcatum* (bupleurum), *Zingiber officinale* (ginger), *Tilia* spp. (lime flowers)
Sore and/or scratchy throat	Emollient	*Althaea officinalis* (marshmallow), *Glycyrrhiza glabra* (liquorice)
	Astringent (topical)	*Salvia officinalis* (sage), *Commiphora molmol* (myrrh), *Euphrasia officinalis* (eyebright)
	Lymphatic	*Phytolacca decandra* (poke root), *Echinacea* spp. (echinacea), *Calendula officinalis* (calendula), *Iris versicolor* (blue flag)
	Respiratory antiseptic (topical)	*Salvia officinalis* (sage), *Thymus vulgaris* (thyme), *Commiphora molmol* (myrrh), *Hydrastis canadensis* (goldenseal)
	Anti-inflammatory	*Glycyrrhiza glabra* (liquorice), *Aloe* spp. (aloe juice), *Calendula officinalis* (calendula), *Commiphora molmol* (myrrh), *Euphrasia officinalis* (eyebright) Quercetin, eicosapentaenoic acid, docosahexaenoic acid
	Topical anaesthetic	*Piper methysticum* (kava), *Syzygium aromaticum* (clove)

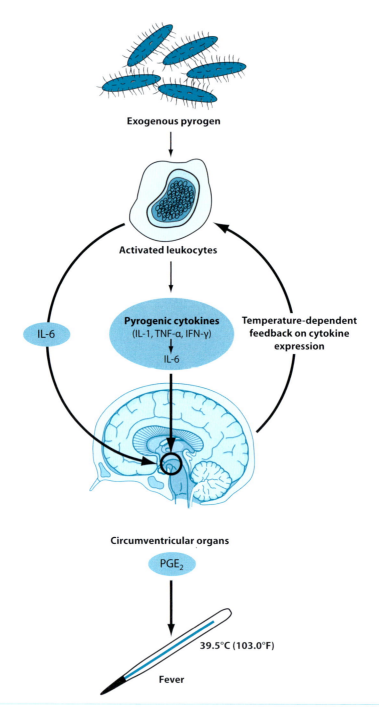

Figure 6.1 Hypothetical model for the febrile response. IL indicates interleukin; TNF, tumour necrosis factor; IFN, interferon; and PGE$_2$, prostaglandin E2.[46]

suppression of the serum neutralising antibody response, and increased nasal signs and symptoms.[53]

An open, randomised, prospective clinical trial compared an aggressive fever treatment strategy (650 mg paracetamol every 6 hours for fever > 38.5°C and cooling blanket added if > 39.5°C) with a permissive strategy (treatment reserved for fever > 40°C only) in stable but critically ill patients. The aggressive treatment group had a higher number of infections compared with the permissive treatment group and a slightly higher rate of antibiotic use. No significant difference in the length of ICU stay was observed. However, the study was ceased prematurely due to safety concerns, after interim analysis revealed an excess mortality rate of 16% (seven of 44) in the aggressive group compared with 3% (one of 38) in the permissive group.[47]

Naturopathic management of fever

This has led some researchers to suggest that fever suppression may be potentially harmful, and that treating moderate fever with antipyretic or direct cooling therapies may be counterproductive.[54] Key pyrogenic cytokines have also demonstrated immune-potentiating capabilities that may in theory enhance resistance to infection, lending credence to the idea of fever as beneficial.[55]

However, the potentially life-threatening nature of fever also needs to be emphasised and respected. Full use should be made of current medical understanding and diagnostic techniques to ensure the fever is not related to a serious condition. Close monitoring of the fever should also be employed, to ensure it stays within an acceptable range (up to 38.9°C),[55] although this can vary in significance depending on whether the fever is deemed to be continuing to rise (the patient feels chilled, indicating they have not reached the new temperature set point) or has reached a peak and has started to fall (the patient feels hot).[55]

According to traditional herbal principles, first line treatments for fever have a 'normalising' effect, being regarded as mildly heating **diaphoretics**. Herbal examples of these include *Achillea millefolium*, *Verbena officinalis*, *Hyssopus officinalis*, *Tilia europaea*, *Sambucus nigra*, *Eupatorium perfoliatum*, *Thymus vulgaris*, *Nepeta cataria*, *Tanacetum vulgare*, *Melissa officinalis*, *Oxalis acetosella* and *Polygonum bistorta*.[41,43]

It is possible that a fever may require enhancement if it is considered that it is not adequately materialising, and sufficient effort has also been made to ensure there is no underlying pathology or life-threatening infection.[41,43] Here moderately warming/**circulation-stimulating remedies** such as *Cinnamomum zeylanicum*, *Allium sativum* and *Elettaria cardamomum* can be used readily. Stronger heating remedies like *Capsicum* spp., *Zingiber officinale* and *Armoracia rusticana* require additional care as they can prove more stimulating to the fever process.[41]

Just as there may be reason to enhance a fever, it is possible that it may need to be controlled. In this instance **cooling bitters** are recommended, for example *Taraxacum officinale*, *Cinnamomum cassia*, *Gentiana lutea* and *Andrographis paniculata*.[41,43]

One trial found that **zinc** supplementation resolved fever 3.1 times more rapidly in 2- to 24-month-old boys.[56] It is suggested that this nutrient is most beneficial in treating fever when the patient has sub-optimum zinc serum levels (see Table 6.6 for a review of the evidence).

Address pathogens

For a discussion of the role of antimicrobials, antivirals and antifungal agents in respiratory illness, refer to Chapter 8 on congestive respiratory illness.

Immune modulation—humoral and cellular immune system

Any factor which depletes immune function may predispose a person to develop a RTI, and those who suffer immune insufficiency, such as the elderly, those with co-existent disease, and the immunocompromised are particularly at risk of recurrent or severe infection.[57]

The causes of lowered innate and adaptive immune resistance are multiple and dynamic in interaction, and immune resistance varies throughout life[58] (see 'Immunity'). The innate homeostasis of individual immune response is influenced by genes, stress, diet, environmental influences, age and prior infection or inflammatory events.[58]

Adequate host defence mechanisms play a role in the symptom severity and clinical outcome of URTIs. While both specific and humoral immunity are important in host response to rhinoviral infection, it seems that the innate response is dominant early after infection, and modulates the symptomatic presentation.[9] This is also the division that is responsible for immunosurveillance of pathogens, and for preventing initial entry.[59] Thus, it is important to strengthen this general defence mechanism.

Antigen-specific humoral and cellular immune responses to URTI are elicited, but are generally not detectable until after symptoms have abated.[9] Thus, enhancement of these systems is more relevant with regard to prevention of re-infection.

Vitamin C has been shown to reduce the incidence and improve the outcome of a number of infections, including RTI.[19] A Cochrane review suggests that vitamin C supplementation is consistently associated with a modest reduction in the duration and severity of colds.[60] The results were most positive in those trials using high doses of 8000 mg daily or more. This intervention works on a number of pathways, although not all of the mechanisms are completely understood.[61,62] Vitamin C is known to be a regulator of redox and metabolic checkpoints that organise the activation and continued survival of immune cells.[19] Ingestion of buffered vitamin C has been shown to significantly enhance both natural killer cells' numbers and activity,[63] and may also enhance T- and B-cell function, suggesting benefits for adaptive immunity and prophylaxis.[63]

Vitamin C may also ameliorate symptoms via its influences on cytokine production, as it inhibits the expression of IL-6 in particular.[64] Other studies show effects on phagocyte function, production of interferon and gene expression of monocyte adhesion molecules, thereby enhancing immune function.[16,61,65]

Nitric oxide (NO) production by epithelial cells has shown a clear role in the body's antiviral responses[9] and reduces epithelial cell release of cytokines and chemokines induced by viral infections.[66] Vitamin C has demonstrated the ability in cell lines to increase NO production, and thus may aid in viral clearance and symptom reduction via this mechanism.[67]

Arginine, the physiological precursor for NO, may also be a novel supplement consideration in this area.[68]

One of the most widely used immune-modulating nutrients is **zinc**. Low levels of this mineral affect almost all aspects of innate and adaptive immunity. It is crucial for the development and function of natural killer cells, phagocytes, macrophages and neutrophils and lack predisposes a person to lymphocytopenia, reduced type 1 T helper (Th1) cells, and decreased thymic function.[16,69–71] Prolonged states of deficiency effectively 'reprogram' the immune system, by increasing glucocorticoid secretion, which accelerates pre-T-cell and pre-B-cell apoptosis.[72] Zinc is also essential for cytokine production and secretion.[16,69–71]

Several studies have demonstrated that zinc administration (up to 30 mg) is effective to ameliorate symptoms, shorten duration and decrease incidence of respiratory infections.[19,73] In children, preventative zinc supplementation (at varying doses) may decrease episodes of RTI by approximately 15%, increasing to 25% in a zinc-deficient population.[74,75] The most bioavailable forms of zinc supplementation appear to be glycinates, gluconates and zinc-enriched yeast.[76–78]

Reviews conclude that the effectiveness of zinc lozenges remains to be established. About half of studies seem to indicate beneficial effects, but a number of these fail to meet rigorous design criteria.[79–81] Zinc nasal gel, however, has shown efficacy in reducing the duration of cold symptoms.[82]

Quercetin may be a useful additional supplement in acute respiratory illness. It seems to exert antiviral effects via Th1:Th2 modulation, encouraging the production of Th1-derived cytokine INF-γ, which eliminates or blocks viral replication in infected cells.[83] Studies suggest that doses of up to 1000 mg/day may protect athletes from URTI in the period of immune depletion following heavy exertion.[84,85] The mechanism seems to be directly antiviral, rather than correction of immune dysregulation.[59] There is some evidence that quercetin supplementation may decrease expression of IL-8[86]—possibly reducing nasal inflammation in the common cold. In influenza, it may protect the lung from the damaging free radicals generated in the disease process.[87]

Low levels of **vitamin A** cause a wide range of immunological defects, and may predispose a person to develop respiratory (and other) infections.[16,88] Theoretically, vitamin A should be of benefit in LRTI due to its ability to up-regulate Th1 and down-regulate Th2-mediated immune responses.[89] The nutrient also enhances innate defences by supporting healthy mucosal barriers and the function of macrophages, neutrophils and natural killer cells.[90] However, although a Cochrane review in 2008 found that supplementation of this nutrient could prevent LRTI in retinol-deficient children or those with a poor nutritional status, evidence did not show that it could beneficially affect other LRTI symptoms.[89] One factor which may be responsible for this puzzling result is that many of these studies were megadose studies, and vitamin A supplementation seems more efficacious when administered via frequent low-dosing.[89,90]

The immunological activity of different herbal medicines is being increasingly documented, with labels such as 'immuno-stimulant' and 'immune-enhancer' being ascribed to herbs such as *Echinacea* spp.[91] While 'stimulation' of certain immunological systems does occur, the term 'immuno-modulation' is perhaps more apt, as the modulation of the immune system by phytoconstituents is more complex than a purely 'stimulating' effect. Various plant constituents modulate the humoral and/or the cellular components of the immune system.[92] While up-regulating the humoral immune system (increasing macrophage activity and phagocytosis) is often beneficial in cases of pathogenic challenge or in a deficient immune system, the workings of the cellular immune system are more complex. Some studies show that herbal medicines may 'up' or 'down' regulate varying aspects of the cellular immune system, and in isolation some constituents may modulate cytokines that individually are anti-inflammatory and/or inflammatory.[*]

Herbal medicines modulate a unique combination of immune pathways, with different medicinal plants often used for similar therapeutic outcomes (e.g. acute infection). They express varying biological activities to achieve this effect. Herbal medicines may enhance the activity of immune components that are beneficial in fighting pathogens via increased humoral activity; natural killer cell, leukocyte, selective cytokine and

---

*It should be noted that many in vitro studies focus on specific phytoconstituents' modulation of individual cytokines. This may not reflect the whole plant activity on the overall immune response.

immunoglobulin production; modulation of Th1 and Th2 cells; and/or down-regulation of NF-ϰB and TNF-α[91] (see Table 6.4).

It should be noted that some herbals, for example ***Hemidesmus indicus*** and ***Tylphora indica***, may actually 'suppress' many components of the immune system.[107] While it is advised that these plants be avoided in acute conditions,[40] they have a place in treating disease processes where an 'over-activated' cellular immune system is apparent (see Chapter 28 on autoimmunity). The clinician may find the complexities of the modulation

Table 6.4 Key herbal medicines with immune enhancing/modulating properties

PHYTOMEDICINE	ACTIONS†	BIOLOGICAL ACTIVITY	MEDICINAL USES
Andrographis paniculata[95–100]	Immune enhancing Antiviral Antipyretic	Andrographolides:‡ Inhibits NF-ϰB and COX-2 ↑ Phagocytosis, WBC count ↓ TNF-α, GM-CSF ↓ IL-2, IFN-y production	Common cold/flu Nasopharyngeal infections/inflammations Fever Hepatic conditions
Uncaria tomentosa[91,101]	Immune modulating Anti-inflammatory	Oxindoles:‡ ↓ NF-ϰB activation ↓ TNF-α production ↑ IL-6 ↓ IL-1 Modulates lymphocytes Enhances phagocytosis	Chronic infections Inflammatory conditions Autoimmune disease Adjuvant treatment of cancer
Eleutherococcus senticosus[102–104]	Immune tonic Tonic Adaptogen	Eleuthrosides:‡ ↑ Lymphocyte and T-cell production ↑ NK activity and production ↑ Phagocytosis ↑ COX-2 inhibition ↑ IL-1, IL-6 activity	Weakened immunity Chronic infections Convalescence Fatigue
Astragalus membranaceus[91,104,105]	Immune tonic Tonic Adaptogen Cardiotonic	Astragalosides and flavonoids:‡ ↑ Leukocyte production, phagocytosis ↑ Mononuclear, NK cells ↓ IL-6, PGE_2, ↑ IgG, IgM, IgE Improved T4/T8 ratios	Weakened immunity Chronic infections Convalescence
Panax ginseng[91,104]	Tonic Adaptogen Immune tonic Anti-carcinogenic	Ginsenosides:‡ ↑ NK, IL-2 ↑ Phagocytotic activity ↑ T-cell, T helper production Modulates IFN-y, TNF-α	Fatigue Convalescence Weakened immunity Adjuvant treatment of cancer
Ganoderma spp.[106]	Immune enhancing Anti-inflammatory Anti-tumoral	Polysaccharides:‡ Macrophage activating ↑ NK, B lymphocytes ↑ IL-12	Chronic infections or inflammation Adjuvant treatment of cancer

†*Key relevant traditional or modern-validated actions*
‡*Regarded as the main constituent responsible for activity*
Note: See Appendix 10 for extra phytomedicine such as Echinacea *spp.*

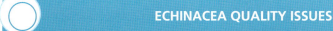

ECHINACEA QUALITY ISSUES

Alkylamides have been found to be most active immune-enhancing constituents in *Echinacea* spp., with a combination of *E. purpurea* and *E. angustifolia*[108–110] enhancing the bioavailability of these compounds. Combining the two extracts provides a protective effect on the alkylamides from *E. angustifolia*, as alkyamides from *E. purpurea* protect them from liver metabolism via the P450 pathway.[109] In order to obtain the highest amounts of these active constituents, not only is the species important, but also the plant part. Research has identified the following differences in the alkylamide content (mg/g) of the various parts of *E. purpurea*: flower 2.7, leaf 0.2, rhizome 5.7 and root 1.7.[111] This would suggest that the rhizome is the preferable plant part to use, though a synergy has been shown between the alkylamides from the aerial parts and the root of *E. purpurea*.[112] Thus, a combination of root and herb tinctures may also provide enhanced immunomodulatory and anti-inflammatory effects.

Finally, the effectiveness of *Echinacea* spp. is also dose-dependent, and a thorough understanding of the therapeutic dosage range is imperative when prescribing the herb. It is important to significantly increase the dose prescribed in the presence of an acute infection. Failure to do this can contribute to echinacea not being as clinically effective as possible, even when good quality botanical product is used.

Any one of the above may be a confounding factor in research, providing insight into why some negative trial results have emerged.

of individual immune components by herbal medicines to be complex and confusing. However, while in vitro and in vivo studies assist in the understanding of mechanisms of action, the key clinical principle is always to prescribe in relation to traditional usage and evidence from human clinical trials.

Three main species of **Echinacea** are used medicinally: *E. palladia, E. purpurea and E. angustifolia*. There is a long history of *Echinacea* spp. use in infectious conditions, and both *E. purpurea* and *E. angustifolia* were used by the eclectics for respiratory illness such as catarrh and chronic bronchitis.[113] Given the quality issues noted in the side-bar, the only relevant studies are those which use the correct plant part at reasonable doses.

Echinacea spp. exert a strong inhibitory effect in vitro on the expression of IL-6 and IL-8 expression by bronchial cells infected with a number of common respiratory pathogens.[40,114] This helps ameliorate URTI symptoms, and is effective both prophylactically *and* symptomatically.[40]

Meta-analyses and reviews of *Echinacea* spp. efficacy have shown differing results, as, in general, they have not screened studies for use of a particular plant part. One recent meta-analysis included a subgroup of standardised products, and found that these generated reductions in the incidence of infection by 58%, and symptom duration 1.4 days.[115] Patients who were given a mix of aerial part and root tincture in addition to vitamin C and propolis showed an 86% decrease in incidence of common cold.[115,116]

Andrographis paniculata is used in Ayurvedic medicine to treat a range of illnesses including influenza, pneumonia and bronchitis.[117] Studies demonstrate reasonably strong evidence that doses of up to 6 g per day may reduce symptom severity and duration when administration is begun within 36 to 48 hours of the onset of URTI.[118,119] Some trials indicate that the effect may be dose-dependent, increasing in effectiveness with higher quantities of andrographolides.[119,120] There is also preliminary evidence indicating a protective effect against infection.[121] In one study, very low doses (200 mg/day) produced a relative risk of URTI contraction 2.1 times lower in the active group than in placebo by the third month.[118] Adverse effects appear minimal, although the herb should be used with caution in pregnancy, bleeding disorders, and with patients taking hypoglycaemic or antiplatelet medication.[118,121] It should be noted that high doses can occasionally lead to gastric discomfort, anorexia and, in extreme cases, vomiting.[42] One way to mitigate this when prescribing high doses is to give smaller doses more frequently.

In comparison to *A. paniculata*, **Astragalus membranaceus** is considered more specific for chronic or recurrent infection, and in instances of immune depletion. In traditional Chinese medicine, it is used for 'all diseases caused by "insufficient qi", typically those manifesting in weakness, fatigue, and vulnerability to infection'.[104,122] Clinically, *A. membranaceus* improves lymphocyte function in both immune-depressed and healthy patients.[104] While no clinical studies examining the use of this botanical agent in respiratory illness could be found thus far, centuries of traditional use and demonstrated immune stimulating activity suggest that it would be of benefit in treating and preventing URTI.

Sambucus nigra has strong traditional indications for respiratory tract diseases.[123] Constituents in the berries neutralise the spikes on a number of enveloped viruses, including Influenza types A and B, rendering them unable to enter cells and replicate.[5,124] They also have an ability to modulate cytokine expression in vitro, and thus potentially enhance phagocytic activity and chemotaxis for clearance of infection.[125,5] This immunomodulary action has also been demonstrated in a number of human trials. Fifteen millilitres of syrup containing *S. nigra* (38% standardised *S. nigra* extract, with other non-active ingredients) administered twice daily produces effective inhibition of the influenza viruses,[124,126] causing symptom duration and severity to decline significantly, with nearly 90% of the *S. nigra* group experiencing 'complete cure' within 2 or 3 days (compared to 6 days in the other group).[126]

For further information and other herbs with immune-stimulating activity refer to Table 6.3. Any one of these may be of use in treating RTI presentations, depending upon the patient. Their use should be guided by the indications suggested.

Preventing respiratory infections and the role of herbal 'tonics' and adaptogens

All traditional healing systems, and variants of complementary and alternative medicine (CAM) recognise a concept of 'vitalism', or a vital force that sustains a person.[127,128] This is at once greater than, and in a different form to, the physical and chemical interactions of the human being.[129,130] This is the concept referred to variously as *prana*, Qi, vital force, life force and universal intelligence, among other names.[129] In its naturopathic form, the concept of *vis medicatrix naturae* ('the healing power of nature') positions the practitioner as facilitator of this energy.[130,131] When it is allowed to flow unhindered, the being exists in a state of optimal functioning, wellbeing or 'vitality'.

Many traditional medical systems incorporate use of treatments in order to maintain the vitality of the body, or keep it 'in tune'.[127] In the Malaysian and Indonesian systems, these are called *jamu*, in Ayurvedia, they are *rasayanas* (for rejuvenation), and in Russia the term *toniziruyuzhie sredstva* literally translates to 'tonic substances'.[127] In the Western tradition, they are referred to as adaptogens or tonics. The general understanding of these remedies is that they are plants containing 'biologically active substances which … induce a state of … increase[d] resistance to … aversive assaults which threaten internal homeostasis'.[128]

In modern life, there are many obstacles to attaining and maintaining a state of ultimate wellness, but much can be done to move closer towards it. A healthy diet and lifestyle, with regular amounts of moderate exercise and low stress levels, contribute to a strong and healthy individual who is resistant to infection and disease.

Traditionally, **immune tonics** were used to fortify the immune system in infection or immune challenge from pathogens, or to 'tonify' and restore the immune system if deemed deficient.[41] A state of dysregulation was perceived to exist in people with recurrent infections, or presenting with symptoms such as a lingering cough, or unresolved infection. In traditional Chinese medicine this is seen as Qi (vital force) deficiency, and the patient often appears with a pale face and tongue, a weak pulse, fatigue and shortness of breath.[135]

The concept of an immune tonic implies a degree of bidirectionality. While immune stimulants/modulators may, for example, encourage the up-regulation of bodily processes (such as an increase in natural killer cell function), they do not possess the ability to down-regulate this function in cases of overactivity. Thus, they are unidirectional. A true immune tonic expresses an ability to restore the immune system to balance no matter which way it departs from homeostasis.[136] A good example is *Echinacea* spp., which exhibits the ability to regulate and balance T helper cell function, with differing actions depending upon the existing state (basal or stimulated) of the immune response.[137] Thus, an immune tonic is a true balancer of dysregulated immune function. Beneficial immune tonic herbs include *Astragalus membranaceus*, *Eleutherococcus senticosus*, *Panax ginseng*, *Ganoderma* spp. and *Echinacea* spp.

There is sometimes controversy over the use of certain herbs for either 'acute' or 'chronic' conditions. A core naturopathic principle is to first use immune enhancers/modulators to assist in the elimination of the pathogen, and follow this with a tonic to strengthen immunity. For example, the use of *Echinacea* spp. and *Andrographis paniculata* for an acute cold/flu would initially be employed, followed by *Astragalus membranaceus* and *Eleutherococcus senticosus* to tonify. However, it is not always so clear cut. Evidence does not preclude the long-term use of immune modulators in chronic conditions as they may be beneficial in preventing infection and RTIs.[138] Also, the use of tonics is contraindicated in most acute cases, as a strong stimulating effect can

KEEPING IT SIMPLE

Often it is the most basic elements of lifestyle and care that are the most effective in treatment and prevention of infection:
- adequate clean (filtered) water
- fresh air
- exposure to (safe levels of) sunshine
- regular exercise
- balanced diet
- rest is vital—adults should be advised to get at least 8 hours' sleep a night, in addition to adequate relaxation during the waking hours; this should be increased in the case of acute infection
- the 'healing relationship'—practitioner empathy significantly predicts the duration and severity of symptoms of illness[133]
- strong interpersonal relationships and social networks
- a positive attitude to life[134] and a strong sense of self-worth.

lead to more florid immune/inflammatory responses and promote a short-term worsening of the condition/symptoms. However, as an exception to the rule, these may traditionally be prescribed in cases of acute cold/flu where the person's energy is so low they cannot fight the pathogen (presenting with marked fatigue, shortness of breath and daytime sweating).[138]

Psychoneuroimmunology, adrenal and nervine tonics

Psychoneuroimmunology is the study of the interactions between the central nervous system, the autonomic and endocrine systems, and the immune system.[139,144] Research demonstrates that stress, depression, anxiety, insomnia and other nervous conditions common in today's society may all have detrimental effects on immune function.[134,145,146] Epidemiological data have long shown a link between life stress and higher likelihood of infectious and inflammatory disease,[148] but it is only relatively recently that the mechanisms behind this connection have begun to be elucidated. It is likely that the effect is mediated by hormones of the hypothalamus-pituitary-adrenal (HPA) axis (see Chapter 15 on adrenal fatigue).[140,133] Generally, these hormones are immune suppressing, and even the transient cortisol spike after intensive exertion may increase susceptibility to URTI.[146] Animal studies illustrate that early-life stress is likely to promote lifelong immune dysregulation.[147] Prolonged psychological stress results in chronic exposure to these hormones, and may predispose a person to lowered immunity and repeated infection.

Additionally, viral illnesses and infections are, in themselves, physiologically stressful, as they induce concomitant activation of the HPA axis, and may favour the evolution of psychological illnesses.[148] Thus, there is a clear role for adrenal support where patients suffer from both repeated infection/poor immunity and chronic or high levels of stress.

This is an area of overlap with the previous treatment goal—boosting vitality and immune resistance. The key distinction in the decision of which actions and interventions to use depends upon the amount of stress, tension and nervous system compromise existing in a patient. If these are a core cause of immune depletion, then adrenal tonics and nervines are indicated. However, if the patient's vitality is weakened more by lifestyle considerations such as a poor diet and a lack of sleep, then adaptogens and immune tonics may be more appropriate. In many cases, both will need to be used.

Useful nutrients include **vitamin C** and **zinc.** Human and animal studies suggest that vitamin C supplementation may be beneficial in reducing circulating cortisol levels both post-exercise and in situations of psychosocial stress.[145,148] It is also an important cofactor for both adrenal medulla and adrenal cortex hormone synthesis, and will be rapidly depleted in situations of over-activity and secretion.[149] Zinc deficiency, rather than impairing adrenal function, directly leads to HPA activation and chronically high circulating levels of glucocorticoids.[73] In populations at risk

EFFECTS OF HORMONES ON IMMUNITY

High levels of corticotropin-releasing hormone (CRH) may lead to vigorous declines in innate and cellular immune responses.[140]
Glucocorticoids:[141–143]
- suppress maturation, differentiation and proliferation of all immune cells
- decrease circulating levels of IL-1 and TNF (protective cytokines)
- decrease the capacity of antigen-presenting cells to provoke appropriate T-cell responses.

of low levels of zinc, this mineral may be useful to mediate HPA overactivity. Given that stress also predisposes many patients to poor digestion and absorption of nutrients, a deficiency may be present despite an adequate diet. Zinc can be toxic at high levels, and so a zinc test should be employed judiciously before supplementation.

Of the botanical adrenal tonics available, *Eleutherococcus senticosus*, *Glycyrrhiza glabra*, *Rehmannia glutinosa*, *Bupleurum falcatum*, *Rhodiola rosea*, *Panax ginseng* and *Withania somnifera* all demonstrate activity on the adrenal glands or hormones. *Eleutherococcus senticosus* is native to Russia and northern Asia and has been used in traditional Chinese medicine use since 190 AD and, more recently, in Russia as an adaptogen.[103,151] Clinical trials demonstrate that *Eleutherococcus senticosus* elicits a biphasic stress response from the adrenal glands, raising cortisol levels when they are too low, and reducing them in elevated states.[152] This may be due to an increased binding of the natural ligands to receptors involved in the feedback systems of stress hormones.[152] It is suggested to inhibit catechol-O-methyl transferase, an enzyme which normally catalyses the degradation of stress hormones and, in doing so, prolongs their action in the body. This activates the negative feedback loop, lowering glucocorticoid secretion, and thus potentially diminishing the immune suppressive effects of stress.

Glycyrrhiza glabra and *Rehmannia glutinosa* may have similar action on cortisol, delaying its breakdown and hence, eventually, lowering the levels expressed.[153,154] The Ayurvedic rasayana *Withania somnifera* also demonstrates activity on the adrenal glands, and an ability to reduce adrenal hypertrophy and circulating levels of glucocorticoids.[155–157] In doing so, it improves the chronic stress-induced decrease of the T-lymphocyte population (CD3+, CD4+/CD8+ T-cells).[155–157] Finally, early experimental evidence suggests that *Rhodiola rosea* also may reduce secretion of CRF, and prevent depletion of adrenal hormones in chronic stress.[158,159]

Panax ginseng has renowned adaptogenic and tonic activity, which is suspected to be due to activity on the adrenal glands.[160–162] In chronic stress, the herb has demonstrated the ability to normalise adrenal gland weight and serum corticosteroid levels via restoration of regular HPA feedback cycles.[163] Restoration of regular feedback loops will decrease abnormally high levels of cortisol that may depress immune function. *Panax ginseng* also increases adrenal capacity, thus toning the organs and promoting normal functioning.[164] Caution needs to be applied when using *Panax ginseng* as there is potential for overstimulation, and concomitant use with caffeine, nicotine or other stimulants should be avoided.[165]

Traditionally, **nervine tonics** such as *Avena sativa*, *Scutellaria lateriflora* and *Hypericum perforatum* are employed to nourish and strengthen the nervous system in cases of stress and nervous debility.[41] *Avena sativa* may be given green or as seed—each has slightly different actions, but both are nervine tonics.[42] The fresh green juice has demonstrated efficacy in reducing nicotine cravings and assisting in smoking cessation,[166] possibly through a stress-relieving, anxiolytic activity. *Scutellaria lateriflora* also has a history of use, and demonstrated clinical efficacy as a nervine tonic.[167–169] Finally, *Hypericum perforatum,* best known for its antidepressant activity, has traditionally been suggested to be of 'value in nervous disorders'.[167] Doses between 300 and 1200 mg have shown clinical efficacy in reducing symptoms of many stress-related disorders including depression,[170] premenstrual syndrome[171] and anxiety (see Section 3 on the nervous system).

Correction of digestive function

The gastrointestinal tract plays a key role in immune function (see Section 1 on the gastrointestinal system). Not only can hypochlorhydria and malabsorption lead to key nutrient deficiencies, but they can also predispose a patient to increased intestinal permeability (leaky gut), which then contributes to systemic immune dysregulation via gut associated lymphatic tissue (GALT) dysfunction. This can then disrupt the mucosal immunity of extra-gastrointestinal tissues including the respiratory tract.[172,173]

Altered intestinal microflora may also contribute to immune deficiency, and may be a further underlying cause of recurrent URTIs. **Probiotic supplementation** with *Lactobacillus GG*, *L. casei rhamnosus*, *Lactobacillus plantarum*, *Lactobacillus rhamnosus* and *Bifidobacterium lactis* has been shown to be useful in controlling respiratory infection.[174–176] A recent meta-analysis of 14 trials has also reported that supplementation of a number of different strains of probiotics may reduce the symptoms and duration of respiratory tract infection.[177]

INTEGRATIVE MEDICAL CONSIDERATIONS

Homoeopathy

Homoeopathic treatment has been shown to be more cost-effective than conventional drug therapy in recurrent respiratory infections.[178] Individualised treatment may also be more efficacious at preventing URTI in the paediatric population.[179]

The homoeopathic remedy Oscillococcinum has evidence of mild effectiveness in reducing duration and severity of URTI, though no evidence of a preventive role.[180,181] Individualised homoeopathy also has evidence of effectiveness in treatment of URTI,[179] though this appeared to be equally effective when using self-administered acute remedies as opposed to classical homoeopathic consultations (see Table 6.5).[182]

Acupuncture

Most of the studies using acupuncture as a treatment method have been undertaken in China—and to a lesser extent Japan—and therefore many published results are unavailable in English.[183] Additionally, acupuncture trials are complicated by the difficulty of practising sham acupuncture as placebo treatment.[184]

In traditional Chinese medicine, URTI may be viewed as pathogenic invasion of wind (wind-cold or wind-heat) into the lung.[185] The studies available do show benefit in the use of this treatment in respiratory infections, but not as prophylaxis.[186] Acupuncture manipulation on the neck produces a significant decrease in the symptoms of the common cold, potentially via immune system activation.[184,186–188]

 Case Study

A 45-year-old woman presents with an **acute common cold**. Her symptoms include **nasal catarrh**, **mild fever** and **fatigue**. She has a history of **repeated upper respiratory tract infections** for which antibiotics have been regularly prescribed. She has a high-pressure job, and works long hours, which causes her to suffer from **stress and tension**.

SUGGESTIVE SYMPTOMS

- Sore throat
- Nasal catarrh
- Mild fever
- Fatigue
- Sneezing
- GIT disturbance

Example treatment

The patient presents with discomfort due to a range of acute symptoms. Therefore the initial treatment focus needs to be on symptomatic relief. Not only is this the patient's priority, but, in meeting her needs, the practitioner will engender trust. Building upon

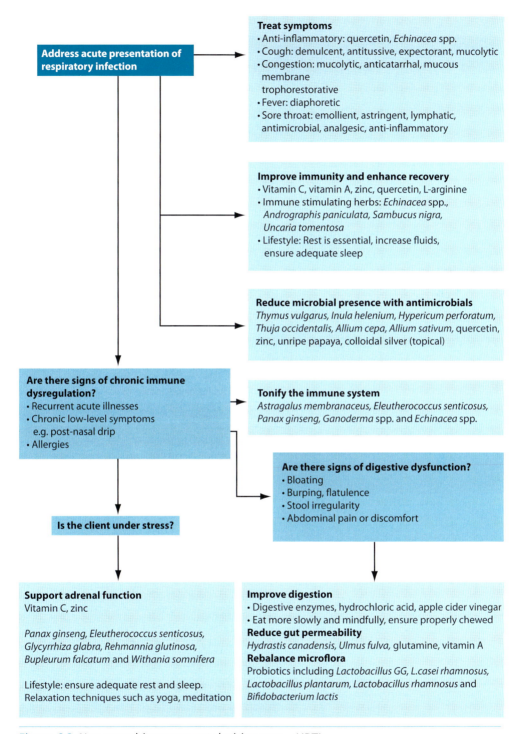

Address acute presentation of respiratory infection

Treat symptoms
- Anti-inflammatory: quercetin, *Echinacea* spp.
- Cough: demulcent, antitussive, expectorant, mucolytic
- Congestion: mucolytic, anticatarrhal, mucous membrane trophorestorative
- Fever: diaphoretic
- Sore throat: emollient, astringent, lymphatic, antimicrobial, analgesic, anti-inflammatory

Improve immunity and enhance recovery
- Vitamin C, vitamin A, zinc, quercetin, L-arginine
- Immune stimulating herbs: *Echinacea* spp., *Andrographis paniculata, Sambucus nigra, Uncaria tomentosa*
- Lifestyle: Rest is essential, increase fluids, ensure adequate sleep

Reduce microbial presence with antimicrobials
Thymus vulgarus, Inula helenium, Hypericum perforatum, Thuja occidentalis, Allium cepa, Allium sativum, quercetin, zinc, unripe papaya, colloidal silver (topical)

Are there signs of chronic immune dysregulation?
- Recurrent acute illnesses
- Chronic low-level symptoms e.g. post-nasal drip
- Allergies

Tonify the immune system
Astragalus membranaceus, Eleutherococcus senticosus, Panax ginseng, Ganoderma spp. and *Echinacea* spp.

Are there signs of digestive dysfunction?
- Bloating
- Burping, flatulence
- Stool irregularity
- Abdominal pain or discomfort

Is the client under stress?

Support adrenal function
Vitamin C, zinc

Panax ginseng, Eleutherococcus senticosus, Glycyrrhiza glabra, Rehmannia glutinosa, Bupleurum falcatum and *Withania somnifera*

Lifestyle: ensure adequate rest and sleep. Relaxation techniques such as yoga, meditation

Improve digestion
- Digestive enzymes, hydrochloric acid, apple cider vinegar
- Eat more slowly and mindfully, ensure properly chewed

Reduce gut permeability
Hydrastis canadensis, Ulmus fulva, glutamine, vitamin A

Rebalance microflora
Probiotics including *Lactobacillus GG, L.casei rhamnosus, Lactobacillus plantarum, Lactobacillus rhamnosus* and *Bifidobacterium lactis*

Figure 6.2 Naturopathic treatment decision tree—URTI

Table 6.5 The most common homoeopathic treatments in URTI[7–9]

REMEDY	INDICATION
Aconite	Used at first sign of cold/flu (first 12 hours). Accompanied by restlessness, fear, thirst. Dry, hoarse cough.
Allium Cepa	Colds with clear, runny mucous. Burning discharge. Acute catarrhal inflammation of mucous membranes.
Arsenicum Album	Flu with tossing and turning, restlessness, anxiety and desire for sips of water. Difficulty breathing.
Belladonna	Sudden onset of symptoms. When hot, dry and thirstless.
Byronia Alba	Flu with irritability and tension. Thirst, headache and aching bones are present. Symptoms worse for movement. Excessive dryness of mucous membranes.
China Officinalis	Recurrent URTI.
Eupatorium Perfoliatum	URTI that make the chest feel sore, with arthralgia and myalgia. Thirst and cough are present. Chronic cough.
Gelselsium	URTI due to overwork, exhaustion or anticipation.
Gripp-Heel	Influenza, influenzal infections and other feverish infectious diseases.
Hepar Sulphuricum	Used for a left-sided sore throat. Croupy, choking or strangling cough.
Kali Bichromium	With mucus that is stringy and tough.
Nux Vomica	Nasal congestion at night that becomes watery (possibly burning) during the day. Patient is impatient and irritable.
Oscillococcinum	Influenza and influenza-like symptoms.
Pulsatilla	With thick yellow mucus. Unable to breathe easily.
Rhus Toxicodendron	With symptoms of stiffness and restlessness after exertion. Worse in cold weather.

this facet of the patient/practitioner relationship will be more likely to lead to compliance in the longer-term management of the condition.

Echinacea spp. was chosen for its immune-enhancing and immune-modulating properties. The root blend is superior in this case as the alkylamides in *E. purpurea* appear to protect those in *E. angustifolia* from hepatic metabolism, thus enhancing their effect.

Andrographis paniculata combines well with echinacea, and is considered specific for acute infections, as it has a rapid onset of action.

Euphrasia officinalis is astringent, anticatarrhal, anti-inflammatory and a mucous-membrane tonic that may be beneficial in treating respiratory conditions with excess mucus.

Sambucus nigra is included for its antiviral properties, as well anti-catarrhal and diaphoretic properties.

Avena sativa (green) is included as a nerve tonic and general tonic as it is probable that stress is a contributing factor to her repeated infections and lowered vitality.

Hydrastis canadensis is included for its mucous-membrane trophorestorative and anticatarrhal properties; its antimicrobial, antibacterial, anti-inflammatory actions will also be of assistance. Unfortunately it cannot be included in the main mixture on account of the tannins in *Sambucus nigra* (see the 'Tannins and alkaloids' box). It can be prescribed as either a simplex extract, or tablet.

Double the regular dose of the main herbal mixture is prescribed in order to effectively treat the acute condition. It is also considered better to dose more regularly rather than in higher quantities, as it maintains a more consistent level of active ingredients in the body throughout the day. As the person is acutely unwell, it should be recommended that they stay home and rest. In this situation, taking herbs six times a day is not as much of an inconvenience as it would otherwise be.

Herbal formulas

Echinacea root blend* 1:2	20 mL
Euphrasia officinalis 1:2	20 mL
Andrographis paniculata 1:2	20 mL
Sambucus nigra 1:2	20 mL
Avena sativa (green) 1:2	20 mL
	100 mL

5 mL every 4 hours (Q4H) in a little water or juice

Herbal tablet

Hydrastis canadensis 1:3
2 mL BD away from main mixture, or 500 mg tablet t.d.s. away from main mixture

Nutritional prescription

Zinc amino acid chelate 25 mg b.d.
Vitamin C + bioflavonoids 1 g t.d.s.
Zinc and vitamin C
Suck one lozenge every 3 hours/p.r.n.
* *E. purpurea* 60%, *E. angustifolia* 40%

Dietary and lifestyle modification (traditional wisdom)
- Vegetable broths, bean and vegetable stews, rice congee, black rice pudding, homemade chicken soup (with the whole carcass from organic chicken).
- Hot lemon drinks with fresh grated ginger (and/or garlic) and raw honey.
- One traditional recipe calls for the whole lemon to be juiced (skin and all), then added to hot water with honey and brandy.

TANNINS AND ALKALOIDS—TROUBLE BREWING?

If tannins and alkaloids are mixed in a liquid extract prescription, a muddy precipitate is observed to form. It is considered that this renders the alkaloids less available for absorption and consequently it is recommended that these not be mixed in a formula.[41]

The main alkaloid-containing herb of concern is *Hydrastis canadensis*,[190] as berberine and hydrastine (the alkaloid components) are considered important actives. If these precipitate and are not bioavailable, then the herb may be inactive.

Tannin-rich herbs to be aware of are *Agrimonia eupatoria*, *Camellia sinensis*, *Filipendula ulmaria*, *Geranium maculatum*, *Rubus idaeus*,[190] *Albizzia lebbeck*, *Cinnamomum zeylanicum*, *Matricaria recutita*, *Rhodiola rosea*, *Mentha piperita*, *Rosmarinus officinalis*, *Hypericum perforatum*, *Sambucus nigra*, *Thymus vulgaris* and *Prunus serotina*.

- Avoid eating too many dairy products as they are commonly considered to be mucus-forming. (Refer to the discussion in Chapter 8, 'Congestive respiratory disorders'.)
- Rest is essential. It must be stressed to the patient that even though they may start to feel better after a day or so (depending upon the severity of the acute infection) they should not go straight back work. It is strongly recommended that the patient takes adequate time to recover fully.
- During the acute and convalescent stage of illness, extra sleep is likely to be required by the patient. This should be encouraged, as the patient (especially if they are stressed and busy) may not see this as a valuable use of time.
- Hydration is important during acute illness, particularly if there are fever and resultant sweating. Moreover, when people work in high-pressure industries, or are always engaged, they can forget very simple activities such as maintaining adequate fluid intake.

Expected outcomes and follow-up protocols

Once the initial stages of the illness have eased, the dose of the main herbal mixture can be reduced to 5 mL three times each day. It is important that the initial prescription is maintained for at least a week after symptoms appear to have resolved. After this, treatment should be altered to address chronic or longer-term concerns. At this stage the practitioner should address the chronic underlying aspects of the condition—GIT dysregulation and chronic stress. Immune support should be continued, but move from an acute response to support with immune tonics. As discussed above, adaptogens may be beneficial after the cessation of the acute infection in order to enhance vitality and, in conjunction with a nervine tonic, assist bodily adaptation to stress. Gastrointestinal tract repair is indicated at this stage to address continued immune depletion, particularly due to the history of regular antibiotic prescriptions. *Echinacea purpurea/angustifolia* root blend can be continued in light of the long-standing immune dysregulation. *Astragalus membranaceus* can also be commenced to rebuild immune integrity and restore vitality. It has adaptogenic properties in addition to being an immune tonic. *Scutellaria lateriflora* will support the nervous system by decreasing the overall level of anxiety, and subsequent stress responses. *Rhodiola rosea* and *Withania somnifera* are useful as adrenal tonics and adaptogens. They will assist in balancing chronically elevated cortisol levels, and support the correction of immune dysregulation. *Hydrastis canadensis* is continued (as a tablet due to the tannin content of *Rhodiola rosea*) to assist with repair of the GIT mucosa.

Long-term dietary suggestions for supporting healthy immune function

Herbs and nutritional supplements are important to assist the patient restore a state of homeostatic balance. However, once this is reached, it is desirable that the patient be able to maintain a balanced and vital state through healthy dietary and lifestyle choices. While there are many components to an ideal diet, some foods and nutrients are particularly useful for immune function. A number of these are set out below:

- garlic, onion and shallots, which contain antimicrobial compounds that differ in efficacy according to their method of preparation. Fresh garlic has the strongest activity; however, most of this action is lost after 5 minutes of cooking whereas shallots maintain their potency well when heated,[190] so if using garlic in cooking add it as late in the process as possible, or use it raw, and consider using shallots more often in cooking.

Table 6.6 Review of the major evidence

INTERVENTION	KEY LITERATURE	SUMMARY OF RESULTS
Vitamin C	**Meta-analysis and reviews** Douglas et al. 2000[191] Hemilä 2004[193] Douglas et al. 2004[192] Douglas et al. 2007[60] Hemilä and Louhiala 2007[194]	• Prophylactic use of at least 0.2 g/day is beneficial, with a reduction in cold duration of 8% for adults and 13.6% for children.[60] • Evidence does not, at this stage, show that vitamin C prophylaxis reduces common cold incidence in the general population.[60] • In populations exposed to short periods of extreme physical or cold stress or both, prophylactic use reduces incidence of common cold by 45–91%.[60,193] • Prophylactic use seems useful to prevent pneumonia, especially in populations with low serum levels.[194]
	Trials Anderson et al. 1974[195] Anderson et al. 1975[196] Anderson et al. 1980[197] Heuser & Vojdani 1997[63] Carrillo et al 2008[146]	• Use as acute treatment in pneumonia seems beneficial, especially in populations with low serum levels.[195,196] • Use as an acute treatment in coryza is not as convincing as trials are lacking, and most show no difference to placebo.[60] Positive trials are detailed below: - Reduction in cold duration has been shown in treatment with 8 g/day.[195] - 1.5 g/day for the first day of the common cold and 1 g/day for the following 4 days have been shown to have a significant effect on cold symptoms.[196,197] • Enhances natural killer cell numbers and activity by up to 10 times, and enhances T- and B-cell function.[63] • Reduces circulating cortisol levels after 12 days of 500 mg t.d.s. supplementation.[146,150]
Zinc	**Meta-analysis and reviews** Marshall 2000[81] Wintergerst, et al 2006[19] Caruso et al. 2007[79] Marshall 2007[80]	• The overall trials of zinc on common cold report conflicting results.[19,79–81] • In about half of studies found, zinc lozenges seem to have beneficial effects on naturally acquired colds. However, many of these studies are poorly designed, so more research is needed.[79–81] (*Note*: The latter Cochrane study[80] seems to have been withdrawn.) • Trials of oral supplementation (up to 30 mg) reduces pneumonia incidence in adults and children by 41% and 26% respectively.[19] • Deficiency may increase susceptibility to infection.[19]
	Trials Mahalanabis et al. 2004[56] Hirt et al 2007[82]	• Zinc nasal gel reduces duration of cold symptoms when taken within 24 hours of onset.[82] • Zinc supplementation resolved fever 3.1 times more rapidly in 2- to 24-month-old boys. This population may have been zinc deficient.[56]

(Continued)

Table 6.6 Review of the major evidence *(Continued)*

INTERVENTION	KEY LITERATURE	SUMMARY OF RESULTS
Echinacea spp.	**In vitro** Sharma et al 2009[40] Sharma et al. 2009[114]	• Inhibition of rhinovirus induced secretion of IL-6 and IL-8.[40] • Inhibition of viral growth and the secretion of pro-inflammatory cytokines.[114]
	Meta-analysis Shah et al. 2007[115] Schoop et al. 2006[198]	• In 14 unique studies, echinacea decreased the odds of developing the common cold by 58% and the duration of a cold by 1.4 days.[115] • The likelihood of experiencing a clinical cold was 55% higher with placebo than with echinacea.[197]
	Clinical trial O'Neil et al. 2008[199]	• Over 8 weeks of treatment the echinacea group experienced fewer sick days, but the result was not significant against a placebo of parsley.[199] This may be partly due to the health benefits of parsley, and an inert placebo would have been preferable.
Andrographis paniculata	**Literature review** Kligler et al. 2006[118]	• Andrographis is as effective in treatment of URI most likely via anti-inflammatory or immunomodulatory properties.[118]
	Systematic review Poolsup et al. 2004[119] Coon & Ernst 2004[121]	• One review of four studies with 433 patients in total showed *Andrographis paniculata* extract to be more effective than placebo and an appropriate alternative treatment of uncomplicated acute upper respiratory tract infection.[119] • Systematic literature searches collectively suggest that *Andrographis paniculata* is superior to placebo in alleviating the subjective symptoms of uncomplicated upper respiratory tract infection.[121] • There is also preliminary evidence of a preventative effect.[121]

Acupuncture	**Reviews**
	Kawakita et al. 2008[186]
	Suzuki et al 2009[183]
		• Most of the literature is in Chinese or Japanese, making a thorough review of the evidence difficult.[183]
		• Rigorous trial design is complicated by the difficulty of supplying a placebo equivalent.[183]
		• Overall, the available reviews suggest that:[186]
		  - acupuncture is effective for treating common cold symptoms
		  - there is lack of convincing evidence to recommend Japanese acupuncture or moxibustion for prevention of common cold
		  - the studies reviewed had several limitations, so further research is advisable.

	Trial Kawakita et al. 2004[184]	One trial showed that fewer symptoms of common cold were reported by a group receiving acupuncture treatment compared to placebo.[184]

- foods rich in vitamin A, C and E, including carrots, spinach, cabbage, kale, red bell peppers, mustard greens, oranges, melons, the green leafy vegetables, sunflower seeds and almonds
- the minerals selenium and zinc, commonly found in nuts, seeds and mushrooms, calf's liver and fish
- omega-3 fatty acids: flax seeds, walnuts and cold-water fish such as salmon.

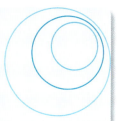

KEY POINTS

- Treatment should address the presenting symptoms of infection in addition to underlying causes.
- Support the body/mind to combat the pathogen, then tonify after the acute condition has resolved.
- Suggest lifestyle changes to support recovery where necessary, for example increased rest and sleep, water, dietary modification.
- Observe GIT symptoms, as dysfunction of this system may be an important contributing factor to impaired immunity.

Further reading

Cunningham-Rundles S, et al. Mechanisms of nutrient modulation of the immune response. J Allergy Clin Immunol 2005;115(6):1119–1128.

Murray M.T. A comprehensive review of vitamin C. American Journal of Natural Medicine 1996;3: 8–21.

Spelman K, et al. Modulation of cytokine expression by traditional medicines: a review of herbal immunomodulators. Altern Med Rev. Jun 2006;11(2):128–150.

References

1. Heikkinen T, Jarvinen A. The common cold. Lancet 2003;361(9351):51–59.
2. Mackay IM. Human rhinoviruses: the cold wars resume. J Clin Virol 2008;42(4):297–320.
3. Meissner HC. Reducing the impact of viral respiratory infections in children. Pediatr Clin North Am 2005;52(3):695–710, v.
4. Kuiken T, Taubenberger JK. Pathology of human influenza revisited. Vaccine 2008;26Suppl. 4:D59–D66.
5. Roxas M, Jurenka J. Colds and influenza: a review of diagnosis and conventional, botanical, and nutritional considerations. Altern Med Rev 2007;12(1):25–48.
6. Wardwell L, et al. Nutrient intake and immune function of elderly subjects. J Am Diet Assoc 2008;108(12):2005–2012.
7. Hemming VG. Viral respiratory diseases in children: classification, etiology, epidemiology, and risk factors. J Pediatr 1994;124(5 Pt 2):S13–S16.
8. Sloots TP, et al. Emerging respiratory agents: new viruses for old diseases? J Clin Virol 2008;42(3):233–243.
9. Proud D. Upper airway viral infections. Pulm Pharmacol Ther 2008;21(3):468–473.
10. Arruda E, et al. Frequency and natural history of rhinovirus infections in adults during autumn. J Clin Microbiol 1997;35(11):2864–2868.
11. Beutler B, et al. Genetic dissection of innate immunity to infection: the mouse cytomegalovirus model. Curr Opin Immunol 2005;17(1):36–43.
12. Leonard WJ. Genetic effects on immunity: editorial overview. Current Opinion in Immunology 2000;12(4):465–467.
13. Mouton D, et al. Genetic factors of immunity against infection. Ann Inst Pasteur Immunol 1985;136D(2):131–141.
14. Cohen S. Psychological stress and susceptibility to upper respiratory infections. Am J Respir Crit Care Med 1995;152(4 Pt 2):S53–S58.
15. Cashat-Cruz M, et al. Azpiri M. Respiratory tract infections in children in developing countries. Semin Pediatr Infect Dis 2005;16(2):84–92.
16. Cunningham-Rundles S, et al. Mechanisms of nutrient modulation of the immune response. J Allergy Clin Immunol 2005;115(6):1119–1128; quiz 1129.
17. Villamor E, Fawzi WW. Effects of vitamin A supplementation on immune responses and correlation with clinical outcomes. Clin Microbiol Rev 2005;18(3):446–464.
18. Schaible UE, Kaufmann SH. Malnutrition and infection: complex mechanisms and global impacts. PLoS Med 2007;4(5):e115.
19. Wintergerst ES, et al. Immune-enhancing role of vitamin C and zinc and effect on clinical conditions. Ann Nutr Metab 2006;50(2):85–94.
20. Trakatellis A. et al. Pyridoxine deficiency: new approaches in immunosuppression and chemotherapy. Postgrad Med J 1997;73(864):617–622.
21. Arredondo M, Nunez MT. Iron and copper metabolism. Mol Aspects Med 2005;26(4–5):313–327.
22. Glynn A, et al. Immune cell counts and risks of respiratory infections among infants exposed pre- and postnatally to organochlorine compounds: a prospective study. Environ Health 2008;7:62.
23. Kostka T, et al. Physical activity and upper respiratory tract infections. Int J Sports Med 2008;29(2):158–162.
24. Neiman D. Exercise and immunity: clinical studies. Psychoneuroimmunology. 4th edn. 2007:661–673.
25. Johnson C, Eccles R. Acute cooling of the feet and the onset of common cold symptoms. Fam Pract 2005;22(6):608–613.

26. Falagas ME, et al. Effect of meteorological variables on the incidence of respiratory tract infections. Respir Med 2008;102(5):733–737.
27. Zhu Z, et al. Rhinovirus stimulation of interleukin-6 in vivo and in vitro. Evidence for nuclear factor kappa B-dependent transcriptional activation. J Clin Invest 1996;97(2):421–430.
28. Turner RB, et al. Association between interleukin-8 concentration in nasal secretions and severity of symptoms of experimental rhinovirus colds. Clin Infect Dis 1998;26(4):840–846.
29. Mayhew M. Treatment of the common cold: the evidence. Journal for Nurse Practitioners 2008;4(1):61–63.
30. Woo T. Pharmacology of cough and cold medicines. J Pediatr Health Care 2008;22(2):73–79; quiz 80–82.
31. Arroll B. Common cold. Clin Evid 2005(13):1853–1861.
32. Gwaltney JM. Viral respiratory infection therapy: historical perspectives and current trials. Am J Med 2002;112Suppl 6A:33S–41S.
33. Arroll B. Non-antibiotic treatments for upper-respiratory tract infections (common cold). Respir Med 2005;99(12):1477–1484.
34. Arroll B. Antibiotics for upper respiratory tract infections: an overview of Cochrane reviews. Respir Med 2005;99(3):255–261.
35. Spurling G, et al. Delayed antibiotics for respiratory infections. Cochrane Database Syst Rev 2007;(3):CD004417.
36. Ram F, et al. Antibiotics for exacerbations of chronic obstructive pulmonary disease. Cochrane Database Syst Rev 2006;(2):CD004403.
37. Nicholson KG, et al. Efficacy and safety of oseltamivir in treatment of acute influenza: a randomised controlled trial. Neuraminidase Inhibitor Flu Treatment Investigator Group. Lancet 2000;355(9218):1845–1850.
38. Kim BH, et al. Quercetin 3-O-beta-(2'-galloyl)-glucopyranoside inhibits endotoxin LPS-induced IL-6 expression and NF-kappa B activation in macrophages. Cytokine 2007;39(3):207–215.
39. Liu J, et al. The inhibitory effect of quercetin on IL-6 production by LPS-stimulated neutrophils. Cell Mol Immunol 2005;2(6):455–460.
40. Sharma M, et al. Echinacea as an antiinflammatory agent: the influence of physiologically relevant parameters. Phytother Res 2009;23(6):863–867.
41. Mills S, Bone K. Principles and practice of phytotherapy. Edinburgh: Churchill Livingstone, 2000.
42. Bone KM. A clinical guide to blending liquid herbs. Philadelphia: Churchill Livingstone, 2003.
43. Scientific Committee of the British Herbal Medical Association. British herbal pharmacopoeia. Bournemouth: British Herbal Medicine Association, 1983.
44. Fisher CP. Materia medica of western herbs for the southern hemisphere. Auckland: CP Fisher, 1996.
45. Osiecki H. The nutrient bible. 6th edn. Eagle Farm: Bio Concepts Publishing, 2004.
46. Mackowiak PA. Concepts of fever. Arch Intern Med 1998;158(17):1870–1881.
47. Schulman CI, et al. The effect of antipyretic therapy upon outcomes in critically ill patients: a randomized prospective study. Surg Infect (Larchmt) 2005;6(4):369–375.
48. Dinarello C, Porat R. Fever and rash. In: Fauci AS, et al., ed. Harrison's Principles of Internal Medicine. New York: McGraw-Hill Companies, Inc. 2008.
49. Bryant RE, et al. Factors affecting mortality of gram-negative rod bacteremia. Arch Intern Med 1971;127(1):120–128.
50. Weinstein MI, et al. Spontaneous bacterial peritonitis: a review of 28 cases with emphasis on improved survival and factors influencing prognosis. American Journal of Medicine 1978;64(4):592–598.
51. Doran T, et al. Acetaminophen: more harm than good for chicken pox? Journal of Pediatrics 1989;114(6):1045–1048.
52. Stanley ED, et al. Increased viral shedding with aspirin treatment of rhinovirus infection. JAMA 1975;231(12):1248–1251.
53. Graham NM, et al. Adverse effects of aspirin, acetaminophen, and ibuprofen on immune function, viral shedding, and clinical status in rhinovirus-infected volunteers. J Infect Dis 1990;162(6):1277–1282.
54. Laupland KB. Fever in the critically ill medical patient. Crit Care Med 2009;37(7 Suppl):S273–S278.
55. Dinarello C. Endogenous pyrogens: the role of cytokines in the pathogenesis of fever. In Mackowiak PA, ed. Fever: basic mechanisms and management. New York: Raven Press, 1997:23–47.
56. Mahalanabis D, et al. Randomized, double-blind, placebo-controlled clinical trial of the efficacy of treatment with zinc or vitamin A in infants and young children with severe acute lower respiratory infection. Am J Clin Nutr 2004;79(3):430–436.
57. Canton R, et al. Respiratory tract infections: at-risk patients who are they? Implications for their management with levofloxacin. Int J Antimicrob Agents 2006;28 Suppl 2:S115–S127.
58. Wissinger E, et al. Immune homeostasis in the respiratory tract and its impact on heterologous infection. Semin Immunol 2009;21(3):147–155.
59. Nieman DC. Immunonutrition support for athletes. Nutr Rev 2008;66(6):310–320.
60. Douglas R, et al. Vitamin C for preventing and treating the common cold. Cochrane Database Syst Rev 2007;18(3):CD000980.
61. Hemilä H. Vitamin C respiratory infections and the immune system. Trends Immunol 2003;24(11):579–580.
62. Hemilä H, Douglas RM. Vitamin C and acute respiratory infections. Int J Tuberc Lung Dis 1999;3(9):756–761.
63. Heuser G, Vojdani A. Enhancement of natural killer cell activity and T and B cell function by buffered vitamin C in patients exposed to toxic chemicals: the role of protein kinase-C. Immunopharmacol Immunotoxicol 1997;19(3):291–312.
64. Hartel C, et al. Effects of vitamin C on intracytoplasmic cytokine production in human whole blood monocytes and lymphocytes. Cytokine 2004;27(4–5):101–106.
65. Rayment SJ, et al. Vitamin C supplementation in normal subjects reduces constitutive ICAM-1 expression. Biochem Biophys Res Commun 2003;308(2):339–345.
66. Proud D. Nitric oxide and the common cold. Curr Opin Allergy Clin Immunol 2005;5(1):37–42.
67. Mizutani A, et al. Ascorbate-dependent enhancement of nitric oxide formation in activated macrophages. Nitric Oxide 1998;2(4):235–241.
68. Coman D, et al. New indications and controversies in arginine therapy. Clin Nutr 2008;27(4):489–496.
69. Fraker PJ. Roles for cell death in zinc deficiency. J Nutr 2005;135(3):359–362.
70. Fraker PJ, et al. The dynamic link between the integrity of the immune system and zinc status. J Nutr 2000;130(5S Suppl):1399S–1406S.
71. Prasad AS. Clinical, immunological, anti-inflammatory and antioxidant roles of zinc. Exp Gerontol 2008;43(5):370–377.
72. Fraker PJ, King LE. Reprogramming of the immune system during zinc deficiency. Annu Rev Nutr 2004;24:277–298.
73. Sazawal S, et al. Zinc supplementation reduces the incidence of acute lower respiratory infections in infants and preschool children: a double-blind, controlled trial. Pediatrics 1998;102(1 Pt 1):1–5.
74. Brown KH, et al. Preventive zinc supplementation among infants, preschoolers, and older prepubertal children. Food Nutr Bull 2009;30(1 Suppl):S12–S40.

75. Roth DE, et al. Acute lower respiratory infections in childhood: opportunities for reducing the global burden through nutritional interventions. Bull World Health Organ 2008;86(5):356–364.

76. Gandia P, et al. A bioavailability study comparing two oral formulations containing zinc (Zn bis-glycinate vs. Zn gluconate) after a single administration to twelve healthy female volunteers. Int J Vitam Nutr Res 2007;77(4):243–248.

77. Siepmann M, et al. The pharmacokinetics of zinc from zinc gluconate: a comparison with zinc oxide in healthy men. Int J Clin Pharmacol Ther 2005;43(12):562–565.

78. Tompkins TA, et al. Clinical evaluation of the bioavailability of zinc-enriched yeast and zinc gluconate in healthy volunteers. Biol Trace Elem Res 2007;120(1–3):28–35.

79. Caruso TJ, et al. Treatment of naturally acquired common colds with zinc: a structured review. Clin Infect Dis 2007;45(5):569–574.

80. Marshall I. WITHDRAWN: Zinc for the common cold. Cochrane Database Syst Rev 2006;(3):CD001364.

81. Marshall I. Zinc for the common cold. Cochrane Database Syst Rev 2000;(2):CD001364.

82. Hirt M, et al. Zinc nasal gel for the treatment of common cold symptoms: a double-blind, placebo-controlled trial. Ear Nose Throat J 2000;79(10):778–782.

83. Nair MP, et al. The flavonoid, quercetin, differentially regulates Th-1 (IFNgamma) and Th-2 (IL4) cytokine gene expression by normal peripheral blood mononuclear cells. Biochim Biophys Acta 2002;1593(1):29–36.

84. Nieman DC, et al. Quercetin reduces illness but not immune perturbations after intensive exercise. Med Sci Sports Exerc 2007;39(9):1561–1569.

85. Davis JM, et al. Quercetin reduces susceptibility to influenza infection following stressful exercise. Am J Physiol Regul Integr Comp Physiol 2008;295(2):R505–R509.

86. Nieman DC, et al. Quercetin's influence on exercise-induced changes in plasma cytokines and muscle and leukocyte cytokine mRNA. J Appl Physiol 2007;103(5):1728–1735.

87. Kumar P, et al. Effect of quercetin supplementation on lung antioxidants after experimental influenza virus infection. Exp Lung Res 2005;31(5):449–459.

88. Cameron C, et al. Neonatal vitamin A deficiency and its impact on acute respiratory infections among preschool Inuit children. Can J Public Health 2008;99(2):102–106.

89. Chen H, et al. Vitamin A for preventing acute lower respiratory tract infections in children up to seven years of age. Cochrane Database Syst Rev 2008;(1):CD006090.

90. Stephensen CB. Vitamin A, infection, and immune function. Annu Rev Nutr 2001;21:167–192.

91. Spelman K, et al. Modulation of cytokine expression by traditional medicines: a review of herbal immunomodulators. Altern Med Rev 2006;11(2):128–150.

92. Huang CF, et al. The immunopharmaceutical effects and mechanisms of herb medicine. Cell Mol Immunol 2008;5(1):23–31.

93. Barrett B. Medicinal properties of echinacea: a critical review. Phytomedicine 2003;10(1):66–86.

94. Mishima S, et al. Antioxidant and immuno-enhancing effects of Echinacea purpurea. Biol Pharm Bull 2004;27(7):1004–1009.

95. Abu-Ghefreh AA, et al. In vitro and in vivo anti-inflammatory effects of andrographolide. Int Immunopharmacol 2009;9(3):313–318.

96. Burgos RA, et al. Andrographolide inhibits IFN-gamma and IL-2 cytokine production and protects against cell apoptosis. Planta Med 2005;71(5):429–434.

97. Shen YC, et al. Andrographolide prevents oxygen radical production by human neutrophils: possible mechanism(s) involved in its anti-inflammatory effect. Br J Pharmacol 2002;135(2):399–406.

98. Hidalgo MA, et al. Andrographolide interferes with binding of nuclear factor-kappaB to DNA in HL-60-derived neutrophilic cells. Br J Pharmacol 2005;144(5):680–686.

99. Naik SR, Hule A. Evaluation of immunomodulatory activity of an extract of andrographolides from Andographis paniculata. Planta Med 2009;75(8):785–791.

100. Qin LH, et al. Andrographolide inhibits the production of TNF-alpha and interleukin-12 in lipopolysaccharide-stimulated macrophages: role of mitogen-activated protein kinases. Biol Pharm Bull 2006;29(2):220–224.

101. Laus G. Advances in chemistry and bioactivity of the genus Uncaria. Phytother Res 2004;18(4):259–274.

102. Drozd J, et al. Estimation of humoral activity of Eleutherococcus senticosus. Acta Pol Pharm 2002;59(5):395–401.

103. Bleakney TL. Deconstructing an adaptogen: Eleutherococcus senticosus. Holist Nurs Pract 2008;22(4):220–224.

104. Block KI, Mead MN. Immune system effects of echinacea, ginseng, and astragalus: a review. Integr Cancer Ther 2003;2(3):247–267.

105. Prieto JM, et al. Influence of traditional Chinese anti-inflammatory medicinal plants on leukocyte and platelet functions. J Pharm Pharmacol 2003;55(9):1275–1282.

106. Zhou X, et al. Ganodermataceae: natural products and their related pharmacological functions. Am J Chin Med 2007;35(4):559–574.

107. Bone K. Clinical applications of Ayurvedic and Chinese herbs. 1996. Warwick: Phytotherapy Press.

108. Matthias A, et al. Permeability studies of alkylamides and caffeic acid conjugates from echinacea using a Caco-2 cell monolayer model. J Clin Pharm Ther 2004;29(1):7–13.

109. Matthias A, et al. Echinacea alkylamide disposition and pharmacokinetics in humans after tablet ingestion. Life Sci 2005;77(16):2018–2029.

110. Agnew LL, et al. Echinacea intake induces an immune response through altered expression of leucocyte hsp70, increased white cell counts and improved erythrocyte antioxidant defences. J Clin Pharm Ther 2005;30(4):363–369.

111. Perry NB, et al. Alkylamide levels in Echinacea purpurea: a rapid analytical method revealing differences among roots, rhizomes, stems, leaves and flowers. Planta Med 1997;63(1):58–62.

112. Chicca A, et al. Synergistic immunomopharmacological effects of N-alkylamides in Echinacea purpurea herbal extracts. Int Immunopharmacol 2009;9(7 8):850–858.

113. Felter HW, Lloyd JU. King's American dispensatory. Online. Available: http://www.henriettesherbal.com/eclectic/kings/extracta

114. Sharma M, et al. Induction of multiple pro-inflammatory cytokines by respiratory viruses and reversal by standardized echinacea, a potent antiviral herbal extract. Antiviral Res 2009;83:165–170.

115. Shah SA, et al. Evaluation of echinacea for the prevention and treatment of the common cold: a meta-analysis. Lancet Infect Dis 2007;7(7):473–480.

116. Cohen HA, et al. Effectiveness of an herbal preparation containing echinacea propolis and vitamin C in preventing respiratory tract infections in children: a randomized, double-blind, placebo-controlled multicenter study. Arch Pediatr Adolesc Med 2004;158(3):217–221.

117. Williamson E, ed. Major herbs of Ayurveda. London: Churchill Livingstone, 2002.

118. Kligler B, et al. Andrographis paniculata for the treatment of upper respiratory infection: a systematic review by the Natural Standard Research Collaboration. Explore (NY) 2006;2(1):25–29.

119. Poolsup N, et al. *Andrographis paniculata* in the symptomatic treatment of uncomplicated upper respiratory tract infection: systematic review of randomized controlled trials. J Clin Pharm Ther 2004;29(1):37–45.

120. Thamlikitkul V, et al. Efficacy of *Andrographis paniculata* Nees for pharyngotonsillitis in adults. J Med Assoc Thai 1991;74(10):437–442.

121. Coon JT, Ernst E. *Andrographis paniculata* in the treatment of upper respiratory tract infections: a systematic review of safety and efficacy. Planta Med 2004;70(4):293–298.

122. Brush J, et al. The effect of *Echinacea purpurea, Astragalus membranaceus* and *Glycyrrhiza glabra* on CD69 expression and immune cell activation in humans. Phytother Res 2006;20(8):687–695.

123. Boericke W. Boericke's Materia Medica. 1901.

124. Zakay-Rones Z, et al. Inhibition of several strains of influenza virus in vitro and reduction of symptoms by an elderberry extract (*Sambucus nigra* L.) during an outbreak of influenza B Panama. J Altern Complement Med 1995;1(4):361–369.

125. Barak V, et al. The effect of Sambucol, a black elderberry-based natural product, on the production of human cytokines: I. Inflammatory cytokines. Eur Cytokine Netw 2001;12(2):290–296.

126. Zakay-Rones Z, et al. Randomized study of the efficacy and safety of oral elderberry extract in the treatment of influenza A and B virus infections. J Int Med Res 2004;32(2):132–140.

127. Davydov M, Krikorian AD. *Eleutherococcus senticosus* (Rupr. & Maxim.) Maxim. (Araliaceae) as an adaptogen: a closer look. J Ethnopharmacol 2000;72(3):345–393.

128. Kannur DM, et al. Screening of anti-stress properties of herbal extracts and adaptogenic agents. Pharmacognosy Reviews 2008;2(3):95–101.

129. Coulter ID, Willis EM. The rise and rise of complementary and alternative medicine: a sociological perspective. MJA 2004;180:587–589.

130. Evans S. Changing the knowledge base in western herbal medicine. Soc Sci Med 2008;67(12):2098–2106.

131. Whorton JC. Nature cures: the history of alternative medicine in America. New York: Oxford University Press, 2004.

132. Rakel DP, et al. Practitioner empathy and the duration of the common cold. Fam Med 2009;41(7):494–501.

133. Kemeny ME, Schedlowski M. Understanding the interaction between psychosocial stress and immune-related diseases: a stepwise progression. Brain Behav Immun 2007;21(8):1009–1018.

134. Maciocia G. The foundations of Chinese medicine. Singapore: Churchill Livingstone, 1989.

135. Mowery DB. Herbal tonic therapies. New York: Wings Books, 1993.

136. Matthias A, et al. Echinacea alkylamides modulate induced immune responses in T-cells. Fitoterapia 2008;79(1):53–58.

137. Shah S, et al. Evaluation of echinacea for the prevention and treatment of the common cold: a meta-analysis. Lancet Infect Dis 2007;7(7):347–348.

138. Maciocia G. The practice of Chinese medicine: the treatment of diseases with acupuncture and Chinese herbs. London: Churchill Livingstone, 1994.

139. Strausbaugh H, Irwin M. Central corticotropin-releasing hormone reduces cellular immunity. Brain Behav Immun 1992;6(1):11–17.

140. DeRijk R, et al. Exercise and circadian rhythm-induced variations in plasma cortisol differentially regulate interleukin-1 beta (IL-1 beta), IL-6, and tumor necrosis factor-alpha (TNF alpha) production in humans: high sensitivity of TNF alpha and resistance of IL-6. J Clin Endocrinol Metab 1997;82(7):2182–2191.

141. Singh A, et al. Lymphocyte subset responses to exercise and glucocorticoid suppression in healthy men. Med Sci Sports Exerc 1996;28(7):822–828.

142. Moser M, et al. Glucocorticoids down-regulate dendritic cell function in vitro and in vivo. Eur J Immunol 1995;25(10):2818–2824.

143. Irwin MR. Human psychoneuroimmunology: 20 years of discovery. Brain Behav Immun 2008;22(2):129–139.

144. Kainuma E, et al. Association of glucocorticoid with stress-induced modulation of body temperature, blood glucose and innate immunity. Psychoneuroendocrinology 2009. In press.

145. Kemeny M. Emotions and the immune system. In: Ader R, ed. Psychoneuroimmunology. San Diego: Elsevier Academic Press, 2007.

146. Carrillo AE, et al. Vitamin C supplementation and salivary immune function following exercise-heat stress. Int J Sports Physiol Perform 2008;3(4):516–530.

147. Avitsur R, et al. Role of early stress in the individual differences in host response to viral infection. Brain Behav Immun 2006;20(4):339–348.

148. Gibb J, et al. Neurochemical and behavioral responses to inflammatory immune stressors. Front Biosci (Schol Ed) 2009;1:275–295.

149. Satterlee DG, et al. Vitamin C amelioration of the adrenal stress response in broiler chickens being prepared for slaughter. Comp Biochem Physiol A Comp Physiol 1989;94(4):569–574.

150. Patak P, et al. Vitamin C is an important cofactor for both adrenal cortex and adrenal medulla. Endocr Res 2004;30(4):871–875.

151. Grieve M. A modern herbal. New York: Dover, 1931.

152. Gaffney BT, et al. *Panax ginseng* and *Eleutherococcus senticosus* may exaggerate an already existing biphasic response to stress via inhibition of enzymes which limit the binding of stress hormones to their receptors. Med Hypotheses 2001;56(5):567–572.

153. Kato H, et al. 3-Monoglucuronyl-glycyrrhetinic acid is a major metabolite that causes licorice-induced pseudoaldosteronism. J Clin Endocrinol Metab 1995;80(6):1929–1933.

154. Zhang RX, et al. *Rehmannia glutinosa*: review of botany, chemistry and pharmacology. J Ethnopharmacol 2008;117(2):199–214.

155. Bhattacharya SK, Muruganandam AV. Adaptogenic activity of *Withania somnifera*: an experimental study using a rat model of chronic stress. Pharmacol Biochem Behav 2003;75(3):547–555.

156. Kaur P, et al. Effect of 1-oxo-5beta 6beta-epoxy-witha-2-ene-27-ethoxy-olide isolated from the roots of *Withania somnifera* on stress indices in Wistar rats. J Altern Complement Med 2003;9(6):897–907.

157. Kour K, et al. Restoration of stress-induced altered T cell function and corresponding cytokines patterns by Withanolide A. Int Immunopharmacol Int Immunopharmacol 2009;9(10):1137–1144.

158. Perfumi M, Mattioli L. Adaptogenic and central nervous system effects of single doses of 3% rosavin and 1% salidroside *Rhodiola rosea* L. extract in mice. Phytother Res 2007;21(1):37–43.

159. Kelly GS. *Rhodiola rosea*: a possible plant adaptogen. Altern Med Rev 2001;6(3):293–302.

161. Blumenthal M, et al, eds. Herbal medicine: expanded Commission E monographs (English translation). Austin: Integrative Medicine Communications, 2000.

160. Tachikawa E, Kudo K. Proof of the mysterious efficacy of ginseng: basic and clinical trials: suppression of adrenal medullary function in vitro by ginseng. J Pharmacol Sci 2004;95(2):140–144.

162. Nocerino E, et al. The aphrodisiac and adaptogenic properties of ginseng. Fitoterapia 2000;71(Suppl 1):S1–A5.

163. Rai D, et al. Anti-stress effects of *Ginkgo biloba* and *Panax ginseng*: a comparative study. J Pharmacol Sci 2003;93(4):458–464.

164. Fulder SJ. Ginseng and the hypothalamic-pituitary control of stress. Am J Chin Med 1981;9(2):112–118.
165. Braun L, Cohen M. Herbs and natural supplements: an evidence-based guide. 2nd edn. Sydney: Churchill Livingstone, 2007.
166. Anand CL. Effect of *Avena sativa* on cigarette smoking. Nature 1971;233(5320):496.
167. Felter H. The eclectic materia medica pharmacology and therapeutics. 1922. Online. Available: http://www.swsbm.com/FelterMM/Felters.html
168. Cook W. The Physiomedical Dispensatory. 1896. Online. Available: http://medherb.com/cook/home.htm
169. Wolfson P, Hoffmann DL. An investigation into the efficacy of *Scutellaria lateriflora* in healthy volunteers. Altern Ther Health Med 2003;9(2):74–78.
170. Kasper S, et al. Superior efficacy of St John's wort extract WS 5570 compared to placebo in patients with major depression: a randomized, double-blind, placebo-controlled, multi-center trial [ISRCTN77277298]. BMC Med 2006;4:14.
171. Stevinson C, Ernst E. A pilot study of *Hypericum perforatum* for the treatment of premenstrual syndrome. BJOG 2000;107(7):870–876.
172. Fasano A. Physiological pathological and therapeutic implications of zonulin-mediated intestinal barrier modulation: living life on the edge of the wall. Am J Pathol 2008;173(5):1243–1252.
173. Lamblin C, et al. [The common mucosal immune system in respiratory disease]. Rev Mal Respir 2000;17(5):941–946.
174. Hatakka K, et al. Effect of long term consumption of probiotic milk on infections in children attending day care centres: double blind randomised trial. BMJ 2001;322(7298):1327.
175. Lin JS, et al. Different effects of probiotic species/strains on infections in preschool children: A double-blind randomized controlled study. Vaccine 2009;27(7):1073–1079.
176. Pregliasco F, et al. A new chance of preventing winter diseases by the administration of synbiotic formulations. J Clin Gastroenterol 2008;42 Suppl 3 Pt 2:S224–S233.
177. Vouloumanou EK, et al. Probiotics for the prevention of respiratory tract infections: a systematic review. Int J Antimicrob Agents 2009;34(3):197:.e1–197.e10.
178. Rossi E, et al. Cost-benefit evaluation of homeopathic versus conventional therapy in respiratory diseases. Homeopathy 2009;98(1):2–10.
179. Steinsbekk A, et al. Homeopathic care for the prevention of upper respiratory tract infections in children: a pragmatic, randomised, controlled trial comparing individualised homeopathic care and waiting list controls. Complement Ther Med 2005;13(4):231–238.
180. Vickers A, Smith C. Homoeopathic Oscillococcinum for preventing and treating influenza and influenza-like syndromes. Cochrane Database Syst Rev 2006;(3):CD001957.
181. Jaber R. Respiratory and allergic diseases: from upper respiratory tract infections to asthma. Prim Care 2002;29(2):231–261.
182. Steinsbekk A, et al. An exploratory study of the contextual effect of homeopathic care. A randomised controlled trial of homeopathic care vs. self-prescribed homeopathic medicine in the prevention of upper respiratory tract infections in children. Prev Med 2007;45(4):274–279.
183. Suzuki M, et al. Research into acupuncture for respiratory disease in Japan: a systematic review. Acupunct Med 2009;27(2):54–60.
184. Kawakita K, et al. Preventive and curative effects of acupuncture on the common cold: a multicentre randomized controlled trial in Japan. Complement Ther Med 2004;12(4):181–188.
185. Zhou ZY, Jin HD, et al. Clinical manual of Chinese herbal medicine and acupuncture. Oxford: Churchill Livingstone, 1997.
186. Kawakita K, et al. Do Japanese style acupuncture and moxibustion reduce symptoms of the common cold? Evid Based Complement Alternat Med 2008;5(4):481–489.
187. Sato T, et al. Acupuncture stimulation enhances splenic natural killer cell cytotoxicity in rats. Jpn J Physiol 1996;46(2):131–136.
188. Ye F, et al. Effects of electro-acupuncture on T cell subpopulations, NK activity, humoral immunity and leukocyte count in patients undergoing chemotherapy. J Tradit Chin Med 2007;27(1):19–21.
189. Pengelly A. The constituents of medicinal plants. 2nd edn. Crows Nest: Allen & Unwin, 2004.
190. Amin M, Kapadnis BP. Heat stable antimicrobial activity of *Allium ascalonicum* against bacteria and fungi. Indian J Exp Biol 2005;43(8):751–754.
191. Douglas RM, et al. Vitamin C for preventing and treating the common cold. Cochrane Database Syst Rev 2000;(2):CD000980.
192. Douglas RM, et al. Vitamin C for preventing and treating the common cold. Cochrane Database Syst Rev 2004;(4):CD000980.
193. Hemilä H. Vitamin C supplementation and respiratory infections: a systematic review. Mil Med 2004;169(11):920–925.
194. Hemilä H, Louhiala P. Vitamin C for preventing and treating pneumonia. Cochrane Database Syst Rev 2007;(1):CD005532.
195. Anderson TW, Suranyi G, Beaton GH. The effect on winter illness of large doses of vitamin C. Can Med Assoc J 1974;111(1):31–36.
196. Anderson TW, et al. Winter illness and vitamin C: the effect of relatively low doses. Can Med Assoc J 1975;112(7):823–826.
197. Anderson R, et al. The effects of increasing weekly doses of ascorbate on certain cellular and humoral immune functions in normal volunteers. Am J Clin Nutr 1980;33(1):71–76.
198. Schoop R, et al. Echinacea in the prevention of induced rhinovirus colds: a meta-analysis. Clin Ther 2006;28(2):174–183.
199. O'Neil JH, et al. Effects of echinacea on the frequency of upper respiratory tract symptoms: a randomized, double-blind, placebo-controlled trial. Ann Allergy Asthma Immunol 2008;100(4):384–388.

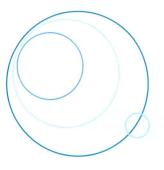

7
Asthma

David Casteleijn
ND, RN, MHSc
Tessa Finney-Brown
ND

OVERVIEW AND AETIOLOGY

Asthma is a chronic inflammatory disorder of the airways and may be classed as atopic (extrinsic) or intrinsic.[1] It is marked by recurrent attacks of paroxysmal dyspnoea with wheeze, due to spasmodic contraction of the bronchi.[1,2] Key indicative symptoms include wheeze, cough, shortness of breath, chest tightness and sputum production.[3] The signs and symptoms of asthma may be subtle, and some children present with atypical features such as recurrent respiratory tract infections, seasonal asthma and night-time cough. Often symptoms will present or worsen in relation to certain triggers.[3]

The most common theory of asthma development proposes that the condition is the result of multicellular inflammation driven by airway hyperresponsiveness, with airway remodelling and potentially permanent bronchial obstruction.[4,5] This inflammation is due to the recruitment and activation of mast cells, macrophages, dendritic cells, neutrophils and eosinophils with resultant cellular infiltration and airway inflammation.[4,5] With the activation of such cells, preformed and generated cytokines and growth factors are released, resulting in the remodelling of the airways with amplified goblet cell

ASTHMA TRIGGERS[2,3]

- Inhaled allergens (animal dander or fur, dust mites, fungi, pollen)
- Inhaled irritants (tobacco smoke, air pollution)
- Occupational exposure to dust, chemicals, fumes, or aerosols of industrial material
- Cold air
- Changes in weather
- Exercise
- Viral infection
- Stress, or high levels of emotion
- Menstrual cycles

production, smooth muscle hypertrophy and deposition of extracellular proteins.[6] The inflammatory mediators also induce changes in the noradrenergic and parasympathetic nervous systems that may lead to bronchial hyperresponsiveness.[5]

It is postulated that allergen exposure in genetically predisposed individuals leads to T helper type 2 (Th2) proliferation. Th2 cells stimulate B-lymphocytes to produce specific IgE antibodies, which then activate an inflammatory cascade upon subsequent exposure to the allergen (see Figure 7.1).[7]

In general, infants are born with a disposition towards pro-allergic and pro-inflammatory Th2 immune responses, but early childhood exposure to infections and endotoxins shifts the body towards a predominance of Th1 responses, which suppress Th2 cells and induce tolerance.[8] The hygiene hypothesis suggests that in developed countries, the trend towards smaller families,[9] cleaner environments[10] and early use of vaccinations and antibiotics may deprive children of these Th2-suppressing, tolerance-inducing exposures, partly explaining the continuous increase in asthma prevalence in developed countries.[8] It should be noted that, in contrast to this hypothesis, certain studies have identified a pathogenic role for viral respiratory infection in the development of asthma in atopic infants.[11]

In exercise-induced (intrinsic) asthma, bronchoconstriction seems to be stimulated by moisture loss from the respiratory tract and increased airway cooling due to an increase in ventilation.[12] However, despite the lack of identifiable allergenic triggers, immune dysregulation, in the form of inappropriate IgE production and activated T-cells, still seems to be a feature.[13]

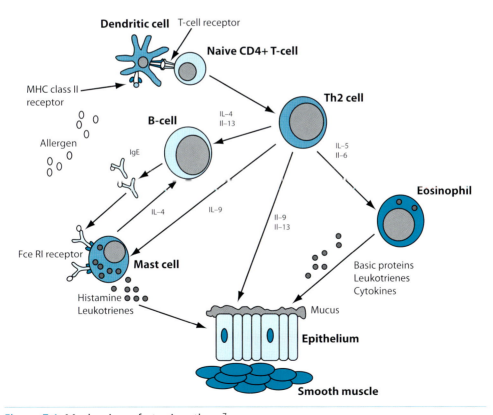

Figure 7.1 Mechanism of atopic asthma[7]

RISK FACTORS

Familial, genetic and environmental factors

Having first-degree relatives with a history of asthma, or a personal or family history of atopy, is a risk factor for the condition.[1] Atopic responsiveness is inherited, and genes have been identified that influence bronchial hyperresponsiveness, even in the absence of allergies.[14,15]

The environment also affects asthma development, particularly during early childhood. Breastfeeding during the neonatal period seems to prevent the development of atopy, perhaps as a desensitisation response to continual oral intake of the allergen.[16,17] However, antigen exposure later in infancy seems to promote atopic responses.[14] This may partially explain why the early introduction of formula seems to lead to an increase in child body mass index (BMI) and early asthma and atopy.[18] Childhood exposure to air pollution has been found to be associated with the development of persistent wheeze and atopy in children living in urban environments.[19] Paracetamol use in infancy has also been associated with an increased risk of current wheeze in young children.[20]

Digestive and dietary factors

Gastrointestinal symptoms appear to be common in children with asthma;[21] and an increased prevalence of increased intestinal permeability and cytokines in patients with asthma may support naturopathic theory that leaky gut is associated with the condition.[22,23]

Gastro-oesophageal reflux has been recognised as a common trigger of asthma,[24] via oesophageal acid-induced reflex bronchoconstriction, or microaspiration of acid. A connection has also been made between hypochlorhydria and bronchial asthma.[25] This correlation may be the result of inadequate protein digestion,[26] increasing atopic allergic reactions. It may also cause poorer nutrient absorption in general,[26] affecting the development of atopy and/or bronchial hyperresponsiveness through various deficiencies.

Dietary intake also plays a role in atopic asthma. Nutrient deficiencies, in particular of vitamins D and E, magnesium, potassium, vitamin C and fatty acids, are associated with asthma.[27-29] Poor maternal diet has been correlated with a rise in asthma at the ages of 2 and 5 years.[28] Asthma is also known to have a number of dietary triggers such as specific 'allergenic' foods or food additives.[30,31] Hen's eggs, cow's milk, soy, wheat, tree nuts, peanuts, fish and shellfish, monosodium glutamate (MSG), tartrazine and sulfites have all been implicated.[29]

Antibiotic use in the first year of life is associated with an increased risk of wheeze in New Zealand children,[20] suggesting that dysbiosis may be a risk factor. This theory is supported by evidence showing that atopic infants have higher levels of i-caproic acid (a marker of *Clostridium difficile*) and lower populations of lactobacilli, bifidobacteria and *Bacteroides* than non-atopic children.[32]

Stress

Stress is a well-known asthma trigger, but it may also play a role in pathogenesis.[2,3,33] Parental divorce or separation, exposure to violence and severe disease of a family member all increase the risk of developing atopic conditions.[34] Lower socioeconomic status is associated with elevated levels of stress and threat perception, as well as heightened production of IL-5 and IL-13 and higher eosinophil counts in children with asthma.[35] Children from this background are more likely to develop asthma, and exhibit poorer health outcomes.[36,37] Anxiety disorders and asthma are also common comorbidities, but the exact relationship is unclear.[38]

Metabolic syndrome

Abdominal obesity and hypertension are both components of metabolic syndrome that increase the risk of asthma-like symptoms.[39] Epidemiological studies show that, generally, people with asthma tend to be heavier than those without—a relationship that is more consistent in adults than children.[32] Additionally, the risk of asthma seems to increase as body mass index (BMI) rises.[40] As both obesity and asthma begin in early life, some researchers have proposed common predisposing factors including genetics, early life weight gain, low physical activity, prenatal diet and nutrition, altered intestinal microflora and adipocytokines.[32]

CONVENTIONAL TREATMENT

There is a lack of international consensus on conventional diagnosis and treatment, with a significant number of children continuing to suffer symptoms despite current treatment.[41] Patient attitudes towards medical professionals and asthma treatment have been found to predict the degree of asthma control a patient is likely to achieve with conventional therapies.[42]

The National Asthma Education and Prevention Program (NAEPP) proposes a stepwise approach to the management of asthma, based upon severity.[3] Medications fall into two categories: short-acting agents designed to relieve airway obstruction in an acute exacerbation, and longer-term prevention therapy:[40]

- Inhaled short-acting β2-agonists (SABA), as short-term reliever therapy, act to dilate the bronchioles.
- Inhaled corticosteroids (ICS) are recommended as prevention therapy. They reduce hyperresponsiveness of the airways, reduce inflammatory cell migration and block late-stage allergic responses. These drugs reduce exacerbation risk and impairment of functioning, but do not seem to modify disease progression or severity.
- A leukotriene receptor antagonist (LTRA) may be considered as an alternative to ICS in some patients in order to combat the increased airway inflammation via modulation of leukotriene mediators released from mast cells, eosinophils and basophils.

Table 7.1 Stepwise management of asthma[40]

STAGE	ASTHMA SYMPTOMS	RECOMMENDATION
1	Mild, intermittent	• No daily medication • Exacerbations: short-acting β2-agonist or inhaled glucocorticoid as needed
2	Mild, persistent	• Low-dose inhaled glucocorticoids daily • Additional treatments may include cromolyn, leukotriene modifier, nedocromil or sustained-release theophylline • Exacerbations: short-acting β2-agonist as needed
3	Moderate, persistent	• Low to medium dose glucocorticoids ± long-acting β2-agonist daily • Alternative: leukotriene modifier or theophylline instead of β2-agonists • Exacerbations: short-acting β2-agonist as needed
4	Severe, persistent	• Medium-high dose glucocorticoid + long-acting β2-agonist daily • If needed, additional oral glucocorticoids • Exacerbations: short-acting β2-agonist as needed

- Cromolyn sodium and nedocromil stabilise mast cells and interfere with chloride channel function, and may be used as additional preventive therapy if needed. They may also be used before exercise or unavoidable exposure to known allergens.
- Long-acting β2-agonists (LABA) have a duration of bronchodilation for up to 12 hours and are useful as preventers.
- Sustained-release theophylline is a mild to moderate bronchodilator.

KEY TREATMENT PROTOCOLS

The main role of naturopathic treatment is to prevent acute exacerbations and ultimately address the chronic aspects of asthma. It is essential to remember (and remind the patient) that asthma attacks may be life-threatening and should always be taken seriously. Any severe acute exacerbation requires urgent medical assistance.

A symptom diary and elimination diet are useful tools to identify trigger factors (see Chapter 5 on food intolerance and allergy). Once known, these should be avoided wherever possible. With time, and naturopathic treatment (including diges-

> **NATUROPATHIC TREATMENT AIMS**
> - Identify allergic triggers and encourage avoidance.
> - Modulate the immune response appropriately.
> - Reduce airway hypersensitivity.
> - Enhance brochodilation.
> - Promote expectoration if required.
> - Correct underlying digestive dysregulation:
>   - GIT dysbiosis
>   - increased intestinal permeability.
> - Support the nervous system to reduce the stress response.

tive repair and immune support), the patient may be well enough that certain factors cease to be problematic. As the underlying mechanism of airway obstruction is inflammation, a key priority is to manage the inflammatory response with anti-inflammatory, antiallergic and immune-modulating substances, and reduce airway hypersensitivity. On a symptomatic level, respiration will be most efficient and uncomplicated when the bronchioles are clear. Bronchodilation and expectoration are central actions to open the airways and promote symptom-free ventilation. Given the sizeable role of digestive dysfunction in the aetiogenesis of asthma, once symptoms are stabilised, better control and prevention may then be established by redressing intestinal permeability and dysbiosis.

Dampen the inflammatory cascade

Reducing pulmonary inflammation in asthma will improve symptoms and assist in moderating disease progression. A number of herbal agents demonstrate anti-inflammatory actions specific to asthma. **Boswellia serrata** inhibits 5-lipoxygenase,[43] a key cytokine implicated in asthmatic inflammation. Seventy per cent of patients treated with *B. serrata* showed improvement in their asthma symptoms, as opposed to 27% of controls.[44] The anti-inflammatory, antioxidant and antiviral activity of curcumin in **Curcuma longa** has been effective in treating airway hyperresponsiveness in allergic inflammatory diseases.[45,46] The oil of this botanical is also significantly active in removing sputum, relieving cough and preventing asthma,[47] and phytochemicals derived from *C. longa* may interrupt the action of NF-κB (which induces inflammation) and diminish Th2 responses, with a concurrent reduction in asthmatic symptoms.[48] **Zingiber officinale** may also inhibit the release of prostaglandins,[49] suppress Th2-mediated immune responses[50] and inhibit airway contraction, possibly via blockade of plasma membrane Ca^{2+} channels.[51]

Dietary supplementation with **omega-3 fatty acids**, **zinc** and **vitamin C** significantly improved asthma control, pulmonary function tests and pulmonary inflammatory markers in children with moderately persistent bronchial asthma.[52] Benefits from essential fatty acids may be derived as far back as fetal development, with research showing that adequate maternal intake corresponds with lower rates of asthma in offspring (see Figure 7.2).[53] The ingestion of 2.7 g of omega-3 polyunsaturated fatty acids for the last 10 weeks of pregnancy was shown to have a significant protective effect against the development of asthma in offspring by the age of 16 years.[54]

Omega-3 fatty acids may also be beneficial in direct treatment, as 3.2 g EPA and 2.2 g DHA daily for 3 to 10 weeks reduces inflammatory markers, pulmonary compromise (fall in FEV_1) by nearly 80% and bronchodilator use by up to 20% in exercise-induced asthma.[55,56]

In the airways of asthmatics, inflammation is often associated with increased generation of reactive oxygen species and free radical damage.[57] Thus the antioxidants **vitamins A**, **C** and **E** may be useful. By reducing the effect of the reactive oxygen species

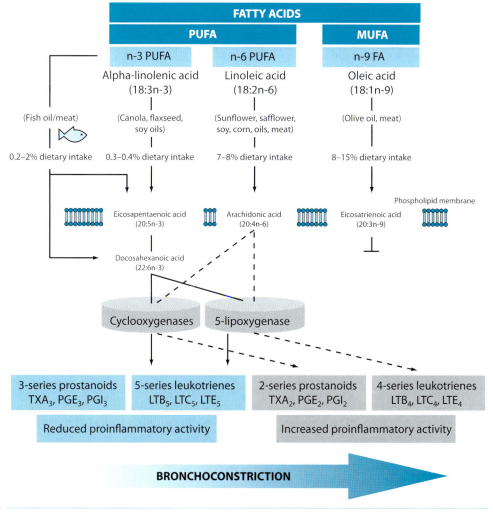

Figure 7.2 Metabolism of fatty acids, and their contribution to inflammatory asthma responses

produced in the inflammatory process, these modulate the development of asthma and the impairment of pulmonary function.[57] Vitamin C supplementation demonstrates a protective effect against exercise-induced airway narrowing in asthmatic subjects.[58] Serum levels of the **antioxidants** alpha and beta carotene have also been positively correlated to lung function and FEV_1 and FVC in epidemiological studies.[59,60]

Quercetin has the ability to inhibit inflammatory cytokine and chemokine production in acute and chronic inflammatory conditions.[61,62] High levels of this flavonoid are found in onions, apples, blueberries, curly kale, hot peppers, green and black tea and broccoli.[63,64]

In asthma, platelet activating factor (PAF) is released in response to exposure to allergens and induces an inflammatory airway response.[65] It is a potent bronchoconstrictor,[66] and elicits pulmonary and bronchial oedema, leading to airway obstruction and difficulty breathing.[67] While pharmaceutical PAF antagonists have not displayed absolute therapeutical efficacy alone, they may be a useful part of a combined treatment strategy.[68]

Ginkgo biloba is best known for its well-demonstrated neurological effects.[69,70] However, it has also shown activity as a PAF antagonist, exerting an anti-inflammatory action and reducing airway hyperresponsiveness and bronchospasm.[71] The most active constituents appear to be quercetin and the ginkgolides, in particular ginkgolide B.[72] Some researchers also suggest that *G. biloba* may modulate lymphocyte activation in asthma,[73] and in murine models of asthma the herb appears to impede the disease progress by alleviating all established chronic histological changes of lung except smooth muscle thickness.[74] Glycyrrhizae from ***Glycyrrhiza glabra*** has also demonstrated ability to inhibit PAF production by human neutrophils in a dose-dependent manner.[75] ***Allium cepa*** exerts antiasthmatic and anti-PAF effects through its thiosulfinate content. In one study, allergen-induced asthma attacks were almost completely inhibited by an *A. cepa* extract.[76] Thus, there may be potential for garlic, onions and shallots to be included in dietary management of asthma.

Immune regulation

Immune dysregulation is a key feature of atopic asthma (and perhaps intrinsic asthma – see above). Strengthening immune resistance generally, rebalancing T-cell levels and restoring immune homeostasis in the lung may decrease sensitisation to allergens and triggers.[7] In addition, viral infections are known to worsen asthma symptoms,[3] and immune enhancement will help to prevent these.

Herbal immune modulators such as *Echinacea angustifolia* may be beneficial in supporting the body's natural resistance to infection and is particularly efficacious in prophylaxis/treatment of upper respiratory tract infections.[77] In addition to its significant immune enhancing properties,[78] *Andrographis paniculata* may also be anti-inflammatory via inhibition of the NF-κB pathway.[79] *Astragalus membranaceus* has good traditional evidence as an immune-enhancing herb, and may potentially play a specific role in treating allergic asthma.[80] Also useful is *Picorrhiza kurroa*, which helps to prevent allergen- and PAF-induced bronchial obstruction.[76] General **immune supportive nutrients** are vitamin C, vitamin A, zinc and selenium (for further immune modulators, refer to Chapter 6 on infectious respiratory disease).

Allergy management

Albizzia lebbeck stabilises mast cell membranes in murine models, suggesting that it may inhibit histamine release in allergenic asthma.[81] This herb appears to deliver best results in asthma of less than 2 years' duration.[82] ***Scutellaria baicalensis*** contains various flavonoids that suppress eotaxin—a chemokine associated with recruitment of eosinophils to sites of allergic inflammation—indicating a theoretical mechanism for its traditional use in asthma.[83] The flavonoid baicalin was associated with significant reductions in inflammatory mediators in patients with bronchial asthma and was five to 10 times more potent than the antiallergic drug azalestine.[84]

In severe cases, the practitioner may consider **immunosuppressive herbs**, such as *Tylophora indica* or *Hemidesmus indicus*, but caution is urged with regard to dosage, and the patient should be monitored closely. (For protocol on using these herbs, see Chapter 28 on autoimmunity.) Four small, early studies using *T. indica* for short periods indicate beneficial effects (such as increased peak expiratory flow rate and ventilatory capacity).[85–87]

In addition to an anti-inflammatory role, **quercetin** is useful for its anti-allergic qualities. In animal models it reduced the production of IL-4 (a Th2 cytokine) and increased the production of IFN-γ (a Th1 cytokine), potentially indicating a T-cell regulatory effect.[88] Dietary intake of **antioxidant nutrients** such as vitamin A, C, E and selenium may also help to regulate this balance. Supplementation of vitamin E and selenium are reported to promote Th1 differentiation.[89–93]

Enhance brochodilation

A key priority for the practitioner is to facilitate the ease of ventilation, and remove airway obstruction. This will reduce the symptoms of asthma caused by bronchospasm and constriction.

Adhatoda vasica is considered a specific for asthma, and is generally thought to be safe for long-term treatment.[94] The alkaloids in *A. vasica* have been compared to theophylline for their bronchodilator and antiasthmatic actions,[95] as they exhibit pronounced protection against allergen-induced bronchial obstruction.[76] ***Euphorbia* spp.** are also considered a reliable antiasthmatic, particularly in spasmodic forms of the condition. These promote expectoration, allay cough[96] and have antiproliferative properties.[97]

Forskolin from ***Coleus forskohlii*** has been shown to increase the levels of cAMP in cells, making it a natural bronchodilator.[98] In a model using guinea pig trachea, it showed efficacy in reducing antigen-induced constriction;[99] and in early trials it improved forced expiratory volume and decreased airway resistance in male asthmatics.[100] Other useful bronchospasmolytics and bronchodilators with traditional evidence are ***Grindelia camporum*** and ***Glycyrrhiza glabra***.[101,102]

Magnesium is also a renowned bronchodilator. It antagonises the movement of calcium across cell membranes, decreasing the uptake and release of the mineral in bronchial smooth muscle, and leading to relaxation and dilation of the airways.[103] In acute situations, magnesium sulfate administered intravenously or via a nebuliser appears to be effective in improving the pulmonary function of asthmatics.[104,105] In a short-term trial, 400 mg of magnesium was added to a low-magnesium diet for 3 weeks, producing an improvement in symptom scores.[106] In asthmatic children, 300 mg/day for 2 months produced reduced bronchial and skin hyperreactivity to known antigens, in addition to fewer asthma exacerbations and less medication use.[107]

Tea, **yerba maté** and **coffee**[108] are all agents that may be useful in bronchodilation. The pharmaceutical agent theophylline was derived from tea, and the caffeine that these agents contain may improve lung function for up to 4 hours in people with asthma.[109]

Promote expectoration if required
Refer to Chapter 8 on congestive respiratory disorders.

Digestive connection

The development of asthma has been variously linked to increased digestive permeability,[23] oesophageal reflux[110] and dysbiosis,[111,112] making these the key areas to address.

Inflammation may be attenuated, and the healing of the mucosal lining facilitated, by interventions including vitamin A,[113] glutamine[114,115] and *Aloe vera*.[116] Improving overall digestive capacity involves the use of **herbal bitters** such as *Gentiana lutea* or *Peumus boldus* and **warming digestives** such as *Zingiber officinale* or *Cinnamomum cassia* in association with enzyme therapy.[96,117–119]

With dysbiosis, the aim is to reduce overgrowth of detrimental strains of microflora and enhance beneficial strains, following a protocol known colloquially as a 'weed, seed and feed'. In various animal models, **probiotic** strains significantly reduce IgE production, airway hyperresponsiveness and/or inflammatory infiltration of the lungs (see the box below).[120]

For complete protocol and treatment suggestions, refer to the section on the digestive system.

Diet and lifestyle modification

Dietary modification

An elimination diet may be the most successful method of identifying allergens in asthmatic patients (see Figure 5.1 for the elimination diet protocol).[122] Egg, shellfish, tree nuts and peanuts are the foods most associated with immediate onset, while those most commonly associated with delayed onset are milk, chocolate, wheat, citrus and food colourings.[123]

A diet high in sodium may be associated with more severe asthma symptoms in some patients (see Figure 7.3),[124] and fast food intake is directly correlated with asthma risk.[125]

It has been suggested that oxidative stress may contribute to respiratory pathologies, particularly asthma.[126–128] A reduced intake of antioxidant-rich foods induces a worsening of asthma symptoms, and antioxidants are often lower in patients with asthmatic or respiratory distress.[129,130] **Antioxidant-rich diets** are associated with reduced asthma prevalence[121] and improved respiratory function.[131]

Antioxidant supplementation with 50 mg vitamin E and 250 mg vitamin C daily has been found to modulate the effects of pollution on children with asthma.[132] Improved beta-carotene levels are associated with a lower incidence of asthma,[133] and improved FEV_1.[59] Lycopene supplementation has been linked with reduced airway neutrophil influx.[130] These relationships do not automatically imply a causal relationship and may instead be used as a marker of healthy diets more broadly. This is confirmed by epidemiological evidence that suggests that eating a **Mediterranean-style diet**, with high levels of fresh fruit, vegetables, omega-3 fatty acid and nuts, may reduce asthma risk in children by up to 80%.[134,135] The inclusion of **omega-3 fatty acids** should be a key priority.[108] An avoidance of heavy meals at night has also been proposed in order to manage asthma.[136]

POTENTIALLY USEFUL PROBIOTIC STRAINS[121]

- *Lactobacillus plantarum* ATCC 8014
- *L. reuteri* ATCC 23272 LGG
- *Bifidobacterium animalis* sp. *lactis* Bb-12
- *L. acidophilus* L92
- *L. fermentum* CP34

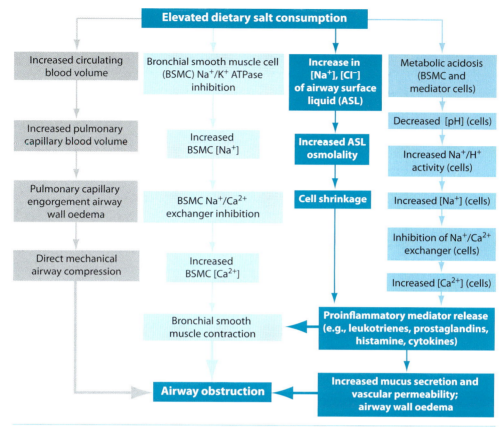

Figure 7.3 The mechanisms by which salt may contribute to airway obstruction and worsening of asthma symptoms[108]

Lifestyle advice

The association between asthma symptom severity and stress is strong. It is thought that stress exacerbates the immune reactions responsible for airway inflammation in asthma,[137] indicating that relaxation therapies may be of particular use. **Meditation**,[138] **tai chi**[139] and **yoga**[140–143] have shown efficacy in this area. The benefits of these therapies may be partly related to their focus on breathing exercises. The yogic science of **pranayama** is designed to promote deep breathing, expand the lungs and reduce stress. These exercises may help reduce histamine response to allergens, produce decreases in FEV_1, peak expiratory flow rate, symptom score and inhaler use, and improve quality of life indexes.[144–147] The interventions have little or no effect on lung physiology and are presumed to have a secondary or indirect effect on the condition due in part to their relaxation effects.

Journalling about stressful experiences not previously disclosed to others has been associated with a 13% improvement in lung function,[148] and may be a useful adjunct to treatment.

Regular **exercise** increases overall quality of life for asthmatics,[149] an approach which seems particularly relevant in children.[150–152] Maintenance of a healthy weight is important, as asthma prevalence has a positive association with obesity[153] and weight loss in overweight patients results in the improvement of asthma symptoms.[154]

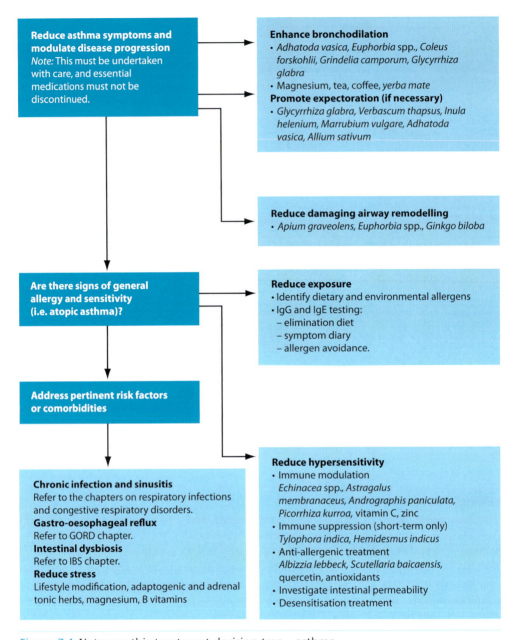

Figure 7.4 Naturopathic treatment decision tree—asthma

INTEGRATIVE MEDICAL CONSIDERATIONS
Buteyko

The **Buteyko** breathing technique—which involves making breathing shallow and slow – has demonstrated an ability to reduce medication use and produce improvements in quality of life scores in patients with asthma.[155–158]

Acupuncture

Acupuncture is useful for the asthmatic patient, and has been used for thousands of years to treat lung dysfunction.[159] Approaches generally address excessive or **deficient Qi** in the respiratory system.[159] Reports suggest that it can decrease symptom severity and improve lung function (at least in the short term),[159,160] with an immediate bronchodilatory effect, and improvements in FEV after even one treatment.[161] A Cochrane review of the English-language evidence determined that more research is needed to make a definitive conclusion.[162]

Homoeopathy

Homoeopathic treatments for asthma may include Arsenicum Album, Kali Carbonicum, Natrum Sulphuricum and Aconite.[33] It is difficult to judge the effectiveness of treatment from a clinical evidence base, as the nature of homoeopathy is that it prescribes so specifically for individuals, and trials are usually conducted with a singular intervention. A Cochrane review found that there was insufficient evidence to reliably assess the role of homoeopathy in asthma treatment.[162] However, some individual trials (including the use of allergen isopathy) have yielded promising results on lung function and subjective symptoms.[147]

Case Study

A 46-year-old male presents with recent diagnosis and onset of **asthma**. He is currently taking inhaled corticosteroids and bronchodilators. His asthma is **made worse by aspirin**, **certain food additives** and **stress**. In addition, he suffers from **indigestion** and **heart burn**.

SUGGESTIVE SYMPTOMS

- Shortness of breath
- Difficulty breathing
- Wheezing
- Respiratory catarrh
- Tightness of chest

Example treatment

This patient's asthma appears to have an atopic basis, as it has associations to aspirin and food additives. Allergy is associated with an inflammatory immune response, which provokes the release of additional inflammatory mediators (such as histamine and platelet activating factor), intensifying initial bronchoconstriction. To address this facet of the presentation, it is essential to modulate the immune response and dampen the inflammatory cascade.

Stress has been demonstrated to cause significant exacerbation of inflammation, so addressing the patient's heightened stress response is an important objective in this case.

A clear connection between digestive dysfunction and bronchoconstriction has been established. Additionally, chronic digestive dysregulation often contributes to immune dysregulation and may predispose the patient to allergies. While the above actions will ease asthmatic flare-ups, direct symptom relief is also required and to this end specific bronchodilators need to be prescribed.

Herbal and nutritional prescription

Albizzia lebbeck is included in the formula due to its antiallergenic properties, and demonstrated specific effectiveness in asthma of recent (less than 2 years) diagnosis.

Adhatoda vasica and *Euphorbia* spp. exhibit bronchodilatory properties.

Astragalus membranaceus is an immune-enhancing agent and tonic, and may be used in this case as there is no apparent acute infection. As an adaptogen it will assist in modulation of the patient's stress response.

Glycyrrhiza glabra is a soothing demulcent employed to treat the mucous membranes, and as a result a secondary antitussive. Like *A. membranaceus*, this herb is adaptogenic and an adrenal tonic, and will support the patient through exposure to external stressors.

Gentiana lutea provides a bitter principle, and is included to address his digestive underactivity (which may be involved in the pathogenesis of his asthma).

Boswellia serrata is prescribed in tablet form (as a resin, it is not ideal to be administered in extract form). The botanical has solid evidence in the treatment of asthma by exerting an anti-inflammatory activity, which is synergistically enhanced by its combination with *Curcuma longa* and *Zingiber officinale*, both of which are also demonstrated anti-inflammatories.

Magnesium is included for its muscle-relaxing properties, using a combination

Herbal treatment	
Albizzia lebbeck 1:2	25 mL
Adhatoda vasica 1:2	15 mL
Euphorbia spp. 1:2	10 mL
Astragalus membranaceus 1:2	30 mL
Glycyrrhiza glabra 1:1	15 mL
Gentiana lutea 1:2	5 mL
	100 mL
Boswellia serrata	2.0 g
Curcuma longa	2.0 g
Zingiber officinale	300 mg
Combined in tablet form: 2 tablets t.d.s	
	Orotalel citrate combination 400 mg b.d.
	3:2 g EPA/day
	2:2 g DHA/day

Nutritional treatment
Magnesium
Omega-3 fatty acids

of forms to enhance absorption and bioavailability. Doses at the higher end of the supplementary range are recommended in the initial stage of treatment in order to overcome the effects of a chronic deficiency. The dose will be reduced as the treatment phase moves from acute response to long-term management.

Omega-3 fatty acids are included due to marked anti-inflammatory effects.

Expected outcomes and follow-up protocols

The above prescription should produce significant improvements within days. It is suggested that this treatment be maintained for a number of weeks. Once the patient appears stable, treatment can move towards addressing the underlying causes of the condition. Naturopathically, these may be considered to include chronic immune dysregulation as a result of long-term gastrointestinal dysbiosis, and, potentially, increased gut permeability. (See the section on the digestive system.) In addition to the formula *Hydrastis canadensis* may be added to the formula to enhance repair of the GIT and support the action of the prebiotic fibre supplement. *Avena sativa* (green) may be included as nervous system support once *G. glabra* and *A. lebbeck* are removed from the formula. Substitution is necessary due to concerns with long-term use and hypertension (*G. glabra*). The patient should continue with the *Boswellia* combination tablet, decreased to b.d. rather than t.d.s., with the magnesium combination reduced to 400 mg per day, and continue the omega-3 supplementation at the initial dose, while taking a prebiotic supplement to promote digestive function.

Table 7.2 Review of the major evidence

INTERVENTION	KEY LITERATURE	SUMMARY OF RESULTS
Vitamin C	**Meta-analysis** Kaur, Rowe & Arnold 2009[163]	Meta-analysis found evidence from trials insufficient due to the fact that trials were small, designs varied and reporting was poor.[163]
	Reviews Bielory et al. 1994[164] Hatch 1995[165] Monteleone & Sherman 1997[31]	Reviews concluded variously that:[164,165,31] • role of vitamin C was unclear due to lack of evidence • vitamin C showed efficacy in reversing or improving asthma symptoms in a majority of trials • vitamin C may have a short-term protective effect on airway responsiveness.
	RCTs Romieu et al. 2002[132] Fogarty et al. 2006[166] Tecklenburg et al. 2007[58]	Individual RCTs show: • a significant attenuation of post-exercise bronchoconstriction[58] • modest corticosteroid-sparing effects[166] • combined with vitamin E, vitamin C improves FEF and PEF in asthmatics by protecting lungs from the effects of inhaled pollutants.[132]
	Cross-sectional and longitudinal studies Schwartz & Weiss 1994[167] Britton et al. 1995[168] Grievink et al. 1998[169] McKeever et al. 2002[170] Gilliland et al. 2003[170]	Epidemiologically:[167–171] • higher dietary intake of nutrient associated with increased lung capacity and decreased respiratory symptoms • low intake associated with pulmonary deficit.
Boswellia serrata	**In vitro** Ammon et al. 1991[172] Ammon et al. 1993[43]	• Boswellic acids inhibit LT synthesis by binding to 5-lipoxygenase.[172] • Blocks 5-hydroxyeicosatetraenoic acid (5-HETE) and leukotriene B4 (LTB4) synthesis, which are responsible for bronchoconstriction.[172]
	Animal studies Singh & Atal 1986[173]	It is non-toxic and non-ulcer forming.[173]
	Clinical trials Gupta et al. 1998[44]	In RCT, it improved asthma symptoms in 70% of treated patients vs 27% in controls. Dosage was 300 mg of resin t.d.s. for 6 weeks.[44]
Ginkgo biloba	**In vitro** Mahmoud et al. 2000[73] Vogensen et al. 2003[174]	• Reduces PAF activity, thus modulating the allergic and inflammatory reactions in atopic asthma.[174] • Modulates lymphocyte cytokine production, potentially altering allergic inflammatory response.[73]
	Animal studies Babayigit et al. 2009[74]	Reduces all chronic histological signs of pathological airway remodelling except smooth muscle thickness.[74]
	Clinical trials Li , Zhang & Yang 1997[71] Tang et al. 2007[175]	• Decreases inflammatory cytokine Interleukin-5 in sputum of asthmatics.[175] • Reduces airway hyperresponsiveness and bronchospasm.[71] • Concentrated gingko leaf liquor produced significant clinical improvement in FEV_1 at 8 weeks.[71]

(Continued)

Table 7.2 Review of the major evidence *(Continued)*

INTERVENTION	KEY LITERATURE	SUMMARY OF RESULTS
Breathing exercises	**Buteyko** Bowler, Green & Mitchell 1998[158] Opat et al. 2000[156] Cooper et al. 2003[155] McHugh et al. 2003[176] Cowie et al. 2008[157]	• Regular use of Buteyko breathing over 4 weeks to 6 months reduces asthma symptoms and bronchodilator use and increases quality of life.[155–158,176] • In one trial patients were also able to reduce inhaled corticosteroid treatment by 50% and β2-agonist use by 85% after 6 months.[176] • Buteyko breathing does not seem to alter bronchial responsiveness or lung function.[155]

	Pranayama
	Nagendra & Nagarathna 1986[177]
	Singh et al. 1990[147]
	Vedanthan et al. 1998[140]
		• Asthmatics practising yogic techniques, including pranayama (or pranayama solely) on a regular basis exhibit:[147,177,140]
		   – better exercise tolerance
		   – a trend towards less β2-agonist use
		   – a trend towards improvement in FEV_1, peak expiratory flow rate, symptom score, and inhaler use
		   – reduced FEV_1 decrease in responsive to histamine.
		• Older studies show that up to 66% of patients may be able to stop or reduce corticosteroid treatment with regular practice.[177]

Acupuncture	**Reviews** Leake & Broderick 1999[160] McCarney et al. 2004[178] Ngai & Jones 2006[159]	• Cochrane review suggests that more evidence is required to reach definitive conclusion.[178] • Given the method of treatment it is difficult to find a suitable placebo, complicating trial design. • Other reviews suggest that treatment can decrease symptom severity and improve lung function, at least in the short term.[159,160]
	RCTs Biernacki & Peake 1998[179] Chu et al. 2007[161]	Trials show immediate bronchodilating effect, and ability to improve quality of life and reduce bronchodilator medication.[161,179]

Note: RCT = randomised controlled trial

KEY POINTS

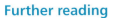

• Acute asthma is a medical emergency and requires immediate referral.
• Patients should be strongly counselled about not stopping conventional treatments for asthma in the acute phase of treatment.
• Patients should be informed that they need to ensure they continue to carry acute treatment medication with them at all times.
• Observe for signs of digestive dysbiosis and treat appropriately.
• While it is pertinent to identify and remove obvious reactive triggers, the aim of naturopathic treatment is to treat the underlying causes of hyperreactivity. With time, not all triggers may need to be avoided. True allergic reactions, however, are likely to persist.

Further reading

Borchers AT, et al. Probiotics and immunity. J Gastroenterol 2009;44(1):26–46.

Mickleborough TD. A nutritional approach to managing exercise-induced asthma. Exerc Sport Sci Rev 2008;36(3):135–144.

von Mutius E, et al. Exposure to endotoxin or other bacterial components might protect against the development of atopy. Clin Exp Allergy 2000;30:1230–1234.

References

1. Barnes P. Asthma. In: Fauci AS, et al., ed. Harrison's principles of internal medicine. New York: McGraw-Hill Companies, Inc., 2008.
2. McCunney RJ. Asthma, genes, and air pollution. J Occup Environ Med 2005;47(12):1285–1291.
3. National Asthma Education and Prevention Program. Guidelines for the diagnosis and management of asthma. In: National Asthma Education and Prevention Program Expert Panel Report 3. Washington: National Institutes of Health, 2007.
4. Anderson GP. Endotyping asthma: new insights into key pathogenic mechanisms in a complex, heterogeneous disease. Lancet 2008;372(9643):1107–1119.
5. Linzer JFS. Review of asthma: pathophysiology and current treatment options. Clin Pediatr Emer Med 2007;8(2):87–95.
6. Holgate ST, et al. Epithelial-mesenchymal interactions in the pathogenesis of asthma. J Allergy Clin Immunol 2000;105(2 Pt 1):193–204.
7. Ryanna K, et al. Regulatory T cells in bronchial asthma. Allergy 2009;64(3):335–347.
8. Beers MH, et al. Merck manual of diagnosis and therapy. 18th edn. West Point: Merck & Co., Inc., 2006.
9. Strachan D. Hay fever, hygiene, and household size. BMJ 1989;299:1259–1260.
10. Braun-Fahrländer C, et al. Exposure to farming environment during the first year of life protects against the development of asthma and allergy. Am J Respir Crit Care Med 2001;163:A157.
11. Kusel MM, et al. Early-life respiratory viral infections, atopic sensitization, and risk of subsequent development of persistent asthma. J Allergy Clin Immunol 2007;119(5):1105–1110.
12. Carlsen KH, Carlsen KC. Exercise-induced asthma. Paediatr Respir Rev 2002;3(2):154–160.
13. Jayaratnam A, et al. The continuing enigma of non-atopic asthma. Clin Exp Allergy 2005;35(7):835–837.
14. Kay AB. Allergy and allergic diseases. First of two parts. N Engl J Med 2001;344(1):30–37.
15. Holgate ST, et al. The genetics of asthma: ADAM33 as an example of a susceptibility gene. Proc Am Thorac Soc 2006;3(5):440–443.
16. Friedman NJ, Zeiger RS. The role of breast-feeding in the development of allergies and asthma. J Allergy Clin Immunol 2005;115(6):1238–1248.
17. Verhasselt V, et al. Breast milk-mediated transfer of an antigen induces tolerance and protection from allergic asthma. Nat Med 2008;14(2):170–175.
18. Oddy WH, Sherriff JL. Breastfeeding, body mass index, asthma and atopy in children. Asia Pac J Public Health 2003;15(Suppl):S15–S17.
19. Salvi S. Health effects of ambient air pollution in children. Paediatr Respir Rev 2007;8(4):275–280.
20. Mitchell EA, et al. Cross-sectional survey of risk factors for asthma in 6–7-year-old children in New Zealand: International Study of Asthma and Allergy in Childhood Phase Three. J Paediatr Child Health 2009;45(6):375–383.
21. Caffarelli C, et al. Gastrointestinal symptoms in patients with asthma. Arch Dis Child 2000;82(2):131–135.
22. Hijazi Z, et al. Intestinal permeability is increased in bronchial asthma. Arch Dis Child 2004;89(3):227–229.
23. Benard A, et al. Increased intestinal permeability in bronchial asthma. J Allergy Clin Immunol 1996;97:1173–1178.
24. Peterson KA, et al. The role of gastroesophageal reflux in exercise-triggered asthma: a randomized controlled trial. Dig Dis Sci 2009;54(3):564–571.
25. Gonzalez H, Ahmed T. Suppression of gastric H2-receptor mediated function in patients with bronchial asthma and ragweed allergy. Chest 1986;89(4):491–496.
26. Kelly G. Hydrochloric acid: physiological functions and clinical implications. Altern Med Rev 1997;2(2):116–127.
27. Litonjua AA, Weiss ST. Is vitamin D deficiency to blame for the asthma epidemic? J Allergy Clin Immunol 2007;120(5):1031–1035.
28. Seaton A. From nurture to nature – the story of the Aberdeen asthma dietary hypothesis. QJM 2008;101(3):237–239.
29. Roberts G, Lack G. Food allergy and asthma – what is the link? Paediatr Respir Rev 2003;4(3):205–212.
30. Ozol D, Mete E. Asthma and food allergy. Curr Opin Pulm Med 2008;14(1):9–12.
31. Monteleone C, Sherman AR. Nutrition and asthma. Arch Intern Med 1997;157(1).23–34.
32. Litonjua AA, Gold DR. Asthma and obesity: common early-life influences in the inception of disease. J Allergy Clin Immunol 2008;121(5):1075–84;quiz 1085–1086.
33. Dupler D. Asthma. In: Krapp KL, ed. The Gale encyclopedia of alternative medicine. Farmington Hills: Gale Group, 2001:126–132.
34. Williams DR, et al. Social determinants: taking the social context of asthma seriously. Pediatrics 2009;123 Suppl 3:S174–S184.
35. Chen E, et al. Socioeconomic status and inflammatory processes in childhood asthma: the role of psychological stress. J Allergy Clin Immunol 2006;117(5):1014–1020.
36. Claudio L, et al. Socioeconomic factors and asthma hospitalization rates in New York City. J Asthma 1999;36(4):343–350.
37. Ernst P, et al. Socioeconomic status and indicators of asthma in children. Am J Respir Crit Care Med 1995;152(2):570–575.
38. Goodwin RD. Asthma and anxiety disorders. Adv Psychosom Med 2003;24:51–71.
39. Lee EJ, et al. Asthma-like symptoms are increased in the metabolic syndrome. J Asthma 2009;46(4):339–342.
40. Beuther DA, Sutherland ER. Overweight, obesity, and incident asthma: a meta-analysis of prospective epidemiologic studies. Am J Respir Crit Care Med 2007;175:661–666.
41. Bisgaard H, Szefler S. Prevalence of asthma-like symptoms in young children. Pediatr Pulmonol 2007;42(8):723–728.
42. Jones CA, et al. Predicting asthma control using patient attitudes toward medical care: the REACT score. Ann Allergy Asthma Immunol 2009;102(5):385–392.
43. Ammon HP, et al. Mechanism of antiinflammatory actions of curcumine and boswellic acids. J Ethnopharmacol 1993;38(2–3):113–119.
44. Gupta I, et al. Effects of *Boswellia serrata* gum resin in patients with bronchial asthma: results of a double-blind, placebo-controlled, 6-week clinical study. Eur J Med Res 1998;3(11):511–514.
45. Ram A, et al. Curcumin attenuates allergen-induced airway hyperresponsiveness in sensitized guinea pigs. Biol Pharm Bull 2003;26(7):1021–1024.
46. Kobayashi T, et al. Curcumin inhibition of *Dermatophagoides farinea*-induced interleukin-5 (IL-5) and granulocyte macrophage-colony stimulating factor (GM-CSF) production by lymphocytes from bronchial asthmatics. Biochem Pharmacol 1997;54(7):819–824.
47. Li C, et al. Effect of turmeric volatile oil on the respiratory tract. Zhongguo Zhong Yao Za Zhi 1998;23(10):624–625.
48. Kurup VP, et al. Immune response modulation by curcumin in a latex allergy model. Clin Mol Allergy 2007;25(5):1.
49. Mascolo N, et al. Ethnopharmacologic investigation of ginger (I). J Ethnopharmacol 1989;27(1–2):129–140.
50. Berthe Ahui ML, et al. Ginger prevents Th2-mediated immune responses in a mouse model of airway inflammation. Int Immunopharmacol 2008;8(12):1626–1632.
51. Ghayur MN, et al. Ginger attenuates acetylcholine-induced contraction and Ca^{2+} signaling in murine airway smooth muscle cells. Can J Physiol Pharmacol 2008;86(5):264–271.

52. Biltagi MA, et al. Omega-3 fatty acids, vitamin C and Zn supplementation in asthmatic children: a randomized self-controlled study. Acta Paediatr 2009;98(4):737–742.

53. Salam M, et al. Maternal fish consumption during pregnancy and risk of early childhood asthma. J Asthma 2005;42(6):513–518.

54. Olsen SF, et al. Fish oil intake compared with olive oil intake in late pregnancy and asthma in the offspring: 16 y of registry-based follow-up from a randomized controlled trial. Am J Clin Nutr 2008;88(1):167–175.

55. Mickleborough TD, et al. Fish oil supplementation reduces severity of exercise-induced bronchoconstriction in elite athletes. Am J Respir Crit Care Med 2003;168(10):1181–1189.

56. Arm JP, et al. Effect of dietary supplementation with fish oil lipids on mild asthma. Thorax 1988;43(2):84–92.

57. Riccioni G, et al. Antioxidant vitamin supplementation in asthma. Ann Clin Lab Sci 2007;37(1):96–101.

58. Tecklenburg SL, et al. Ascorbic acid supplementation attenuates exercise-induced bronchoconstriction in patients with asthma. Respir Med 2007;101(8):1770–1778.

59. Grievink L, et al. Serum carotenoids, alpha-tocopherol, and lung function among Dutch elderly. Am J Respir Crit Care Med 2000;161(3 Pt 1):790–795.

60. Guizhou Hu, Cassano PA. Antioxidant nutrients and pulmonary function: the Third National Health and Nutrition Examination Survey (NHANES III). Am J Epidemiol 2000;151(10):975–981.

61. Geraets L, et al. Dietary flavones and flavonoles are inhibitors of poly(ADP-ribose)polymerase-1 in pulmonary epithelial cells. J Nutr 2007;137(10):2190–2195.

62. Lim M, et al. Topical antimicrobials in the management of chronic rhinosinusitis: a systematic review. Am J Rhinol 2008;22(4):381–389.

63. Erdman Jnr JW, et al. Flavonoids and heart health: proceedings of the ILSI North America Flavonoids Workshop, May 31–June 1, 2005, Washington, DC. J Nutr 2007;137(3 Suppl 1):718S–737S.

64. Manach C, et al. Bioavailability and bioefficacy of polyphenols in humans. I. Review of 97 bioavailability studies. Am J Clin Nutr 2005;81(1 Suppl):230S–242S.

65. Kaplan M, et al. Use of herbal preparations in the treatment of oxidant-mediated inflammatory disorders. Complement Ther Med 2007;15(3):207–216.

66. Hsieh KH. Effects of PAF antagonist, BN52021, on the PAF-, methacholine-, and allergen-induced bronchoconstriction in asthmatic children. Chest 1991;99:877–882.

67. Page CP. The role of platelet-activating factor in asthma. J Allergy Clin Immunol 1988;81(1):144–152.

68. Kasperska-Zajac A, et al. Platelet-activating factor (PAF): a review of its role in asthma and clinical efficacy of PAF antagonists in the disease therapy. Recent Pat Inflamm Allergy Drug Discov 2008;2(1):72–76.

69. Mix JA, Crews WD. A double-blind, placebo-controlled, randomized trial of Ginkgo biloba extract EGb 761 in a sample of cognitively intact older adults: neuropsychological findings. Hum Psychopharmacol 2002;17:267–277.

70. Kennedy DO, et al. The dose-dependent cognitive effects of acute administration of Ginkgo biloba to healthy young volunteers. Psychopharmacol 2000;151:416–423.

71. Li M, et al. Effects of Ginkgo leaf concentrated oral liquor in treating asthma. Chung Kuo Ching Hsi I Chieh Ho Tsa Chih 1997;17(4):216–218.

72. Shi C, et al. Protective effects of Ginkgo biloba extract (EGb761) and its constituents quercetin and ginkgolide B against beta-amyloid peptide-induced toxicity in SH-SY5Y cells. Chem Biol Interact 2009;181(1):115–123.

73. Mahmoud F, et al. In vitro effects of ginkgolide B on lymphocyte activation in atopic asthma: comparison with cyclosporin A. Jap J Pharmacol 2000;83(3):241–245.

74. Babayigit A, et al. Effects of Ginkgo biloba on airway histology in a mouse model of chronic asthma. Allergy Asthma Proc 2009;30(2):186–191.

75. Nakamura T, et al. Effects of saiboku-to (TJ-96) on the production of platelet-activating factor in human neutrophils. Ann N Y Acad Sci 1993;685:572–579.

76. Dorsch W, Wagner H. New antiasthmatic drugs from traditional medicine? Int Arch Allergy Appl Immunol 1991;94(1–4):262–265.

77. Barrett B. Medicinal properties of echinacea: a critical review. Phytomedicine 2003;10(1):66–68.

78. Poolsup N, et al. Andrographis paniculata in the symptomatic treatment of uncomplicated upper respiratory tract infection: systematic review of randomized controlled trials. J Clin Pharm Ther 2004;29(1):37–45.

79. Bao Z, et al. A novel antiinflammatory role for andrographolide in asthma via inhibition of the nuclear factor-kappaB pathway. Am J Res Cri Care Med 2009;179(8):657–665.

80. Shen HH, et al. Astragalus membranaceus prevents airway hyperreactivity in mice related to Th2 response inhibition. J Ethnopharmacol 2008;116(2):363–369.

81. Johri RK, et al. Effect of quercetin and Albizzia saponins on rat mast cell. Indian J Physiol Pharmacol 1985;29(1):43–46.

82. Bone KM. A clinical guide to blending liquid herbs. Philadelphia: Churchill Livingstone, 2003.

83. Nakajima T, et al. Inhibitory effect of baicalein, a flavonoid in scutellaria root, on eotaxin production by human dermal fibroblasts. Planta Med 2001;67(2):132–135.

84. Niitsuma T, et al. Effects of absorbed components of saiboku-to on the release of leukotrienes from polymorphonuclear leukocytes of patients with bronchial asthma. Methods Find Exp Clin Pharmacol 2001;23(2):99–104.

85. Shivpuri DN, et al. A crossover double-blind study on Tylophora indica in the treatment of asthma and allergic rhinitis. J Allergy 1969;43(3):145–150.

86. Shivpuri DN, et al. Treatment of asthma with an alcoholic extract of Tylophora indica: a cross-over, double-blind study. Ann Allergy 1972;30(7):407–412.

87. Thiruvengadam KV, et al. Tylophora indica in bronchial asthma (a controlled comparison with a standard anti-asthmatic drug). J Indian Med Assoc 1978;71(7):172–176.

88. Park HJ, et al. Quercetin regulates Th1/Th2 balance in a murine model of asthma. Int Immunopharmacol 2009;9(3):261–267.

89. Broome CS, et al. An increase in selenium intake improves immune function and poliovirus handling in adults with marginal selenium status. Am J Clin Nutr 2004;80(1):154–162.

90. Zheng K, et al. Effect of dietary vitamin E supplementation on murine nasal allergy. Am J Med Sci 1999;318(1):49–54.

91. Han SN, et al. Vitamin E supplementation increases T helper 1 cytokine production in old mice infected with influenza virus. Immunology 2000;100(4):487–493.

92. Malmberg KJ, et al. A short-term dietary supplementation of high doses of vitamin E increases T helper 1 cytokine production in patients with advanced colorectal cancer. Clin Cancer Res 2002;8(6):1772–1778.

93. Jeong DW, et al. Protection of mice from allergen-induced asthma by selenite: prevention of eosinophil infiltration by inhibition of NF-kappa B activation. J Biol Chem 2002;277(20):17871–17876.

94. Claeson U, et al. Adhatoda vasica: a critical review of ethnopharmacological and toxicological data. J Ethnopharmacol 2000;72(1–2):1–20.

95. Williamson E. Major herbs of Ayurveda. London: Churchill Livingstone, 2002.

96. Felter HW, Lloyd JU. King's American dispensatory. Online. Available: http://www.henriettesherbal.com/eclectic/kings/extracta.

97. Chaabi M, et al. Anti-proliferative effect of Euphorbia stenoclada in human airway smooth muscle cells in culture. J Ethnopharmacol 2007;109(1):134–139.

98. Laurenza A, et al. Forskolin: a specific stimulator of adenylyl cyclase or a diterpene with multiple sites of action? Trends Pharmacol Sci 1989;10(11):442–447.

99. Burka JF, Paterson NA. A comparison of antigen-induced and calcium ionophore A23187 induced contraction of isolated guinea pig trachea. Can J Physiol Pharmacol 1981;59(10):1031–1038.

100. Lichey I, et al. Effect of forskolin on methacholine-induced bronchoconstriction in extrinsic asthmatics. Lancet 1984;2(8395):167.

101. Scientific Committee of the British Herbal Medicine Association. British herbal pharmacopoeia. Bournemouth: British Herbal Medicine Association, 1983.

102. Liu B, et al. Isoliquiritigenin, a flavonoid from licorice, relaxes guinea-pig tracheal smooth muscle in vitro and in vivo: role of cGMP/PKG pathway. Eur J Pharmacol 2008;587(1–3):257–266.

103. Jaber R. Respiratory and allergic diseases: from upper respiratory tract infections to asthma. Prim Care 2002;29(2):231–261.

104. Rowe B, et al. Magnesium sulfate is effective for severe acute asthma treated in the emergency department. West J Med 2000;172(2):96.

105. Blitz M, et al. Inhaled magnesium sulfate in the treatment of acute asthma. Cochrane Database Syst Rev 2005(4):CD003898.

106. Hill J, et al. Investigation of the effect of short-term change in dietary magnesium intake in asthma. Eur Respir J 1997;10(10):2225–2229.

107. Gontijo-Amaral C, et al. Oral magnesium supplementation in asthmatic children: a double-blind randomized placebo-controlled trial. Eur J Clin Nutr 2007;61(1):54–60.

108. Mickleborough TD. A nutritional approach to managing exercise-induced asthma. Exerc Sport Sci Rev 2008;36(3):135–144.

109. Bara AI, Barley EA. Caffeine for asthma. Cochrane Database Syst Rev 2001;(4):CD001112.

110. Harding SM. Gastroesophageal reflux and asthma: insight into the association. J Allergy Clin Immunol 1999;104 (2 Pt 1):251–259.

111. Fukuda S, et al. Allergic symptoms and microflora in schoolchildren. J Adolesc Health 2004;35(2):156–158.

112. Noverr MC, Huffnagle GB. The microflora hypothesis of allergic diseases. Clin Exp Allergy 2005;35(12):1511–1520.

113. McCullough FS, et al. The effect of vitamin A on epithelial integrity. Proc Nutr Soc 1999;58(2):289–293.

114. Scheppach W, et al. Effect of free glutamine and alanyl-glutamine dipeptide on mucosal proliferation of the human ileum and colon. Gastroenterology 1994;107(2):429–434.

115. Ban K, Kozar RA. Enteral glutamine: a novel mediator of PPARgamma in the postischemic gut. J Leukoc Biol 2008;84(3):595–599.

116. Hamman JH. Composition and applications of Aloe vera leaf gel. Molecules 2008;13(8):1599–1616.

117. Speisky H, Cassels BK. Boldo and boldine: an emerging case of natural drug development. Pharmacol Res 1994;29(1):1–12.

118. Ali BH, et al. Some phytochemical, pharmacological and toxicological properties of ginger (Zingiber officinale Roscoe): a review of recent research. Food Chem Toxicol 2008;46(2):409–420.

119. Low Dog T. A reason to season: the therapeutic benefits of spices and culinary herbs. Explore (NY) 2006;2(5):446–449.

120. Borchers AT, et al. Probiotics and immunity. J Gastroenterol 2009;44(1):26–46.

121. Hodge L, et al. Assessment of food chemical intolerance in adult asthmatic patients. Thorax 1996;51:805–809.

122. Ogle K, Bullocks J. Children with allergic rhinitis and/or bronchial asthma treated with elimination diet: a five year follow-up. Ann Allergy 1980;44:273–278.

123. Carey O, et al. Effect of alterations of dietary sodium on the severity of asthma in men. Thorax 1993;48(7):714–718.

124. Wickens K, et al. Fast foods—are they a risk factor for asthma? Allergy 2005;60(12):1537–1541.

125. Rahman I, et al. Oxidant and antioxidant balance in the airways and airway diseases. Eur J Pharmacol 2006;533(1–3):222–239.

126. Wood L, et al. Lipid peroxidation as determined by plasma isoprostanes is related to disease severity in mild asthma. Lipids 2000;35(9):967–974.

127. Wood LG, et al. Biomarkers of lipid peroxidation, airway inflammation and asthma. Eur Respir J 2003;21(1):177–186.

128. Misso N, et al. Plasma concentrations of dietary and nondietary antioxidants are low in severe asthma. Eur Respir J 2005;26:257–264.

129. Wood LG, et al. Lycopene-rich treatments modify noneosinophilic airway inflammation in asthma: proof of concept. Free Radic Res 2008;42(1):94–102.

130. Patel B, et al. Dietary antioxidants and asthma in adults. Thorax 2006;61:388–393.

131. Schünemann H, et al. The relation of serum levels of antioxidant vitamins C and E, retinol and carotenoids with pulmonary function in the general population. Am J Respir Crit Care Med 2001;163(5):1246–1255.

132. Romieu I, et al. Antioxidant supplementation and lung functions among children with asthma exposed to high levels of air pollutants. Am J Respir Crit Care Med 2002;166(5):703–709.

133. Rubin R, et al. Relationship of serum antioxidants to asthma prevalence in youth. Am J Respir Crit Care Med 2004;169(3):393–398.

134. Chatzi L, et al. Protective effect of fruits, vegetables and the Mediterranean diet on asthma and allergies among children in Crete. Thorax 2007;62(8):677–683.

135. Castro-Rodriguez JA, et al. Mediterranean diet as a protective factor for wheezing in preschool children. J Pediatr 2008;152(6):823–828.

136. Singh V, et al. Barriers in the management of asthma and attitudes towards complementary medicine. Respiratory Med 2002;96(10):835–840.

137. Chen E, Miller G. Stress and inflammation in exacerbations of asthma. Brain Behav Immun 2007;21(8):993–999.

138. Wilson A, et al. Transcendental meditation and asthma. Respiration 1975;32(1):74–80.

139. Chang Y, et al. Tai chi chuan training improves the pulmonary function of asthmatic children. J Microbiol Immunol Infect 2008;41(1):88–95.

140. Vedanthan P, et al. Clinical study of yoga techniques in university students with asthma: a controlled study. Allergy Asthma Proc 1998;19(1):3–9.

141. Manocha R, et al. Sahaja yoga in the management of moderate to severe asthma: a randomised controlled trial. Thorax 2002;57(2):110–115.

142. Nagarathna R, Nagendra H. Yoga for bronchial asthma: a controlled study. Br Med J 1985;291(6502):1077–1079.

143. Galantino M, et al. Therapeutic effects of yoga for children: a systematic review of the literature. Pediatr Phys Ther 2008;20(1):66–80.

144. Thomas M, et al. Breathing exercises for asthma: a randomised controlled trial. Thorax 2009;64(1):55–61.

145. Holloway E, West R. Integrated breathing and relaxation training (the Papworth method) for adults with asthma in primary care: a randomised controlled trial. Thorax 2007;62(12):1039–1042.

146. von Steinaecker K, et al. Pilot study of breathing therapy in groups for patients with bronchial asthma [in German]. Forsch Komplementmed 2007;14(2):86–91.

147. Singh V, et al. Effect of yoga breathing exercises (pranayama) on airway reactivity in subjects with asthma. Lancet 1990;335(8702):1381–1383.

148. Smyth J, et al. Effects of writing about stressful experiences on symptom reduction in patients with asthma or rheumatoid arthritis: a randomized trial. JAMA 1999; 281(14):1304–1309.

149. Lucas SR, Platts-Mills TA. Physical activity and exercise in asthma: relevance to etiology and treatment. J Allergy Clin Immunol 2005;115(5):928–934.

150. Bonsignore M, et al. Effects of exercise training and montelukast in children with mild asthma. Med Sci Sports Exerc 2008;40(3):405–412.

151. Fanelli A, et al. Exercise training on disease control and quality of life in asthmatic children. Med Sci Sport Exerc 2007;39(9):1474–1480.

152. Welsh L, et al. Effects of physical conditioning on children and adolescents with asthma. Sport Med 2005;35(2): 127–141.

153. Beuther D, Sutherland E. Overweight, obesity, and incident asthma: a metaanalysis of prospective epidemiologic studies. Am J Respir Crit Care Med 2007;175:661–666.

154. Eneli I, et al. Weight loss and asthma: a systematic review. Thorax 2008;63(8):671–678.

155. Cooper S, et al. Effect of two breathing exercises (Buteyko and pranayama) in asthma: a randomised controlled trial. Thorax 2003;58(8):674–679.

156. Opat A, et al. A clinical trial of the Buteyko breathing technique in asthma as taught by a video. J Asthma 2000;37(7):557–564.

157. Cowie R, et al. A randomised controlled trial of the Buteyko method as an adjunct to conventional management of asthma. Respir Med 2008;102(5):726–732.

158. Bowler S, et al. Buteyko breathing techniques in asthma: a blinded randomised controlled trial. Med J Aust 1998;169(11–12).575–578.

159. Ngai S, et al. A short review of acupuncture and bronchial asthma – western and traditional Chinese medicine concepts. Hong Kong Physiotherapy J 2006;24:28–38.

160. Leake RB, Broderick J. Treatment efficacy of acupuncture: a review of the research literature. Integr Med 1999;1(3):107–115.

161. Chu KA, et al. Acupuncture therapy results in immediate bronchodilating effect in asthma patients. J Chin Med Assoc 2007;70(7):265–268.

162. McCarney RW, et al. An overview of two Cochrane systematic reviews of complementary treatments for chronic asthma: acupuncture and homoeopathy. Respir Med 2004;98(8):687–696.

163. Kaur B, et al. Vitamin C supplementation for asthma. Cochrane Database Syst Rev 2009;(1):CD000993.

164. Bielory L, Gandhi R. Asthma and vitamin C. Ann Allergy 1994;73(2):89–96: quiz 96–100.

165. Hatch GE. Asthma, inhaled oxidants, and dietary antioxidants. Am J Clin Nutr 1995;61(3 Suppl): 625S–630S.

166. Fogarty A, et al. Corticosteroid sparing effects of vitamin C and magnesium in asthma: a randomised trial. Respir Med 2006;100(1):174–179.

167. Schwartz J, Weiss ST. Relationship between dietary vitamin C intake and pulmonary function in the First National Health and Nutrition Examination Survey (NHANES I). Am J Clin Nutr 1994;59(1):110–114.

168. Britton JR, et al. Dietary antioxidant vitamin intake and lung function in the general population. Am J Respir Crit Care Med 1995;151(5):1383–1387.

169. Grievink L, et al. Dietary intake of antioxidant (pro)-vitamins, respiratory symptoms and pulmonary function: the MORGEN study. Thorax 1998;53(3):166–171.

170. McKeever TM, et al. Prospective study of diet and decline in lung function in a general population. Am J Respir Crit Care Med 2002;165(9):1299–1303.

171. Gilliland FD, et al. Children's lung function and antioxidant vitamin, fruit, juice, and vegetable intake. Am J Epidemiol 2003;158(6):576–584.

172. Ammon HP, et al. Inhibition of leukotriene B4 formation in rat peritoneal neutrophils by an ethanolic extract of the gum resin exudate of *Boswellia serrata*. Planta Med 1991;57(3):203–207.

173. Singh GB, Atal CK. Pharmacology of an extract of salai guggal ex-*Boswellia serrata*, a new non-steroidal anti-inflammatory agent. Agents Actions 1986;18(3–4): 407–412.

174. Vogensen SB, et al. Preparation of 7-substituted ginkgolide derivatives: potent platelet activating factor (PAF) receptor antagonists. J Med Chem 2003;46(4):601–608.

175 Tang Y, et al. The effect of *Ginkgo biloba* extract on the expression of PKCalpha in the inflammatory cells and the level of IL-5 in induced sputum of asthmatic patients. J Huazhong Univ Sci Technolog Med Sci 2007;27(4): 375–380.

176. McHugh P, et al. Buteyko breathing technique for asthma: an effective intervention. N Z Med J 2003; 116(1187):U710.

177. Nagendra HR, Nagarathna R. An integrated approach of yoga therapy for bronchial asthma: a 3–54-month prospective study. J Asthma 1986;23(3):123–137.

178. McCarney RW, et al. Acupuncture for chronic asthma. Cochrane Database Syst Rev 2004;(1):CD000008.

179. Biernacki W, Peake MD. Acupuncture in treatment of stable asthma. Respir Med 1998;92(9):1143–1145.

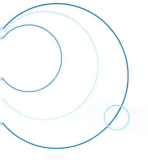

Congestive respiratory disorders

David Casteleijn,
ND, RN, MHSc
Tessa Finney-Brown
ND

OVERVIEW AND AETIOLOGY

Congestive respiratory disorders are conditions that present with mucus build-up in the upper and/or lower respiratory tract. Rhinitis and sinusitis are the most common upper respiratory expression of congestion. Sinusitis is an inflammatory condition of one or more of the four paired paranasal sinuses.[1] The condition may be classified by symptom duration (acute if < 4 weeks, chronic if > 12 weeks) or by aetiology (viral, bacterial, fungal or non-infectious).[1,2] Chronic sinusitis is one of the most common long-term illnesses in the United States of America, where it affects approximately 14% of the population.[3,4]

Sinusitis presents with clinical features including:[1,2]

- nasal drainage and congestion (it may be difficult to distinguish bacterial sinusitis from preceding viral upper respiratory tract infection (URTI), since both can be associated with thick, purulent or discoloured nasal discharge)
- headache
- facial pain or pressure that is worse when bending over or supine
- tenderness over affected sinus (particularly with maxillary infection).

Sinusitis is usually bacterial in origin. Common organisms include *Streptococcus pneumoniae, Haemophilus influenzae, Streptococcus pyogenes,* other streptococci and *Neisseria* spp.[1,5]

Lower respiratory congestion is usually associated with an acute infection, or chronic obstructive process, either reversible (such as asthma) or non-reversible (such as chronic obstructive airways disease (COAD).[6]

RISK FACTORS

Key factors in the development of sinusitis are sinus obstruction and/or impaired ciliary clearance of secretions. Inflammatory polyps were found to be a cause of chronic frontal sinusitis (requiring frontal sinus surgery) in 53% of sinus surgery cases.[5,7] Other local conditions that predispose children to rhinosinusitis include an URTI, swimming and diving, enlarged and infected adenoids, vasomotor disturbance leading to obstruction of drainage and deflection of the nasal septum.[8]

Chronic sinusitis is often a concomitant presentation with other forms of respiratory atopy, such as allergic rhinitis,[9] and suppressive treatment of hay fever is hypothesised to lead to the development of chronic sinus inflammation.

Dietary factors are often suggested to contribute to excess mucus production. Dairy, wheat and corn have been proposed to promote a more globular mucus, disable sinus drainage and promote antigen exposure.[10] While certain individuals may be predisposed to inflammatory responses with certain foods, the concept that some foods are universally mucus-promoting is an oversimplification of the process.[11] In people who believe this, however, the consumption of such products does dispose them to greater subjective respiratory symptoms,[11] demonstrating a potential psychosomatic component. (For risk factors for lower respiratory tract (LRT) congestion, see Chapter 6 on respiratory infections and immune insufficiency and Chapter 7 on asthma.)

CONVENTIONAL TREATMENT

The predominant conventional treatment of sinusitis centres on antibiotics to control infection and corticosteroids to reduce acute inflammation.[10,12] Adjunctive treatments include topical and oral decongestants and antihistamines to reduce mucosal blood flow, decrease tissue oedema and perhaps enhance drainage of secretions from the sinus ostia.[10,12] In chronic or unresponsive cases, nasal endoscopic surgery may assist in clearance of the sinuses, and restoration of mucociliary activity.[13]

While antibiotics are frequently prescribed, a Cochrane review of 49 studies concluded that they produced insignificant cure rates, with only a small treatment effect on patients in a primary care setting.[14] (For conventional treatment of LRT congestion, see Chapter 6 on respiratory infections and immune insufficiency and Chapter 7 on asthma.)

KEY TREATMENT PROTOCOLS

As congestive respiratory disorders differ significantly from one another (for example, COAD and allergic rhinitis), general treatment protocols will require adaptation to suit the individual presentation. However, for all of these conditions, an overwhelming priority will be the reduction of congestion and easing of airway blockage with the use of mucolytic and anticatarrhal herbs and nutrients. Obstruction may also be eased by reducing inflammation and, in LRT disorders, enhancing bronchodilation. If there is a cough, this may be relieved and/or used to assist airway clearance.

> ### NATUROPATHIC TREATMENT AIMS
> - Reduce congestion (clear the paranasal sinuses or bronchioles).
> - Reduce bacterial colonisation.
> - Support immune response.
> - Support the integrity of the mucous membranes.
> - If chronic, support elimination via the lymphatic system.
> - Use tonifying protocols after acute infection is cleared.

Acute immune support and reduction of pathogens will also be necessary in the acute infection. If congestion is chronic or repeated, then longer-term immune tonics and adaptogens should be used in order to strengthen the resistance of the individual. In forms of congestion linked to atopy, antiallergic substances and those which modulate hypersensitivity can be useful.

Often in chronic conditions, there are underlying factors to be addressed. Digestive disturbance or general lymphatic stagnation may play a role in exacerbating and/or perpetuating the complaint.

Whenever there is an overproduction of catarrh, the respiratory mucous membranes will be stressed and compromised. Trophorestoratives and nutritive support are essential to nourish these back to health. Their strength is vital as they are one of the few body surfaces exposed continually to the external environment, and play a large role in first-line innate immune defence.

Reduce congestion in the sinuses and airways

Blocked sinuses: steam inhalations, heat therapy and nasal irrigation

With chronic sinusitis it is important to liquefy the congested secretions in an effort to clear the sinus passages. **Herbal mucolytics** act to thin out mucosal secretions and make them easier to expel.[15] *Trigonella foenum-graecum*[16] is particularly useful, especially as a hot infusion, with the heat and steam being an integral part of the process. It is important to warn your patient that they should expect a nasal discharge to result, so they can plan the best time for the intervention. If they know, they are also less likely to take antihistamines, which would suppress the desired effect. Other mucolytic herbs to consider are *Foeniculum vulgare, Allium cepa, Armoracia rusticana* and *Allium sativum*.[17,18]

An additional category of herbs applied in the case of sinus congestion are upper respiratory tract **anticatarrhals**, such as *Euphrasia* spp., *Plantago lanceolata*, *Sambucus nigra* and *Hydrastis canadensis*.[18] Anticatarrhals differ from mucolytics in that their action involves the reduction of mucus production, rather than simply breaking it down to expel.[19] Few well-designed clinical trials were found to substantiate the effectiveness of these interventions, but they have a history of traditional use.[18,20] *H. canadensis* is traditionally contraindicated in acute inflammatory conditions of the mucous membranes but may be used in subacute or chronic conditions.[18] A combination of *Gentiana lutea, Primula veris, Rumex* spp., *Sambucus nigra* and *Verbena officinalis* is approved by Commission E to treat sinusitis and seems to exert mucolytic or anticatarrhal, antiviral and anti-inflammatory effects in a number of trials.[21,22]

Nutritional mucolytics may also be very useful when included in a supplement regimen. **N-acetylcysteine** (NAC) is perhaps the most researched and broadly used mucolytic.[23,24] The sulfhydryl group works to cleave disulphide bonds in mucous glycoproteins, making nasal secretions easier to expel.[25] NAC has demonstrated the ability to increase the mucociliary clearance rate by 35%, in comparison to no effect by placebo.[26]

Proteolytic enzymes, including bromelain, may also be useful. Proteolytic enzymes show an ability to break down the naked peptide region of mucous glycoproteins when applied topically.[25] There have been questions surrounding the bioavailability of these agents upon oral ingestion, but studies show that ingestion of the compounds leads to appreciable increases in their serum concentration.[28,29,30] In a number of trials

POSSIBLE FENUGREEK ALLERGY

One study has found that fenugreek seed powder may contain a number of potential allergenic proteins. In most cases, this reactivity seems to be due to cross-reactivity with peanut sensitisation.[19,2] While true fenugreek allergy is unlikely to be a concern, practitioners should be aware of the potential for cross-reactivity when using this mucolytic agent in patients with peanut allergies.

conducted on patients with chronic sinusitis or allergic rhinitis, the administration of bromelain (in addition to individualised conventional treatment) produced significant improvements in parameters including nasal mucosal inflammation, overall symptoms, breathing difficulties and nasal discomfort.[30–32]

One of the longer-standing traditional remedies for blocked sinuses and nasal congestion has been the inhalation of steam. Often this is with an additive (see below). Studies are mixed on the use of hot, moist air alone, with some positive trials[33,34] and others showing no effect greater than room-temperature air.[35,36]

The 'old wives' tale' cure of **chicken soup** may not be such a myth. The inhalation of hot air (from hot water) is known to help clear nasal congestion,[35,36] but research has shown that hot chicken soup is more effective than hot water.[37] The addition of aromatic spices and culinary herbs will also help to open up the nasal passages and clear secretions.[38] As an additional benefit, the liquid component inhibits neutrophil migration, possibly helping reduce symptoms in infection.[38]

The use of botanicals may improve therapeutic effectiveness of steam inhalation. For example Commission E supports the use of inhalation of *Matricaria recutita* for inflammation and irritation of the respiratory tract.[21] The **essential oils** of *Cinnamomum zeylanicum*, *Thymus vulgaris*, *Mentha piperita*, *Perilla frutescens*, *Cymbopogon* spp. and *Eucalyptus* spp. have demonstrated antibacterial activity against common respiratory pathogens through vapour contact, and thus may also be of use.[39–41] One of the most common inhalants is eucalyptus oil; when administered via inhalation or as a chest rub, it has demonstrated ability to reduce nasal congestion and improve breathing function in those with respiratory infection.[40,42] A German product combining **cineol**, **limonene** and **alpha-pinene** also has great efficacy in treating purulent mucosinusitis.[43] These are constituents of many essential oils including *Mentha piperita*, citrus oils, *Anethum graveolens*, *Pinus* spp., *Piper nigrum*, *Eucalyptus* spp. and *Melaleuca cajuputi*.[44] Other common inhalations include *Mentha piperita*, *Lavandula* spp., *Pinus sylvestris*, *Melaleuca alternifolia* and *Rosmarinus officinalis*.[45] As an extension of this principle, local application of heat more generally has also been shown to alleviate the symptoms of allergic rhinitis.[46,47]

Nasal irrigation is another natural method of clearing sinus congestion. The origins of this technique lie in yogic and homoeopathic traditions.[48,49] **Jala neti** is a Hatha yoga technique of pouring water in through one nostril using a neti pot so that it pours out the other. The method is believed to be an essential part of health maintenance, and is recommended three or four times a week.[50,51] There are a number of positive trials of nasal irrigation among people with allergic rhinitis or chronic sinusitis.[52] A Cochrane review in 2007 reported that nasal irrigation could improve the symptoms of chronic rhinosinusitis in the majority of patients, with few adverse effects.[49] Benefits are derived not solely from the initial mechanical clearance of the airways, but also due to the physiological benefits of topical **saline (sodium chloride)**, which has been proposed to improve mucus clearance, enhance ciliary beat activity, remove antigens, biofilm or inflammatory mediators, and to be protective of the mucous membranes.[49] **Sodium bicarbonate** is also mucolytic in nature and may therefore be useful in nasal irrigation.[53]

One method of nasal irrigation is suggested in Figure 8.1, but there are many slight variations, and it is recommended that the practitioner become comfortable with their chosen technique themselves first before recommending it to others. It should also be noted that bulb syringe irrigators have been found to be a potential source of contamination in rhinosinusitis,[54] so attempts should be made to ensure the cleanliness of the equipment and procedure.

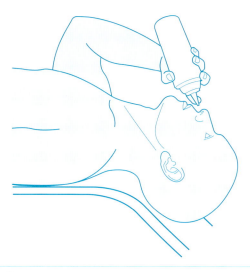

Figure 8.1 Nasal irrigation

HOW TO PERFORM NASAL IRRIGATION

1. Lie on a bed with head extended off the end of the bed or over bathtub or sink.
2. Direct saline solution into the right nostril.
3. Slowly release the saline solution to comfortably fill nasal and sinus cavities.
4. Repeat in left nostril directing the nozzle towards the left ear.
5. Remain in this position for 2 minutes.
6. Turn the head to the side and allow the saline solution to release.
7. Return to an upright position.
8. If necessary, gently blow your nose when you have finished.

Phlegm and cough

With regards to mucus congestion and cough, a number of different treatment strategies may be used. Dry (non-productive) or particularly severe coughs can benefit from suppression with an antitussive agent. Otherwise, although it may be annoying, it is best not to suppress the productive cough reflex, as it helps to clear infectious organisms from the airways.[55]

Expectorants may enhance a productive cough, allowing greater clearance of abnormal and thick phlegm and mucus. This will assist the removal of pathogens, speeding recovery and decreasing the fatiguing effort required to cough. The majority of expectorants fall into one of two categories:

1. stimulating expectorants, which provoke cough by reflex irritation of the upper digestive tract membranes[56]
2. warming expectorants, which increase blood flow to the respiratory mucosa, provide reflex stimulation of the upper digestive lining and alter the mucopolysaccharides constituents of mucus, making it runnier and easier to expel.[57]

Mucolytics and anticatarrhals may also be of use where there is a great deal of phlegm, mucus and/or congestion present. These agents will help to reduce catarrhal congestion of the upper or lower respiratory system. As with mucolytic pharmaceuticals, their mechanism of action is not fully understood, but they may act by altering the mucopolysaccharide structure of mucus, decreasing its elasticity or viscosity.[24]

Herbal medicines with demulcent action may help to reduce a cough if it is a reflex response to hyperactive or irritated receptors in the oropharynx.[55] Treatments used in Western herbal traditions for productive cough include *Thymus vulgaris*, *Glycyrrhiza glabra*, *Lobelia inflata* and *Polygala senega*.[21] Additionally, *Verbascum thapsus*, *Tussilago farfara* and *Althaea officinalis* are marked demulcents and antitussives indicated for dry or unproductive coughs.[21] Some herbs, such as *Prunus serotina*, are primary antitussives; however, caution needs to be applied when prescribing these as they can suppress a cough despite there being mucus to expectorate. This may potentially exacerbate an acute respiratory infection.

Glycyrrhiza glabra is approved by Commission E to treat upper respiratory catarrh and cough.[21] In addition to its expectorant and antitussive actions, *G. glabra* has anti-inflammatory, immune-enhancing and mucoprotective effects, the traditional reason behind its use in respiratory tract infections. The herb has demonstrated antitussive effects in animal studies, most likely due to the component liquiritin and its metabolite, liquiritigenin.[58] *Thymus vulgaris* has been used successfully in a large trial for the treatment of bronchial cough.[59] It demonstrates an ability to improve mucociliary clearance in vivo, although the mechanism remains to be elucidated.[60] In conjunction with the herbs *Sambucus nigra*, *Primula veris*, *Rumex acetosa*, *Verbena officinalis*, *T. vulgaris* and *Gentiana lutea*, the extract demonstrated ability to reduce the frequency of symptomatic coughing fits.[61,62] It is also traditionally recommended for use in respiratory tract infections as an extract or gargle due to its antimicrobial and antitussive qualities.[21,57,63]

In the case of productive cough, *Inula helenium* is another key herb to use, due to its combined effects as a stimulating expectorant and antibacterial agent.[64] Given that it contains a high level of mucilage, it also contributes to soothing the mucous membranes, thus covering a wide range of the required therapeutic actions. It is also a respiratory spasmolytic that is well tolerated in long-term therapy.[59] Traditional eclectic texts purport *Althaea officinalis* to be useful in the case of catarrh or irritated mucous membranes.[17,65] The polysaccharide constituent has demonstrated inhibition of coughs caused by laryngopharangeal and tracheobronchial irritation.[66] New research indicates a relatively pronounced antibacterial effect (stronger than that of *Thymus vulgaris*) on various strains of *E. coli*, exerted via inhibition of microbial metabolism.[67] *Althaea officinalis* is more indicated for an irritating than a congestive cough.[21]

Adhatoda vasica is mentioned in the Vedas for treatment of a number of respiratory illnesses, and is also listed in the *Pharmacopoeia of India*.[68] Extracts of the aerial parts administered orally exhibit the ability to inhibit both mechanical and chemically induced coughs.[68] When this treatment was combined with *Echinacea* spp. and *Eleutherococcus senticosus* extracts in clinical trials, it produced additive benefits in treating URTI.[69] Patients showed greater improvement in many of the parameters tested, including severity of coughing, frequency of coughing, efficacy of mucus discharge in the respiratory tract, nasal congestion and general feeling of sickness.[69]

Inhaled preparations containing menthol, such as **eucalyptus oil,** have shown the ability to significantly increase tracheobronchial clearance of mucus from the lungs[70] and help to reduce cough.[71]

As discussed above, **nutritional mucolytic** agents such as **N-acetylcysteine** and **proteolytic enzymes** may be useful in LRT congestion. Dietary treatment should also be employed. *Allium* spp. is an antimicrobial, expectorant, mucolytic and anti-inflammatory agent.[57] The respiratory system is one of the main systems to benefit from the antimicrobial action of its volatile oil, as it is excreted from the lungs. Culinary herbs such as *Pimpinella*

CHRONIC OBSTRUCTIVE AIRWAYS DISEASE

Overview
Chronic obstructive airways disease (COAD) or chronic obstructive pulmonary disease (COPD) includes emphysema and chronic bronchitis. Unlike asthma, the airflow obstruction is only partially reversible, and the disease process is progressive and irreversible.[72] Airflow obstruction is usually associated with abnormal inflammation of the airways, parenchyma and pulmonary vasculature in response to chronic inhalation of noxious particles or gases.[5,72,73]

COAD is diagnosed when a patient has spirometry readings of:
- FEV_1/FVC^* of less than or equal to 70%
- FEV_1 of less than or equal to 80% after administration of a bronchodilator[72] and symptoms that may include cough, dyspnoea, wheezing and sputum or mucus production.[4]

The major risk factors include:[72,74]
- smoking (this is the major environmental factor)
- heavy exposure to occupational dusts and chemicals (vapours, irritants and fumes)
- indoor/outdoor air pollution
- genetic factors
- repeated/severe respiratory infections.

Treatment protocols
- Support smoking cessation.[75]
- Reduce/remove exposure to irritants.
- Reduce mucus congestion.
- Reduce airway inflammation and constriction.
- Support the mucous membranes.
- Improve immunity and address any acute infection.
- Support special needs nutritionally–adequate caloric intake and protein intake,[76] possibly a high-fat, low-carbohydrate diet.[77,78,79]

CAM interventions
Mucolytics and anticatarrhals: *Trigonella foenum-graecum, Plantago lanceolata, Hydrastis canadensis, Foeniculum vulgare, Allium cepa, Armoracia rusticana, Allium sativum,* N-acetylcysteine, [80,23,81] bromelain, trypsin, papain and aromatic inhalants.[82]

Anti-inflammatory: *Boswellia serrata, Curcuma longa, Zingiber officinale,* omega-3 fatty acids, quercetin, fish, antioxidant foods (fruit and vegetables) [83–85,27] and possibly antioxidant nutrients,[7,86,87] *Camellia sinensis.*[85]

Bronchodilating: *Adhatoda vasica, Euphorbia* spp., *Coleus forskohlii, Grindelia camporum, Glycyrrhiza glabra,* magnesium[88] (dietary and supplemental).

Acute immune enhancement (in the case of infection): vitamin C, vitamin A, zinc, quercetin, *Echinacea* spp., *Andrographis paniculata, Picorrhiza kurroa, Uncaria tomentosa*

Immune tonics (during chronic stages where there is no acute infection): *Astragalus membranaceus, Eleutherococcus senticosus, Withania somnifera* and *Echinacea* spp. may be used throughout both periods of remission and exacerbation.

Mucous membrane trophorestoratives: *Hydrastis canadensis,* vitamins A and C, zinc, selenium, adequate protein intake.[89]

FEV₁ = forced expiratory volume, FVC = forced expiratory vital capacity

anisum, Foeniculum vulgare, Trigonella foenum-graecum and *Zingiber officinale* are warming expectorants and can be incorporated into treatment, either in food or as hot beverages.[57]

Reduce microbial colonisation

Herbal antimicrobials (encompassing antivirals, antibacterials and antifungals) differ from some pharmaceutical products in that they usually exert a biocidal or bacteriostatic effect on the pathogen rather than being directly cytotoxic. Biocidal agents act via a number of mechanisms, at a number of different target sites in the cell. The combined overall activity seems to result in the bactericidal death of the microbe.[90] According to Maillard, when used at lower doses, biocides exert a bacteriostatic effect, inhibiting the growth and colonisation of a pathogen.[90] Although more research is needed in the area, it seems that herbal agents (given at the right doses) exert a bacteriostatic, rather than a cytotoxic or even biocidal, effect.

While there are many individual constituents which have been identified as antimicrobial, whole plant extracts seem to be more efficacious at clearing pathogens due to synergism between components.[91] For further information on plant compounds and their antimicrobial efficacy, see Table 8.1.

In the case of respiratory infections, antimicrobials are useful to address the primary infection, inhibiting further replication of the causative organism and additionally to prevent secondary infection. However, they are unlikely to 'cure' an infection when used alone. Rather, they are most effective when combined with other botanicals, such as those with immune-modulating activity.

Antimicrobial herbs traditionally recommended for the respiratory system are *Allium sativum, Inula helenium, Hydrastis canadensis* and *Thymus vulgaris*. The essential oil of *Thymus vulgaris* exhibits some of the most pronounced antimicrobial effects of herbs that have been scientifically evaluated. It contains a multitude of compounds with activity against microorganisms, including thymol, carvacrol, luteolin and linalool.[91,92] The combined effect of these is more potent than the individual constituents alone, illustrating the importance of using whole plant extracts for the most rapid antimicrobial effects.[91] When tested against a number of the most common bacterial respiratory pathogens, *T. vulgaris* oil exhibited marked inhibitory effects on bacterial cell growth.[93] The two other oils with marked significant action against these pathogens were *Cinnamomum zeylanicum* and *Syzygium aromaticum*.[93] It is interesting to note that these effects were just as strong in antibiotic multi-resistant strains of bacteria, suggesting a role for increasing use of botanical agents in clearing respiratory infection.[93] When combined with either primrose herb or ivy leaf extract, *T. vulgaris* shows marked efficacy in treating the symptoms and shortening the duration of acute bronchitis, an effect which is likely to be due in part to its antimicrobial action.[62,63,94]

Inula helenium also exhibits antimicrobial activity in vitro, but clinical trials of the herb are sorely lacking.[65] Among its constituents, *I. helenium* contains thymol derivatives, and thus, at least in theory, some of the results of research with thyme oil may be extrapolated.[95] Among the most potent **antivirals** in the herbal repertory are *Hypericum perforatum* and *Thuja occidentalis*. The hypericin component of *H. perforatum* is especially active against enveloped viruses, such as HIV and herpes simplex while *T. occidentalis* has a broader spectrum of viricidal targets.[96] When *T. occidentalis* is given in combination with *Baptisiae tinctoriae* radix, *E. purpureae* radix and *E. pallidae* radix, the mixture exhibits ability to inhibit Influenza A virus pathology in animals.[97] One widely available antimicrobial is *Allium sativum*.[98] It has demonstrated activity against a number of bacteria, fungi and viruses implicated in respiratory

Table 8.1 Plant constituents and their antimicrobial effects (adapted from [109])

CONSTITUENT CLASS	SUBCLASS	ANTIMICROBIAL EFFECTS	EXAMPLES
Phenolics	Simple phenols	Substrate deprivation Membrane disruption[110,111]	*Picorrhiza kurroa*[45]
	Phenolic acids	Cell membrane interaction as protonophores?[112]	*Amphipterygium adstringens Arctostaphylos uva-ursi Anacardium pulsatilla Matricaria recutita*[45,109,12]
	Quinones	Bind to adhesions Complex with cell wall Weaken cell membrane Inactivate enzymes[109,113]	Coenzyme Q10[45]
	Flavonoids	Bind to adhesins[114,115]	*Camellia sinensis*[109]
	Flavones	Complex with cell wall Inactivate enzymes Inhibit HIV reverse transcriptase[116–118,119]	*Zingiber officinale Piper solmsianum*[75,117]
	Flavonols[120]	Action on the cytoplasmic membrane causing bacterial aggregation[121]	Quercetin[45]
	Tannins	Bind to proteins Bind to adhesins Enzyme inhibition Substrate deprivation Complex with cell wall Membrane disruption Metal ion complexation[109,122,123]	*Potentilla* spp. *Arctium lappa Rhamnus purshiana Eucalyptus* globules *Melissa officinalis Thymus vulgaris*[109,123]
	Coumarins	Interaction with eucaryotic DNA (antiviral activity)[109]	*Carum carvi*[109]
Terpenoids, essential oils		Membrane disruption[124]	*Capsicum* spp. *Melaleuca* spp. *Berberis vulgaris Syzygium aromaticum Armoracia rusticana Mentha piperita Rosmarinus officinalis Thymus vulgaris Curcuma longa*[45,109]
Alkaloids		Intercalate into cell wall and/or DNA[109,125–127]	*Piper nigrum Hydrastis canadensis Mahonia aquifolia*[109]
Lectins and polypeptides		Block viral fusion or adsorption Form disulfide bridges[109,128,129]	*Phytolacca decandra Viscum album Urtica dioica Juglans nigra*[45]
Polyacetylenes[130]			*Arctium lappa*[109]

infection, with some of its most potent constituents being allicin and allitridin.[99–102] In a recent trial, intranasal garlic powder was shown to decrease the likelihood of contracting an airborne infection while travelling.[103]

Increasing food intake of shallots (*Allium ascalonicum*), garlic and onions (*Allium cepa*) will also provide the active **organosulfur compounds** and exert an antimicrobial effect, and be beneficial in treating respiratory infection.[98,104,105] These foods will be at their most potent fresh or as close to fresh as possible.[105] Other nutrients and foods that exhibit bacteriostatic qualities are **zinc** and **unripe papaya**.[106,107]

If considering a topical throat spray or gargle, suspended nanoparticles of **zinc** and **silver colloidal** may be useful, as they demonstrate antimicrobial (bacteriostatic and bactericidal) efficacy against a range of organisms including *Enterococcus faecalis*, *Staphylococcus* spp., *Streptococcus pyogenes*, *Pseudomonas aeruginosa* and *Escherichia coli*.[107,108]

Support immune response

In congestive respiratory disorders, it is important to identify the cause, as this will affect what type of immune modulation is necessary. In cases of infection or an altered immune response the practitioner should boost general immunity and, if allergies are present or contributing, then give antiallergic agents. In asthma, immune modulation of T-cell ratios may be necessary. Chronic diseases will very likely benefit from immune tonics.

Pelargonium sidoides has been found to be significantly superior to placebo in the treatment of acute rhinosinusitis[131] with decreased debilitating symptoms and faster recovery. The activity of this herb is likely to be due to moderate antimicrobial activity and marked immune modulating activity, including an ability to alter the release of tumour-necrosis factor (TNF-α) and nitric oxide.[132]

Vitamin C has proven efficacious in the treatment of chronic sinusitis and allergic rhinitis. As a nutrient, it enhances both innate and adaptive components of the immune system, including natural killer cells, T-cells and B-cells.[133] It is also antiallergic, in that it stabilises mast cells and inhibits histamine release.[134] Levels of ascorbic acid, vitamin E, copper and zinc were found to be lower in children with chronic rhinosinusitis than in controls without the condition.[135] Treatment of allergic rhinitis with an ascorbic acid solution intranasally three times daily has been shown to reduce symptoms in up to 74% of treated subjects. They experienced a decrease in nasal secretions, blockage and oedema.[136]

Allergic concerns may also be treated with *Urtica dioica*, which may inhibit inflammation, ironically, through its histamine content, which inhibits leukotriene formation.[137] The herb has demonstrated success in treating allergic rhinitis, with all treated patients in a randomised controlled trial (RCT) reporting improved global assessments.[138] Other antiallergic agents include quercetin and the herbs *Albizzia lebbeck* and *Scutellaria baicalensis*. (Refer to Chapter 6 on respiratory infections and immune insufficiency and Chapter 7 on asthma for review of the evidence.)

Support the integrity of the mucous membranes

Continual goblet cell activation and mucus production may compromise the mucosal linings of the airways. This necessitates support of the mucous membranes themselves through herbal **mucous membrane trophorestoratives** and nutritionally with **collagen supportive nutrients**. *Hydrastis canadensis* and *Euphrasia* spp. are traditionally indicated for the support of mucosal surfaces in the body, especially in the upper respiratory tract.[18,64] At present, no pharmacological research or clinical trials have been found to substantiate these effects.

Nutrients that are important in the healing of wounds and help to support the integrity of collagen, epithelium and mucous membranes are vitamins A and C, lysine, proline and zinc. In addition to its antioxidant role, **vitamin C** is required for the conversion of proline and lysine to hydroxyproline and hydroxylysine so that they may be incorporated into collagen structures.[113] **Zinc** is a cofactor for RNA and DNA polymerase, meaning that it is essential for DNA replication, repair and cell proliferation.[139] It also stimulates reepithelialisation, fibroblast proliferation and is involved with collagen synthesis,[139,140] and thus is essential for the correct structure of the airways. **Copper** is also essential for collagen and elastin cross-linking.[139]

Vitamin A is essential for the strength and health of the mucous membranes and epithelial integrity.[141,142] It assists 'normal endodermal differentiation as well as maintaining balanced cell proliferation, differentiation and apoptosis'.[143] Studies have repeatedly demonstrated the beneficial effects of vitamin A supplementation on gastrointestinal mucosa,[144] and the benefits may be extrapolated to also apply to the respiratory mucosa.

Support elimination via the lymphatic system

The idea of lymphatic cleansing is a traditional naturopathic approach to many chronic congestive conditions, including respiratory, musculoskeletal and skin disorders. The beneficial herbal actions are *lymphatic and alterative*, and herbs such as *Phytolacca decandra, Echinacea* spp., *Urtica* spp., *Galium aparine* and *Calendula officinalis* are viable options.[20]

INTEGRATIVE MEDICAL CONSIDERATIONS

Yoga

Participation in yoga programs may be of benefit in congestive disorders. After participating in a specially adapted program, elderly COAD sufferers were able to tolerate more activity without dyspnoea-related distress and improved functional performance.[145] One session of yogic breathing techniques alone may produce favourable respiratory changes in sufferers.[146]

Acupuncture

A review[147] examined seven high-quality RCTs and concluded that there was sufficient evidence to recommend acupuncture for improving symptoms of perennial rhinitis. Vasomotor rhinitis has also been shown to respond favourably to acupuncture–patients in a recent trial showed significant improvement in nasal sickness score both over baseline and in comparison to controls given sham acupuncture.[148]

In COAD, acupuncture may be useful due to its ability to reduce disease-related dyspnoea.[149,150] Acu-TENS also produces increased FEV and decreased dyspnoea in patients compared to controls, even after a single 45-minute session.[151]

Reflexology and massage

An early trial into reflexology treatment of COAD shows some moderate improvements, perhaps relating to the increased relaxation felt by patients.[152] In a small trial of five patients treated with twenty 4-weekly treatments of neuromuscular release massage therapy, four of these experienced increases in thoracic gas volume, peak flow and FVC.[153]

Aromatherapy

Aromatherapy is most useful in these conditions when used as an inhaled preparation. Most of the beneficial essential oils have been covered above.

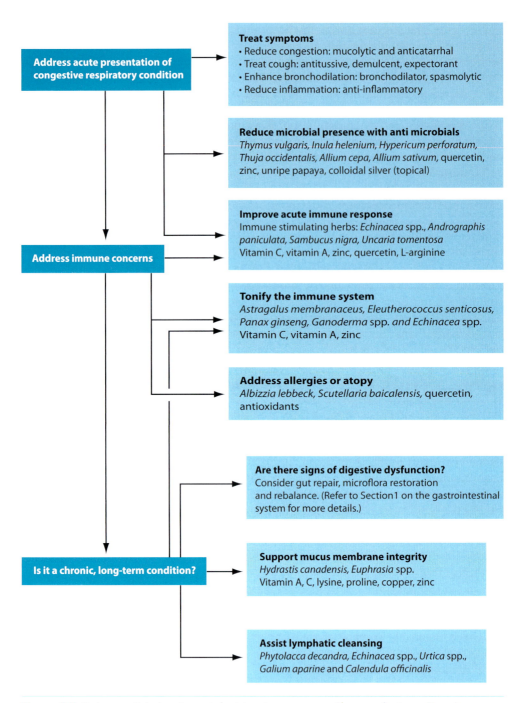

Figure 8.2 Naturopathic treatment decision tree—congestive respiratory disorders

Case Study

A 32-year- old male presents with **constant nasal congestion** and **sinus pressure**, which 'comes and goes' in severity but has been ongoing for at least 2 years. The pressure and associated facial pain are **aggravated by bending over or lying down**, with an **underlying dull headache**. He presents with an **acute flare-up with a nasal discharge that is thick and yellow-coloured**. The patient has a **history of regular prescriptions of antibiotics** and **use of antihistamines**.

SUGGESTIVE SYMPTOMS

- Thick and discoloured mucus (suggesting bacterial colonisation)
- Frontal and maxillary pressure and pain
- Recurrent flare-ups

Example treatment

Naturopathically, the primary aim is to aid the removal of mucous congestion, which acts as a reservoir for infection. The patient will need to agree to, and be fully informed about, this process as there is likely to be a period of increased discomfort while the mucus is liquefied and expelled. A key priority is to help the patient avoid the use of antihistamines, as these may prevent the long-term resolution of the condition by drying up the secretions and maintain or even encourage the pathogenic reservoir.

Immune enhancement and antimicrobial actions are also required. Once the acute infection has eased, long-term management will need to address the underlying causes of immune dysregulation, most likely related to altered colonic microflora and increased GIT permeability.

Herbal and nutritional prescription

Warm *Trigonella foenum-graecum* infusion taken t.d.s. may be beneficial as a mucolytic and anticatarrhal. Raw honey can be added to assist with taste if needed. This may be made by steeping 10 g of fenugreek seeds in boiling water for 5 minutes, or adding 5 mL of the herbal extract to boiling water. This remedy will liquefy mucosal secretions and clear the nasal passages, removing the reservoir for chronic infection.

Echinacea root blend (60/40) was chosen for its immune modulating properties, which assist in modulating a potentially over-responsive immune system.

Being astringent, anticatarrhal, anti-inflammatory, and a mucous membrane tonic, *Euphrasia officinalis* is particularly useful to control the excess production of mucus.

Foeniculum vulgare synergistically enhances the mucolytic action of *Trigonella foenum-graecum*, clearing congestion and

Herbal formula

Echinacea root blend* 1:2	20 mL
Euphrasia officinalis 1:2	20 mL
Foeniculum vulgare 1:2	15 mL
Pelargonium sidoides 1:5	20 mL
Albizzia lebbeck 1:2	25 mL
	100 mL

5 mL t.d.s. in a little water or juice.

Herbal infusion

Trigonella foenum-graecum as a hot infusion t.d.s.

Nutritional prescription

Tablet formulation containing betacarotene, vitamin D3, papain, pancreatin and *Allium sativum*
2 tablets t.d.s. during the initial stage of treatment
*E. purpurea 60%; E. angustifolia 40%

removing the microbial reservoir. Additionally, it addresses infection directly, via its anti-bacterial action.

Pelargonium sidoides has confirmed action in rhinosinusitis, reducing the symptoms and enhancing resolution of the condition. It is antimicrobial and a marked immune modulator.

Albizzia lebbeck is an antiallergic herb to reduce the need for antihistamine medication.

Betacarotene, a vitamin A precursor and antioxidant, helps repair damaged cells of the mucous membranes. It also reduces membrane sensitivity to various irritants.

Papain and pancreatin digest mucus accumulations, break up immune complexes and provide anti-inflammatory activity. Combined with the mucolytic garlic, this combination is effective at breaking down sinus congestion.

Lifestyle and dietary advice

The patient should be advised to maintain or increase fluid intake to assist with hydration of the mucous membranes. In the case of any acute infection, it is important to rest and avoid excess stress in order to enhance the body's healing capacity. Onions and garlic and shallots can be emphasised in the diet, as they have strong antimicrobial activity. Garlic in particular needs to be used raw, and, if used in cooking, heated for less than 5 minutes where possible. Shallots, however, appear to retain their antimicrobial activity after significant heating for long periods. Chicken soup has also demonstrated mucolytic and antimicrobial properties, and is an easy way to encourage increased fluid intake.

Any allergenic foods should be avoided. Some practitioners may wish to advise the avoidance of foods that are commonly considered 'mucus causing' or inflammatory (for example, wheat, dairy products and sugar). The regular use of nasal irrigation techniques with clean equipment may assist in clearing chronic infection, and preventing further acute exacerbations of sinusitis. It is important to educate the patient on the effects of the medication they may use for the condition. Antibiotic overuse may lead to gastrointestinal dysbiosis and contribute to antibiotic-resistant pathogens, while antihistamines may suppress symptoms and contribute to chronicity of a condition. Regardless, there is a time and place for these medications, and the patient should be advised to weigh up the facts in each situation and make their own decision.

Expected outcomes and follow-up protocols

In the above case, the acute infection is expected to be addressed within the week of treatment. If the patient's infection worsens, then referral for antibiotic treatment may be advised (although it is desirable to avoid this). In this case, the process of treatment and prevention can start after the infection has been removed. After the acute infection is addressed, the treatment process may take months for him to be 'sinusitis-free'. It will take time for the inflammatory process to desist, and for the nasomaxillary mucosa and architectural structures to repair. Due to this the patient must be advised to endure the process, as flare-ups may occur even after months of treatment.

The use of mucous membrane trophorestoratives (for example, *Hydrastis canadensis*) and tonics (for example, *Astragalus membranaceus* and *Eleuthrococcus senticosus*) may be of assistance in preventing a flare-up after the acute infection has abated.[58] Signposts of recovery include reduction of the severity and the frequency of the sinusitis. Over time sinus pain and tenderness should decline and the infectious flare-ups should abate.

Table 8.2 Review of the major evidence

INTERVENTION	KEY LITERATURE	SUMMARY OF RESULTS
N-acetylcysteine (NAC)	**In vitro** Sheffner et al. 1964[154] Rhee et al. 1999[53]	In vitro, decreases the viscosity and elasticity of mucopu-rulent nasal mucus and tracheobronchial secretions.[154,53]
	Meta-analyses and reviews Grandjean et al. 2000[23] Stey et al. 2000[82] Sadowska et al. 2007[155]	• Prolonged NAC administration results in fewer acute exacerbations of bronchopulmonary disease.[23] • Reduces the risk of exacerbations and improves symptoms in patients with chronic bronchitis when given orally for 12–24 weeks.[82] • At dosages used in COAD treatment, it reduces exacerbation rate and limits the number of hospitalisation days, but has little or no influence on lung function parameters.[155]
	Clinical trials Todisco et al. 1985[26]	NAC increases mucociliary clearance in people with slow mucociliary clearance. These people are in a higher risk category for congestive bronchopulmonary disease.[26]
Thymus vulgaris	**In vitro** Fabio et al. 2007[93] Iten et al. 2009[91]	• Demonstrated antimicrobial activity against a number of common respiratory pathogens.[93] • The effects of *Thymus vulgaris* extract are more potent than isolated constitutents.[91]
	Animal studies Wienkötter et al. 2007[60]	In animal studies, improves mucociliary clearance by an unknown mechanism.[60]
	Clinical trials Büechi et al. 2005[156] Kemmerich 2007[61] Kemmerich et al. 2007[62] Marzian 2007[94]	Clinical trials have all used the herb as part of a combination formula, whereby it reduces the frequency of symptomatic cough.[61,62,94,156]
Proteolytic enzymes	**Review** Majima 2002[25]	Split the peptide bond of naked mucous glycoprotein when applied topically.[25]
	Clinical trials Seltzer 1967[30] Ryan 1967[31] Taub 1967[32]	Clinical trials are quite old, but demonstrate that bromelain may decrease: • nasal inflammation • breathing difficulties • overall symptoms • nasal discomfort in allergic rhinitis and sinusitis.[30–32]
Nasal irrigation	**Review** Harvey et al. 2007[49]	Nasal lavage with saline, or additional sodium hypochlorite, is well tolerated, with only minor side effects.[49]
	Clinical trials Rabago et al. 2002[52] Rabago et al. 2005[157] Rabago et al. 2006[158] Raza et al. 2008[159]	It improves symptoms of: • nasal obstruction • posterior nasal discharge • headache • nasal endoscopic grading of oedema • erythema • purulent discharge • nasal crusts • nasal airway resistance • concomitant allergic rhinitis, asthma or polyposis.[52,157–159]

(Continued)

Table 8.2 Review of the major evidence *(Continued)*

INTERVENTION	KEY LITERATURE	SUMMARY OF RESULTS
Inhalation of essential oils	Much of the literature in this area is in German or Russian.	
	In vitro Cowan 1999[109] Inouye et al. 2001[39] Fabio et al. 2007[93]	Many plant constituents, especially essential oils, show marked antimicrobial activity.[93, 109, 39]
	Reviews Lim et al. 2008[160]	Systemic review shows that topical antimicrobial agents appear effective in the treatment of chronic rhinosinusitis.[160]
	Clinical trials Federspil et al. 1997[43] Meister 1999[82] Matthys et al. 2000[161] Hasani et al. 2003[70]	Trials demonstrate: • Improvement of mucociliary clearance from the lungs of patients with chronic bronchitis after inhalation of aromatics.[70] • Decreased symptoms of mucopurulent sinusitis.[43] • More rapid regression of acute bronchitis.[161] • Protection against acute exacerbation of chronic bronchitis.[82]

KEY POINTS

- Congestive disorders present in a variety of forms.
- They may be infectious or non-infectious and all require some form of immune support.
- Encourage the avoidance of antihistamines where possible.
- Liquefy and remove the secretions that can be a reservoir for infection.
- Once the initial symptoms have been controlled, address the underlying causes.
- Consider a tonifying protocol once acute exacerbations have ceased.

Further reading

Helms S, Miller A. Natural treatment of chronic rhinosinusitis. Altern Med Rev 2006;11(3):196–207.

Cowan MM. Plant products as antimicrobial agents. Clin Microbiol Rev 1999;12(4):564–682.

Smit HA, et al. Dietary influences on chronic obstructive lung disease and asthma: a review of the epidemiological evidence. Proc Nutr Soc 1999;58(2):309–319.

References

1. Rubin MG, et al. Infections of the upper respiratory tract. In: Fauci AS, et al., ed. Harrison's principles of internal medicine. New York: McGraw-Hill Companies, Inc., 2008.
2. Piccirillo JF. Clinical practice. Acute bacterial sinusitis. N Engl J Med 2004;351(9):902–910.
3. Van Cauwenberge P, Watelet JB. Epidemiology of chronic rhinosinusitis. Thorax 2000;55(Suppl 2):S20–S21.
4. Celli BR, MacNee W. Standards for the diagnosis and treatment of patients with COPD: a summary of the ATS/ERS position paper. Eur Respir J 2004;23(6):932–946.
5. Rabe KF, et al. Global strategy for the diagnosis, management, and prevention of chronic obstructive pulmonary disease: GOLD executive summary. Am J Respir Crit Care Med 2007;176(6):532–555.
6. National Asthma Education and Prevention Program. Guidelines for the diagnosis and management of asthma. In: National Asthma Education and Prevention Program Expert Panel Report 3. Washington: National Insititutes of Health, 2007.
7. Han JK, et al. Various causes for frontal sinus obstruction. Am J Otolaryngol 2009;30(2):80–82.
8. Benjamin B. Sinusitis in children–general considerations. Int J Pediatr Otorhinolaryngol 1983;5(3):281–284.
9. Spector SL. The role of allergy in sinusitis in adults. J Allergy Clin Immunol 1992;90(3 Pt 2):518–520.
10. Helms S, Miller A. Natural treatment of chronic rhinosinusitis. Altern Med Rev 2006;11(3):196–207.
11. Wuthrich B, et al. Milk consumption does not lead to mucus production or occurrence of asthma. J Am Coll Nutr 2005;24(6): (Suppl) 547S–555S.

12. Slavin RG, et al. The diagnosis and management of sinusitis: a practice parameter update. J Allergy Clin Immunol 2005;116(6) (Suppl):S13–S47.

13. Lanza DC, Kennedy DW. Current concepts in the surgical management of chronic and recurrent acute sinusitis. J Allergy Clin Immunol 1992;90(3 Pt 2):505–510:discussion 511.

14. Ahovuo-Saloranta A, et al. Antibiotics for acute maxillary sinusitis. Cochrane Database Syst Rev 2008;(2):CD000243.

15. Rogers DF. Mucoactive agents for airway mucus hypersecretory diseases. Respir Care 2007;52(9):1176–1193: discussion 1193–1197.

16. Wichtl M, ed. Herbal drugs and phytopharmaceuticals: a handbook for practice on a scientific basis. 3rd edn. Stuttgart: Medpharm GmbH Scientific Publishers, 2004.

17. Felter HW, Lloyd JU. King's American dispensatory. Online. Available: http://www.henriettesherbal.com/eclectic/kings/extracta

18. Agency EM. Community Monograph on *Foeniculum vulgare*. London: EMEA Committee on Herbal Medicinal Products, 2007.

19. Bone KM. A clinical guide to blending liquid herbs. Philadelphia: Churchill Livingstone, 2003.

20. Mittman P. Ask the experts. Severe recurring sinusitis. Explore (NY) 2005;1(6):495–496.

21. Blumenthal M, et al. eds. Herbal medicine: expanded Commission E Monographs (English translation). Austin: Integrative Medicine Communications 2000.

22. Guo R, et al. Herbal medicines for the treatment of rhinosinusitis: a systematic review. Otolaryngol Head Neck Surg 2006;135(4):496–506.

23. Grandjean EM, et al. Efficacy of oral long-term N-acetylcysteine in chronic bronchopulmonary disease: a meta-analysis of published double-blind, placebo-controlled clinical trials. Clin Ther 2000;22(2):209–221.

24. Henke MO, Ratjen F. Mucolytics in cystic fibrosis. Paediatr Respir Rev 2007;8(1):24–29.

25. Majima Y. Mucoactive medications and airway disease. Paediatr Respir Rev 2002;3(2):104–109.

26. Todisco T, et al. Effect of N-acetylcysteine in subjects with slow pulmonary mucociliary clearance. Eur J Respir Dis(Suppl) 1985;139:136–141.

27. Rautalahti M, et al. The effect of alpha-tocopherol and beta-carotene supplementation on COPD symptoms. Am J Respir Crit Care Med 1997;156(5):1447–1452.

28. Maurer HR. Bromelain: biochemistry, pharmacology and medical use. Cell Mol Life Sci 2001;58(9):1234–1245.

29. Castell JV, et al. Intestinal absorption of undegraded proteins in men: presence of bromelain in plasma after oral intake. Am J Physiol 1997;273(1 Pt 1):G139–G146.

30. Seltzer AP. Adjunctive use of bromelains in sinusitis: a controlled study. Eye Ear Nose Throat Mon 1967;46(10):1281–1288.

31. Ryan RE. A double-blind clinical evaluation of bromelains in the treatment of acute sinusitis. Headache 1967;7(1):13–17.

32. Taub SJ. The use of bromelains in sinusitis: a double-blind clinical evaluation. Eye Ear Nose Throat Mon 1967;46(3):361–362 passim.

33. Ophir D, Elad Y. Effects of steam inhalation on nasal patency and nasal symptoms in patients with the common cold. Am J Otolaryngol 1987;8(3):149–153.

34. Tyrrell D, et al. Local hyperthermia benefits natural and experimental common colds. BMJ 1989;298:1280–1283.

35. Forstall G, et al. Effect of inhaling heated vapor on symptoms of the common cold. JAMA 1994;271(14):1109–1111.

36. Macknin M, et al. Effect of inhaling heated vapor on symptoms of the common cold. JAMA 1990;264:989–991.

37. Saketkhoo K, et al. Effects of drinking hot water, cold water, and chicken soup on nasal mucus velocity and nasal airflow resistance. Chest 1978;74(4):408–410.

38. Rennard BO, et al. Chicken soup inhibits neutrophil chemotaxis in vitro. Chest 2000;118(4):1150–1157.

39. Inouye S, et al. Screening of the antibacterial effects of a variety of essential oils on respiratory tract pathogens, using a modified dilution assay method. J Infect Chemother 2001;7(4):251–254.

40. Burrows A. The effects of camphor, eucalyptus and menthol vapour on nasal resistance to airflow and nasal sensation. Acta Otolaryngol 1983;96:157–163.

41. Shubina L, et al. [Inhalations of essential oils in the combined treatment of patients with chronic bronchitis]. Vrach Delo 1990;5:66–67.

42. Food and Drug Administration. Over the counter drugs: monograph for OTC nasal decongestant drug products. Fed Reg 1994;41:38408–38409.

43. Federspil P, et al. [Effects of standardized Myrtol in therapy of acute sinusitis—results of a double-blind, randomized multicenter study compared with placebo]. Laryngorhinootologie 1997;76(1):23–27.

44. Pengelly A. The constituents of medicinal plants. 2nd edn. Crows Nest: Allen & Unwin, 2004.

45. Purchon N. Nerys Purchon's handbook of aromatherapy. 2nd edn. Sydney: Hodder Headline Australia, 1999.

46. Yerushalmi A, et al. Treatment of perennial allergic rhinitis by local hyperthermia. Proc Natl Acad Sci 1982;79(15):4766–4769.

47. Elad Y, et al. Effects of elevated intranasal temperature on subjective and objective findings in perennial rhinitis. Ann Otol Rhinol Laryngol 1988;97(3):259–263.

48. Burton MJ, et al. Extracts from the Cochrane Library: Nasal saline irrigations for the symptoms of chronic rhinosinusitis. Otolaryngol Head Neck Surg 2007;137(4):532–534.

49. Harvey R, et al. Nasal saline irrigations for the symptoms of chronic rhinosinusitis. Cochrane Database Syst Rev 2007;(3):CD006394.

50. Jefferson W. The neti pot for better health. Summertown: Healthy Living Publications, 2005.

51. VanEs HA. Beginning yoga. Antioch: letsdoyoga.com.

52. Rabago D, et al. Efficacy of daily hypertonic saline nasal irrigation among patients with sinusitis: a randomized controlled trial. J Fam Pract 2002;51(12):1049–1055.

53. Rhee C, et al. Effects of mucokinetic drugs on rheological properties of reconstituted human nasal mucus. Arch Otolaryngol. Head Neck Surg 1999;125:101–105.

54. Williams GB, et al. Are bulb syringe irrigators a potential source of bacterial contamination in chronic rhinosinusitis? Am J Rhinol 2008;22(4):399–401.

55. Ziment I. Herbal antitussives. Pulm Pharmacol Ther 2002;15(3):327–333.

56. Gunn J. The action of expectorants. BMJ 1927;2:972–975.

57. Mills S, Bone K. Principles and practice of phytotherapy. Edinburgh: Churchill Livingstone, 2000.

58. Kamei J, et al. Pharmacokinetic and pharmacodynamic profiles of the antitussive principles of *Glycyrrhizae* radix (licorice), a main component of the Kampo preparation Bakumondo-to (Mai-men-dong-tang). Eur J Pharmacol 2005;507(1–3):163–168.

59. Ernst E, et al. [Acute bronchitis: effectiveness of Sinupret. Comparative study with common expectorants in 3,187 patients] Fortschr Med 1997;115(11):52–53.

60. Wienkotter N, et al. The effect of thyme extract on beta2-receptors and mucociliary clearance. Planta Med 2007;73(7):629–635.

61. Kemmerich B. Evaluation of efficacy and tolerability of a fixed combination of dry extracts of thyme herb and primrose root in adults suffering from acute bronchitis with productive cough. A prospective, double-blind, placebo-controlled multicentre clinical trial. Arzneimittelforschung 2007;57(9):607–615.

62. Kemmerich B, et al. Efficacy and tolerability of a fluid extract combination of thyme herb and ivy leaves and matched placebo in adults suffering from acute bronchitis with productive cough. A prospective, double-blind, placebo-controlled clinical trial. Arzneimittelforschung 2006;56(9):652–660.

63. Scientific Committee of the British Herbal Medical Association. British herbal pharmacopoeia. Bournemouth: British Herbal Medicine Association, 1983.

64. Deriu A, et al. Antimicrobial activity of *Inula helenium* L. essential oil against Gram-positive and Gram-negative bacteria and *Candida* spp. Int J Antimicrob Agents 2008;31(6):588–590.

65. Felter HW. The eclectic materia medica. Pharmacology and therapeutics. 1922.

66. Nosal'ova G, et al. [Antitussive action of extracts and polysaccharides of marsh mallow (*Althea officinalis* L., var. *robusta*)]. Pharmazie 1992;47(3):224–226.

67. Watt K, et al. The detection of antibacterial actions of whole herb tinctures using luminescent *Escherichia coli*. Phytother Res 2007;21(12):1119–1193.

68. Dhuley JN. Antitussive effect of *Adhatoda vasica* extract on mechanical or chemical stimulation-induced coughing in animals. J Ethnopharmacol 1999;67(3):361–365.

69. Narimanian M, et al. Randomized trial of a fixed combination (KanJang) of herbal extracts containing *Adhatoda vasica*, *Echinacea purpurea* and *Eleutherococcus senticosus* in patients with upper respiratory tract infections. Phytomedicine 2005;12(8):539–547.

70. Hasani A, et al. Effect of aromatics on lung mucociliary clearance in patients with chronic airways obstruction. J Altern Complement Med 2003;9(2):243–249.

71. Morice AH, et al. Effect of inhaled menthol on citric acid induced cough in normal subjects. Thorax 1994;49(10):1024–1106.

72. Pauwels RA, et al. Global strategy for the diagnosis, management, and prevention of chronic obstructive pulmonary disease: National Heart, Lung, and Blood Institute and World Health Organization Global Initiative for Chronic Obstructive Lung Disease (GOLD): executive summary. Respir Care 2001;46(8):798–825.

73. Barnes PJ. Mechanisms in COPD: differences from asthma. Chest 2000;117(2)(Suppl):10S–14S.

74. Radin A, Cote C. Primary care of the patient with chronic obstructive pulmonary disease—part 1: frontline prevention and early diagnosis. Am J Med 2008;121(7)(Suppl):S3–S12.

75. White P. COPD: Challenges and opportunities for primary care. Respiratory Medicine: COPD Update 2005;1:43–52.

76. Brug J, et al. Dietary change, nutrition education and chronic obstructive pulmonary disease. Patient Educ Couns 2004;52(3):249–257.

77. Frankfort JD, et al. Effects of high- and low-carbohydrate meals on maximum exercise performance in chronic airflow obstruction. Chest 1991;100(3):792–795.

78. Angelillo VA, et al. Effects of low and high carbohydrate feedings in ambulatory patients with chronic obstructive pulmonary disease and chronic hypercapnia. Ann Intern Med 1985;103(6 (Pt 1)):883–885.

79. Efthimiou J, et al. Effect of carbohydrate rich versus fat rich loads on gas exchange and walking performance in patients with chronic obstructive lung disease. Thorax 1992;47(6):451–456.

80. Sadowska AM, et al. Role of N-acetylcysteine in the management of COPD. Int J Chron Obstruct Pulmon Dis 2006;1(4):425–434.

81. Stey C, et al. The effect of oral N-acetylcysteine in chronic bronchitis: a quantitative systematic review. Eur Respir J 2000;16(2):253–262.

82. Meister R, et al. Efficacy and tolerability of myrtol standardized in long-term treatment of chronic bronchitis. A double-blind, placebo-controlled study. Study Group Investigators. Arzneimittelforschung 1999;49(4):351–358.

83. Smit HA, et al. Dietary influences on chronic obstructive lung disease and asthma: a review of the epidemiological evidence. Proc Nutr Soc 1999;58(2):309–319.

84. Britton J, Knox A. Respiratory medicine. No cures but some advances. Lancet 1997;350(Suppl 3):SIII24.

85. Celik F, Topcu F. Nutritional risk factors for the development of chronic obstructive pulmonary disease (COPD) in male smokers. Clin Nutr 2006;25(6):955–961.

86. Hu G, Cassano PA. Antioxidant nutrients and pulmonary function: the Third National Health and Nutrition Examination Survey (NHANES III). Am J Epidemiol 2000;151(10):975–981.

87. Fujimoto S, et al. Effects of coenzyme Q10 administration on pulmonary function and exercise performance in patients with chronic lung diseases. Clin Investig 1993;71(8)(Suppl):S162–S166.

88. Bhatt SP, et al. Serum magnesium is an independent predictor of frequent readmissions due to acute exacerbation of chronic obstructive pulmonary disease. Respir Med 2008;102(7):999–1003.

89. Faeste CK, et al. Allergenicity and antigenicity of fenugreek (*Trigonella foenum-graecum*) proteins in foods. J Allergy Clin Immunol 2009;123(1):187–194.

90. Maillard JY. Bacterial target sites for biocide action. Symp Ser Soc Appl Microbiol 2002(31):16S–27S.

91. Iten F, et al. Additive antimicrobial effects of the active components of the essential oil of *Thymus vulgaris*–chemotype Carvacrol. Planta Med 2009:In press.

92. Lopez-Lazaro M. Distribution and biological activities of the flavonoid luteolin. Mini Rev Med Chem 2009;9(1):31–59.

93. Fabio A, et al. Screening of the antibacterial effects of a variety of essential oils on microorganisms responsible for respiratory infections. Phytother Res 2007;21(4):374–377.

94. Marzian O. [Treatment of acute bronchitis in children and adolescents. Non-interventional postmarketing surveillance study confirms the benefit and safety of a syrup made of extracts from thyme and ivy leaves]. MMW Fortschr Med 2007;149(11):69–74.

95. Stojakowska A, et al. Thymol derivatives from a root culture of *Inula helenium*. Z Naturforsch C 2004;59(7–8):606–608.

96. Miskovsky P. Hypericin—a new antiviral and antitumor photosensitizer: mechanism of action and interaction with biological macromolecules. Curr Drug Targets 2002;3(1):55–84.

97. Bodinet C, et al. Effect of oral application of an immunomodulating plant extract on Influenza virus type A infection in mice. Planta Med 2002;68(10):896–900.

98. Low Dog T. A reason to season: the therapeutic benefits of spices and culinary herbs. Explore (NY) 2006;2(5):446–449.

99. Zhen H, et al. Experimental study on the action of allitridin against human cytomegalovirus in vitro: Inhibitory effects on immediate-early genes. Antiviral Res 2006;72(1):68–74.

100. Adeleye IA, Opiah L. Antimicrobial activity of extracts of local cough mixtures on upper respiratory tract bacterial pathogens. West Indian Med J 2003;52(3):188–190.

101. Luo DQ, et al. Anti-fungal efficacy of polybutylcyanoacrylate nanoparticles of allicin and comparison with pure allicin. J Biomater Sci Polym Ed 2009;20(1):21–31.

102. Liu ZF, et al. Experimental study on the prevention and treatment of murine cytomegalovirus hepatitis by using allitridin. Antiviral Res 2004;61(2):125–128.

103. Hiltunen R, et al. Preventing airborne infection with an intranasal cellulose powder formulation (Nasaleze travel). Adv Ther 2007;24(5):1146–1153.

104. Amin M, Kapadnis BP. Heat stable antimicrobial activity of *Allium ascalonicum* against bacteria and fungi. Indian J Exp Biol 2005;43(8):751–754.

105. Al-Waili NS, et al. Effects of heating, storage, and ultra-violet exposure on antimicrobial activity of garlic juice. J Med Food 2007;10(1):208–212.

106. Osato JA, et al. Antimicrobial and antioxidant activities of unripe papaya. Life Sci 1993;53(17):1383–1389.

107. Jones N, et al. Antibacterial activity of ZnO nanoparticle suspensions on a broad spectrum of microorganisms. FEMS Microbiol Lett 2008;279(1):71–76.

108. Djokic S. Synthesis and antimicrobial activity of silver citrate complexes. Bioinorg Chem Appl 2008:436–458.

109. Cowan MM. Plant products as antimicrobial agents. Clin Microbiol Rev 1999;12(4):564–582.

110. Peres MT, et al. Chemical composition and antimicrobial activity of *Croton urucurana* Baillon (Euphorbiaceae). J Ethnopharmacol 1997;56(3):223–226.

111. Toda M, et al. The protective activity of tea catechins against experimental infection by *Vibrio cholerae* O1. Microbiol Immunol 1992;36(9):999–1001.

112. Castillo-Juarez I, et al. Anti-*Helicobacter pylori* activity of anacardic acids from *Amphipterygium adstringens*. J Ethnopharmacol 2007;114(1):72–77.

113. Alves DS, et al. Membrane-related effects underlying the biological activity of the anthraquinones emodin and barbaloin. Biochem Pharmacol 2004;68(3):549–561.

114. Perrett S, et al. The plant molluscicide *Millettia thonningii* (Leguminosae) as a topical antischistosomal agent. J Ethnopharmacol 1995;47(1):49–54.

115. Rojas A, et al. Screening for antimicrobial activity of crude drug extracts and pure natural products from Mexican medicinal plants. J Ethnopharmacol 1992;35(3):275–283.

116. Brinkworth RI, et al. Flavones are inhibitors of HIV-1 proteinase. Biochem Biophys Res Commun 1992;188(2):631–637.

117. Sookkongwaree K, et al. Inhibition of viral proteases by Zingiberaceae extracts and flavones isolated from *Kaempferia parviflora*. Pharmazie 2006;61(8):717–721.

118. Ono K, et al. Inhibition of reverse transcriptase activity by a flavonoid compound, 5,6,7-trihydroxyflavone. Biochem Biophys Res Commun 1989;160(3):982–987.

119. Taniguchi M, Kubo I. Ethnobotanical drug discovery based on medicine men's trials in the African savanna: screening of east African plants for antimicrobial activity II. J Nat Prod 1993;56(9):1539–1546.

120. Li M, Xu Z. Quercetin in a lotus leaves extract may be responsible for antibacterial activity. Arch Pharm Res 2008;31(5):640–644.

121. Cushnie TP, et al. Aggregation of *Staphylococcus aureus* following treatment with the antibacterial flavonol galangin. J Appl Microbiol 2007;103(5):1562–1567.

122. Haslam E. Natural polyphenols (vegetable tannins) as drugs: possible modes of action. J Nat Prod 1996;59(2):205–215.

123. Tomczyk M, Latte KP. *Potentilla*–a review of its phytochemical and pharmacological profile. J Ethnopharmacol 2009;122(2):184–204.

124. Cichewicz RH, Thorpe PA. The antimicrobial properties of chile peppers (*Capsicum* species) and their uses in Mayan medicine. J Ethnopharmacol 1996;52(2):61–70.

125. Atta-ur R, Choudhary MI. Diterpenoid and steroidal alkaloids. Nat Prod Rep 1995;12(4):361–379.

126. Freiburghaus F, et al. Evaluation of African medicinal plants for their in vitro trypanocidal activity. J Ethnopharmacol 1996;55(1):1–11.

127. Houghton PJ, et al. Antiviral activity of natural and semisynthetic chromone alkaloids. Antiviral Res 1994;25(3–4):235–244.

128. Meyer JJ, et al. Antiviral activity of galangin isolated from the aerial parts of *Helichrysum aureonitens*. J Ethnopharmacol 1997;56(2):165–169.

129. Zhang Y, Lewis K. Fabatins: new antimicrobial plant peptides. FEMS Microbiol Lett 1997;149(1):59–64.

130. Kokoska L, Janovska D. Chemistry and pharmacology of *Rhaponticum carthamoides*: A review. Phytochemistry 2009;70(7):842–855.

131. Bachert C, et al. Treatment of acute rhinosinusitis with the preparation from *Pelargonium sidoides* EPs 7630: a randomized, double-blind, placebo-controlled trial. Rhinology 2009;47(1):51–58.

132. Lizogub VG, et al. Efficacy of a pelargonium sidoides preparation in patients with the common cold: a randomized, double blind, placebo-controlled clinical trial. Explore (NY) 2007;3(6):573–584.

133. Heuser G, Vojdani A. Enhancement of natural killer cell activity and T and B cell function by buffered vitamin C in patients exposed to toxic chemicals: the role of protein kinase-C. Immunopharmacol Immunotoxicol 1997;19(3):291–312.

134. Murray MT. A comprehensive review of Vitamin C. American Journal of Natural Medicine 1996;3:8–21.

135. Unal M, et al. Serum levels of antioxidant vitamins, copper, zinc and magnesium in children with chronic rhinosinusitis. J Trace Elem Med Biol 2004;18(2):189–192.

136. Podoshin L, et al. Treatment of perennial allergic rhinitis with ascorbic acid solution. Ear Nose Throat J 1991;70(1):54–55.

137. Flamand N, et al. Histamine-induced inhibition of leukotriene biosynthesis in human neutrophils: involvement of the H2 receptor and cAMP. Br J Pharmacol 2004;141(4):552–561.

138. Mittman P. Randomized, double-blind study of freeze-dried *Urtica dioica* in the treatment of allergic rhinitis. Planta Med 1990;56(1):44–47.

139. Demling RH. Nutrition, anabolism, and the wound healing process: an overview. Eplasty 2009;9:e9.

140. Barbul A, Purtill WA. Nutrition in wound healing. Clin Dermatol 1994;12(1):133–140.

141. Ross AC, Ternus ME. Vitamin A as a hormone: recent advances in understanding the actions of retinol, retinoic acid, and beta carotene. J Am Diet Assoc 1993;93(11):1285–1290;quiz 1291–1292.

142. Osiecki H. The nutrient bible. 6th edn. Eagle Farm: Bio concepts Publishing, 2004.

143. Kohlmeier M. Nutrient metabolism. Oxford: Elsevier, 2003.

144. McCullough FS, et al. The effect of vitamin A on epithelial integrity. Proc Nutr Soc 1999;58(2):289–293.

145. Donesky-Cuenco D, et al. Yoga therapy decreases dyspnea-related distress and improves functional performance in people with chronic obstructive pulmonary disease: a pilot study. J Altern Complement Med 2009;15(3):225–234.

146. Pomidori L, et al. Efficacy and tolerability of yoga breathing in patients with chronic obstructive pulmonary disease: a pilot study. J Cardiopulm Rehabil Prev 2009;29(2):133–137.

147. Lee MS, et al. Acupuncture for allergic rhinitis: a systematic review. Ann Allergy Asthma Immunol 2009;102(4):269–279;quiz 279–281, 307.

148. Fleckenstein J, et al. Impact of acupuncture on vasomotor rhinitis: a randomized placebo-controlled pilot study. J Altern Complement Med 2009;15(4):391–398.

149. Suzuki M, et al. The effect of acupuncture in the treatment of chronic obstructive pulmonary disease. J Altern Complement Med 2008;14(9):1097–1105.

150. Jobst K, et al. Controlled trial of acupuncture for disabling breathlessness. Lancet 1986;2(8521–8522):1416–1419.

151. Lau KS, Jones AY. A single session of Acu-TENS increases FEV$_1$ and reduces dyspnoea in patients with chronic obstructive pulmonary disease: a randomised, placebo-controlled trial. Aust J Physiother 2008;54(3):179–184.

152. Wilkinson IS, et al. A randomised-controlled trial examining the effects of reflexology of patients with chronic obstructive pulmonary disease (COPD). Complement Ther Clin Pract 2006;12(2):141–147.

153. Beeken JE, et al. The effectiveness of neuromuscular release massage therapy in five individuals with chronic obstructive lung disease. Clin Nurs Res 1998;7(3):309–325.

154. Sheffner AL, et al. The in vitro reduction in viscosity of human tracheobronchial secretions by acetylcysteine. Am Rev Respir Dis 1964;90:721–729.

155. Sadowska AM, et al. Antioxidant and anti-inflammatory efficacy of NAC in the treatment of COPD: discordant in vitro and in vivo dose-effects: a review. Pulm Pharmacol Ther 2007;20(1):9–22.

156. Buechi S, et al. Open trial to assess aspects of safety and efficacy of a combined herbal cough syrup with ivy and thyme. Forsch Komplementarmed Klass Naturheilkd 2005;12(6):328–332.

157. Rabago D, et al. The efficacy of hypertonic saline nasal irrigation for chronic sinonasal symptoms. Otolaryngol Head Neck Surg 2005;133(1):3–8.

158. Rabago D, et al. Qualitative aspects of nasal irrigation use by patients with chronic sinus disease in a multimethod study. Ann Fam Med 2006;4(4):295–301.

159. Raza T, et al. Nasal lavage with sodium hypochlorite solution in *Staphylococcus aureus* persistent rhinosinusitis. Rhinology 2008;46(1):15–22.

160. Lim M, et al. Topical antimicrobials in the management of chronic rhinosinusitis: a systematic review. Am J Rhinol 2008;22(4):381–389.

161. Matthys H, et al. Efficacy and tolerability of myrtol standardized in acute bronchitis. A multi-centre, randomised, double-blind, placebo-controlled parallel group clinical trial vs. cefuroxime and ambroxol. Arzneimittelforschung 2000;50(8):700–711.

Section 3 Cardiovascular system

The cardiovascular system is essential for life, penetrating throughout the body with its counterpart, the central nervous system. The cardiovascular system consists of an intricate network of arteries, veins and capillaries, which pump blood throughout the body, delivering life-sustaining oxygen and nutrients and removing metabolic waste.

Cardiovascular disease accounts for the highest mortality and morbidity rate in the developed world. The organ systems involved in cardiovascular system disorders observed in clinical practice include the heart (left ventricular hypertrophy, endocardial scarring, congestive heart failure and coronary insufficiency); the large and medium sized arteries (accelerated atherosclerosis, aneurysm formation—with or without dissection); the brain (ischaemia, haemorrhagic and thrombotic infarction); and the kidneys (nephrosclerosis, with or without renal failure). Due to this, the treatment approach to cardiovascular system diseases is underpinned by the understanding of the systemic link between the cardiovascular and renal systems.

Of the known cardiovascular risk factors, hypertension is the most prevalent, with many cases remaining either undiagnosed or untreated. Approximately half of all untreated cases of hypertension develop end-organ damage over a period of 7–10 years; preventive or expedient treatment is therefore vital. Atherosclerosis also remains a major cause of death and premature disability in developed societies. Hardening and damage of the coronary arteries may cause myocardial infarction and angina pectoris, and in the central nervous system it may provoke strokes and transient ischaemic attacks. In the peripheral arteries atherosclerosis is associated with intermittent claudication and gangrene, jeopardising limb viability, and potentially causing renal artery stenosis in the kidneys. Patients should be advised that atherogenesis does not generally occur in a smooth, linear fashion and typically occurs over a period of many years—usually decades. This again cements the importance of holistic preventive strategies to be used early, in conjunction with corrective treatment and management.

Cardiovascular conditions can be positively influenced by lifestyle modifications such as reducing risk factors (such as alcohol, being overweight or smoking) and promoting healthy behaviours—including diet and exercise. Epidemiological evidence has demonstrated that the 'Mediterranean diet' has a cardioprotective effect, so the recommendation of incorporating into the patient's diet garlic, red wine, complex carbohydrates, fruits, vegetables and olive oil (in addition to deep-sea fatty fish) is always a good starting point. Various nutritional interventions, including omega-3 fatty acids, vitamins B, C and E and minerals such as zinc, calcium and magnesium, have been shown to have positive effects on cardiovascular system health. Botanical medicines such as *Crataegus oxyacantha* also have evidentiary support. Educating patients that these are non-static, chronic conditions that may progress as they age is also paramount. The heart has traditionally been associated with emotion and many treatments aimed at improving emotional and psychological wellbeing will also be of benefit.

Naturopathic medicine has at its disposal a variety of effective specific interventions depending on the cardiovascular system condition. Such interventions may focus on increasing diuresis, promoting a vascular protective effect, altering lipid profile and effecting an anxiolytic/relaxant response. Principal protocols to assist in the management of venous conditions usually involve increasing microcirculation and improving vascular integrity. When treating cardiovascular conditions practitioners need to remind their patients that, even though wholesale changes can produce significant short to medium term health benefits, they need to view all treatment as a long-term solution that should be integrated into their lifestyle.

This section will focus on those conditions expected to be most commonly encountered in contemporary clinical naturopathic practice, as well as focusing on treatment principles that may significantly reduce the risk of a person developing acute cardiovascular events.

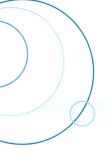

9

Atherosclerosis and dyslipidaemia

Michael Alexander
ND, BPharm

EPIDEMIOLOGY AND AETIOLOGY

The association between elevated serum cholesterol and coronary heart disease (CHD) was first reported in the 1930s, and subsequent large epidemiologic studies confirmed the strong relationship between serum cholesterol and CHD.[1–3] Current predictions estimate that by the year 2020 cardiovascular diseases, notably atherosclerosis, will become the leading global cause of total disease burden.[4] Lipoprotein disorders or dyslipidaemias are common and are an important risk factor for coronary artery disease and all types of atherosclerotic vascular disease.[5] Cardiovascular risk was found to be positively associated with low-density lipoprotein (LDL-C) levels and inversely with high density lipoprotein (HDL-C) levels.[6] The relationship between fasting serum triglyceride (TG) and cardiovascular risk has been confounded by the inverse association between TG and HDL-C, as well as by the association of TG with other risk factors such as diabetes mellitus and body mass (see Table 9.1).[6] Triglycerides alone are now considered an important independent predictor of cardiovascular risk.[1]

Atherosclerosis affects various regions of the circulation and will present with unique clinical symptoms depending on the particular vascular bed affected. In coronary arteries it causes myocardial infarction and angina, whereas stroke and transient cerebral ischaemia can occur when it is present in the arteries of the nervous system.[2,7] In the peripheral circulation it can result in intermittent claudication and gangrene, which can jeopardise limb viability.[4]

Atherogenesis or the pathogenesis of atherosclerosis usually occurs over decades in a discontinuous fashion with relative periods of quiescence punctuated with periods of rapid evolution.[3] The eventual clinical manifestation may be chronic, as is the case in angina, or acute, such as a heart attack or stroke or sudden death. Regardless, individuals may live with atherosclerosis and experience no symptoms or reduced life expectancy and morbidity.

The 'fatty streak' represents the initial lesion, usually due to focal increases in the density of lipoproteins within the region of the intima of a blood vessel; hence the reason for vigilance in maintaining low levels of these particles in the bloodstream.[8] The

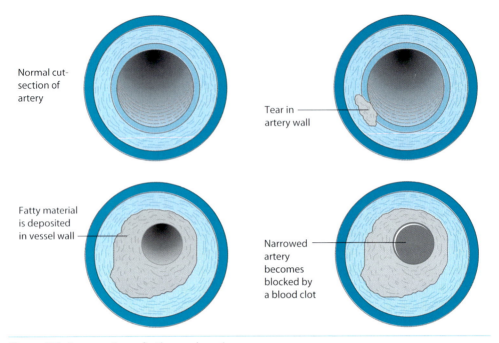

Figure 9.1 Progression of atherosclerosis

lipoproteins often associate with glycosaminoglycans in the arterial extracellular matrix and become more 'fixed' in the vasculature. These lipoprotein macromolecules undergo oxidative modifications, giving rise to hydroperoxides, lysophospholipids, oxysterols and aldehydic breakdown products.[4] Constituents of oxidatively modified LDL-C can augment expression of leukocyte adhesion molecules, recruiting leukocytes and macrophages into the area, which undergoes inflammation.[9]

Areas of inflammation produce altered laminar flow in the arteries affected, and reduce the production of nitric oxide, which is locally both vasodilatory and anti-inflammatory. The inflammatory process eventually penetrates or tears the endothelial layer with the products of lipoprotein oxidation, inducing cytokines and tumour necrosis factor alpha (TNF-α) released from the vascular cell walls.[4] Once inside the walls of the artery mononuclear phagocytes mature into macrophages and become foam cells.

The cytokines and TNF-α produce growth factors that induce the smooth muscle to produce local growth factors such as platelet-derived growth factor and fibroblast growth factors.[9] This fibro-fatty material recruits more smooth muscle cells into the intima from the tunica media layer of the vessel. At this point transforming growth factor beta (TGF-β), amongst other mediators, stimulates collagen production by the smooth muscle cells transforming the fatty streak into a more fibrous smooth-muscle cell and extracellular-rich lesion.[4] In addition to this process products of blood coagulation and thrombosis contribute to athroma evolution, which justifies the alternative term for the process, 'atherothrombosis' (see Figure 9.1).

Unfortunately the prevalence of traditional risk factors is almost as high in those without cardiovascular disease as in subsequently affected individuals.[1] Recently, several novel key biomarkers have been implicated in the pathology of atherosclerosis. There are several, but the more commonly researched include C-reactive protein (CRP), homocysteine (Hcy) and indicators of oxidative stress.[8,10]

Table 9.1 Common secondary causes of dyslipidaemia

CAUSE	EFFECT ON LIPID PROFILE
Hypothyroidism Nephrotic syndrome Cholestasis Anorexia nervosa	Increased LDL-C
Type 2 diabetes Obesity Renal impairment Smoking	Increased TG and/or decreased HDL-C
Alcohol use Oestrogen use	Increased TG, HDL-C may increase rather than decrease; cardiovascular risk may not be increased

Source: Therapeutic Guidelines (Cardiovascular).[17]

C-reactive protein (CRP)

CRP is a calcium-binding pentameric protein consisting of five identical, non-covalently linked 23-kDa subunits.[1] It is present in trace amounts in humans and appears to have been highly conserved over hundreds of millions of years. It is synthesised primarily by hepatocytes in response to activation of several cytokines, such as interleukins 1 and 6, and TNF-α.[1] In healthy people in the absence of active inflammatory states, CRP levels are usually below 1 mg/L. CRP is expressed in atherosclerotic plaque and may enhance expression of local adhesion molecules, increase expression of endothelial plasminogen activation inhibitor 1, reduce endo-thelial nitric oxide bioactivity and alter low-density lipoprotein (LDL) cholesterol by macrophages.[10]

Homocysteine (Hcy)

The homocysteine theory of arteriosclerosis attributes one of the underlying causes of vascular disease to elevation of blood homocysteine concentrations as the result of dietary, genetic, metabolic, hormonal or toxic factors.[11] Dietary deficiency of vitamin B6 and folic acid and absorptive deficiency of vitamin B12, which result from tradi-tional food processing or abnormal absorption of B vitamins, are important factors in causing elevations in blood homocysteine.[11,10] It is believed that homocysteinylation of lipoproteins increases their atherogenicity and hence their cytotoxic effects on endothe-lial tissue.[12] It is hypothesised that oxidative stress and methylative modification is the mechanism by which Hcy is pro-atherosclerotic.[13]

Oxidative stress

Endothelial dysfunction is the initial step in the pathogenesis of atherosclerosis.[14,15] Nitric oxide (NO) plays an important role in the regulation of vascular tone and the suppression of smooth muscle cell proliferation. An increase in oxidative stress inac-tivates NO, impairing endothelium-dependent vasodilation and creating endothelial dysfunction.[16] Dyslipidaemia may be primary or secondary. The secondary causes are shown in Table 9.1, and should be looked for in patients and treated appropriately. If secondary causes have been excluded, primary dyslipidaemia due to genetic and envi-ronmental (particularly dietary) factors is diagnosed.[17]

RISK FACTORS

The general risk factors applicable to atherosclerosis relate to lifestyle choices and genetics. Overall estimates of the heritability of myocardial infarction, one of the major clinical outcomes of atherosclerosis, have varied widely, ranging from very little to greater than 50%.[18,19] It is important to note that heritability varies from population to population. In populations in which the environment is relatively homogeneous, for example in Iceland, genetics will tend to predominate, whereas in populations exhibiting large environmental differences, for example in Los Angeles, genetics are relatively less important.[1] The known risk factors for atherosclerosis generally exhibit very significant heritability estimates as well (see Figure 9.2). Smoking and alcohol consumption as well as a diet rich in refined sugars and saturated fats will adversely influence the condition (see the box below).[20] Hypertension, diabetes and obesity have a pronounced negative influence on the disease.[1] Exercise is also a significant factor.[3] In women the protective effects of oestrogen are greatly diminished in menopause.[1] There are several medical conditions that drastically increase the risk associated with this condition, and all of these may cause altered blood fat profiles as secondary to their primary condition.

The influence of environmental factors on lipoprotein metabolism and cardiovascular disease has been dramatically revealed by comparisons of different populations.[3] Studies have shown that intrauterine under-nutrition is associated with obesity and other detrimental metabolic characteristics in adulthood.[1] In particular under-nutrition

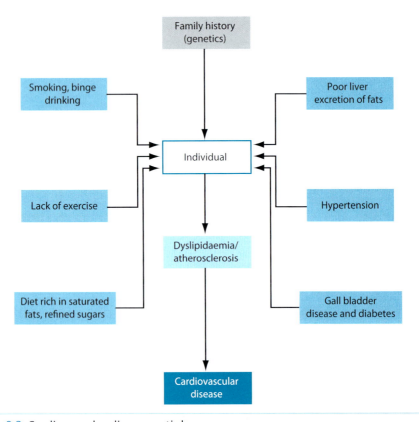

Figure 9.2 Cardiovascular disease aetiology

GENETIC AND ENVIRONMENTAL RISK FACTORS FOR CARDIOVASCULAR DISEASE[1]

Risk factors with a significant genetic component (h^2)
Total cholesterol (40–60%)
High-density-lipoprotein cholesterol (45–75%)
Total triglycerides (40–80%)
Body mass index (25–60%)
Systolic blood pressure (30–70%)
Diastolic blood pressure (30–65%)
Lipoprotein(a) levels (90%)
Homocysteine levels (45%)
Type 2 diabetes (40–80%)
Fibrinogen (20–50%)
C-reactive protein (~40%)
Myeloperoxidase
Carotid intima-media thickness (~40%)
Gender (100%)
Environmental risk factors
Smoking
Diet
Exercise
Infection
Fetal environment
Air pollution (particulates)

was associated with a premature onset of neonatal leptin surge, which appears to be involved in the formation of the energy-regulation circuits in the hypothalamus that affect metabolism in adults.[1]

CONVENTIONAL TREATMENT

The assessment of dyslipidaemia involves the measurement of fasting total cholesterol (TC), high density lipoprotein (HDL-C), low-density lipoprotein (LDL-C) and triglyceride (TG).[10] Fasting usually takes place from midnight prior to the blood test.

Dyslipidaemia is treated in cases of:
• LDL-C elevation and/or mild to moderate hypertriglyceridaemia (see Table 9.2), particularly if associated with reduced HDL-C (increases the risk of cardiovascular disease)
• TG exceeding 10 mmol/L (increases the risk of pancreatitis).

The question that needs to be addressed in relation to dyslipidaemia is: who should in fact be treated and when? Tables 9.3 and 9.4 list the current Australian medical protocols. The aim of treatment is to reduce the progression of atherosclerosis and improve survival rates of individuals. An even more important aim is to prevent myocardial infarct (heart attack) and stroke in patients with established cardiovascular disease. A reduction in triglyceride levels should prevent the occurrence of pancreatitis in susceptible individuals as well. Common pharmacological interventions are listed in Table 9.5.

Table 9.2 Target lipid levels

LDL-C < 2.5 mmol/L (< 2.0 mmol/L for high-risk patients with existing cardiovascular disease)
Total cholesterol < 4.0 mmol/L
HDL-C > 1.0 mmol/L
Triglycerides < 1.5 mmol/L

These target levels are adapted from the National Heart Foundation of Australia/Cardiac Society of Australia and New Zealand position statement on lipid management, 2005.

Source: Therapeutic Guidelines (Cardiovascular).[17]

Table 9.3 Patients at increased risk and warranting therapy, based on their fasting lipid levels

PATIENT CHARACTERISTICS	LIPID LEVEL (FASTING)
Diabetes mellitus, but the patient is not in the 'very high risk' category (see below).	Total cholesterol > 5.5 mmol/L
Aboriginal or Torres Strait Islander Hypertension	Total cholesterol > 6.5 mmol/L or total cholesterol > 5.5 mmol/L and HDL cholesterol < 1 mmol/L
HDL cholesterol < 1 mmol/L	Total cholesterol > 6.5 mmol/L
Familial hypercholesterolaemia identified by: • DNA mutation or • tendon xanthomas in the patient or their first- or second-degree relative Family history of coronary heart disease: • which has become symptomatic before the age of 60 years in one or more first degree relatives or • which has become symptomatic before the age of 50 years in one or more second degree relatives	If aged 18 years or less at treatment initiation: • LDL cholesterol > 4 mmol/L If aged more than 18 years at treatment initiation: • LDL cholesterol > 5 mmol/L or • total cholesterol > 6.5 mmol/L or • total cholesterol > 5.5 mmol/L and HDL cholesterol < 1 mmol/L
Patients not already identified who are: • male aged 35 to 75 years or • postmenopausal women aged up to 75 years	Total cholesterol > 7.5 mmol/L or triglyceride > 4 mmol/L
Patients not already identified	Total cholesterol > 9 mmol/L or triglyceride > 8 mmol/L

Source: Therapeutic Guidelines (Cardiovascular).[17]

KEY TREATMENT PROTOCOLS

Plasma total homocysteine (Hcy) has been associated with cardiovascular risk in multiple large-scale epidemiological studies, and it has been considered as an independent risk factor for atherosclerosis.[21] Evidence indicates that although mild hyper-Hcy may be regarded as a minor risk factor for CHD in low-risk patients, it can play a role in triggering new events in patients with known CHD, also by interacting with the

NATUROPATHIC TREATMENT AIMS

• Alter lipid profile via diet (reduced saturated/trans fats).
• Modify lifestyle.
• Exercise.
• Reduce excess homocysteine levels where appropriate.
• Reduce levels of C-reactive protein.

Table 9.4 Patients in the 'very high risk' category warranting therapy regardless of their fasting lipid levels

The following patients are in the 'very high risk' category, regardless of their fasting lipid levels:
• patients with symptomatic coronary heart, cerebrovascular, or peripheral vascular disease
• patients with diabetes mellitus who:
  – are aged 60 years or more, or
  – are Aboriginal or Torres Strait Islander, or
  – have microalbuminuria (urinary albumin excretion rate of > 20 µg/minute, or urinary albumin to creatinine ratio of > 2.5 [males], > 3.5 [females])
• patients who have a family history of premature coronary heart disease (one or more first degree relatives symptomatic before the age of 45 years, or two or more first degree relatives symptomatic before the age of 55 years).

Source: Therapeutic Guidelines (Cardiovascular).[17]

Table 9.5 Pharmacological treatment of dyslipidaemia

DRUG	BENEFIT	DISADVANTAGE
Statin	Reduces LDL-C by 30–50%. Best tolerated	Reduces coenzyme Q10
Bile-acid binding resin	Reduces LDL-C by 15–25%	Poorly tolerated, may worsen hypertriglyceridaemia
Nicotinic acid	Reduces LDL-C by 15–30%, triglycerides by 25–40%. Increases HDL-C by 20–35%	Causes severe flushing, which limits use
Ezetimibe	Reduces LDL-C by 18%. Well tolerated	Generally not used alone
Fibrate	Reduces LDL-C by 18%,* and triglycerides by 40–80%. Increases HDL-C by 10–30%	*Can increase LDL-C in some instances.

Source: Taken from Australian Medicines Handbook.[45]

'classical' CV risk factors.[21] The administration of vitamins **B6** (300 mg/day) and **B12** (250 µg/day) and **folic acid** (10 mg/day) over a 120-day period reduced plasma Hcy levels by 24%; this in turn resulted in a 28.5% reduction in coronary risk.[22] In a study of 23 patients with angiographically proven coronary artery disease, daily dosing with a multivitamin containing 0.65 mg folic acid, 150 mg alpha-tocopherol, 150 mg ascorbic acid, 12.5 mg beta-carotene and 0.4 mg B12 produced a 28% reduction in Hcy and a decrease in in vitro LDL oxidation of 39%.[23] However, in patients with stable coronary artery disease, Hcy-lowering therapy with B vitamins does not affect levels of inflammatory markers (CRP and soluble CD4 ligands CD40L) associated with atherogenesis.[24] After two months treatment with oral folic acid in 16 patients with insulin-dependent diabetes, plasma Hcy fell by 25%, however there was no difference in endothelial function or markers of oxidant stress.[25] There was however both a reduction in Hcy levels and an increase in endothelial function in a study of 60 patients receiving either 5 mg of folic acid or 600 mg of **N-acetylcysteine**.[26] Of interest is a small study in which 12 patients with coronary artery disease underwent therapy with high dose (10 mg daily) folic acid therapy. Whereas resting myocardial blood flow remained unchanged, stress myocardial blood flow and coronary flow reserve increased significantly along with reduction in Hcy.[27] **Phenolic compounds** from extra virgin olive oil (hydroxytyrosol, homovanillyl alcohol, caffeic acid and ferulic acid) in vivo significantly reduced homocysteine-induced endothelial dysfunction.[28]

C-reactive protein (CRP)

C-reactive protein (CRP) is an inflammatory protein that may play a role in the pathogenesis of atherosclerosis. Evidence now suggests that a single nucleotide polymorphism that results in the CRP-757C allele may be responsible for an increase in the intima thickness in the carotid arteries of cardiovascular patients.[29] Loss of body fat has a positive correlation with lower CRP levels. A study of 33 obese subjects over 20 weeks showed a 35% reduction in CRP levels only after significant loss of body fat; this reduction was maintained for the duration of the study.[30] In epidemiological trials high fibre intakes have consistently been associated with reduction in cardiovascular disease risk and CRP levels. A data synthesis of seven clinical trials reported significantly lower CRP concentrations in six of them in the vicinity of 25–54% through increased dietary fibre consumption with dosages ranging between 3.3 and 7.8 g/MJ.[31] Inflammatory reactions in coronary plaques play an important role in the pathogenesis of acute atherothrombotic events. The association of serum CRP with the incidence of first major coronary heart disease (CHD) event was studied in 936 men.[32] The results indicated that there was a prognostic significance to raised CRP and CHD events.[32] Antioxidants may play a role in reducing levels of CRP. **Vitamin C** supplementation at 515 mg daily reduced CRP levels by 24%.[33] **Alpha-tocopherol** (vitamin E) supplementation (especially at higher doses) in human subjects and animal models has been shown to be both antioxidant and anti-inflammatory, decreasing C-reactive protein (CRP) and the release of pro-inflammatory cytokines such as chemokines IL-8 and PAI-1.[34]

Oxidative stress

Oxidative stress plays a pivotal role in atherogenesis, and some antioxidants, such as **lipoic acid**, can have an effect on attenuating dyslipidaemia. Supplementation with lipoic acid induced decreases in lipid peroxidation, plasma cholesterol, triacylglycerols and low-density lipoprotein cholesterol, and an increase in high-density lipoprotein in mice fed a high fat diet.[35] Similarly, rabbits on a high-cholesterol diet had significantly lower levels of LDL-C and total cholesterol when given 4.2 mg/kg of lipoic acid daily.[36] It is posited that lipoic acid reduces oxidative stress by increasing free radical scavenger enzyme expression in the cell.[35] A combination of omega-3 fatty acids, vitamin E, gamma oryzanol and niacin produced significant improvements in lipid profiles in a study amongst 57 participants.[37] In mice **vitamin E** has a modest effect at best on experimental atherosclerosis, and only in situations of severe vitamin E deficiency.[38] However, the benefits of vitamin E may be due to its effects on smooth muscle proliferation. Cell culture studies have shown that alpha-tocopherol brings about inhibition of smooth muscle cell proliferation. This takes place via inhibition of protein kinase C activity. Alpha-tocopherol also inhibits LDL-induced smooth muscle cell proliferation and protein kinase C activity.[39] Forty-four patients undergoing outpatient treatment for atherosclerosis with simvastatin 10 mg were administered 90 mg of **coenzyme Q10** for 12 weeks. The positive effects of coenzyme Q10 were particularly expressed in relation to the antiatherogenic fraction of cholesterol, which increased by 23%. The index of atherogenicity decreased by 27%. At the background of coenzyme Q10 treatment 30% reduction in plasma lipoperoxide levels occurred, demonstrating the potentially independent role of coenzyme Q10 in the positive modification of oxidative stress.[40] A study of 21 patients using 60 mg of coenzyme Q10 alone demonstrated its potentially independent role in the positive modification of oxidative stress, antiatherogenic fraction of the lipid profile, atherogenic ratio and platelet aggregatability.[41]

Polygonum multiflorum stilbene-glycoside is a water-soluble fraction of *Polygonum multiflorum*, a traditional Chinese herbal medicines, and has protective effects on the cardiovascular system. Rabbits fed for 12 weeks on a high-cholesterol diet and *Polygonum multiflorum* stilbene-glycoside had a decrease in the atherosclerotic lesioned area of 43% when given 50 mg/kg, and 60% when given 100 mg/kg.[42] This was possibly due to reductions in intercellular adhesion molecule-1 protein and the vascular endothelial growth factor.

Cocoa is rich in plant-derived flavonoids, which have a therapeutic benefit in atherosclerosis. In humans, flavonol-rich cocoa counteracts lipid peroxidation and therefore lowers the plasma level of F2-isoprostanes, markers of in vivo lipid peroxidation, and plasma levels of oxidised LDL in hypercholesterolaemic patients.[43]

Alteration of lipid profile with natural products

Nicotinic acid, or niacin, has established efficacy for the treatment of dyslipidaemia, but the clinical use of niacin has been limited by cutaneous flushing, a well-recognised associated adverse effect. Flushing has been cited as the main reason for the discontinuation of niacin therapy, estimated at rates as high as 25–40%.[44] It has good LDL- and triglyceride-lowering effects and produces a marked increase in HDL (typically reduces LDL by 15–30% and triglycerides by 25–40%, and increases HDL by 20–35%).[45] Niacin promotes angiographic regression when used in combination with other drugs that lower LDL cholesterol and can reduce cardiovascular risk in patients with coronary heart disease.[46] The *Therapeutic Guidelines*[17] recommend daily dosing of 500 mg slowly increasing to 3 g daily.

Policosanol is a mixture of higher primary aliphatic alcohols purified from sugarcane wax with cholesterol-lowering effects proven in patients with type II hypercholesterolaemia and dyslipidaemia due to type 2 diabetes mellitus.[47] A once-daily dose of 5 mg has been shown to reduce LDL-C by 32.6% after 12 weeks as well as improve lipid ratios in a cohort of adolescents.[47] The effects of policosanol were compared to those of lovastatin in patients with dyslipidaemia and type 2 diabetes in a randomised double-blind study. A daily dose of 10 mg of policosanol for 8 weeks lowered LDL-C by 29.9%, TC by 21.1% and TGs by 13.6%.[48] Policosanol (10 mg/day) was slightly more effective than lovastatin (20 mg/day) in reducing the LDL-C/HDL-C and total cholesterol/HDL-C ratios, in increasing HDL-C levels and in preventing LDL oxidation.[48] However a double-blind, randomised, placebo-controlled trial amongst 70 patients contradicted previous evidence. The addition of 10 mg policosanol daily to a dietetic regimen failed to produce any significant change in BMI, TC, HDL-C, LDL-C and TG plasma levels.[49] In a double-blind, randomised, placebo-controlled trial of 68 patients with primary hypercholesterolaemia, a daily dose of policosanol 20 mg over 8 weeks did not produce any significant change in the parameters mentioned above.[50]

Allium sativum (garlic) and many of its preparations have been widely recognised as effective in the prevention and treatment of atherosclerosis and other risk factors for cardiovascular disease. Studies have suggested a multitude of physiological effects, including inhibition of platelet activity and increased levels of antioxidant enzymes.[51] Garlic has been shown to inhibit the enzymes involved in lipid synthesis, decrease platelet aggregation, prevent lipid peroxidation of oxidised erythrocytes and LDL, increase antioxidant status, and inhibit angiotensin-converting enzyme.[52] A small study involving the administration of 600 mg fish oil with 500 mg garlic oil daily concluded that the total cholesterol, low-density lipoprotein, serum triglyceride, very low-density lipoprotein and the total cholesterol:high-density lipoprotein ratio decreased by 20%, 21%, 37%, 36.7% and 23.4%, respectively, and the high-density lipoprotein increased by 5.1% after 60 days of supplementation.[53] A single-blind, placebo-controlled study concluded after 6 weeks of garlic supplementation that TC, LDL-C and TG all decreased by 12.1%, 17.3% and 6.3% respectively, while HDL-C rose by 15.7%. In newly diagnosed dyslipidaemia in type 2 diabetics, 600 mg of garlic daily resulted in 12.03% reduction in total cholesterol, 17.99% reduction in LDL-C as well as an 8.81% increase in HDL-C levels.[54] Long-term results, however, may not be as promising. In its evidence report on garlic, the Agency for Health Care Research and Quality reviewed 37 randomised trials and found that garlic preparations lowered total cholesterol by small amounts in the short term, but no reduction was observed at 6 months.[51]

The principal **essential fatty acids** in fish oil are eicosapentaenoic acid (EPA) and docosahexaenoic acid (DHA).[55] Fish oil has been reported to have anti-inflammatory and immunosuppressive effects, and EPA competitively inhibits synthesis of thromboxane A2. Both EPA and DHA interfere with prostaglandin synthesis in platelets and blood vessels, resulting in decreased platelet activity.[55]

The beneficial effect of dietary fish oil on plasma triglycerides is thought to be related to the high quantities of omega-3 polyunsaturated fatty acids found in many types of fish.[17] In an attempt to further explain the mechanism of action of fish oil, a study of a fish oil-rich diet administered to apolipoprotein E-deficient mice resulted in reduced adhesion molecule expression in atherosclerotic lesions.[56] Because these molecules are involved in lesion progression, the effect of fish oil may explain the observed decrease in atherogenesis. There is now considerable evidence that omega-3 fatty acid treatment at the prescription strength of 4 g/day effectively and safely lowers triglyceride levels and increases low-density lipoprotein size, as well as affecting high-density lipoprotein metabolism.[57] Daily doses of > 6 capsules are required to reduce triglyceride concentrations for brands where a 1 g capsule contains 300 mg of omega-3 fatty acids (180 mg eicosapentaenoic acid and 120 mg docosahexaenoic acid).[45]

Cocoa butter, a fat derived from cocoa plants and found predominantly in dark chocolate, contains an average of 33% monounsaturated oleic acid and 33% stearic acid.[43] In hypertensive patients, daily consumption of 100 g flavonoid-rich chocolate over 2 weeks led to a significant 12% reduction of serum total and LDL cholesterol levels. Moreover, cocoa appears to inhibit LDL oxidation.[43]

Promoting liver choleresis

Bile acids and their salts are essential in the management of cholesterol levels. They are synthesised from cholesterol in the liver. There are three groups: primary (cholic and chenodeoxycholic acids and their salts); secondary, made from the action of bacteria on primary bile salts (deoxycholate and lithocholate); and tertiary, the result of modifications of secondary bile salts (sulfate ester of lithocholate, ursodeoxycholate and 7-β-epimer of chenodeoxycholate).[58] Saponins have been implicated in interference with the absorption of cholesterol, bile acids and fats and have shown potential in the reduction of blood cholesterol levels.[58] Their cholesterol-lowering effect may also be linked to their binding of bile salts and increasing their faecal excretion.

Choleretics stimulate bile production by hepatocytes and most have effective cholagogue properties as well.[58] One such compound is *Cynara scolymus*. A study of 75 normal and moderately hypercholesterolaemic volunteers reduced plasma cholesterol

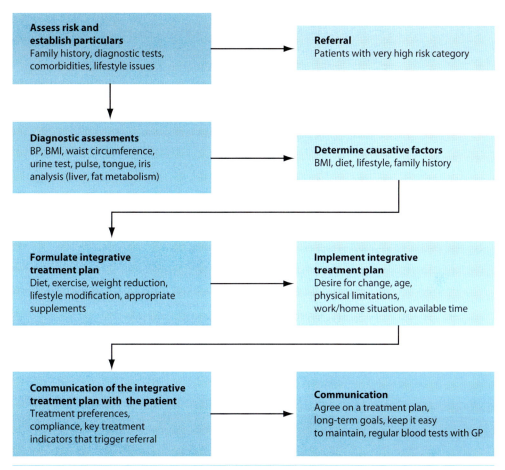

Figure 9.3 Naturopathic treatment decision tree—atherosclerosis and dyslipidaemia

by 4.2% with daily intake of *C. scolymus* of 1280 mg daily for 12 weeks.[59] In 2004 an in vitro study of an artichoke leaf extract increased the activity of an endothelial nitric oxide synthase (eNOS) promoter.[60] The compounds thought responsible were the flavonoids luteolin and cynaroside, with the activity suspected to occur through an increase in eNOS gene transcription.[60] Apart from this choleretic activity *C. scolymus* has long been known for its antioxidant ability. The antioxidant activity of the herbal medicine was confirmed by its in vitro inhibition of LDL oxidation in rats. It also raised levels of glutathione peroxidase activity.[61] A methanolic extract of *C. scolymus* was found to suppress serum triglyceride elevation in olive loaded mice, with the components responsible identified as sesquiterpenes (cynaropicrin, aguerin B and grosheimin) together with new sesquiterpene glycosides (cynarascolosides A, B and C).[62] ***Curcuma comosa*** is an indigenous plant of Thailand, and has been traditionally and widely used as an anti-inflammatory agent for the treatment of postpartum uterine bleeding and uterine inflammation.[63] The administration of an ethyl acetate extract to hypercholesterolaemic hamsters (0–500 mg/kg for 7 days) resulted in a decrease in both plasma triglyceride and cholesterol levels in a dose-dependent manner.[64] Plasma HDL-C was increased and LDL-C was reduced; there is also a choleretic effect.[64]

INTEGRATIVE MEDICAL CONSIDERATIONS

Current evidence tentatively supports yoga, acupuncture and traditional Chinese medicine in the treatment of cardiovascular disease. Yoga retarded progression and increased regression of coronary atherosclerosis in patients with severe coronary artery disease.[65] Acupuncture and moxibustion improved the plaque of carotid atherosclerosis, so as to alleviate and prevent the development of ischaemic cerebrovascular disease.[66] A study of the press needle technique repeated 200 times up to four times a day showed a reduction in triglycerides, homocysteine and CRP.[67] A small study (40 patients) showed the return to normal levels of plasma endothelin, nitric oxide and raised apoprotein after treatment with collateral circulation in a limb affected by atherosclerosis increased significantly as well.[68]

Case Study

A 62-year-old woman is seeking treatment options after being diagnosed with **atherosclerosis** via angiography and stress testing. She is not obese and is a non-smoker. She was also diagnosed with **high cholesterol** after a blood test: **triglycerides (fasting) 2.0, total cholesterol 7.1 mmol/L, HDL 2.0 mmol/L and LDL 4.2 mmol/L.**

SUGGESTIVE SIGNS AND SYMPTOMS

Atherosclerosis	Dyslipidaemia
Hardening of the arterial tissue (revealed by medical tests)	Fasting blood levels of: • triglycerides ≥ 1.7 mmol/L • total cholesterol ≥ 5.5 mmol/L • HDL-C (M) ≤ 0.9 mmol/L (W) ≤ 1.0 mmol/L • LDL-C ≥ 3.4 mmol/L

Example treatment

Prescription

As a minimum all patients should be given dietary advice. This includes enriching their diet with a good source of fibre, both soluble and insoluble, between 10 and 60 g daily.[69,70] Smoking should be ceased,[71,33] and alcohol intake should be reduced to a moderate level (1–2 glasses of wine daily) at a minimum.[72] Binge drinking, particularly with beer and spirits, should be discouraged. The optimal level of exercise is the equivalent of 30 minutes daily of an intensity at 65–80% peak oxygen consumption.[73,74] *Cynara scolymus* is beneficial as an antioxidant and choleretic.[59,61] It reduced the oxidative effects on plasma lipids at the same time as reducing their levels.[62] The effect on nitric oxide adds a vasodilator dimension to its actions.[60] *Allium sativum* is beneficial for both its anti-thrombotic activity and its ability to modify lipid components, in raising HDL-C levels and reducing both TG and LDL-C fractions in the blood.[54,52] *Crataegus oxyacantha* possesses many cardiovascular benefits, particularly the ability to reduce resting diastolic blood pressure and heart rate as well as potent antioxidant activity. Coenzyme Q10 has a

Herbal prescription

Cynara scolymus tablets 1 x 4 g b.d.
Allium sativum tablets 1 x 2 g b.d.
Crataegus oxyacantha tablets 1 x 1 g b.d.

Nutritional prescription

Coenzyme Q10 100 mg daily
Policosanol 10 mg b.d.
Omega-3 fish oil 3 g b.d.

positive effect in reducing oxidative stress as well as other antiatherogenic effects.[40,41] Policosanol has a more definite therapeutic application, particularly in reducing the more harmful blood fat fractions such as LDL-C, TG and total cholesterol (TC).[47,48] Fish oil is prescribed to modify plasma lipid profiles to increase HDL-C levels while reducing LDL-C and TG fractions at the same time.[57,45] Its ability to reduce platelet aggregation makes it particularly good for patients at risk of infarction and stroke. The liquids available to practitioners may contain almost 2.8 g of omega-3 fatty acids per 5 mL; this makes it easy to use doses of approximately 6 g (equivalent to 6 × 1000 mg capsules) daily. At this level profound changes may occur to blood lipid profiles.

Dietary and lifestyle modification

Irrespective of whether an individual is in a high-risk category, dietary treatment should be the first line of therapy for dyslipidaemia. Naturally most protocols are centred on fat reduction and an increase in fibre intake. The National Cholesterol Education Program Adult Treatment Panel III (ATP III)[75] recommends a low saturated fat diet with nutritional supplementation (fish oil, oat bran or plant sterol). These diets generally lowered total cholesterol TC (7–18%) and LDL-C (7–15%) concentrations respectively.[75] Intake of dietary fibre lowers plasma lipids. Soluble fibre lowers serum TC and LDL-C without significant alteration in serum HDL-C and TG.[70] Subjects taking 45 g of oats daily as part of a low caloric diet for 6 weeks had significant reductions in both total cholesterol and LDL-C.[69] A trial in 2008 compared a low-fat diet with a very low carbohydrate diet. Each diet provided around 1500 kcal daily and around 20–30 g protein. The diets differed in the amount of carbohydrate, being 12% for the low-carbohydrate diet and 56% for the low fat diet. The low-carbohydrate diet was higher in fats, particularly omega-6 fatty acids. The very low carbohydrate diet resulted in profound alterations in fatty acid composition and reduced inflammation compared to a low-fat diet, as well as reducing atherosclerosis.[76]

Lifestyle advice includes alcohol and smoking reduction. The importance of smoking as a risk factor for coronary heart disease is beyond doubt. Free radicals in cigarette smoke cause oxidative damage to proteins, DNA and lipids, contributing to the pathobiology of atherosclerosis, heart disease and cancer. As an exercise to estimate the magnitude of risk reduction, a review of 20 independent studies was undertaken.[71] Cessation of smoking was associated with a substantial reduction in risk of all-cause mortality among patients with CHD of 36%.[71] Both active and passive smoking raise plasma levels of CRP.[33] This causes oxidative damage to vascular endothelium via raised plasma fats. Light to moderate alcohol intake is known to have cardioprotective properties; however, the magnitude of protection depends on other factors and may be confined to some subsets of the population.[72] This cardioprotective effect seems to be larger among middle-aged and elderly adults than young adults. The levels of alcohol at which the risk of CHD is lowest and the levels of alcohol at which the risk of CHD exceeds the risk among abstainers are lower for women than for men. There is evidence to suggest that wine may have more beneficial effects than beer and distilled spirits, with drinking patterns producing greater risk reduction through steady versus binge drinking.[72]

At the patient's age, a vigorous exercise program is recommended to be based on her physical ability (after medical consultation). Exercise is well known to have positive effects on lipid levels. A 2002 study attempted to ascertain the level of exercise required to produce optimal benefits. A level of exercise equivalent to jogging 32.0 km per week at 65 to 80% of peak oxygen consumption resulted in greater improvements than did the lower amounts of exercise, which were the equivalent of jogging

Table 9.6 Review of the major evidence

INTERVENTION	METHODOLOGY	RESULT	COMMENT
Lipoic acid[35]	Mice were randomly assigned to one of three groups ($n = 8$). One group was fed a normal diet and two groups were fed with a high-fat diet (21.45% fat, w/w). After 6 wk, plasma lipid level and antioxidant status were examined.	High-fat diet resulted in alterations in lipid profiles and a depressed antioxidant defence system. Lipoic acid up-regulated the expression of genes related to beta-oxidation and free radical scavenger enzymes, whereas those involved in cholesterol synthesis were down-regulated.	Lipoic acid can prevent: • high-fat diet-induced dyslipidaemia by modulating lipid metabolism, by increasing beta-oxidation and decreasing cholesterol synthesis, and • oxidative stress by increasing those of free radical scavenger enzyme gene expression.
Exercise on CHD and lipids[73]	Systematic review from approximately 4500 individuals in earlier meta-analyses to 8440 (7683 contributing to the total mortality outcome).	Pooled effect produced a 27% reduction in all-cause mortality. Total cardiac mortality was reduced by 31%. Reduction in total cholesterol and LDL.	It is not clear from this review whether exercise only or a comprehensive cardiac rehabilitation intervention is more beneficial.
Combined dietary supplementation[37]	57 dyslipidaemic volunteers were randomly assigned to receive: placebo, PUFA n-3 and vitamin E, the same as B plus gamma-oryzanol and niacin. Lipid profile, reactive oxygen species, total antioxidant capacity, vitamin E, IL1-beta) TNF-α and thromboxane B2 were determined at baseline (t_0) and after 4 months (t_1).	All dyslipidaemic subjects showed, at baseline, oxidative stress and after 4 months all biochemical markers improved significantly in groups treated with dietary supplementation.	Combining different compounds, which protect each other and act together at different levels of the lipid chain production, improves lipid profile, inflammatory and oxidative status, allowing the dose of each compound to be reduced under the threshold of its side effects.
Allium sativum (garlic)[54]	12 week randomised, single-blind, placebo-controlled study on type 2 diabetic patients with newly diagnosed dyslipidaemia ($n = 70$). Given 300 mg garlic twice daily (1.3% allicin).	After 12 weeks the garlic-treated group had a significant reduction in total cholesterol, LDL-C. HDL cholesterol was significantly increased. No significant difference in triglyceride levels.	Garlic significantly reduced serum total cholesterol and LDL cholesterol and moderately raised HDL cholesterol as compared to placebo.
Cynara scolymus (artichoke leaf extract)[59]	75 adult volunteers took randomised 1280 mg of standardised artichoke leaf extract or placebo daily for 12 weeks.	Total plasma cholesterol decreased by 4.2%.	Artichoke leaf extract consumption resulted in a modest but favourable, statistically significant reduction in plasma cholesterol after 12 weeks.

19.2 km a week at 65 to 80% of peak oxygen consumption and the equivalent of walking 19.2 km per week at 40 to 55% of peak oxygen consumption. All three interventions were superior to the control condition in all 11 lipid variables.[74] In the National Cholesterol Education Program mentioned above, exercise intervention increased HDL-C levels (5–14%) and lowered TG levels (4–18%) respectively.[75] A meta-analysis of studies on the effect of exercise on identifiable risk factors in 8440 patients indicated a pooled effect estimate for total mortality reduction of 27%.[73] As well as this, there was a significant net reduction in total cholesterol of –0.57 mmol/L and LDL-C –0.51 mmol/L respectively.[73]

Expected outcomes and follow-up protocols

In treating a patient with atherosclerosis the aim is to minimise or prevent the long-term sequelae of the condition. Each patient must be assessed for both their cardiovascular risk and their treatment benefit. Medical practitioners routinely divide patients up by sex, decade of life, whether they have diabetes and whether they have hypertension (providing a 5-year risk level). It is prudent to encourage high-risk patients to seek medical advice immediately and consider pharmaceutical intervention. All other patients can be treated in a stepped manner.

All patients of varying risk levels should be given dietary advice; however, obese patients should be seen weekly and given strict dietary guidelines with the aim to reduce weight by at least 2 kg monthly. All other patients can be seen fortnightly for the first month to work out any treatment problems, and then monthly, since body and blood changes take months to occur. Blood pressure readings should be routinely performed at each visit given the comorbidity relationship to the condition. The only way to clinically determine therapeutic outcomes with atherosclerosis is through blood examination, which ideally should be performed every 6 months. So it is best to work with the patient and their medical practitioner.

As there is no mention in the above case of hypertension or obesity, and only mildly elevated blood fats, it is acceptable to begin treatment as mentioned. It would be prudent to see the patient monthly as daily/weekly therapeutic benefits would not usually be obvious. The fact that she presents with clinical signs confirmed via angiography and stress testing indicates that treatment without pharmacological medicine could only realistically be allowed for 3 months, after which a second round of blood tests would need to be ordered. If there was no change in her blood fat status then she should be referred to her medical practitioner for shared treatment.

KEY POINTS

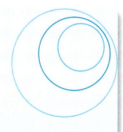

- Atherosclerosis and dyslipidaemia are chronic conditions that need to be consistently treated.
- Small changes in blood lipid levels may have significant effects on health.
- Consider the effect of comorbidities on cardiovascular health.
- Blood-test monitoring is the only guarantee of assessing treatment outcomes.

Further reading

McCully KS. Homocysteine, vitamins and vascular disease prevention. Am J Clin Nutr 2007;86(5):1563S–1568S.

Therapeutic guidelines, cardiovascular (version 5). Online. Available: http://etg.hcn.net.au/. Accessed 23 April 2009.

Topol EJ, et al. Textbook of cardiovascular medicine. 3rd edn. Lippincott Williams & Wilkins, 2007.

References

1. Topol EJ, ed. Textbook of cardiovascular medicine. 3rd edn. Philadelphia: Lippincott Williams & Wilkins, 2007.
2. Peck MD, Ai AL. Cardiac conditions. J Gerontol Soc Work 2008;50 Suppl 1:13–44.
3. Vanuzzo D, et al. [Cardiovascular risk and cardiometabolic risk: an epidemiological evaluation]. G Ital Cardiol (Rome) 2008;9(4 Suppl 1):6S–17S.
4. Harrison's principles of internal medicine. Online [cited 2009, June 2]. Available: http://www.accessmedicine.com/content.aspx?aID=2872140&searchStr=atherosclerosis.
5. Arora S, Nicholls SJ. Atherosclerotic plaque reduction: blood pressure, dyslipidemia, atherothrombosis. Drugs Today (Barc) 2008;44(9):711–718.
6. Rizzo M, et al. Atherogenic dyslipidemia and oxidative stress: a new look. Transl Res 2009;153(5):217–223.
7. Easton JD, et al. Definition and evaluation of transient ischemic attack: a scientific statement for healthcare professionals from the American Heart Association/American Stroke Association Stroke Council; Council on Cardiovascular Surgery and Anesthesia; Council on Cardiovascular Radiology and Intervention; Council on Cardiovascular Nursing; and the Interdisciplinary Council on Peripheral Vascular Disease. The American Academy of Neurology affirms the value of this statement as an educational tool for neurologists. Stroke 2009;40(6):2276–2293.
8. Sobenin IA, et al. [Reduction of cardiovascular risk in primary prophylaxy of coronary heart disease]. Klin Med (Mosk) 2005;83(4):52–55.
9. Rodriguez G, et al. [Role of inflammation in atherogenesis]. Invest Clin 2009;50(1):109–129.
10. Liapis CD, et al. What a vascular surgeon should know and do about atherosclerotic risk factors. J Vasc Surg 2009;49(5):1348–1354.
11. McCully KS. Homocysteine, vitamins and vascular disease prevention. Am J Clin Nutr 2007;86(5):1563S–1568S.
12. Ferretti G, et al. Homocysteinylation of low-density lipoproteins (LDL) from subjects with Type 1 diabetes: effect on oxidative damage of human endothelial cells. Diabetic Med 2006;23(7):808–813.
13. Su J, et al. A comparative study on pathogenic effects of homocysteine and cysteine on atherosclerosis. Wei Sheng Yan Jiu 2009;38(1):43–46.
14. Harrison DG, Gongora MC. Oxidative stress and hypertension. Med Clin North Am 2009;93(3):621–635.
15. Roberts CK, Sindhu KK. Oxidative stress and metabolic syndrome. Life Sci 2009;84(21–22):705–712.
16. Higashi Y, et al. Endothelial function and oxidative stress in cardiovascular diseases. Circ J 2009;73(3):411–418. [Epub 2009, Feb 4].
17. Therapeutic guidelines, cardiovascular (version 5). Online. Available: http://etg.hcn.net.au/. Accessed 23 April 2009.
18. Cottart CH, et al. [Biology of arterial ageing and arteriosclerosis.]. C R Biol 2009;332(5):433–447.
19. Roy H, et al. Molecular genetics of atherosclerosis. Hum Genet 2009;125(5–6):467–491.
20. Walker C, Reamy BV. Diets for cardiovascular disease prevention: what is the evidence? Am Fam Physician 2009;79(7):571–578.
21. Cesari M, et al. Homocysteine-lowering treatment in coronary heart disease. Curr Med Chem Cardiovasc Hematol Agents 2005;3(4):289–295.
22. Garces PA, et al. [Lowering plasma homocysteine with vitamins B6, B12, and folic acid. Effect on lipids concentration in patients with secondary hyperlipoproteinemia type IV, with and without Lovastatin treatment]. Arch Latinoam Nutr 2006;56(1):36–42.
23. Bunout D, et al. Effects of supplementation with folic acid and antioxidant vitamins on homocysteine levels and LDL oxidation in coronary patients. Nutrition 2000;16(2):107–110.
24. Bleie O, et al. Homocysteine-lowering therapy does not affect inflammatory markers of atherosclerosis in patients with stable coronary artery disease. J Intern Med 2007;262(2):244–253.
25. Wotherspoon F, et al. The effect of oral folic acid upon plasma homocysteine, endothelial function and oxidative stress in patients with type 1 diabetes and microalbuminuria. Int J Clin Pract 2008;62(4):569–574.
26. Yılmaz H, et al. Effects of folic acid and N-acetylcysteine on plasma homocysteine levels and endothelial function in patients with coronary artery disease. Acta Cardiol 2007;62(6):579–585.
27. Graf S, et al. 13N-ammonia rest/stress PET: folic acid improves global coronary vasoreactivity in coronary artery disease patients with normal or elevated homocysteine levels. Nuklearmedizin 2006;45(6):248–253.
28. Manna C, et al. Olive oil phenolic compounds inhibit homocysteine-induced endothelial cell adhesion regardless of their different antioxidant activity. J Agric Food Chem 2009;57(9):3478–3482.
29. Ben-Assayag E, et al. Association of the -757T>C polymorphism in the CRP gene with circulating C-reactive protein levels and carotid atherosclerosis. Thromb Res 2009;24(4):458–462.
30. Belza A, et al. Effect of diet-induced energy deficit and body fat reduction on high-sensitive CRP and other inflammatory markers in obese subjects. Int J Obes (Lond) 2009;33(4):456–464.
31. North CJ, et al. The effects of dietary fibre on C-reactive protein, an inflammation marker predicting cardiovascular disease. Eur J Clin Nutr 2009;63(8):921–933.
32. Koenig W, et al. C-reactive protein, a sensitive marker of inflammation, predicts future risk of coronary heart disease in initially healthy middle-aged men: results from the MONICA (Monitoring Trends and Determinants in Cardiovascular Disease) Augsburg Cohort Study, 1984 to 1992. Circulation 1999;99(2):237–242.
33. Block G, et al. Plasma C-reactive protein concentrations in active and passive smokers: influence of antioxidant supplementation. J Am Coll Nutr 2004;23(2):141–147.
34. Singh U, Devaraj S, Vitamin E. inflammation and atherosclerosis. Vitam Horm 2007;76:519–549.
35. Yang RL, et al. Lipoic acid prevents high-fat diet-induced dyslipidemia and oxidative stress: a microarray analysis. Nutrition 2008;24(6):582–588.
36. Amom Z, et al. Lipid lowering effect of antioxidant alpha-lipoic acid in experimental atherosclerosis. J Clin Biochem Nutr 2008;43(2):88–94.

37. Accinni R, et al. Effects of combined dietary supplementation on oxidative and inflammatory status in dyslipidemic subjects. Nutr Metab Cardiovasc Dis 2006;16(2): 121–127.

38. Suarna C, et al. Protective effect of vitamin E supplements on experimental atherosclerosis is modest and depends on preexisting vitamin E deficiency. Free Radic Biol Med 2006;41(5):722–730.

39. Kartal Ozer N, et al. Molecular mechanisms of cholesterol or homocysteine effect in the development of atherosclerosis: role of vitamin E. Biofactors 2003;19(1–2):63–70.

40. Chapidze GE, et al. [Combination treatment with coenzyme Q10 and simvastatin in patients with coronary atherosclerosis]. Kardiologiia 2006;46(8):11–13.

41. Chapidze G, et al. Prevention of coronary atherosclerosis by the use of combination therapy with antioxidant coenzyme Q10 and statins. Georgian Med News 2005;118:20–25.

42. Yang PY, et al. Reduction of atherosclerosis in cholesterol-fed rabbits and decrease of expressions of intracellular adhesion molecule-1 and vascular endothelial growth factor in foam cells by a water-soluble fraction of Polygonum multiflorum. J Pharmacol Sci 2005;99(3):294–300.

43. Corti R, et al. Cocoa and cardiovascular health. Circulation 2009;119:1433–1441.

44. Davidson M. Niacin use and cutaneous flushing: mechanisms and strategies for prevention. Am J Cardiol 2008;101(8 Suppl. 1):S14–S19.

45. Australian medicines handbook. Adelaide: Australian Medicines Handbook Pty Ltd, 2009.

46. Berra K. Clinical update on the use of niacin for the treatment of dyslipidemia. J Am Acad Nurse Pract 2004;16(12):526–534.

47. Castano G, et al. A randomized, double-blind, placebo-controlled study of the efficacy and tolerability of policosanol in adolescents with type II hypercholesterolemia. Curr Ther Res Clin Exp 2002;63(4):286–303.

48. Castano G, et al. Effects of policosanol and lovastatin on lipid profile and lipid peroxidation in patients with dyslipidemia associated with type 2 diabetes mellitus. Int J Clin Pharmacol Res 2002;22(3–4):89–99.

49. Francini-Pesenti F, et al. Sugar cane policosanol failed to lower plasma cholesterol in primitive, diet-resistant hypercholesterolemia: a double blind, controlled study. Complement Ther Med 2008;16(2):61–65.

50. Francini-Pesenti F, et al. Effect of sugar cane policosanol on lipid profile in primary hypercholesterolemia. Phytother Res 2008;22(3):318–322.

51. Mansoor GA. Herbs and alternative therapies in the hypertension clinic. Am J Hypertens 2001;14:971–975.

52. Rahman K, Lowe GM. Garlic and cardiovascular disease: a critical review. J Nutr 2006;136(3 Suppl):736S–740S.

53. Jeyaraj S, et al. Effect of combined supplementation of fish oil with garlic pearls on the serum lipid profile in hypercholesterolemic subjects. Indian Heart J 2005;57(4): 327–331.

54. Ashraf R, et al. Effects of garlic on dyslipidemia in patients with type 2 diabetes mellitus. J Ayub Med Coll Abbottabad 2005;17(3):60–64.

55. Tassoni D, et al. The role of eicosanoids in the brain. Asia Pac J Clin Nutr 2008;17(Suppl 1):220–228.

56. Casos K, et al. Atherosclerosis prevention by a fish oil-rich diet in apoE(–/–) mice is associated with a reduction of endothelial adhesion molecules. Atherosclerosis 2008;201(2):306–317.

57. Goldberg RB, Sabharwal AK. Fish oil in the treatment of dyslipidemia. Curr Opin Endocrinol Diabetes Obes 2008;15(2):167–174.

58. Mills S, Bone K. Principles and practice of phytotherapy. St Louis: Churchill Livingstone, 2000.

59. Bundy R, et al. Artichoke leaf extract (Cynara scolymus) reduces plasma cholesterol in otherwise healthy hypercholesterolemic adults: a randomized, double blind placebo controlled trial. Phytomedicine 2008;15(9):668–675.

60. Li H, et al. Flavonoids from artichoke (Cynara scolymus L.) up-regulate endothelial-type nitric-oxide synthase gene expression in human endothelial cells. J Pharmacol Exp Ther 2004;310(3):926–932.

61. Jimenez-Escrig A, et al. In vitro antioxidant activities of edible artichoke (Cynara scolymus L.) and effect on biomarkers of antioxidants in rats. J Agric Food Chem 2003;51(18):5540–5545.

62. Shimoda H, et al. Anti-hyperlipidemic sesquiterpenes and new sesquiterpene glycosides from the leaves of artichoke (Cynara scolymus L.): structure requirement and mode of action. Bioorg Med Chem Lett 2003;13(2):223–228.

63. Jantaratnotai N, et al. Inhibitory effect of Curcuma comosa on NO production and cytokine expression in LPS-activated microglia. Life Sci 2006;78(6):571–577.

64. Piyachaturawat P, et al. Reduction of plasma cholesterol by Curcuma comosa extract in hypercholesterolaemic hamsters. J Ethnopharmacol 1999;66(2):199–204.

65. Manchanda SC, et al. Retardation of coronary atherosclerosis with yoga lifestyle intervention. J Assoc Physicians India 2000;48(7):687–694.

66. Wang WZ, et al. [Clinical study on acupuncture and moxibustion for treatment of plaque of carotid atherosclerosis]. Zhongguo Zhen Jiu 2005;25(5):312–314.

67. Omura Y, et al. Anatomical relationship between traditional acupuncture point ST 36 and Omura's ST 36 (True ST 36) with their therapeutic effects: 1) inhibition of cancer cell division by markedly lowering cancer cell telomere while increasing normal cell telomere, 2) improving circulatory disturbances, with reduction of abnormal increase in high triglyceride, L-homocystein, CRP, or cardiac troponin I, T in blood by the stimulation of Omura's ST 36–Part 1. Acupunct Electrother Res 2007;32(1–2):31–70.

68. Wang C, et al. [Clinical study on treatment of atherosclerosis obliterans by integrated traditional Chinese and Western medicine]. Zhongguo Zhong Xi Yi Jie He Za Zhi 2000;20(11):828–830.

69. Saltzman E, et al. An oat-containing hypocaloric diet reduces systolic blood pressure and improves lipid profile beyond effects of weight loss in men and women. J Nutr 2001;131(5):1465–1470.

70. Mia MA, et al. Dietary fibre and coronary heart disease. Mymensingh Med J 2002;11(2):133–135.

71. Critchley JA, Capewell S. Smoking cessation for the secondary prevention of coronary heart disease. Cochrane Database Syst Rev 2003;(4):CD003041.

72. Tolstrup J, Gronbaek M. Alcohol and atherosclerosis: recent insights. Curr Atheroscler Rep 2007;9(2):116–124.

73. Jolliffe J, et al. Exercise-based rehabilitation for coronary heart disease. Cochrane Database Syst Rev 2001;(1):CD003316.

74. Kraus WE, et al. Effects of the amount and intensity of exercise on plasma lipoproteins. N Engl J Med 2002;347(19):1483–1492.

75. Varady KA, Jones PJ. Combination diet and exercise interventions for the treatment of dyslipidemia: an effective preliminary strategy to lower cholesterol levels? J Nutr 2005;135(8):1829–1835.

76. Forsythe CE, et al. Comparison of low fat and low carbohydrate diets on circulating fatty acid composition and markers of inflammation. Lipids 2008;1:65–77.

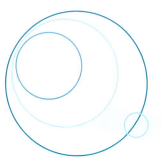

10
Hypertension and stroke

Michael Alexander
ND, BPharm

EPIDEMIOLOGY AND AETIOLOGY

Hypertension or high blood pressure (BP) is a *sustained* rise in *resting* blood pressure. Persistent systolic blood pressure (≥ 140 mmHg) and diastolic blood pressure (≥ 90 mmHg) is considered 'hypertension'.[1] It is very common, affecting approximately one-third of the population. Hypertension is an important risk factor in coronary heart disease and in cerebrovascular accident or 'stroke', and may also lead to kidney failure and left ventricular failure or 'heart failure'.[2,3] Hypertension with no known cause (primary) is the most common (90%), and hypertension with an identified cause (secondary) can be due to kidney disease (the most common cause), coarctation of the aorta, endocrine diseases and pregnancy.[1] Diagnosis is by sphygmomanometry, usually over three consecutive visits to a medical doctor.[4]

Left ventricular hypertrophy usually develops in response to some factor, such as high blood pressure, that requires the left ventricle to work harder. As the workload increases, the walls of the chamber grow thicker, lose elasticity and eventually may fail to pump with as much force as a healthy heart.[5] Left ventricular hypertrophy presents with increased risk of heart disease, including heart attack, heart failure, irregular heartbeats (arrhythmia) and sudden cardiac arrest.[6]

The term 'stroke' encompasses a heterogenous group of cerebrovascular disorders. Ischaemic stroke or cerebral infarction accounts for 80–85% of all strokes and typically presents as a sudden, painless, focal neurological deficit with preserved consciousness.[1,2] Haemorrhagic stroke accounts for 15–20% of all strokes, and presents as an acute focal neurological deficit, but continues to worsen as the haematoma expands, with headache and altered consciousness resulting.[5]

RISK FACTORS

Genetics, social behaviour and diet all have a role to play in this multifactorial condition (see Figure 10.1).[7] The risk of high blood pressure increases with age, and is more prevalent in middle-aged men and postmenopausal women.[8] It develops at an earlier age in black ethnicity than it does in Caucasians and is influenced by family history. Although

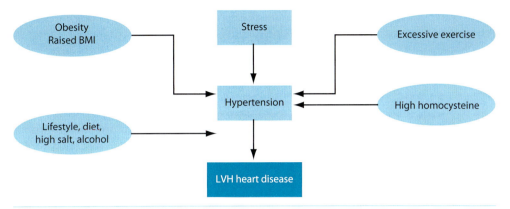

Figure 10.1 Risk factors for hypertension

the long-term effect of stress on blood pressure is not well understood, chronic stress can lead to transient rises of significant hypertension.[9] Dietary factors that may affect hypertension include high levels of salt, reduced levels of potassium, and heavy drinking. Apart from alcohol, other social behaviours such as smoking and physical inactivity have long-term detrimental effects on blood pressure.[10]

CONVENTIONAL TREATMENT

The initial medical treatment in non-life-threatening hypertension centres on weight loss and dietary changes.[11] Patients are encouraged to increase the level of fruits and vegetables in their diet, while concurrently reducing salt and alcohol intake. These interventions, combined with regular aerobic exercise, can reduce systolic blood pressure by 6–10 mmHg.[12]

If the hypertension is high (> 140/90 mmHg) on several occasions or unresponsive to lifestyle modification, then drug therapy is instigated.[1] For uncomplicated hypertension, unless there is a contraindication or a specific indication for another drug, then the order of consideration is:
- ACE inhibitor, or
- a dihydropyridine calcium channel blocker, or
- if 65 or older, a thiazide diuretic (low dose).[12]

For all patients, treatment aims to reduce BP to < 140/90 mm Hg; for those with a kidney disorder or diabetes, the goal is < 130/80 mm Hg or as near this level as tolerated. Even the elderly and frail can tolerate a diastolic BP as low as 60 to 65 mm Hg well without an increase in cardiovascular events.[1]

KEY TREATMENT PROTOCOLS

Unlike orthodox medicine that categorises most hypertension as primary or idiopathic, a naturopathic approach assumes that there exists a definite cause–effect relationship, even in primary (idiopathic) hypertension. Differing hypertension prevalence among certain population and age groups is partially

NATUROPATHIC TREATMENT AIMS
- Reduce stress and advise relaxation techniques.
- Focus on attaining a healthy weight (body mass index).
- Give dietary advice.
- Encourage graded exercise.
- Modify homocysteine levels.
- Support key organs of assistance (kidneys).

due to differences in the intake of certain nutrients. Sustained raised blood pressure is positively associated with higher sodium, alcohol and protein intakes, and is inversely associated with potassium, calcium and magnesium intake.[13] Due to this, dietary and lifestyle measures are of primary focus in treating hypertension.

Stress reduction

The stress response increases sympathetic nervous activity, which can adversely affect the cardiovascular system (see Chapter 15 on adrenal fatigue). Cardiovascular disease is due in part to stress-induced mechanisms mediated primarily through increased adrenergic stimulation.[5] These stress-induced mechanisms include elevations in serum lipids, alterations in blood coagulation, atherogenesis, vascular changes in hypertension and myocardial ischaemia.[9]

It is difficult to quantify the extent to which stress influences cardiovascular health; however, there are causal relationships between stress and pathophysiological behaviours that in turn have detrimental effects on health, including hypertension. A study over 7 years with 6576 subjects clearly indicated that stress led to increased consumption of alcohol, smoking and a reduction in physical activity.[14] A small Indian study in 2008 of 77 individuals looked at the short-term effect of a comprehensive but brief lifestyle intervention with **yoga** on their subjective wellbeing. The group included healthy individuals as well subjects with hypertension, coronary artery disease and diabetes mellitus. The results suggested that the stress management program made an appreciable contribution to primary disease prevention.[15]

Interventions for coronary heart disease-prone behaviour patterns have proven successful. A large study was found to support the effect of therapeutic lifestyle changes on hypertension (see Table 10.2 at the end of the chapter for a review of the evidence).[10] *Valeriana officinalis* may have a positive effect on anxiety and stress, as well as on vasospastic activity.[16] It is believed that the relaxing effect of *V. officinalis* is related to the level of valerenic acid, a sesquiterpenic acid, which specifically modulates certain GABA-α receptors and activity.[17] A 2007 study found ethanolic extracts of valerian to be as effective as nifedipine in their 'anticoronaryspastic' activity against cardiovascular disease.[18] Another sesquiterpene isolated from *Magnolia grandifolia* flower petals produced a statistically significant decrease in coronary vascular resistance on the Langendorff isolated perfused heart.[19] *Passiflora incarnata* was as effective as oxazepam in the treatment of generalised anxiety disorder, with low incidence of impairment of job performance[20] (see Section 5 on the endocrine system and Section 4 on the nervous system).

Arterial elasticity and integrity

Age-related changes in the arterial system begin in the 1930s and accelerate through midlife.[5] Increased collagen deposition and weakened vascular elastin result in altered elasticity, distensibility and dilatation.[5] Stiffening of the central arteries results in higher wave velocities and augmentation of systolic arterial pressure.[5] In a double-blind, randomised and placebo controlled clinical study, 26 overweight hypertensive patients were given 3 g of **omega-3 fish oil** daily for 8 weeks.[21] After 8 weeks' follow-up, the large artery elasticity in the fish-oil group, compared with its baseline, had significantly improved. A small study of 28 middle-aged men and women undertaking a randomised, double-blind trial of 400 IU of **vitamin E** daily for 8 weeks improved arterial compliance by 44% in 12 out of 14 subjects.[22] Antioxidants, such as **bioflavonoids**, enhance endothelial nitric oxide (NO) synthase expression and subsequent NO release from endothelial cells; this is important in arterial vasodilation. Pycnogenol, an extract of bark from ***Pinus pinaster*** (French maritime pine) consists of a concentrate of water-soluble polyphenols. Pycnogenol contains the bioflavonoids catechin and taxifolin, as well as phenolcarbonic acids. Pycnogenol augments endothelium-dependent vasodilation by increasing NO production in the vascular wall.[23]

Dietary flavonoids, such as quercetin and epicatechin, can augment nitric oxide status and reduce endothelin-1 concentrations, and may thereby improve endothelial function.[24] **Cocoa** is rich in plant-derived flavonoids. In the Zutphen Elderly Study, a cohort of 470 elderly men revealed that cocoa intake was inversely related to blood pressure. A small amount of dark chocolate daily (6 g) in the evening significantly reduced mean systolic blood pressure by 2.9 ± 1.6 mmHg and diastolic blood pressure by 1.9 ± 1.0 mmHg.[25] Although still debated, a range of potential mechanisms through which flavonols and cocoa might exert their benefits on cardiovascular health include activation of NO and antioxidant anti-inflammatory and antiplatelet effects, which in turn might improve endothelial function, lipid levels, blood pressure, insulin resistance and eventually clinical outcome.[25] It was also shown that homocysteine-lowering therapy improved small arterial elasticity in diabetic patients treated with high-dose metformin.[26]

Magnesium plays a role in a number of chronic disease-related conditions, including hypertension. Magnesium acts as a calcium channel antagonist, stimulates production of vasodilator prostacyclins and nitric oxide and alters vascular responses to vasoactive agonists.[27] It may also play a role in metabolic syndrome and raised serum lipid profiles. Interestingly, it has a more profound effect when added to the diet than it does when supplemented.[28]

Most of the herbal treatments for hypertension probably act as peripheral vasodilators.[1] One of the most useful herbs is ***Crataegus oxyacantha***; its leaves, flowers and fruits contain such biologically active substances as flavonoids and catechins, which appear to be related to *C. oxyacantha* antioxidant effects.[29] As well as reducing high blood pressure this herb has a trophic effect on heart muscle.[31] Other studies have shown that *C. oxyacantha* reduces resting heart rate and mean diastolic blood pressure during exercise and increases the perfusion of the myocardium through revascularisation.[29] This is important because left ventricular heart failure is often caused by prolonged hypertension.[1] In a pilot study where 500 mg of *Crataegus oxyacantha* extract was taken daily for 10 weeks, there were promising results on the diastolic component of mild hypertension among subjects.[30]

Vasopressin and diuresis

Diuretics have long been used to treat hypertension in general practice. Technically, a 'diuretic' is an agent that increases urine volume, while a 'natriuretic' causes an increase in renal sodium excretion. Because natriuretics almost always also increase water excretion, they are usually called diuretics.[31] Generally, diuretics should be initiated at the lowest effective dose of the class chosen. Problems that may occur with both short- and long-term use of diuretics include hyponatraemia, hypokalaemia, metabolic alkalosis and increased uric acid levels. Carbohydrate metabolism is frequently disturbed, with resultant hyperglycaemia and insulin resistance.[32] A review of the scientific evidence associated with herbal diuretics showed promising results.[31] One such herb that exhibits diuretic effects is ***Taraxacum officinale***. It is important that the leaves are used, as they have high levels of potassium.[31] The effect of an aqueous extract of ***Phyllanthus amarus*** administered intravenously on male normotensive rabbits produced a fall in mean diastolic, systolic and arterial pressure.[33] Methyl brevifolincarboxylate isolated from the leaves of *Phyllanthus niruri* showed a vasorelaxant effect on rat aortic rings. It exhibited slow relaxation activity against norepinephrine-induced contractions of rat aorta with or without endothelium.[34] A single oral administration of a 5% aqueous extract of *Phyllanthus sellowianus* (400 mg/kg body weight) produced significant increases in urinary excretion in test animals.[35] ***Clerodendron trichotomum*** has been traditionally used for the treatment of hypertension in China, Korea and Japan. An ethanolic extract produced the following phenylpropanoid glycosides: acteoside, leucosceptoside A, martynoside, acteoside isomer and isomartynoside. These glycosides displayed significant angiotensin-converting enzyme inhibition.[36]

Body mass index

Obesity and hypertension are highly correlated;[37] however, the concept of ideal body weight may raise more questions than it answers. The body mass index (BMI) attempts to create a statistical framework that can be used as a clinical tool to assess 'normal, healthy' human weight. While the method may provide an understanding of ideal weight for individuals of varying heights, it does not take into account muscle mass and body frame.

The body mass index (BMI) is a ratio:

$$\frac{\text{weight of individual (kg)}}{(\text{height of individual in metres})^2}$$

The results of BMI are categorised in Table 10.1.

In the Physician's Health Study,[37] raised BMI over an 8-year period correlated with an increased risk of cardiovascular disease in 13,230 middle-aged men. Women are not immune to the effects of BMI on hypertension. Caucasian women with a BMI > 30 kg/m^2 had a significantly greater risk of CVD mortality than women with a 'normal' BMI.[39] This was particularly so in women below the age of 60 years.[39] A BMI > 30 plus any two of triglycerides ≥ 1.7 mmol/L, HDL < 1.03, BP ≥ 130/85 mmHg and fasting glucose ≥ 5.6 mmol/L is considered to be metabolic syndrome[40] (discussed further in Chapter 16 on diabetes). As there is a continuous linear relationship between excess body fat blood pressure and the prevalence of hypertension,[31] weight loss to achieve normal BMI should always be attempted.

Homocysteine (Hcy)

As mentioned previously, over-exercise as well as deficiency of folic acid, vitamin B6 and/or vitamin B12 can result in elevated total plasma homocysteine concentrations (tHcy), which is considered to be a risk factor for vascular disease.[41] As discussed in Chapter 9 on atherosclerosis, there is considerable evidence to suggest that Hcy plays a significant role in the pathology of cardiovascular disease. Elevated levels of Hcy may

Table 10.1 BMI chart

BMI (KG/M²)	WEIGHT CATEGORY
Less than 18.5	Underweight
18.5 to 24.9	Healthy
25 to 29.9	Overweight
30 or higher	Obese

Source: 'Understanding body mass index'.[38]

be related to the cause of isolated systolic hypertension in some individuals, and in nor-motensive older adults is an independent risk factor for atherosclerosis.[41] Some antihy-pertensive medications, such as candesartan and amlodipine, were effective in reducing cellular oxidative stress, but this effectiveness was reduced when the patient also had raised Hcy levels.[42] Experimentally increasing plasma Hcy concentrations by methio-nine loading rapidly impairs both conduit and resistance vessel endothelial function in healthy humans. Endothelial dysfunction in conduit and resistance vessels may under-lie the reported associations between Hcy, atherosclerosis and hypertension. Increased oxidant stress appears to play a pathophysiological role in the deleterious endothelial effects of Hcy.[43]

A 'healthy' **vegetarian diet** may be considered a healthy choice for hypertensive indi-viduals, due to its effect on the reduction of saturated fats and general beneficial effects on weight. However 66% of vegans and vegetarians in a group of Austrian cohorts had considerably lower levels of vitamins B2 and B12; these led to excessive levels of Hcy.[44] Raised Hcy levels can be relatively easily reduced by daily supplementation of vitamins B6 and B12 and folate.[45]

Prevention and treatment of stroke

A great concern of chronic hypertension is stroke.[5] *Ginkgo biloba*, a Chinese traditional medicine, is widely used in the treatment of acute ischaemic stroke in China.[46] Its effi-cacy, however, is uncertain. A Cochrane review of 10 trials produced mixed results.[47] Whereas it has been shown that *G. biloba* extract leads to a significant increase in cere-bral blood flow and glucose uptake into brain tissue, there was no convincing evidence, from trials of sufficient methodological quality, to support the routine use of *G. biloba* to promote recovery after stroke.[47] A more recent trial in wild mice produced more encouraging results. A Ginkgo extract, EGb761, administered orally to mice produced 50.9% less neurological dysfunction and 48.2% smaller infarct volumes than non-treated mice after cerebral infarct (stroke).[48] Part of the positive result was attributed to its ability to induce haem oxygenase.[48] It is interesting to note that a recent study examining the effects of a *G. biloba* extract on the distal left anterior descending coro-nary artery blood flow and plasma nitric oxide and endothelin-1 levels in patients with coronary artery disease produced encouraging results. The treatment led to an increase of artery blood flow as well as an alteration in the nitric oxide/endothelin-1 ratio, which produced a beneficial result.[49]

There is evidence to support the use of **acupuncture** in stroke victims. Issues such as spasticity and anxiety are commonplace amongst sufferers. Poststroke anxiety neurosis was successfully relieved with acupuncture in 82.35% of patients in a small trial of 34 individuals.[50] A trial of 131 patients with spastic hemiplegia received two 30-day treatment regimens involving traditional acupuncture treatment.[51] Acupuncture was effective in reducing spastically increased muscle tone and motor neuron excitability in spastic hemiplegia and could improve spastic states in stroke patients. A study in the poststroke rehabilitation wards of five UK hospitals using acupuncture with electrical stimulation over 4 weeks produced a negative result, with acupuncture failing to pro-duce a benefit over placebo.[52] A Cochrane review of 31 trials involving the organised inpatient care for stroke victims indicated that patients who receive this care are more likely to survive their stroke, return home and become independent in looking after themselves.[53] While current evidence is not entirely supportive, more study needs to be done in this area to ascertain if there is a role for complementary medicines in managing or preventing stroke.

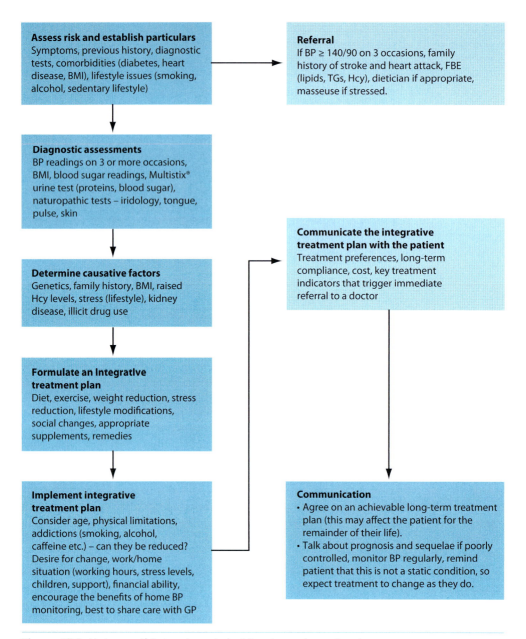

Assess risk and establish particulars
Symptoms, previous history, diagnostic tests, comorbidities (diabetes, heart disease, BMI), lifestyle issues (smoking, alcohol, sedentary lifestyle)

Referral
If BP ≥ 140/90 on 3 occasions, family history of stroke and heart attack, FBE (lipids, TGs, Hcy), dietician if appropriate, masseuse if stressed.

Diagnostic assessments
BP readings on 3 or more occasions, BMI, blood sugar readings, Multistix® urine test (proteins, blood sugar), naturopathic tests – iridology, tongue, pulse, skin

Communicate the integrative treatment plan with the patient
Treatment preferences, long-term compliance, cost, key treatment indicators that trigger immediate referral to a doctor

Determine causative factors
Genetics, family history, BMI, raised Hcy levels, stress (lifestyle), kidney disease, illicit drug use

Formulate an Integrative treatment plan
Diet, exercise, weight reduction, stress reduction, lifestyle modifications, social changes, appropriate supplements, remedies

Implement integrative treatment plan
Consider age, physical limitations, addictions (smoking, alcohol, caffeine etc.) – can they be reduced? Desire for change, work/home situation (working hours, stress levels, children, support), financial ability, encourage the benefits of home BP monitoring, best to share care with GP

Communication
• Agree on an achievable long-term treatment plan (this may affect the patient for the remainder of their life).
• Talk about prognosis and sequelae if poorly controlled, monitor BP regularly, remind patient that this is not a static condition, so expect treatment to change as they do.

Figure 10.2 Naturopathic treatment decision tree—hypertension

INTEGRATIVE MEDICAL CONSIDERATIONS

The influence of stress in cardiovascular disease should not be underestimated. In fact it has been shown in clinical trials that unchecked long-term stress can be a contributing factor in hypertension.[54] Massage therapists have suggested that their therapy elicits the relaxation response and therefore can decrease BP and hypertension.[54] This is also dependent upon the type of massage, having greatest effect with relaxing (Swedish) massage.[55] Regular massage therapy has been shown to reduce long-term hypertension.

If the individual's stress stems from environmental factors (such as work, home life and financial problems), then referral to a counsellor or psychologist may be a consideration. Some patients may prefer to obtain dietary advice from a dietician or a qualified nutritionist.

Practitioners may also consider referral to an acupuncturist. However, a review of randomised clinical trials (RCTs) produced inconclusive results for this therapy, and revealed most studies to have poor methodology and small sample sizes.[56] There is some evidence to suggest that acupuncture increases circulation by increasing the number of capillaries, thereby improving capillary density, decreasing venous and arterial blood stasis as well as reducing blood viscosity and haematocrit, resulting in improved circulation through the reduction of peripheral resistance.[29] Acupuncture is also thought to decrease the rate of renin secretion by the kidneys.[29] Yoga, an integral part of Ayurveda, has been shown to be useful to patients with heart disease and hypertension.[57] Yoga may reduce anxiety, promote wellbeing and improve quality of life. Its safety profile is solid, but its use as a complementary therapeutic regimen under medical supervision may still be appropriate.[30] Tai chi or other gentle martial art forms for stress reduction and general wellbeing may also be beneficial.

Case Study

A 53-year-old male overweight patient presents to the clinic after a diagnosis with **hypertension**. He originally saw his doctor because he had **dizziness** on and off for several weeks with **headache and fatigue** that he thought was an infection. An ECG has revealed that he also has **slight left ventricular hypertrophy**. He has concerns because **his father died of a stroke when he was 49**. He is also a social smoker.

SUGGESTIVE SYMPTOMS

- Dizziness
- Flushed face
- Headache
- Fatigue
- Fourth heart sound

Example treatment
Prescription

The herbal formula is designed to exert a hypotensive action via smooth muscle relaxation, vasodilation and stress reduction (*Valeriana* spp., and *Crataegus oxyacantha*).[31,17,29] Magnesium also indirectly produces vasodilation.[27] A diuretic effect may occur via *Taraxacum officinale*.[31] *Ginkgo biloba* may be of benefit in improving circulation and enhancing vascular integrity.[47–49] Omega-3 fish oil can be taken at a dose of 6 capsules daily (1000 mg fish oil per capsule), to increase arterial elasticity.[21] Vitamin B6 in a daily dose of 100 mg daily and vitamin B12 in a dose of 1000 μg daily will assist healthy homocysteine metabo-

Herbal prescription	
Valeriana officinalis 1:2	25 mL
Crataegus oxyacantha 1:2	25 mL
Ginkgo biloba 2:1	25 mL
Taraxacum officinale leaf 1:2	25 mL
7 mL b.d.	100 mL

Nutritional prescription
Magnesium chelate 200 mg b.d. (400 mg elemental Mg daily)
Omega-3 fish oil 3 g b.d.
Vitamin B2, B6, B5 100 mg of each daily
Folic acid 500 μg/B12 1000 μg 1 daily

lism.[41,44,45] It may be appropriate to use a sublingual form of B12 to overcome the low levels of intrinsic factor that may preclude gut absorption. Folic acid can be taken in a daily dose of 500 μg. *Allium sativum* can also be prescribed or increased in the diet to augment the hypotensive action of the prescription.

Dietary and lifestyle modifications
Diet
Naturopaths may consider embracing the findings of the Dietary Approaches to Stop Hypertension (DASH) Collaborative Research Group. In this study of 459 adults, groups were assigned one of two diets for 8 weeks.[58] The first included raised levels of fruit and vegetables, and the second a combined diet, which was the same diet with added low-fat dairy products and reduced total fat. The group eating more fruit and vegetables had reductions of 2.8 mmHg (systolic) and 1.1 mmHg (diastolic). The group on the combined diet had even greater reductions of 5.5 mmHg (systolic) and 3 mmHg (diastolic).[58] It is assumed that salt plays an important role in the inactivation of nitric oxide synthase in endothelial cells of arteries, causing a reduction in elasticity and an increase in pressure.[59] Females of an older age are the most sensitive to the hypertensive effects of dietary sodium, so sodium consumption should be monitored in this population.[60] Although the effects of caffeine on BP are considered to be temporary, a reduction in caffeine intake may be beneficial.

Exercise
There is strong epidemiological and experimental evidence to support a positive link between the lowering of BP and exercise. Aerobic exercise that uses large muscle groups for 20–60 minutes a day for a minimum of 3 days a week is advisable.[1] It is interesting to note, however, that exercise over 758 minutes a week (108 minutes per day) increases methionine metabolism, which also increases its amino acid metabolic intermediate homocysteine (Hcy), known to increase cardiovascular risk.[61] Strength training has also been shown to reduce arterial blood pressure in a small study of 10 participants with type 2 diabetes co-morbidity.[62]

GRADED EXERCISE

It is important to remember that optimal exercise activity should be implemented in a graded fashion, under the direction of an exercise physiologist and/or medical practitioner.

Expected outcomes and follow-up protocols
The outcomes affecting future protocols can be broadly divided into two groups: those that are objective (measurable) and those that are subjective.

The measurable outcomes that have the greatest influence on treatment regimen are:
- weight and BMI
- blood pressure (it is recommended that the patient buy a basic automated blood pressure monitor); this should be augmented with BP and pulse readings at each consultation
- full blood examination through their doctor, which would provide information about other risk factors that should be considered in all vascular disease (blood fats, insulin levels, and so on).

The patient in this case is already in contact with a medical practitioner, and given his family history it would be prudent to ensure that he maintains his contact and has regular blood test reviews. This is especially important since he is overweight and has a family history of stroke, which is usually associated with dyslipidaemia. The patient is strongly advised to reduce his weight to a healthier level and stop smoking. He also needs to adopt an exercise program, which will have beneficial effects on both his weight and stress.

Of the subjective outcomes, those associated with satisfaction of treatment and reduction in stress, as well as with feelings of empowerment, are the most significant to take note of. After an initial consultation it would then be prudent to have a weekly follow-up for a month, then fortnightly return visits for another month, then four more monthly visits. At this 6-month point of treatment, if there are encouraging signs that there has been significant weight loss (assume an average of 0.5–1 kg/month) and good blood pressure control (BP ≤ 130/80 in ≥ 80% of monitor readings), then follow-up consultations could be extended to 6 months between visits.

Table 10.2 Review of the major evidence

INTERVENTION	METHODOLOGY	RESULT	COMMENT
B6, B12, folic acid combination[45]	Randomised, placebo, double-blind controlled trial ($n = 220$). Measured total plasma homocysteine and serum methylmalonic acid (MMA) of elderly women over 6 months.	Median concentrations of serum cobalamin, serum folate and erythrocyte folate increased significantly and tHcy and alpha-EAST activity (indicative of improved status of vitamin B6) coefficient decreased significantly in the supplemented group. Median MMA concentration of the supplemented group was significantly lower than that of the placebo group after the intervention	6-month supplementation including physiological dosages of B vitamins improved the status of these nutrients and reduced tHcy in presumed healthy elderly women.
Strength training program[62]	An ambulatory 24-hour BP-monitoring (ABPM) ($n = 10$). The ABPM equipment (oscillometric Model Mobil-O-Graph CE 0434) was applied before and after 4-month training period. Routine HbA_{1c} levels were measured using standard techniques.	Significant reduction of mean arterial BP (from 93.8 ± 19.2 to 90.6 ± 14.3 mmHg; $p > 0.01$) after a 4-month ST (–3.4% mmHg)	Significant reduction of mean arterial BP after a 4-month strength training, measured by the ABPM system.
Study of stress on cardiovascular disease (CVD) risk.[14]	6576 subjects (ages 50.9 ± 13.1 years). Measured: • psychological stress (12-item version of the General Health Questionnaire) • behavioural (smoking, alcohol, physical activity) • pathophysiological (CRP, fibrinogen, total HDL-C, obesity, hypertension). Observed CVD events.	Cigarette smoking, physical activity, alcohol intake, C-reactive protein and hypertension were independently associated with psychological distress. 223 incident CVD events (63 fatal) over an average follow-up of 7.2 years	The association between psychological distress and CVD risk is largely explained by behavioural processes. Therefore, treatment of psychological distress, aiming to reduce CVD risk, should primarily focus on health behaviour change.

(Continued)

Table 10.2 Review of the major evidence *(Continued)*

INTERVENTION	METHODOLOGY	RESULT	COMMENT
Therapeutic lifestyle changes (TLCs)[10]	2478 subjects. Evaluated at baseline and after 6 months after participation in community TLCs (exercise training, nutrition, weight management, stress management and smoking cessation).	Baseline BP (125 ± 8/79 ± 3 mmHg) decreased by 6 ± 12/3 ± 3 mm Hg ($p \leq 0.001$), with 952 subjects (38.4%) normalising their BP ($p \leq 0.001$). In subjects with a baseline systolic BP of 120 to 139 mm Hg ($n = 2,082$), systolic BP decreased by 7 ± 12 mm Hg ($p \leq 0.001$). In subjects with a baseline diastolic BP of 80 to 89 mm Hg ($n = 1504$), diastolic BP decreased by 6 ± 3 mm Hg ($p \leq 0.001$). Subjects with a baseline body mass index (BMI) < 30 kg/m^2 had a greater reduction in BP than those with a BMI $\geq$ 30 kg/m^2.	Supports the effectiveness of TLC on cardiovascular parameters in a real-world setting.
Omega 3 fish oil[21]	Double-blind, randomised and placebo-controlled clinical study ($n = 52$). 26 in placebo group, 26 assigned 3 g fish oil daily. 8 weeks follow-up.	Large artery elasticity in the fish oil group was significantly improved (C(1): 15.5 ± 1.5 vs 12.8 ± 3.7 mL mm Hg^{-1} × 10). No effect in placebo.	Fish oil supplementation improves large arterial elasticity; no effect on BP in overweight hypertensive patients.

KEY POINTS

- Hypertension has multifactorial pathogenesis, and requires a multifaceted treatment.
- Blood pressure monitoring by the patient is an important aspect of treatment.
- Hypertension rarely exists without other co-morbidities, so investigation is necessary.
- Be prepared to adjust treatment over time, as hypertension is a chronic condition that will change in the patient over time.

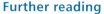

Further reading

Appel LJ, et al. A clinical trial of the effects of dietary patterns on blood pressure. DASH Collaborative Research Group. N Engl J Med 1997;336(16):1117–1124.

Chang Q, et al. Hawthorn. J Clin Pharmacol 2002;42(6):605–612.

Lawes CM, et al. Blood pressure and coronary heart disease: a review of the evidence. Semin Vasc Med 2002;2(4):355–368.

Mahady GB. *Ginkgo biloba* for the prevention and treatment of cardiovascular disease: a review of the literature. J Cardiovasc Nurs 2002;16(4):21–32.

References

1. The Merck Manual's online medical library. Online. Available: http://www.merck.com/mmpe/sec07/ch071/ch071a.html. Accessed 28 September 2008.
2. Easton JD, et al. Definition and evaluation of transient ischemic attack: a scientific statement for healthcare professionals from the American Heart Association/American Stroke Association Stroke Council; Council on Cardiovascular Surgery and Anesthesia; Council on Cardiovascular Radiology and Intervention; Council on Cardiovascular Nursing; and the Interdisciplinary Council on Peripheral Vascular Disease. The American Academy of Neurology affirms the value of this statement as an educational tool for neurologists. Stroke 2009;40(6):2276–2293.
3. Vardaxis NJ. Pathology for the health sciences. South Melbourne: MacMillan Education Australia, 1996:106.
4. Padwal RS, et al. The 2009 Canadian Hypertension Education Program recommendations for the management of hypertension: part 1 – blood pressure measurement, diagnosis and assessment of risk. Can J Cardiol 2009;25(5):279–286.
5. Textbook of cardiovascular medicine. Online. Available: http://ovidsp.tx.ovid.com. Accessed 15 February 2009.
6. The Mayo Clinic. Online. Available: http://www.mayoclinic.com/health/left-ventricular-hypertrophy/DS00680. Accessed 1 November 2008.
7. Murphy BP, et al. Hypertension and myocardial ischemia. Med Clin North Am 2009;93(3):681–695.
8. The Mayo clinic. Online. Available: http://www.mayoclinic.com/health/high-blood-pressure/DS00100/DSECTION = risk-factors. Accessed 5 October 2008.
9. Engler MB, Engler MM. Assessment of the cardiovascular effects of stress. J Cardiovasc Nurs 1995;10(1):51–63.
10. Bavikati VV, et al. Effect of comprehensive therapeutic lifestyle changes on prehypertension. Am J Cardiol 2008;102(12):1677–1680.
11. Khan NA, et al. The 2009 Canadian Hypertension Education Program recommendations for the management of hypertension: part 2 – therapy. Can J Cardiol 2009;25(5):287–298.
12. Australian Medicines Handbook. Online. Available: http://amh.hcn.net.au/view.php. Accessed 15 April 2009.
13. Suter P, et al. Nutritional factors in the control of blood pressure and hypertension. Nutr Clin Care 2002;5(1):9–19.
14. Hamer M, et al. Psychological distress as a risk factor for cardiovascular events: pathophysiological and behavioural mechanisms. J Am Coll Cardiol 2008;52(25):2163–2165.
15. Sharma R, et al. Effect of yoga based lifestyle intervention on subjective wellbeing. Indian J Physiol Pharmacol 2008;52(2):123–131.
16. Sarris J. Herbal medicines in the treatment of psychiatric disorders: a systematic review. Phytother Res 2007;21(8):703–716.
17. Trauner G, et al. Modulation of GABAA receptors by valerian extracts is related to the content of valerenic acid. Planta Med 2008;74(1):19–24.
18. Circosta C, et al. Biological and analytical characterization of two extracts from Valeriana officinalis. J Ethnopharmacol 2007;112(2):361–367.
19. Del Valle-Mondragon, et al. Coronary vasodilator activity of vulgarenol, a sesquiterpene isolated from Magnolia grandiflora, and its possible mechanism. Phytother Res 2009;23(5):666–671.
20. Akhondzadeh S, et al. Passionflower in the treatment of generalized anxiety: a pilot double-blind randomized controlled trial with oxazepam. J Clin Pharm Ther 2001;26(5):363–367.
21. Wang S, et al. Fish oil supplementation improves large arterial elasticity in overweight hypertensive patients. Eur J Clin Nutr 2008;62(12):1426–1431.
22. Mottram P, et al. Vitamin E improves arterial compliance in middle-aged men and women. Atherosclerosis 1999;145(2):399–404.
23. Nishioka K, et al. Pycnogenol, French maritime pine bark extract, augments endothelium-dependent vasodilation in humans. Hypertension Res 2007;30(9):775–780.
24. Loke WM, et al. Pure dietary flavonoids quercetin and (–)–epicatechin augment nitric oxide products and reduce endothelin-1 acutely in healthy men. Am J Clin Nutr 2008;88(4):1018–1025.
25. Corti R, et al. Cocoa and cardiovascular health. Circulation 2009;119:1433–1441.
26. Mashavi M, et al. Effect of homocysteine-lowering therapy on arterial elasticity and metabolic parameters in metformin-treated diabetic patients. Atherosclerosis 2008;199(2):362–367.
27. Sontia B, Touyz RM. Magnesium transport in hypertension. Pathophysiology 2007;14(3–4):205–211.
28. Champagne C. Magnesium in hypertension, cardiovascular disease, metabolic syndrome, and other conditions: a review. Nutr Clin Pract 2008;23(2):142–151.
29. Sutherland JA. Selected complementary methods and nursing care of the hypertensive patient. Holist Nurs Pract 2001;15(4):4–11.
30. Walker AF, et al. Promising hypotensive effect of hawthorn extract: a randomized double-blind pilot study of mild, essential hypertension. Phytotherapy Res 2002;16(1):48–54.
31. Katzung, BG. Basic and clinical pharmacology. 10th edn. 2007. Online. Available: http://online.statref.com/Document/Document.aspx?docAddress = TIFOA7l8O5e5XA5c4bAs3A%3d%3d&Scroll = 1&Index = 0&SessionId = F5A72EKGPYHLJMJM. Accessed 30 May 2009.
32. Topol EJ, ed. Textbook of cardiovascular medicine. 3rd edn. 2007. Online. Available: http://ovidsp.tx.ovid.com/spa/ovidweb.cgi?&S = ELFHFPFONJDDONNMNCFLDFPJPKDHAA00&Link + Set = S.sh.18%7c1%7csl_10. Accessed 30 May 2009.
33. Amaechina FC, Omogbai EK. Hypotensive effect of aqueous extract of the leaves of Phyllanthus amarus Schum and Thonn (Euphorbiaceae). Acta Pol Pharm 2007;64(6):547–552.
34. Iizuka T, et al. Vasorelaxant effects of methyl brevifolincarboxylate from the leaves of Phyllanthus niruri. Biol Pharm Bull 2006;29(1):177–179.
35. Hnatyszyn O, et al. Diuretic activity of an aqueous extract of Phyllanthus sellowianus. Phytomedicine 1999;6(3):177–179.
36. Kang DG, et al. Angiotensin converting enzyme inhibitory phenylpropanoid glycosides from Clerodendron trichotomum. J Ethnopharmacol 2003;89(1):151–154.
37. Bowman TS, et al. Eight-year change in body mass index and subsequent risk of cardiovascular disease among healthy non-smoking men. Prev Med 2007;45(6):436–441.
38. AccessMedicine. Understanding body mass index. Postgraduate Medicine;117(2). Online. Available: http://www.accessmedicine.com/patientEd.aspx?aID = 857710&searchStr = body+mass+index+procedure. Accessed 25 February 2009.
39. Abell JE, et al. Age and race impact the association between BMI and CVD mortality in women. Public Health Rep 2007;122(4):507–512.
40. Longmore, et al. Oxford handbook of clinical medicine. 7th edn. Oxford: Oxford University Press, 2007:198.
41. Sutton-Tyrrell K, et al. High homocysteine levels are independently related to isolated systolic hypertension in older adults. Circulation 1997;96(6):1745–1749.
42. Muda P, et al. Effect of antihypertensive treatment with candesartan or amlodipine on glutathione and its redox status, homocysteine and vitamin concentrations in patients with essential hypertension. J Hypertension 2005;23(1):105–112.

43. Kanani PM, et al. Role of oxidant stress in endothelial dysfunction produced by experimental hyperhomocyst(e)inemia in humans. Circulation 1999;100(11):1161–1168.

44. Majchrzak D, et al. B-vitamin status and concentrations of homocysteine in Austrian omnivores, vegetarians and vegans. Ann Nutr Metab 2006;50(6):485–491.

45. Wolters M, et al. Effect of multivitamin supplementation on the homocysteine and methylmalonic acid blood concentrations in women over the age of 60 years. Eur J Nutr 2005;44(3):183–192.

46. Di Renzo G. *Ginkgo biloba* and the central nervous system. Fitoterapia 2000;71(Suppl. 1):S43–S47.

47. Zeng X, et al. *Ginkgo biloba* for acute ischaemic stroke. Cochrane Database Syst Rev 2005;(4):CD003691. Online. Available: doi: 10.1002/14651858.CD003691.pub2.

48. Saleem S, et al. *Ginkgo biloba* extract neuroprotective action is dependent on heme oxygenase 1 in ischemic reperfusion brain injury. Stroke 2008;39(12):3389–3396.

49. Wu YZ, et al. *Ginkgo biloba* extract improves coronary artery circulation in patients with coronary artery disease: contribution of plasma nitric oxide and endothelin-1. Phytother Res 2008;22(6):734–739.

50. Wu P, Liu S. Clinical observation on post-stroke anxiety neurosis treated by acupuncture. J Tradit Chin Med 2008;28(3):186–188.

51. Zhao JG, et al. Effect of acupuncture treatment on spastic states of stroke patients. J Neurol Sci 2009;276(1–2):143–147.

52. Hopwood V, et al. Evaluating the efficacy of acupuncture in defined aspects of stroke recovery: a randomised, placebo controlled single blind study. J Neurol 2008;255(6):858–866.

53. Stroke Unit Trialists' Collaboration. Organised inpatient (stroke unit) care for stroke. Cochrane Database Syst Rev 2007;(4):CD000197. Online. Available: doi: 10.1002/14651858.CD000197.pub2.

54. Olney CM. The effect of therapeutic back massage in hypertensive persons: a preliminary study. Biol Res Nurs 2005;7(2):98–105.

55. Camron JA, et al. Changes in blood pressure after various forms of therapeutic massage: a preliminary study. J Altern Complement Med 2006;12(1):65–70.

56. Lee H, et al. Acupuncture for lowering blood pressure: systematic review and meta-analysis. Am J Hypertens 2009;22(1):122–128.

57. Mamtani R, Mamtani R. Ayurveda and yoga in cardiovascular disease. Cardiol Rev 2004;12(5):155–162.

58. Appel LJ, et al. A clinical trial of the effects of dietary patterns on blood pressure. DASH Collaborative Research Group. N Engl J Med 1997;336(16):1117–1124.

59. Li J, et al. Salt inactivates endothelial nitric oxide synthase in endothelial cells. J Nutr 2009;139(3):447–451.

60. He J, et al. Gender difference in blood pressure responses to dietary sodium intervention in the GenSalt study. J Hypertens 2009;27(1):48–54.

61. Joubert LM, Manore MM. The role of physical activity level and B-vitamin status on blood homocysteine levels. Med Sci Sports Exerc 2008;40(11):1923–1931.

62. Strasser B, et al. The benefit of strength training on arterial blood pressure in patients with type 2 diabetes mellitus measured with ambulatory 24-hour blood pressure systems. Wien Med Wochenschr 2008;158(13–14):379–384.

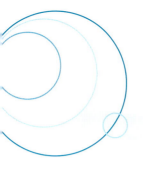

11
Chronic venous insufficiency

Matthew Leach
ND, RN, PhD

AETIOLOGY AND EPIDEMIOLOGY

Chronic venous insufficiency (CVI) is a pathological disorder of the venous system, characterised by impaired venous blood flow in the lower limbs. The condition is manifested by pathological changes to the skin, subcutaneous tissue and vascular tissue.[1] These manifestations, which can range from mild to severe, can be grouped into symptomatic complaints, such as leg heaviness, discomfort and pruritus, or advanced physical signs, including leg oedema, ochre pigmentation and lipodermatosclerosis. The condition, which is a precursor to varicose veins and venous leg ulceration, is not uncommon, affecting between 0.1% and 17% of men, and from 0.2% to 20% of women.[1]

This chronic and sometimes disabling disorder is believed to originate from an episode of macrovascular injury, which may be attributed to lower limb surgery, trauma, deep vein thrombosis (DVT) or pregnancy. This insult to the venous system can lead to valvular incompetence, venous reflux (or retrograde blood flow), ambulatory venous hypertension, venous wall dilatation and a subsequent rise in capillary filtration. As well as contributing to the formation of interstitial oedema, increased capillary filtration may also lead to localised hypoxia, malnutrition and eventual tissue destruction (see Figure 11.1). The extravasation of fibrinogen and the consequent formation of pericapillary cuffs, and the intraluminal trapping of leucocytes and subsequent release of toxic metabolites, proteolytic enzymes and tissue necrosis factor alpha (TNF-α)[2] are some of the mechanisms linking elevated capillary filtration pressure to changes in tissue perfusion and local architecture. The extravasation of fibrinogen and leucocyte products into pericapillary tissue may also mediate inflammation, suggesting that CVI may be a disease of chronic inflammation.[2]

RISK FACTORS

Many risk factors, both modifiable and non-modifiable, are claimed to be responsible for the pathogenesis of venous insufficiency. Occupations requiring periods of prolonged standing (such as nurses, flight attendants and factory workers) have been observed across a number of studies to have a higher prevalence and severity of CVI and varicose veins.[1]

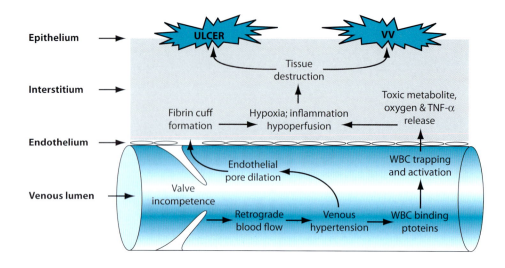

VV = varicose vein

Figure 11.1 The pathiophysiology of chronic venous insufficiency[5]

This could be attributed in part to excessive lower limb venous congestion secondary to reduced calf-muscle pump activity. Evidence linking other modifiable risk factors to chronic venous insufficiency, such as obesity, smoking, constipation, hormone therapy and hypertension, has been inconsistent however.[1]

In terms of non-modifiable risk factors, both family history and increasing age appear to be associated with an increased risk of CVI.[1] Advancing age is also correlated with an increased prevalence of varicose veins[1] and venous leg ulceration.[3] While female gender has been associated with an increased risk of varicose veins[1] and venous leg ulceration,[4] there is conflicting evidence regarding the link between sex and CVI risk.

CONVENTIONAL TREATMENT

There are a number of different approaches to the management of CVI. Two approaches often recommended in conventional practice are compression therapy and surgery. Compression therapy is advocated in conventional practice as it helps to reduce leg oedema, venous reflux, venous hypertension and lipodermatosclerosis, while improving deep vein blood flow velocity, capillary clearance, calf-muscle pump function, venous refilling time and venous ejection volume.[5] Compression therapy targets a number of processes associated with the pathogenesis of venous insufficiency, with a meta-analysis of 11 randomised controlled trials (n = 1453) finding compression therapy (10–15 mmHg) to be significantly more effective than low grade compression, placebo stockings and no treatment at reducing the symptoms of CVI, including lower limb oedema and discomfort.[6] These results need to be interpreted with caution, however, given the heterogeneous populations and diverse assessment techniques used in these studies. It is also possible that the reported effectiveness of compression therapy may not reflect that observed in clinical practice due to the poor level of compliance observed with this treatment. Some of the reasons for the poor adherence to compression therapy may relate to the long duration of therapy, the visible appearance of the stockings, associated discomfort, skin reactions, and the cost and maintenance of the therapy.[7]

The surgical restoration or removal of diseased vessels also may be advised in the overall management of chronic venous insufficiency. The array of surgical techniques that may be recommended include sclerotherapy, venous ligation and stripping, endovenous laser treatment, phlebectomy and valvuloplasty. Evidence from a meta-analysis of three randomised controlled trials (RCTs) suggests that venous ligation and valvuloplasty may be more effective than ligation alone in improving ambulatory venous pressure and quality of life.[8] Another meta-analysis of three RCTs found subfascial endoscopic perforator vein surgery (SEPS) to be significantly more effective than conventional surgery at reducing venous ulcer recurrence, wound infection and length of hospital stay in patients with CVI.[9] It is not clear from either of these reviews, however, whether the benefits of these techniques outweigh the risks and costs of surgery, and whether these approaches are relatively more effective (both economically and clinically) than the conservative management of CVI.

KEY TREATMENT PROTOCOLS

One of the core principles of naturopathic practice is to identify the underlying aetiology of the presenting condition. While some measures may be put in place to prevent macrovascular injury (such as adequate hydration and mobilisation), prevention of venous insufficiency may not always be possible, given that many individuals only present to their practitioner after CVI is well established. The naturopath can, however, target a number of mechanisms to prevent further progression of venous insufficiency, such as chronic inflammation, enzymatic degradation and oxidative damage.

NATUROPATHIC TREATMENT AIMS
- Identify the underlying cause of the venous insufficiency.
- Improve venous vessel tone and integrity.
- Improve venous haemodynamics.
- Alleviate unpleasant symptoms of venous insufficiency.
- Prevent further progression of venous insufficiency.
- Educate the patient about appropriate lifestyle choices.

Venous integrity
Enzymatic degradation
The abnormal venous tone observed in chronic venous insufficiency may be linked to an increase in lysosomal enzyme activity, as evidenced by the elevated levels of these enzymes in patients with CVI,[10] and in the exudate of venous ulcers.[11] The lysosomal enzymes hyaluronidase and elastase are believed to be responsible for this extravascular and extracellular matrix degradation,[12] and the subsequent increase in capillary permeability and oedema formation. It is therefore hypothesised that a reduction in lysosomal enzyme activity could decrease the symptoms of CVI by restoring venous elasticity and contractility through improvements in collagen biosynthesis[10] and proteoglycan recovery.[12]

The **saponins** and sapogenins of *Hedera helix* and *Aesculus hippocastanum* have been shown to inhibit hyaluronidase activity in vitro,[12] whereas *Ruscus aculeatus* saponins,[12] rutin[13] and grape seed procyanidins[14] have been found to inhibit elastase activity in vitro. By attenuating overactive lysosomal enzyme activity, these compounds may shift the equilibrium between proteoglycan synthesis and degradation, towards net synthesis. This reduction in enzyme activity against capillary wall mucopolysaccharides may improve vessel wall integrity and subsequently reduce oedema formation.[15–17] Although the saponins appear to be responsible for the anti-exudative and vascular-tightening effect of several of these plant extracts, the effect of other constituents (such as the flavonoids) cannot be dismissed.

Oxidative damage

Another process implicated in the pathogenesis of CVI is oxidative injury. This process involves the peroxidation of venous lipids, production of oxygen free radicals[18-19] and consequent destruction of lipids, proteins, collagen, proteoglycan and hyaluronic acid.[20] Agents that exhibit significant antioxidant activity may interrupt this cascade of events and, as a result, preserve venous tissue and improve venous integrity.

Many **phlebotonic agents** exhibit good antioxidant activity in experimental models, particularly free radical scavenging activity, including *Aesculus hippocastanum* horse chestnut seed extract (HCSE),[18] *Centella asiatica* flavonoids,[21] *Vaccinium myrtillus* extract,[22] grape seed extract, pine bark extract,[23] quercetin and rutin.[24] When the active-oxygen scavenging activity of 65 plant extracts were compared in vitro, HCSE and *Hamamelis virginiana* demonstrated the greatest antioxidant activity. Both extracts were found to be more potent than ascorbic acid and α-tocopherol in scavenging superoxide anions, but less effective than ascorbic acid in scavenging hydroxyl radicals and inhibiting singlet-oxygen generation.[19] As an indicator of cell protection, Masaki et al.[19] explored the effect that the plant extracts had on fibroblast survival. HCSE, witch hazel and English oak (*Quercus robur*) were the most protective, increasing fibroblast survival at least threefold. As fibroblasts are a key source of collagen, elastin, proteoglycans and matrix metalloproteinases,[11] increasing fibroblast survival is likely to improve venous integrity.

There is a large body of evidence to support the use of HCSE in the management of mild to moderate CVI. A Cochrane review of 17 RCTs found orally administered HCSE (standardised to 50–150 mg aescin daily, and administered for 20 days to 16 weeks (mean = 6 weeks)) to be more effective than placebo, and as effective as other phlebotonic agents, at reducing leg pain, oedema, pruritus, leg volume and ankle and calf circumference in patients with mild to moderate CVI.[25] As for severe or advanced cases of CVI, it appears that HCSE may not be as effective.[26]

Inflammation

Chronic inflammation is another contributing factor in the development of CVI. It is hypothesised that the manifestation of venous hypertension leads to widened capillary pore diameter, causing intravascular components such as fibrinogen, erythrocytes and α_2-macroglobulin to be leached into the interstitium.[2] These potent chemoattractants up-regulate the expression of intracellular adhesion molecule 1 (ICAM-1) and, together with increased platelet reactivity,[27] increase the expression of platelet-derived growth factor (PDGF) and vascular endothelial growth factor (VEGF). These growth factors trigger leucocyte migration. Once recruited, the white blood cells secrete or activate transforming growth factor-β_1 (TGF-β_1). Since TGF-β_1 has been located in pericapillary cuffs, it is believed that this growth factor may be responsible for tissue remodelling and fibrosis, as well as capillary angiogenesis, increased capillary tortuosity and density.[2] This factor may therefore contribute to some of the defining features of CVI, including varicose veins and lipodermatosclerosis. The increased expression of ICAM-1,[28-30] TGF-β_1,[31] PDGF and VEGF[32] in the dermis of patients with CVI lends some support to this sequelae of events.

Venotonic agents exhibiting antiinflammatory activity may attenuate the progression of CVI through a number of different pathways. Aescin (from HCSE)[33] and

Ruscus aculeatus extract,[34] for instance, both inhibit histamine-induced vascular permeability in vivo, an important step in the pathogenesis of CVI. Aescin,[33] grape seed extract[35] and *Vaccinium myrtillus* anthocyanosides[36] have also been shown to inhibit carrageenan-induced paw oedema, another measure of acute anti-inflammatory activity. French maritime pine bark extract (Pycnogenol™), on the other hand, exhibits anti-inflammatory activity by inhibiting nuclear factor kappa B (NFκB) and the proinflammatory cytokine interleukin-1 (IL-1);[37] whereas rutin and quercetin reduce inflammation by inhibiting the secretion of TNF-α, IL-1, IL-6, IL-8 and immunoglobulin E-induced histamine release.[38] Apart from grape seed extract,[39] however, few of these agents have yet been found to inhibit the key chemical mediators of CVI pathogenesis, including PDGF, VEGF, ICAM-1 and TGF-β_1.

The body of mechanistic data that supports many of these aforementioned treatments is supported by a growing body of clinical evidence. Many of these studies have, however, used complex formulations. This is problematic as it is almost impossible to extrapolate the effect of an individual agent from the effect of a complex formulation. Thus, when reviewing the best available evidence for these treatments, only those studies using monopreparations were included (see Table 11.1). In brief, evidence from RCTs indicate *Ruscus aculeatus* extract is statistically significantly superior to placebo in reducing leg volume, ankle and leg girth, and leg heaviness, fatigue and tension;[40] titrated extracts of *Centella asiatica* are significantly more effective than placebo at reducing ankle circumference and oedema,[41] lower leg volume[42] and leg heaviness and oedema;[43] Pycnogenol™ is significantly more effective than placebo at reducing leg heaviness and subcutaneous oedema;[44–45] and red vine leaf extract is statistically significantly superior to placebo at reducing calf circumference.[46–47]

INTEGRATIVE MEDICAL CONSIDERATIONS

The naturopathic management of CVI can be complemented by a range of conventional treatments, including compression therapy and surgery. Both of these approaches have already been described in detail under 'Conventional treatment'. In more advanced cases of venous insufficiency (such as venous leg ulceration), other members of the health-care team will need to be involved in the patient's care, including a nurse (for wound management) and vascular surgeon (for clinical review, surgical intervention and/or monitoring of vascular function). Other interventions that may be integrated into the patient's management plan are massage and reflexology. While massage may help to alleviate venous congestion, and thus may be theoretically justified as a treatment for CVI, there is still uncertainty about the safety and clinical effectiveness of massage in chronic venous insufficiency.

Reflexology

Reflexology is a tactile therapy that manipulates specific points in the hands, feet and/ or ears to initiate a reflex or physiological response in distant organs and tissues. A single-blind RCT tested whether this treatment may be effective in CVI by randomly allocating 55 healthy pregnant women with foot oedema to one of three groups: relaxation foot reflexology, lymphatic foot reflexology and rest.[48] Up to four 15-minute treatments were provided, though the mean number of visits in each group was not clear. The study found no statistically significant difference between groups in mean ankle and foot circumference measurements over time. While all groups demonstrated a significant reduction in pain, discomfort and tiredness, it is not clear if these symptoms related to the overall pregnancy or to CVI specifically. Thus, at this point in time, it is uncertain whether reflexology would be useful in alleviating the symptoms of venous insufficiency.

Table 11.1 Review of the major evidence

INTERVENTION	KEY LITERATURE	SUMMARY OF RESULTS	COMMENT
Centella asiatica (gotu kola) (multiple RCTs)	Cesarone et al. 2001[42] De Sanctis et al. 2001[41] Pointel et al. 1987[43]	Titrated extracts of *Centella asiatica* (60–180 mg / day) were more effective than placebo at reducing ankle circumference and oedema at 4 weeks, lower leg volume at 6 weeks, and leg heaviness and oedema at 8 weeks.	It is not yet clear if the long-term use of high-dose *C. asiatica* is safe or effective in CVI.
French maritime bark extract (Pycnogenol™) (multiple RCTs)	Arcangeli 2000[44] Petrassi et al. 2000[45]	French maritime bark extract (300 mg/day) was more effective than placebo at reducing leg heaviness and subcutaneous oedema at 8 weeks.	Changes in venous haemodynamics were not consistent between the two studies.
Horse chestnut seed extract (HCSE) (Cochrane review)	Pittler & Ernst 2006[25]	HCSE (standardised to 50–150 mg aescin daily, and administered for 20 days to 16 weeks) was more effective than placebo, and as effective as other phlebotonic agents, at reducing leg pain, oedema, pruritus, leg volume, and ankle and calf circumference in patients with mild to moderate CVI.	The saponins in HCSE may cause gastric irritation and/or nausea in some individuals. Enteric-coated HCSE formulations may reduce the risk of these adverse events.
Red vine leaf extract (RVLE) (multiple RCTs)	Kalus et al. 2004[46] Kiesewetter et al. 2000[47]	Red vine leaf extract (360–720 mg/day) was more effective than placebo at reducing calf circumference at 6 and 12 weeks.	Changes in ankle circumference were not consistent between the two studies.
Ruscus aculeatus (Butcher's broom) (RCT)	Vansheidt et al. 2002[40]	*Ruscus aculeatus* extract was more effective than placebo at reducing leg volume, ankle and leg girth, and leg heaviness, fatigue and tension at 12 weeks.	All study participants were women. Therefore, these findings may not be applicable to men.

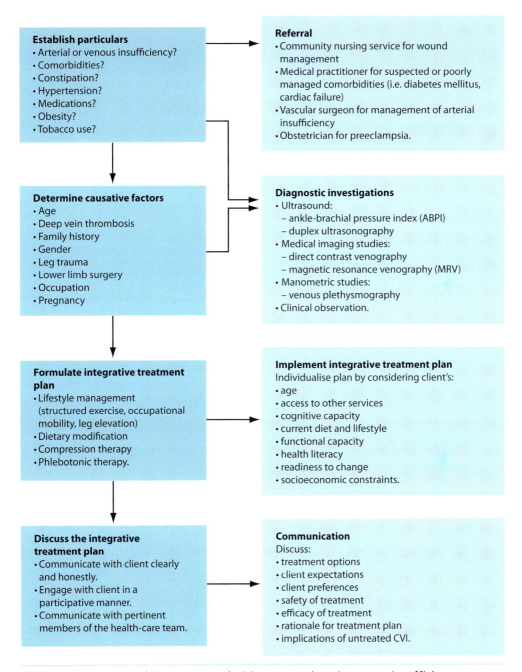

Establish particulars
• Arterial or venous insufficiency?
• Comorbidities?
• Constipation?
• Hypertension?
• Medications?
• Obesity?
• Tobacco use?

Referral
• Community nursing service for wound management
• Medical practitioner for suspected or poorly managed comorbidities (i.e. diabetes mellitus, cardiac failure)
• Vascular surgeon for management of arterial insufficiency
• Obstetrician for preeclampsia.

Determine causative factors
• Age
• Deep vein thrombosis
• Family history
• Gender
• Leg trauma
• Lower limb surgery
• Occupation
• Pregnancy

Diagnostic investigations
• Ultrasound:
  – ankle-brachial pressure index (ABPI)
  – duplex ultrasonography
• Medical imaging studies:
  – direct contrast venography
  – magnetic resonance venography (MRV)
• Manometric studies:
  – venous plethysmography
• Clinical observation.

Formulate integrative treatment plan
• Lifestyle management (structured exercise, occupational mobility, leg elevation)
• Dietary modification
• Compression therapy
• Phlebotonic therapy.

Implement integrative treatment plan
Individualise plan by considering client's:
• age
• access to other services
• cognitive capacity
• current diet and lifestyle
• functional capacity
• health literacy
• readiness to change
• socioeconomic constraints.

Discuss the integrative treatment plan
• Communicate with client clearly and honestly.
• Engage with client in a participative manner.
• Communicate with pertinent members of the health-care team.

Communication
Discuss:
• treatment options
• client expectations
• client preferences
• safety of treatment
• efficacy of treatment
• rationale for treatment plan
• implications of untreated CVI.

Figure 11.2 Naturopathic treatment decision tree—chronic venous insufficiency

Case Study

A 68-year-old woman presents with a 15-year history of **bilateral lower limb heaviness, discomfort** and **mild pitting pedal oedema**. The symptoms were relieved 6 years ago following bilateral lower limb venous ligation and stripping, but have returned in the last 12 months. **Underlying cardiovascular, lymphatic and renal disease have been excluded**.

SUGGESTIVE SYMPTOMS

- Leg heaviness
- Lipodermatosclerosis
- Ochre pigmentation
- Oedema
- Pain/discomfort

- Pruritus
- Skin dryness
- Varicose veins
- Venous leg ulceration

Example treatment

Herbal and nutritional prescription

Once the underlying causes of the CVI have been identified, and measures introduced to address the causes (where possible), the naturopath should focus their attention on the pathological processes of the disease. Agents with venotonic activity, as well as antioxidant, anti-inflammatory, antienzymatic and antioedema effects, would be most desirable in this case. Interventions that exhibit more than one of these actions and, more importantly, have

Herbal prescription	
Aesculus hippocastanum 1:2	25 mL
Centella asiatica 1:1	30 mL
Ruscus aculeatus 1:2	35 mL
Zingiber officinale 1:2	10 mL
	100 mL

Dose: 7 mL b.d. (before meals)

Nutritional prescription
Mixed bioflavonoids (including 500 mg rutin, 500 mg hesperidin and 500 mg quercetin) b.d.

demonstrable clinical efficacy in patients with CVI should be afforded the highest priority in the naturopathic management of venous insufficiency. Examples of interventions that fulfil these criteria include horse chestnut seed extract, *Ruscus aculeatus*, *Vaccinium myrtillus*, *Centella asiatica*, French maritime pine bark extract, red vine leaf extract and grape seed extract. Many of these agents have been included in the herbal prescription outlined on the right. The inclusion of mixed bioflavonoids (as a nutritional prescription) is based on theoretical evidentiary support only–specifically, data from mechanistic studies.[24,38]

Dietary and lifestyle advice

Many lifestyle changes may be recommended in the management of CVI. However, much of this advice is based on theoretical or pathophysiological rationale. In fact, many lifestyle factors (smoking, obesity, constipation, physical inactivity) have not been shown conclusively to increase the risk of CVI. There is also insufficient evidence linking the modification of these risk factors to clinical improvements in venous insufficiency. There is weak evidence, however, to suggest that lower limb elevation and prescribed exercise may be helpful in CVI.

Leg elevation is often recommended to people with CVI to help reduce lower limb venous pressure, leg discomfort and oedema. Although lower limb elevation (to 30 cm above heart level) has been shown to enhance microcirculatory flow velocity in liposclerotic skin of patients with chronic venous insufficiency,[49] it is uncertain whether leg elevation offers any significant clinical benefit to patients with CVI. Given that many

HAEMORRHOIDS

Overview
The underlying causes of haemorrhoidal disease are similar to that of varicose veins. As the portal venous system contains no valves, factors that increase venous congestion in the region—including intraabdominal pressure from causes such as strained defecation, pregnancy, cirrhosis of the liver or standing or sitting for prolonged periods of time—can hasten haemorrhoid formation.[51–53] Haemorrhoids are common and tend to develop between the ages of 20 and 50 years–in the Western world they are extremely common and half of all people will experience them by the time they reach 50 years of age.[53]

Internal haemorrhoids are a complex of dilated blood vessels, including branches of the superior haemorrhoidal artery and veins of the internal haemorrhoidal venous plexus.

Bleeding is the first (and, in many people, only) symptom of haemorrhoids—the word itself means 'flow of blood'. Other symptoms may include itching and irritation, prolapsed, mucoid discharge, incomplete bowel evacuation and pain.

Conventional treatment
Treatment for the removal of haemorrhoids revolves around a number of surgical options: rubber band ligation, cryotherapy and sphincterotomy.[51–53] However, treatment in conventional medicine is increasingly focused towards prevention. The most common cause of haemorrhoids is constipation due to lack of fibre. Accordingly, conventional treatment centres around the promotion of a soft, bulky stool through dietary modification and/or supplementation.[52] Topical treatment for pruritus ani or pain may also be recommended, most often in the form of steroid or anaesthetic medication.[53]

CAM interventions
Nutrition clearly needs to be considered. With overwhelming evidence to support increased fibre in the diet, appropriate dietary adjustments should be suggested. However, supplementation with bulking agents such as *Ulmus fulva* or *Plantago ovata* husks may also be beneficial. Supplementation with *Plantago ovata* husks is approved by Commission E for relieving constipation in haemorrhoids.[15]

A warm sitz bath may also be an effective and non-invasive treatment for haemorrhoids, most likely due to mechanisms involving relaxation of the internal anal sphincter.[54]

The internal use of herbs and nutrients for varicose veins and venous insufficiency suggested earlier in the chapter will be equally well indicated in restoring venous integrity in haemorrhoid treatment. Herbal medicines may be useful both internally and topically. However, few trials of herbal or clinical nutritional treatment in haemorrhoids exist. In one double-blind, placebo-controlled trial, internal use of *Aesculum hippocastanum* (equivalent to 40 mg aescin three times daily) for 6 days or more was found to relieve symptoms (82% compared to 32% with placebo) and reduce swelling (87% versus 38% with placebo) in 72 patients with acute symptamatic haemorrhoids.[17]

Topical therapy in most instances will provide only temporary relief of symptoms. Astringent therapy may be beneficial in restoring venous tone and has been traditionally used for this purpose.[15,55] Astringent ointments containing *Hamamelis virginiana*, for instance, have been shown in clinical studies to be beneficial in alleviating the symptoms of haemorrhoids, demonstrating similar efficacy to conventional topical applications.[56,57] Other topical herbs that have been used include *Matricaria recutita* and *Calendula officinalis*.

patients experience some relief of symptoms following lower limb elevation, there is no reason why this practice should not be recommended at this point in time.

A structured exercise program also may be recommended to individuals with CVI in order to facilitate calf-muscle pump function and reduce venous congestion. Findings from a small RCT (n = 31) showed that a supervised calf-muscle strength exercise program, together with compression hosiery, significantly improved mean venous ejection fraction at 6 months when compared to control. Between-group differences in venous reflux, venous severity scores and quality of life, however, were not statistically significant.[50] Nevertheless, given that long periods of standing may contribute to the pathogenesis of CVI, it is probable that a structured exercise program may still be useful in preventing the onset and/or progression of the disease.

Dietary modification is a central feature of the naturopathic prescription. Even though there is a paucity of clinical evidence to justify dietary modification in CVI management, the potential benefit of this approach should not be overlooked. It is possible that many of the pathological processes of CVI, such as inflammation and oxidation, may be attenuated by reducing the dietary intake of saturated, omega-6 and *trans*-fatty acids, and by increasing the consumption of foods high in omega-3 fatty acids (such as salmon), flavonoids (such as onion) and procyanidins (such as berries).

Expected outcomes and follow-up protocols

For the 68-year-old woman presenting with CVI (as outlined at the beginning of this section), it is unlikely that this chronic condition will ever be cured. The naturopathic treatment approach may, however, prevent further progression of the disease by attenuating the pathogenesis of CVI, and, in turn, prevent the development of more serious pathologies, including varicose veins and venous leg ulceration. If the patient adheres to the naturopathic treatment plan (herbal and nutritional prescriptions, and dietary and lifestyle advice), a clinically significant reduction in CVI manifestations (such as leg heaviness, discomfort and oedema) should be evident within 3 or 4 weeks. If no clinical improvement is observed within this period of time, one of the extracts in the herbal prescription can be substituted with *Vaccinium myrtillus*, French maritime pine bark extract, red vine leaf extract or grape seed extract. Alternatively, the herbal formulation may be replaced with high dose, enteric-coated HCSE (standardised to 150 mg aescin daily). If the patient continues to be unresponsive to naturopathic treatment after 12 weeks, the patient should be referred to a vascular surgeon for review.

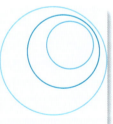

KEY POINTS
- CVI is a chronic and often disabling disorder of the lower limbs.
- The treatment of CVI should focus primarily on addressing and resolving the underlying cause, and pathological processes, of the condition.
- The naturopathic management of CVI should give preference to agents with venotonic, anti-inflammatory, antioxidant, antienzymatic and antioedema activity, particularly those with demonstrable clinical efficacy in persons with CVI.
- Patients with advanced CVI should be referred for compression therapy, surgery, wound management and/or further assessment where applicable.

Further reading

Pappas PJ, et al. Causes of severe chronic venous insufficiency. Seminars in Vascular Surgery 2005;18:30–35.

White JV, Ryjewski C. Chronic venous insufficiency. Perspectives in Vascular Surgery & Endovascular Therapy 2005;17(4):319–327.

References

1. Beebe-Dimmer JL, et al. The epidemiology of chronic venous insufficiency and varicose veins. Annals of Epidemiology 2004;15:175–184.
2. Pappas PJ, et al. Causes of severe chronic venous insufficiency. Seminars in Vascular Surgery 2005;18:30–35.
3. Baker S, Stacey M. Epidemiology of chronic leg ulcers in Australia. Australian & New Zealand Journal of Surgery 1994;64(4):258–261.
4. Callam M, et al. Chronic ulcer of the leg: clinical history. British Medical Journal 1987;294(6584):1389–1391.
5. Leach MJ. Making sense of the venous leg ulcer debate: a literature review. Journal of Wound Care 2004;13(2):52–57.
6. Amsler F, Blattler W. Compression therapy for occupational leg symptoms and chronic venous disorders – a meta-analysis of randomised controlled trials. European Journal of Vascular and Endovascular Surgery, 2008;35(3):366–372.
7. Raju S, et al. Use of compression stockings in chronic venous disease: patient compliance and efficacy. Annals of Vascular Surgery 2008;21(6):790–795.
8. Hardy SC, et al. Surgery for deep venous incompetence. Cochrane Database of Systematic Reviews 2004;(3).
9. Luebke T, Brunkwall J. Meta-analysis of subfascial endoscopic perforator vein surgery (SEPS) for chronic venous insufficiency. Phlebology 2009;24(1):8–16.
10. Kreysel H, et al. A possible role of lysosomal enzymes in the pathogenesis of varicosis and the reduction in their serum activity by Venostasin. VASA 1983;12(4):377–382.
11. Schultz G, Mast B. Molecular analysis of the environment of healing and chronic wounds: cytokines, proteases, and growth factors. Wounds 1998;10(Supp F):1F–9F.
12. Facino R, et al. Anti-elastase and anti-hyaluronidase activities of saponins and sapogenins from *Hedera helix, Aesculus hippocastanum*, and *Ruscus aculeatus*: factors contributing to their efficacy in the treatment of venous insufficiency. Archiv der Pharmazie 1995;328(10):720–724.
13. Selloum L, et al. Anti-inflammatory effect of rutin on rat paw oedema, and on neutrophils chemotaxis and degranulation. Experimental & Toxicologic Pathology 2003;54(4):313–318.
14. Carini M, et al. Procyanidins from *Vitis vinifera* seeds inhibit the respiratory burst of activated human neutrophils and lysosomal enzyme release. Planta Medica 2001;67(8):714–717.
15. Blumenthal M, ed. The complete German Commission E monographs: therapeutic guide to herbal medicines. Austin: American Botanical Council, 1998.
16. Gruenwald J, et al. PDR for herbal medicines. Montvale: Medical Economics Company, 2000.
17. Sirtori C. Aescin: pharmacology, pharmacokinetics and therapeutic profile. Pharmacological Research 2001;44(3):183–193.
18. Guillaume M, Padioleau F. Veinotonic effect, vascular protection, antiinflammatory and free radical scavenging properties of horse chestnut extract. Arzneimittel Forschung 1994;44(1):25–35.
19. Masaki H, et al. Active-oxygen scavenging activity of plant extracts. Biological & Pharmaceutical Bulletin 1995;18(1):162–166.
20. Yeoh S. The influence of iron and free radicals on chronic leg ulceration. Primary Intention 2000;8(2):47–55.
21. Zheng CJ, Qin LP. Chemical components of *Centella asiatica* and their bioactivities. Journal of Chinese Integrative Medicine 2007;5(3):348–351.
22. Faria A, et al. Antioxidant properties of prepared blueberry (*Vaccinium myrtillus*) extracts. Journal of Agricultural & Food Chemistry 2005;53(17):6896–6902.
23. Busserolles J, et al. In vivo antioxidant activity of procyanidin-rich extracts from grape seed and pine (Pinus maritima) bark in rats. International Journal for Vitamin & Nutrition Research 2006;76(1):22–27.
24. Zhang J, et al. Free radical scavenging and cytoprotective activities of phenolic antioxidants. Molecular Nutrition & Food Research 2006;50(11):996–1005.
25. Pittler MH, Ernst E. Horse chestnut seed extract for chronic venous insufficiency. Cochrane Database of Systematic Reviews 2006;(1): CD003230.
26. Leach MJ, et al. Clinical efficacy of horsechestnut seed extract in the treatment of venous ulceration. Journal of Wound Care 2006;15(4):159–167.
27. Lu X, Chen Y, Huang Y, Li W, Jiang M. Venous hypertension induces increased platelet reactivity and accumulation in patients with chronic venous insufficiency. Angiology 2006;57(3):321–329.
28. Ciuffetti G, et al. Circulating leucocyte adhesion molecules in chronic venous insufficiency. VASA 1999;28(3):156–159.
29. Peschen M, et al. Expression of the adhesion molecules ICAM-1, VCAM-1, LFA-1 and VLA-4 in the skin is modulated in progressing stages of chronic venous insufficiency. Acta Dermato-Venereologica 1999;79(1):27–32.
30. Wilkinson LS, et al. Leukocytes: their role in the etiopathogenesis of skin damage in venous disease. Journal of Vascular Surgery 1993;17:669–675.
31. Pappas PJ, et al. Dermal tissue fibrosis in patients with chronic venous insufficiency is associated with increased transforming growth factor-β1 gene expression and protein production. Journal of Vascular Surgery 1999;30(6):1129–1145.
32. Peschen M, et al. Increased expression of platelet-derived growth factor receptor alpha and beta and vascular endothelial growth factor in the skin of patients with chronic venous insufficiency. Archives of Dermatological Research 1998;290(6):291–297.
33. Matsuda H, et al. Effects of escins Ia, Ib, IIa, and IIB from Horse chestnut, the seeds of *Aesculus hippocastanum* L., on acute inflammation in animals. Biological & Pharmaceutical Bulletin 1997;20(10):1092–1095.
34. Bouskela E, et al. Possible mechanisms for the inhibitory effect of *Ruscus* extract on increased microvascular permeability induced by histamine in hamster cheek pouch. Journal of Cardiovascular Pharmacology 1994;24(2):281–285.
35. Greenspan P, et al. Antiinflammatory properties of the muscadine grape (*Vitis rotundifolia*). Journal of Agricultural & Food Chemistry 2005;53(22):8481–8488.
36. Lietti A, et al. Studies on *Vaccinium myrtillus* anthocyanosides. I. Vasoprotective and antiinflammatory activity. Arzneimittel Forschung 1976;26(5):829–832.
37. Cho KJ, et al. Effect of bioflavonoids extracted from the bark of *Pinus maritima* on proinflammatory cytokine interleukin-1 production in lipopolysaccharide-stimulated RAW 264.7. Toxicology & Applied Pharmacology 2000;168(1):64–71.
38. Park HH, et al. Flavonoids inhibit histamine release and expression of proinflammatory cytokines in mast cells. Archives of Pharmaceutical Research 2008;31(10):1303–1311.
39. Wen W, et al. Grape seed extract inhibits angiogenesis via suppression of the vascular endothelial growth factor receptor signalling pathway. Cancer Prevention Research 2008;1(7):554–561.

40. Vanscheidt W, et al. Efficacy and safety of a Butcher's broom preparation (*Ruscus aculeatus* L. extract) compared to placebo in patients suffering from chronic venous insufficiency. Arzneimittel Forschung 2002;52(4):243–250.

41. De Sanctis MT, et al. Treatment of edema and increased capillary filtration in venous hypertension with total triterpenic fraction of *Centella asiatica:* a clinical, prospective, placebo-controlled, randomized, dose-ranging trial. Angiology 2001;52(Suppl 2):S55–S59.

42. Cesarone MR, et al. Microcirculatory effects of total triterpenic fraction of *Centella asiatica* in chronic venous hypertension: measurement by laser Doppler, TcPO2–CO2, and leg volumetry. Angiology 2001;52(Suppl 2):S45–S48.

43. Pointel JP, et al. Titrated extract of *Centella asiatica* (TECA) in the treatment of venous insufficiency of the lower limbs. Angiology 1987;38(1, Pt 1):46–50.

44. Arcangeli P. Pycnogenol in chronic venous insufficiency. Fitoterapia 2000;71(3):236–244.

45. Petrassi C, et al. Pycnogenol in chronic venous insufficiency. Phytomedicine 2000;7(5):383–388.

46. Kalus U, et al. Improvement of cutaneous microcirculation and oxygen supply in patients with chronic venous insufficiency by orally administered extract of red vine leaves AS 195: a randomised, double-blind, placebo-controlled, crossover study. Drugs in R&D 2004;5(2):63–71.

47. Kiesewetter H, et al. Efficacy of orally administered extract of red vine leaf AS 195 (folia vitis viniferae) in chronic venous insufficiency (stages I-II). A randomized, double-blind, placebo-controlled trial. Arzneimittel Forschung 2000;50(2):109–117.

48. Mollart L. Single-blind trial addressing the differential effects of two reflexology techniques versus rest, on ankle and foot oedema in late pregnancy. Complementary Therapies in Nursing and Midwifery 2003;9(4):203–208.

49. Abu-Own A, et al. Effect of leg elevation on the skin microcirculation in chronic venous insufficiency. Journal of Vascular Surgery 1994;20(5):705–710.

50. Padberg FT, et al. Structured exercise improves calf muscle pump function in chronic venous insufficiency: a randomized trial. Journal of Vascular Surgery 2004;39(1):79–87.

51. Chong PS, Bartolo DC. Hemorrhoids and fissure in ano. Gastroenterol Clin North Am 2008;37(3):627–644.

52. Acheson AG, Scholefield JH. Management of haemorrhoids. BMJ 2008;336(7640):380–383.

53. Murtagh J. General practice. Sydney: McGraw-Hill, 2006.

54. Shafik A. Role of warm-water bath in anorectal conditions. The 'thermosphincteric reflex'. J Clin Gastroenterol 1993;16(4):304–308.

55. Scientific Committee of the British Herbal Medical Association. British herbal pharmacopoeia. Bournemouth: British Herbal Medicine Association, 1983.

56. Drug therapy of hemorrhoids. Proven results of therapy with a hamamelis containing hemorrhoid ointment. Results of a meeting of experts. Fortschr Med 1991;116(Supp):1–11.

57. Knoch HG, et al. Ointment treatment of 1st degree hemorrhoids. Comparison of the effectiveness of a phytogenic preparation with two new ointments containing synthetic drugs. Fortschr Med 1992;110(8):135–138.

Section 4 Nervous system

The nervous system is inextricably linked with all bodily systems, and has an interaction with every disease and health condition. Nervous impulses govern the nervous system, which is a complex network of cells that communicate information by means of electrochemical signals.

The psychological aspect of the nervous system differentiates this system from all others. Neuronal communication conveys information from the environment and facilitates the emotional and mental experience of it. The mind has a potent effect on a person's perceived wellbeing; this affects all aspects of health or disease. The field of psychoneuroimmunology concerns the study of the effect the mind has on the immune function and other systems. In essence, a positive health mental state will enhance the body's ability to heal itself, while a poor mental state will impede healing. This process involves a complex dynamic between the nervous, endocrine and immune systems.

Common conditions treated by naturopaths specifically involving the nervous system include psychiatric disorders, insomnia, headaches, herpes zoster, neuralgia and pain. Other conditions not so commonly treated are Alzheimer's disease, Huntington's disease, epilepsy, Bell's palsy, multiple sclerosis, Parkinson's disease and central nervous system (CNS) disorders. With respect to the specific treatment of nervous system conditions, the influence of stress (on lifestyle, work and relationships), diet, exercise and spiritual dynamics should be explored through the case-taking process.

Nervous system conditions are treated in naturopathy by means of a range of interventions including herbal medicine, nutrients, dietary modification, manual therapy, exercise, aromatherapy and psychological support. Nutrients that are involved in nervous system function include omega-3 fatty acids, B vitamins (including folate and B12), vitamin C and amino acids. These therapies and interventions may provide benefit by potentially modulating neuronal communication, thereby affecting neuroreceptor binding and activity, and altering neurotransmitter formation and activity, hence regulating and enhancing neural transmission to the cells and organs throughout the body. Herbal medicines are particularly adept at modulating neurological activity due to some constituents' ability to bind with neuroreceptor sites and modulate neurotransmission. Common actions can involve stimulating or sedating CNS activity, and regulating or supporting the healthy function of the hypothalamic pituitary adrenal axis.

A key protocol in treating most nervous system conditions is to assess the systemic relationship with other systems, and conversely the effect of other health conditions on the nervous system and psychological state of the patient. The clinician, via thorough case taking, should always assess the basic psychological state of the patient and the effect this may be having on other health conditions. The focus of this section is on psychological disorders, as these conditions are prevalent and have a marked influence on health and wellbeing. It should be noted that dementia and cognitive decline are covered in Chapter 32, but conditions such as epilepsy are outside the scope of this text.

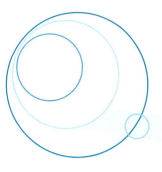

12
Clinical depression

Jerome Sarris
ND, MHSc, PhD

CLASSIFICATION, EPIDEMIOLOGY AND AETIOLOGY

Depression is associated with normal emotions of sadness and loss, and can be seen as part of the natural adaptive response to life's stressors. True 'clinical depression', however, is a disproportionate ongoing state of sadness, or absence of pleasure, that persists after the exogenous stressors have abated. Clinical depression is commonly characterised by either a low mood, or a loss of pleasure, in combination with changes in, for example, appetite, sleep and energy, and is often accompanied by feelings of guilt or worthlessness or suicidal thoughts.[1] The *Diagnostic and Statistical Manual of Mental Disorders* (DSM-IV) classifies 'Major Depressive Disorder' (MDD) as a clinical depressive episode that lasts longer than 2 weeks, and is uncomplicated by recent grief, substance abuse or a medical condition.[2] Depression presents a significant socioeconomic burden, with the condition being projected by the year 2020 to effect the second greatest increase in morbidity after cardiovascular disease.[3] The lifetime prevalence of depressive disorders varies depending on the country, age, sex and socioeconomic group, and approximates about one in six people.[4,5] The 12-month prevalence of MDD is approximately 5–8%, with women approximately twice as likely as men to experience an episode.[4,5]

The pathophysiology of MDD is complex, and to date no unified theory explaining the biological cause exists.[1] The main premise concerning the biopathophysiology of MDD centres on monoamine impairment, involving:[6–10]

- dysfunction in monoamine expression and receptor activity, or a lowering of monoamine production
- secondary messenger system malfunction, for example G proteins or cyclic AMP
- neuroendocrinological abnormality concerning hyperactivity of the hypothalamic–pituitary–adrenal axis (HPA axis), which increases serum cortisol and thereby subsequently reduces brain-derived neurotropic factor (BDNF) and neurogenesis
- impaired endogenous opioid function
- changes in GABAergic and/or glutamatergic transmission, and cytokine or steroidal alterations
- abnormal circadian rhythm.

From a holistic perspective, the biological causes of depression are unique to the individual, and can be viewed biochemically as varying impairment of monoamine

THE FOUR HUMORS

A traditional view of depression terms the condition 'melancholia'. This is based on the humoral model, which depicts four 'humors' (choleric, sanguine, phlegmatic and melancholic).[17]

Depression falls under the auspices of the melancholic humor, being embodied as 'black bile'.

The liver from an energetic perspective in traditional Western folkloric medicine and from traditional Chinese medicine is considered to be the organ primarily involved with depression, and is seen to regulate emotions.[17,18]

Western medicine views the liver purely from a biomedical perspective, and research has not yet been conducted to examine any correlation between liver function/health and depression.

activity, homocysteine, cortisol and BDNF, and inflammatory interactions. Psychologically, cognitive and behavioural causes (or manifestations) of MDD are also commonly present in variations of negative or erroneous thought patterns, or schemas, impaired self-mastery, challenged social roles, and depressogenic behaviours or lifestyle choices.[11–13]

Several biological and psychological models theorising the causes of depression have been proposed (reviewed below). The predominant biological model of depression in the last 60 years is the monoamine hypothesis.[14] Other key biological theories involve the homocysteine hypothesis,[15] and the inflammatory cytokine depression theory.[8] A prominent psychological model is the stress-diathesis model, which promulgates the theory that a combination of vulnerabilities (genetic, parenting, health status and cognitions) are exploited by a life stressor, for example relationship break-up, job loss and family death.[13,16] These stressful events may trigger a depressive disorder. Some scholars have advanced the theory of a biopsychosocial model, which aims to understand depression in terms of a dynamic interrelation between the biological, psychological and social causes (discussed later).[12]

RISK FACTORS

Various factors that increase the risk of MDD exist, and such an episode may in turn cause certain health disorders/issues. Genetic vulnerability may play an important part in the development of MDD. Genetic studies have revealed that polymorphisms relevant to monoaminergic neurotransmission exist in some people who experience MDD.[19] Recent hypotheses suggest that genes related to neuroprotective/toxic/trophic processes, and to the overactivation of the hypothalamic–pituitary axis may be involved in the pathogenesis of MDD.[19] Early life events or proximal stressful events increase the risk of an episode.[20] Twin studies provide evidence of the effect of environmental stressors on depression and many studies have revealed that a range of stressful events are involved, affecting remission and relapse of the disorder. Recurrence of depressive episodes and early age at onset present with the greatest familial risk.[21] Current evidence suggests that the primary risk factors involved in MDD are a complex interplay of genetics and exposure to depressogenic life events.

DEPRESSION: AT-RISK GROUPS[4,5,22]

- Females
- Younger people
- Previously married or unmarried people (especially for men)
- Unemployed or under financial pressure
- People with disabilities
- Possibly those living in large urban areas
- Major health conditions (especially cardiovascular disease)
- Obesity/metabolic disorders
- Chronic insomnia
- Alcohol/drug abuse or dependency

A consistent theme revealed by epidemiological data is that females have higher rates of MDD than men, approximating two times higher in some community samples.[4] This is associated with a higher risk of first onset, and not due to differential persistence or recurrence. It appears that hormonal factors are not responsible (for example, oestrogen levels, pregnancy or the use of oral contraceptives). Biological vulnerabilities and environmental psychosocial factors appear to be responsible for the increased incidence of depression among women. Initial psychosocial triggers may occur in early teen years upon the onset of puberty, whereby gender difference markedly presents. As Kessler states,[23] it is conceivable that MDD presents more commonly in females due to social and psychological influences, such as sex-role differences and an intrinsic propensity to ruminate. Another methodological possibility is that men's depression may present with irritability rather than anhedonia, and as depression scales place less weight on irritability this may skew the results.

Practitioners should be aware of the existence of conditions that commonly co-occur with MDD. People who are clinically depressed have a far greater risk of having co-occurring generalised anxiety, sleep disorders and substance abuse or dependency.[23] It should be noted that these conditions may cause MDD and may also result from MDD. Depression is also often misdiagnosed as 'unipolar' when in fact it is the presentation of the depressive phase of 'bipolar' depression.[24] Appropriate screening needs to occur in patients presenting with depression. Initial questioning should assess the length and frequency of previous and current episodes, the severity, what triggers an episode, and whether they think about death regularly or have felt so low lately that they have considered suicide. Assessment should also include a drug and alcohol screen in addition to reviewing their sleep pattern and level of anxiety and stress. To assess any bipolarity of the depression, it is important to determine whether they have ever experienced several days or more of feeling very happy or 'high' in addition to behavioural changes such as a decreased need for sleep, rapidity of cognition or ideas, and any increases in planning, spending money or sexual drive (the bipolar spectrum discussed further below).[24] Appropriate referral in the case of suspected alcohol/substance abuse or dependency or bipolar disorder is recommended, as complementary or alternative medicine (CAM) currently lacks evidence as a primary intervention in these areas (although CAM may be adjuvantly beneficial).

SUICIDE

- Screen for presence of a clearly articulated plan to suicide, any preparations being made, and any past serious attempts.
- If patient is suicidal, refer immediately to an emergency department of a hospital for psychiatric assessment.
- Extreme caution should be observed for patients who in light of a recent suicidal disposition suddenly appear happy with no clear reason (they may be at peace with their decision to suicide).
- Initial antidepressant use may increase risk of suicide. Be especially aware of antidepressant use in adolescents.

CONVENTIONAL TREATMENT

Current medical treatment strategies for MDD primarily involves synthetic antidepressants (for example, tricyclics, monoamine oxidase inhibitors or selective serotonin reuptake inhibitors), and psychological interventions (for example, cognitive behavioural therapy (CBT), interpersonal therapy (IPT) and behavioural therapy (BT)).[1,25] Medical treatment guidelines usually involve options such as providing counselling, CBT or IPT for mild depression, antidepressants and/or CBT for moderate depression, and antidepressants and ECT (and possibly hospitalisation) for severe depression.[26,27] As only 30–40% of people achieve a satisfactory response to first-line antidepressant prescription, and approximately 40% do not achieve remission after several antidepressant prescriptions, further pharmacotherapeutic developments are currently being pursued.[14,28] Future novel antidepressant mechanisms of action may involve modulating cytokines, secondary messengers, and glucocorticoid, opioid, dopaminergic or melatoninergic pathways.[9]

KEY TREATMENT PROTOCOLS

From a clinical perspective, the goal of treating MDD is to ameliorate the depression as safely and quickly as possible. Suicide is a great concern, and is a devastating potential consequence of MDD. If suicidal ideation is significant, or if self-harm is a distinct possibility at any stage, referral to a medical practitioner or to an emergency ward of hospital for immediate psychiatric assessment is crucial. The socioeconomic cost of untreated MDD is massive, and treated depression reduces the burden on health-care systems.[29] Evidence advocates early intervention to effectively treat MDD, to enhance remission, and thereby subsequently decrease human suffering and socioeconomic burden.[29]

NATUROPATHIC TREATMENT AIMS
- Reduce depression and improve mood.
- Improve energy level.
- Promote positive balanced cognition.
- Encourage beneficial lifestyle changes.
- Educate about depressogenic factors and create a plan to combat them.

Although medical research has not currently advanced to the state of tailoring pharmacotherapy prescriptions to individual neurochemical or genetic profiles, 'whole-system' naturopathic diagnosis and treatment has an advantage in being able to prescribe in an individualised manner. First, in order to treat depression effectively, it helps to understand the psychological and biological factors that are involved. Causes of depression are multifaceted, and individual presentations vary markedly. Because of this, tailoring the prescription for the individual may assist in compliance and recovery. Causative factors can be classified into pre-existing 'vulnerabilities' to depression, which may be 'triggered' by a stressor (commonly a series of stressors or one key event), then 'maintaining' factors may exacerbate or prolong the episode.

Several herbal medicines are particularly adept at affecting neuroreceptor binding and activity to achieve an antidepressant effect. Herbal medicines used to treat mental health disorders usually have central nervous system or endocrine-modulating activity.[6] Common actions can involve monoamine activity modulation, stimulation or sedation of central nervous system activity, and regulation or support of healthy hypothalamic pituitary adrenal axis function (see Table 12.1).[30]

Biopsychosocial model of depression

The most suitable model consistent with the holistic paradigm is a biopsychosocial model.[12] The essence of the model is that the cause of depression is multifactorial, with many interrelated influences involved in its growth. Genetics and biochemistry (biological), cognitions and personality traits (psychological), environmental factors (environmental) and social interactions (sociological) all affect the level of a person's 'vulnerability' to a depressive disorder, which is commonly triggered by chronic or acute stressors. Protective factors are considered to be good genetics, balanced positive cognitions, healthy interpersonal relations and social support, and spirituality.[11,31]

A balanced and integrative naturopathic treatment plan needs to address all aspects concerning the biopsychosocial model. Herbal, nutraceutical and dietary prescription can modulate the biological component of depression; psychological therapies and counselling support is advised to reconfigure negative cognitions, resolve underlying issues, and build resilience; and social concerns (for example, healthy work, lifestyle, exercise, rest balance, and sufficient family/friend/community interaction) should also be addressed. Depression may provide a context for developing meaning from the experience, thereby promoting spiritual growth. Displayed below is a model developed

Table 12.1 Nervous system herbal medicine actions[30]

TRADITIONAL ACTION	PROPOSED MECHANISMS	APPLICATIONS
Nervines (tonics, stimulants)	HPA-modulation, beta-adrenergic activity	Depression, fatigue, convalescence
Adaptogens, thymoleptics, antidepressants, tonics	Monoamine interactions HPA-modulation	Depression, fatigue, convalescence
Anxiolytics, hypnotics, sedatives	GABA or adenosine-receptor binding or modulation	Anxiety disorders, insomnia
Antispasmodics, analgesics	Calcium/sodium channel modulation Substance P or enkephalin effects	Muscular tension (dysmenorrhoea, irritable bowel syndrome, headaches), visceral spasm, pain
Cognitive enhancers	Cholinergic activity Acetylcholine esterase inhibition	Cognitive decline, dementia

by the author for treating depression: the ALPS model (see Figure 12.1). This treatment model is based on the biopsychosocial model, outlining specific strategies for treating depression holistically. The model advocates a combined approach of antidepressant agents (natural or synthetic); lifestyle adjustments such as dietary improvement, and reduction of alcohol and caffeine, and increased relaxation and exercise; psychological interventions; and improved social functioning and integration.

Monoamine hypothesis

The monoamine hypothesis concerns the theory that depression is primarily caused by dysregulation of serotonin, dopamine and noradrenaline pathways (receptor activity and density, neurotransmitter production and neurochemical transport and transmission).[9] Herbal and nutritional/dietary modulation may be helpful in modulating monoaminergic transmission. To date, the phytotherapy with the most evidence of monoamine modulation is ***Hypericum perforatum***. Enough human clinical trials have been conducted for several meta-analyses to be conducted (see Table 12.2). All meta-analyses have revealed that *H. perforatum* provides a significant antidepressant effect compared to placebo, and an equivalent efficacy compared to synthetic antidepressants. *H. perforatum* has demonstrated several beneficial effects on modulating monoamine transmission. Although initial in vitro experiments suggested monoamine oxidase-inhibition by *H. perforatum*, further conducted experiments have not confirmed this activity.[32] In vivo and in vitro studies have, however, revealed non-selective inhibition of the neuronal reuptake of serotonin, dopamine and norepinephrine.[33] This activity is likely to occur in part via modulation of neurotransmitter transport systems (for example, via Na^+ gradient membranes). Increased dopaminergic activity in the prefrontal cortex has been documented.[34] A decreased degradation of neurochemicals and a sensitisation of and increased binding to various receptors (for example, GABA, glutamate and adenosine) have also been observed.[35–37] It should be noted that some of the pharmacodynamic studies used intraponeal rather than oral administration; caution in extrapolating to humans is advised.

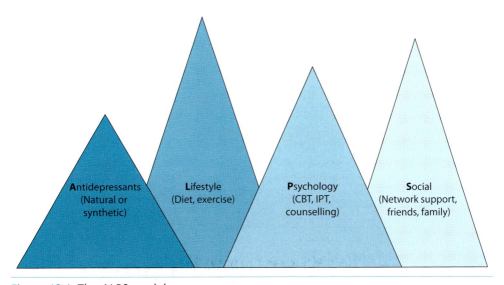

Figure 12.1 The ALPS model

Aside from *H. perforatum,* **Rhodiola rosea** and **Crocus sativus** currently possess the most evidence as monoamine and neuroendocrine modulators, and have provided preliminary human clinical evidence of efficacy in treating MDD.[38,39] *R. rosea* is a stimulating adaptogen, which possesses antidepressant, anti-fatigue and tonic activity.[39,40] A 6-week, phase III, three-arm randomised controlled trial (RCT) involving 91 subjects comparing *R. rosea* SHR-5 standardised extract (680 mg and 340 mg/day) with placebo demonstrated significant dose-dependent improvement on depression.[41] It should be noted that the effect size was small, with a low response in comparison to a very low placebo response (usually there is a 20–50% reduction of depression in a placebo group); further studies need to be conducted to confirm efficacy. The phytochemicals salidroside, rosvarin, rosarin, rosin and tyrosol are considered to be the active constituents.[42] In animal models, *R. rosea* has been documented to increase noradrenaline, dopamine and serotonin in the brainstem and hypothalamus, and to increase the blood–brain permeability to neurotransmitter precursors.[43] *Crocus sativus* is developing clinical evidence as an effective antidepressant (reviewed later). Crocin and safranal are currently regarded as the constituents responsible for *C. sativus*'s antidepressant action.[38] The mechanisms responsible for the antidepressant actions are purported to be mediated via reuptake inhibition of dopamine, norepinephrine and serotonin, and NMDA receptor antagonism.[38] Safranal is posited to exert selective GABA-α agonism, and possible opioid receptor modulation, as demonstrated via intracerebroventricular administration in an animal model.[44]

Other herbal medicines that have been documented to exert monoamine modulation include *Bacopa monnieri, Ginkgo biloba, Panax ginseng* and *Convolvulus pluricaulis*; however, to date insufficient clinical trials have confirmed antidepressant effects in humans.[45,46]

HPA-axis modulation

In the last two decades, cortisol has achieved increased attention in the study of the pathogenesis of depression. Substantial evidence exists for the role of cortisol and the HPA axis in depression.[47] Postmortem studies and cerebral spinal fluid sampling have found that corticotrophin-releasing hormone (CRF) can be elevated in samples from depressed patients.[48] A combination of vulnerability factors (genetic, age and early life events) and precipitating factors (psychological, physiological stressors, substance misuse and comorbid disease) may provoke an increase in CRF. This stimulates the secretion of adrenocorticotropin hormone (ACTH), and subsequent cortisol release from the adrenal glands (see Section 5 on the endocrine system). In vitro and animal models have demonstrated that HPA-axis dysfunction and increased cortisol attenuate the production of BDNF in the brain.[9] BDNF is an important growth factor that nourishes nerve cells, and lower BDNF is correlated with depressive states.[1,19] Synthetic antidepressants and electroconvulsive therapy appear to regulate the HPA axis and increase the production of BDNF.[47] In animal models, hypericin and the flavonoid derivatives have demonstrated to down-regulate plasma ACTH and corticosterone levels.[31] In particular, an animal model demonstrated that 8 weeks of **H. perforatum** or hypericin administration decreased the expression of genes involved in the regulation of the HPA axis, and significantly decreased levels of CRH mRNA by 16–22% in the hypothalamic paraventricular nucleus (PVN) and serotonin 5-HT(1A) receptor mRNA by 11–17% in the hippocampus. Human studies have, however, found that *H. perforatum* increases salivary and serum cortisol levels.[49,50] Importantly, while in vivo studies have shown that synthetic antidepressants can increase BDNF, *H. perforatum* does not prevent a decrease in stress-reduced BDNF.[51] It should be noted that while evidence does suggest that HPA modulation does occur with *H. perforatum* administration, the complex pharmacodynamics of the effect has not been fully elucidated to date, with variables such as differing human or animal models, stress study methodology and types of *H. perforatum* extracts obfuscating the conclusion.

Herbal adaptogens and tonics may play a beneficial role in modulating ACTH (refer further to Section 5 on the endocrine system). Stimulating adaptogens such as *Eleutherococcus senticosus*, *Schisandra chinensis* and *Rhodiola rosea* have demonstrated significant adaptogenic effects, posited as occurring from HPTA modulation.[42] Although *E. senticosus*, *S. chinensis* and other adaptogens such as *Panax ginseng* and *Withania somnifera* have not demonstrated specific antidepressant activity, they may provide a supportive role in depressive presentations with HPA-axis dysregulation.

Homocysteine hypothesis

The homocysteine hypothesis centres on the theory that genetic and environmental factors elevate levels of homocysteine, which in turn provokes changes in neuronal architecture and neurotransmission, resulting in depression.[15,52] The sulfur compound homocysteine (formed from methionine) has been demonstrated to be directly toxic to neurons, and can induce DNA strand breakage. Higher serum levels of homocysteine have been noted in depressive populations compared to healthy controls.[52] Metabolism of homocysteine to **S-adenosyl methionine (SAMe)** or back to methionine requires folate, B6 and B12. Folate is involved with the methylation pathways in the 'one-carbon' cycle, and is responsible for the metabolism and synthesis of various monoamines.[52] Folate is also most notably involved with the synthesis of SAMe, an endogenous antidepressant formed from homocysteine. Folate deficiency is implicated in causing increased homocysteine levels, and has been consistently demonstrated in depressive populations and in poor responders to antidepressants.[53,54] Folate deficiency has been reported in approximately one-third of people suffering from depressive disorders.[54] Finally, a correlation has been discovered between methylenetetrahydrofolate reductase (a folate-metabolising enzyme) polymorphisms and depression, indicating a genetic link.[55]

Several studies exist assessing the antidepressant effect of **folic acid** in humans with concomitant antidepressant use.[1,56,57] All of these studies yielded positive results with regard to enhancing antidepressant response rates or increasing the onset of response. An example of folic acid's antidepressant activity is reflected in a controlled study using 500 µg of folic acid or placebo adjuvantly with 20 mg fluoxetine in 127 subjects with a Hamilton Depression Rating Scale (HDRS) of ≥ 20.[57,58] The study demonstrated a statistically significant reduction after 10 weeks on the HDRS for women. This effect was not, however, replicated in the male sample. Along with a good dietary intake of folate-rich leafy vegetables or folic acid supplementation, a multivitamin high in B vitamins (especially B6 and B12) may assist in reducing homocysteine, and maintaining adequate levels of SAMe. This will also assist in maintenance of energy production, adrenal function and the creation of neurotransmitters.

Inflammatory factors causing depression

A cytokine-mediated pro-inflammatory event has been considered as a factor involved with the pathophysiology of MDD.[8] Studies have demonstrated that otherwise healthy patients with depression have presented with activated inflammatory pathways.[59] It has been posited that pro-inflammatory cytokines produced from inflammation may influence neuroendocrine function via entry through the 'leaky regions' of the brain (for example, the circumventricular organs), and subsequent modulation of cytokine specific transport molecules, or cytokine stimulation of vagal afferent fibres.[8] Modulation of both CRT and neurotransmitters is known to be effected by cytokines. The main pro-inflammatory cytokines implicated in depressogenesis centres on IFN-α producing IL-1β, IL-6 and TNF-α cytokines (see Chapter 28 on autoimmunity). In laboratory studies, animals exposed to a variety of stressors have demonstrated an increase in these pro-inflammatory cytokines. Synthetic antidepressants have been shown to inhibit the production of various inflammatory cytokines, and to stimulate the production of anti-inflammatory cytokines.[8] Although in its infancy, nascent research is evolving towards developing synthetic medicines that modulate cytokines with a regard to ameliorating depression.[9]

Attenuation of pro-inflammatory cytokines may be of benefit in individuals who present with either a preceding or comorbid inflammatory condition, or a chronic latent infection. Appropriate screening to determine any infections, or inflammatory process, with reference to the chronology of the onset of depression is advised. If an association is plausible, herbal medicines and nutrients that dampen the inflammatory cascade and attenuate the production of pro-inflammatory cytokines may be advised (see Section 2 on the respiratory system and and Section 1 on the gastrointestinal system). In brief, herbal and nutritional medicines that may potentially benefit the treatment of pro-inflammatory evoked MDD include ***Albizzia* spp.**, ***Echinacea* spp.**, **vitamin C** and **bioflavonoids**, and **zinc**. *Albizzia* spp. (in particular *A. lebbeck*) have been documented to exert anti-inflammatory and antiallergic activity.[60] In addition to this activity, anxiolytic and antidepressant effects have been demonstrated in animal models, and in the case of *Albizzia julibrissan*, the plant curiously is known as 'happy bark' in traditional Chinese medicine.[61–63]

Aside from the previously mentioned herbal and nutritional medicines, **omega-3 fatty acids** also have a role in reducing inflammation-based MDD.[59] Epidemiological studies have demonstrated that a rise in depressive symptoms may be correlated with lower dietary omega-3 fish oil (eicosapentaenoic acid (EPA) and docosahexaenoic acid (DHA)).[64–67] Studies have also demonstrated that people with depression have a tendency towards a higher ratio of serum arachidonic acid to essential fatty acids, and an overall lower serum level of omega-3 compared to healthy controls.[59,68–70] Urbanised Western cultures tend to have a far higher ratio of dietary omega-6 oils compared to omega-3 oils, and this has been regarded as a possible factor in the rise of depression over the last several decades.[64,67] The pathophysiology occurring from a pro-omega-6 diet may involve an increased promotion of inflammatory eicosanoids, a lessening of BDNF and a decrease in neuronal cell membrane fluidity and communication.[67,71] Evidence currently suggests that omega-3 fatty acids exert antidepressant activity via beneficial effects on neurotransmission.[72] This may occur via modulation of neurotransmitter (norepinephrine, dopamine and serotonin) reuptake, degradation, synthesis and receptor binding.[73,74] Animal models have demonstrated that omega-3 fatty acids increase serotonin and dopamine concentrations in the frontal cortex, and that a diet deficient in the nutrient decreases catecholamine synthesis.[73,75,76] A recent human clinical trial demonstrated a significant increase in plasma concentrations of norepinephrine in healthy humans.[74]

Several human clinical trials have been conducted assessing the efficacy of EPA, DHA or a combination of both of these essential fatty acids.[77] Clinical evidence regarding the use of essential fatty acids as a monotherapy is equivocal, with a mixture of positive and negative trials (see Table 12.2 at the end of the chapter for a review of the evidence).

ADDITIONAL THERAPEUTIC OPTIONS

S-adenosyl methionine (SAMe)
- It is an endogenous compound produced from methionine and various methylators (e.g. B6, B12 and folate) in the body.[80]
- It serves as a necessary methyl donor of methyl groups involved with the metabolism and synthesis of neurotransmitters.[81,82]
- In vivo studies have consistently shown that SAMe possesses antidepressant activity.[2] Many human clinical trials using SAMe in MDD have been conducted, and all have revealed beneficial antidepressant effects, and comparable effects to synthetic antidepressants.[83–88] Studies, however, are heterogenous in terms of dosage, trial length and methodology.[80]
- Most clinical studies involved parenteral or intramuscular injections of SAMe, rather than oral preparations.[82]
- Considering pharmacokinetic variability between administration techniques, oral preparations may not provide the same effect.
- SAMe should be used with caution in patients with a history of (hypo)mania due to concerns over switching from unipolar depression to mania.
- SAMe is expensive and the cost may be prohibitive for some people.

L-tryptophan
- It is an essential monoamine precursor required for the synthesis of serotonin.[89,90] L-tryptophan has been studied extensively as an antidepressant.
- Although many positive studies exist, only one RCT of sufficient methodological rigour exists. An RCT involving 115 participants with depression comparing L-tryptophan to placebo, an L-tryptophan-amitriptyline combination or amitryptyline demonstrated that the amino acid was equally as effective to the antidepressants and superior to placebo.[91]
- Eight controlled adjuvancy studies using L-tryptophan with antidepressants provide encouraging evidence. Tryptophan augmentation was found to be effective in increasing the antidepressant response with phenezine sulfate,[92] clomipramine,[93,94] tranylcypromine[95] and fluoxetine.[96] However, other clinical studies using tricyclics discovered no additional benefit compared to placebo.[97–100]
- Evening dosing of L-tryptophan (with relevant cofactors such as B6 and B12, folate and magnesium), taken with fructose and without protein, may have a role in treating depression, especially with co-occurring insomnia.
- Always take amino acids without food to avoid competitive absorption with other amino acids, and prescribe them with the relevant cofactors. Use caution in high dosage and with antidepressants (potential serotonin syndrome).

***Crocus sativus* (saffron)**
- Saffron is a Persian traditional plant medicine with reputed antidepressant activity.
- Clinical trials comparing the herbal medicine with synthetic agents, imipramine and fluoxetine have demonstrated equal efficacy.[101–103]
- Extracts standardised to exert antidepressant action are usually standardised for at least 5% safranal. Crocin and safranal are currently regarded as the constituents responsible for the antidepressant activity.[104–105]
- No definitive safety data currently exist. Traditional knowledge of adverse reactions includes nausea, vomiting and diarrhoea.[38] Clinical trials have detailed anxiety, tachycardia, nausea, dyspepsia and changes in appetite as possible side effects.[104–105]

This may in part be due to many studies using olive oil as an 'inert' control, and some studies using higher DHA to EPA ratios or DHA alone.[78] Clinical trials using essential fatty acids adjuvantly with antidepressants have provided positive evidence of additional increased reduction of depression level.[79] Current evidence supports the use of essential fatty acids adjuvantly with antidepressants, in cases of deficiency or if comorbid cardiovascular or inflammatory disorders are present.

The mood spectrum versus categorical diagnosis

Naturopathic diagnosis of mood disorders reflects the holistic psychiatric medicine model, whereby individuals present with unique presentation of MDD, often oscillating between varying levels of depression and anxiety, and sometimes present with peaks of hypomania (for example, increased mental activity, socialisation, work and planning, and decreased sleep). An advantage of naturopathic practice is that prescriptions can be altered to flexibly accommodate the natural rhythm of mood disorders. While it is more applicable to treat the patient holistically (not just 'the depression'), if the condition is viewed in terms of a discrete medical diagnosis, then specific treatment protocols and prescriptions can be instigated (see Figure 12.3).

- The concept of the 'mood spectrum', advocated by academics such as Akiskal, Angst, Cassano and Benazzi, promotes the theory that depressive presentations occur along a continuum, rather than existing as specific discrete diagnostic categories.[106,107]
- Evidence supports the idea that unipolar depression and bipolar II depression occur across a spectrum, with 30% of MDD patients experiencing various bipolar symptoms (for example, agitation, racing thoughts and decreased sleep).[106]
- Individual depressive subtype classifications (for example, melancholic, atypical and co-thymic) are diagnostically unstable, with studies showing that people with mood disorders commonly move between various depressive presentations.[107]
- The effect of seasonal influence on MDD should also be considered. While seasonal affective disorder (SAD) is a specific type of depressive disorder, low light and cold weather may exacerbate non-SAD diagnosed depression.[108] Although evidence specifically supports light therapy only in treating SAD, exposure to morning sunlight is a commonsense recommendation. Sunlight intuitively lifts the mood, and causes increased serotonin turnover in the brain.[109]

INTEGRATIVE MEDICAL CONSIDERATIONS

As detailed above, an integrative treatment plan should ideally be provided. Other treatments include acupuncture and psychological interventions. If the patient is unresponsive to CAM treatment (after 2–4 weeks of treatment), the prescription should be altered or additional interventions provided. Synthetic antidepressants may be required if the depressive episode worsens and suicidal ideation is present, or if symptoms persist after several prescription modifications to non-response.

Acupuncture and massage

The use of acupuncture to treat depressive disorders has been documented in traditional Chinese medicine (TCM) texts.[110] In TCM the two main organs (energetically) involved in depression are the liver and the heart.[18] Two primary patterns of depression are diagnosed in TCM: 'Stagnation of Liver Qi' (excess pattern) and 'Deficiency of Qi, Blood, or Kidney Jing' (deficient pattern).[110] In principle, physical activity and exercise are regarded to 'Move Qi and Blood', thereby alleviating 'Stagnation', and to 'Tonify Qi'

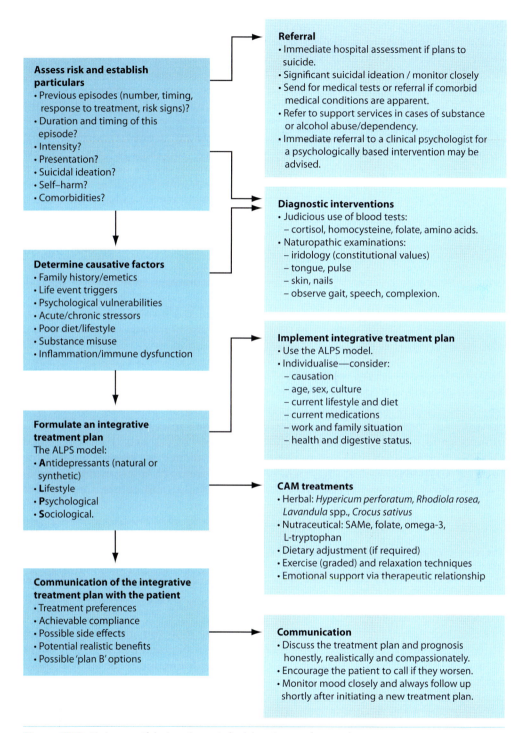

Assess risk and establish particulars
- Previous episodes (number, timing, response to treatment, risk signs)?
- Duration and timing of this episode?
- Intensity?
- Presentation?
- Suicidal ideation?
- Self–harm?
- Comorbidities?

Referral
- Immediate hospital assessment if plans to suicide.
- Significant suicidal ideation / monitor closely
- Send for medical tests or referral if comorbid medical conditions are apparent.
- Refer to support services in cases of substance or alcohol abuse/dependency.
- Immediate referral to a clinical psychologist for a psychologically based intervention may be advised.

Diagnostic interventions
- Judicious use of blood tests:
  – cortisol, homocysteine, folate, amino acids.
- Naturopathic examinations:
  – iridology (constitutional values)
  – tongue, pulse
  – skin, nails
  – observe gait, speech, complexion.

Determine causative factors
- Family history/emetics
- Life event triggers
- Psychological vulnerabilities
- Acute/chronic stressors
- Poor diet/lifestyle
- Substance misuse
- Inflammation/immune dysfunction

Implement integrative treatment plan
- Use the ALPS model.
- Individualise—consider:
  – causation
  – age, sex, culture
  – current lifestyle and diet
  – current medications
  – work and family situation
  – health and digestive status.

Formulate an integrative treatment plan
The ALPS model:
- **A**ntidepressants (natural or synthetic)
- **L**ifestyle
- **P**sychological
- **S**ociological.

CAM treatments
- Herbal: *Hypericum perforatum, Rhodiola rosea, Lavandula* spp., *Crocus sativus*
- Nutraceutical: SAMe, folate, omega-3, L-tryptophan
- Dietary adjustment (if required)
- Exercise (graded) and relaxation techniques
- Emotional support via therapeutic relationship

Communication of the integrative treatment plan with the patient
- Treatment preferences
- Achievable compliance
- Possible side effects
- Potential realistic benefits
- Possible 'plan B' options

Communication
- Discuss the treatment plan and prognosis honestly, realistically and compassionately.
- Encourage the patient to call if they worsen.
- Monitor mood closely and always follow up shortly after initiating a new treatment plan.

Figure 12.2 Naturopathic treatment decision tree—depression

(lung and spleen), thereby improving energy and vigour. A review of eight small-randomised controlled trials confirmed that acupuncture could significantly reduce the severity of depression on the HDRS or Beck Depression Scale.[111] However, no significant effect of active acupuncture was found on the response rate or remission rate. Another review[112] found a total of four RCTs meeting a minimum standard of methodological rigour (for example, a randomised sample and control groups used). Results of these studies revealed significant effects on reducing depression versus non-specific or sham acupuncture, and equivocal efficacy to tricyclic antidepressants. In one study, although acupuncture was equally effective to massage and sham acupuncture, only the true acupuncture provided sustained antidepressant effects. Acupuncture has been documented to interact with opioid pathways, and substances which modulate these pathways have been shown to have antidepressant activity.[9,113,114] Other possible antidepressant mechanisms of action include the increased release of serotonin and norepinephrine, and CRT and cortisol modulation.[113]

Massage may also be of benefit in improving mood and reducing depression. Studies of varying methodological rigour have shown that massage increases relaxation, decreases stress and elevates the mood.[115] A rigorous review of massage techniques in treating clinical depression commented that, while positive studies exist, a lack of evidence from RCTs does not support this intervention.[116] While evidence currently does not support massage as a primary monotherapy in treating MDD, use of massage adjuvantly can be advised, especially in cases of co-occurring muscular tension.

Psychological intervention

As outlined under the ALPS model, psychological intervention is an important component in treating MDD. Guidelines support the use of psychological interventions such as cognitive behavioural therapy (CBT) and interpersonal therapy (IPT) in mild depression rather than synthetic medication.[27] CBT and IPT are accepted psychological interventions, both having equal evidence of efficacy in treating MDD.[25] CBT involves learning cognitive skills to 'reprogram' erroneous or negative thought patterns with positive balanced cognitions, and to institute positive behavioural modifications.[117] The theory is based on the concept that a person's negative, critical, erroneous thought patterns provoke deleterious emotional and physiological responses. By intervening before this cascade occurs, and establishing a positive balanced inner dialogue, this spiral can be avoided. IPT focuses on identifying problematic social situations that are depressogenic, and developing interpersonal techniques (such as social skills) to manage interpersonal relationships.[117] By increasing confidence and competency in managing social interactions, a robust self-esteem may develop.

Other techniques, such as teaching problem-solving skills to identify and deal with depressogenic triggers, may be of assistance. Finally, it is important to assist the patient to identify external triggers that may cause an episode (for example, the anniversary of a death, or a change in weather), and help them to formulate a 'pro-euthymic' plan to combat this. Naturopaths may learn basic skills in teaching CBT and IPT, and a caring humanistic approach should always be present. However, for skilled psychological intervention, referral to a clinical psychologist or highly trained counsellor is advised.

Adjuvant CAM treatments with antidepressants

If the patient is taking antidepressant medication, adjuvancy options are recommended (see Sarris et al.[118] for a review). Adjuvant strategies with antidepressants involve combining an additional thymoleptic intervention to directly increase the antidepressant effect, or use a supplementary therapy to enhance activity, or reduce side effects by a synergistic interaction. Such prescription should be discussed between the physician and naturopath, and be closely monitored. The evidence regarding combining synthetic antidepressants and herbal medicines is currently unknown. Potential exists in combining antidepressant herbal medicines to increase the therapeutic effect in absent or partial responders to synthetic antidepressants. Consideration of serotonin syndrome or switching to bipolar (hypo) mania should, however, be given. Co-administration of herbal medicines may also have a potential role in addressing individual presentations or comorbid features of

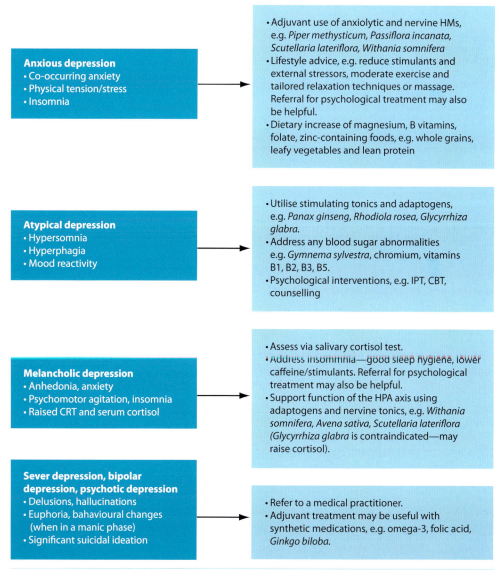

Figure 12.3 Psychiatric diagnostic depressive presentations and example treatment options[2,100,130]

depression (see Figure 12.3), or to reduce side effects of antidepressants. Note the following:

- Strong evidence exists for combining **SAMe**, **L-tryptophan**, **folic acid or omega-3** with SSRIs or tricyclic antidepressants to increase response or speed the onset of action.[79]
- Novel adjuvant prescription includes the use of aromatic or bitter herbs such as *Zingiber officinale* or *Cynara scolymus* to reduce nausea and relieve dyspepsia.[119,120]
- Co-occurring fatigue could potentially be reduced via co-administration of adaptogens such as *Rhodiola rosea*[39] or *Panax ginseng*.[121]
- Insomnia and irritability could be treated via herbal anxiolytics such as *Passiflora incanata*[122] or *Piper methysticum*.[123]
- Sexual dysfunction may be alleviated in some patients by using *Ginkgo biloba*,[124–126] although not all studies show positive results.[128]
- The occurrence of hepatotoxicity could be potentially reduced by using antioxidant hepatics such as *Silybum marianum* or *Schisandra chinensis*.[129]

Case Study

A 28-year-old female presents with persistent **low mood**. She says that for the last few months she **lacks motivation,** and has **lost pleasure** in activities that she usually enjoys. Her **energy is very low** and says she **just wants to sleep**. Her diet is poor, lacking in leafy vegetables and fish.

SUGGESTIVE SYMPTOMS

- Persistent low mood
- Loss of pleasure in work and hobbies
- Weight and appetite change
- Sleep disturbance, Insomnia
- Altered cognitions (guilt, low self-worth, suicidal ideation)
- Psychomotor agitation or slowness
- Fatigue

Example treatment
Herbal and nutritional prescription

In the above case, the primary prescriptive protocol is to provide an antidepressant action to treat the depression. The co-occurring manifestations of fatigue, amotivation and hypersomnia can be addressed via stimulating tonics and adaptogens. In the above case, a dysregulation of serotonin may be responsible for the low mood; norepinephrine dysregulation may affect amotivation, hypersomnia and fatigue; while dopamine dysregulation may be responsible for anhedonia. *Hypericum perforatum*, *Rhodiola rosea* and *Lavandula angustifolia* should aid in the elevation of her mood. *Panax ginseng*, *Rhodiola rosea* and *Glycyrrhiza glabra* will assist in

Herbal formula	
Hypericum perforatum 1:2	25 mL
Rhodiola rosea 2:1	25 mL
Lavandula angustifolia 1:2	20 mL
Panax ginseng 1:1	15 mL
Glycyrrhiza glabra 1:1	15 mL
7.5 mL morning and afternoon	100 mL 100 mL

Nutritional prescription
Omega-3 fish oil 3 tablets (3 g) 2× day
Multivitamin 1 per day (high in B vitamins and folic acid)

enhancing adrenal activity and invigorating her energy and motivation.[101] Omega-3 may be of benefit in treating her depression (especially if she is deficient in it), and a multivitamin high in folate will provide the nutrients involved in the manufacture and transmission of neuroreceptors, while assisting the methylation pathway.

Dietary and lifestyle advice

Dietary programs designed to treat depression have to date not been rigorously evaluated. Although evidence supporting specific dietary advice is currently absent, a basic balanced diet (see Section 1 on the gastrointestinal system) including foods rich in a spectrum of nutrients can be recommended. Foods rich in folate, omega-3, tryptophan, B and C vitamins, zinc and magnesium are necessary for the production of neurotransmitters and neuronal communication.[77] These include whole grains, lean meat, deep-sea fish, green leafy vegetables, coloured berries and nuts (walnuts, almonds).[65,130]

General lifestyle advice should focus on encouraging a balance between meaningful work, adequate rest and sleep, judicious exercise, positive social interaction and pleasurable hobbies. Behavioural therapy techniques have shown positive effects on reducing depression by training the person to reduce or better manage stressful situations, and to increase pleasurable activities that enhance self-esteem and self-mastery. If substance or alcohol dependence or misuse is apparent, supportive advice on curtailing this, or appropriate referral, should be communicated (see the case in Chapter 13 on chronic generalised anxiety for more detail).

Exercise or physical activity

Increasing physical activity is advised in cases of underactivity. Associations between greater physical activity and improved mood and wellbeing have been documented,[131] and several RCTs support exercise as effective in managing MDD. A meta-analysis of 11 treatment-outcome studies of exercise on the treatment of depression showed a significant effect in favour of physical exercise compared with control conditions (routine care, wait list, meditation/relaxation or low-intensity exercise).[132] A very large average effect size was obtained with all but two studies obtaining superior results from exercise than from control. However, many of these studies had methodological failings (for example, not using blind assessment or intention-to-treat analyses). Research strongly suggests that anabolic exercise of high intensity is more effective than low intensity.[133] The biological antidepressant effects of exercise include a beneficial modulation of the HPA axis, increased expression of 5-HT, and increased levels of circulating testosterone (which may have a protective effect against depression).[134] Evidence also exists for the use of yoga to reduce depression and improve mood. A review documented five RCTs using various types of yoga to treat MDD.[135] While the studies reviewed all concluded positive results, the methodologies were poorly reported and thereby no firm conclusion can be reached. It is worthwhile highlighting that certain types of yoga may actually have greater antidepressant effect. 'Mindfulness' in exercise techniques such as yoga may potentially have greater efficacy than low-intensity, low-focus yoga, although evidence does not currently confirm this theory.[136]

Evidence for the type and amount of exercise for the management of MDD, currently favours anabolic over aerobic activity to gain the greatest benefits, and the intensity needs to be moderate to high and performed two or three times per week.[133] Caveats exist regarding exercise prescription for MDD. Depression may be worsened if the person is unable to meet expectations, potentially promoting a sense of failure and guilt. This may be more likely to occur in severe MDD, especially where psychomotor retardation, hypersomnia, somnolescence, marked fatigue or anhedonia are present. Exercise plans should be instituted after a medical assessment, and initially commenced at a low intensity to allow for physical and psychological adaptation to occur to the new stimulus.

Table 12.2 Review of the major evidence

INTERVENTION	KEY LITERATURE	SUMMARY OF RESULTS	COMMENT
St John's wort (*Hypericum perforatum*)	**Meta-analyses** Linde et al. 2005[137] Roder et al. 2004[138] Werneke et al. 2004[139] Whiskey et al. 2001[140]	**Relative risk: SJW versus placebo on HDRS** 1.71 (1.40–2.09)[137] 1.52 (1.28–1.75)[138] 1.73 (1.40–2.14)[139] 1.98 (1.49–2.62[140] **Relative risk: SJW vs. synthetics on HDRS** 0.96 (0.85–1.08)[138] 1.00 (0.90–1.11)[140]	SJW consistently demonstrates greater efficacy than placebo in treating MDD. Efficacy is equal to synthetic antidepressants. Lower hyperforin extracts are advised to minimise drug interactions.
Omega-3 fish oil	**Meta-analyses and reviews** Lin & Su 2007[77] Appleton et al. 2006[66]	Two meta-analyses of nine and eight studies respectively revealed positive results (effect size $d = 0.61$; $d = 0.73$). Most positive studies included were 'adjuvant' trials. Several recent equivocal RCTs using monotherapy omega-3 exist.[78]	The balance of evidence suggests limited efficacy as a monotherapy for MDD. Recommend in deficient states, or in comorbid inflammatory conditions or CVD, or adjuvantly with antidepressants.
Folic acid	**Monotherapy RCTs** Currently no robust studies exist using folic acid in MDD. Several adjuvancy studies using antidepressants and folic acid exist (see Taylor et al. 2004 for a review).[53]	Antidepressant augmentation with folate may increase response rate increases and efficacy in treating MDD. Subjects with lower folate levels are more likely to have a delayed response by on average 1.5 weeks.	In cases of folate deficiency supplementation can be cautiously recommended with antidepressants to potentially ↑ response and efficacy. May be more efficacious in females than males. Caution should be observed in pernicious anaemia (addition of B12 required).
L-tryptophan	**Systematic review and meta-analysis** Shaw et al. 2002[141] Positive augmentation studies by Coppen et al. 1963,[95] Glassman & Platman 1969,[92] and Walinder et al. 1976.[94]	Tryptophan augmentation with MAOIs, SSRIs and some TCAs is effective in increasing the antidepressant response. No difference occurred compared to placebo with other tricyclics. High dosage may cause adverse reactions, e.g. GIT complaints, nausea or serotonin syndrome.	May be of use in subjects taking antidepressants, in tryptophan deficiency, or in depression caused by serotonergic pathway dysregulation.
S-adenosyl methionine (SAMe)	**Meta-analysis and reviews** Several monotherapy RCTS, and adjuvant studies exist: Williams et al. 2005[82] Papakostas et al. 2003[81] Bottiglieri et al. 1994[142]	Intramuscular and oral augmentation of SAMe with antidepressants has demonstrated ↑ response and remission rates. May enhance response in antidepressant non-responders.	Parenteral administration may be more efficacious than oral administration. May interact with serotonergic antidepressants. Caution in bipolar patients to avoid switching to mania. Expense may be a caveat.

(Continued)

Table 12.2 Review of the major evidence *(Continued)*

INTERVENTION	KEY LITERATURE	SUMMARY OF RESULTS	COMMENT
Physical Interventions (aerobic exercise, weights, yoga, massage)	**Key studies or reviews** See Sarris et al. 2008 for a review.[143] Exercise: Lawlor Hopker 2001[132] Running: Doyne et al. 1987[144] Weights: Dunn et al. 2001[133] Yoga: Pilkington et al. 2005[135] Massage: Coelho et al. 2008[116]	Aerobic exercise, weights and yoga more effective in reducing depression compared with no treatment or wait list control. Large effect size noted in Lawlor & Hopker 2001[132] meta-analysis ($d = 1.42$, 95% CI: 0.92–1.93). Most studies support massage as a mood-improving intervention. Currently there is a lack of high quality evidence.	All modes of physical activity have antidepressant effects. Higher-intensity exercise and weights appear to have the greatest antidepressant effect.

Expected outcomes and follow-up protocols

In the above case, reduction of depression and a return towards euthymia is expected within a month of commencing treatment. A depressive episode will commonly remit within 6 months (even without treatment due to the natural rhythmicity of MDD), although maintaining factors and the number of previous episodes may affect complete remission. Many people will have their depression alleviated simply by taking the step to seek treatment, making lifestyle adjustments, and from the interpersonal therapeutic relationship with the practitioner. If the depressive episode persisted and suicidality was still absent, a change of prescription would be warranted. Additional interventions such as SAMe or L-tryptophan augmentation may be helpful. If the condition worsened then medical referral would be advised. Depressive episodes are often diagnostically unstable, and thereby the patient should be monitored carefully to modulate the prescription according to any changes in symptoms. Changes that may occur include bipolar elements, anxiety, insomnia or changes in appetite, energy and cognition. After the depressive symptoms remit, treatment should be continued for 3–6 months to enhance the chance of remission.

KEY POINTS
- Depression is a condition that should be treated early and assertively.
- An integrated individualised treatment approach such as ALPS is recommended.
- Carefully monitor the prescription's effect and any change in suicidal ideation.
- If depression persists or worsens, refer appropriately.

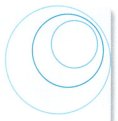

Further reading

Belmaker RH, Agam G. Major depressive disorder. N Engl J Med 2008;358(1):55–68.

Sarris J. Herbal medicines in the treatment of psychiatric disorders: a systematic review. Phytother Res 2007;21(8):703–716.

Sarris J, et al. Major depressive disorder and nutritional medicine: A review of monotherapies and adjuvant treatments. Nutrition Reviews 2009;67(3):125–131.

Werneke U, et al. Complementary medicines in psychiatry: Review of effectiveness and safety. Br J Psychiatry 2006;188:109–121.

References

1. Belmaker RH, Agam G. Major depressive disorder. N Engl J Med 2008;358(1):55–68.
2. American Psychiatric Association. Diagnostic and statistical manual of mental disorders. 4th edn. Arlington: American Psychiatric Association, 2000.
3. WHO. Mental and neurological disorders. Depression. 2006. Online. Available: http://www.who.int/mental_health/management/depression/definition/en/.
4. Kessler RC, et al. The epidemiology of major depressive disorder: results from the National Comorbidity Survey Replication (NCS-R). JAMA 2003;289(23):3095–3105.
5. Alonso J, et al. Prevalence of mental disorders in Europe: results from the European Study of the Epidemiology of Mental Disorders (ESEMeD) project. Acta Psychiatr Scand Suppl 2004;420(420):21–27.
6. Antonijevic IA. Depressive disorders – is it time to endorse different pathophysiologies? Psychoneuroendocrinology 2006;31(1):1–15.
7. Ressler KJ, Nemeroff CB. Role of serotonergic and noradrenergic systems in the pathophysiology of depression and anxiety disorders. Depress Anxiety 2000;12(Suppl 1):2–19.
8. Raison CL, et al. Cytokines sing the blues: inflammation and the pathogenesis of depression. Trends Immunol 2006;27(1):24–31.
9. Hindmarch I. Expanding the horizons of depression: beyond the monoamine hypothesis. Hum Psychopharmacol 2001;16(3):203–218.
10. Plotsky PM, et al. Psychoneuroendocrinology of depression. Hypothalamic-pituitary-adrenal axis. Psychiatr Clin North Am 1998;21(2):293–307.
11. Southwick SM, et al. The psychobiology of depression and resilience to stress: implications for prevention and treatment. Annu Rev Clin Psychol 2005;1:255–291.
12. Molina J. Understanding the biopsychosocial model. Int'l J Psychiatry in Medicine 1983;13(1):29–36.
13. Haeffel GJ, Grigorenko EL. Cognitive vulnerability to depression: exploring risk and resilience. Child Adolesc Psychiatr Clin N Am 2007;16(2):435–448, x.
14. Berton O, Nestler EJ. New approaches to antidepressant drug discovery: beyond monoamines. Nat Rev Neurosci 2006;7(2):137–151.
15. Folstein M, et al. The homocysteine hypothesis of depression. Am J Psychiatry 2007;164(6):861–867.
16. Kessler RC. The effects of stressful life events on depression. Annu Rev Psychol 1997;48:191–214.
17. Culpeper N. Culpeper's complete herbal. Hertfordshire: Wordsworth Editions Ltd, 1652.
18. Maciocia G. The foundations of Chinese medicine. Singapore: Churchill Livingstone, 1989.
19. Levinson DF. The genetics of depression: a review. Biol Psychiatry 2006;60(2):84–92.
20. Tennant C. Life events, stress and depression: a review of recent findings. Aust N Z J Psychiatry 2002;36(2):173–182.
21. Paykel E. Life events and affective disorders. Acta Psychiatr Scand Suppl. 2003;418:61–66.
22. Australian Bureau of Statistics. Mental health in Australia: a snapshot. Australian Bureau of Statistics, 2004.
23. Kessler RC, et al. Prevalence, severity, and comorbidity of 12-month DSM-IV disorders in the National Comorbidity Survey Replication. Arch Gen Psychiatry 2005;62(6):617–627.
24. Miklowitz DJ, Johnson SL. The psychopathology and treatment of bipolar disorder. Annu Rev Clin Psychol 2006;2:199–235.
25. Parker G, Fletcher K. Treating depression with the evidence-based psychotherapies: a critique of the evidence. Acta Psychiatr Scand 2007;115(5):352–359.
26. Ellen S, et al. Depression and anxiety: pharmacological treatment in general practice. Aust Fam Physician 2007;36(4):222–228.
27. Ellis P. Australian and New Zealand clinical practice guidelines for the treatment of depression. Aust N Z J Psychiatry 2004;38(6):389–407.
28. Warden D, et al. The STAR*D Project results: a comprehensive review of findings. Curr Psychiatry Rep 2007;9(6):449–459.
29. Donohue J, Pincus H. Reducing the societal burden of depression: a review of economic costs, quality of care and effects of treatment. Pharmacoeconomics 2007;25(1):7–24.
30. Spinella M. The psychopharmacology of herbal medicine: plant drugs that alter mind, brain and behavior. Cambridge: MIT Press, 2001.
31. Schotte CK, et al. A biopsychosocial model as a guide for psychoeducation and treatment of depression. Depress Anxiety 2006;23(5):312–324.
32. Butterweck V, Schimdt M. St John's wort: role of active compounds for its mechanism of action and efficacy. Wien Med Wochenschr 2007;157(13–14):356–361.
33. Muller WE. Current St John's wort research from mode of action to clinical efficacy. Pharmacol Res 2003;47:101–109.
34. Yoshitake T, et al. Hypericum perforatum L (St John's wort) preferentially increases extracellular dopamine levels in rat prefrontal cortex. Br J Pharmacol 2004;142(3):414–418.
35. Butterweck V. Mechanism of action of St John's wort in depression: what is known? CNS Drugs 2003;17(8):539–562.
36. Zanoli P. Role of hyperforin in the pharmacological activities of St John's Wort. CNS Drug Rev 2004;10(3):203–218.
37. Mennini T, Gobbi M. The antidepressant mechanism of Hypericum perforatum. Life Sci 2004;75(9):1021–1027.
38. Schmidt M, et al. Saffron in phytotherapy: pharmacology and clinical uses. Wien Med Wochenschr 2007;157(13–14):315–319.
39. Kelly GS. Rhodiola rosea: a possible plant adaptogen. Altern Med Rev 2001;6(3):293–302.
40. Kucinskaite A, et al. [Experimental analysis of therapeutic properties of Rhodiola rosea L. and its possible application in medicine]. Medicina (Kaunas) 2004;40(7):614–619.
41. Darbinyan V, et al. Clinical trial of Rhodiola rosea L. extract SHR-5 in the treatment of mild to moderate depression. Nord J Psychiatry 2007;61(5):343–348.
42. Panossian A. Stimulating effect of adaptogens: an overview with particular reference to their efficacy following single dose administration. Phytother Res 2005;19:819–838.
43. Kucinskaite A, et al. Evaluation of biologically active compounds in roots and rhizomes of Rhodiola rosea L. cultivated in Lithuania. Medicina (Kaunas) 2007;43(6):487–494.
44. Hosseinzadeh H, Sadeghnia HR. Protective effect of safranal on pentylenetetrazol-induced seizures in the rat: involvement of GABAergic and opioids systems. Phytomedicine 2007;14(4):256–262.
45. Sarris J. Herbal medicines in the treatment of psychiatric disorders: a systematic review. Phytother Res 2007;21(8):703–716.
46. Kumar V. Potential medicinal plants for CNS disorders: an overview. Phytother Res 2006;20(12):1023–1035.
47. Pariante C, et al. Do antidepressants regulate how cortisol affects the brain? Psychoneuroendocrinology 2003;29:423–447.
48. Mitchell AJ. The role of corticotropin releasing factor in depressive illness: a critical review. Neurosci Biobehav Rev 1998;22(5):635–651.
49. Schule C, et al. Neuroendocrine effects of Hypericum extract WS 5570 in 12 healthy male volunteers. Pharmacopsychiatry 2001;34(Suppl 1):S127–S133.
50. Franklin M, et al. Effect of sub-chronic treatment with Jarsin (extract of St John's wort, Hypericum perforatum) at two dose levels on evening salivary melatonin and cortisol concentrations in healthy male volunteers. Pharmacopsychiatry 2006;39(1):13–15.

51. Butterweck V, et al. St John's wort, hypericin, and imipramine: a comparative analysis of mRNA levels in brain areas involved in HPA axis control following short-term and long-term administration in normal and stressed rats. Mol Psychiatry 2001;6(5):547–564.

52. Bottiglieri T, et al. Homocysteine, folate, methylation, and monoamine metabolism in depression. J Neurol Neurosurg Psychiatry 2000;69(2):228–232.

53. Taylor MJ, et al. Folate for depressive disorders: systematic review and meta-analysis of randomized controlled trials. J Psychopharmacol 2004;18(2):251–256.

54. Morris DW, et al. Folate and unipolar depression. J Altern Complement Med 2008;14(3):277–285.

55. Bjelland I, et al. Folate, vitamin B12, homocysteine, and the MTHFR 677C→T polymorphism in anxiety and depression: the Hordaland Homocysteine Study. Arch Gen Psychiatry 2003;60(6):618–626.

56. Godfrey PS, et al. Enhancement of recovery from psychiatric illness by methylfolate. Lancet 1990;336(8712): 392–395.

57. Coppen A, Bailey J. Enhancement of the antidepressant action of fluoxetine by folic acid: a randomised, placebo controlled trial. J Affect Disord 2000;60(2):121–130.

58. Hamilton M. A rating scale for depression. J Neurol Neurosurg Psychiatry 1960;23:56–62.

59. Dinan T, et al. Investigating the inflammatory phenotype of major depression: focus on cytokines and polyunsaturated fatty acids. J Psychiatr Res 2009;43(4):471–476.

60. Johri RK, et al. Effect of quercetin and *Albizzia* saponins on rat mast cell. Indian J Physiol Pharmacol 1985;29(1):43–46.

61. Kim JH, et al. Antidepressant-like effects of *Albizzia julibrissin* in mice: involvement of the 5-HT1A receptor system. Pharmacol Biochem Behav 2007;87(1):41–47.

62. Chintawar SD, et al. Nootropic activity of *Albizzia lebbeck* in mice. J Ethnopharmacol 2002;81(3):299–305.

63. Une HD, et al. Nootropic and anxiolytic activity of saponins of *Albizzia lebbeck* leaves. Pharmacol Biochem Behav 2001;69(3–4):439–444.

64. Sanchez-Villegas A, et al. Mediterranean diet and depression. Public Health Nutr 2006;9(8A):1104–1109.

65. Appleton KM, et al. Depressed mood and n-3 polyunsaturated fatty acid intake from fish: non-linear or confounded association? Soc Psychiatry Psychiatr Epidemiol 2007;42(2):100–104.

66. Appleton KM, et al. Effects of n-3 long-chain polyunsaturated fatty acids on depressed mood: systematic review of published trials. Am J Clin Nutr 2006;84(6):1308–1316.

67. Parker G, et al. Omega-3 fatty acids and mood disorders. Am J Psychiatry 2006;163:969–978.

68. Maes M, et al. Fatty acid composition in major depression: decreased omega 3 fractions in cholesteryl esters and increased C20: 4 omega 6/C20:5 omega 3 ratio in cholesteryl esters and phospholipids. J Affect Disord 1996;38(1):35–46.

69. Adams PB, et al. Arachidonic acid to eicosapentaenoic acid ratio in blood correlates positively with clinical symptoms of depression. Lipids 1996;31(Suppl):S157–S161.

70. Edwards R, et al. Omega-3 polyunsaturated fatty acid levels in the diet and in red blood cell membranes of depressed patients. J Affect Disord 1998;48(2–3): 149–155.

71. Tassoni D, et al. The role of eicosanoids in the brain. Asia Pac J Clin Nutr 2008;17(Suppl 1):220–228.

72. Williams AL, et al. Do essential fatty acids have a role in the treatment of depression? J Affect Disord 2006; 93(1–3):117–123.

73. Chalon S, et al. Dietary fish oil affects monoaminergic neurotransmission and behavior in rats. J Nutr 1998;128(12):2512–2519.

74. Hamazaki K, et al. Effect of omega-3 fatty acid-containing phospholipids on blood catecholamine concentrations in healthy volunteers: a randomized, placebo-controlled, double-blind trial. Nutrition 2005;21(6):705–710.

75. Chalon S. Omega-3 fatty acids and monoamine neurotransmission. Prostaglandins Leukot Essent Fatty Acids 2006;75(4–5):259–269.

76. Delion S, et al. Alpha-Linolenic acid dietary deficiency alters age-related changes of dopaminergic and serotoninergic neurotransmission in the rat frontal cortex. J Neurochem 1996;66(4):1582–1591.

77. Lin PY, Su KP. A meta-analytic review of double-blind, placebo-controlled trials of antidepressant efficacy of omega-3 fatty acids. J Clin Psychiatry 2007;68(7):1056–1061.

78. Sarris J, et al. Major depressive disorder and nutritional medicine: a review of monotherapies and adjuvant treatments. Nutr Reviews 2009;67(3):125–131.

79. Werneke U, et al. Complementary medicines in psychiatry: review of effectiveness and safety. Br J Psychiatry 2006;188:109–121.

80. Papakostas GI, et al. The relationship between serum folate, vitamin B12, and homocysteine levels in major depressive disorder and the timing of improvement with fluoxetine. Int J Neuropsychopharmacol 2005;8(4): 523–528.

81. Papakostas GI, et al. S-adenosyl-methionine in depression: a comprehensive review of the literature. Curr Psychiatry Rep 2003;5(6):460–466.

82. Williams AL, et al. S-adenosylmethionine (SAMe) as treatment for depression: a systematic review. Clin Invest Med 2005;28(3):132–139.

83. Alpert JE, et al. S-adenosyl-L-methionine (SAMe) as an adjunct for resistant major depressive disorder: an open trial following partial or nonresponse to selective serotonin reuptake inhibitors or venlafaxine. J Clin Psychopharmacol 2004;24(6):661–664.

84. Pancheri P, et al. A double-blind, randomized parallel-group, efficacy and safety study of intramuscular S-adenosyl-L-methionine 1,4-butanedisulphonate (SAMe) versus imipramine in patients with major depressive disorder. Int J Neuropsychopharmacol 2002;5(4):287–294.

85. Salmaggi P, et al. Double-blind, placebo-controlled study of S-adenosyl-L-methionine in depressed postmenopausal women. Psychother Psychosom 1993;59(1): 34–40.

86. Agnoli A, et al. Effect of s-adenosyl-l-methionine (SAMe) upon depressive symptoms. J Psychiatr Res 1976;13(1):43–54.

87. Berlanga C, et al. Efficacy of S-adenosyl-L-methionine in speeding the onset of action of imipramine. Psychiatry Res 1992;44(3):257–262.

88. Rosenbaum JF, et al. The antidepressant potential of oral S-adenosyl-l-methionine. Acta Psychiatr Scand 1990;81(5):432–436.

89. Hood SD, et al. Acute tryptophan depletion. Part I: rationale and methodology. Aust N Z J Psychiatry 2005;39(7):558–564.

90. Roiser J, et al. The subjective and cognitive effects of acute phenylalanine and tyrosine depletion in patients recovered from depression. Neuropsychopharmacology 2005;30:775–785.

91. Byerley WF, et al. 5-Hydroxytryptophan: a review of its antidepressant efficacy and adverse effects. J Clin Psychopharmacol 1987;7(3):127–137.

92. Glassman AH, Platman SR. Potentiation of a monoamine oxidase inhibitor by tryptophan. J Psychiatr Res 1969;7(2):83–88.

93. Nardini M, et al. Treatment of depression with L-5-hydroxytryptophan combined with chlorimipramine, a double-blind study. Int J Clin Pharmacol Res 1983;3(4):239–250.

94. Walinder J, et al. Potentiation of the antidepressant action of clomipramine by tryptophan. Arch Gen Psychiatry 1976;33(11):1384–1389.

95. Coppen A, et al. Potentiation of the antidepressive effect of a monoamine-oxidase inhibitor by tryptophan. Lancet 1963;1(7272):79–81.

96. Levitan RD, et al. Preliminary randomized double-blind placebo-controlled trial of tryptophan combined with fluoxetine to treat major depressive disorder: antidepressant and hypnotic effects. J Psychiatry Neurosci 2000;25(4):337–346.

97. Shaw DM, et al. Tricyclic antidepressants and tryptophan in unipolar depression. Psychol Med 1975;5(3):276–278.

98. Thomson J, et al. The treatment of depression in general practice: a comparison of L-tryptophan, amitriptyline, and a combination of L-tryptophan and amitriptyline with placebo. Psychol Med 1982;12(4):741–751.

99. Ayuso Gutierrez JL, et al. [Tryptophan and amitriptyline in the treatment of depression (double blind study)]. Actas Luso Esp Neurol Psiquiatr Cienc Afines 1973;1(3):471–476.

100. Mills S, Bone K. Principles and practice of phytotherapy. London: Churchill Livingstone, 2000.

101. Akhondzadeh S, et al. Comparison of Crocus sativus L. and imipramine in the treatment of mild to moderate depression: a pilot double-blind randomized trial [ISRCTN45683816]. BMC Complement Altern Med 2004;4:12.

102. Noorbala AA, et al. Hydro-alcoholic extract of Crocus sativus L. versus fluoxetine in the treatment of mild to moderate depression: a double-blind, randomized pilot trial. J Ethnopharmacol 2005;97(2):281–284.

103. Akhondzadeh S, et al. Comparison of petal of Crocus sativus L. and fluoxetine in the treatment of depressed outpatients: a pilot double-blind randomized trial. Prog Neuropsychopharmacol Biol Psychiatry 2007;30(2):439–442.

104. Akhondzadeh S, et al. Crocus sativus L. in the treatment of mild to moderate depression: a double-blind, randomized and placebo-controlled trial. Phytother Res 2005;19(2):148–151.

105. Moshiri E, et al. Hesameddin Abbasi S, Akhondzadeh S. Crocus sativus L. (petal) in the treatment of mild-to-moderate depression: a double-blind, randomized and placebo-controlled trial. Phytomedicine 2006;13(9–10):607–611.

106. Benazzi F. Is there a continuity between bipolar and depressive disorders? Psychother Psychosom 2007;76(2):70–76.

107. Cassano GB, et al. Conceptual underpinnings and empirical support for the mood spectrum. Psychiatr Clin North Am 2002;25(4):699–712,v.

108. Magnusson A, Partonen T. The diagnosis, symptomatology, and epidemiology of seasonal affective disorder. CNS Spectr 2005;10(8):625–634;quiz 621–614.

109. Lambert GW, et al. Effect of sunlight and season on serotonin turnover in the brain. Lancet 2002;360(9348):1840–1842.

110. Maciocia G. The practice of Chinese medicine: the treatment of diseases with acupuncture and Chinese herbs. London: Churchill Livingstone, 1994.

111. Wang H, et al. Is acupuncture beneficial in depression: a meta-analysis of 8 randomized controlled trials? J Affect Disord. 2008;111(2–3):125–134.

112. Leo RJ, Ligot JS Jr. A systematic review of randomized controlled trials of acupuncture in the treatment of depression. J Affect Disord 2007;97(1–3):13–22.

113. Cabyoglu MT, et al. The mechanism of acupuncture and clinical applications. Int J Neurosci 2006;116(2):115–125.

114. Wang SM, et al. Acupuncture analgesia: I. The scientific basis. Anesth Analg 2008;106(2):602–610.

115. Garner B, et al. Pilot study evaluating the effect of massage therapy on stress, anxiety and aggression in a young adult psychiatric inpatient unit. Aust N Z J Psychiatry 2008;42(5):414–422.

116. Coelho HF, et al. Massage therapy for the treatment of depression: a systematic review. Int J Clin Pract 2008;62(2):325–333.

117. Markowitz JC. Evidence-based psychotherapies for depression. J Occup Environ Med 2008;50(4):437–440.

118. Sarris J, et al. Adjuvant use of nutritional and herbal medicines with antidepressants, mood stabilizers and benzodiazepines. J Psychiatr Res 2009;44(1):32–41.

119. Chrubasik S, et al. Zingiberis rhizoma: a comprehensive review on the ginger effect and efficacy profiles. Phytomedicine 2005;12(9):684–701.

120. Holtmann G, et al. Efficacy of artichoke leaf extract in the treatment of patients with functional dyspepsia: a six-week placebo-controlled, double-blind, multicentre trial. Aliment Pharmacol Ther 2003;18(11–12):1099–1105.

121. Narimanian M, et al. Randomized trial of a fixed combination (KanJang) of herbal extracts containing Adhatoda vasica, Echinacea purpurea and Eleterococcus senticosus in patients with upper respiratory tract infections. Phytomedicine 2005;12(8):539–547.

122. Miyasaka LS, et al. Passiflora for anxiety disorder. Cochrane Database Syst Rev 2007;(1):CD004518.

123. Pittler MH, Ernst E. Kava extract for treating anxiety. Cochrane Database Syst Rev 2006;(1):CD003383.

124. Mahady GB. Ginkgo biloba for the prevention and treatment of cardiovascular disease: a review of the literature. Journal of Cardiovascular Nursing 2002;16(4):21.

125. Zhou W, et al. Clinical use and molecular mechanisms of action of extract of Ginkgo biloba leaves in cardiovascular diseases. Cardiovasc Drug Rev. Winter 2004;22(4):309–319.

126. Cohen AJ, Bartlik B. Ginkgo biloba for antidepressant-induced sexual dysfunction. J Sex Marital Ther 1998;24(2):139–143.

127. Wheatley D. Triple-blind, placebo-controlled trial of Ginkgo biloba in sexual dysfunction due to antidepressant drugs. Hum Psychopharmacol 2004;19(8):545–548.

128. Kang BJ, et al. A placebo-controlled, double-blind trial of Ginkgo biloba for antidepressant-induced sexual dysfunction. Hum Psychopharmacol 2002;17(6):279–284.

129. Saller R, et al. An updated systematic review of the pharmacology of silymarin. Forsch Komplement Med 2007;14(2):70–80.

130. Osiecki H. The physician's handbook of clinical nutrition. 5th edn. Brisbane: Bioconcepts Publishing, 1998.

131. Brosse AL, et al. Exercise and the treatment of clinical depression in adults: recent findings and future directions. Sports Med 2002;32(12):741–760.

132. Lawlor DA, et al. The effectiveness of exercise as an intervention in the management of depression: systematic review and meta-regression analysis of randomised controlled trials. BMJ (Clinical Research Ed.) 2001;322(7289):763–767.

133. Dunn AL, et al. Exercise treatment for depression: efficacy and dose response. American Journal Of Preventive Medicine 2005;28(1):1–8.

134. McIntyre RS, et al. Calculated bioavailable testosterone levels and depression in middle-aged men. Psychoneuroendocrinology 2006;31:1029–1035.

135. Pilkington K, et al. Yoga for depression: the research evidence. Journal Of Affective Disorders 2005;89(1–3):13–24.

136. Tsang HW, et al. Effects of mindful and non-mindful exercises on people with depression: a systematic review. Br J Clin Psychol 2008;47(Pt 3):303–322.

137. Linde K, Knuppel L. Large-scale observational studies of hypericum extracts in patients with depressive disorders – a systematic review. Phytomedicine 2005;12(1–2):148–157.

138. Roder C, et al. [Meta-analysis of effectiveness and tolerability of treatment of mild to moderate depression with St. John's Wort]. Fortschr Neurol Psychiatr 2004;72(6):330–343.
139. Werneke U, et al. How effective is St John's wort? The evidence revisited. J Clin Psychiatry 2004;65(5): 611–617.
140. Whiskey E, et al. A systematic review and meta-analysis of *Hypericum perforatum* in depression: a comprehensive clinical review. Int J Clin Psychopharm 2001;16: 239–252.
141. Shaw K, et al. Tryptophan and 5-hydroxytryptophan for depression. Cochrane Database Syst Rev 2002;(1):CD003198.
142. Bottiglieri T, Hyland K. S-adenosylmethionine levels in psychiatric and neurological disorders: a review. Acta Neurol Scand Suppl 1994;154:19–26.
143. Sarris J, et al. Depression and exercise. Journal of Complementary Medicine 2008;3:48–50, 61.
144. Doyne EJ, et al. Running versus weight lifting in the treatment of depression. Journal of Consulting and Clinical Psychology 1987;55(5):748–754.

13

Chronic generalised anxiety

Jerome Sarris
ND, MHSc, PhD

CLASSIFICATION, EPIDEMIOLOGY AND AETIOLOGY

Generalised anxiety disorder (GAD) is diagnosed in people with excessive worry and anxiety, which the person finds difficult to control. Somatic complaints and sleeping problems often accompany the anxiety. According to DSM-IV diagnostic criteria, in addition to uncontrollable worrying, there must also be at least three of six somatic symptoms (restless, fatigue, concentration problems, irritability, tension or sleep disturbance), occurring for a period of at least 6 months.[1] For a diagnosis of GAD to be reached, significant distress or impaired functioning from the condition must be present. As in MDD, a number of exclusion criteria must also be ruled out (for example, symptoms must not be confined to features of another mental disorder or due to substance use or general medical conditions). Occasional worry and situational anxiety is a normal human experience; true chronic generalised anxiety is a disorder whereby the worrying becomes self-perpetuating and uncontrollable, has a number of distressing somatic features and causes marked impairment of work or social functioning. It should be noted that the diagnosis of GAD is fairly restrictive in terms of the requirement of a long duration and multiple somatic symptoms. As the condition commonly waxes and wanes, the DSM-IV diagnosis may be excessively restrictive in clinical practice.[2] A utilitarian diagnosis may involve a period of anxiety or worry that is bothersome to the patient and has occurred for longer than 2 weeks. It is also worth considering that in some people GAD may reflect 'trait anxiety'—that is, a person whose personality archetype is that of a chronic worrier.

Anxiety disorders are second only to MDD as the most commonly diagnosed psychiatric conditions in primary care,[3] with GAD being present in 22% of primary care patients who complain of anxiety problems.[4] Consistent with the DSM-IV manual's description of the 1-year prevalence of GAD as approximately 3%,[1] a sample of 10,641 Australians interviewed in 1997 had a 1-month prevalence of 2.8% and a 12-month prevalence of 3.6%.[5] Lifetime prevalence of GAD is approximated at around 5–6%.[4] Anxiety symptoms are endemic in depression,[6] and true comorbidity of depressive and anxious conditions commonly occurs.[7,8] Studies have revealed that approximately 60–80% of patients with GAD will suffer from a mood disorder within their lifetimes.[9,10] Pure GAD (without other comorbid psychiatric disorders) exists at around 25%.[4] The socioeconomic burden of GAD is immense, with sufferers more likely than any other patient group to make frequent medical appointments and use medical resources. In a study of 36,435 GAD patients aged 18 to 64 identified from a claims database, the average total healthcare costs per patient was US$7451.[10] Patients with comorbid depression were found to have on average 10% higher costs. As in the case of major depressive disorder, only approximately 40% of sufferers seek treatment and 60% will achieve full or partial remission for over 5 years.[11]

The pathophysiology of GAD is still uncertain. It appears that GAD has a strong underlying genetic component, which may be triggered into expression by environmental factors.[12] Current evidence indicates that the neurobiological influence involves abnormalities of serotonergic, noradrenergic and GABAergic transmission, which is reflected in the efficacy of selective serotonin reuptake inhibitors (SSRIs) and serotonin and noradrenalin reuptake inhibitors (SNRIs) and benzodiazepines, which modulate the previously mentioned pathways, respectively.[13] Although still not understood, the main neurocircuitry involved in the panic, fear and anxiety response in humans appears to involve the prefrontal cortex, the hippocampus and the amygdala.[14] Psychological causes may also exist, for instance a specific cognitive bias to increased attention and misinterpretation of ambiguous stimuli, which are perceived as threatening.[11]

RISK FACTORS

Several risk factors and protective factors exist for GAD (see Figure 13.1). The primary risk factor for developing GAD appears to be genetic.[12] Significant familial aggregation also exists, with a strong correlation between the sufferer and a first-order relative with the disorder.[15] An anxiogenic familial environment appears also to contribute to the development of the pathology, although the data suggest that genetics are the dominant

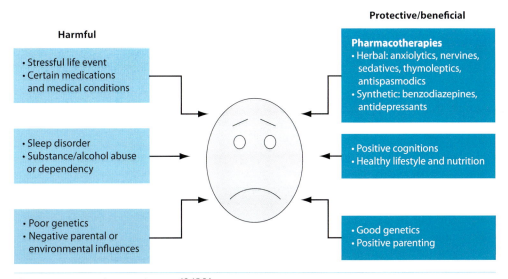

Harmful

- Stressful life event
- Certain medications and medical conditions

- Sleep disorder
- Substance/alcohol abuse or dependency

- Poor genetics
- Negative parental or environmental influences

Protective/beneficial

Pharmacotherapies
- Herbal: anxiolytics, nervines, sedatives, thymoleptics, antispasmodics
- Synthetic: benzodiazepines, antidepressants

- Positive cognitions
- Healthy lifestyle and nutrition

- Good genetics
- Positive parenting

Figure 13.1 Anxiety and stress[12,15,24]

factor.[12] Women are twice more likely to experience GAD than men, and a diagnosis of GAD is uncommon in children and adolescents with the incidence of GAD greatly increasing later in life (onset is usually after 25 years of age).[15] As discussed above, comorbidity with depression is common, so it is salient to do a screening for GAD when depressive symptomatology is present. Comorbidity with other psychiatric disorders is more common than not, with an estimated 90% of GAD patients having one or more disorders such as social phobia, panic disorder, obsessive-compulsive disorder and bipolar depression.[16] In fact, the diagnosis of GAD may be seen as a risk factor for the development of these other psychiatric disorders and also of alcohol and substance abuse disorders.[17]

CONVENTIONAL TREATMENT

Medical treatment of anxiety disorders primarily focuses on pharmaceutical and psychological interventions. Pharmacotherapies include synthetic anxiolytics (for example, benzodiazepines, pre-gabalin, β-blockers and buspirone), and antidepressants (for example, tricyclics, monoamine oxidase inhibitors and SSRIs/SNRIs).[18] Current evidence supports the use of both antidepressants and benzodiazepines, with some studies indicating that paroxetine and venlafaxine are the preferable choices. Several issues are present with respect to treatment of anxiety disorders with benzodiazepines. Common side effects include sedation, motor disturbance and cognitive interference (due to GABA-$\alpha_{1,2}$ agonism), while long-term treatment (> 2 weeks) may cause dependence and withdrawal issues.[18,19] Abrupt cessation of benzodiazepines may cause rebound symptoms such as insomnia, agitation and digestive disturbance, and the patient's anxiety may return to an even higher level than before treatment.[19] Psychological interventions include a variety of cognitive, behavioural and interpersonal techniques.[11] Combination approaches using psychological and pharmacotherapy treatments are commonly recommended; also, evidentiary support does not currently endorse this approach over using each as a monotherapy.[20] The combination does, however, seem to make sense, as pharmacotherapies such as benzodiazepines (or natural alternatives such as *Piper methysticum*) may elicit an immediate benefit while psychology techniques have been shown to lessen the chance of relapse over the long term.[11,20]

KEY TREATMENT PROTOCOLS

As outlined in the naturopathic treatment aims box, anxiety disorders need to be treated both symptomatically and systemically (as in the case of depression). Initially, thorough case taking is necessary to determine the causes, onset and duration of the episode, the level of impairment, comorbidities, and their individual presentation. With respect to causes, practitioners should ask about any potential trigger that makes them anxious, their cognitive state and any potentially anxiogenic factors—caffeine, alcohol and illicit drugs, pharmaceuticals, poor sleep pattern or excessive work to rest ratio. Anxiety-reducing herbal pharmacotherapies may be useful as an initial

NATUROPATHIC TREATMENT AIMS

- Reduce anxiety, worrying and somatic symptoms.
- Support and normalise adrenal function.
- Regulate HPA-axis activity.
- Teach 'worry management' techniques.
- Encourage stress management via lifestyle changes.
- Improve diet and reduce stimulants.
- Prevent or lessen chance of relapsing anxiety.

treatment to ameliorate anxiety. Psychological intervention also at this time may be beneficial by working on interpersonal and behavioural skills, and the elimination of anxiogenic self-talk. It is also worth noting that a depressive phase often occurs after an episode of GAD,[21] so patient education and prevention strategies are vital. The final main protocol in treating GAD is to educate the patient about self-help interventions they can use to better manage their stress. The use of bibliotherapy, massage, aroma-therapy and exercise, and the adoption of calming euthymic activities or hobbies, may also be beneficial (these are reviewed below). While individually each of the aforementioned interventions may possess limited evidence, or have a small clinical effect, the use of many of these self-help techniques in the context of an overall lifestyle pattern may provide a sustained healing effect.

Although the goal is to use evidence-based treatments, it is encouraging to know that any therapeutic interface will commonly promote an anxiolytic effect. Evidence reveals that sufferers of GAD commonly experience other presentations of anxiety such as panic attacks and social phobias.[23] Because of this, thorough case taking needs to be employed to assess for any comorbidities. Panic attacks are a severe manifestation of anxiety, and their co-occurrence with GAD or MDD indicates a more severe condition, resulting in a potentially poorer prognosis and more demanding treatment protocol. In the case of comorbid social phobia, behavioural and interpersonal issues need to be explored via an appropriate psychological intervention. As detailed below, several theories and models exist.

GABA pathways and the limbic system

The key biological pathway involved in the presentation and modulation of anxiety disorders involves gamma aminobutyric acid (GABA).[11] GABAergic neurones and receptors are involved in the main mode of inhibitory transmission in the central nervous system, and these innervations densely occupy parts of the anxiety/fear-modulating corticolimbic system such as the hippocampus and amgydala.[25] GABA-α receptors are the principal target of benzodiazepines, exerting affects such as anxiolysis, sedation and anticonvulsant effects.[13] Stimulation of GABAergic pathways also modulates the release of several key neurochemicals (for example, noradrenaline, serotonin and dopamine), although the exact effects are still disputed. Herbal medicines may exert GABA-modulating activity; however, no definitive GABA-$\alpha_{1,2}$ modulation has been demonstrated to date in humans by any herbal medicines. Valerenic acid from ***Valeriana officinalis*** has, however, demonstrated GABA-A receptor (β3 subunit) agonism; this mechanism has been identified as an important pharmacodynamic action responsible for the plant's anxiolytic and hypnotic action.[26]

The phytotherapy that has received the greatest attention regarding GABAergic activity is ***Piper methysticum*** (kava). Current evidence indicates that kavalactones (the resinoid lipid-soluble constituents found primarily in the root and stem) modulate GABA activity via alteration of lipid membrane structures, and sodium channel alteration, rather than by significant GABA-$\alpha_{1,2}$ agonism.[27–29] Importantly, this activity in animal models was found to occur in the anxiety/fear modulating hippocampus and amygdala. Other neuromodulatory activity effecting anxiolysis are considered to involve

Placebo response is endemic in sufferers of anxiety, with approximately 25% receiving marked benefit from a placebo (dummy) intervention![22]

a down-regulation of β-adrenergic activity and MAO-B inhibition.[30] Interestingly, inhibition of the re-uptake of noradrenaline in the prefrontal cortex has been demonstrated in animal models.[30] This facilitates kava's unique effect of enhancing mental acuity while relaxing the body and calming the mind. This effect is of a distinct advantage compared to alcohol and benzodiazepines, which cause deleterious cognitive effects. Another advantage of using kava in anxiety disorders is that kavalactones have also demonstrated relaxation of muscular contractibility via modulation of sodium and calcium channels.[31] Somatic tension is a common occurrence in anxiety disorders.[11]

Strong evidence supports the use of kava in treating anxiety disorders. A Cochrane review of 12 randomised, double-blind, controlled trials of rigorous methodology using kava mono-preparations (60 mg–280 mg of kavalactones) in anxious conditions revealed positive results in favour of the phytomedicine.[32] A meta-analysis of seven homogenous trials using the Hamilton anxiety scale[33] (HAMA) demonstrated that kava reduced anxiety significantly compared to placebo. This effect was supported by another meta-analysis based on six placebo-controlled, randomised trials using a standardised kava extract WS1490 in anxiety (assessed via HAMA).[34] Medicinal use of kava is currently restricted in the European Union, and Canada over hepatotoxicity.[35] The World Health Organization (WHO) has recommended research into 'aqueous' extracts of the plant to establish its safety and efficacy in treating anxiety disorders.[35] This is in preference to previous acetonic or ethanolic extracts, which may be implicated in hepatotoxic reactions. A recent clinical trial sought to assess the effects of an aqueous extract of kava (see the box below).

Other herbal medicines that may affect anxiolysis via limbic system interaction with evidence from human studies include *Passiflora incarnata*, *Scutellaria lateriflora*, *Melissa officinalis* and *Ginkgo biloba*. *Passiflora incarnata* has traditional usage in the treatment of anxiety and neurosis.[37] A Cochrane review of *P. incarnata* in the treatment of anxiety included two randomised controlled trials (RCTs) that met inclusion criteria with a total of 198 participants.[38] One, a study comparing *P. incarnata* extract (90 mg/day) to the benzodiazepine mexazolam (1.5 mg/day), revealed no statistical differences in outcome. A trend towards advantage of phytomedicine over the

THE KAVA ANXIETY DEPRESSION SPECTRUM STUDY (KADSS)[36]

- This was a 3-week placebo-controlled, double-blind, crossover trial involving 60 adult participants with elevated stable anxiety and varying levels of depressive symptoms.
- Participants were prescribed 5 kava tablets per day: 2 tablets morning, 2 tablets after lunch, and 1 tablet in the evening (250 mg of kavalactones/day).
- The aqueous extract of kava reduced participants' HAMA anxiety score in the first controlled phase by –9.9 (CI: 7.1, 12.7) compared to –0.8 (CI: –2.7, 4.3) for placebo, and in the second controlled phase by –10.3 (CI: 5.8, 14.7) compared to +3.3 (CI: –6.8, 0.2).
- The pooled effect of kava compared to placebo across phases was highly significant with a very strong effect size. Pooled analyses also revealed highly significant relative reductions in BAI anxiety and MADRS depression scores.
- The extract was found to be safe, with no serious adverse effects, and no clinical hepatotoxicity.

benzodiazepines was noted with respect to decreased sedation and job performance. The other trial included in the review, a pilot RCT using *P. incarnata* extract on 36 patients with GAD, demonstrated equivalent efficacy of the HM with oxazepam (30 mg/day) in reducing anxiety.[39] The herb was determined to cause fewer side effects.[40] A recent study using *P. incarnata* (500 mg) in a controlled study involving 60 patients with preoperative anxiety (90 minutes before surgery) revealed significantly lower anxiety (assessed via a numerical rating scale) in the active group than in the control group.[41] No significant differences occurred between other psychological variables, for example recovery and psychomotor function.

The fragrant herbal medicine ***Melissa officinalis*** has traditional usage as a mild sedative and an antispasmodic.[37,42] A double-blind, placebo-controlled, randomised, balanced crossover experiment involving 18 participants using two separate single doses of a standardised *M. officinalis* extract (300 mg, 600 mg) and placebo showed that acute dosing of the herbal medicine demonstrated a significant increase in self-rated calmness on a Defined Intensity Stressor Simulation (DISS) test.[43] A subsequent crossover RCT using a standardised *M. officinalis* and *Valeriana officinalis* product in 24 healthy volunteers demonstrated that a 600 mg dose of the combination lowered anxiety levels compared to control on the DISS.[44]

Scutellaria lateriflora is a traditional anxiolytic herbal medicine that has been used to treat a variety of nervous system disorders in Native American and eclectic medicine.[37] In an animal maze test model, the herb displayed anxiolytic effects, with the compounds baicalin and baicalein purported to be involved in this activity via GABA-α binding.[45] A double-blind, placebo-controlled crossover study of 19 healthy adults demonstrated that *S. lateriflora* dose-dependently reduced symptoms of anxiety and tension after acute administration compared to control.[40] It should be noted that the methodology of this trial was weak and further research is required to confirm the herb's efficacy.

While ***Ginkgo biloba*** is primarily studied for neuromodulatory activity for the treatment of cognitive conditions, studies have documented mood modulation in cognitively impaired subjects.[46] A 2006 RCT involving 82 subjects with GAD using *G. biloba* EGb 761 extract (480 mg or 240 mg per day) or placebo for 4 weeks revealed a significant dose-dependent reduction of HAMA over placebo in the 480 mg/day and the 240 mg/day *G. biloba* groups.[47]

Eschscholtzia californica, ***Zizyphus jujuba*** and ***Valeriana*** spp. are other plant medicines with encouraging activity; however, to date no human clinical studies have been conducted using these as monotherapies to treat anxiety disorders. Studies are required to validate these traditional uses. *Eschscholtzia californica* promisingly exerts binding affinity to GABA receptors, with flumazenil (a benzodiazepine receptor antagonist) suppressing these sedative and anxiolytic effects.[48] Animal models have revealed that the jujubosides in *Zizyphus jujuba* inhibit glutamate-mediated pathways (excitory pathway) in the hippocampus.[49] Other studies using suanzoaren (a traditional Chinese medicine formula containing *Z. jujuba* as the principal herbal medicine) in animal models have demonstrated modulation of central monoamines and limbic system interaction.[50,51]

Magnesium has an important role in neurological activity, and deficiency of the nutrient may cause neuropathologies.[52] Magnesium ions regulate calcium ion flow in neuronal calcium channels, helping to regulate neuronal nitric oxide production.[53] The deficit of neuronal magnesium ions may be induced by stress hormones, excessive dietary calcium and dietary deficiencies of magnesium.[53] Studies using animal models have demonstrated that magnesium deficiency can cause depression and anxiety-like behaviour. After magnesium administration to deficient animals, anxiolytic activity was demonstrated in mice during elevated plus maze and forced swim tests.[54] Magnesium appears to exert its anxiolytic effect by the involvement of the NMDA/glutamate pathway, and this activity may involve the glycine(B) sites.[55] Interaction between magnesium and benzodiazepine/GABA-α receptors may also be involved in producing anxiolytic-like activity.[56] A preliminary controlled study for the relief of mild premenstrual symptoms using combinations of magnesium, vitamin B6, magnesium and vitamin B6, and placebo for one menstrual cycle in 44 women showed no overall difference between individual treatments.[57] Further specific subanalyses, however, showed a significant effect of 200 mg/day Mg + 50 mg/day vitamin B6 on reducing anxiety-related premenstrual symptoms (nervous tension, mood swings, irritability or anxiety). Although encouraging, the design of the study and the modest results preclude a firm conclusion of efficacy.

Endocrinological factors

Although not entirely understood yet, the endocrine system has a distinct role in stress and anxiety, with HPA-axis hyperactivation being regarded as a prime component in chronic anxiogenesis.[58] CAM interventions that modulate the HPA axis may have a role in treating stress and anxiety (see Section 5 on the endocrine system). Among CAM interventions that may provide HPA-axis modulation are herbal 'adaptogens' and 'tonics', including *Withania somnifera* and *Rhodiola rosea*. **Withania somnifera** is classified in Ayurvedic medicine as a 'rasayana', a medicine used to enhance physical and mental performance and ward off disease.[59] The plant has been adopted recently into Western herbal materia medica for its use in nervous system and endocrine disorders.[42] An animal study observed adaptogenic effects of *W. somnifera* in a stress-inducing procedure, via the attenuation of stress-related parameters (cortisol levels, mental depression and sexual dysfunction).[60] The purported active constituents, the glycowithanolides, were administered orally in an animal model once daily for 5 days, and were discovered to induce an anxiolytic effect comparable to that produced by lorazepam relevant tests (elevated plus maze, social interaction and feeding latency in an unfamiliar environment tests).[61]

Rhodiola rosea may also have a place in treating generalised anxiety, especially if presenting with fatigue and cardiovascular problems. A small pilot trial used a standardised *R. rosea* (Rhodax®) formulation in 10 participants with diagnosed generalised anxiety disorder. Participants received 340 mg of Rhodax® in two divided doses for a period of 10 weeks.[62] Results demonstrated a significant drop on the Hamilton Anxiety Scale. Although baseline levels on the Hamilton Depression Rating Scale were low, a statistically significant response also occurred on this outcome measure. While this study yielded a positive outcome, the uncontrolled design and small sample temper confidence in the results. A caveat that should be observed by clinicians using *R. rosea* root for anxious presentations is that the herb has (dose-dependently) been found to cause anxiety, irritability and insomnia in some people.

The biological and energetic role of the 'heart'

Crataegus oxyacantha has traditional use as a phytomedicine to treat cardiovascular complaints and is considered to have heart-tonifying properties.[63] *Crataegus* spp. is usually prescribed in phytomedicine for cardiovascular complaints, an arena in which it possesses robust evidence of efficacy.[64,65]

Emerging data indicate a use in anxiety, especially where somatic cardiovascular symptoms present (for example, palpitations or tachycardia). An RCT administering 500 mg of hawthorn extract to 36 mildly hypertensive patients measured in a secondary outcome a non-significant trend towards reduction of anxiety, compared with placebo.[69]

THE HEART AND ANXIETY

- The connection between cardiovascular conditions and anxiety has evidence.[66]
- Cardiovascular disease may cause anxiety or vice versa.[66]
- A somatic effect of anxiety is heart palpitations and tachycardia.[15]
- This reflects traditional knowledge of the heart–emotion/mental connection.[67,68]

In a later double-blind, randomised, placebo-controlled trial involving participants presenting with mild-moderate GAD (assessed via DSM-III-R) 264 adults were prescribed two tablets containing fixed quantities of ***Crataegus oxyacantha*** (300 mg), ***Eschscholtzia californica*** (80 mg) and **magnesium** (300 mg elemental) twice daily for 3 months.[70] Total and somatic HAMA scores, subjective patient-rated anxiety and physician's Clinical Global Impressions scale were used as outcome measures. The results demonstrated that the formula markedly ameliorated anxiety in comparison to placebo as determined by HAMA and subjectively assessed anxiety.

INTEGRATIVE MEDICAL CONSIDERATIONS

As in all psychiatric disorders, an integrative approach is advised in managing GAD. Aside from judicious prescription of complementary or synthetic pharmacotherapies and the recommendation of psychological interventions, options such as massage, acupuncture and an exercise and relaxation program may be of additional benefit. A key integrative management technique of chronic anxiety is to screen, or refer for assessment, alcohol or substance abuse or dependency issues and other comorbid medical and psychiatric disorders.

Muscular relaxation therapy

The therapeutic technique of progressive muscle relaxation, developed by Jacobson in 1938, reduces anxiety and stress by first tensing a muscle and then releasing that tension.[71] By releasing physical tension the sympathetic nervous system-activated 'flight or flight' response may be reduced. This technique may be of value in GAD, which commonly presents with somatic tension. Aside from the physiological relaxation that ensues from progressive muscle relaxation, the technique may have additional anxiolytic benefits by focusing the person's mind away from worries, and allowing them to develop a sense of self-mastery over their anxiety. Evidence supports the use of muscular relaxation therapy techniques to reduce anxiety and tension. A review of 60 studies concluded that these techniques are as effective as pharmacologic and cognitive techniques.[72] A review of the effect sizes from five controlled studies revealed a moderate pooled effect size.

Psychological intervention

As documented in the previous depression chapter, various psychological techniques including cognitive and/or behavioural therapy and interpersonal techniques may be of benefit in treating GAD. Some people may be 'wired to worry' via genetic and/or familial upbringing. Although the understanding of people with trait anxiety is limited, it is possible that CAM and pharmaceutical interventions may be only of supportive

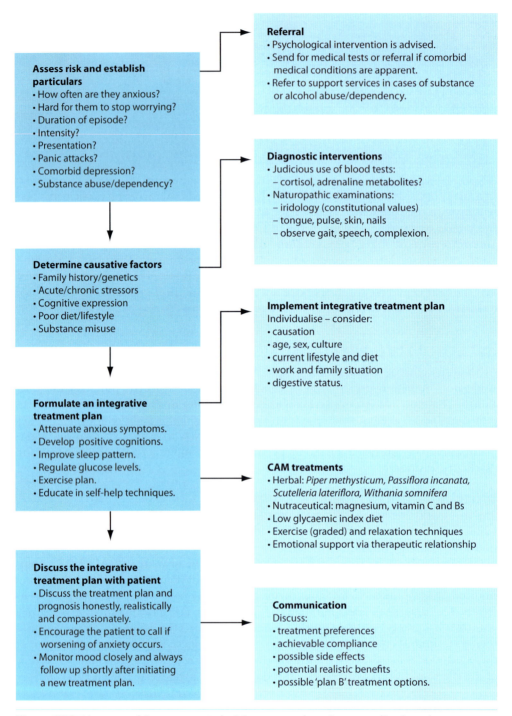

Assess risk and establish particulars
- How often are they anxious?
- Hard for them to stop worrying?
- Duration of episode?
- Intensity?
- Presentation?
- Panic attacks?
- Comorbid depression?
- Substance abuse/dependency?

Referral
- Psychological intervention is advised.
- Send for medical tests or referral if comorbid medical conditions are apparent.
- Refer to support services in cases of substance or alcohol abuse/dependency.

Diagnostic interventions
- Judicious use of blood tests:
  – cortisol, adrenaline metabolites?
- Naturopathic examinations:
  – iridology (constitutional values)
  – tongue, pulse, skin, nails
  – observe gait, speech, complexion.

Determine causative factors
- Family history/genetics
- Acute/chronic stressors
- Cognitive expression
- Poor diet/lifestyle
- Substance misuse

Implement integrative treatment plan
Individualise – consider:
- causation
- age, sex, culture
- current lifestyle and diet
- work and family situation
- digestive status.

Formulate an integrative treatment plan
- Attenuate anxious symptoms.
- Develop positive cognitions.
- Improve sleep pattern.
- Regulate glucose levels.
- Exercise plan.
- Educate in self-help techniques.

CAM treatments
- Herbal: *Piper methysticum, Passiflora incanata, Scutelleria lateriflora, Withania somnifera*
- Nutraceutical: magnesium, vitamin C and Bs
- Low glycaemic index diet
- Exercise (graded) and relaxation techniques
- Emotional support via therapeutic relationship

Discuss the integrative treatment plan with patient
- Discuss the treatment plan and prognosis honestly, realistically and compassionately.
- Encourage the patient to call if worsening of anxiety occurs.
- Monitor mood closely and always follow up shortly after initiating a new treatment plan.

Communication
Discuss:
- treatment preferences
- achievable compliance
- possible side effects
- potential realistic benefits
- possible 'plan B' treatment options.

Figure 13.2 Naturopathic treatment decision tree—chronic generalised anxiety

value in people who are wired to worry. Techniques that modify anxiogenic behaviours, such as hyperventilation, and assist patients to understand how their thoughts may affect their anxiety and how to alter these cognitive patterns, may reduce the intensity and frequency of the anxiety. While practitioners are encouraged to refer to clinical psychologists or a qualified counsellor they can still employ a 'person-centred' approach (empathy, active listening and genuineness) to the therapeutic encounter. A Cochrane meta-analysis was conducted involving 22 controlled studies (1060 participants) using psychological interventions to treat GAD.[73] Results based on a subsection of 13 studies using cognitive behavioural therapy (CBT) found the technique to be more effective than 'treatment as usual' or 'wait list' control in achieving a reduction of anxiety. However, six studies comparing CBT against basic supportive therapy revealed no significant difference in clinical response at post-treatment. Psychological therapies based on CBT or interpersonal supportive principles are effective treatments in reducing anxiety.

Acupuncture

A meta-analysis of the efficacy of acupuncture in the treatment of anxiety and anxiety disorders included 12 controlled trials of sufficient methodological standard.[74] All trials reported positive findings, but the reports lacked many basic methodological details. Evidence of studies involving perioperative anxiety was generally supportive of acupuncture. Acupuncture, and in particular auricular (ear) acupuncture, was found to be more effective than acupuncture at sham points. The authors note, however, that most results were based on subjective measures and blinding could not be guaranteed. An example of a controlled study of auricular acupuncture involved 67 people with pre-dental operation anxiety using controls, intranasal midazolam, placebo acupuncture, and no treatment.[75] The auricular acupuncture group and the midazolam group were significantly less preoperatively anxious compared to the placebo acupuncture group measured on the Spielberger State-Trait Anxiety Inventory X1.[76] Scientific research has found that acupuncture increases a number of central nervous system hormones (adrenocorticotropin hormone, beta-endorphins, serotonin and noradrenaline).[77,78]

Comorbid presentation of other anxiety disorders

As previously discussed, comorbidity of GAD with other anxiety disorders is the rule, not the exception. Other psychiatric disorders such as depression (unipolar and bipolar), social phobia, panic disorder, obsessive-compulsive disorder (OCD), post-traumatic distress disorder and attention deficit hyperactivity disorder (ADHD) commonly co-exist.[79,80] As in the case of major depressive disorder, GAD sufferers with comorbid mental disorders have increased psychological and social impairment, require more treatment and present with a poorer prognosis.[23] While specific diagnosis is the domain of psychiatrists and psychologists, it is important that practitioners take a methodical case study to determine more detail beyond the presentation of 'anxiety'. As illustrated in the box, an initial presentation of 'stress' or 'anxiety' may be confused with other disorders, for example a depressive disorder, bipolar (hypo)mania, ADHD or OCD or social phobia, or may co-present with other disorders, for example panic disorder.

If the patient presents with an obvious bipolar disorder, delusions or self-harm/suicidality, referral to a medical practitioner or to psychiatric assessment is advised. In the case of co-occurring social phobia, OCD or ADHD, CAM interventions currently do not have firm evidentiary support (although they may have a beneficial adjuvant role). Psychological support to assist in behavioural and cognitive modification may be helpful as part of an integrative solution.

MENTAL DISORDERS CO-OCCURRING WITH GAD*

Unipolar depression: Persistent low mood or lack of pleasure in combination with changes in sleep patterns, appetite, self-esteem, sexual drive, motivation and possible suicidal ideation

Bipolar (hypo)mania: Hypomania—a distinct period of elevated, expansive or irritable mood lasting > 4 days in addition to an increase in signs such as ↑ self-esteem/goal-oriented activity/grandiosity/pleasurable activities, ↓ need for sleep. Mania—the previous signs plus possible hospitalisation, psychotic features, marked social impairment

Social phobia: Significant anxiety provoked by exposure to social or performance situations, leading to avoidance of social situations

Panic disorder: Regular experience of panic attacks (acute anxiety and fear with signs and symptoms such as tachycardia, sweating, rapid breathing, fear of 'losing control' and persistent worry about another panic attack occurring). This causes distress and interferes with social and work functioning.

Obsessive-compulsive disorder: Persistent chronic compulsive or obsessive thoughts or activities. Compulsions cause anxiety and are allayed by repetitive actions. It must cause distress and social or work impairment, be noticeable by others and be time consuming.

ADHD: Several signs of inattention, hyperactivity and/or impulsiveness such as poor focus, poor self-control, difficulty sitting still and difficulty controlling speech. Must first occur before the age of 7 years.

*Modified from DSM-IV diagnostic criteria[1]

Managing comorbid alcohol and substance abuse or dependence

A common occurrence with anxiety disorders (and depression) is the over-representation of these disorders by sufferers of alcohol or substance overuse.[81,82] Practitioners should be aware of this as the overuse needs to be addressed sufficiently before the anxiety disorder can be treated. A basic diagnostic guideline involves differentiating alcohol or drug 'abuse' from 'dependence'. In the former there is a significant pattern of overuse leading to distress or social or work impairment within a 12-month period, and illegal and dangerous activities, and violence; the latter has additional issues such as tolerance, withdrawal, difficulty reducing use and excessive time spent on pursuing the use.[1] Alcohol abuse and dependency is common in Western society with a US epidemiological study involving a sample of 43,093 adults revealing that the 12-month prevalence was 17.8% and 12.5% for these disorders, respectively.[83]

Substance abuse and dependence is a serious problem throughout the world, with alcohol and tobacco being the most commonly abused substances.[84] The research and development of pharmacotherapies to treat these have medical, social and economical significance:

- Recent preliminary studies have reported potential therapeutic effects for *Hypericum perforatum* in smoking cessation, prickly pear extract in the prevention of alcohol hangover and magnesium as an adjunct to methadone treatment.[85]
- Other clinical studies have reported negative findings for *Ginkgo biloba* as an adjunctive treatment for cocaine dependence, *Cynara scolymus* as a prevention of alcohol

hangover, and acupuncture for alcohol withdrawal.[85] Drug dependence (nicotine included) causes a powerful maladaptive effect on the mesolimbic areas of the brain (depending on substance) via various pathways: dopaminergic, opioid, serotinerigc and glutaminergic.[86] It is likely that in cases of regular abuse that CAM interventions may provide only a supportive role in addition to psychological support, pharmaceutical prescription and abstinent recovery over time, due to marked neurological change.

- Various herbal and nutritional medicines considered to have anecdotal use in substance use disorders such as *Valeriana* spp., *Hypericum perforatum*, *Avena sativa* and magnesium do not have to date any robust clinical evidence.
- A review[84] revealed, however, that preliminary in vivo evidence exists for *H. perforatum* in alcohol and nicotine dependence.
- Animal models have shown that in ethanol withdrawal *H. perforatum* (50 and 100 mg/kg) produced some significant inhibitory effects on tremor and audiogenic seizures during the withdrawal period.[87]
- Another study using *H. perforatum* extracts in a genetically induced animal model of alcoholism HP Ze 117 (10–40 mg/kg) dose-dependently reduced alcohol intake in a 12-h limited access period.[88]
- *H. perforatum* may be an interesting adjunct for the treatment of alcoholism, but human trials are required to determine the clinical relevance. Overall, at this stage there remains insufficient evidence to support the use of natural and complementary therapies as a primary intervention for substance use disorders. Further clinical trials are required to clarify the potential role of particular agents.

Case Study

A 62-year-old male presents with **chronic anxiety**. He says that over the last 10 months he **constantly worries** about anything and everything, and **finds it difficult to stop worrying**. He says he has lately been suffering from sore **aching muscles** and **regular heart palpitations**. His diet consists mainly of processed foods, is high in sugars and is devoid of whole grains, nuts, fruit and vegetables.

SUGGESTIVE SYMPTOMS

- Persistent excessive worry (> 6 months)
- Restlessness, unable to relax
- Poor concentration, poor memory
- Sore muscles, tension headaches
- Heart palpitations, dizziness
- Sweating (not due to heat)
- Hyperthermia
- Fatigue
- Insomnia

Example treatment
Herbal and nutritional prescription

The herbal prescription is designed to primarily exert anxiolytic, nervine tonic and adaptogenic activity.[63] *Piper methysticum* is used as the premier anxiety-reducing herbal medicine. *Passiflora incarnata* and *Scutellaria lateriflora* will augment this effect. *Withania somnifera* will provide a non-stimulating adaptogenic tonic action. The use of *Crataegus oxyacantha* for the above case will address the cardiovascular presentation of the anxiety (palpitations) and may provide a supplementary anxiolytic activity. Magnesium prescription may be of benefit as an anxiolytic, as his diet is low in the mineral. A multivitamin high in B vitamins may be of benefit in assisting to restore proper adrenal and neurochemical activity.

Dietary and lifestyle advice

Dietary programs designed to treat depression have to date not been rigorously evaluated. Although evidence supporting specific dietary advice is currently absent, a basic balanced diet (see Section 1 on the gastrointestinal system) with foods rich in individual nutrients such as folate, omega-3, tryptophan, B and C vitamins, zinc and magnesium can be recommended. These foods include whole grains, lean meat, deep-sea fish, green leafy vegetables, coloured berries and nuts (walnuts and almonds).[52] A low glycaemic index diet may be beneficial in stabilising blood sugar

> **Herbal prescription**
>
> | *Withania somnifera* 1:1 | 40 mL |
> | *Passiflora incarnata* 1:2 | 25 mL |
> | *Scutellaria lateriflora* 1:2 | 20 mL |
> | *Crataegus oxyacantha* 1:2 | 15 mL |
> | 7.5 mL b.d. | 100 mL |
>
> *Piper methysticum* (50 mg kavalactones) 2 tablets 2 x day
>
> **Nutritional prescription**
>
> Magnesium amino acid chelate (100 mg elemental) 2 tablets 2 × day
> Multivitamin 1 per day (high in B vitamins and folic acid)

levels, which may in turn reduce the 'fight or flight' response of low blood sugar levels (see Section 5 on the endocrine system).

General lifestyle advice should focus on encouraging a balance between meaningful work, adequate rest and sleep, judicious exercise, positive social interaction and pleasurable hobbies. Behavioural therapy techniques have shown positive effects in reducing anxiety by training the person to reduce or better manage stressful situations, and to increase pleasurable activities. These may enhance self-esteem and self-mastery, and increase physical and mental wellbeing. With respect to sleep, insomnia is common in anxiety sufferers (see Chapter 14 on insomnia) and treating this is of primary importance as poor sleep may in turn deleteriously affect neuroendocrine balance and subsequently exacerbate the anxiety. Removal of caffeine from the person's diet is a vital component to reduce anxiety and improve sleep.[89] Caffeine causes arousal, hypervigilance and possible anxiogenesis in certain individuals via stimulation of β-adrenergic receptors and up-regulation of noradrenalin and dopamine; additionally, adenosine receptor antagonism interferes with sleep.[90] 'Decaffeinated' coffee and tea products still provide for the experience to be had without the sweaty palms and heart palpitations.

Exercise or physical activity

Physical activity is anecdotally regarded as having a positive effect on reducing stress and anxiety, with people often participating in activities such as walking, swimming, cycling doing yoga or going to the gym in order to improve their wellbeing. A recent meta-analysis conducted to examine the effects of exercise on anxiety included 49 studies and showed an overall moderate effect size, indicating larger reductions in anxiety among exercise groups than no-treatment control groups.[91] A non-significant trend towards a dose-dependent effect for moderate exercise occurred, while both lower and higher intensity exercise appears less effective. Exercise was found to have a stronger effect than stress management and education, while it was shown as having similar effects to CBT and a slightly less efficacy than pharmacotherapies. Caution should be adopted with anxious people who present with respiratory or cardiovascular symptoms, as these symptoms may be exacerbated with exercise and this in turn may increase anxiety. In some cases respiratory distress may also provoke a panic attack. Graded exercise programs that may be appropriate for anxiety may involve either aerobic or anabolic exercise for a minimum of 20 minutes three to five times per week.

ADDITIONAL PRESCRIPTIVE OPTIONS

Massage
- Massage therapy has been used extensively by many cultures for millennia for a variety of curative purposes.
- Theories of massage therapy's mechanism of action involve the 'gate control theory of pain reduction' (whereby manual pressure creates a stimulus that interferes with the pain signal), promotion of parasympathetic nervous system activity, stimulation of serotonergic and endorphin activity, reduction of somatic tension; and via interpersonal attention.[92]
- Evidence supports the acute application of massage therapy to reduce state anxiety, and the use of multiple treatments over time to reduce trait anxiety.[93]
- A meta-analysis involving 37 controlled studies (using various massage therapy techniques in various health applications) revealed that massage therapy significantly reduced both state and trait anxiety.[94] A moderate effect size was demonstrated for state anxiety, and a moderate-strong effect size for trait anxiety.
- Many confounding variables exist with respect to these studies. Massage therapy techniques and practitioner training level vary markedly, as well as the length of the treatment, the body parts massaged and environment and gender factors.

Aromatherapy
- Aromatherapy is the art and science of using essential oils as an inhalation or dermal application to promote health.
- The use of aromatherapy may provide a place as an adjuvant lifestyle intervention.
- The volatile constituents responsible for purported anxiolytic activity include linalool, linalyl acetate, geraniol; plants rich in these constituents include lavender, lemon balm, neroli, rose and ylang ylang.[95]
- Essential oils exert activity via postdermal or inhalant application crossing the blood–brain barrier and via limbic effects stimulated by subjective pleasant experience from aromas.
- While substantive in vitro and in vivo evidence exists for the use of various essential oils to reduce stress markers, there is a paucity of human clinical studies to support their use. Although essential oils such as *Lavender* spp. have been shown in animal studies to possess an anxiolytic profile,[96] controlled studies do not currently support the use of essential oils in anxiety disorders.
- An example involves an RCT on 313 patients undergoing radiotherapy randomly assigned either carrier oil with fractionated oils, carrier oil only, or pure essential oils of lavender, bergamot and cedarwood (administered by inhalation concurrently with radiation treatment).[97]
- Although there were no significant differences in depression outcomes, HAMA scores were actually significantly lower at treatment completion in the carrier oil only group (placebo) compared with either of the volatile oil arms.
- Another controlled, prospective study consisting of a sample of 118 patients evaluated the use of aromatherapy to reduce anxiety prior to scheduled investigative surgical procedures.[98] The control group was given an inert oil (placebo) for inhalation, and the experimental group inhaled lavender. There was no statistical difference in state anxiety levels post-treatment between the lavender and control group.

ADDITIONAL PRESCRIPTIVE OPTIONS *(Continued)*

Meditation
- Meditative techniques have been documented to reduce the arousal state and may also ameliorate anxiety symptoms.
- A Cochrane review conducted included two randomised controlled studies of sufficient methodological rigour.[99] Both studies were of moderate quality and used active control comparisons (another type of meditation, relaxation, biofeedback or anxiolytic drugs).
- In one study transcendental meditation showed a reduction in anxiety symptoms and electromyography scores comparable with biofeedback and relaxation therapy. Another study compared kundalini yoga with relaxation/mindfulness meditation. Assessment on the Yale-Brown Obsessive Compulsive Scale[100] showed no statistically significant difference between groups.
- The evidence concludes that transcendental meditation is comparable with other kinds of relaxation therapies in reducing anxiety, and kundalini yoga does not show significant effectiveness in treating obsessive-compulsive disorders compared with relaxation or meditation. The small numbers of studies included in this review, however, do not permit any conclusions to be drawn on the effectiveness of meditation therapy for anxiety disorders.

Expected outcomes and follow-up protocols

In the above case the patient's anxiety is expected to abate shortly after the commencement of kava, which has a quick onset of activity. The prognosis is better if the course of anxiety is not complicated by comorbid mental disorders or substance abuse, or if there is a history of anxiety.[23] The integrative approach involving psychological, dietary/nutraceutical, lifestyle and herbal intervention should offer a sustained benefit if compliance is maintained. Kava should only be prescribed in

KAVA AND THE LIVER

Liver toxicity has been documented from kava usage, and the plant was banned in 2002 in certain countries.[35]

Hepatotoxicity caused by European kava products may in part be due to a commercial cost-motivated preference for the aerial parts and root or stem peelings, which contain the alkaloid pipermethystine, and due to the use of non-traditional solvents (ethanol and acetone).[35]

There are various possible causes of hepatotoxicity from kava: a possible interaction with drugs or alcohol, the inhibition of CYP P450 (perhaps especially in the presence of a genetic insufficiency of CYP P450 2D6), reduction of liver glutathione content (or other enzymes needed to metabolise kavalactones) or inhibition of cyclooxygenase enzyme activity.[101,102]

The use of a water soluble extract of the peeled rootstock of a 'Noble' cultivar of kava may be the solution.[103]

The advice is to use kava away from alcohol and drugs, and within therapeutic dosage range. An occasional liver function test is also advised if regularly consuming the plant.

short-term, intermittent courses with occasional liver function tests being conducted to monitor for the rare occurrence of liver dysfunction (see the box for kava safety issues).

If after 2 weeks of the prescription minimal benefit occurred, kava could be withdrawn and the herbal prescription modified to include other potential anxiolytics, for example *Rhodiola rosea*, *Melissa officinalis*, *Bacopa monnieri*, *Valeriana officinalis* or *Ginkgo biloba*. Additional psychological interventions may also be of assistance—behavioural or social-based models to examine and aid in the management of the external triggers of the anxiety.

Table 13.1 Review of the major evidence

INTERVENTION	KEY LITERATURE	SUMMARY OF RESULTS	COMMENT
Piper methysticum	Pittler et al. 2003 Cochrane review[32] Witte et al. 2005[34] Meta-analysis 6 RCTs	$n = 345$ HAMA 5.0 point reduction over placebo (95% CI: 1.1–8.8) $n = 345$ OR = 3.3 (success rate) (95% CI: 2.09–5.22)	Significant anxiolysis occurred with *P. methysticum* over placebo in both meta-analyses.
Exercise	Wipfli et al. 2008[91] 49 RCTs Long & van Stavel 1995[104] 40 controlled studies	Moderate effect size (0.48) Small–moderate effect size	Exercise groups showed a greater reduction than other forms of exercise. Adults with higher stress baseline may have greater benefit.
Acupuncture	Pilkington et al. 2007[74] 12 controlled trials 6 on generalised anxiety disorder	Positive results in all studies	Overall most studies included had poor methodology. No studies included assessing other anxiety disorders, e.g. OCD, panic disorder.
Relaxation therapy	Jorm et al. 2004[72] 60 RCTs	Effect sizes from 5 controlled studies revealed a moderate pooled effect size of $d = 0.49$ (Glass effect size technique)	Good evidence but needs to be conducted by a person trained in relaxation techniques.
Meditation	Krisanaprakornkit et al. 2008 Cochrane review[99] 2 RCTs	Insufficient controlled studies to make any firm conclusion	More studies are required to assess different types of meditation.
Massage	Moyer et al. 2004[94] 37 RCTs	A moderate effect size; state anxiety $g = 0.37$ Moderate-strong effect size for trait anxiety $g = 0.75$	Practitioner training level varied markedly, as well as the length of the treatment, body parts massaged, and environment and gender factors.

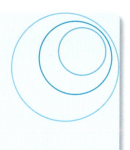

KEY POINTS

- 'Stress' in patients should be further screened for anxiety disorders.
- Chronic worry needs to not be dismissed as a personality trait—it could be GAD.
- The first responsibility is to provide to reduce acute suffering, especially in panic disorder.
- Check for co-occurring substance/alcohol abuse or dependence, depression and insomnia.

Further reading

Jorm AF , et al Rodgers B, Blewitt KA. Effectiveness of complementary and self-help treatments for anxiety disorders. Med J Aust 2004;181(7 Suppl):S29–S46.

Nutt DJ, et al. Generalized anxiety disorder: comorbidity, comparative biology and treatment. Int J Neuropsychopharmacol 2002;5(4):315–325.

Sarris J, et al. The Kava Anxiety Depression Spectrum Study (KADSS): a randomized placebo-controlled crossover study using an aqueous extract of *Piper methysticum*. Psychopharmacology (Berl) 2009;205(3): 399–407.

Tyrer P, Baldwin D. Generalised anxiety disorder. Lancet 2006;368(9553):2156–2166.

References

1. American Psychiatric Association. Diagnostic and statistical manual of mental disorders. 4th edn. Arlington: American Psychiatric Association, 2000.
2. Shearer SL. Recent advances in the understanding and treatment of anxiety disorders. Prim Care 2007;34(3): 475–504,v–vi.
3. Antai-Otong D. Current treatment of generalized anxiety disorder. J Psychosoc Nurs Ment Health Serv 2003;41(12):20–29.
4. Wittchen HU. Generalized anxiety disorder: prevalence, burden, and cost to society. Depress Anxiety 2002;16(4):162–171.
5. Hunt C, et al. DSM-IV generalized anxiety disorder in the Australian National Survey of Mental Health and Well-Being. Psychol Med 2002;32(4): 649–659.
6. Kessler RC, et al. The epidemiology of major depressive disorder: results from the National Comorbidity Survey Replication (NCS-R). JAMA 2003;289(23):3095–3105.
7. Hunt C, et al. Generalized anxiety disorder and major depressive disorder comorbidity in the National Survey of Mental Health and Well-Being. Depress Anxiety 2004;20(1):23–31.
8. Sartorius N, et al. Depression comorbid with anxiety: results from the WHO study on psychological disorders in primary health care. Br J Psychiatry Suppl 1996;(30): 38–43.
9. Gorwood P. Generalized anxiety disorder and major depressive disorder comorbidity: an example of genetic pleiotropy? Eur Psychiatry 2004;19(1):27–33.
10. Zhu B, et al. The cost of comorbid depression and pain for individuals diagnosed with generalized anxiety disorder. Nerv Ment Dis 2009;197(2):136–139.
11. Tyrer P, Baldwin D. Generalised anxiety disorder. Lancet 2006;368(9553):2156–2166.
12. Hettema JM, et al. A review and meta-analysis of the genetic epidemiology of anxiety disorders. Am J Psychiatry 2001;158(10):1568–1578.
13. Baldwin DS, Polkinghorn C. Evidence-based pharmacotherapy of generalized anxiety disorder. Int J Neuropsychopharmacol 2005;8(2):293–302.
14. Bremner J. Brain imaging in anxiety disorders. Future Drugs 2004;4(2):275–284.
15. Nutt DJ, et al. Generalized anxiety disorder: comorbidity, comparative biology and treatment. Int J Neuropsychopharmacol 2002;5(4):315–325.
16. Dunner DL. Management of anxiety disorders: the added challenge of comorbidity. Depress Anxiety 2001;13(2):57–71.
17. Kessler RC. The epidemiology of pure and comorbid generalized anxiety disorder: a review and evaluation of recent research. Acta Psychiatr Scand Suppl 2000;(406):7–13.
18. Rickels K, Rynn M. Pharmacotherapy of generalized anxiety disorder. J Clin Psychiatry 2002;63(Suppl 14):9–16.
19. Chouinard G. Issues in the clinical use of benzodiazepines: potency, withdrawal, and rebound. J Clin Psychiatry 2004;65(Suppl 5):7–12.
20. Bandelow B, et al. Meta-analysis of randomized controlled comparisons of psychopharmacological and psychological treatments for anxiety disorders. World J Biol Psychiatry 2007;8(3):175–187.
21. Kessler RC, et al. Co-morbid major depression and generalized anxiety disorders in the National Comorbidity Survey follow-up. Psychol Med 2008;38(3): 365–374.
22. Martin JL, et al. Benzodiazepines in generalized anxiety disorder: heterogeneity of outcomes based on a systematic review and meta-analysis of clinical trials. J Psychopharmacol 2007;21(7):774–782.
23. Nutt D, et al. Generalized anxiety disorder: a comorbid disease. Eur Neuropsychopharmacol 2006;16(Suppl 2):S109–S118.
24. Mellman TA. Sleep and anxiety disorders. Psychiatr Clin North Am 2006;29(4):1047–1058;abstract x.
25. Millan M. The neurobiology and control of anxious states. Prog Neuropsychobiol 2003;70:83–244.
26. Benke D, et al. GABA(A) receptors as in vivo substrate for the anxiolytic action of valerenic acid, a major constituent of valerian root extracts. Neuropharmacology 2009;56(1):174–181.
27. Davies LP, et al. Kava pyrones and resin: studies on GABAA, GABAB and benzodiazepine binding sites in rodent brain. Pharmacol Toxicol 1992;71(2):120–126.
28. Yuan CS, et al. Kavalactones and dihydrokavain modulate GABAergic activity in a rat gastric-brainstem preparation. Planta Med 2002;68(12):1092–1096.

29. Magura EI, et al. Kava extract ingredients, (+)-methysticin and (+/–)-kavain inhibit voltage-operated Na(+)-channels in rat CA1 hippocampal neurons. Neuroscience 1997;81(2):345–351.

30. Singh YN, Singh NN. Therapeutic potential of kava in the treatment of anxiety disorders. CNS Drugs 2002;16(11):731–743.

31. Martin HB, et al. Kavain attenuates vascular contractility through inhibition of calcium channels. Planta Med 2002;68(9):784–789.

32. Pittler MH, Ernst E. Kava extract for treating anxiety. Cochrane Database Syst Rev 2006;(1):CD003383.

33. Hamilton M. The assessment of anxiety states by rating. Br J Med Psychol 1959;32(1):50–55.

34. Witte S, et al. Meta-analysis of the efficacy of the acetonic kava-kava extract WS1490 in patients with non-psychotic anxiety disorders. Phytother Res 2005;19(3):183–188.

35. Coulter D. Assessment of the risk of hepatotoxicity with kava products. Geneva: WHO appointed committee, World Health Organization, 2007.

36. Sarris J, et al. The Kava Anxiety Depression Spectrum Study (KADSS): a randomized, placebo-controlled, cross-over trial using an aqueous extract of *Piper methysticum*. Psychopharmacology (Berl) 2009; 205(3):399–407.

37. Felter HW, Lloyd JU. King's American dispensatory. Online. Available: http://www.henrietteherbal.com/eclectic/kings/extracta

38. Miyasaka LS, et al. Passiflora for anxiety disorder. Cochrane Database Syst Rev 2007;(1):CD004518.

39. Akhondzadeh S, et al. Passionflower in the treatment of generalized anxiety: a pilot double-blind randomized controlled trial with oxazepam. J Clin Pharm Ther 2001;26(5):363–367.

40. Wolfson P, Hoffmann DL. An investigation into the efficacy of *Scutellaria lateriflora* in healthy volunteers. Altern Ther Health Med 2003;9(2):74–78.

41. Movafegh A, et al. Preoperative oral Passiflora incarnata reduces anxiety in ambulatory surgery patients: a double-blind, placebo controlled study. Anesth Analg 2008;106(6):1728–1732.

42. Bone K. A clinical guide to blending liquid herbs: herbal formulations for the individual patient. St Louis: Churchill Livingstone, 2003.

43. Kennedy DO, et al. Attenuation of laboratory-induced stress in humans after acute administration of *Melissa officinalis* (lemon balm). Psychosom Med 2004;66(4):607–613.

44. Kennedy DO, et al. Anxiolytic effects of a combination of *Melissa officinalis* and *Valeriana officinalis* during laboratory induced stress. Phytother Res 2006;20(2):96–102.

45. Awad R, et al. Phytochemical and biological analysis of skullcap (*Scutellaria lateriflora* L.): a medicinal plant with anxiolytic properties. Phytomedicine 2003;10(8):640–649.

46. Scripnikov A, et al. Effects of *Ginkgo biloba* extract EGb 761 on neuropsychiatric symptoms of dementia: findings from a randomised controlled trial. Wien Med Wochenschr 2007;157(13–14):295–300.

47. Woelk H, et al. *Ginkgo biloba* special extract EGb 761((R)) in generalized anxiety disorder and adjustment disorder with anxious mood: a randomized, double-blind, placebo-controlled trial. J Psychiatr Res 2007;41(6):472–480.

48. Rolland A, et al. Neurophysiological effects of an extract of *Eschscholzia californica* Cham. (Papaveraceae). Phytother Res 2001;15(5):377–381.

49. Zhang M, et al. Inhibitory effect of jujuboside A on glutamate-mediated excitatory signal pathway in hippocampus. Planta Med 2003;69(8):692–695.

50. Hsieh MT, et al. Suanzaorentang, an anxiolytic Chinese medicine, affects the central adrenergic and serotonergic systems in rats. Proc Natl Sci Counc Repub China B 1986;10(4):263–268.

51. Hsieh MT, et al. Effects of Suanzaorentang on behavior changes and central monoamines. Proc Natl Sci Counc Repub China B 1986;10(1):43–48.

52. Osiecki H. The physician's handbook of clinical nutrition. 5th edn Brisbane: Bioconcepts publishing, 1998.

53. Eby GA, et al. Rapid recovery from major depression using magnesium treatment. Med Hypotheses 2006;67(2):362–370.

54. Spasov AA, et al. [Depression-like and anxiety-related behaviour of rats fed with magnesium-deficient diet]. Zh Vyssh Nerv Deiat Im I P Pavlova 2008,58(4).476–485.

55. Poleszak E, et al. NMDA/glutamate mechanism of magnesium-induced anxiolytic-like behavior in mice. Pharmacol Rep 2008;60(5):655–663.

56. Poleszak E. Benzodiazepine/GABA(A) receptors are involved in magnesium-induced anxiolytic-like behavior in mice. Pharmacol Rep 2008;60(4):483–489.

57. De Souza MC, et al. A synergistic effect of a daily supplement for 1 month of 200 mg magnesium plus 50 mg vitamin B6 for the relief of anxiety-related premenstrual symptoms: a randomized, double-blind, crossover study. J Womens Health Gend Based Med 2000;9(2):131–139.

58. Arborelius L, et al. The role of corticotropin-releasing factor in depression and anxiety disorders. J Endocrinol 1999;160(1):1–12.

59. Rege NN, et al. Adaptogenic properties of six rasayana herbs used in Ayurvedic medicine. Phytother Res 1999;13(4):275–291.

60. Bhattacharya SK, et al. Adaptogenic activity of Withania somnifera: an experimental study using a rat model of chronic stress. Pharmacol Biochem Behav 2003;75(3):547–555.

61. Bhattacharya SK, et al. Anxiolytic-antidepressant activity of Withania somnifera glycowithanolides: an experimental study. Phytomedicine 2000;7(6):463–469.

62. Bystritsky A, et al. A pilot study of Rhodiola rosea (Rhodax) for generalized anxiety disorder (GAD). J Altern Complement Med 2008;14(2):175–180.

63. Mills S, et al. Principles and practice of phytotherapy. London: Churchill Livingstone, 2000.

64. Rigelsky JM, et al. Hawthorn: pharmacology and therapeutic uses. Am J Health Syst Pharm 2002;59(5):417–422.

65. Pittler MH, et al. Hawthorn extract for treating chronic heart failure: meta-analysis of randomized trials. Am J Med 2003;114(8):665–674:1.

66. Peck MD, Ai AL. Cardiac conditions. J Gerontol Soc Work 2008;50(Suppl 1):13–44.

67. Culpeper N. Culpeper's complete herbal. Hertfordshire: Wordsworth Editions Ltd, 1652.

68. Maciocia G. The foundations of Chinese medicine. Singapore: Churchill Livingstone, 1989.

69. Walker AF, et al. Promising hypotensive effect of hawthorn extract: a randomized double-blind pilot study of mild, essential hypertension. Phytother Res 2002;16(1):48–54.

70. Hanus M, et al. Double-blind, randomised, placebo-controlled study to evaluate the efficacy and safety of a fixed combination containing two plant extracts (Crataegus oxyacantha and Eschscholtzia californica) and magnesium in mild-to-moderate anxiety disorders. Curr Med Res Opin 2004;20(1):63–71.

71. Conrad A, et al. Muscle relaxation therapy for anxiety disorders: it works but how? Journal of Anxiety Disorders 2007;21:243–264.

72. Jorm AF, et al. Effectiveness of complementary and self-help treatments for anxiety disorders. Med J Aust 4 2004;181(7 Suppl):S29–S46.

73. Hunot V, et al. Psychological therapies for generalised anxiety disorder. Cochrane Database Syst Rev 2007;24(1):CD001848.

74. Pilkington K, et al. Acupuncture for anxiety and anxiety disorders—a systematic literature review. Acupunct Med 2007;25(1–2):1–10.

75. Karst M, et al. Auricular acupuncture for dental anxiety: a randomized controlled trial. Anesth Analg 2007;104(2):295–300.

76. Spielberger C, et al. STAI manual for the State-Trait Anxiety Inventory. Palo Alto: Consulting Psychologists Press, 1970.

77. Samuels N, et al. Acupuncture for psychiatric illness: a literature review. Behav Med 2008;34(2):55–64.

78. Cabyoglu MT, et al. The mechanism of acupuncture and clinical applications. Int J Neurosci 2006;116(2):115–125.

79. Kessler RC, et al. Prevalence, severity, and comorbidity of 12-month DSM-IV disorders in the National Comorbidity Survey Replication. Arch Gen Psychiatry 2005;62(6):617–627.

80. Biederman J, et al. Comorbidity of attention deficit hyperactivity disorder with conduct, depressive, anxiety, and other disorders. American Journal of Psychiatry 1991;148(5):564–577.

81. Hasin D, et al. Substance use disorders: Diagnostic and Statistical Manual of Mental Disorders, fourth edition (DSM-IV) and International Classification of Diseases, tenth edition (ICD-10). Addiction 2006;101(Suppl 1):59–75.

82. Cargiulo T. Understanding the health impact of alcohol dependence. Am J Health Syst Pharm 2007;64(5 Suppl 3):S5:11.

83. Hasin DS, et al. Prevalence, correlates, disability, and comorbidity of DSM-IV alcohol abuse and dependence in the United States: results from the National Epidemiologic Survey on Alcohol and Related Conditions. Arch Gen Psychiatry 2007;64(7):830–842.

84. Uzbay TI. Hypericum perforatum and substance dependence: a review. Phytother Res 2008;22(5):578–582.

85. Dean AJ. Natural and complementary therapies for substance use disorders. Curr Opin Psychiatry 2005;18(3):271–276.

86. Feltenstein MW, et al. The neurocircuitry of addiction: an overview. Br J Pharmacol 2008;154(2):261–274.

87. Coskun I, et al. Attenuation of ethanol withdrawal syndrome by extract of Hypericum perforatum in Wistar rats. Fundam Clin Pharmacol 2006;20(5):481–488.

88. De Vry J, et al. Comparison of hypericum extracts with imipramine and fluoxetine in animal models of depression and alcoholism. Eur Neuropsychopharmacol 1999;9(6):461–468.

89. Smith A. Effects of caffeine on human behavior. Food Chem Toxicol 2002;40(9):1243–1255.

90. Nehlig A, et al. Caffeine and the central nervous system: mechanisms of action, biochemical, metabolic and psychostimulant effects. Brain Res Brain Res Rev 1992;17(2):139–170.

91. Wipfli BM, et al. The anxiolytic effects of exercise: a meta-analysis of randomized trials and dose-response analysis. J Sport Exerc Psychol 2008;30(4):392–410.

92. Bender TS, et al. The effect of physical therapy on beta-endorphin levels. European Journal Of Applied Physiology 2007;100(4):371–382.

93. Kuriyama H, et al. Immunological and psychological benefits of aromatherapy massage. Evid Based Complement Alternat Med 2005;2(2):179–184.

94. Moyer C, et al. A meta-analysis of massage therapy research. Psychol Bull 2004;130(1):3–18.

95. Perry N, et al. Aromatherapy in the management of psychiatric disorders. CNS Drugs 2006;20(4):257–280.

96. Bradley BF, et al. Anxiolytic effects of Lavandula angustifolia odour on the Mongolian gerbil elevated plus maze. J Ethnopharmacol 2007;111(3):517–525:22.

97. Graham PH, et al. Inhalation aromatherapy during radiotherapy: results of a placebo-controlled double-blind randomized trial. J Clin Oncol 2003;21(12):2372–2376.

98. Muzzarelli L, et al. Aromatherapy and reducing preprocedural anxiety: a controlled prospective study. Gastroenterol Nurs 2006;29(6):466–471.

99. Krisanaprakornkit T, et al. Meditation therapy for anxiety disorders. Cochrane Database Syst Rev 2006;(1):CD004998.

100. Goodman W. The Yale-Brown Obsessive Compulsive Scale. Arch Gen Psychiatry 1989;46:1006–1011.

101. Anke J, et al. Pharmacokinetic and pharmacodynamic drug interactions with Kava (Piper methysticum Forst. f.). J Ethnopharmacol 2004;93(2–3):153–160.

102. Clouatre DL. Kava kava: examining new reports of toxicity. Toxicol Lett 2004;150(1):85–96.

103. Sarris J, et al. wort: current evidence for use in mood and anxiety disorders. J Altern Complement Med 2009;15(8):827–836.

104. Long B, et al. Effects of exercise training on anxiety: a meta-analysis. Journal of Applied Sport Psychology 1995;7:167–189.

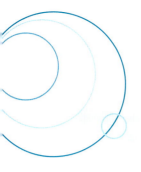

14
Insomnia

Jerome Sarris
ND, MHSc, PhD

AETIOLOGY, CLASSIFICATION AND EPIDEMIOLOGY

Periods of sleep disturbance due to acute stress or environmental change are common human experiences. The diagnostic DSM-IV classification of chronic primary insomnia is differentiated from an acute occurrence of insomnia, requiring the disorder to be a major health complaint, presenting with over 1 month of persistent problems in initiating or maintaining sleep, or having non-restorative sleep.[1] Furthermore, for this diagnosis to be met the sleep disturbance must cause significant distress or impairment in social, occupational functioning, be exclusive of other disorders (such as other sleep or psychiatric disorders), and not due to medications, drugs, alcoholism or a general medical condition. Insomnia may be secondary (caused by) another medical condition, from medicines, recreational drugs or alcohol consumption, or be from environmental factors such as altitude, jet lag, poor bedding, excess light or noise. Because of this a thorough assessment is required to establish the particulars of the cause. It is estimated that 25% of chronic insomnia can be classified as 'primary', with approximately 75% due to the aforementioned causes.[2] Interestingly, people who experience 'transient' insomnia (< 1 month), usually from an environmental change, acute social stressors or the loss of a loved one, usually experience daytime sleepiness during this period; a person with chronic insomnia usually does not feel sleepy, and instead may feel 'hyperstimulated' even after 4–6 hours' sleep.[2]

Parameters measuring sleep outcomes involve evaluating total sleep time, sleep latency (how long it takes to get to sleep) and wake time after sleep onset.[3] Little regard in present research is given to next-day functioning or improved outcomes in comorbid psychiatric or medical disorders. These remain areas of significance in enhancing outcomes in sleep disorders.

The prevalence of general sleep disturbance experienced by people over a year is estimated at approximately 85%, while the estimate of diagnosed chronic insomnia is estimated at around 10%.[2] As in the case of other psychiatric disorders, women have a slightly higher incidence of primary insomnia.

The pathophysiology behind sleep disorders appears to involve:[4–7]
- hyperarousal of the neuroendocrine system caused by abnormalities in circadian rhythm (involving clock genes, melatonin secretion and adenosine receptors)
- GABA pathway dysregulation

- endocrine factors (HPA-axis/cortisol hyperactivation)
- excitory pathways involving glutamate and aspartate.

Prolonged poor 'sleep hygiene' may cause behavioural conditioning towards 'expecting' to have bad sleep.[8] This is reflected in the fact that population surveys indicate that of the 50% of people who have sleep difficulties, between 20% and 36% report the duration is greater than 1 year.[9] 'Sleep hygiene' is a term used to describe lifestyle interventions that assist with preparation for sleep. Aspects of good sleep hygiene focus on replacing stimulating activities with restful and quiescent activities (or non-activities) to establish a regulated circadian rhythm (this is discussed further below). Beyond the socioeconomic cost, the subjective effect of chronic sleep disturbance often involves the person experiencing a low mood or anxiety (this may not meet diagnostic threshold), fatigue or daytime somnolence, poor concentration or memory, tension headaches and digestive disturbances.[10]

RISK FACTORS AND ECONOMIC IMPACT

The elderly, female gender, shift workers, chronic-pain sufferers and people with co-occurring medical conditions or psychiatric disorders (especially depression and anxiety) are at greater risk of developing chronic insomnia (see the box below).[4] A sedentary life and reduced exposure to sunlight may also contribute to sleep disorders. Elderly populations frequently report that they perceive a poorer quality of sleep, commonly that they have interrupted sleep, wake early or feel inadequately rested.[11] Interestingly, studies show that, statistically, the elderly sleep similar hours to younger counterparts, and that the reduction of qualitative sleep experience is actually due to comorbid health issues or medications, not to do with 'being old'.[11] Chronic experience of pain increases the risk of insomnia, with a study revealing that 44% of people with chronic pain had co-existing insomnia.[11] Furthermore, the more severe the level of pain was, the greater the percentage who experienced insomnia.

With respect to major depressive disorder, a study[12] showed that patients with chronic insomnia had an increased risk of a major depressive disorder of 1.6 times higher than subjects with good sleep; if the insomnia was maintained for a year the risk was 40 times as high! Sleep disturbance is a frequent symptom of depression, and a strong causal link exists between insomnia and depression.[11] It is likely that this is bimodal; that is, insomnia can cause depression and vice versa. Furthermore, epidemiological data have shown that approximately 40% of chronic insomniacs suffer from another comorbid psychiatric disorder.[10,13] The cost that sleep disorders cause is immense, with an estimate of direct cost of insomnia in the United States of America approximating US$13.93 billion in 1999.[14] Interestingly, most of this cost was service-based (especially for nursing home costs) and only a fraction was from

CONDITIONS CAUSING CHRONIC SLEEP DISTURBANCE[15,16]

Medical conditions
Cancer, congestive heart failure, HIV/AIDS, stroke, benign prostatic hypertrophy, hyperthyroidism, renal disease, gastro-oesophageal reflux, psychiatric disorders
Other abnormal events
Restless leg syndrome, respiratory distress, headaches, panic attacks, pain

DRUGS THAT MAY CAUSE INSOMNIA[11,15]

Alcohol, stimulants (nicotine, caffeine, amphetamines), stimulating antidepressants, ADHD psychostimulants, corticosteroids, thyroxin, calcium channel blockers, bronchodilators, beta-blockers, decongestants, anticholinergic agents, oral contraceptive pills

prescriptive costs. While prescriptive drug use is prevalent in insomniacs for the treatment of the disorder, medications for other conditions may also cause insomnia (see the box above).[11,15]

It should be noted that while the previously mentioned risk factors may cause sleep disorders chronic sleep disturbances may also in turn cause a variety of physical and mental conditions.[9,17] The most concerning link with chronic insomnia is that evidence indicates that people with poor sleep or < 6 hours per night have a significantly greater risk of: [3]

- developing cardiovascular disorders (such as hypertension and hypercholesterolaemia)
- metabolic disorders (increase in weight and blood sugar level, insulin resistance, increased cortisol level and decreased human growth hormone)
- a higher incidence than healthy sleepers of experiencing more accidents, higher work absenteeism and lower productivity, and higher health-care costs.[10]

Sleep disorders and headaches

Sleep, or lack thereof, is regarded as being able to both provoke and relieve headache.[18] Epidemiological research has associated sleep disorders with more frequent and severe headaches. Clinical research correlates specific headache diagnoses with chronobiological sleep-pattern disturbance, implicating similar neurochemical processes between the two disorders.[19] Chronic daily morning headache patterns are particularly suggestive of sleep disorders, including sleep-related breathing disorders, insomnia, circadian rhythm disorders and parasomnias.[18]

CONVENTIONAL TREATMENT

Sage advice when treating transient insomnia should be to establish the underlying causes, initiate good sleep hygiene changes, commence (or refer) an appropriate psychological intervention and offer lifestyle and prescriptive advice.[15] The medical 'quick fix' is usually the use of pharmaceutical hypnotics as the primary first-line pharmacotherapy to treat chronic insomnia.[20] The use of benzodiazepines such as diazepam (or its metabolites) or non-benzodiazepine hypnotics such as zolpidem or zopiclone are preferred currently over older barbiturates which can cause death in cases of overdose.[20] Although benzodiazepines are relatively safe medications, concerns exist over dependency, and currently most guidelines endorse only short-term use.[21]

Sedating antidepressants, for example mirtazepine or fluvoxamine, may also be prescribed, especially in cases of comorbid depression.[20] In some cases the use of sedating antipsychotic or tricyclic medication may also be employed. Opiates also have soporific effects, and may be indicated in cases of chronic pain with insomnia. Melatonin (an endogenous hormone secreted by the pineal gland) is also prescribed in some countries, especially to treat sleep disturbance, especially if caused by jet lag.[22] A novel

SHIFT-WORK SLEEP DISORDER[23,24]

Shift workers are especially at risk of developing a sleep disorder. The experience of clinically significant excessive sleepiness or insomnia associated with work (during normal nocturnal sleep time) has important safety implications and socioeconomic, medical and quality-of-life consequences.

Treatment protocols may involve using stimulant therapy and bright light upon waking, and hypnotic agents upon retiring. To date no CAM interventions have been rigorously assessed in real-life situations to manage shift-work sleep disorders. The best treatment is to avoid shift work if possible!

melatoninergic agent called agomelatine, a melatonin 1,2 receptor agonist and serotonin $5HT_{2c}$ receptor agonist (at stage IV clinical trials), may in the future be used as a non-addictive hypnotic with anxiolytic properties.[25] Referral for psychological interventions such as cognitive modification or behavioural adjustments may also be recommended in primary care.[26]

KEY TREATMENT PROTOCOLS

Circadian rhythm modulation

The primary circadian 'clock' in humans is located in the suprachiasmatic nuclei in the hypothalmus; these cells govern the daily biological rhythm over a cycle lasting approximately 24 hours and 11 minutes.[5] The wake/sleep cycle is influenced externally by light and dark, with exposure to light increasing the secretion of serotonin, while darkness increases the secretion of melatonin. The circadian rhythm governs internal temperature changes, sleep and

NATUROPATHIC TREATMENT AIMS

- Assess the causes of the sleep disorder.
- Educate on good sleep hygiene practices.
- Regulate circadian rhythm, HPA function and GABAergic activity.
- Regulate and support the nervous system.
- Encourage beneficial lifestyle changes.
- Appropriately address external stressors, e.g. relationship or job factors.

eating patterns. Human clock genes have been identified as being involved with various sleep disorders.[5] Future gene therapy may target the expression of these clock genes to effectively reset the circadian rhythm. In the meantime, the use of interventions that modulate the circadian rhythm and the use of sleep hygiene techniques such as 'sleep restriction' and 'light therapy' may assist in readjusting the circadian rhythm.

Another neurological factor involved in sleep is the endogenous compound adenosine. This inhibitory compound and the adenosine receptor binding sites are a homeostatic sleep factor responsible for mediating the REM cycle (see Figures 14.1 and 14.2).[27] **Adenosine** can potently inhibit cholinergic neurons that are involved with cortical arousal, and during periods of prolonged wakefulness adenosine accumulates in certain parts of the brain and promotes the transition from a wake state to a sleep state.[7] This is considered to be one of the factors involved in the theory of 'sleep debt', in which sleep deprivation over days accrues a chronological sleep debt (a build-up of adenosine), which then prompts a period of increased sleep to make up for loss. Caffeine antagonises adenosine receptors, thereby increasing wakefulness (see the lifestyle advice section below).[28] The compound adenosine would appear to be a potential hypnotic substance;

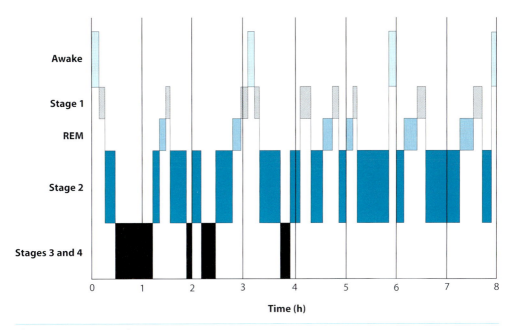

Figure 14.1 REM cycle

as discussed above, endogenous adenosine is responsible for modulating the wake-sleep cycle via binding to adenosine (A1) and (A2) receptors. A literature search reviewing clinical evidence of this product revealed no clinical evidence, however, this remains an area of potential exploration.

Humulus lupulus is used in Europe extensively in sleep formulations to promote sleep. The bitter herb is regarded by the eclectics as a useful remedy for imparting sedative and hypnotic actions.[29] While animal and in vitro models do not currently support sedative or anxiolytic activity, hypnotic effects involving melatoninergic and GABAergic modulation have been documented.[30] *Humulus lupulus* combines well with *Valeriana* spp. root, demonstrated by a fixed valerian–hop combination (Ze 91019) found to reduce sleep latency and waking time compared to placebo in 30 subjects after 2 weeks of treatment.[31] Another randomised controlled trial (RCT) comparing the combination to placebo and diphenhydramine revealed less conclusive results.[32] The 4-week study involving 184 adults with mild insomnia showed none or only minor improvements of subjective sleep parameters compared to placebo, with most outcomes being similar between all three groups. It is possible that the inclusion of 'mild' insomniacs diluted the response from the herbal combination. In vitro studies indicate that hops–valerian preparations invoke hypnotic activity via agonising adenosine, melatonin and serotonin receptors.[33–35]

Valeriana officinalis has a rich folkloric tradition of use in conditions of restlessness, hysteria, nervous headache and mental depression,[29,36] with Pliny regarding the powder of the root as effective in cases of spasms causing pain.[37] Energetically *Valeriana* spp. root was regarded by Dioscorides as possessing warming properties;[37] this is reflected in the pungent aroma of the essential oils (valerenal, iso/valerianic acid) and terpenes (valerenic acid).[38] The use of *Valeriana* spp. in prescriptions needs to be monitored due to this 'heating' effect, which can evoke stimulation and restlessness (the eclectics classified valerian as a 'cerebral stimulant').[29,39] A systematic review and meta-analysis included 16 eligible RCTs involved a total of 1093 patients.[38] The results revealed that on six studies with a dichotomous outcome of sleep quality ('improved' or

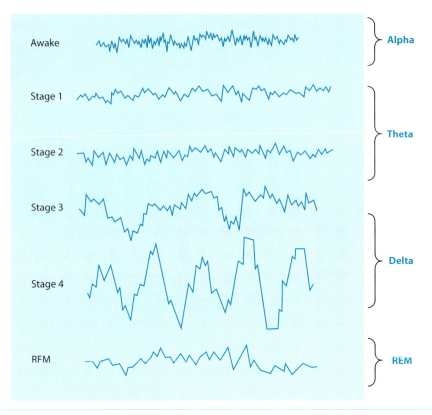

Figure 14.2 Brain waves

'not improved') a statistically significant benefit occurred. Nine out of 16 studies did not, however, have positive outcomes in regard to improvement of sleep quality. It should be noted that many studies included in the review involved combinations of valerian with other herbal medicines (for example *Piper methysticum* or *H. lupulus*), differing outcome scales, dosages and participant populations, and eight trials had small sample sizes. Because of this, currently the evidence does not firmly support the use of valerian as a stand-alone hypnotic.

A 2001 clinical trial demonstrated that *V. edulis* improved sleep architecture over *V. officinalis* by diminishing waking episodes and improving delta sleep.[40] This is an important difference with respect to addressing 'maintenance insomnia'. *Valeriana* spp. have demonstrated some clinical evidence in enhancing sleep parameters when used for periods of >2 weeks, and acute administration appears to have only minor effect.[31,41,42] The mechanism of action regarding *Valeriana* spp. hypnotic effect is posited as involving an increase in REM stage and delta sleep,[40,41] mediated by GABA-A receptor (β3 subunit) agonism,[43] and adenosine 1, benzodiazepine and serotonin 5-HT (1A) receptor agonism.[33,35,44] Commission E and the World Health Organization support the use of valerian for restlessness and sleep disorders,[45] but more robust clinical trials are required to provide firm endorsement.

Vitex agnus-castus, although used commonly for hormonal and menstrual irregularities,[46] may exert a novel melatoninergic activity. While to date no human clinical trials exist testing *V. agnus-castus* in insomnia, a study of 20 healthy human males demonstrated a significant dose-dependent increase of melatonin secretion using 120 mg, 240 mg, 480 mg of the extract per day compared to placebo for 14 days.[47]

Hypothalamus-pituitary-adrenal axis (HPA) hyperarousal

Chronic primary insomnia has been characterised by a state of biopsychological arousal, which is counter to a lowering of body temperature, blood pressure and cortisol (see Figure 14.3).[4] Elevations of circulating catecholamines, adrenocorticotropic hormone and cortisol production, raised metabolic rate and core body temperature and overactive beta EEG frequency have been documented in this hyperstimulated state responsible for chronic insomnia.[4] Interestingly, this mirrors various presentations of melancholic depression (anxiety, psychosocial unresponsiveness and early morning waking), and the common link (an overactive HPA axis) could explain the link between depression and insomnia (see the depression chapter, and Section 5 on the endocrine system).[13,48] Herbal medicines that regulate HPA-axis activity and exercise may have role in treating insomnia. **Withania somnifera** is regarded as an anxiolytic, adaptogen and nervine trophorestorative, used to assist in reducing mental tension and revitalise body/mind.[49] *W. somnifera* is classed as a 'rasayana' in Ayurvedic medicine, and is used to promote physical and mental health.[50] Animal studies have confirmed its efficacy in the treatment of chronic stress and anxiety,[50,51] with the glycowithanolides regarded as the active constituents, exerting a GABA-mimetic activity.[49,50] To date no RCTs exist examining the herb for use in insomnia, so caution should be adopted when extrapolating from the minor in vitro and in vivo evidence. **Other herbal medicines** that may exert a HPA-axis modulating effect include *Rhodiola rosea*, *Panax ginseng* (its use in the evening due to its stimulatory properties should be limited) and *Eleutherococcus senticosus*.[39,52]

Exercise and physical activity are advised to assist in balancing the function of the HPA axis. Regular graded physical exercise may promote relaxation and raise core body temperature, this activity potentially benefiting the sleep pattern.[53] Exercise also addresses weight gain and obesity, which are factors that increase the occurrence of sleep disorders. A Cochrane review found that, in one trial involving a sample of 43 elderly participants with insomnia, exercise improved sleep onset latency, total sleep and quality of sleep.[54]

The GABAergic system

As discussed previously in the anxiety case, GABA has a role in the inhibitory effect on neurological activity by attenuating hyperarousal in both mood and sleep disturbance. GABA-α receptors play a crucial role in the initiation and maintenance of non-REM sleep (deep sleep).[6] Furthermore, in cases of comorbid anxiety, interventions that modulate GABA activity may have a role in reducing anxiety, which in turn may ameliorate insomnia. The use of **GABA modulating phytotherapies** such as *Scutellaria lateriflora*, *Passiflora incarnata* and *Piper methysticum* may be of benefit in treating insomnia. *S. lateriflora* was regarded by eclectic physicians and physiomedicalists as a 'truly valuable medicine' used to treat nervous excitability, restlessness or wakefulness (see the anxiety chapter for evidence).[29,36] *P. incarnata* has a history of use by. Europeans and Native Americans for its hypnotic and anxiolytic action (see the anxiety chapter for evidence).[29] It should be noted that while both *S. lateriflora* and *P. incarnata* have documented anxiolytic activity, it does not necessarily confer a hypnotic effect. The use of the herbs may play an adjuvant synergistic role with hypnotic interventions, especially if comorbid anxiety is apparent.

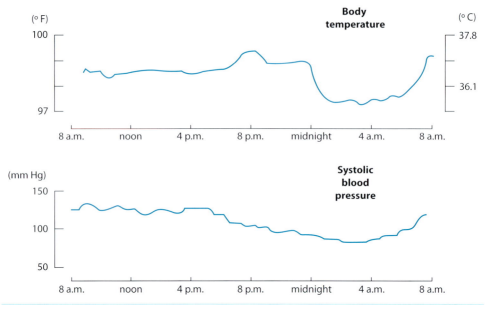

Figure 14.3 Body temperature and systolic blood pressure cycle

P. methysticum is a well documented GABA-modulator that has solid evidence as an effective anxiolytic. It may be of benefit in anxious insomnia, and to date one specific study has examined the plant in this presentation. A 4-week RCT using 200 mg of a standardised extract of kava in 61 patients explored the effect on anxious participants with comorbid insomnia.[55] Via a sleep questionnaire, the results revealed that, compared to placebo, the extract improved the quality of sleep and the recuperative effect after sleep. A 5-week RCT has also been conducted to explore the use of *P. methysticum* on benzodiazepine withdrawal. A standardised WS® 1490 *P. methysticum* extract was used on 40 subjects with chronic anxiety and a long history of benzodiazepine use.[56] Subjects were tapered off their benzodiazepines over the first 2 weeks, while the kava was titrated from 50 mg up to 300 mg by the end of week 1. *P. methysticum* produced a statistically significant reduction in anxiety on the Hamilton anxiety scale[57] (a 7.5 point decrease over placebo at week 5), and the Benfindlichkeits-Skala subjective wellbeing scale.[58] Importantly, aside from some subjects experiencing withdrawal symptoms, no negative reactions (such as increased sedation) occurred during the first week of adjuvant *P. methysticum* use. Furthermore, five subjects in the *P. methysticum* group displayed adverse symptoms from benzodiazepine withdrawal compared with 10 in the placebo group. During a follow-up study, nine out of 14 subjects who were switched from *P. methysticum* to placebo experienced recurrence of anxiety. A qualitative study conducted by Sarris et al. (2009: in submission) exploring the experiences of people taking kava in a clinical trial revealed that in addition to the plant improving participants' mood and anxiety levels, some participants detailed beneficial effects on sleep markers.

INTEGRATIVE MEDICAL CONSIDERATIONS

Various integrative options exist for treating insomnia. Referral for appropriate psychological interventions and for an exercise program or relaxation techniques (and possibly acupuncture) may be of assistance. Sleep clinics are usually available in large cities. These

SLEEP APNOEA AND SNORING[59]

- Sleep apnoea is caused by abnormalities in the anatomy and physiology of the pharynx and upper airway muscle dilator, and in the stability of ventilatory control, which cause pharyngeal collapse during sleep. Obstructive sleep apnoea can be diagnosed from a history of snoring and daytime sleepiness, and via a physical examination and overnight polysomnography. People with sleep apnoea are rarely aware of having difficulty breathing, even upon awakening.
- Snoring is a common presentation of obstructive sleep apnoea, and is the result of vibration of respiratory structures (the uvula and soft palate) causing a sound due to obstructed air movement. Aside from structural issues, the causes of snoring may also involve obesity, smoking and use of alcohol and CNS-depressant medications.
- Treatment usually involves lifestyle changes such as avoiding alcohol or muscle relaxants, losing weight and quitting smoking. Sleeping at a 30-degree elevation of the upper body may also be of benefit. 'Breathing machines' (delivering continuous positive airway pressure) can be used in severe cases that are unresponsive to lifestyle interventions. Surgical procedures may also assist. To date no CAM products have strong evidentiary support in treating apnoea or snoring.
- A novel study assessed the use of didgeridoo playing on daytime sleepiness and other outcomes in 25 patients with moderate obstructive sleep apnoea syndrome and snoring.[60] Participants undertook didgeridoo lessons and daily practice at home with standardised instruments for 4 months. In the didgeridoo group, daytime sleepiness improved significantly and partners reported less sleep disturbance compared with the control group.

clinics may perform EEG tests observing the person's sleep latency and arousal level during sleep, and other nocturnal factors such as sleep apnoea. Sleep hygiene techniques may also be taught at these clinics.

Psychological intervention

A review of the psychological and behavioural treatments of insomnia by Morin et al.[26] of 37 controlled studies involving 2246 subjects concluded that these techniques produced reliable changes in several sleep parameters, and that these improvements were well-sustained over time. Five main evidence-based psychological and behavioural treatments exist in the management of insomnia:

1. *Stimulus control therapy* involves the patient going to bed only when sleepy, getting out of bed when not sleepy, using the bed only for sleeping and arising from bed at the same time every day
2. *Sleep restriction therapy* involves the patient curtailing the time in bed to the average time the person sleeps; for example, if they sleep only 6 out of 8 hours in bed, then they should reduce the time in bed to 6 hours and work up to 8 hours
3. *Relaxation training* involves the patient using techniques to reduce somatic and psychological stress via muscular relaxation, imagery or meditation
4. *Sleep hygiene education* involves instruction on health practices to enhance sleep, for example exercise, diet, substance use and environmental factors (light, noise, temperature, bed quality, removal of bedside clocks)

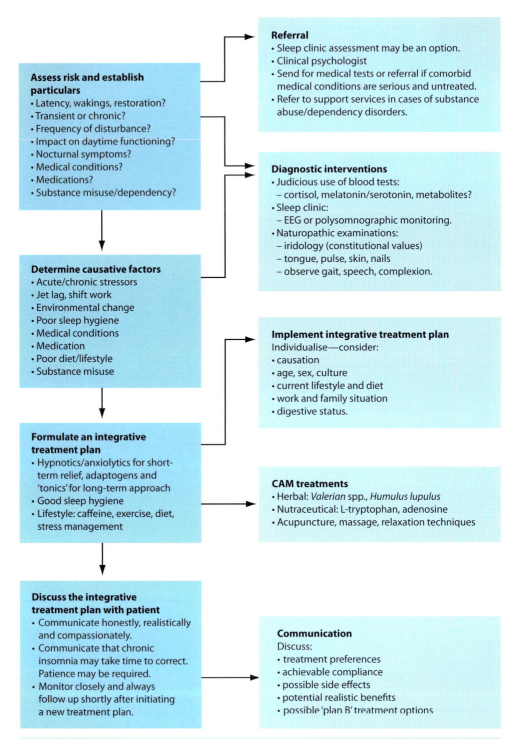

Assess risk and establish particulars
- Latency, wakings, restoration?
- Transient or chronic?
- Frequency of disturbance?
- Impact on daytime functioning?
- Nocturnal symptoms?
- Medical conditions?
- Medications?
- Substance misuse/dependency?

Referral
- Sleep clinic assessment may be an option.
- Clinical psychologist
- Send for medical tests or referral if comorbid medical conditions are serious and untreated.
- Refer to support services in cases of substance abuse/dependency disorders.

Diagnostic interventions
- Judicious use of blood tests:
  - cortisol, melatonin/serotonin, metabolites?
- Sleep clinic:
  - EEG or polysomnographic monitoring.
- Naturopathic examinations:
  - iridology (constitutional values)
  - tongue, pulse, skin, nails
  - observe gait, speech, complexion.

Determine causative factors
- Acute/chronic stressors
- Jet lag, shift work
- Environmental change
- Poor sleep hygiene
- Medical conditions
- Medication
- Poor diet/lifestyle
- Substance misuse

Implement integrative treatment plan
Individualise—consider:
- causation
- age, sex, culture
- current lifestyle and diet
- work and family situation
- digestive status.

Formulate an integrative treatment plan
- Hypnotics/anxiolytics for short-term relief, adaptogens and 'tonics' for long-term approach
- Good sleep hygiene
- Lifestyle: caffeine, exercise, diet, stress management

CAM treatments
- Herbal: *Valerian* spp., *Humulus lupulus*
- Nutraceutical: L-tryptophan, adenosine
- Acupuncture, massage, relaxation techniques

Discuss the integrative treatment plan with patient
- Communicate honestly, realistically and compassionately.
- Communicate that chronic insomnia may take time to correct. Patience may be required.
- Monitor closely and always follow up shortly after initiating a new treatment plan.

Communication
Discuss:
- treatment preferences
- achievable compliance
- possible side effects
- potential realistic benefits
- possible 'plan B' treatment options

Figure 14.4 Naturopathic treatment decision tree—insomnia

5. *Cognitive therapy* involves the patient challenging and changing their erroneous beliefs about sleep. Cognitive therapy may assist some sleep sufferers that form erroneous beliefs about their sleep pattern. They may catastrophise by thinking thoughts such as 'I can never get to sleep', or 'I need a sleeping pill to sleep'. They may also present with a trait of being a chronic worrier, and may be kept up by an overactive internal dialogue (if so, the naturopath needs to screen for generalised anxiety disorder). While evidence supports these interventions, more studies are required to evaluate the effect on morbidity outcomes such as daytime fatigue and cognitive functioning.

Acupuncture

A Cochrane review and meta-analysis of acupuncture and acupressure in the treatment of insomnia has been conducted.[61] Seven trials met sufficient methodological rigour for inclusion and included 590 participants. Conventional needle acupuncture, acupressure, auricular magnetic and seed therapy, and transcutaneous electrical acupoint stimulation were evaluated. Results revealed that acupuncture and acupressure may help to improve sleep quality scores when compared to control or compared to no treatment. The authors note that the efficacy of acupuncture or its variants was inconsistent between studies for many sleep parameters, such as sleep onset latency, total sleep duration and wake after sleep onset. The combined result from three RCTs evaluating subjective insomnia improvement, however, revealed that acupuncture or its variants was no more effective than control. Although promising, the small numbers of heterogenous and methodologically poor RCTs do not strongly support the use of any form of acupuncture for the treatment of insomnia.

Case Study

A 62-year-old male reports that his **sleeping pattern is poor**. He has a **long sleep latency** (1 hour to get to sleep) and **wakes during the night**. He has a stressful job and present relationship difficulties. Due to getting only between 5 and 6 hours sleep per night he is drinking coffee throughout the day to stay awake. Complicating matters, he also complains that he suffers from **regular migraine headaches**, which he says affects his sleep (see Figure 14.5).

SUGGESTIVE SYMPTOMS

- *Latency*: Difficulty falling asleep
- *Maintenance*: Broken sleep, or early morning waking, or reduced overall hours of sleep
- *Non-restorative sleep*: A feeling that sleep is unrefreshing or light; daytime consequences such as fatigue present as a result

Example treatment
Herbal and nutritional prescription

As part of an integrative approach, the use of hypnotic, anxiolytic and adaptogenic actions in the formula should aid in the restoration of sleep. *Withania somnifera* is prescribed as a sedative and adaptogen; *Valeriana officinalis*, *Humulus lupulus* and *Vitex agnus-castus* are prescribed to exert a hypnotic activity.[30,38,39] The use of two doses in the evening is important. The initial dose will exert a hypnotic and anxiolytic effect that will prepare the body/mind for sleep. The next dose 1 hour before sleep will boost serum levels of the constituents, and in combination with good sleep hygiene techniques should facilitate sleep. Although currently only possessing theoretical evidentiary support, the use of adenosine phosphate tablets may aid in the modulation of the circadian rhythm.[27] The use of L-tryptophan or melatonin may also be options (see 'Additional therapeutic options' below).

To address his migraines, as detailed in Figure 14.5, the implementation of a diet reducing the consumption of common food triggers (such as dietary amines, MSG and nitrates) may be of benefit. Magnesium may be beneficial in reducing the frequency of the attacks.[62] *Tanacetum parthenium* has a history of traditional use for the treatment of migraine. While this may be a potential therapeutic option for the patient, two RCTs have revealed no efficacy in treating migraine headaches beyond placebo.[63]

Current evidence for CAM interventions for migraine is mixed. More research is required to firmly endorse the listed treatments.

Herbal formula	
Withania somnifera 1:1	30 mL
Valeriana officinalis 1:2	25 mL
Passiflora incarnata 1:2	20 mL
Humulus lupulus 1:2	15 mL
Vitex agnus-castus 1:2	10 mL
7.5 mL b.d.	100 mL
(early evening and 1 hour before bedtime)	

Nutritional prescription

Magnesium elemental 300 mg b.d.
Adenosine 100 mg
2 tablets sublingually
1 hour before bedtime

Sleep hygiene and dietary and lifestyle advice

General lifestyle advice should focus on good sleep hygiene techniques (see Figure 14.6).[8] The key techniques revealed by sleep researchers focus primarily on limiting exposure to the bed (sleep restriction)—that is, the patient having only a limited time to sleep, and getting up at a set time in the morning regardless of quality or quantity of sleep.[8] This should in time regulate the circadian rhythm. Patients should also be advised not to 'force' sleep. If sleep does not occur within 20 minutes, then they should get up and focus the mind on an activity until they feel tired (still minimising light and mental activity). The other mainstay is to reduce exposure to light prior to sleep, and increase exposure to morning sunlight upon waking. It is also best to avoid excessive daytime naps as this may disturb the circadian rhythm.

Further sleep hygiene advice includes stimulus control: avoidance of stimulating activity and stimulants close to sleep (for example, smoking, caffeine and stimulating TV or books),[66] and adequate sleep preparation (for example, aromatherapy baths, relaxing reading material, gentle lovemaking and positive calming mental cognition). Avoidance of excess energetically 'heating' foods (such as alcohol, garlic, chillies and curries) may also be of assistance,[67] while the diet (or supplementation) may provide the nutrients required for the creation and regulation of adrenal hormones and psychoactive neurotransmitters (B vitamins, magnesium, calcium and vitamin C) helps support healthy functioning of the nervous system.[68] Although evening meal portions should not be excessive (this may cause rebound hypoglycaemia), sufficient calorific intake is required to avoid waking up due to hunger. Some people find a warm milk drink helpful in initiating sleep; this may be due to the effect of calcium.[69] Finally, moderating a busy work schedule is desirable to allow for regular exercise and relaxation to reduce stress levels.

The most obvious advice is to cut down or eliminate caffeine consumption. Caffeine is antagonistic to adenosine receptors and will interfere with circadian rhythm.[28]

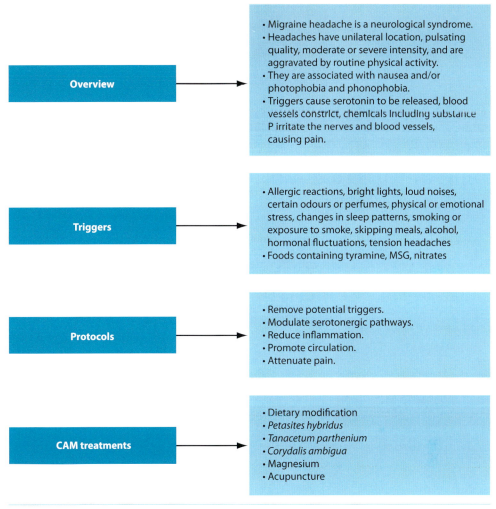

Overview
- Migraine headache is a neurological syndrome.
- Headaches have unilateral location, pulsating quality, moderate or severe intensity, and are aggravated by routine physical activity.
- They are associated with nausea and/or photophobia and phonophobia.
- Triggers cause serotonin to be released, blood vessels constrict, chemicals including substance P irritate the nerves and blood vessels, causing pain.

Triggers
- Allergic reactions, bright lights, loud noises, certain odours or perfumes, physical or emotional stress, changes in sleep patterns, smoking or exposure to smoke, skipping meals, alcohol, hormonal fluctuations, tension headaches
- Foods containing tyramine, MSG, nitrates

Protocols
- Remove potential triggers.
- Modulate serotonergic pathways.
- Reduce inflammation.
- Promote circulation.
- Attenuate pain.

CAM treatments
- Dietary modification
- *Petasites hybridus*
- *Tanacetum parthenium*
- *Corydalis ambigua*
- Magnesium
- Acupuncture

Figure 14.5 Migraine headaches[62,64,65]

The half-life of caffeine is approximately 4–6 hours and in women taking the oral contraceptive pill it may be greatly increased (see the anxiety chapter for more detail).[28] Pharmacokinetically, the caffeine from a cup of coffee drunk at 1 p.m can be still in the system by sleep time at 11 p.m., so avoidance of caffeine after lunch may be prudent. Patients may also be advised to keep a sleep diary over 2 weeks to record their sleep patterns. This may provide more diagnostic detail, and allow for a more thorough critique of their sleep hygiene. A 'worry diary' can also be an added component, with patients writing down before they sleep anything on their minds. This technique may help the person 'let go' of these concerns, leaving them on paper to be addressed the following day.

With respect to dietary change to address his migraines, various potential 'migraine-triggering' food groups can be removed and re-challenged (see Chapter 5 on food intolerance). Below is a list of common culprits that may provoke a migraine attack:
- milk
- wheat
- cheese

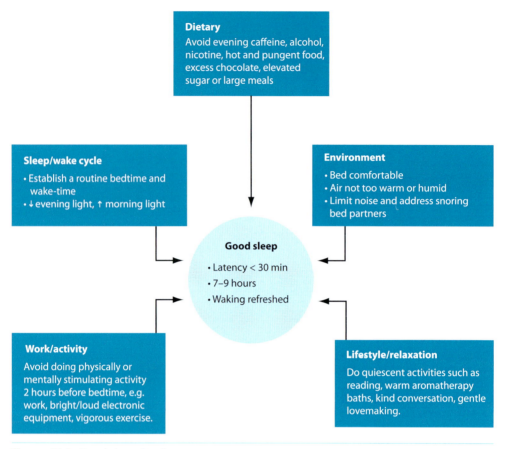

Figure 14.6 Good sleep hygiene

- chocolate
- nuts
- egg
- wine, alcohol
- MSG
- nitrite-containing foods
- fruits.

Additional therapeutic options

- L-tryptophan is used by the body to convert into serotonin. This neurochemical plays a role in non-REM deep sleep and its depletion has been shown in depression and insomnia.[70]
- As reviews by Hartmann[70] and Boman[71] detail, the weight of evidence (animal and human studies) indicates that L-tryptophan produces an increase in sleepiness and a decrease in sleep latency.
- These authors comment that the best results seem to occur in cases of mild insomnia with long sleep latency, and in the absence of comorbid medical or psychiatric disturbance.
- The prescriptive use of the amino acid may be restricted in some countries (such as Australia), but safe and reliable sources of L-tryptophan or 5-HT taken within

Table 14.1 Review of the major evidence

INTERVENTION	KEY LITERATURE	SUMMARY OF RESULTS	COMMENT
Valerian and hops (Reviews)	*Valerian*: Bent et al. 2006[38] *Hops*: Zanoli & Zavatti 2008[30]	Inconclusive evidence for valerian or hops individually in the treatment of insomnia. May be effective in some individuals if used long-term (> 2 weeks).	The combination of valerian and hops may be synergistically more effective Use caution with valerian in people with 'heat' signs, and with hops in people with depression.
L-tryptophan (Reviews)	Boman 1988[71] Hartmann 1982[70]	Good supportive evidence for use in insomnia. Better for milder types of sleep disturbance, or for long sleep latency.	Use caution in cases of co-prescription with antidepressants. Stay within prescriptive guidelines and use only reputable products.
Melatonin (Meta-analysis)	Buscemi et al. 2005[72]	Positive evidence supporting the use of melatonin in reducing sleep latency. Lacks evidence in treating other sleep markers, e.g. duration and quality.	Product quality can be a significant issue. In some countries the sale of melatonin may be restricted.
Acupuncture (Cochrane review)	Cheuk et al. 2007[61]	Tentatively supportive evidence; may improve subjective quality of sleep.	Only use qualified acupuncturists Use caution in cases of needle phobia, which may increase distress in some people.

recommended dosage should not present with any high level of risk (see a health professional for exact prescriptive advice).

- Melatonin at oral doses of 1–2 mg may be of benefit in decreasing sleep latency.[72]
- *Zizyphus jujuba*, *Eschscholzia californica*, *Melissa officinalis* and *Scutellaria lateriflora* are herbal medicines with purported sedative and anxiolytic properties, and these may provide other prescriptive options for the sleep formula. However, more studies are required to validate efficacy (see the anxiety case for a review of the evidence).
- The use of other interventions for insomnia in adults, such as exercise programs, aromatherapy and music therapy, although they may be helpful in some individuals, currently do not have any robust evidentiary support.[17,73]

Expected outcomes and follow-up protocols

In the above case the patient's insomnia is expected to be ameliorated within the week. Chronic insomniacs have a poor prognosis and the prognosis is worse if it is complicated by comorbid mental disorders and substance abuse.[74] An integrative approach involving sleep hygiene education, psychological, dietary/nutraceutical, lifestyle and herbal intervention should offer a sustained benefit if compliance is maintained. If after 2 weeks of the prescription minimal benefit has occurred, the herbal prescription can be modified to include other hypnotics and anxiolytics such as *Eschscholzia californica*, *Melissa officinalis* and *Bacopa monnieri*.[29,75] Melatonin or L-tryptophan may also be used if the patient is non-responsive to the initial prescription. Additional psychological interventions (behavioural or social-based models) may also be of assistance to examine and aid in the management of the external triggers of the stress and insomnia. The key is to advise the person to be patient and not to 'force' the sleep process, to be disciplined if following sleep restriction techniques (no daytime napping and a regular waking time), maintain good sleep hygiene and try to address any psychosocial social factors impacting sleep. With regard to the patient's migraines, his headaches may take longer to abate, and if no change was occurring after several weeks of treatment with dietary adjustment and herbal and nutritional prescription, use of *Tanacetum parthenium* and *Petasites hybridus* and referral for acupuncture may be advised. It is likely that the migraines will be mitigated when the patient's sleep pattern improves.

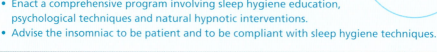

KEY POINTS

- Try to determine the causes of the insomnia and the current sleep hygiene status.
- Assess, monitor and if required refer any substance use issues, medical or psychiatric conditions.
- Enact a comprehensive program involving sleep hygiene education, psychological techniques and natural hypnotic interventions.
- Advise the insomniac to be patient and to be compliant with sleep hygiene techniques.

Further reading

Sateia M, Nowell PD. Insomnia. Lancet 2004;364(9449):1959–1973.

Roth T, Roehrs T. Insomnia: epidemiology, characteristics, and consequences. Clinical Cornerstone: Chronic Insomnia 2003;5(3):5–15.

References

1. American Psychiatric Association. Diagnostic and statistical manual of mental disorders. 4th edn. Arlington: American Psychiatric Association, 2000.
2. Roth T, Roehrs T. Insomnia: epidemiology, characteristics, and consequences. Clinical Cornerstone: Chronic Insomnia 2003;5(3):5–15.
3. Krystal AD, Roth T. Definitions, measurements, and management in insomnia. Journal of Clinical Psychiatry 2004;65:5–7.
4. Roth T, et al. Insomnia: pathophysiology and implications for treatment. Sleep Medicine Reviews 2007;11(1):71–79.
5. Piggins HD. Human clock genes. Annals of Medicine 2002;34(5):394–400.
6. Lancel M. Role of GABA(A) receptors in the regulation of sleep: initial sleep responses to peripherally administered modulators and agonists. Sleep 1999;22(1):33–42.
7. Strecker RE, et al. Another chapter in the adenosine story. Sleep 2006;29(4):426–428.
8. Stepanski EJ, Wyatt JK. Use of sleep hygiene in the treatment of insomnia. Sleep Medicine Reviews 2003;7(3):215–225.
9. Krystal AD. The changing perspective on chronic insomnia management. Journal of Clinical Psychiatry 2004;65:20–25.
10. Roth T. Measuring treatment efficacy in insomnia. Journal of Clinical Psychiatry 2004;65:8–12.
11. Benca RM, et al. Special considerations in insomnia diagnosis and management: depressed, elderly, and chronic pain populations. Journal of Clinical Psychiatry 2004;65:26–35.
12. Ford D, Kamerow D. Epidemiologic study of sleep disturbances and psychiatric disorders: an opportunity for prevention? JAMA 1989;262:1479–1484.
13. Roth T. Insomnia as a risk factor for depression. International Journal of Neuropsychopharmacology 2004;7: S34–S35.
14. Walsh JK. Clinical and socioeconomic correlates of insomnia. Journal of Clinical Psychiatry 2004;65:13–19.
15. Ramakrishnan K, Scheid DC. Treatment options for insomnia. American Family Physician 2007;76(4):517–526.
16. Sateia MJ, et al. Evaluation of chronic insomnia. Sleep 2000;23(2):243–308.
17. Sateia MJ, Nowell PD. Insomnia. Lancet 2004; 364(9449):1959–1973.
18. Rains JC, et al. Sleep and headaches. Curr Neurol Neurosci Rep 2008;8(2):167–175.
19. Rains JC, Poceta JS. Headache and sleep disorders: review and clinical implications for headache management. Headache 2006;46(9):1344–1363.
20. Tariq SH, Pulisetty S. Pharmacotherapy for insomnia. Clinics in Geriatric Medicine 2008;24(1):93–105.
21. Rickels K, Rynn M. Pharmacotherapy of generalized anxiety disorder. J Clin Psychiatry 2002;63(Suppl 14):9–16.
22. Cajochen C, et al. Role of melatonin in the regulation of human circadian rhythms and sleep. Journal of Neuroendocrinology 2003;15(4):432–437.
23. Schwartz JR, Roth T. Shift work sleep disorder: burden of illness and approaches to management. Drugs 2006;66(18):2357–2370.
24. Hein H. [The sleep apnoea syndromes: alternative therapies]. Pneumologie 2004;58(5):325–329.
25. Lemoine P, et al. Improvement in subjective sleep in major depressive disorder with a novel antidepressant, agomelatine: randomized, double-blind comparison with venlafaxine. J Clin Psychiatry 2007;68(11):1723–1732.

26. Morin CM, et al. Psychological and behavioral treatment of insomnia: update of the recent evidence (1998–2004). Sleep 2006;29(11):1398–1414.

27. Basheer R, et al. Adenosine and sleep-wake regulation. Prog Neuropsychobiol 2004;73:379–396.

28. Nehlig A, et al. Caffeine and the central nervous system: mechanisms of action, biochemical, metabolic and psychostimulant effects. Brain Res Brain Res Rev 1992; 17(2):139–170.

29. Felter HW, Lloyd JU. King's American dispensary. Online. Available: http://www.henriettesherbal.com/eclectic/kings/extracta

30. Zanoli P, Zavatti M. Pharmacognostic and pharmacological profile of *Humulus lupulus* L. Journal of Ethnopharmacology 2008;116:383–396.

31. Fussel A, et al. Effect of a fixed valerian-hop extract combination (Ze 91019) on sleep polygraphy in patients with non-organic insomnia: a pilot study. Eur J Med Res 2000;5(9):385–390.

32. Morin C, et al. Valerian-hops combination and diphenhydramine for treating insomnia: a randomized placebo-controlled clinical trial. Sleep 2005;28(11):1465–1471.

33. Abourashed EA, et al. In vitro binding experiments with a valerian, hops and their fixed combination extract (Ze91019) to selected central nervous system receptors. Phytomedicine 2004;11(7–8):633–638.

34. Muller CE, et al. Interactions of valerian extracts and a fixed valerian-hop extract combination with adenosine receptors. Life Sci 2002;71(16):1939–1949.

35. Schellenberg R, et al. The fixed combination of valerian and hops (Ze91019) acts via a central adenosine mechanism. Planta Med 2004;70(7):594–597.

36. Cook W. The physiomedical dispensatory. Online. Available: http://www.ibiblio.org/herbmed/eclectic/cook/main.htm. Accessed 10 October 2005.

37. Culpeper N. Culpeper's complete herbal. Hertfordshire: Wordsworth Editions Ltd, 1652.

38. Bent S, et al. Valerian for sleep: a systematic review and meta-analysis. American Journal of Medicine 2006;119:1005–1012.

39. Mills S, Bone K. Principles and practice of phytotherapy. London: Churchill Livingstone, 2000.

40. Herrera-Arellano A, et al. Polysomnographic evaluation of the hypnotic effect of Valeriana edulis standardized extract in patients suffering from insomnia. Planta Med 2001;67(8):695–699.

41. Donath F, et al. Critical evaluation of the effect of valerian extract on sleep structure and sleep quality. Pharmacopsychiatry 2000;33(2):47–53.

42. Gutierrez S, et al. Assessing subjective and psychomotor effects of the herbal medication valerian in healthy volunteers. Pharmacol Biochem Behav 2004;78(1):57–64.

43. Benke D, et al. GABA(A) receptors as in vivo substrate for the anxiolytic action of valerenic acid, a major constituent of valerian root extracts. Neuropharmacology 2009;56(1):174–181.

44. Schumacher B, et al. Lignans isolated from valerian: identification and characterization of a new olivil derivative with partial agonistic activity at A(1) adenosine receptors. J Nat Prod 2002;65(10):1479–1485.

45. Blumenthal M, et al, eds. The ABC clinical guide to herbs. Austin: American Botanical Council, 2004.

46. Wuttke W, et al. Chaste tree *(Vitex agnus-castus)* – pharmacology and clinical indications. Phytomedicine 2003;10(4):348–357.

47. Dericks-Tan JS, et al. Dose-dependent stimulation of mel atonin secretion after administration of *agnus castus*. Exp Clin Endocrinol Diabetes 2003;111(1):44–46.

48. Ayuso-Gutierrez JL. Depressive subtypes and efficacy of antidepressive pharmacotherapy. World J Biol Psychiatry 2005;6(Suppl 2):31–37.

49. Mishra LC, et al. Scientific basis for the therapeutic use of *Withania somnifera* (ashwagandha): a review. Altern Med Rev 2000;5(4):334–346.

50. Bhattacharya SK, et al. Anxiolytic-antidepressant activity of *Withania somnifera* glycowithanolides: an experimental study. Phytomedicine 2000;7(6):463–469.

51. Bhattacharya SK, Muruganandam AV. Adaptogenic activity of *Withania somnifera:* an experimental study using a rat model of chronic stress. Pharmacol Biochem Behav 2003;75(3):547–555.

52. Kelly GS. *Rhodiola rosea:* a possible plant adaptogen. Altern Med Rev 2001;6(3):293–302.

53. Atkinson G, Davenne D. Relationships between sleep, physical activity and human health. Physiol Behav 2007;90(2–3):229–235.

54. Montgomery P, Dennis J. Physical exercise for sleep problems in adults aged 60+. Cochrane Database Syst Rev 2002;(4):CD003404.

55. Lehrl S. Clinical efficacy of kava WS 1490 in sleep disturbances associated with anxiety disorders. Results of a multicenter, randomized, placebo-controlled, double-blind clinical trial. J Affect Disord 2004;78:101–110.

56. Malsch U, Kieser M. Efficacy of kava-kava in the treatment of non-psychotic anxiety, following pretreatment with benzodiazepines. Psychopharmacology (Berl) 2001;157:277–283.

57. Hamilton M. The assessment of anxiety states by rating. Br J Med Psychol 1959;32(1):50–55.

58. CIPS. Internationale Skalen fur die Psychiatrie. Gottingen: Beltz, 1996.

59. Malhotra A, White DP. Obstructive sleep apnoea. Lancet 2002;360(9328):237–245.

60. Puhan MA, et al. Didgeridoo playing as alternative treatment for obstructive sleep apnoea syndrome: randomised controlled trial. BMJ 4 2006;332(7536):266–270.

61. Cheuk DKL, et al. Acupuncture for insomnia. Cochrane Database syst Rev 2007;(3):CD005472.

62. Rios J, Passe MM. Evidenced-based use of botanicals, minerals, and vitamins in the prophylactic treatment of migraines. J Am Acad Nurse Pract 2004;16(6):251–256.

63. Pittler MH, et al. Feverfew for preventing migraine. Cochrane Database Syst Rev 2000;(3):CD002286.

64. Silberstein SD. Migraine. Lancet 2004;363(9406):381–391.

65. Griggs C, Jensen J. Effectiveness of acupuncture for migraine: critical literature review. J Adv Nurs 2006;54(4):491–501.

66. Jefferson CD, et al. Sleep hygiene practices in a population-based sample of insomniacs. Sleep 2005;28(5): 611–615.

67. Maciocia G. The foundations of Chinese medicine. Singapore: Churchill Livingstone, 1989.

68. Haas EM. Staying healthy with nutrition. Berkeley: Celestial Arts, 1992.

69. Werbach M. Nutritional influences on illness. 2nd edn. Tarzana: Third Line Press, 1996.

70. Hartmann E. Effects of L-tryptophan on sleepiness and on sleep. J Psychiatr Res 1982;17(2):107–113.

71. Boman B. L-tryptophan: a rational anti-depressant and a natural hypnotic? Aust N Z J Psychiatry 1988;22(1): 83–97.

72. Buscemi N, et al. The efficacy and safety of exogenous melatonin for primary sleep disorders. A meta-analysis. J Gen Intern Med 2005;20(12):1151–1158.

73. Lazic SE, Ogilvie RD. Lack of efficacy of music to improve sleep: a polysomnographic and quantitative EEG analysis. International Journal of Psychophysiology 2007;63(3):232–239.

74. Nutt D, et al. Generalized anxiety disorder: a comorbid disease. Eur Neuropsychopharmacol 2006;16(Suppl 2): S109–S118.

75. Bone K. A clinical guide to blending liquid herbs: herbal formulations for the individual patient. St Louis: Churchill Livingstone, 2003.

Section 5 Endocrine system

The main function of the endocrine system is to achieve internal homeostasis. The system consists of tissues (endocrine and exocrine glands) that produce and secrete hormones. The endocrine glands differ from exocrine glands in that they are ductless and secrete their hormones directly into the bloodstream. This allows the endocrine system to influence any cell, tissue or organ that has receptors specific to the particular hormone to read its 'message'. Modulation of the endocrine system is slow to take effect, unlike the nervous system, which responds with alacrity. Because of this, the treatment of endocrine diseases requires a longer, more sustained therapeutic approach.

Hormones are sensitive to the chemical environment in which they operate and any changes therein, and various complex feedback loops ensure homeostasis and stability. For example, once cortisol has been released as a response to stress, the very nature of high cortisol levels in the blood reduces the amount of triggering hormone, ACTH; this returns the system to baseline. Due to the complex nature of hormones and their target sites, endocrine hormones may also influence the hormones of other systems. For example, the nervous system is intricately linked with the endocrine system and this interface is readily observed in the science of neuroendocrinology, the study of how nervous activity affects endocrine response and vice versa. Interventions that modulate neurological activity therefore have an effect on endocrine activity.

Herbal medicine actions that effect this response include adaptogens, nervine tonics, antidepressants and stimulants. Botanicals that have this effect usually are rich in triterpenoid or steroidal saponins or alkaloids, or certain volatile compounds such as terpenes. Nutrients that play a potential role in supporting neuroendocrine activity are the vitamins B1, B2, B3, B5 and C; calcium; and magnesium.

In naturopathic practice, most commonly encountered hormone dysregulations are related to the thyroid, adrenal, pancreatic or gonadal glands. Significant hormonal conditions seen clinically include non-insulin-dependent diabetes (NIDD) and thyroid disorders. However, patients will often present to a naturopath with an array of symptoms that may seem vague and unrelated, perhaps manifesting as weight issues or fatigue (often involving hypothalamic–pituitary–adrenal axis dysregulation). These 'warning signs' could be part of a metabolic hormonal disturbance, which may be diagnosable via a medical test, or may be subclinical (though still having a marked effect on health). Hormones often work in concert with each other, and when one is out of balance it may affect other endocrine organs. For example, NIDD may have an overarching effect on various other systems such as the cardiovascular, and may manifest as a complex 'metabolic disorder' rather than a specific condition.

This section focuses on the hormones from the adrenal, pancreatic and thyroid glands: the stress-mediating hormones, the blood sugar regulating hormone, and the thyroid hormones. A special consideration should be given to other connecting chapters in Section 4 on the nervous system and Chapter 35 on chronic fatigue syndrome.

15
Adrenal exhaustion

Tini Gruner
ND, MSc, PhD

AETIOLOGY

Stress

Hans Selye, in 1935, was the first to develop a theory of stress. When he imposed different types of physical stressors on rats he discovered that, regardless of the kind of stressor, the same physiological response was the result: hypertrophied adrenal glands, atrophied lymphatic organs (lymph nodes, spleen and thymus) and bleeding gastric ulcers. These symptoms developed over time. He called this the 'general adaptation syndrome' (GAS), stating 'stress is the nonspecific response of the body to any demand made upon it'.[1] This requires adjustment or adaptation to a new situation.

From his observations he hypothesised three stages: alarm, resistance and exhaustion. The alarm stage was characterised by hormonal changes such as increased sympathetic nervous system (SNS) activity, with its typical fight or flight response and noradrenaline secretions, and up-regulated cortisol. In the resistance stage the body had adapted to the stressor, the above symptoms had disappeared and body metabolism had returned to normal. In the exhaustion stage the stress triad of hypertrophied adrenals, atrophied lymph organs and gastric ulcers were noticed, together with an initial increase in cortisol, which later declined to below normal. Only in this stage, with severe stress over prolonged periods of time, did the body lose its ability to cope and eventually death ensued. However, in general the physiological changes mentioned above were thought of as being protective to ensure the animal's survival.[1,2] Therefore, stress is actually a positive occurrence needed for protection (readiness for action when in danger, increased immune particles when injured). It becomes pathological only if it is protracted or uncontrolled.[3–5]

Physiologically, a stressor causes disruptions in homeostasis, leading to neural and endocrine changes known as the 'stress response' or 'stress cascade' (Figure 15.1).[6,7] Mental and emotional stressors stimulate the hypothalamus via the limbic system (the hippocampus and amygdala),[6–8] whereas physical and physiological processes, such as injury or hypoglycaemia, can stimulate the hypothalamus directly.

The first (and immediate) reaction to a stressor is caused by imbalances in the central nervous system (CNS) through overstimulation of the SNS and suppression of the parasympathetic nervous system (PNS). The SNS stimulates the adrenal medulla to secrete the catecholamines noradrenaline and adrenaline. They are produced from

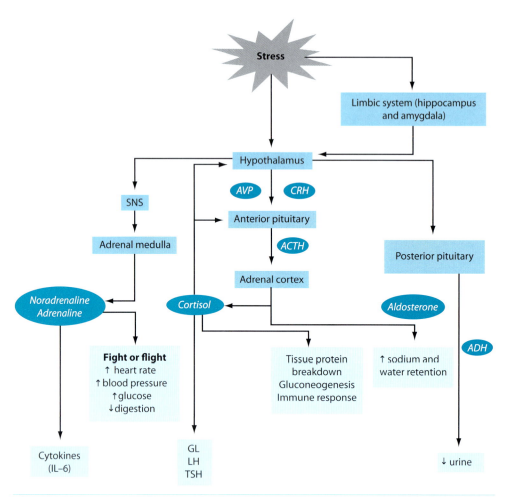

Figure 15.1 The stress cascade. Solid arrows indicate stimulation and dotted arrows indicate inhibition. AVP = arginine vasopression, CRH = corticotrophin–releosing hormone, ACTH = adrenocorticotrophic system, SNS = sympathetic nervous system, ADH = antidiuretic hormone.

phenylalanine and hence tyrosine (Figure 15.2). These hormones lead to heightened alertness to quickly judge a situation regarding its potential danger. Blood pressure, breathing and heart rate are accelerated for fight or flight, for which glycogenolysis (release of glycogen from the liver) provides the extra fuel. Endorphins are released to dampen pain from a potential injury. Digestion, relaxation and sleep are suppressed. In other words, the body is prepared for swift action needed for survival.[3,6,9,10]

Stimulation of the anterior pituitary gland is achieved through secreting corticotrophin releasing hormone (CRH), and to a lesser extent arginine vasopressin (AVP), which leads to the release of adrenocorticotropic hormone (ACTH). ACTH triggers the release of vast amounts of cortisol glucocorticoid and moderate amounts of aldosterone (a mineral corticoid) from the adrenal cortex. Both these hormones are made (a minerale certicoid) from cholesterol (Figure 15.3).

Under normal circumstances cortisol levels are highest in the morning and lowest in the evening. Its physiological actions control carbohydrate, protein and fat metabolism, and it inhibits prostaglandin synthesis and contributes to emotional stability.

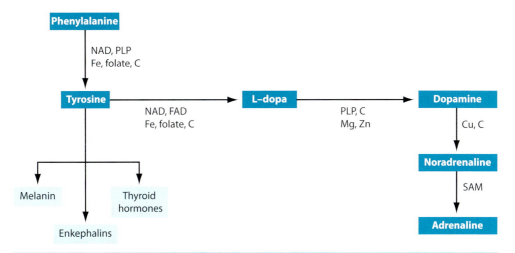

Figure 15.2 Catecholamine production

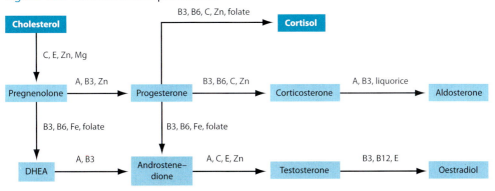

Figure 15.3 Steroid hormone production with nutrient cofactors

In stress, however, cortisol levels in blood are elevated, triggering an increase in protein breakdown and mobilisation of fatty acids (gluconeogenesis) in order to provide glucose for the fight or flight response. This results in a hyperglycaemic state in the liver with peripheral hypoglycaemia, temporarily leading to moderate insulin resistance. High cortisol also decreases lymphocyte and eosinophil counts, effectively dampening any inflammation or immune response.[2,6,7] Moreover, elevated glucocorticoids influence reproduction, growth and thyroid functions by inhibiting gonadotropin-releasing hormone (GnRH) and luteinising hormone (LH), growth hormone (GH) and thyroid-stimulating hormone (TSH), respectively.[6] As a result, these functions are suppressed because the body deems them to be of minor importance in the face of an acute stressor.[6,11–14]

Cortisol, adrenaline and glucagon all have the ability to raise blood glucose levels. Due to their hyperglycaemic action they have a catabolic effect on the body. Cortisol is involved in replenishing depleted energy stores; hence it converts food into glycogen and fat, and initiates hunger. Adrenaline increases mental alertness, blood pressure, breathing and heart rate, muscle tone, glycogenolysis and the release of endorphins. Simultaneously, it down-regulates appetite, digestion, elimination, relaxation and sleep.[3] Glucagon opposes insulin by mediating the release of glucose from storage.

The second hormone released by the adrenal cortex—aldosterone—retains sodium and water in the body. In addition, stimulation of the posterior pituitary gland by the hypothalamus results in antidiuretic hormone (ADH) secretion. The combined result of these actions is fluid retention and increased blood volume, which can lead to increased blood pressure.[2]

The secretion and interplay of the stress hormones will vary, depending on the type, intensity and duration of the stressor as well as its hormonal regulation.[15,16] High amounts of circulating cortisol will, via negative feedback loops, shut off the release of hormones from the hypothalamus and anterior pituitary glands. Therefore, once the acute stressor has subsided, the stress cascade abates and the physiology of the organism returns to normal. The individual becomes more resilient as a result of successful adaptation to a new situation in which wear and tear are minimised.[17] This memory is stored in the hippocampus and readily accessible when a similar stressful situation arises, so the learning from the first event can guide the (re)actions when it recurs. The role of the amygdala is to retain the emotional impact of the stressor and, together with the hippocampus, will ensure a better memory of an emotionally charged event. Both cortisol and adrenaline are needed for this memory to happen.[3] Thus mind and body can both be strengthened from a stressful experience, becoming more resilient to future stressors.

Distress

If, however, stress is chronic or intense and exceeds the person's mental and physical resources, it becomes distress. This is the case in adrenal exhaustion which corresponds to the final stage of Selye's GAS. The circulating hormones will not return to their normal levels and initially stay in a state of hyperarousal.[6,8] As a result, CRH, AVP and ACTH are no longer inhibited via negative feedback (leading to dysregulation of the HPA axis), target organs become overstimulated, receptors possibly become desensitised and tissue damage ensues.[4] This 'wear and tear' or 'cost' of adaptation or allostasis has been termed 'allostatic load'. It is implicated in numerous disease processes[4,18–20] and has been associated with an energy-deficiency state of the body.[14] It is mediated by adrenaline and cortisol. Both hormones actually serve to imprint the stressful event into long-term memory, but prolonged action will cause damage to the part of the brain that should shut them off. This in turn leads to higher levels of these hormones circulating in the blood ('cortisol resistance'), which can do more damage to the brain, especially the hippocampus. High levels of cortisol have been linked to the conditions outlined in Table 15.1.

However, with time there is a blunted response before cortisol levels will decline or the diurnal rhythm will flatten.[20] With lowered cortisol levels, endogenous glucose production is compromised, and sugar and stimulant cravings are likely as a consequence of the resultant hypoglycaemia. If untreated, this can lead to adrenal burnout and chronic fatigue.[34] The results of low cortisol are shown in Table 15.2.

The flow-on effect of these disturbances in neurotransmitters and stress hormones can lead to exhausted serotonin levels as well, potentially resulting in anxiety and sleep disturbances. The precursor of serotonin is tryptophan (Figure 15.4). The established link between carbohydrate cravings and depression is thought to be due to its tryptophan-increasing properties,[42,43] with mood-elevating results.[44]

Agitation and anxiety can also be caused by glutamatergic activation. Note that the precursor for both the inhibitory and the excitatory pathways is the same amino acid: glutamine (Figure 15.5). If zinc or vitamin B6 are in short supply then adequate amounts of GABA, the inhibitory neurotransmitter, cannot be formed. Instead, glutamate, the excitatory neurotransmitter, accumulates, leading to the above-mentioned symptoms.[45]

Table 15.1 Chronic diseases caused by high cortisol[3]

HORMONAL DYSREGULATION	DISORDER
General effects	Addictions, alcoholism and obsessive-compulsive disorders[21-23] anorexia nervosa[24] Cushing's syndrome[7]
Lowered serotonin levels	Anxiety, panic disorder and melancholic depression[5,6,25-27]
High cytokines leading to oxidative stress	Neurological diseases[27-29] Overtraining syndrome in athletes[30]
Suppression of immune function	Infections[31,32]
↑ bone demineralisation	Reduction in bone mass and osteoporosis[6,27]
↑ storage of fat around abdomen → ↑ gluconeogenesis from protein (loss of muscle mass) to meet energy demands → ↑ insulin → ↑ cortisol → ↑ eating energy-dense foods → ↑ storage of fat	Visceral adiposity, insulin resistance and loss of glycaemic control[6,8,27,33,34] Metabolic syndrome[35,36]
Shrivelling of dendrites → destruction of neurons → ↓ neurogenesis → cerebral ischaemia → ↓ hippocampus size	Impaired memory and loss of cognitive function, acceleration of ageing[28]
Impaired conversion of T_4 to T_3	Thyroid dysfunction[6]
Dysregulation of reproductive hormones[37]	Hormonal disturbances[6,13]

Table 15.2 Chronic diseases caused by low cortisol (insufficient HPA response to stress)[3]

HORMONAL DYSREGULATION	DISORDER
General	Addison's disease[7] Hypopituitarism[38] Hypothyroidism[6]
Unresponsive HPA, low (exhausted) cortisol levels and blunted response to exercise, disturbances in serotonergic neurotransmission and AVP	Chronic fatigue syndrome, fibromyalgia[26,34,39] Atypical (flat) depression[26] Inflammatory conditions[40]
Flat cortisol rhythm Burnout → loss of regulation in limbic system → brain damage and atrophy	Poor mental performance[20,41] Non-melancholic depression[3]
Depleted adrenaline Hypoarousal	Non-melancholic depression[3]

Testing for adrenal exhaustion

Adrenal exhaustion is a vague term that is not generally used in medicine. 'Adrenal fatigue' has been used to describe hypoadrenia. It is therefore important to assess HPA axis dysregulation before treatment is instigated.[46] The tests in Table 15.3 have been shown to be useful in diagnosing HPA axis dysregulation. The information gleaned from these tests will indicate not only the level of cortisol excess or depletion but also any concomitant health conditions that may have developed as a result of stress, such as insulin resistance, hypopituitarism and inflammation.

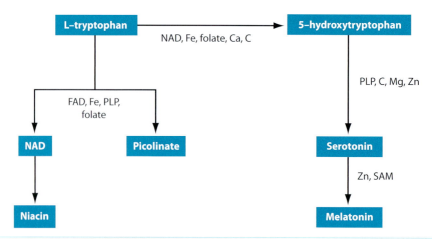

Figure 15.4 Production of serotonin

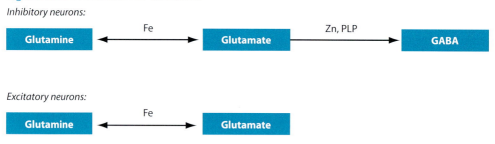

Figure 15.5 Production of GABA

RISK FACTORS

While the SNS is responsible for arousal, for fight and flight, the PNS facilitates rest, relaxation and healing (repair), it slows heart rate and promotes digestion and elimination. Neurotransmitters activated by the SNS include adrenaline and noradrenaline, whereas acetylcholine is the predominant neurotransmitter of the PNS. In a healthy state there is balance between the SNS and PNS. However, during stress the SNS is dominant, suppressing the actions of the PNS. This can lead to digestive and sleep disturbances and agitation.[49] Repercussions of this may include reduced absorption of nutrients through diminished production of digestive juices, anxiety and further drain on energy through lack of restful sleep.

The use of stimulants such as coffee increases the stress response and adrenal output, as shown by elevated catecholamines, notably adrenaline, in urine.[50,51] If coffee is used as a pick-me-up without having an effect, leading to increasingly greater consumption, it begs the question as to whether adrenaline production ability has been exhausted. This kind of stimulation may therefore hasten the decline in adrenal function, thus being a stressor in its own right. Adrenal exhaustion can be the result of multiple stressors, each of them not being enough to cause HPA dysfunction. However, the additive effects (if not addressed) can weaken the system to such an extent that other health problems could arise, such as chronic fatigue, clinical depression, hypothyroidism, inflammatory and autoimmune conditions, and hormonal disturbances, as outlined in Table 15.2.

Table 15.3 Pathology tests for evaluating stress markers[47]

TEST	TISSUE	COMMENTS
Cortisol	Serum	Cortisol is diurnal—it is highest in the morning at 6 to 8 a.m. and drops throughout the day, with lowest levels occurring around midnight. Therefore, tests should be performed at around 8 a.m. and again at 4 p.m., with the morning readings close to the maximum and the afternoon values closer to the lower end of the reference range.
	Urine	24 hour readings indicate whether adequate amounts of cortisol have been produced overall.
	Saliva	Several readings can be taken throughout the day to determine the diurnal variation.
ACTH	Serum	ACTH needs to be present to stimulate cortisol release and is therefore following the same diurnal variation as cortisol. If both cortisol and ACTH are low, an ACTH stimulation test should be performed to determine whether cortisol is low because of lack of ACTH.
ACTH stimulation	Serum	A synthetic form of ACTH (cosyntropin) is injected after taking a blood sample for baseline cortisol measurements. Blood samples are taken in half-hourly intervals for the following 1–2 hours. If cortisol is still low, adrenal exhaustion or Addison's disease (primary hypoadrenalism) is the likely cause. If cortisol levels are within the normal range, then the problem lies with inadequate ACTH secretion (hypopituitarism or secondary hypoadrenalism).
GTT (glucose tolerance test)	Serum	A 3-hour glucose tolerance test can be performed, with half-hourly measurements of glucose, insulin and cortisol. If hypoglycaemia is present, then cortisol levels should increase to activate glucose release from glycogen stores. Both the hypoglycaemia and low cortisol in response are indicative of adrenal exhaustion.
ITT (insulin tolerance test)	Serum	This test is usually used for identifying patients with growth hormone (GH) deficiency, but it has also been used to determine HPA status.[48] Hypoglycaemia is induced by the IV infusion of insulin and/or arginine. Blood samples for growth hormone, glucose and cortisol are taken at regular intervals for 90 minutes. However, this test is contraindicated in cases of low basal plasma cortisol.
Inflammatory markers	Serum	ESR, CRP, homocysteine and antibodies should all be tested, as low cortisol reduces the ability of the body to control inflammatory processes.
Electrolytes	Serum	Altered aldosterone levels due to mineralocorticoid insufficiency (as part of glucocorticoid insufficiency) can lead to imbalances in electrolytes, notably sodium.
Aldosterone	Blood and urine	Aldosterone can be altered due to adrenal pathology. However, this test is mainly used to diagnose hyperaldosteronism and may not be relevant in this scenario.

(Continued)

Table 15.3 Pathology tests for evaluating stress markers[47] *(Continued)*

TEST	TISSUE	COMMENTS
Lipid studies	Serum	Cortisol is made in the body from cholesterol. Further, in an insulin-resistant state it is likely that triglycerides and possibly LDL are elevated, with insufficient amounts of HDL.
Viruses	Serum	To rule out any viral causes of fatigue.

DIAGNOSIS

Adrenal exhaustion is diagnostically based on a holistic naturopathic diagnosis, and should be distinguished from conventional medical diagnoses such as Addison's disease, clinical depression and chronic fatigue syndrome.

CUSHING'S DISEASE[52]

Excess glucocorticoid production in adrenal cortex due to either excess treatment with corticosteroids or malignancy, causing disturbance in carbohydrate, protein and fat metabolism

Symptoms

Increased blood glucose

Abdominal obesity

Sarcopenia

Muscle loss and weakness, wasted extremities

Osteoporosis

Hypertension due to Na+ and fluid retention

Bruising and stretch marks

Increased facial and body hair growth

ADDISON'S DISEASE[52]

Lack of cortisol production by the adrenal cortex , mostly due to destruction of the adrenal cortex by autoimmunity, leading to abnormalities in blood glucose and blood volume, and skin pigmentation due to uninhibited ACTH and melatonin-stimulating hormone

Symptoms

Skin pigmentation

↓ blood pressure

↓ Na+ and ↑ K+

↓ blood glucose, especially when fasting, to the point of hypoglycaemic symptoms

Circulatory problems due to reduced blood volume

CONVENTIONAL TREATMENT

The diagnosis of adrenal exhaustion is not often made in conventional medicine, and if it is made, it is from a different perspective to what naturopaths consider. Primary hypoadrenalism (Addison's disease) is rare. If it is part of an autoimmune endocrine disease,[53] where adrenal function has been maintained through endogenous up-regulation of corticotropic hormone stimulation, treatment may not be required. If secondary hypoadrenalism has been diagnosed, glucocorticoids are the drugs of choice,[54,55] with mineralocorticoids if needed.[56] DHEA has been trialled, with mixed results.[56,57] Apart from the removal of the adrenals like in Cushing's syndrome, hypoadrenalism is mainly recognised in the medical literature as being the result of brain injury,[58] tumours, endocrine disorders or critical illness,[59,60] where adrenal crisis has either happened or may be imminent.[61] In any case, the diagnosis seems to be thought of only at a very late stage.[53] Where naturopaths use the diagnosis of adrenal exhaustion, conventional treatment would therefore focus on the symptoms, with antidepressants being the most likely prescription.[62–64] Other interventions may include beta-blockers[65,66] and glutamatergic agents.[63] Novelty treatments trialled are glucocorticoid receptor antagonists and atrial natriuretic peptide receptor agonists.[64]

KEY TREATMENT PROTOCOLS

In adrenal exhaustion, hormones such as cortisol and adrenaline are generally low, resulting in a blunted stress response. Patients commonly complain about lack of enjoyment in life, such as the inability to look forward to a pleasurable event. The overall impression is one of endogenous depression (although this does not exclude external triggers as well). There is energy depletion on a cellular level, coupled with lack of neurotransmitter precursors and/or cofactors.

The aim of treatment is to repair suboptimally functioning cells, thus increasing the energy and wellbeing in the patient. Since the HPA axis is stimulated by mental and emotional as well as physical events, giving the patient resources requires not only support with nutrients but also teaching better coping strategies.[46]

> **NATUROPATHIC TREATMENT AIMS**
> - Reduce strain on the HPA axis.
> - Increase energy.
> - Increase physical and emotional stamina and sense of wellbeing.
> - Resource body and mind to be able to deal with stressors:
>   - low glycaemic load diet
>   - elimination of stimulant use
>   - nutritional supplements to replete metabolic pathways (cortisol and – neurotransmitter synthesis)
>   - adaptogens
>   - counselling and social contact.
> - Strengthen taxed systems via phytotherapy.
> - Explore ways of feeling supported in a new environment.

Modulation of the HPA axis

The HPA axis activates and is inactivated by cortisol (Figure 15.1).[67] In the case of low cortisol, the negative feedback is impaired, leading to dysregulation of other stress hormones. Diet, lifestyle and thought patterns have a key influence on the HPA axis. Adjusting these are the primary concerns as they will need to be the first line of defence for future stressors. Herbs have been used traditionally to modulate the nervous system and the stress response.

Diet

Reduction or avoidance of stimulants such as tea and coffee, so commonly used to keep up alertness and functioning in today's hectic life, will prevent further drain on the adrenals. These beverages can be replaced with decaffeinated coffee or tea, herb teas and filtered water. The change is best done slowly to reduce the risk of caffeine withdrawal symptoms such as headache and further fatigue.[51]

Stress is often accompanied by carbohydrate cravings, which can lead to blood sugar imbalances, especially if they are high in sugar and refined starches. Fruit is best limited to two pieces a day as it may increase glycaemic load. Whole grains are preferable due to their fibre content, thus slowing down the release of sugar,[68] and their B vitamin content. B vitamins are essential in the Krebs cycle for energy production.[45] Carbohydrates are commonly craved during stress due to their tryptophan-serotonin enhancing qualities.[42,43] This partially explains the weight gain experienced by some people when under stress.[43] High cortisol is also known to lead to weight increases and potentially to metabolic syndrome,[69,70] although in adrenal exhaustion cortisol is usually low (depleted). High-protein foods and snacks for amino acids, especially fish as the latter also contributes to a favourable EFA balance, may decrease carbohydrate cravings while at the same time providing the necessary amino acids as precursors for neurotransmitter synthesis. Protein powders can be used in smoothies to provide additional amino acids for neurotransmitter production and to help reduce hypoglycaemic episodes.

Lifestyle

Balance of work, relaxation and sleep, socialising, physical activities and daily chores is difficult to achieve in modern life. However, it is important to be aware of a person's commitments and how these influence their life. Chronic stress has been linked to premature death,[71] and social support networks are related to positive states of health and reduced disease burden.[72]

The importance of physical activity cannot be underestimated. Since the body is geared up for action when under stress ('fight or flight'), exercise is a potent tool to bring stress hormones back under control.[73] Regular physical activity has been shown to help in reducing stress, depression and anxiety.[74]

Herbal medicines

One of the most important herbal remedies acting on cortisol is **Glycyrrhiza glabra**. *G. glabra*, especially its active constituent glycyrrhetinic acid, is a potent inhibitor of 11 beta-hydroxysteroid dehydrogenase (which converts active cortisol to inactive cortisone),[75,76] thus increasing the amount of circulating cortisol.[77–79] It is therefore ideally suited to cases of low cortisol, such as in adrenal exhaustion although contraindicated in the 'alarm' or 'adaptation' stress phase. However, care needs to be taken as *G. glabra* can lead to pseudoaldosteronism by binding to mineralocorticoid receptors, thus promoting sodium and fluid retention as well as potassium loss, potentially leading to hypertension.[80] It is therefore not recommended in liver and kidney disease. A diet high in potassium and low in sodium is recommended if *G. glabra* is used long-term.[81]

Further, herbs with anxiolytic, sedative, adaptogenic and memory-enhancing properties[82–84] may be indicated in HPA-axis dysregulation. In order to treat specific diseases arising from allostatic load, many more herbs (such as anti-inflammatory and immune-modulating herbs) are available and need to be carefully selected to match the condition of the patient. The information on the following herbs has been taken from several textbooks[81–83,85–89] as well as some additional references stated in the text below.

Anxiolytics and sedative herbs

These herbs are indicated for states of anxiety, restlessness and difficulty falling or staying asleep. Concomitant use of barbiturates, benzodiazepines or narcotics is not recommended as this could potentiate the effect, leading to increased drowsiness.

For mild forms of anxiety and restlessness, **Matricaria recutita** could be useful.[81] It is a mild sedative and generally safe. However, it should not be taken at the same time as iron supplements. Care should be taken when a patient is on anticoagulants. In rare cases allergies have been reported. Alternatively, **Melissa officinalis**, a safe herb with a subtle lemon taste, could be used as a mild nervine and antispasmodic.[81] Both herbs are suitable for children.

If a stronger action is desirable, **Valeriana spp.** should be considered. *Valeriana officinalis* and *Valeriana edulis* are both used, with the former having higher levels of terpenes and the latter higher levels of valepotriates.[81] They improve sleep quality without morning drowsiness or impairment of concentration or reaction time and are therefore preferable to drug treatment.[90] In a blinded, randomised crossover study with *V. officinalis*, *V. edulis* has shown stronger effects.[91] Both have nervine and soporific actions and combine well with **Humulus lupulus** *M. recutita* and *M. officinales* for sleep disorders with anxiety and restlessness.[90] These herbs are safe, but long-term use of valerian can lead to insomnia. On rare occasions, valerian can have a stimulating effect in some people and should therefore be avoided.

Passiflora incarnata has been used for any kind of nervous system disorders, from headaches, irritability and restlessness to insomnia.[90] It has similar actions to hops and valerian and could be used in their place or combined with them. Alternatively, **Scutellaria lateriflora** could be prescribed due to its trophorestorative and nervine properties.

Lavandula angustifolia is another safe herb that is used for anxiety, restlessness and insomnia. It has antidepressant and mood-enhancing qualities. *L. angustifolia* could potentially have an addictive effect with some antidepressants.

Piper methysticum is an excellent remedy for sleeplessness. It has anxiolytic, antispasmodic and soporific qualities. In recent years alcohol and acetone extracts of kava have been withdrawn in some countries (including Australia) due to severe liver damage in rare cases,[92] possibly due to mitochondrial toxicity.[93] Traditionally, watery extracts were used with no adverse effects,[94] and *P. methysticum* produced in the traditional way is now available again in tablet form. Nonetheless, caution is indicated in patients with liver disease. Due to its possible dopamine antagonism it should not be used for patients with Parkinson's disease. Other contraindications include the use of non-steroidal anti-inflammatory drugs and alcohol; it should not be given to children or patients with endogenous depression.

In the Chinese tradition **Zizyphus jujuba var. spinosa** has been used for Yin deficiency and as a Qi tonic. Apart from its hypnotic and sedative qualities it is prescribed for irritability and to prevent sweating, especially at night. In addition, it can reduce heart palpitations and hypertension.[90] It may augment the effects of corticosteroids.

Adaptogens

Adaptogens have been defined as 'herbal preparations used to increase attention and endurance during fatigue and to reduce or prevent stress-induced impairments of neuroendocrine or immune function'.[95] Three categories of adaptogenic activity have been identified: regulating the stress response via the HPA axis, antioxidant action and modulating the central nervous system.[11] Several herbs, as shown below, have increased physical and mental stamina.[11,96] This class of herbs is therefore ideally suited to treat adrenal exhaustion.

Perhaps the strongest of the adaptogenic herbs is ***Panax ginseng***. It has a long tradition as a tonic in China, Japan, Korea and Russia. In the West, it is used to combat mental or physical fatigue and stress, and to enhance energy, wellbeing and performance.[79,97–99] It is used as an adrenal tonic, antidepressant, adaptogen and immuno-modulator. It is not recommended for diabetes as it may potentiate the actions of oral hypoglycaemic drugs and insulin. Further, it may decrease the effectiveness of warfarin or cause symptoms of oestrogen excess. Long-term use or high amounts may cause overstimulation.

Due to the limited resources of *P. ginseng*, Russians have investigated ***Eleutherococcus senticosus*** and found it to be the most important substitute for *P. ginseng*.[100] *E. senticosus* has shown non-specific body resistance to stress and fatigue.[101] It has similar properties to *P. senticosus*, in that it is an adaptogenic, a tonic and an immune modulator, and has anabolic qualities. It has been suggested that a threshold exists: when stress hormones are high *E. senticosus* will have a lowering effect, and if stress hormones are low they will be enhanced.[12] This herb is generally safe but may give falsely elevated test results for digoxin and hypertension.

Another adaptogen from the ginseng family is ***Panax quinquefolium***. It has tonic, immune-modulating and anti-inflammatory properties, combats stress and enhances the nervous and immune systems.[102] Both *P. quinquefolium* and *P. ginseng* can elevate cortisol levels due to its effect on the HPA axis.[103] Research in mice has resulted in normalising dopamine, noradrenaline and 5-hydroxytryptophan after chronic unpredictable stress when *P. quinquefolium* was given at an oral dose of 200 mg/kg, but not at 100 mg/kg.[104]

A much gentler, yet just as patent, adaptogen is ***Withania somnifera***. Its many qualities include a regulatory effect on the HPA axis by exerting a positive influence on the endocrine, nervous and cardiovascular systems. Main actions are adaptogenic, mildly sedative, anti-stress, immunomodulatory, trophorestorative, anti-inflammatory, anti-oxidant and rejuvenating.[11,84,97,105,106] Application includes convalescing after illness, fatigue and weakness.[79]

The Russian herb ***Rhodiola rosea*** belongs to the key adaptogenic herbs.[11,84,96,107] It has been used traditionally to alleviate symptoms of anxiety, insomnia and depression. Clinical trials have corroborated these findings.[108–111] *R. rosea* has been found to relieve fatigue,[112] increase work and exercise performance,[96,113] increase physical fitness and decrease mental fatigue in stressful situations.[114] It has therefore been used in asthenic conditions (conditions of weakness and debility, decline in function)[109] and chronic stress.[115] Apart from the actions described here there are many more benefits to be gained from this herb,[107,116] but they are beyond the scope of this chapter.

Other herbs with adaptogenic activity and stress control include ***Rehmannia glutinosa***,[81] ***Ocimum sanctum***,[84,117] ***Ginkgo biloba***[118] and ***Bacopa monnieri***.[119] The last two are also used for increasing cognitive function and concentration.[81]

Homoeopathy

In naturopathy in general and homoeopathy in particular, stress is not necessarily deemed 'bad', but only becomes 'negative' if it dominates our lives.[120,121] Homoeopathy has been used to treat stress and adrenal exhaustion, but remedies depend on the personal characteristics of the patient. The remedies are prescribed singly or in combination, and methods of determining the remedy include questionnaires, repertorisation and muscle testing.[122] The following remedies have been used in anxiety, where the symptom picture agrees: Arsenicum Album (Ars), Gelsemium (Gels), Argentum Nitricum (Arg-n), Lycopodium (Lyc) and Sulphur (Sulph).[123]

Nourishing depleted adrenals and reducing strain on HPA axis

A healthy diet, coupled with a balanced lifestyle and regular exercise, will help to settle imbalances in the stress cascade. To replenish depleted adrenals and neurotransmitters and nourish compromised physiology, select nutritional supplements could be indicated.

Nutritional supplements

To support depleted adrenal glands, nutrients such as **B vitamins** and **vitamin C** are essential. B vitamins and **coenzyme Q10** are cofactors in the Krebs cycle and oxidative phosphorylation (electron transport chain), respectively, which can be compromised (as is seen particularly in chronic fatigue syndrome). These nutrients may therefore be needed to increase energy production. **Magnesium** is a cofactor in energy production and needed for glucose regulation. It is best given with an organic ligand such as citrate for optimal bioavailability.[124,125]

Phenylalanine and **tyrosine** are precursors for dopamine, noradrenaline and adrenaline synthesis. Reduced dopamine levels have been implicated in impaired reward/punishment processing.[126,127] Precursors for serotonin and melatonin synthesis are tryptophan or 5-hydroxytryptophan (5HTP).[128] **Glutamine** is needed for GABA production.[45] Vitamins B2, B3 and B6 (ideally in the form of pyridoxyl 5-phosphate—PLP), folate, vitamins B12 and C, and minerals **iron**, **copper**, **calcium** and **zinc** are needed as cofactors for neurotransmitter synthesis (see Figures 15.2, 15.4 and 15.5). In depression, it may well be the synergy of these neurotransmitters and their cofactors that is unbalanced.[126] Ensuring their optimal supply in cellular metabolism seems mandatory for resilience to stress.

At a dose of 1500 mg/day vitamin C has reduced adrenaline, cortisol and anti-inflammatory peptides in stress,[129] thus showing a lowered stress response and allostatic load. Most animals (except primates, guinea pigs, fruit bats and some birds) produce their own vitamin C from glucose in response to a stressor, indicating that this vitamin is indeed essential for mounting an effective stress response.[45]

With high SNS and low PNS activity, digestion can be compromised due to suppression of digestive enzymes. When symptoms indicative of indigestion are reported by the patient, hydrochloric acid, pepsin and pancreatic enzymes with every meal may be indicated. These measures are taken in order to optimise digestive capacity.

With low digestive capacity, vitamin B12 absorption will also be affected due to insufficient or absent intrinsic factor.[130] It can be administered either as sublingual troches or by intramuscular injection by a health-care provider qualified to do so. Vitamin B12 plays an essential role in lowering homocysteine and providing methyl groups for neurotransmitter functioning.[131] Lack of vitamin B12 and folate have been linked to depression,[131] with vitamin B12 termed the 'master key' as it influences so many different systems. It may be needed even when serum levels appear normal.[132] Both nutrients are involved in **S-adenosyl methionine** (SAM or SAMe—SAMe is the brand name for SAM) production and are therefore crucial for methyl transfer. SAMe has been used quite successfully for depression.[128] Endogenously, it is made from homocysteine and requires vitamin B12, folate and adenosine as cofactors. If homocysteine is low methionine or SAMe need to be given as a substrate for methyl groups. SAM is the universal methyl donor and is needed for a range of metabolic reactions, including neurotransmitter production (see Figures 15.2 and 15.4, last step).

Omega-3 fatty acids have been indicated in depression[128] and are needed to support a healthy nervous system and brain function. Due to their anti-inflammatory properties they also dampen stress-induced cytokine activation.[133] Further, antioxidants such as vitamins A, C and E, the minerals selenium and zinc, as well as bioflavonoids, coenzyme Q10 and glutathione are required in higher amounts to combat free-radical damage and oxidative stress.[134–136]

Coenzyme Q10 (CoQ10) tends to be low when cortisol is low.[137] (Abnormal thyroid function can have an influence on CoQ10 levels and should be ruled out.)

The amino acids L-lysine and L-arginine have been shown to enhance ACTH, cortisol, adrenaline and noradrenaline levels in response to psychosocial stress and anxiety.[138]

INTEGRATIVE MEDICAL CONSIDERATIONS

Patients may respond well to talking about their problems if stress is due to known life circumstances. Sharing with friends or family members may help putting stress factors into perspective. Group therapy for depression may give a sense of not being alone with one's problems.

Mindfulness meditation[141,142] attempts to foster greater awareness of thought processes in the 'here and now' in order to increase coping ability. A meta-analysis has found that mindfulness-based stress reduction is indeed able to assist patients in dealing with both mental and physical stressors.[143] Other forms of meditation can be powerful adjuncts to positive thinking, as well as being able to reduce anxiety and pain, and to promote healing.[144]

Cognitive-behavioural therapy has been investigated and found to be a powerful instrument in stress-related health problems such as anxiety, depression, phobias and panic, anorexia and distress. Effects seen were comparable or superior to antidepressants and similar to other behavioural therapies.[145]

Other means to help with problem solving include imagery and creative visualisation.[73] Art and music therapy[146] have been shown to reduce stress, anxiety and pain. Spiritual or pastoral counselling may be needed if the stress is manifesting on the spiritual level.[147] Light therapy has been used successfully for depression,[128] especially for seasonal affective disorders.[3]

Acupuncture has been evaluated for its effect on stress modulation in connection with endothelial dysfunction. It was found that highly hypnotisable subjects responded much better to the procedure than less hypnotisable ones. The researchers concluded that the psychological state of the patient needs to be taken into account when choosing a relaxation method.[148] However, acupuncture may be beneficial to restore energy flows to depleted systems, notably the adrenals and the nervous system.

Massage (with or without aromatherapy),[149,150] reiki[151] and others[152] are means to reduce tension in the musculoskeletal as well as the nervous system due to stress. Touch is one of the most ancient ways of healing and has shown beneficial effects for anxiety and depression.[150] Progressive muscular relaxation, where sequential muscle groups are first tensed and then relaxed, is used to invoke a relaxation response.[73]

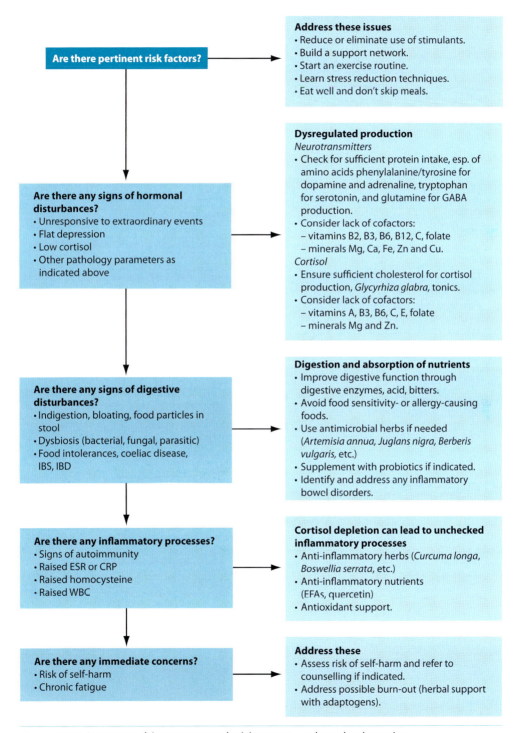

Are there pertinent risk factors?

Address these issues
• Reduce or eliminate use of stimulants.
• Build a support network.
• Start an exercise routine.
• Learn stress reduction techniques.
• Eat well and don't skip meals.

Are there any signs of hormonal disturbances?
• Unresponsive to extraordinary events
• Flat depression
• Low cortisol
• Other pathology parameters as indicated above

Dysregulated production
Neurotransmitters
• Check for sufficient protein intake, esp. of amino acids phenylalanine/tyrosine for dopamine and adrenaline, tryptophan for serotonin, and glutamine for GABA production.
• Consider lack of cofactors:
  – vitamins B2, B3, B6, B12, C, folate
  – minerals Mg, Ca, Fe, Zn and Cu.
Cortisol
• Ensure sufficient cholesterol for cortisol production, *Glycyrhiza glabra*, tonics.
• Consider lack of cofactors:
  – vitamins A, B3, B6, C, E, folate
  – minerals Mg and Zn.

Are there any signs of digestive disturbances?
• Indigestion, bloating, food particles in stool
• Dysbiosis (bacterial, fungal, parasitic)
• Food intolerances, coeliac disease, IBS, IBD

Digestion and absorption of nutrients
• Improve digestive function through digestive enzymes, acid, bitters.
• Avoid food sensitivity- or allergy-causing foods.
• Use antimicrobial herbs if needed (*Artemisia annua, Juglans nigra, Berberis vulgaris,* etc.)
• Supplement with probiotics if indicated.
• Identify and address any inflammatory bowel disorders.

Are there any inflammatory processes?
• Signs of autoimmunity
• Raised ESR or CRP
• Raised homocysteine
• Raised WBC

Cortisol depletion can lead to unchecked inflammatory processes
• Anti-inflammatory herbs (*Curcuma longa, Boswellia serrata,* etc.)
• Anti-inflammatory nutrients (FFAs, quercetin)
• Antioxidant support.

Are there any immediate concerns?
• Risk of self-harm
• Chronic fatigue

Address these
• Assess risk of self-harm and refer to counselling if indicated.
• Address possible burn-out (herbal support with adaptogens).

Figure 15.6 Naturopathic treatment decision tree—adrenal exhaustion

CORTISOL EXCESS

- During a sustained alarm stress phase (adaptation phase), cortisol output is increased and this may deleteriously affect many systems, causing a variety of health disorders (detailed above in the aetiology section).
- People with excess cortisol may present with a comorbid clinical picture involving psychiatric disorders (especially melancholic depression, insomnia), poor immunity, hormonal or metabolic disturbance (such as abdominal obesity and insulin resistance) and cardiovascular problems (particularly hypertension and dyslipidaemia).[139]
- Cortisol levels can be confirmed via a serum, urinary or salivary cortisol test.
- Treatment protocols involve using interventions that reduce cortisol production and serum levels.
- CAM interventions include:
  - lifestyle changes to reduce stress, improve sleep and reduce stimulants
  - herbal medicines that may reduce cortisol, including *Rehmannia glutinosa*[81] and *Panax ginseng*[140]
  - regulation of CRH and HPA axis, achieved by adaptogens due to their very nature to increase stress hormones if they are too low and decrease these hormones if they are too high[11,12]
  - nutrients that may regulate HPA function and may be beneficial in reducing cortisol include vitamin C.[129]
- *Glycyrrhiza glabra* should be avoided in cases of cortisol excess. It may increase glucocorticoid levels and worsen the patient's condition.

Case Study

A 35-year-old female presents with **gradual onset of tiredness** over the past year. Prior to this she had been **working long hours** in a corporate enterprise before her husband was offered an interstate job. She found the transit difficult as she **lost her support system** of family and friends.

Currently, she is struggling to hold down her full-time job as company secretary, and at home her husband now does most of the housework. In order to cope with work she **retires at 8 p.m. and wakes at 7 a.m. unrefreshed**. She feels there is **less enjoyment in her life**. At work she **cannot concentrate** and **tends to forget** even routine activities. She **craves sweet** and **starchy foods** (leading to some weight gain) and **drinks 10–12 cups of coffee a day** in order to stay somewhat alert. A psychiatric assessment has ruled out major depressive disorder, and medical tests have not revealed any major pathology.

SUGGESTIVE SYMPTOMS

- Tiredness
- Waking unrefreshed
- Weight gain
- Depression

- Lack of concentration
- Memory loss
- Stimulant use

Confirming the diagnosis

This patient has been exposed to a number of stress factors, including a demanding job in the past, a shift to another state and loss of her personal support system. She has used stimulants, such as coffee, and carbohydrate-rich foods in order to increase adrenal

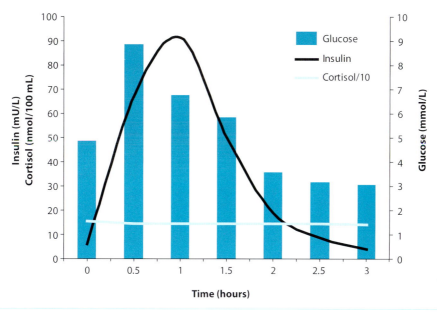

Figure 15.7 Glucose tolerance test demonstrating insulin resistance and unresponsive cortisol to hypoglycaemia

output and energy levels, in an attempt to feel better. At the time of the consultation these means of 'self-medication' did not have the desired effect any more.

The obvious diagnosis for this patient is adrenal exhaustion. To verify this, the following tests were requested: multiple biochemical analysis (MBA) including liver function test (LFT) and CRP, a full blood count (FBC) including ESR, homocysteine and its cofactors folate (in RBC) and vitamin B12 (active B12—holotranscobalamin II), cortisol at 8 a.m. and 4 p.m., ACTH at 8 a.m., lipid studies and glucose tolerance (as outlined above).

The diagnosis of adrenal exhaustion was confirmed by low urea (indicative of reduced protein intake and/or absorption), low cortisol both morning and afternoon, high to normal homocysteine and low to normal vitamin B12 (indicative of impaired methylation), high cholesterol and borderline high triglycerides. GTT revealed elevated insulin with delayed response to glucose (indicative of mild insulin resistance), followed by hypoglycaemia. Cortisol was low with no noticeable change throughout and unresponsive to a below normal glucose level (Figure 15.7). All other parameters were normal.

Example treatment

The following options were discussed with the patient:

- *social*: make an effort to mix with people, e.g. join a club or local group, invite the neighbours.
- *physical activity*: find an enjoyable exercise and do this at least five times a week.
- *physical therapies*: treat herself to a regular massage.
- *mind therapies*: find someone to talk to (husband, friend, workmate) who would not judge her for what she said.
- *miscellaneous therapies*: find a hobby she enjoyed doing.

At the first consultation, the patient was given advice on diet changes, as outlined above. In order to increase omega-3 fatty acids she was advised to have five fish meals a week. A smoothie with protein powder, to be consumed once a day in addition to her regular meals, was recommended. Emphasis was on low glycaemic load and additional protein for better glucose sugar balance and increased nutrients, especially amino acids as precursors for neurotransmitter synthesis.

Lifestyle options were discussed. As a result, the patient and her husband decided to join a local dance group to combine exercise with social outings. At work she was going to join some colleagues for their daily 20-minute walk at lunchtime. The idea of meditation did not appeal to her but she agreed to set aside 15 minutes at the end of each day for reflection and journalising.

Herbal treatment

To strengthen her system overall, with particular focus on the adrenal glands and low moods, a herbal formula was prescribed containing *Rhodiola rosea* to increase mental and physical stamina,[107,115] *Glycyrrhiza glabra* to increase cortisol and adrenal output,[77,80] *Hypericum perforatum* to decrease the reuptake of dopamine and noradrenaline[153] (see also the section on the nervous system) and *Bacopa monnieri* to increase concentration and memory.[119,154]

Nutritional treatment

Additionally, nutritional supplements were prescribed to replenish cellular nutrient depletion. Tyrosine was given to increase dopamine–adrenaline synthesis,[45] and to improve mood and the ability to experience pleasure.[126] B vitamins with PLP and high amounts of folate and vitamin B12 were given to increase Krebs cycle cofactors for energy production[45] and to provide essential nutrients for methylation.[131,155–157] Further, CoQ10 was added for energy production in the electron transport chain,[45,137] and magnesium (as citrate)[124] due to its role in the Krebs cycle[45] and for blood glucose regulation.[158]

Herbal formula	
Rhodiola rosea 2:1	30 mL
Glycyrrhiza glabra 1:1	15 mL
Hypericum perforatum 1:2	20 mL
Bacopa monnieri 1:2	35 mL
5 mL b.d.	100 mL
Nutritional prescription	
Tyrosine 500 mg t.d.s.	
B complex with PLP, high folate and B12 1 tablet b.d.	
CoQ10 100 mg/day	
Magnesium (as citrate) 300 mg/day	

Expected outcomes and follow-up protocols

As can be seen from the list of possible treatments (detailed under the 'Key treatment protocols' section), both herbally and nutritionally, there is scope for changing the treatment should the current prescription fail to produce the desired results (improved mood, energy and coping ability). In cases like the one described here, both physical and mental/emotional symptoms are present and need to be taken into consideration in the design of a treatment plan. The connection between psychological, neurological and endocrine symptoms is now well established in disciplines such as psychoneuro-endocrinology.[159] This patient should respond very favourably to treatment, due to her own commitment and her husband's support. Neither the dietary changes, nor the prescriptions nor the increased social activities on their own would have resulted in the great improvement seen in this case. Willingness to change both attitudes and habits has been the recipe for success. However, in longer-standing problems (as is the case in chronic fatigue), cellular metabolism is further compromised with potential oxidative damage to the brain, as well as the development of a range of chronic diseases.[5,17] Treatment in that case would be more comprehensive and extended over a longer time span.

Allostatic load can be modified and even reversed. People who can ward off allostatic load best tend to have the following attributes: a positive mental attitude, acceptance of themselves and others, fulfilling relationships yet are able to retain their own autonomy, beliefs and principles which they defend, the ability to create and shape their own environment conducive to their needs for health and happiness, a purpose in life and a sense of personal growth. They can pursue their goals and realise their potential.[3] They have good nutritional status and a balanced lifestyle. In short, they are well resourced mentally and physically to withstand stress.

Table 15.4 Review of the major evidence

INTERVENTION	METHODOLOGY	RESULT	COMMENT
Diet[42]	Comparative study 22 high stress prone (HS), 23 low stress prone (LS) subjects submitted to stressful situations and high CHO/low protein or low CHO/high protein diets	Only in uncontrollable stress in HS subjects, the high CHO/low protein diet reduced stress parameters.	The results were attributed to the CHO-rich diet being high in tryptophan. However, the long-term effects of a CHO-rich diet could be dysglycaemia, potentially leading to insulin resistance and metabolic syndrome (which is a known flow-on effect of stress).[160]
Meditation[144]	8 weeks 2 hours/day 2-arm (intervention and waiting list)	Significant improvements on 8 measures of health outcome on stress and mental health at 8 weeks, and at 19 weeks	Since this trial was an open study a placebo effect cannot be ruled out.
Pharmaton®[161] (multivitamin and mineral formulation with *Panax ginseng*)	RCT 42 days, 2-arm ($n = 232$)	Fatigue scores reduced from 9.3 to 2.8 in Pharmaton group and from 9.5 to 3.7 in the placebo group	Although there is a significant effect of Pharmaton, there also appears to be a highly significant placebo effect.
Panax ginseng[162]	RCT 12 weeks ($n = 60$, aged 22–80) 200 mg extract (≈ 1 g root)	Significant improvements in visual and auditory reaction times and recovery from physical exercise	Several trials have shown no benefit over placebo regarding performance; this could be due to their shorter duration. However, most trials done on athletes have shown improvements in stamina.[163]

(Continued)

Table 15.4 Review of the major evidence *(Continued)*

INTERVENTION	METHODOLOGY	RESULT	COMMENT
Panax ginseng[164]	RCT 16 weeks, 2-arm (*n* = 193 active, *n* = 191 placebo) postmenopausal women	Significant improvements in psychological general wellbeing, depression and health	Postmenopausal symptoms did not improve, ruling out a hormonal effect of *Panax.*
Eleutherococcus senticosus[165]	RCT 8 weeks, 2-arm (*n* = 20, aged ≥ 65 years, hypertensive) – 300 mg/day dry extract Short form—36 health survey version 2 (SF-36v2) at baseline, weeks 4 and 8	Significant differences in social functioning between treatment and placebo groups at 4 weeks but not at 8 weeks. No difference in blood pressure	Long-term use seems to attenuate the benefits.
Rhodiola rosea[108]	Pilot study 10 weeks, 1-arm (*n* = 10, aged 34–55 years) – 340 mg/day	Significant improvements in generalised anxiety disorder as measured by the Hamilton Anxiety Rating Scale (HARS).	This is a rather small study and will need to be corroborated in a larger trial.
Rhodiola rosea[111]	RCT 6 weeks, 3 arms (*n* = 89) – 340 mg – 680 mg – placebo 2 depression scales used	Significant reductions in depression were seen, in particular for insomnia, emotional instability and somatisation (physical symptoms caused by mental or emotional factors).	This shows that *Rhodiola* exerts its therapeutic effects in relatively small doses in a time span comparable to antidepressant drugs. Self-esteem was also measured but did not differ from placebo.
Bacopa monnieri[166]	RCT 6 weeks, 2 arms (*n* = 46) – *Bacopa* extract (300 mg/day) – placebo	Significant improvements in: • inspection time • learning rate • memory consolidation. Decrease in forgetting rate	Although the study focused on learning and memory, a significant decrease in anxiety was also noted.
Tyrosine[127]	RCT—crossover 1 dose either complete or tyrosine-free amino acid mix. Neuropsychological test battery after 5 hours (*n* = 40)	Tyrosine-free group demonstrated sad latency bias consistent with depression	As this was a one dose only trial long-term effects of tyrosine depletion need to be investigated

Note: It is difficult to find evidence in form of RCTs for most of the above-mentioned nutritional and herbal interventions. Herbal treatment has predominantly traditional evidence, and nutrient evidence usually is extrapolated from biochemical pathway studies.

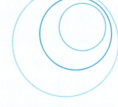

KEY POINTS

- Stress activates the hypothalamus–pituitary–adrenal (HPA) axis and triggers the release of a cascade of hormones and neurotransmitters, notably adrenaline and cortisol.
- With prolonged stress these substances can become exhausted, leading to a gradual decline of adrenal function and neurotransmitters, and finally to a state of adrenal and mental exhaustion.
- This can lead to a range of pathologies that cannot be successfully treated unless the underlying HPA dysregulation has been addressed.
- Practitioners need to discern between the alarm, adaptation and exhaustion phases, and test for the presence of either high or low cortisol levels.
- Treatment needs to focus on both the physical and the mental/emotional aspects of stress.

Further reading

Jefferies W. Safe uses of cortisol. 2nd edn. Springfield: Charles C. Thomas, 1996.

McEwen BS, Lasley EN. The end of stress as we know it. Washington: Dana Press and Joseph Henry Press, 2002.

Wilson J. Adrenal fatigue: the 21st-century stress syndrome. Smart Publications 2002.

References

1. Selye H. Stress without distress. London: Hodder and Stoughton, 1974:27.
2. Thibodeau G, Patton K. Anatomy and physiology. 5th edn. St Louis: Mosby, 2003:Chapter 22.
3. McEwen BS. The end of stress as we know it. Washington: The Dana Press (Joseph Henry Press), 2002.
4. McEwen BS. Interacting mediators of allostasis and allostatic load: towards an understanding of resilience in aging. Metabolism 2003;52(10 Suppl 2):10–16.
5. McEwen BS. Protection and damage from acute and chronic stress: allostasis and allostatic overload and relevance to the pathophysiology of psychiatric disorders. Ann N Y Acad Sci 2004;1032:1–7.
6. Tsigos C, Chrousos GP. Hypothalamic-pituitary-adrenal axis, neuroendocrine factors and stress. J Psychosom Res 2002;53(4):865–871.
7. Miller DB, O'Callaghan JP. Neuroendocrine aspects of the response to stress. Metabolism 2002;51(6 Suppl 1):5–10.
8. Vanitallie TB. Stress: a risk factor for serious illness. Metabolism 2002;51(6 Suppl 1):40–45.
9. Haddad JJ, et al. Cytokines and neuro-immune-endocrine interactions: a role for the hypothalamic-pituitary-adrenal revolving axis. J Neuroimmunol 2002;133(1–2):1–19.
10. Eskandari F, Sternberg EM. Neural-immune interactions in health and disease. Ann N Y Acad Sci 2002;966:20–27.
11. Wilson L. Review of adaptogenic mechanisms: *Eleutherococcus senticosus, Panax ginseng, Rhodiola rosea, Schisandra chinensis* and *Withania somnifera*. Australian Journal of Medical Herbalism 2007;19(3):126–138.
12. Gaffney BT, et al. The effects of *Eleutherococcus senticosus* and *Panax ginseng* on steroidal hormone indices of stress and lymphocyte subset numbers in endurance athletes. Life Sci 2001;70(4):431–442.
13. Cutolo M, et al. Hypothalamic-pituitary-adrenocortical and gonadal functions in rheumatoid arthritis. Ann N Y Acad Sci 2003;992:107–117.
14. Loucks AB, Redman LM. The effect of stress on menstrual function. Trends Endocrinol Metab 2004;15(10):466–471.
15. Gilad GM, Gilad VH. Overview of the brain polyamine-stress-response: regulation, development, and modulation by lithium and role in cell survival. Cell Mol Neurobiol 2003;23(4–5):637–649.
16. Goldstein DS, McEwen B. Allostasis, homeostasis, and the nature of stress. Stress 2002;5(1):55–58.
17. McEwen BS. Sex, stress and the hippocampus: allostasis, allostatic load and the aging process. Neurobiol Aging 2002;23(5):921–939.
18. McEwen BS. Stressed or stressed out: what is the difference? J Psychiatry Neurosci 2005;30(5):315–318.
19. McEwen B, Lasley EN. Allostatic load: when protection gives way to damage. Adv Mind Body Med 2003;19(1):28–33.
20. Abercrombie HC, et al. Flattened cortisol rhythms in metastatic breast cancer patients. Psychoneuroendocrinology 2004;29(8):1082–1092.
21. King A, et al. Attenuated cortisol response to alcohol in heavy social drinkers. Int J Psychophysiol 2006;59(3):203–209.
22. Meyer G, et al. Casino gambling increases heart rate and salivary cortisol in regular gamblers. Biol Psychiatry 2000;48(9):948–953.
23. Lovallo WR. Cortisol secretion patterns in addiction and addiction risk. Int J Psychophysiol 2006;59(3):195–202.
24. Hellhammer J, et al. Allostatic load, perceived stress, and health: a prospective study in two age groups. Ann N Y Acad Sci 2004;1032:8–13.
25. McEwen BS. Early life influences on life-long patterns of behavior and health. Ment Retard Dev Disabil Res Rev 2003;9(3):149–154.
26. Korte SM, et al. The Darwinian concept of stress: benefits of allostasis and costs of allostatic load and the trade-offs in health and disease. Neurosci Biobehav Rev 2005;29(1):3–38.
27. McEwen BS. Mood disorders and allostatic load. Biol Psychiatry 2003;54(3):200–207.
28. Carroll BJ. Ageing, stress and the brain. Novartis Found Symp 2002;242:26–36:discussion –45.

29. Weaver JD, et al. Interleukin-6 and risk of cognitive decline: MacArthur studies of successful aging. Neurology 2002;59(3):371–378.
30. Angeli A, et al. The overtraining syndrome in athletes: a stress-related disorder. J Endocrinol Invest 2004;27(6):603–612.
31. Jefferies WM. Cortisol and immunity. Med Hypotheses 1991;34(3):198–208.
32. Butcher SK, et al. Raised cortisol:DHEAS ratios in the elderly after injury: potential impact upon neutrophil function and immunity. Aging Cell 2005;4(6):319–324.
33. Mechanick JI. Metabolic mechanisms of stress hyperglycemia. J Parenter Enteral Nutr 2006;30(2):157–163.
34. Maloney EM, et al. Chronic fatigue syndrome and high allostatic load. Pharmacogenomics 2006;7(3):467–473.
35. Björntorp P, Rosmond R. The metabolic syndrome—a neuroendocrine disorder? Br J Nutr 2000;83(Suppl 1):S49–S57.
36. Nieuwenhuizen AG, Rutters F. The hypothalamic-pituitary-adrenal-axis in the regulation of energy balance. Physiol Behav 2008;94(2):169–177.
37. Kalantaridou SN, et al. Stress and the female reproductive system. J Reprod Immunol 2004;62(1–2):61–68.
38. Anderson KN, ed. Mosby's medical, nursing and allied health dictionary. 6th edn. St Louis, London: CV Mosby, 2002.
39. Demitrack MA, Crofford LJ. Evidence for and pathophysiologic implications of hypothalamic-pituitary-adrenal axis dysregulation in fibromyalgia and chronic fatigue syndrome. Ann N Y Acad Sci 1998;840:684–697.
40. Harbuz M. Neuroendocrine function and chronic inflammatory stress. Exp Physiol 2002;87(5):519–525.
41. Berridge KC. Motivation concepts in behavioral neuroscience. Physiol Behav 2004;81(2):179–209.
42. Markus R, et al. Effects of food on cortisol and mood in vulnerable subjects under controllable and uncontrollable stress. Physiol Behav 2000;70(3–4):333–342.
43. Takeda E, et al. Stress control and human nutrition. J Med Invest 2004;51(3–4):139–145.
44. Christensen L, Brooks A. Changing food preference as a function of mood. J Psychol 2006;140(4):293–306.
45. Gropper S, et al. Advanced nutrition and human metabolism. 5th edn. Australia: Wadsworth: Cengage Learning, 2009.
46. Anderson DC. Assessment and nutraceutical management of stress-induced adrenal dysfunction. Integrative Medicine: A Clinician's Journal 2008;7(5):18–25.
47. Pagana KD, Pagana TJ. Mosby's manual of diagnostic and laboratory tests. 3rd edn USA: CV Mosby, 2006.
48. Giordano R, et al. Hypothalamus-pituitary-adrenal axis evaluation in patients with hypothalamo-pituitary disorders: comparison of different provocative tests. Clin Endocrinol 2008;68(6):935–941.
49. Thibodeau G, Patton K. Anatomy and physiology. 5th edn. St Louis, London: CV Mosby, 2003.
50. Papadelis C, et al. Effects of mental workload and caffeine on catecholamines and blood pressure compared to performance variations. Brain Cogni 2003;51(1):143–154.
51. Lane JD, et al. Caffeine affects cardiovascular and neuroendocrine activation at work and home. Psychosom Med 2002;64(4):595–603.
52. Crowley IV. An introduction to human disease: pathology and pathophysiology correlations. 6th edn. Sudbury: Jones and Bartlett Publishers, 2004.
53. Giordano R, et al. Corticotrope hypersecretion coupled with cortisol hypo-responsiveness to stimuli is present in patients with autoimmune endocrine diseases: evidence for subclinical primary hypoadrenalism? Eur J Endocrinol 2006;155(3):421–428.
54. Debono M, Ross RJ. Doses and steroids to be used in primary and central hypoadrenalism. Ann Endocrinol (Paris) 2007;68(4):265–267.
55. Barbetta L, et al. Comparison of different regimens of glucocorticoid replacement therapy in patients with hypoadrenalism. J Endocrinol Invest 2005;28(7):632–637.
56. Libè R, et al. Effects of dehydroepiandrosterone (DHEA) supplementation on hormonal, metabolic and behavioral status in patients with hypoadrenalism. J Endocrinol Invest 2004;27(8):736–741.
57. Bhagra S, et al. Dehydroepiandrosterone in adrenal insufficiency and ageing. Curr Opin Endocrinol Diabetes Obes 2008;15(3):239–243.
58. Giordano G, et al. Variations of pituitary function over time after brain injuries: the lesson from a prospective study. Pituitary 2005;8(3–4):227–231.
59. Beishuizen A, Thijs LG. The immunoneuroendocrine axis in critical illness: beneficial adaptation or neuroendocrine exhaustion? Curr Opin Crit Care 2004;10(6):461–467.
60. Marik PE. Adrenal-exhaustion syndrome in patients with liver disease. Intensive Care Med 2006;32(2):275–280.
61. Omori K, et al. Risk factors for adrenal crisis in patients with adrenal insufficiency. Endocr J 2003;50(6):745–752.
62. Ströhle A. [The neuroendocrinology of stress and the pathophysiology and therapy of depression and anxiety]. Nervenarzt 2003;74(3):279–291:quiz 292.
63. Cortese BM, Phan KL. The role of glutamate in anxiety and related disorders. CNS Spectr 2005;10(10):820–830.
64. Ströhle A, Holsboer F. Stress responsive neurohormones in depression and anxiety. Pharmacopsychiatry 2003;36(Suppl 3):S207–S214.
65. Chiericetti SM, et al. Beta-blockers and psychic stress: a double-blind, placebo-controlled study of bopindolol vs lorazepam and butalbital in surgical patients. Int J Clin Pharmacol Ther Toxicol 1985;23(9):510–514.
66. Schweizer R, et al. Effect of two beta-blockers on stress during mental arithmetic. Psychopharmacology 1991;105(4):573–577.
67. De Kloet ER, Derijk R. Signaling pathways in brain involved in predisposition and pathogenesis of stress-related disease: genetic and kinetic factors affecting the MR/GR balance. Ann N YAcad Sci 2004;1032:14–34.
68. Mukherjee A. Fight stress with food. McClatchy-Tribune Business News 2008.
69. Golub MS. The adrenal and the metabolic syndrome. Curr Hypertens Rep 2001;3(2):117–120.
70. Epel E, et al. Are stress eaters at risk for the metabolic syndrome? Ann N Y Acad Sci 2004;1032:208–210.
71. Kopp MS, Rethelyi J. Where psychology meets physiology: chronic stress and premature mortality—the Central-Eastern European health paradox. Brain Res Bull 2004;62(5):351–367.
72. Singer B, et al. Protective environments and health status: cross-talk between human and animal studies. Neurobiol Aging 2005;26(Suppl 1):113–118.
73. Eliopulous C. Invitation to holistic health. Boston: Jones and Bartlett Publishers, 2004.
74. Stear S. Health and fitness series—1. The importance of physical activity for health. J Fam Health Care 2003;13(1):10–13.
75. Duax WL, et al. Steroid dehydrogenase structures, mechanism of action, and disease. Vitam Horm 2000;58:121–148.
76. Kohlmeier M. Nutrient metabolism. Amsterdam: Academic Press, 2003.
77. Braun L, Cohen M. Herbs and natural supplements. 2nd edn. Sydney: Churchill Livingstone, 2007.
78. Kato H, et al. 3-monoglucuronyl-glycyrrhetinic acid is a major metabolite that causes licorice-induced pseudoaldosteronism. J Clin Endocrinol Metab 1995;80(6):1929–1933.
79. Morgan M, Bone K. Herbs with tonic, adaptogenic, adrenal tonic and nervine activity. Phytotherapist Perspectiv 2005:58.
80. Armanini D, et al. History of the endocrine effects of licorice. Exp Clin Endocrinol Diabetes 2002;110(6):257–261.
81. Bone K. A clinical guide to blending liquid herbs. USA: Elsevier, 2003.

82. Blumenthal M. The ABC clinical guide to herbs. Austin: American Botanical Council, 2003.
83. Mills S, Bone K. Principles and practice of phytotherapy. Sydney: Churchill Livingstone, 2000.
84. Rege NN, et al. Adaptogenic properties of six rasayana herbs used in Ayurvedic medicine. Phytother Res 1999;13(4):275–291.
85. Mills S, Bone K. The essential guide to herbal safety. USA: Elsevier, 2005.
86. Kraft K, Hobbs C. Pocket guide to herbal medicine. New York: Thieme, 2004.
87. Basch EM, Ulbricht CE. Natural standard herb and supplement handbook. Boston: Elsevier, 2005.
88. Harkness R, Bratman S. Mosby's handbook of drug-herb and drug-supplement interactions. Sydney: CV Mosby, 2003.
89. Blumenthal M. The complete German Commission E monographs: therapeutic guide to herbal medicines [CD-ROM]. Austin, Texas: American Botanical Council, 1999.
90. Burgoyne B. Herbal treatment of insomnia. Modern Phytotherapist 2002;7(1):12–21.
91. Herrera-Arellano A, et al. Polysomnographic evaluation of the hypnotic effect of *Valeriana edulis* standardized extract in patients suffering from insomnia. Planta Med 2001;67(8):695–699.
92. Teschke R, et al. Kava hepatotoxicity: a European view. N Z Med J 2008;121(1283):90–98.
93. Lüde S, et al. Hepatocellular toxicity of kava leaf and root extracts. Phytomedicine 2008;15(1–2):120–131.
94. Loew D, Gaus W. Kava-Kava: Tragödie einer Fehlbeurteilung. Erfahrungsheilkunde 2003;52(6):386.
95. Bone K. Rhodiola. Clinical Monitor 2008;23:1–2.
96. Panossian A, Wagner H. Stimulating effect of adaptogens: an overview with particular reference to their efficacy following single dose administration. Phytother Res 2005;19(10):819–838.
97. Morgan M. Withania, ginseng: gentle tonic and adaptogenic. Phytotherapist Perspective 2005;59.
98. Beyer I, Rimpler M. Ginseng: Adaptogenität zur Umstimmungstherapie—Teil 2. Biologische Medizin 1996;25(4):151.
99. Beyer I, Rimpler M. Ginseng: Adaptogenität zur Umstimmungstherapie—Teil 1. Biologische Medizin 1996;25(3):98.
100. Baranov AI. Medicinal uses of ginseng and related plants in the Soviet Union: recent trends in the Soviet literature. J Ethnopharmacol 1982;6(3):339–353.
101. Kimura Y, Sumiyoshi M. Effects of various *Eleutherococcus senticosus* cortex on swimming time, natural killer activity and corticosterone level in forced swimming stressed mice. J Ethnopharmacol 2004,95(2–3):447–453.
102. Kitts D, Hu C. Efficacy and safety of ginseng. Public Health Nutr 2000;3(4A):473–485.
103. Nocerino E, et al. The aphrodisiac and adaptogenic properties of ginseng. Fitoterapia 2000;71(Suppl 1):S1–S5.
104. Rasheed N, et al. Involvement of monoamines and proinflammatory cytokines in mediating the anti-stress effects of Panax quinquefolium. J Ethnopharmacol 2008;117(2):257–262.
105. Lindner S. *Withania somnifera*: winter cherry, Indian ginseng, ashwagandha. Australian Journal of Medical Herbalism 1996;8(3):78.
106. Mishra LC, et al. Scientific basis for the therapeutic use of *Withania somnifera* (ashwagandha): a review. Altern Med Rev 2000;5(4):334–346.
107. Morgan M, Bone K. *Rhodiola rosea*—rhodiola. Mediherb Newsletter 2005:47.
108. Bystritsky A, et al. A pilot study of *Rhodiola rosea* (Rhodax) for generalized anxiety disorder (GAD). J Altern Complement Med 2008;14(2):175–180.
109. Kelly GS. *Rhodiola rosea*: a possible plant adaptogen. Altern Med Rev 2001;6(3):293–302.
110. Sarris J. Herbal medicines in the treatment of psychiatric disorders: a systematic review. Phytother Res 2007;21(8):703–716.
111. Darbinyan V, et al. Clinical trial of *Rhodiola rosea* L. extract SHR-5 in the treatment of mild to moderate depression. Nord J Psychiatry 2007;61(5):343–348.
112. Shevtsov VA, et al. A randomized trial of two different doses of a SHR-5 *Rhodiola rosea* extract versus placebo and control of capacity for mental work. Phytomedicine 2003;10(2–3):95–105.
113. De Bock K, et al. Acute *Rhodiola rosea* intake can improve endurance exercise performance. Int J Sport Nutr Exerc Metab 2004;14(3):298–307.
114. Spasov AA, et al. A double-blind, placebo-controlled pilot study of the stimulating and adaptogenic effect of *Rhodiola rosea* SHR-5 extract on the fatigue of students caused by stress during an examination period with a repeated low-dose regimen. Phytomedicine 2000;7(2):85–89.
115. *Rhodiola rosea*. Monograph. Altern Med Rev 2002;7(5):421–423.
116. Brown RP, et al. *Rhodiola rosea*: a phytomedicinal overview. HerbalGram 2002;56:40–52.
117. Morgan M. Holy Basil. Phytotherapist Perspective 2001;19:1–3.
118. Shirai M, et al. Approach to novel functional foods for stress control 5. Antioxidant activity profiles of antidepressant herbs and their active components. J Med Invest 2005;52(Suppl):249–251.
119. Rai D, et al. Adaptogenic effect of *Bacopa monniera* (brahmi). Pharmacol Biochem Behav 2003;75(4):823–830.
120. Dew JM. Homoeopathy and the effects of stress. Homoeopathy 1996;46(3):50.
121. Duelli N. Suffer less from stress: homeopathy can help. Alive: Canadian Journal of Health and Nutrition 2005(271):72–73.
122. King F. Homeopathy. Exploring the hypoadrenia-homeopathy link. Chiropr J 1991;5(11):40.
123. Davidson J, et al. Multivariate analysis of five homoeopathic medicines in a psychiatric population. Br Homoeopath J 1995;84(4):195.
124. Lindberg JS, et al. Magnesium bioavailability from magnesium citrate and magnesium oxide. J Am Coll Nutr 1990;9(1):48–55.
125. Walker AF, et al. Mg citrate found more bioavailable than other Mg preparations in a randomised, double-blind study. Magnes Res 2003;16(3):183–191.
126. Roiser JP, et al. The subjective and cognitive effects of acute phenylalanine and tyrosine depletion in patients recovered from depression. Neuropsychopharmacology 2005;30(4):775–785.
127. McLean A, et al. The effects of tyrosine depletion in normal healthy volunteers: implications for unipolar depression. Psychopharmacology 2004;171(3):286–297.
128. Freeman MP, et al. Selected integrative medicine treatments for depression: considerations for women. J Am Med Women's Assoc 2004;59(3):216–224.
129. Peters EM, et al. Vitamin C supplementation attenuates the increases in circulating cortisol, adrenaline and anti-inflammatory polypeptides following ultramarathon running. Int J Sports Med 2001;22(7):537–543.
130. Rufenacht P, et al. [Vitamin B12 deficiency: a challenging diagnosis and treatment]. Rev Méd Suisse 2008;4(175):2212.
131. Coppen A, Bolander-Gouaille C. Treatment of depression: time to consider folic acid and vitamin B12. J Psychopharmacol 2005;19(1):59–65.
132. Volkov I, et al. Vitamin B12 could be a 'master key' in the regulation of multiple pathological processes. J Nippon Med Sch 2006;73(2):65–69.
133. Kidd P. Th1/Th2 balance: the hypothesis, its limitations, and implications for health and disease. Altern Med Rev 2003;8(3):223–246.

134. Urso ML, Clarkson PM. Oxidative stress, exercise, and antioxidant supplementation. Toxicology 2003;189(1–2):41–54.
135. Mayne ST. Antioxidant nutrients and chronic disease: use of biomarkers of exposure and oxidative stress status in epidemiologic research. J Nutr 2003;133(Suppl 3):933S–940S.
136. Dhanasekaran M, Ren J. The emerging role of coenzyme Q-10 in aging, neurodegeneration, cardiovascular disease, cancer and diabetes mellitus. Curr Neurovasc Res 2005;2(5):447–459.
137. Mancini A, et al. Coenzyme Q10 evaluation in pituitary-adrenal axis disease: preliminary data. Biofactors 2005;25(1–4):197–199.
138. Jezova D, et al. Subchronic treatment with amino acid mixture of L-lysine and L-arginine modifies neuroendocrine activation during psychosocial stress in subjects with high trait anxiety. Nutr Neurosci 2005;8(3):155–160.
139. Putignano P, et al. Tissue-specific dysregulation of 11 beta-hydroxysteroid dehydrogenase type 1 and pathogenesis of the metabolic syndrome. J Endocrinol Invest 2004;27(10):969–974.
140. Tode T, et al. Effect of Korean red ginseng on psychological functions in patients with severe climacteric syndromes. Int J Gynaecol Obstet 1999;67(3):169–174.
141. Adelman EM. Mind-body intelligence: a new perspective integrating eastern and western healing traditions. Holist Nurs Pract 2006;20(3):147–151.
142. Shigaki CL, et al. Mindfulness-based stress reduction in medical settings. J Clin Psychol Med Settings 2006;13(3):209–216.
143. Grossman P, et al. Mindfulness-based stress reduction and health benefits—a meta-analysis. J Psychosom Res 2004;57(1):35–43.
144. Oman D, et al. Passage meditation reduces perceived stress in health professionals: a randomized, controlled trial. J Consult Clin Psychol 2006;74(4):714–719.
145. Butler AC, et al. The empirical status of cognitive-behavioral therapy: a review of meta-analyses. Clin Psychol Rev 2006;26(1):17–31.
146. Pratt RR. Art, dance, and music therapy. Phys Med Rehabil Clin N Am 2004;15(4):827–841.
147. Pronk K. Role of the doctor in relieving spiritual distress at the end of life. Am J Hosp Palliat Care 2005;22(6):419–425.
148. Jambrik Z, et al. Traditional acupuncture does not modulate the endothelial dysfunction induced by mental stress. Int J Cardiovasc Imaging 2004;20(5):357–362.
149. Murakami S, et al. Aromatherapy for outpatients with menopausal symptoms in obstetrics and gynecology. J Altern Complement Med 2005;11(3):491–494.
150. Robson T. An introduction to complementary medicine. Sydney: Allen & Unwin, 2003.
151. Burden B, et al. The increasing use of reiki as a complementary therapy in specialist palliative care. Int J Palliat Nurs 2005;11(5):248–253.
152. Long L, et al. Which complementary and alternative therapies benefit which conditions? A survey of the opinions of 223 professional organizations. Complement Ther Med 2001;9(3):178–185.
153. Rodríguez-Landa JF, Contreras CM. A review of clinical and experimental observations about antidepressant actions and side effects produced by Hypericum perforatum extracts. Phytomedicine 2003;10(8):688–699.
154. Kidd PM. A review of nutrients and botanicals in the integrative management of cognitive dysfunction. Altern Med Rev 1999;4(3):144–161.
155. Miller AL. The methylation, neurotransmitter, and antioxidant connections between folate and depression. Altern Med Rev 2008;13(3):216.
156. Bottiglieri T. Homocysteine and folate metabolism in depression. Prog Neuropsychopharmacol Biol Psychiatry 2005;29(7):1103–1112.
157. Abou-Saleh MT, Coppen A. Folic acid and the treatment of depression. J Psychosom Res 2006;61(3):285–287.
158. Werbach MR. Nutritional strategies for treating chronic fatigue syndrome. Altern Med Rev 2000;5(2):93–108.
159. Vitetta L, et al. Mind-body medicine: stress and its impact on overall health and longevity. Ann N Y Acad Sci 2005;1057:492–505.
160. Brunner EJ, et al. Adrenocortical, autonomic, and inflammatory causes of the metabolic syndrome: nested case-control study. Circulation 2002;106(21):2659–2665.
161. Le Gal M, et al. Pharmaton capsules in the treatment of functional fatigue: a double-blind study versus placebo evaluated by a new methodology. Phytother Res 1996;10(1):49–53.
162. Dorling E, et al. Do ginsenosides influence the performance? Notabene Med 1980;10(5):241–246.
163. Bone K. Ginseng—the regal herb part 2. Mediherb Professional Review 1998;63:1–5.
164. Wiklund IK, et al. Effects of a standardized ginseng extract on quality of life and physiological parameters in symptomatic postmenopausal women: a double-blind, placebo-controlled trial. Swedish Alternative Medicine Group. Int J Clin Pharmacol Res 1999;19(3):89–99.
165. Cicero AF, et al. Effects of Siberian ginseng (Eleuterococcus senticosus Maxim.) on elderly quality of life: a randomized clinical trial. Arch Gerontol Geriatr Suppl 2004(9):69–73.
166. Stough C, et al. The chronic effects of an extract of Bacopa monniera (brahmi) on cognitive function in healthy human subjects. Psychopharmacology 2001;156(4):481–484.

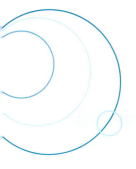

16

Diabetes type 2

Tini Gruner
ND, PhD, MSc

AETIOLOGY

Diabetes type 2, in contrast to type 1, is a lifestyle disease. It has become a public health burden worldwide, leading to premature morbidity and mortality. Abdominal obesity with deranged glucose tolerance (where glucose tissue uptake is impaired) leads to insulin resistance, hyperinsulinaemia, diabetes type 2 and cardiovascular abnormalities such as hypertension, hypertriglyceridaemia, low high-density lipo-proteins (HDL), microvascular lesions and atherosclerosis.[1,2] It is also a risk factor for polycystic ovarian syndrome, sleep apnoea and some hormone-sensitive cancers.[3] It has been aptly called the 'hyperactive fork and hypoactive foot', a 'deadly duet'.[4]

Two commonly encountered mechanisms seem to underlie the development of insulin resistance, leading to metabolic syndrome: high cortisol levels and adiposity. Increases in serum cortisol, such as is seen in stress, lead to gluconeogenesis (often derived from protein, leading to progressive muscle wasting) and therefore increased glucose levels in blood.[5,6] The interconnection of cortisol and glucose could thus be the cause for the progressive nature of the disease.[7] Up-regulation of cortisol due to stress (see also Chapter 15 on adrenal exhaustion) increases glucose and very low density lipoproteins (VLDL) secretion from the liver while inhibiting their reuptake, thus promoting hyperinsulinaemia, insulin resistance and storage of energy in the form of visceral fat.[8,9] Disturbances in the hypothalamic–pituitary–adrenal (HPA) axis not only increase cortisol levels but also enhance immune activation.[10] These disturbances exert their influence on other steroid hormones. Assaying these may give a better understanding of underlying wider-ranging pathology; it may also give clues as to their possible treatment.[11]

Increased inflammatory markers have been noted, linking the signs and symptoms of metabolic syndrome to an inflammatory process.[12] One study[10] hypothesises that the pathoaetiology of metabolic syndrome results from pro-inflammatory cytokines (IL-1, IL-6, TNF-α), due to inflammatory processes or emotional stress, enhancing sympathetic nervous system (SNS) activity, leading to obesity from enhanced feeding activity and increased leptin levels due to neuropeptide Y. A further indicator of inflammation in insulin resistance is an elevation in C-reactive protein (CRP).[13] Genetic links have also been suggested, with glucocorticoid receptor polymorphism.[14] Research echoes all of the above.[15]

Chronic elevations in blood glucose result in glycosylation of red blood cells and other biological substances, leading to oxidative tissue damage. It is suggested that this is the underlying mechanism that results in the common, late complications of diabetes, such as microvascular damage in blood vessels, eyes and kidneys.[16,17] It has been suggested that oxidative stress could also be the cause, not just the result, of this syndrome.[18]

High dietary saturated fat intake, low omega-3 fatty acids and other polyunsaturated fatty acids, alcohol consumption, sedentary lifestyle and mental stress are all promoters of metabolic syndrome. Certain personality types have enhanced sympathetic nervous system activity, with increased secretion of catecholamines, cortisol and serotonin, which all appear to be involved in the pathogenesis of metabolic syndrome.[19,20] It is estimated that approximately 40% of Europeans above the age of 60 years have metabolic syndrome, with rates in the US population climbing to approximately two-thirds.[1,20] Figure 16.1 shows the interdependency of the variables described in the text above.[21]

Metabolism of glucose uptake into the cells and the role of insulin

In most tissues, except hepatic tissue, glucose relies on a transport system called GLUT4 to be able to enter the cell. This system requires insulin for optimal uptake of glucose by muscle and adipose tissue, where insulin enhances the translocation of GLUT4 from the intracellular pool to the cell membrane.[22] The putative metabolic cause for diabetes type 2 lies in suboptimal functioning of these glucose transporters due to insulin resistance.[21]

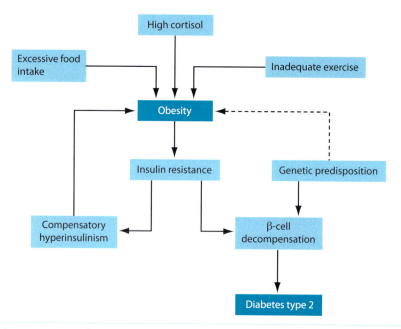

Figure 16.1 Overview of diabetes type 2 aetiology
Source: Adapted from Gropper et al. 2009[21]

It has been found that insulin is more effective in the presence of chromium. The mechanism is not entirely elucidated, but it is suggested that chromium (Cr^{3+}), bound to transferrin, enters the cells via transferrin receptors. Once inside the cell, chromium is released and four chromium ions bind with apochromodulin, forming holochromodulin (often simply called 'chromodulin'). Chromodulin then binds to the insulin receptor, increasing receptor activity.[21] Figures 16.2a and 16.2b illustrate the initial phase of insulin uptake (Figure 16.2a) and the resultant uptake of glucose into the cell (Figure 16.2b), and the role of chromodulin.

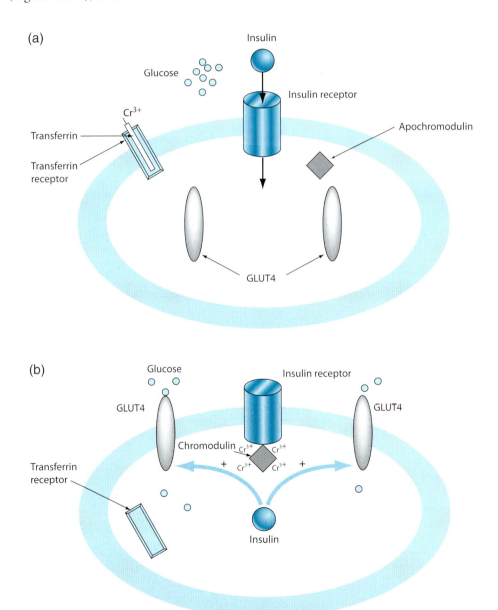

Figure 16.2 (a) Cell activation for glucose uptake (b) Glucose uptake into the cell
Source: Adapted from Devlin[22] and Gropper et al. 2009[21]

Testing for diabetes type 2 and metabolic syndrome

In-house testing comprises blood glucose, urinalysis (dipstick), blood pressure and anthropometric measurements. The latter includes body mass index (BMI*), waist circumference† and body composition measured through skinfold thickness or bioimpedance.[2]

Metabolic syndrome is confirmed when there are abnormalities in three or more of the following:
- elevated fasting glucose
- elevated glucose tolerance test results
- elevated insulin
- increased waist circumference or BMI
- high blood pressure (> 130/85)
- high triglycerides
- low HDL.

Since multiple parameters are involved in diabetes type 2 and metabolic syndrome the combined results of in-house and pathology testing can give conclusive evidence. Table 16.1 shows information on each of the laboratory tests involved.

RISK FACTORS

Stress, a diet high in refined and simple carbohydrates and human-modulated fats, and low in fibre, antioxidants and polyunsaturated fatty acids, especially omega-3, as well as lack of exercise, are the most outstanding contributors to obesity and metabolic syndrome.

This disease process brings with it a number of other risk factors, notably in cardiovascular health. Hypertension and dyslipidaemia are commonly encountered and in fact are part of metabolic syndrome. The derangement of steroid hormones, including sex hormones and dehydroepiandrosterone (see Figure 15.3 in Chapter 15 on adrenal exhaustion) can lead to lack of libido, erectile dysfunction and prostate problems in men, and menstrual irregularities, infertility and exacerbation of hormonal symptoms in females.

Due to the reduced life quality that accompanies any chronic health problem and possibly the decreased feelings of self-worth from being overweight, depression and anxiety should also be considered. Depression may also play a role in the aetiology of stress and metabolic syndrome (see also Chapter 12 on depression).

CONVENTIONAL TREATMENT

It is now commonly accepted that diet and lifestyle need to be considered in order to control this disease.[30] A number of diets have been recommended, with no clear answers as yet (see the discussion below).

In addition, medical treatment aims at regulating blood sugar to gain control of diabetes type 2. The drugs mentioned here are suitable only if there is some function left in the pancreatic β-cells; otherwise insulin needs to be given.

---

*Calculated as weight (in kg)/(height (m))^2. Ideal range is 18.5–25, with values > 30 indicating obesity.
†Ideal range for males is < 102 cm and for females < 88 cm. Measurements above these values constitute abdominal obesity.

Table 16.1 **Pathology tests recommended for suspected diabetes type 2 and metabolic syndrome**[23,24]

TEST	TISSUE	COMMENTS
Fasting glucose	Serum	Values > 6 mmol/L are indicative of diabetes type 2 or metabolic syndrome.
Fasting insulin	Serum	Normal values are 4–10 mU/L.
GTT (glucose tolerance test)	Serum	Commonly, the test is done over 2 hours, with blood samples taken pre-glucose loading and 2 hours after. Values > 7.8 mmol/L post-loading are indicative of DM2. However, this test will not show insulin and cortisol levels, nor the finer details of glucose control. Hence a 3-hour test with half-hourly measurements of glucose, insulin and cortisol is recommended. Insulin should not rise more than eightfold after glucose loading.
Glycosylated haemo-globin (HbA$_{1c}$)	Serum	HbA$_{1c}$ measures long-term glucose control and is an indicator of how well diabetics are managing their disease. Non-diabetic: 2.2–4.8% Good diabetic control: 2.5–5.9% Fair diabetic control: 6–8% Poor diabetic control: > 8%
Cortisol	Serum Urine Saliva	Cortisol is subject to diurnal variations, being highest in the morning and lowest at night. The best time for measuring cortisol levels in serum are early morning and again around 4 p.m. Night-time or 24-hour urinary cortisol, or repeat salivary samples, may be even more advantageous.[25]
Lipid studies	Serum	Triglycerides > 1.81 and 1.52 mmol/L and HDL < 0.75 and 0.91 in males and females, respectively, are indicative of diabetes type 2 or metabolic syndrome.
Liver profile	Serum	Elevations in alanine aminotransferase (ALT) have been found in insulin resistance and metabolic syndrome.[26]
CRP, ESR (inflammatory markers)	Serum	The ideal range of CRP and ESR is < 1. Elevation, even if still within the normal range, is indicative of inflammation, with the level of these markers proportional of the degree of inflammation.
Homocysteine	Serum	Homocysteine is an inflammatory amino acid produced in the methylation cycle. It is commonly elevated in metabolic and heart diseases.[27] Ideal range is < 10.
Active B12	Serum	Active B12 or holotranscobalamin has been termed the best and earliest indicator of impending vitamin B12 deficiency.[28] It needs to be > 35 pmol/L.
Folate	RBC	Folate and vitamin B12 are both needed in the homocysteine-methionine (methylation) cycle. Values differ markedly between laboratories.

(Continued)

Table 16.1 Pathology tests recommended for suspected diabetes type 2 and metabolic syndrome[23,24] *(Continued)*

TEST	TISSUE	COMMENTS
Vitamin D	Serum	Despite the high amount of sunshine, vitamin D deficiency is high in Australia. It is needed for insulin secretion and found to be low in people not receiving much sunlight on their skin.[29] Both the inactive (25-hydroxyvitamin D) and the active (1,25-dihydroxyvitamin D) forms can be measured. Ideal values for vitamins are in the upper half of the reference range.
TSH	Serum	Hypothyroidism is present when thyroid-stimulating hormone is elevated. It may explain some people's inability to lose weight. However, subtle elevations (> 2.5 mIU/L) within the reference range (0.4–5.0 mIU/L) could indicate a 'labouring' thyroid or a pre-hypothyroid state.[30,31]

In the first instance, biguanides (such as metformin) will be prescribed. The supposed mechanisms include reduced gluconeogenesis and increased insulin sensitivity. A possible side effect of this drug is pernicious anaemia. Therefore, vitamin B12 should be measured regularly and, if found to decline or be low, vitamin B12 treatment via monthly intramuscular injections should be initiated.[33]

Sulfonylureas are recommended to enhance the secretion of insulin in response to blood glucose. However, care needs to be taken in patients with liver or kidney disease. They also promote weight gain and are therefore not ideal in metabolic syndrome.

Another treatment option is α-glucosidase inhibitors. This class of drugs reduces the breakdown of carbohydrates in the intestines by inhibiting the enzymes involved in this process, thus reducing the rise in blood sugar levels following a meal. They are therefore useful in obesity. However, the remaining carbohydrates are likely to be fermented in the gastrointestinal tract, leading to unwelcome side effects such as bloating and flatulence.

The glitazones (thiazolidinediones) reduce insulin, but have no direct effect on glucose. Their beneficial action in diabetes type 2 may be the lowering of free fatty acids, thus increasing muscular glucose usage.

Various combinations of these drugs, notably metformin with sulfonylureas, are currently used, particularly when good glucose control (as assessed by HbA$_{1c}$ levels) is not achieved by one drug alone. Only as a last resort will insulin be used for diabetes type 2.

Cardiovascular risk factors are commonly controlled by blood pressure and lipid-lowering medication (see Section 3 on the cardiovascular system).

KEY TREATMENT PROTOCOLS

This needs to be a multi-pronged approach, including stress management, dietary and lifestyle changes, exercise, and nutritional and herbal supplements.

Modify lifestyle and diet

Fat loss, even if it is small, is paramount and has resulted in greater insulin sensitivity, lower blood pressure and improved lipid profile, thus reducing risk factors for both diabetes type 2 and heart disease.[1] A hypocaloric diet rather than a total fast has been advocated, together with physical exercise and reduction in alcohol consumption. These lifestyle changes, although superior to drug treatment, are sometimes difficult to achieve and an extensive health-care program needs to be initiated to prevent relapse.[20] A slow reduction in weight seems to be better to rapid weight-loss diets for lasting success as the weight is more likely to stay off. **Protein** needs to be emphasised as there is often a reduction in lean body mass due to the gluconeogenic effects of raised cortisol.

> **NATUROPATHIC TREATMENT AIMS**
> - Self-motivate to do something about the condition.
> - Reduce stress.
> - Reduce excess body fat.
> - Reduce inflammation.
> - Prevent the development of additional risk factors or reduce them:
>   - heart disease
>   - metabolic syndrome.

There has been much debate regarding the best diet for this condition: high complex-carbohydrate/low-fat (HC/LF) or high-protein/low-carbohydrate diet (HP/LC), or anything in between.[44,45] It is feared that the HP/LC diet may be too high in saturated fats due to its high meat content and hence contribute to increased calorie consumption. Although weight loss after 1 year seems to be the same on either diet, the HC/LF dieters tends to have a better LDL profile. However, the HP/LC diet has led to greater fat loss and improved triglyceride and HDL values.[44,46]

Further, there is evidence that animal fat (in dairy and meat), particularly conjugated linoleic acid, can have a protective effect against obesity, diabetes, heart disease and cancer.[47–50] With the low-fat diet recommendations, apparently people now consume less than half the amount of conjugated linoleic acid needed to reap the benefits.[51] And the beneficial effects of fish consumption, especially those with high omega-3 content, are well known. Another advantage of a low-carbohydrate diet lies in its reduced insulin requirements.

Care needs to be taken, too, with low-fat products, as the fat is often replaced with carbohydrates such as olestra or a similar 'fat substitute'. Believing that this is a low-fat (healthy) food, people may tend to eat more, thus making up the calories. Besides, these

DIABETIC FOOT CARE[43,34]

'Diabetic foot' is the umbrella term for the numerous foot problems in diabetics that arise from arterial complications and peripheral neuropathy. This combination can lead in turn to poor circulation; poor wound healing and eventual ulcer development. Therapies such as corrective footwear, diabetic socks and regular podiatrist review are encouraged, as well as hyperbaric oxygen and various wound management techniques when or if ulceration does occur. However, one of the best patient recommendations may simply be that of increased vigilance—studies suggest that increasing awareness of the issue is effective in reducing serious lesions. Simple tips such as testing shoe tightness with fingers to reduce pressure—which many patients may not be aware of, due to neuropathy— may stave off serious issues in the future. Improving circulation may also reduce the possibility of ulcer formation by improving wound-healing ability. Considering that 10–15% of diabetic patients can expect complications, that over half of diabetic hospital admissions are related to foot complications and that diabetes is the most common reason for medical amputation, these recommendations need to be an integral part of diabetic patient management.

fat replacers also have calories. Carroll claims that this substitution has contributed markedly to the current obesity epidemic.[52] In addition, olestra has been shown to reduce the absorption of fat-soluble vitamins, thus depriving the body further of essential nutrients.[53]

In order to achieve a feeling of satiety without overindulging in calorie-rich foods, **fibre** needs to be an essential dietary constituent of every person attempting to lose weight.[45] Fibre will bind fats and lower the absorption of glucose through delaying gastric emptying. Studies with **psyllium hulls** (*Plantago psyllium*) have shown significant reductions in fasting plasma glucose, cholesterol, LDL and triglycerides, and elevations in HDL.[54] However, care needs to be taken as too much of it will reduce nutrient absorption and can lead to flatulence.

Increase exercise

The positive influence of **exercise** on glucose control cannot be overemphasised,[20] as a plethora of literature on this topic testifies. It facilitates the uptake of glucose into the cells and lowers insulin resistance, apart from the beneficial effect on body composition. Even small daily tasks, such as getting up to change the TV channel or taking the stairs rather than the lift, will be beneficial.[55]

In insulin resistance and diabetes type 2, high levels of fatty acids are stored in skeletal muscle, with exercise being able to reduce this through β-oxidation (fat burning), thus lowering triglycerides and improving glucose control.[56] For people with impaired fasting glucose, before the development of diabetes type 2, even greater benefits can be achieved, as seen in improvements in glycolysis, aerobic metabolism, β-oxidation and mitochondrial biogenesis.[57]

In particular, strength training maximises fat loss and minimises the loss of lean body mass which usually accompanies weight loss diets.[2] Sarcopenia is common in diabetics, particularly in the elderly.[58] Since it is the muscles that use glucose to produce energy, lack of muscle mass further promotes the disease process.

Tai chi has shown to significantly improve glycaemic control and lower triglyceride levels in Chinese diabetic women.[59] In a 6-month trial in Korea those people adhering to the activity schedule experienced much better glucose control and quality of life.[60]

As exercise usually has a glucose-lowering effect, blood glucose needs to be monitored carefully regarding possible hypoglycaemia, and medication may need to be adjusted (see also Chapter 19 on endometriosis).[58]

Increase insulin release and receptor sensitivity, and reduce hyperinsulinaemia

The precursor to diabetes type 2 is insulin resistance and compensatory hyperinsulinaemia. Although insulin is overproduced and secreted by the pancreas it is not facilitating glucose uptake into the cell. Fat loss results in increased insulin sensitivity and should be pursued.[61] Certain nutrients and herbs can aid insulin sensitivity, thus reducing hyperinsulinaemia.

Nutritional interventions

A whole range of vitamins, minerals, amino acids and bioactive substances have been explored in the treatment of diabetes type 2 and insulin resistance. Nutrients which have shown a positive effect include vitamins A, B_1, B_3 and biotin, the minerals calcium, potassium, zinc and manganese and fructo-oligosaccharides. Some amino acids, such as taurine (needed for liver detoxification pathways and control of heart rhythm and blood pressure) and L-arginine (for nitric oxide production to maintain endothelial function) may also help.[3,4,21,38,45] However, there are nutrients that are very specific for diabetes type 2, as demonstrated below.

Most animals produce their own **vitamin C** from glucose. The two molecules are therefore structurally similar, and competition for cellular uptake between vitamin C and glucose has been suggested as a possible mechanism by which this vitamin exerts its positive influence on glucose metabolism. Further, vitamin C is needed to stimulate the release of insulin following glucose ingestion. As little as 500 mg/day has been shown to be effective. Vitamin C also acts as an antioxidant, reduces blood pressure and protects blood vessels.[4]

Chromium is needed to facilitate the entry of glucose into the cells by stimulating insulin uptake and enhancing its activity (Figure 16.2).[21] Supplementation has had a beneficial effect on metabolic syndrome by lowering fasting blood glucose (FBG), postprandial glucose (PPG) and corresponding insulin levels, and by improving insulin sensitivity, HbA_{1c} values and lipid profiles. The recommended dosage is 200–1000 µg/day. Increased benefits have been noted with higher doses.[45,62] Another possible effect of chromium is its action on down-regulating pancreatic β-cell activity, thus increasing glucagon levels.[63]

Magnesium is essential for all reactions requiring energy as it is needed to stabilise ATP. Low levels have been found in cardiovascular disease and diabetes, and in people with high alcohol intake. Normalisation through supplementation up to 400 mg/day has enhanced insulin sensitivity, reduced fasting glucose and improved HbA_{1c}.[21,45,64] Trials with small amounts of magnesium have yielded mixed results. However, reductions in FBG and HbA_{1c}, and increases in postprandial insulin, in glucose uptake and in glucose oxidation have been noted.[62]

Enhanced insulin sensitivity with reductions in FBG, HbA_{1c} and hepatic glucose production, and better insulin-mediated glucose uptake, have been found with **vanadium**.[62] The usual dose is 100 µg/day. Vanadium mimics the action of insulin, as seen by its similar effects on the translocation of GLUT4 to the cell membrane.[21]

Coenzyme Q10 has been shown to reduce blood glucose, hyperinsulinaemia, high blood pressure, triglycerides and lipid peroxidation.[4] Dosage range is 30–120 mg/day. It is particularly important for people on statin drugs as some of these have a depleting effect on this nutrient.[65]

N-acetyl carnitine, made from lysine by methylation, is instrumental in the transport of fatty acids across the mitochondrial membrane for β-oxidation. It is therefore essential for energy production from fat burning.[38] Administration of this nutrient has enhanced glucose uptake, storage and utilisation, and insulin sensitivity.[62] A relatively high amount, ≥ 3 g/day, is needed to achieve these effects.

Vitamin E tends to decrease HbA_{1c}, FBG and PPG.[62]

The bioactive nutrient **α-lipoic acid** is both water and fat soluble and has been shown to enhance cellular glucose uptake and utilisation. The daily amount is up to 1200 mg/day. In conjunction with exercise, this nutrient has shown to enhance glucose transport and insulin signalling in skeletal muscle cells.[66]

Herbal medicines

In diabetes type 2, insulin resistance and metabolic syndrome, a range of herbal supplements have been proven to be of help in blood glucose and insulin regulation.[67] In particular, bitters have been indicated.[68] *Galega officinalis* allegedly increases the action of insulin. Its active ingredient, galegine, was used as a model for metformin.[62,69]

Coccinia indica seems to mimic the action of insulin, *Bauhinia forficata* has been dubbed 'vegetable insulin', **garlic** and **onion** can decrease fasting serum glucose levels as well as exerting a beneficial effect on cardiovascular risk factors, *Opuntia streptacantha* has reportedly insulin-sensitising properties and *Aloe vera* juice has hypoglycaemic effects.[62,69] **Berberis-containing herbs** have shown regulatory effects not only on glucose control but also on cardiovascular pathology.[68] *Coleus forskohlii* has putative beneficial effects on insulin resistance and diabetes type 2. *Inula racemosa* has shown increased insulin sensitivity in an animal model,[3] and *Ocimum sanctum* (holy basil) is effective in lowering FBG, PPG and glucosuria.[62,69] The use of *Cinnamomum cassia* (cinnamon) shows in in vitro studies that it can potentiate the action of insulin.[70]

Gymnema sylvestre has glucose-lowering ability without causing hypoglycaemia. Decreases in FBG, HbA_{1c} and urinary glucose excretion have been found, leading to a reduced need for conventional medication. *G. sylvestre* is thought to delay glucose uptake in the small intestines, and through its restorative action on β-cells the release of insulin from the pancreas has been increased.[62,71] Lipid studies have also shown favourable effects.[70] If given at least 30 minutes before eating, it reduces appetite and the cravings for sweets by anaesthetising the taste buds (1–2 mL/day). Therefore it may aid in weight loss.[69,70] Thus, *G. sylvestre* has the ability to affect a number of factors linked to the aetiology and pathophysiology of diabetes type 2 simultaneously, something that no other single hypoglycaemic agent is able to exert.[72]

The various forms of ginseng (*Panax ginseng* and *P. quinquefolium,* and *Eleutherococcus senticosus*) have beneficial effects in diabetes type 2.[62] Decreases in PPG, FBG and HbA_{1c} have been noted with *P. quinquefolium*.[62,73]

Supplementation with *Trigonella foenum-graecum* carbohydrate has led to lowered FBG, PPG, postprandial insulin, urine glucose and carbohydrate absorption, with modulation of peripheral glucose utilisation, thus increasing glycaemic control.[62,69,70]

Momordica charantia has hypoglycaemic (for both PPG and FBG) and antidiabetic effects. It has the ability to stimulate the pancreas to release insulin; to increase glucose uptake, glycogen synthesis, and glucose oxidation; and to decrease hepatic gluconeogenesis.[62,69,71]

Tinospora cordifolia can avert blood sugar elevation by reducing glycogenolysis (the breakdown of glycogen to form free glucose) from liver and muscle, thus preventing excess lactic acid being converted to glucose in the liver, and increasing glucose utilisation in muscle tissue.[71]

The Indian herb *Salacia oblonga* has been used in trials to treat diabetes and it was found to be as effective as prescription drugs. A maximum of 1000 mg has been used.[74]

Apart from working as an antioxidant by restoring glutathione levels, *Silybum marianum* can lower blood and urinary glucose, and HbA_{1c}. It also has beneficial effects on insulin, lowering its requirement.[62] In other studies, the positive effect was mainly on diabetic complications and lipid parameters.[68]

Reduce immune system activation and inflammation

Inflammation plays an important part in the pathophysiology of chronic and lifestyle-induced disease such as diabetes type 2, and **polyunsaturated fatty acids** (PUFAs) play an important role in regulating pro-inflammatory cytokines.[75,76] Not only the omega-3 but also the omega-6 series have positive effects, leading to anti-inflammatory prostaglandin E3 and E1, respectively. Low levels of γ-linolenic acid have been found in diabetes type 2 due to the reduced activity of the enzymes delta 5 and delta 6 desaturase,[75,77] as insulin is needed for their activation.[78] Research has therefore focused on the beneficial effects of fish oils to bypass these enzymes. In addition to the triglyceride-lowering and anti-inflammatory effects that have been noted with the administration of fish oils,[19,45] reductions in serum lipids, lipoproteins, platelet aggregation and blood pressure, and increases in cell membrane fluidity, have been found.[76,79]

Due to the inflammatory component of metabolic syndrome, antioxidants are paramount. **Vitamin E** has been investigated with mixed results as to its effects on inflammation, diabetes and heart disease.[45] However, antioxidants need to be administered in conjunction with each other, due to their mutual recycling. It is important, too, to use mixed tocopherols, not the synthetic d-α-tocopherol. Further, **N-acetyl cysteine** has shown to have beneficial effects in insulin resistance due to its antioxidant properties[17] and being a cofactor for glutathione production.

Vitamin D plays a role in immunomodulation and insulin secretion. There are correlations between insulin resistance, diabetes type 2 and heart disease, and supplementation of ≥ 1000 IU/day (regardless of body status) has shown to improve these parameters.[6,38,29,80]

Chronic immune activation, as is the case in obesity, increases **tryptophan** breakdown, potentially leading to serotonin deficit and symptoms of mood disorder, depression and impaired satiety. The latter increases caloric intake, especially from carbohydrates, thus perpetuating a vicious circle.[81]

Reduce stress

Stress increases cortisol through HPA axis activation (see Chapter 15 on adrenal exhaustion). Elevated cortisol promotes visceral adiposity, insulin resistance and loss of glycaemic control,[82–85] thus contributing to metabolic syndrome.[15,86] The vicious cycle of visceral fat storage, gluconeogenesis from muscle protein and increased demand for insulin with resultant increase in cortisol promotes carbohydrate cravings, which in turn leads to further abdominal fat gain.

To break this cycle, stress management is paramount. The following herbs do not only have adaptogenic properties with balancing effects on stress hormones; they also have shown direct benefits in treating insulin resistance and diabetes type 2.

Eleutherococcus senticosus is known for its adaptogenic properties during stress. It is used during periods of fatigue and debility. It has shown positive effects on blood pressure, total and LDL cholesterol, triglycerides and glucose. There may be reduction of stress-related symptoms and faster recovery in chronic illness due to increased aerobic metabolism.[70,87] Due to its potential hypoglycaemic effects, diabetics should monitor their blood sugar levels when taking this herb.[73]

Panax ginseng is another adaptogen used in stress, in chronic diseases and to replenish depleted energy stores.[70] The rate of carbohydrate absorption is reduced, with increased glucose uptake, transport and storage in form of glycogen. Insulin secretions can be modulated.[62] Although small drops in blood glucose have been reported, one study[68] claims that further results in diabetes can be achieved only when the herb has been injected.

Prevent/address diabetic complications

Despite medication, chronic elevations and fluctuations in blood glucose in both diabetes type 1 and diabetes type 2 cannot be avoided entirely. Oxidative stress and inflammation have been found not only in diabetic patients but also in obese people and those with insulin resistance. This, plus the increase in free fatty acids and possibly other metabolites, is responsible for the oxidative stress that leads to diabetic complications such as damage to the nerves, the vascular endothelium and the kidneys. Various antioxidant treatments have been used to alleviate oxidative damage and thus delay or prevent these complications.[19,28,29]

Nutritional interventions

Essential fatty acids, including evening primrose oil, can alleviate diabetic complications due to their anti-inflammatory properties (as outlined above).[68,79] **N-acetyl cysteine** has been recommended as being useful to alleviate oxidative stress.[16,17] It is the limiting amino acid for glutathione production, and whey is an excellent source of this nutrient.[88] Supplementation with either whey or N-acetyl cysteine may therefore increase the availability of the endogenous antioxidant glutathione.

Vitamin E improves the action of other antioxidants, especially vitamin C and glutathione. It reduces LDL and the risk of cardiovascular complications of insulin resistance. It may help to preserve pancreatic β-cells. Since vitamin E works closely with **selenium** in endogenous antioxidant systems, the combined use has resulted in greater benefits.[4] Its use in nephropathy has resulted in decreased microalbuminaemia due to reductions in thromboxane A2.[89]

The renin-angiotensin system is crucial in the development of diabetic nephropathy. It is negatively regulated by **vitamin D**, which suppresses renin expression. Research on mice has shown a protective effect of vitamin D on the renal system by modulating the renin-angiotensin system.[90] The active form of vitamin B6, **pyridoxl 5'-phosphate**, has shown in rats to prevent advanced glycation end-products being formed, thus favourably influencing diabetic nephropathy. This may yet prove to be a valuable treatment in this condition for diabetic patients.[91]

The mechanism by which **α-lipoic acid** exerts its benefits in diabetes are thought to be due to its ability to facilitate the translocation of GLUT4 to the cell membrane, in readiness for glucose uptake into the cell.[39] It is especially useful to prevent or reduce diabetic complications resulting from oxidative damage,[92] such as cataract formation, polyneuropathy and damage to blood vessels. As an antioxidant it also helps to recycle other antioxidants, such as vitamins C and E, and glutathione.[4,39,62]

Diabetic neuropathy is characterised by demyelinisation with resultant reductions in nerve conduction velocity.[93] A review[94] found that α-lipoic acid in conjunction with vitamin E reduced diabetic neuropathy and corrected nerve conduction velocity. Although some conflicting data exist regarding what exactly α-lipoic acid improves in diabetic neuropathy, there is no doubt that it does have a beneficial effect in this condition.[95] Its application is safe and effective.[96]

One of the most troublesome symptoms of diabetic neuropathy is pain. **Acetyl L-carnitine** at a daily dose of 1000 mg has been effective in regenerating nerve fibres and significantly reducing pain.[97] Vitamin B12, in its coenzyme form of **methylcobalamin**, has been injected intrathecally (injection into the subarachnoid space) with dramatic improvements in leg pain, heaviness and paraesthesia (tingling, numbness, and pins and needles).[98] This suggests that vitamin B12 deficiency plays a role in diabetic neuropathy.

Herbal medicines

Silybum marianum has been trialled in diabetes type 2 due to its antioxidant profile and beneficial effects on diabetes. An improvement in glycaemic control has been found; this could reduce the risk of diabetic complications.[99,100]

Gymnema sylvestre has wide-ranging actions on blood glucose metabolism and is therefore able to alleviate a range of diabetic complications, including cardiovascular risk factors such as hypertension, hyperlipidaemia and atherosclerosis, and the diabetic complications trio nephropathy, neuropathy and retinopathy, as well as susceptibility to infection and erectile dysfunction.[72]

Leg ulcers are a common complication of diabetes and are often difficult to heal. *Aesculus hippocastanum*, due to its venous toning, antioxidant and anti-inflammatory effects, has been used to treat this condition.[101] Significant improvements have been noted in wound slough and in reduced necessity to change wound dressings.[102,103]

Diabetic retinopathy has been treated with traditional Chinese medicine and antioxidants. Chinese yin-nourishing, kidney-tonifying and blood-activating herbs have been used to enhance blood flow to the eyes, resulting in improved visual acuity.[104] However, there have been no conclusive trials as yet on the use of antioxidants in this condition,[105–107] although it would be reasonable to concur that antioxidants are called for since this condition is the result of oxidative damage.

Similarly, nephropathy is thought to be a result of oxidative stress. Several combinations of **traditional Chinese herbal medicine** remedies to nourish Qi with Western medicine have been used with good results.[108–110] A traditional Chinese medicine formulation to remove blood stasis, stomach heat and heart fire, while supporting the stomach and kidneys, has proven superior to drug treatment.[111] One study used a combination of *Fructus arctii* and *Astragalus membranaceus*, which reduced proteinuria and albuminuria, and improved blood glucose and lipids.[112]

Ginkgo biloba is known as an antioxidant, circulatory stimulant and neuroprotectant,[70] and its use in diabetic nephropathy seems therefore logical. In the early stages of the disease *G. biloba* has been found to be effective in increasing renal function with resultant decreased albuminuria and other improvements.[113,114] Benefits have also been shown with *G. biloba* with respect to intercellular and vascular adhesion molecules.[115]

Address comorbidities

Insulin resistance, diabetes type 2, heart disease and metabolic syndrome are closely related. Due to insulin resistance, the risk of heart disease is increased in diabetes type 2 as part of the metabolic syndrome.[27] Hypertension and dyslipidaemia (high triglycerides, high LDL and low HDL) are part of the symptom picture in metabolic syndrome and need to be addressed conjointly with insulin resistance and diabetes type 2.[1,2] Please refer to Section 3 on the cardiovascular system for more detailed interventions.

Nutritional interventions

Essential fatty acids (EFAs) prevent organ damage in diabetes type 2[42] through their effect on dyslipidaemia and the ability to lower triglycerides, blood pressure and atherogenesis.[76] Brain function has been improved on omega-3 fatty acids,[19] evidenced by the fact that people with diabetes type 2 have reported less depression when supplementing with omega-3 fatty acids. This may be linked to the beneficial effects omega-3 fatty acids have on cardiovascular disease.[116]

Vitamin B12 and **folate** are both needed for the remethylation of homocysteine to methionine (the universal methyl group donor). **Vitamin B6** facilitates the breakdown of homocysteine via the transsulfuration pathway.[21] Together, they are needed to reduce homocysteine levels, which can pose an independent risk factor for heart disease and diabetes type 2.[27] Recent research has cast doubt on the link of homocysteine to heart disease. However, the fact remains that it is also linked to reduced bioavailability of nitric oxide, thus indirectly effecting cardiovascular disease.[117]

A derivative of vitamin B5, **pantethine**, has shown promising results in the prevention of diabetes-induced angiopathy, due to its triglyceride-, lipid- and apolipoprotein-lowering effects.[118] It is particularly useful in dyslipidaemia when this is not amenable to dietary or other means.[119]

> The reader should be aware that the evidence stated under nutritional interventions has been mostly derived from trials where single substances have been used. As is the case with antioxidants, combinations of the above may yield even better results. Nutrients and herbs that match the individual patient's profile best need to be chosen.

Herbal medicines

One of the early manifestations of heart disease is hypertension. This can be improved by *Crataegus monogyna*. This herb has also shown benefits in other areas of heart disease, such as congestive heart failure[70] and decreased cardiac output, circulatory disturbances and arrythmias.[120] *Coleus forskohlii* has blood pressure lowering as well as platelet inhibiting effects.[70]

Trigonella foenum-graecum, apart from its beneficial effects on blood glucose, has been shown to lower atherosclerotic parameters.[70] Similarly, *Cynara scolymus* can reduce hyperlipidaemic parameters such as cholesterol and triglycerides.[70]

INTEGRATIVE MEDICAL CONSIDERATIONS

Relaxation exercises such as meditation have shown beneficial effects not only on mood and depression, but also on insulin receptors and the HPA axis.[19] Since metabolic syndrome is a multifaceted disease a whole range of parameters need to be considered and attended to. Therefore, a close working relationship with the patient's GP would be advisable.

Homoeopathy has been used successfully in cases of diabetes type 2[121] as well as its complications.[122] Although some remedies tend to have a greater positive effect on this disease than others,[123] it is still important to repertorise and thus individualise,[124] as more obscure remedies may be the ones needed for a particular individual.[125,126]

PATHOGENESIS AND CONVENTIONAL TREATMENT FOR DIABETES TYPE 1[34,32,21]

Diabetes type 1 is primarily an autoimmune disease where the β-cells of the pancreas, which produce insulin, are destroyed by leukocyte infiltration.[35] The starting age is usually during childhood or adolescence. The disease is characterised mainly by ketoacidosis with the typical acetone breath, polyuria with resultant thirst, postural hypotension and anorexia due to uncontrolled hyperglycaemia, which interferes with electrolyte and osmotic balance. This is a catabolic disease with elevated glucagon and muscle wasting due to gluconeogenesis, and can lead to coma and death if untreated. Lifelong exogenous insulin by injection is the usual treatment. In recent years the transplant of a whole pancreas or pancreatic islet cells has been trialled, with several patients not requiring insulin for some time after the procedure, but cytotoxic drugs are then needed for life.[30] This treatment is still in its infancy and not yet common practice.

Diagnosis is made from either urine or fasting blood glucose levels. Reference ranges are the same as for diabetes type 2. A glucose tolerance test may be performed to corroborate the results of the urine or blood test. To ascertain long-term control, HbA_{1c} will be measured every 3 to 6 months.

Acute diabetic complications include hypoglycaemia due to too much insulin administration which can lead to coma. Long term complications involve damage to the micro- and macrovascular systems, nervous tissue, skin and eyes and are the result of fluctuations in blood glucose levels that are part of the disease picture. Common conditions include cataracts, retinopathy leading to blindness, nephropathy leading to renal failure, neuropathy, myocardial infarction and stroke, and gangrene of the feet leading to amputations.

TREATMENT PROTOCOLS AND POSSIBLE INTERVENTIONS FOR DIABETES TYPE 1

A nutritious, balanced diet is recommended, with regular meals, and sugar in particular needs to be restricted. The use of artificial sweeteners, so often recommended as sugar substitutes and considered safe for diabetics, may have harmful effects long-term and should be avoided or at least limited.

Vitamin D deficiency has been linked to the pathogenesis of autoimmune diseases, including diabetes type 1.[6,36] Early intervention with vitamin D may be able to arrest the pro-inflammatory cytokine production and thus avoid or alleviate the disease if supplementation is commenced early. Oxidative stress is part of DT1 and its complications, and antioxidants should be considered.[37,38] Lipoic acid is particularly beneficial for the prevention and treatment of diabetic complications.[39] It has also been used, in conjunction with vitamin E, in diabetic neuropathy.[40] For glaucoma and raised intraocular pressure, high dose vitamin C, lipoic acid, vitamin B12, magnesium, melatonin, *Ginkgo biloba* and *Coleus forskohlii* have been suggested.[41] Essential fatty acids have also been shown to play a role in diabetes type 1.[38,42]

The Indian system of Ayurveda has a wide range of herbal medicines for many diseases. In diabetes type 2, **Pterocarpus marsupium** (kino tree) has decreased elevated blood glucose and glycosylated haemoglobin levels.[127]

Other useful modalities and therefore referrals include acupuncture, fitness training (gym), grief counselling and creativity (art and music).

Case Study

A 67-year-old male presents with **inability to stop weight gain**. His last blood test showed a **fasting blood sugar level of 11.3 mmol/L and a cortisol level of 720 nmol/L**. He has put on **20 kg over the past 5 years**, since his wife died of cancer. Most of this weight gain happened since his retirement 2 years ago. He finds it hard to cope on his own; he has isolated himself from his friends and family and spends most of his days at home watching television (for distraction). With **little cooking skills** his meals consist mainly of sandwiches (white bread) with cheese or jam, and biscuits in between. Occasionally he fries an egg or some sausages, or buys some take-aways. **Fluid intake is mainly derived from four cups of coffee a day** (with milk and 2 teaspoons of sugar), two cans of soft drink and three or four cans of beer at night.

SUGGESTIVE SIGNS AND SYMPTOMS

- Hyperglycaemia
- Abdominal obesity
- Lack of exercise
- Hypercortisolism
- High carbohydrate diet
- Moderate to high alcohol intake

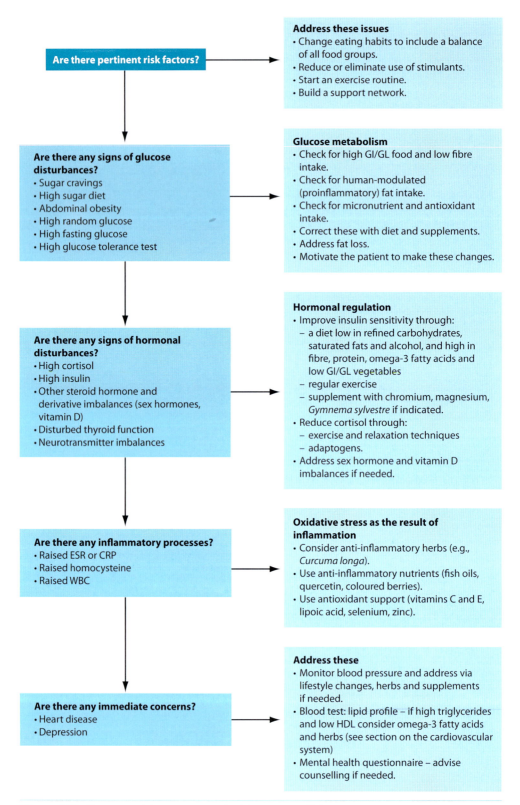

Are there pertinent risk factors?

Address these issues
- Change eating habits to include a balance of all food groups.
- Reduce or eliminate use of stimulants.
- Start an exercise routine.
- Build a support network.

Are there any signs of glucose disturbances?
- Sugar cravings
- High sugar diet
- Abdominal obesity
- High random glucose
- High fasting glucose
- High glucose tolerance test

Glucose metabolism
- Check for high GI/GL food and low fibre intake.
- Check for human-modulated (proinflammatory) fat intake.
- Check for micronutrient and antioxidant intake.
- Correct these with diet and supplements.
- Address fat loss.
- Motivate the patient to make these changes.

Are there any signs of hormonal disturbances?
- High cortisol
- High insulin
- Other steroid hormone and derivative imbalances (sex hormones, vitamin D)
- Disturbed thyroid function
- Neurotransmitter imbalances

Hormonal regulation
- Improve insulin sensitivity through:
  - a diet low in refined carbohydrates, saturated fats and alcohol, and high in fibre, protein, omega-3 fatty acids and low GI/GL vegetables
  - regular exercise
  - supplement with chromium, magnesium, *Gymnema sylvestre* if indicated.
- Reduce cortisol through:
  - exercise and relaxation techniques
  - adaptogens.
- Address sex hormone and vitamin D imbalances if needed.

Are there any inflammatory processes?
- Raised ESR or CRP
- Raised homocysteine
- Raised WBC

Oxidative stress as the result of inflammation
- Consider anti-inflammatory herbs (e.g., *Curcuma longa*).
- Use anti-inflammatory nutrients (fish oils, quercetin, coloured berries).
- Use antioxidant support (vitamins C and E, lipoic acid, selenium, zinc).

Are there any immediate concerns?
- Heart disease
- Depression

Address these
- Monitor blood pressure and address via lifestyle changes, herbs and supplements if needed.
- Blood test: lipid profile – if high triglycerides and low HDL consider omega-3 fatty acids and herbs (see section on the cardiovascular system)
- Mental health questionnaire – advise counselling if needed.

Figure 16.3 Naturopathic treatment decision tree—diabetes type 2

Example treatment

The tentative diagnosis for this patient is hypercortisolism due to prolonged stress, combined with an imbalanced high-glycaemic-index diet, excess alcohol consumption and a sedentary lifestyle, resulting in insulin resistance, diabetes type 2 and metabolic syndrome.

The first consultation, after thorough case taking, physical examination and in-house testing (see Table 16.2), was spent educating the patient about how stress, his diet and his lifestyle have contributed to his current health problems. He knew he was not feeling 100%, but had no idea how much at risk of major health problems he was until his medical practitioner had told him he had diabetes and wanted him to take medication. This was a 'big wake-up call' for him—he had rarely taken medication in his whole life.

It was deemed important to explain the connections between stress, lifestyle and diet in detail and in terms he could relate to. Since he used to be a builder the analogy of mortar and bricks to build a house, and what happens when materials are missing or are of poor quality, was used. This understanding on the part of the patient was considered of utmost importance to achieve compliance.

Treatment options

To reduce stress and elevated cortisol levels, he was advised to:
- develop an interest or hobby that entails mixing with people
- do relaxation exercises.

To reduce elevated glucose levels and obesity, and increase insulin sensitivity, he should:
- drastically reduce alcohol intake
- make dietary changes:
  - eat low glycaemic index/glycaemic load carbohydrates
  - increase protein to 1.5 times ideal body weight/1000
  - avoid refined carbohydrates
  - reduce (ideally eliminate) stimulants
  - increase (filtered) water intake
- take various herbs and nutritional supplements that have shown beneficial effects (see above)

Table16.2 Physical examination at first consultation

MEASUREMENT	ACTUAL	IDEAL
BP	145/90	120/80
Height	1.71 m	Not applicable
Weight	99.5 kg	73 kg
BMI	34	25 (maximum)
Lean body mass	49.5 kg	60 kg
Fat mass	50 kg	13 kg
Urinalysis	Glucose 1+	None

- take up exercise
  - walking (for example, golf)
  - gym (resistance exercises)
  - other forms of exercise to which the patient can commit long-term.

These options were discussed to find out what he could do differently, with emphasis on eliciting realistic ideas from him.

With respect to dietary changes, he agreed to add some apples and carrots to his shopping list. As far as other vegetables were concerned, he did not know how to prepare them. Some healthy pre-packaged as well as take-away meal options were discussed. He was prepared to try some wholemeal bread and buy some cans of fish (in spring water) for his lunch. He had a blender at home and was instructed in how to use this for making daily protein smoothies (containing protein powder and mixed berries for antioxidant support, made up with rice milk).

Nutritional prescription	
Magnesium	200 mg b.d.
Chromium	500 µg b.d.
Antioxidant combination with α-lipoic acid	1 b.d.
Vitamins B6, B12 and folate	1 b.d.
Fish oils: EPA (300 mg) and DHA (200 mg) per capsule	2 b.d.
Vitamin D	5000 IU/day

Herbal prescription	
Curcuma longa 1:1	35 mL
Gymnema sylvestre 1:1	35 mL
Eleutherococcus senticosus 1:2	15 mL
Trigonella foecum-gracum 1:2	15 mL
5 mL t.d.s. before meals	100 mL

He was advised to return to his medical practitioner for some further testing (see above), which he agreed to do.

He was prescribed a range of supplements (see the prescription box), consisting of chromium and magnesium to increase insulin sensitivity and an antioxidant with α-lipoic acid to minimise oxidative damage. To reduce the high homocysteine and ensure optimal methylation, folate and vitamin B12 were given as both vitamin levels were low, together with vitamin B6, which breaks down homocysteine in the trans-sulfuration pathway. His vitamin D status was most likely low because he spent so much time inside. To address this deficiency 5000 IU/day was added. Lastly, fish oils were recommended for cardiovascular and brain health and to reduce inflammation, particularly since in diabetes plant oils are not readily converted to EPA and DHA due to delta 6 desaturase deficiency.

The herbal prescription in form of a tincture included *Curcuma longa* for liver phase I and II detoxification support,[70] and its antioxidant, anti-inflammatory and hypolipidaemic properties. *Gymnema sylvestre* was chosen for its ability to reduce sugar cravings and control blood sugar levels. *Eleutherococcus senticosus* also has the ability to regulate blood sugar as well as blood pressure, apart from its adaptogenic effect on stress. Similarly, *Trigonella foecum-gracum* has positive effects on blood sugar control and cardiovascular parameters.

Expected outcomes and follow-up protocols

As the patient is still a 'young retiree' there is hope that some, if not all, parameters can be improved and perhaps even normalised if he maintains his adherence to the protocols and prescriptions given to him, and if he manages to lose some weight. Counselling and joining a social club for outings could be considered.

In the second consultation the patient brought with him the results of the tests requested previously (Table 16.3). He had started to exercise by playing bowls three times a week. His diet had improved somewhat as he was now eating proper meals (meat, potatoes and vegetables). His beer consumption had gone down to one or two cans per night, and he had replaced soft drinks with water. He also was enjoying the protein smoothies. It was decided that further dietary changes were premature and would probably result in failure.

With these encouraging improvements, and due praise from the practitioner, the next step could be tackled: supplementation. None of these nutrients had been contained in his diet (at time of first consultation), so their levels were expected to be low, further evidenced by his health problems and blood-test results. The supplements prescribed were based on signs and symptoms, diet and lifestyle analysis, and on the test results in Table 16.3 (which showed suboptimal values in most parameters).

The glucose tolerance test results are displayed in Figure 16.4. The test revealed hyperglycaemia, hyperinsulinaemia, hypercortisolism and insulin resistance (the right-shift of the insulin peak to the glucose peak denotes delayed insulin response—that is, insulin resistance). The results were explained to the patient; this made him realise how imbalanced his whole body had become. It meant either medication or compliance with the recommendations of the naturopath. He chose the latter.

There are more possibilities regarding nutrients and herbs, and diet could be further refined. Vitamin B12 may need to be given intramuscularly if the oral supplementation fails to raise this. Decreasing vitamin B12 values may also indicate reduced gastric secretions, as is often the case with high stress as well as with age. In that case digestive

Table 16.3 Pathology test results

TEST	PATIENT RESULTS	REFERENCE RANGE*
ALT	56 U/L	5–40 U/L
Homocysteine	14 µmol/L	0–15 µmol/L, but ideally < 10 µmol/L
Active B12	36 pmol/L	> 35 pmol/L
R/C folate	263 nmol/L	> 250 nmol/L
ESR	25 mm/h	1–30 mm/h, but ideally < 1 mm/h
CRP	8 mg/L	0–10 mg/L, but ideally <1 mg/L
Triglycerides	3.4 mmol/L	0.6–2 mmol/L
HbA$_{1c}$	7.8%	< 6%
HDL	0.9 mmol/L	1.1–1.9 mmol/L, ideally at the upper end
Hydroxycalciferol (vitamin D)	45 nmol/L	50–150 nmol/L, but ideally > 100 nmol/L

*The difference between the reference values given in Table 16.1 and those given here are due to the latter being from the laboratory and the former from the textbook.

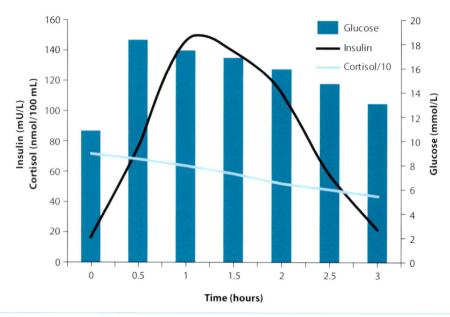

Figure 16.4 Three-hour glucose tolerance test with insulin and cortisol showing hyperglycaemia, hyperinsulinaemia, hypercortisolism and insulin resistance

enzymes (hydrochloric acid, pepsin and pancreatic enzymes) should be added to the regimen.

When the patient returned 4 weeks later he had lost 2 kg. He had been compliant with the instructions given to him and had taken his supplements and herbs assiduously. His diet had further improved as he was now cooking meat, fish and vegetables at home. Instead of drinking beer at night he had one or two glasses of dry red wine.

It was deemed appropriate to talk about low glycaemic index/glycaemic load foods and the balance of macronutrients at this point. He was advised to reduce the carbohydrates (bread and potatoes in particular) and replace them with low glycaemic load vegetables (a handout was given), and to include protein with every meal. It would also be advantageous to replace some of his coffee with green tea, and to use stevia instead of sugar for sweetening.

Again, the patient had been very compliant when he returned 4 weeks later. His weight had gone down a further 3 kg. He was still playing bowls three times a week, and he was going for a walk twice a week with his neighbour. He felt more motivated and had completed many of the small tasks at home. The patient commented that he felt he had a new lease on life.

These positive changes were also reflected in his physical values (Table 16.4). He was delighted and felt encouraged by these results. The prescriptions were repeated and a date for a follow-up consultation made in 3 months.

Table 16.4 Physical examination at fourth consultation

MEASUREMENT	PREVIOUS	ACTUAL	IDEAL
Glucose (fasting)	11.3	7.3 mmol/L	< 6 mmol/L
BP	145/90	135/85	120/80
Weight	99.5 kg	94.5 kg	73 kg
BMI	34	32.3	25 (maximum)
Lean body mass	49.5 kg	50.0 kg	60 kg
Fat mass	50 kg	44.5 kg	13 kg
Urinalysis	Glucose 1+	Glucose ND	None

Table 16.5 Review of the major evidence

INTERVENTION	METHODOLOGY	RESULT	COMMENT
Diet and exercise[128]	Subjects at risk of diabetes type 2 Intervention ($n = 47$) and control ($n = 50$) groups Duration of trial: 1 year	Reductions in total and saturated fat intake, and obesity Increase in physical activity, insulin sensitivity and glucose tolerance	This trial confirms that lifestyle, diet and exercise play a significant role in reducing the risk factors for diabetes type 2.
Tai chi[60]	Subjects with diabetes type 2 Tai chi twice a week for 6 months Those who adhered to program ($n = 31$) compared to those who did not ($n = 31$)	Greater decline in fasting glucose and HbA$_{1c}$, increased diabetic self-care and quality of life in adherence group	Even gentle exercise is sufficient to improve diabetes type 2 parameters.
Aesculus hippocastanum[129]	Triple-blind RCT Patients with leg ulcers Treatment group ($n = 27$) receiving A. hippocastanum Placebo group ($n = 27$)	No difference in wound and pain but improvement in wound slough and frequency of dressing changes	Even those slight improvements increase quality of life. This also leads to reduced costs to the health-care system as fewer visits to medical personnel are needed.
Vitamin B12[98]	Symptomatic diabetic neuropathy ($n = 11$) Monthly intrathecal 2500 µg methylcobalamin injections for several months	Dramatic improvement in paraesthesia, burning pain and heaviness in legs	The symptoms experienced in this group are indicative of vitamin B12 deficiency. Measuring 'active B12' before and after the trial would have been useful.

(Continued)

Table 16.5 Review of the major evidence *(Continued)*

INTERVENTION	METHODOLOGY	RESULT	COMMENT
Silybum marianum[99]	RCT 4-month trial in diabetes type 2 patients (*n* = 51) Treatment group: conventional therapy plus 200 mg *Silymarin* t.d.s. Placebo group: conventional treatment only	Significant decrease in HbA$_{1c}$, FBS, total cholesterol, LDL, and triglycerides with *Silymarin*	*S. marianum* may have acted synergistically with the conventional treatment. It is also a strong antioxidant in its own right, capable of improving the glycaemic profile.
Ginkgo biloba[114]	Randomised trial Patients with early diabetic nephropathy (*n* = 68) Treatment group: conventional treatment + 9.6 mg *G. biloba* extract Placebo group: conventional treatment only Duration: 3 months	Indicators of diabetic nephropathy all improved in the treatment but not in the placebo group	These effects could be due to *G. biloba*'s antioxidant as well as its circulatory stimulation qualities.
Ginkgo biloba[113]	Similar trial to the one above (*n* = 60) Duration: 4 weeks	Decreases in albuminuria excretion rate, improvements in blood lipids, renal function and blood flow No effect on blood pressure and fasting glucose	These two trials corroborate each other's results. Perhaps a longer duration would have also improved blood pressure and glucose.
Policosanol and omega-3 fatty acids[130]	RCT (*n* = 90) 5 weeks on cholesterol-lowering treatment, then omega-3 1 g b.d. + policosanol 5 mg/day or omega-3 1 g b.d. + policosanol 10 mg/day or omega-3 1 g b.d. + placebo for 8 weeks	Significant reductions in LDL and cholesterol and increases in HDL in the policosanol groups Triglycerides were reduced in both the omega-3 only and the omega-3 + policosanol groups.	Lowering triglycerides is of crucial importance as these are paramount to the pathology of diabetes type 2. Policosanol provides additional benefits to omega-3 treatment alone and should be considered where their effect is warranted.
Vitamin E[89]	Open trial Diabetes type 2 with microalbuminaemia (*n* = 19) Diabetes type 2 without microalbuminaemia (*n* = 10) Non-diabetes type 2 subjects without microalbuminaemia (*n* = 10) 1200 IU vitamin E for 4 months	Significant decrease in microalbuminuria and malondialdehyde, indicative of nephroprotection through antioxidant and thromboxane-A2 lowering action of vitamin E	Many of the long-term risks and comorbidities in diabetes type 2 have been linked to oxidation, and combining vitamin E with other antioxidants may have provided even better results.

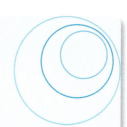

KEY POINTS

- Contributors to diabetes type 2 include:
  - stress
  - high cortisol
  - sedentary lifestyle
  - unbalanced diet.
- Treatment includes:
  - dietary modifications
  - supplementing with chromium, magnesium and lipoic acid
  - utilising herbs that help balance blood glucose, such as:
    - *Gymnema sylvestre*
    - *Trigonella foecum-gracum*
  - exercise
  - stress management if indicated.

Further reading

Bone K. Phytotherapy for diabetes and the key role of *Gymnema.* Modern Phytotherapist 2002;7(1):7–11.

Gropper S, et al. Advanced nutrition and human metabolism. 5th edn. Australia: Wadsworth, Cengage Learning, 2009:276–277.

Kelly GS. Insulin resistance: lifestyle and nutritional interventions. Altern Med Rev 2000;5(2):109–132.

Mota M, et al. The metabolic syndrome—a multifaced disease. Rom J Intern Med 2004;42(2):247–255.

Roberts K, et al. Syndrome X: medical nutrition therapy. Nutr Rev 2000;58(5):154–160.

Shils ME, et al. Modern nutrition in health and disease. Philadelphia: Lippincott Williams & Wilkins, 2006:1004–1066, Chapters 62–65.

Yeh GY, et al. Systematic review of herbs and dietary supplements for glycemic control in diabetes. Diabetes Care 2003;26(4):1277–1294.

References

1. Mota M, et al. The metabolic syndrome—a multifaced disease. Rom J Intern Med 2004;42(2):247–255.
2. Shils ME, et al. Modern nutrition in health and disease. Philadelphia: Lippincott Williams & Wilkins, 2006.
3. Kelly GS. Insulin resistance: lifestyle and nutritional interventions. Altern Med Rev 2000;5(2):109–132.
4. Roberts K, et al. Syndrome X: medical nutrition therapy. Nutr Rev 2000;58(5):154–160.
5. Khani S, Tayek JA. Cortisol increases gluconeogenesis in humans: its role in the metabolic syndrome. Clin Sci 2001;101(6):739–747.
6. Holick MF. Diabetes and the vitamin D connection. Curr Diab Rep 2008;8(5):393–398.
7. Vinson GP. Angiotensin II, corticosteroids, type II diabetes and the metabolic syndrome. Med Hypotheses 2007;68(6):1200–1207.
8. Brindley DN. Role of glucocorticoids and fatty acids in the impairment of lipid metabolism observed in the metabolic syndrome. Int J Obes Relat Metab Dis 1995;19 Suppl 1:S69–S75.
9. Ginsberg HN, et al. Regulation of plasma triglycerides in insulin resistance and diabetes. Arch Med Res 2005;36(3):232–240.
10. Hristova M, Aloe L. Metabolic syndrome—neurotrophic hypothesis. Med Hypotheses 2006;66(3):545–549.
11. Walker BR. Steroid metabolism in metabolic syndrome X. Best Pract Res Clin Endocrinol Metab 2001;15(1):111–122.
12. Pickup JC, et al. NIDDM as a disease of the innate immune system: association of acute-phase reactants and interleukin-6 with metabolic syndrome X. Diabetologia 1997;40(11):1286–1292.
13. Clifton PM. Diet and C-reactive protein. Curr Atheroscler Rep 2003;5(6):431–436.
14. Rosmond R. The glucocorticoid receptor gene and its association to metabolic syndrome. Obes Res 2002;10(10):1078–1086.
15. Björntorp P, Rosmond R. The metabolic syndrome—a neuroendocrine disorder? Br J Nutr 2000;83 Suppl 1:S49–S57.
16. Evans JL, et al. Oxidative stress and stress-activated signaling pathways: a unifying hypothesis of type 2 diabetes. Endocr Rev 2002;23(5):599–622.
17. Evans JL, et al. The molecular basis for oxidative stress-induced insulin resistance. Antioxid Redox Signal 2005;7(7–8):1040–1052.
18. Sebeková K, et al. Association of metabolic syndrome risk factors with selected markers of oxidative status and microinflammation in healthy omnivores and vegetarians. Mol Nutr Food Res 2006;50(9):858–868.
19. Singh RB, et al. Can brain dysfunction be a predisposing factor for metabolic syndrome? Biomed Pharmacother 2004;58 Suppl 1:S56–S68.
20. Wirth A. [Non-pharmacological therapy of metabolic syndrome]. Herz 1995;20(1):56–69.
21. Gropper S, et al. Advanced nutrition and human metabolism. 5th edn. Australia: Wadsworth, Cengage Learning, 2009.
22. Devlin TM. Textbook of biochemistry with clinical correlations. 5th edn. New York: Wiley-Liss, 2002.

23. Pagana KD, Pagana TJ. Mosby's manual of diagnostic and laboratory tests. 3rd edn. USA: CV Mosby, 2006.
24. Upfal J, O'Callaghan J. Your medical tests. what do they really mean? Melbourne: Black Ink, 2001.
25. Pasquali R, et al. The hypothalamic-pituitary-adrenal axis activity in obesity and the metabolic syndrome. Ann N Y Acad Sci 2006;1083:111–128.
26. Schindhelm RK, et al. Liver alanine aminotransferase, insulin resistance and endothelial dysfunction in normotriglyceridaemic subjects with type 2 diabetes mellitus. Eur J Clin Invest 2005;35(6):369–374.
27. Hayden MR, Tyagi SC. Homocysteine and reactive oxygen species in metabolic syndrome, type 2 diabetes mellitus, and atherosclerotropathy: the pleiotropic effects of folate supplementation. Nutr J 2004;3:4.
28. Herbert V, et al. Low holotranscobalamin II is the earliest serum marker for subnormal vitamin B12 (cobalamin) absorption in patients with AIDS. Am J Hematol 1990;34:132–139.
29. Boucher BJ. Inadequate vitamin D status: does it contribute to the disorders comprising syndrome 'X'? [erratum appears in Br J Nutr 1998 Dec;80(6):585]. Br J Nutr 1998;79(4):315–327.
30. Kumar P, Clark M. Clinical medicine. 5th edn. London: W.B. Saunders, 2002.
31. Dickey RA, et al. Optimal thyrotropin level: normal ranges and reference intervals are not equivalent. Thyroid 2005;15(9):1035–1039.
32. Tierney LM, et al. Medical diagnosis and treatment. 44th edn. New York: McGraw-Hill, 2005.
33. MIMS annual. Australian edition. CMPMedica, June 2006.
34. Watkins P. The diabetic foot. BMJ 2003;326(7396):977–979
35. Giarratana N, et al. A vitamin D analog down-regulates proinflammatory chemokine production by pancreatic islets inhibiting T cell recruitment and type 1 diabetes development. J Immunol 2004;173(4):2280–2287.
36. Lips P. Vitamin D physiology. Prog Biophys Mol Biol 2006;92(1):4–8.
37. Chertow B. Advances in diabetes for the millennium: vitamins and oxidant stress in diabetes and its complications. MedGenMed 2004;6(3 Suppl):4.
38. Triggiani V, et al. Role of antioxidants, essential fatty acids, carnitine, vitamins, phytochemicals and trace elements in the treatment of diabetes mellitus and its chronic complications. Endocr Metab Immune Disord Drug Targets 2006;6(1):77–93.
39. Packer L, et al. Molecular aspects of lipoic acid in the prevention of diabetes complications. Nutrition 2001;17(10):888–895.
40. van Dam PS. Oxidative stress and diabetic neuropathy: pathophysiological mechanisms and treatment perspectives. Journal of the Peripheral Nervous System [Article] 2002;7(4):246–248.
41. Head KA. Natural therapies for ocular disorders, part two: cataracts and glaucoma. Altern Med Rev 2001;6(2):141–166.
42. Das UN. Essential fatty acids in health and disease. J Asso Physicians India 1999;47(9):906–911.
43. Giurini J, Lyons T. Diabetic foot complications: diagnosis and management. Int J Low Extrem Wounds 2005;4:171–182.
44. Brehm BJ, D'Alessio DA. Weight loss and metabolic benefits with diets of varying fat and carbohydrate content: separating the wheat from the chaff. Nat Clin Pract Endocrinol Metab [serial on the Internet] 2008;4(3):Online. Available: http://www.medscape.com/viewprogram/8640_pnt.
45. Neff LM. Evidence-based dietary recommendations for patients with type 2 diabetes mellitus. Nutr Clin Care 2003;6(2):51–61.
46. Pelkman CL, et al. Effects of moderate-fat (from monounsaturated fat) and low-fat weight-loss diets on the serum lipid profile in overweight and obese men and women. Am J Clin Nutr 2004;79(2):204–212.
47. Belury MA. Dietary conjugated linoleic acid in health: physiological effects and mechanisms of action. Ann Rev of Nutr 2002;22:505–531.
48. Belury MA, et al. The conjugated linoleic acid (CLA) isomer, t10c12-CLA, is inversely associated with changes in body weight and serum leptin in subjects with type 2 diabetes mellitus. J Nutr 2003;133(1):257S–260S.
49. Gaullier J-M, et al. Supplementation with conjugated linoleic acid for 24 months is well tolerated by and reduces body fat mass in healthy, overweight humans. J Nutr 2005;135(4):778–784.
50. Gaullier J-M, et al. Conjugated linoleic acid supplementation for 1 y reduces body fat mass in healthy overweight humans. Am J Clin Nutr 2004;79(6):1118–1125.
51. Dhiman TR, et al. Factors affecting conjugated linoleic acid content in milk and meat. Crit Rev Food Sci Nutr 2005;45(6):463–482.
52. Carroll J. Attack on the food pyramid. Wall Street Journal 2002:Jun 13;Sect. B.1.
53. Abboud L, Cairns A. Even a diet of fat-free foods can pose a weighty problem. Wall Street Journal 2002:Jun 11;Sect. D.4.
54. Rodríguez-Morán M, et al. Lipid- and glucose-lowering efficacy of Plantago psyllium in type II diabetes. J Diabetes Complications 1998;12(5):273–278.
55. Do Just. It: Diabetes and exercise. Clin Diabetes 2008;26(3):140–141.
56. Turcotte LP, Fisher JS. Skeletal muscle insulin resistance: roles of fatty acid metabolism and exercise. Phys Ther 2008;88(11):1279–1296.
57. Earnest CP. Exercise interval training: an improved stimulus for improving the physiology of pre-diabetes. Med Hypotheses 2008;71(5):752–761.
58. Gulve AE. Exercise and glycemic control in diabetes: benefits, challenges, and adjustments to pharmacotherapy. Phys Ther 2008;88(11):1297–1321.
59. Ying Z, Fu FH. Effects of 14-week Tai Ji Quan exercise on metabolic control in women with type 2 diabetes. Am J Chin Med 2008;36(4):647–654.
60. Song R, et al. Adhering to a t'ai chi program to improve glucose control and quality of life for individuals with type 2 diabetes. J Altern Complement Med 2009;15(6):627–632.
61. Crowley LV. An introduction to human disease: pathology and pathophysiology correlations. 6th edn. Sudbury: Jones and Bartlett Publishers, 2004.
62. Yeh GY, et al. Systematic review of herbs and dietary supplements for glycemic control in diabetes. Diabetes Care 2003;26(4):1277–1294.
63. McCarty MF. Chromium and other insulin sensitizers may enhance glucagon secretion: implications for hypoglycemia and weight control. Med Hypotheses 1996;46(2):77–80.
64. Higdon J. An evidence-based approach to vitamins and minerals. New York: Thieme, 2003.
65. Hargreaves IP, et al. The effect of HMG-CoA reductase inhibitors on coenzyme Q10: possible biochemical/clinical implications. Drug Saf 2005;28(8):659–676.
66. Henriksen EJ, Saengsirisuwan V. Exercise training and antioxidants: relief from oxidative stress and insulin resistance. Exerc Sport Sci Rev 2003;31(2):79–84.
67. Yeh GY, et al. Systematic review of herbs and dietary supplements for glycemic control in diabetes. Diabetes Care 2003;26(4):1277.
68. Mills S, Bone K. Principles and practice of phytotherapy. Sydney: Churchill Livingstone, 2000.
69. Bone K. Phytotherapy for diabetes and the key role of Gymnema. Modern Phytotherapist 2002;7(1):7–11.
70. Bone K. A clinical guide to blending liquid herbs. USA: Elsevier, 2003.
71. Gormley JJ. Herbal approaches to diabetes and hyperglycemia. Better Nutrition 1997;59(10):24.

72. Leach MJ. *Gymnema sylvestre* for diabetes mellitus: a systematic review. J Altern Complement Med 2007;13(9):977–983.

73. Blumenthal M. The ABC clinical guide to herbs. Austin: American Botanical Council, 2003.

74. Anonymous. Diabetes herb as effective as drugs. Better Nutrition 2005;67(5):12.

75. Kapoor R, Huang YS. Gamma linolenic acid: an antiinflammatory omega-6 fatty acid. Curr Pharm Biotechnol 2006;7(6):531–534.

76. Braun L, Cohen M. Herbs and natural supplements. 2nd edn. Sydney: Churchill Livingstone, 2007.

77. König D, et al. Mehrfach ungesättigte Fettsäuren, koronare Herzerkrankung und Diabetes mellitus Typ II—Hinweise fur den Stellenwert von Gamma-Linolensäure. Forsch Komplementärmed 1997;4(2):94.

78. Brenner RR. Hormonal modulation of delta6 and delta5 desaturases: case of diabetes. Prostaglandins Leukot Essent Fatty Acids 2003;68(2):151–162.

79. Malasanos TH, Stacpoole PW. Biological effects of omega-3 fatty acids in diabetes mellitus. Diabetes Care 1991;14(12):1160–1179.

80. Coyne DW. Vitamin D and the diabetic patient. Medscape Nephrology [serial on the Internet]. Online. Available: http://www.medscape.com/viewarticle/573383_print. Accessed 28 April 2008.

81. Brandacher G, et al. Chronic immune activation underlies morbid obesity: is IDO a key player? Curr Drug Metab 2007;8(3):289–295.

82. Tsigos C, Chrousos GP. Hypothalamic-pituitary-adrenal axis, neuroendocrine factors and stress. J Psychosom Res 2002;53(4):865–871.

83. Vanitallie TB. Stress: a risk factor for serious illness. Metabolism 2002;51(6 Suppl 1):40–45.

84. McEwen BS. Mood disorders and allostatic load. Biol Psychiatry 2003;54(3):200–207.

85. Mechanick JI. Metabolic mechanisms of stress hyperglycemia. JPEN J Parenter Enteral Nutr 2006;30(2):157–163.

86. Nieuwenhuizen AG, Rutters F. The hypothalamic-pituitary-adrenal-axis in the regulation of energy balance. Physiol Behav 2008;94(2):169–177.

87. Szolomicki S, et al. The influence of active components of *Eleutherococcus senticosus* on cellular defence and physical fitness in man. Phytother Res 2000;14(1):30–35.

88. Bounous G. Whey protein concentrate (WPC) and glutathione modulation in cancer treatment. Anticancer Res 2000;20(6C):4785–4792.

89. Hirnerová E, et al. [Effect of vitamin E therapy on progression of diabetic nephropathy]. Vnitr Lék 2003;49(7):529–534.

90. Li YC. Vitamin D and diabetic nephropathy. Curr Diab Rep 2008;8(6):464–469.

91. Nakamura S, et al. Pyridoxal phosphate prevents progression of diabetic nephropathy. Nephrol Dial Transplant 2007;22(8):2165–2174.

92. Ruhe RC, McDonald RB. Use of antioxidant nutrients in the prevention and treatment of type 2 diabetes. J Am Coll Nutr 2001;20(5 Suppl):363S–369S;discussion 81S–83S.

93. Tong HI. Influence of neurotropic vitamins on the nerve conduction velocity in diabetic neuropathy. Ann Acad Med Singapore 1980;9(1):65–70.

94. van Dam PS. Oxidative stress and diabetic neuropathy: pathophysiological mechanisms and treatment perspectives. Diabetes Metab Res Rev 2002;18(3):176–184.

95. Foster TS. Efficacy and safety of alpha-lipoic acid supplementation in the treatment of symptomatic diabetic neuropathy. Diabetes Educ 2007;33(1):111–117.

96. Bećić F, et al. [Pharmacological significance of alpha lipoic acid in up to date treatment of diabetic neuropathy]. Med Arh 2008;62(1):45–48.

97. Sima AA, et al. Acetyl-L-carnitine improves pain, nerve regeneration, and vibratory perception in patients with chronic diabetic neuropathy: an analysis of two randomized placebo-controlled trials. Diabetes Care 2005;28(1):89–94.

98. Ide H, et al. Clinical usefulness of intrathecal injection of methylcobalamin in patients with diabetic neuropathy. Clin Ther 1987;9(2):183–192.

99. Huseini HF, et al. The efficacy of *Silybum marianum* (L.) Gaertn. (silymarin) in the treatment of type II diabetes: a randomized, double-blind, placebo-controlled, clinical trial. Phytother Res 2006;20(12):1036–1039.

100. Huseini HF, et al. The clinical trial of *Silybum marianum* seed extract (Silymarin) on type II diabetic patients with hyperlipidemia. Iranian Journal of Diabetes & Lipid Disorders 2004;3:78.

101. Leach M. *Aesculus hippocastanum.* Australian Journal of Medical Herbalism 2001;13(4):136–140.

102. Leach MJ. Evidence-based practice: a framework for clinical practice and research design. Int J Nurs Pract 2006;12(5):248–251.

103. Leach MJ. Integrative health care: a need for change? J Complement Integr Med 2006;3(1):1–11.

104. Deng YP, Xie XJ. [Preliminary study on the treatment of diabetic retinopathy utilizing with nourishing yin, tonifying kidney and blood-activating herbs]. Chinese Journal of Integrated Traditional and Western Medicine 1992;12(5):270.

105. Lopes de Jesus C, et al. Vitamin C and superoxide dismutase (SOD) for diabetic retinopathy. Cochrane Database Syst Rev 2008;(1):CD006695.

106. Millen AE, et al. Relations of serum ascorbic acid and alpha-tocopherol to diabetic retinopathy in the Third National Health and Nutrition Examination Survey. Am J Epidemiol 2003;158(3):225–233.

107. Millen AE, et al. Relation between intake of vitamins C and E and risk of diabetic retinopathy in the Atherosclerosis Risk in Communities Study. Am J Clin Nutr 2004;79(5):865–873.

108. Bian F, et al. [Clinical study on treatment of incipient diabetic nephropathy by integrated traditional Chinese and Western medicine]. Zhongguo Zhong Xi Yi Jie He Za Zhi 2000;20(5):335–337.

109. Zou LH, et al. [Clinical observation on Qidi Yiqi Yangyin Huoxue Recipe in treating diabetic nephropathy at stage III and IV]. Zhongguo Zhong Xi Yi Jie He Za Zhi 2006;26(11):1023–1026.

110. Zhao L, et al. [Integrated treatment of traditional Chinese medicine and western medicine for early- and intermediate-stage diabetic nephropathy]. Nan Fang Yi Ke Da Xue Xue Bao 2007;27(7):1052–1055.

111. Wu S, et al. Treatment of incipient diabetic nephropathy by clearing away the stomach-heat, purging the heart fire, strengthening the spleen and tonifying the kidney. J Tradit Chin Med 2000;20(3):172–175.

112. Wang HY, et al. [Clinical observation on treatment of diabetic nephropathy with compound fructus arctii mixture]. Zhongguo Zhong Xi Yi Jie He Za Zhi 2004;24(7):589–592.

113. Lu J, He H. Clinical observation of *Ginkgo biloba* extract injection in treating early diabetic nephropathy. Chin J Integr Med 2005;11(3):226–228.

114. Zhu HW, et al. [Effect of extract of *Ginkgo biloba* leaf on early diabetic nephropathy]. Zhongguo Zhong Xi Yi Jie He Za Zhi 2005;25(10):889–891.

115. Li XS, et al. [Effect of extract of *Ginkgo biloba* on soluble intercellular adhesion molecule-1 and soluble vascular cell adhesion molecule-1 in patients with early diabetic nephropathy]. Zhongguo Zhong Xi Yi Jie He Za Zhi 2007;27(5):412–414.

116. Pouwer F, et al. Fat food for a bad mood. Could we treat and prevent depression in type 2 diabetes by means of omega-3 polyunsaturated fatty acids? A review of the evidence. Diabet Med 2005;22(11):1465–1475.

117. Romerio SC, et al. Acute hyperhomocysteinemia decreases NO bioavailability in healthy adults. Atherosclerosis 2004;176(2):337–344.
118. Eto M, et al. Lowering effect of pantethine on plasma beta-thromboglobulin and lipids in diabetes mellitus. Artery 1987;15(1):1–12.
119. Arsenio L, et al. Effectiveness of long-term treatment with pantethine in patients with dyslipidemia. Clin Ther 1986;8(5):537–545.
120. Blumenthal M. The complete German Commission E monographs—therapeutic guide to herbal medicines [CD-ROM]. Austin: American Botanical Council, 1999.
121. Paul S. Dare to be non-diabetic. Natl J Homoeopath 2008;10(10):13.
122. Paul S. Homoeopathic approach to diabetes mellitus and its complications. Natl J Homoeopath 2008;10(10):56.
123. Anonymous. Important remedies in diabetes. Homoeopath Update 2000;8(1):40.
124. Bhapkar C. Treat the man, not the disease. Natl J Homoeopath 2008;10(10):48.
125. Hariharan R. The diabetic breakthrough. Natl J Homoeopath 2006;8(2):109.
126. Soldner G, et al. Magnesium chloratum. Merkurstab 2006;59(2):112.
127. Lodha R, Bagga A. Traditional Indian systems of medicine. Ann Acad Med Singapore 2000;29(1):37–41.
128. Corpeleijn E, et al. Improvements in glucose tolerance and insulin sensitivity after lifestyle intervention are related to changes in serum fatty acid profile and desaturase activities: the SLIM study. Diabetologia 2006;49(10):2392–2401.
129. Leach MJ, et al. Clinical efficacy of horsechestnut seed extract in the treatment of venous ulceration. J Wound Care 2006;15(4):159–167.
130. Castano G, et al. Effects of addition of policosanol to omega-3 fatty acid therapy on the lipid profile of patients with type II hypercholesterolaemia. Drugs R D 2005;6(4):207–219.

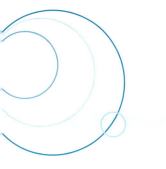

17
Thyroid abnormalities

Tini Gruner
ND, PhD, MSc

AETIOLOGY

The main function of the thyroid is to produce hormones that regulate the metabolic rate of all cells, energy, cell growth and tissue differentiation.[1,2] This is regulated by thyrotropin-releasing hormone (TRH), secreted by the hypothalamus, which activates thyroid-stimulating hormone (TSH), secreted by the pituitary gland, to produce thyroxine (T_4) and triiodothyronine (T_3) (Figure 17.1).[1]

The precursors for thyroid hormone production are tyrosine and iodine. The thyroid gland actively accumulates iodine (~ 60 mg/day) in the form of iodide (I^-), which leads to a much higher concentration in this gland than elsewhere in the body in order to produce T_4 and some T_3. These hormones are then released into the circulation where most are bound to transport proteins. Less than 0.1% are unbound (free T_3 and T_4) and active as hormone. Although the amount of T_4 in the blood exceeds that of T_3 nearly 50-fold, it is T_3 that has much higher biological activity.[3,4] Zinc seems to be needed to facilitate the uptake of the hormone by the cells[5] and favourably affects T_3.[6] Some organs and tissues can convert T_4 to T_3 (mainly liver, kidneys, brain, muscle and brown adipose tissue), with most of the circulating T_3 having been produced peripherally[7] or in the liver. The conversion of T_4 to T_3 is accomplished by 5'-deiodinase which is selenium dependent.[4,8] In the absence of selenium, reverse T_3 (rT_3) is produced; this is metabolically inactive.[9] Figure 17.2 shows the metabolic pathways of T_4 conversion.[4]

Thyroid function not only depends on sufficient precursors (such as iodine and tyrosine) but also on hormone synthesis regulation and the demand for these hormones. Disturbances in any of these can lead to increased TSH production by the pituitary gland with subsequent (non-toxic) goitre formation. This increased thyroid tissue production is an attempt to produce sufficient thyroid hormones in order to maintain normal blood levels. Figure 17.3 illustrates this. However, if the enlarged thyroid gland overproduces thyroid hormones, leading to hyperthyroidism, it is called a 'toxic goitre'.[10]

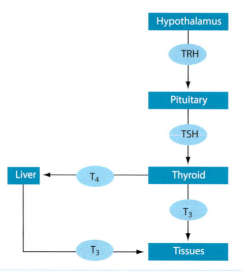

Figure 17.1 Thyroid hormone stimulation

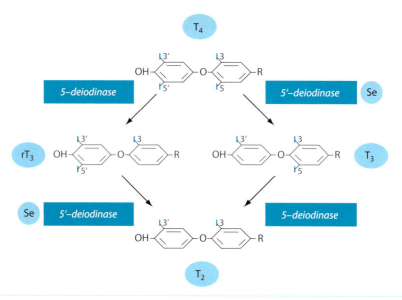

Figure 17.2 Conversion of T_4 to T_3 and catabolism to T_2. The selenium-dependent 5'-deiodinase converts T_4 to the more potent T_3 and further degrades this to T_2. In the absence of selenium the inactive rT_3 is produced; this then accumulates.

Source: Adapted from www.medscape.com/.../38/433856/433856_fig.html

Thyroid antibodies (to thyroglobulin, peroxidase or thyroid receptor) are only raised in the autoimmune forms of hypothyroidism (Hashimoto's disease) and hyperthyroidism (Grave's disease). Gastrointestinal pathogens, through 'molecular mimicry', could be responsible for this.[1,11] Refer to Chapter 28 on autoimmunity for further details.

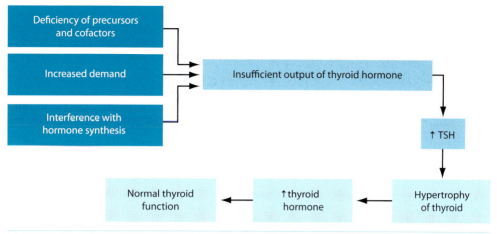

Figure 17.3 Development of goitre
Source: Adapted from Crowley 2004[10]

In hypothyroidism a disturbance in glucose tolerance has been found to be due to decreased sensitivity to insulin, and raised cortisol and free fatty acids.[12] This is not surprising considering that insulin resistance, diabetes type 2, stress (hyper-cortisolism and hyperadrenalism) and hypothyroidism share a number of common signs and symptoms, taking into account the link between the hormones involved in these conditions. Raised cortisol levels with impaired glucagon response were noted when hypoglycaemia was induced in hypothyroid patients.[13] Insulin and glucose control was regained when these patients were given thyroid hormone replacement therapy.[14] Further, hypothyroidism, like insulin resistance and diabetes type 2, leads to inhibition of delta 5 and 6 desaturase, impeding the utilisation of dietary omega-3 and omega-6 fatty acids.[1] A rise in blood pressure has been noted in the hypothyroid state which normalised on thyroid treatment.[15] Conversely, impaired extrathyroidal conversion of T_4 to T_3 has been found in diseases such as heart and liver disease and diabetes type 2, where there is high plasma free fatty acid concentration with no obvious thyroid pathology.[1]

Sick euthyroid syndrome, an underfunctioning thyroid with apparently normal test results, can occur as part of a number of health problems. It has been found, for a variety of reasons, to be part of virtually all severe systemic illnesses, fasting and major operations, affecting T_3, T_4 and rT_3.[16] Treating obese individuals with hypocaloric diets leads to similar thyroid hormone changes as in anorexia, namely decreases in T_3 and T_4 and increases in rT_3. These hormones will normalise with weight normalisation.[17] Certain medications also influence thyroid hormone status by either increasing or decreasing T_4.[7] It is therefore essential to test for these hormones in these situations in order to determine treatment options.

Testing for thyroid function

In hyperthyroidism, T_4 and T_3 levels are elevated, suppressing TSH. In contrast, in primary hypothyroidism TSH tends to be high with T_3 and T_4 being low. In secondary hypothyroidism, however, TSH as well as T_3 and T_4 are low. This latter condition arises from an inability of the pituitary gland to secrete TSH, possibly due to low TRH. By measuring TSH only, this condition can be missed or misinterpreted. Therefore, when there is indication from the symptom picture that thyroid function could be compromised, not only TSH but also T_3 and T_4 should be measured.[18] Table 17.1 gives an overview of the laboratory parameters for each condition, and Table 17.2 shows the reference ranges (which vary somewhat between laboratories) and the ideal ranges of these parameters. In addition, the thyroid should be checked for goitre and nodules by palpation and the latter, if needed, by ultrasound or biopsy.[7]

Laboratory reference values for these parameters encompass 95% of the 'healthy' population, and only when individual values are outside this range will further investigations and possibly therapy be instigated by the doctor. However, in a well-functioning thyroid TSH should be between 0.4 and 2.5 mU/L (otherwise the system is labouring—subclinical hypothyroidism (SCH)—see below), with a therapeutic target range of 0.5 to 2 mU/L.[19,20] The actual hormones should ideally be in the high-normal range. The ratio of T_4 to T_3 has been estimated as 4:1 in healthy thyroid function.[1] Antibodies should be absent and rT_3 should be low.

EPIDEMIOLOGY

Thyroid disorders are much more frequent in women than in men. The overall incidence in Australia is estimated at 5 in 1000 in males and 27 in 1000 in females. No specific figures for hypothyroidism in Australia could be found but in the US populations this

Table 17.1 Thyroid test results for common thyroid disorders

CONDITION	TSH	TOTAL T_4	FREE T_4	T_3
Hyperthyroidism	Suppressed	Increased	Increased	Increased
Hypothyroidism	Increased	Low/low-normal	Low/low-normal	Normal or low
TSH deficiency (secondary hypothyroid)	Low/low-normal	Low/low-normal	Low/low-normal	Normal or low
Sick euthyroid syndrome	Low/low-normal	Slightly low	Slightly low	Slightly low

Source: Adapted from Kumar & Clark, p. 1036[11]

Table 17.2 Reference ranges and ideal ranges of thyroid parameters[2]

PARAMETER	REFERENCE RANGE	IDEAL RANGE
TSH	0.3–5 mU/L	0.4–2.5 mU/L
T_3	2.6–6.0 pmol/L	4–5 pmol/L
T_4	9–19 pmol/L	14–19 pmol/L
rT_3	140–540 pmol/L	< 240 pmol/L
Thyroglobulin AB	< 4 IU/mL	< 1 IU/mL
Peroxidase AB	< 6 IU/mL	< 1 IU/mL
TRAB	< 1 IU/L	< 1 IU/L

AB = antibodies, TRAB = thyroid receptor antibodies

is estimated to be 0.3%.[21] Approximately 10–12 million people in the USA have hypo-thyroidism.[22] In the UK the annual incidence of primary hypothyroidism is estimated to be 0.6 in 1000 for men and 3.5 in 1000 for women. In total, 3% of the population is taking medication for hypothyroidism.[23] In contrast, it is stated that in the US 1–2% of the population is hypothyroid, with a tenfold higher occurrence in women than in men and increasing with age.[3] Including SCH, the figures increase to 4.3–9.5%.[3] Considering that this condition is generally underdiagnosed, at least in its milder form, the incidence would be much higher.

These statistics indicate that there is a large proportion of the population who have SCH. Naturopathy is concerned with life quality and prevention of disease, so recognising an impending disease state gives the practitioner the opportunity to address imbalances before overt signs and symptoms have developed and permanent damage has been done. This not only increases the wellbeing of the patient but it also reduces health-care costs.

An estimated 5–15% of the women of childbearing age have autoimmune thyroid-itis, and the results of going undiagnosed and untreated into a pregnancy include an increased risk of miscarriage, preterm delivery and fetal neurological impairment (such as is seen in cretinism).

RISK FACTORS

Subclinical hypothyroidism

SCH has been characterised by elevated TSH with normal T_3 and T_4.[24,25] There is still debate regarding the significance and possible treatment of SCH. Although treatment with T_4 and/or T_3 has apparently not been shown to provide benefits,[26] withholding treatment may be ill advised. Subtle improvements with early hormonal intervention have been observed, thus warranting thyroid hormone replacement in subclinical manifestations.[27] Most at risk are the elderly and women over the age of 60 years, with increased risk of developing overt hypothyroidism.[25] It is therefore recommended that this population group, people with autoimmune disease and anybody with suggestive symptoms of hypothyroidism be screened.[28] TSH values ranging between 4.5 and 10 mU/L, particularly if antibodies or symptoms are present, may indicate the need for commencement of low-dose T_4 treatment.[29] However, some researchers consider a TSH range up to 20 μU/L (well above the upper limit of the reference range) as the cut-off before instigating therapy.[22]

It is interesting to note that the upper limit of normal for TSH has been reduced from 10 μU/L to between 4 and 5 μU/L during the last decade,[22] with suggestions that this may be further reduced to 2.5 μU/L in the near future. This is based on the observation that 95% of people with normal thyroid function have values under 2.5 μU/L.[20] Suboptimal thyroid function may be due to latent Hashimoto's disease, which could lead, if not addressed early, to overt hypothyroidism.[19,20,22,25] Further, patients with SCH tend to have higher readings of blood pressure, C-reactive protein, homocysteine, cholesterol and LDL, and thus may be presenting with cardiovascular risk factors or disease, including congestive heart failure. Early treatment is therefore recommended;[22] this will also improve long-term life quality by preventing the development of overt hypothyroidism and also reducing the risk factors for cardiovascular disease, not to mention the benefits to the health-care system.

Further, a low T_3 syndrome has been described with increased proinflammatory cytokines, notably IL6, which inhibits 5'-deiodinase. This is commonly seen in congestive heart failure, and T_3 has been shown to be a stronger indicator of all-cause and congestive heart failure mortality than age or dyslipidaemia.[22]

Table 17.3 Iodine reference values[1,32,40]

URINARY IODINE (µG/L)	IODINE NUTRITIONAL STATUS
< 20	Severe deficiency
20–49	Moderate deficiency
50–99	Mild deficiency
100–199	Optimal status
≥ 200	Risk of adverse effects (e.g. hyperthyroidism)

Stress

Stress seems to play a crucial part in thyroid dysregulation and interference with hormone synthesis by triggering the release of corticotropin-releasing hormone, noradrenaline and cortisol. These hormones have an inhibitory influence on TSH secretion and suppress 5'-deiodinase, thus contributing to the suppression of thyroid function[30] (see Chapter 15 on adrenal exhaustion also). The thyroid as well as the adrenal glands requires tyrosine for thyroid hormone and catecholamine synthesis, respectively. Low protein intake and/or impaired protein digestion/use may lead to low tyrosine stores, resulting in low thyroid hormones, especially if this amino acid is required to preferentially produce stress hormones (dopamine, noradrenaline and adrenaline). Urinary cortisol metabolite levels have also been linked to thyroid disorders, both in hypo- and hyperthyroidism, indicative of the influence of stress on thyroid function.[31]

Iodine

Iodine is a common deficiency worldwide, leading to hypothyroidism.[11] It has been found in various parts of Australia (notably Tasmania)[32–36] and New Zealand.[37,38] Often the first visible sign is the development of a goitre. Congenital hypothyroidism, caused by maternal iodine deficiency, leads to mental and physical retardation in infants known as cretinism.[9,39] Iodine reference values, according to the World Health Organization/International Council for the Control of Iodine Deficiency Disorders (WHO/ICCIDD), are given in Table 17.3.

MEDICAL ALERT

Acute exacerbation of hyperthyroid symptoms can occur, called a 'thyroid storm'. It can be brought on by major internal or external stressful events or if hyperthyroidism is inadequately controlled. This condition requires urgent medical attention.[11]

Selenium

Selenium is needed for the conversion of T_4 to T_3 (Figure 17.2). If it is low, the result is not only reduced active thyroid hormone (T_3), but the resultant accumulation of rT_3. Further, rT_3 is also known to block the action of thyroid hormone, thus contributing to hypothyroidism. It is therefore important to measure rT_3, especially with normal T_4 and low T_3 results. Hence, when T_3 is low selenium deficiency should be considered as rT_3 could be elevated.[16] Trauma from injury affects thyroid metabolism with lowered selenium levels, and supplementation with selenium has led to faster normalisation of T_4 and reductions in rT_3.[41] In congenital hypothyroidism, selenium (as selenomethionine) was found to lower TSH and thyroglobulin. It was suggested that the mechanism involved feedback to the hypothalamus–pituitary, thus reducing the stimulation of thyroid tissue and increasing intracellular conversion of T_4 to T_3.[42]

Similarly, in critically ill patients low selenium and T_3 and elevated rT_3 have been found, in addition to low TSH and T_4. However, not only low selenium but also increased cytokine production during inflammation in these patients are responsible for low 5'-deiodinase; this may explain the elevated rT_3. The abnormalities in these parameters have been found to correlate with the severity of the disease.[43] Low T_4 has been attributed to decreases in thyrotropin as well as T_4-binding globulins. Supplementation with T_3, not T_4, has resulted in improvements. The effect of severe systemic illness on thyroid function has been termed 'nonthyroidal illness syndrome' (NTIS).[16]

Mercury

Workers exposed to mercury vapours had a higher risk of hypothyroidism with decreased T_3 and increased rT_3 values, especially if they were also low in iodine.[44]

Molecular mimicry

In hyperthyroidism thyroid hormones are high, suppressing TSH. The increased T_3 and T_4 is evidently due to an antithyroid autoantibody thyroid-stimulating immunoglobulin, which acts like TSH but is not controlled by the same negative feedback mechanism.[10] Certain gram-negative bacteria, such as *Yersinia enterocolitica* and *Escherichia coli*, have been shown to contain TSH binding sites. It could therefore be possible that infection with these organisms could initiate hyperthyroidism through 'molecular mimicry'.[11]

CONVENTIONAL TREATMENT

Hyperthyroidism

Depending on the severity of the disease, hyperthyroidism is treated with drugs that suppress the production of thyroid hormones, radioactive iodine to destroy part or all of the thyroid gland, or surgery to remove some or all of the thyroid. The latter two are likely to require thyroid hormone replacement for life.[11]

In order to make treatment effective but not detrimental to health, in total thyroidectomy a replacement dose of T_4 is usually given at 1.6 µg/kg body weight, with an absorption rate of approximately 65%, resulting in a daily dose of 100–200 µg. It is best taken 1 hour prior to or 2–3 hours after meals. It takes 4–6 weeks for hormone levels to adjust to treatment.[22]

Hypothyroidism

The aim of treatment is to normalise thyroid function, and the treatment of choice for hypothyroidism is levothyroxine sodium (l-T_4). In primary hypothyroidism, optimisation is achieved when TSH levels are 0.5–2 mU/L,[22,45] and in secondary hypothyroidism (where TSH is low) with T_4 and T_3 levels in the upper normal range. When two doses of l-T_4 were compared, one to bring T_4 into the middle and the other into the upper range of normal, the higher dose resulted in lower BMI, cholesterol and LDL.

When the high dose of l-T_4 was combined with liothyronine (l-T_3) at a ratio of 9:1, further benefits were obtained.[22]

This indicates that in certain situations l-T_4 alone is insufficient to return thyroid function to normal. It is estimated that in 10–20% of hypothyroid patients symptoms will persist. This could be due to impaired conversion of T_4 to T_3 (see above under 'Selenium'), a polymorphism in the enzyme 5'-deiodinase,[22] plus several others.[46] Treatment with liothyronine (l-T_3) should therefore be considered when T_4 alone does not improve symptoms or laboratory parameters.[16,22] This is particularly the case in secondary hypothyroidism due to other ill health where there is impaired conversion from T_4 to T_3. In vivo, however, T_3 has a short half-life, leading to supraphysiological peaks without normalisation of TSH. Slow-release formulations are therefore needed.[22]

To overcome the problem regarding when to give T_4 and when T_3, combination preparations are available. However, apart from using the l-T_3 with its half-life problems, the studies done on this have not included measures that indicated the need for T_3.[47] To overcome the instability of T_3, desiccated extract of beef or pork thyroid have been used.[22,45] (Desiccated bovine or porcine thyroid extract is contained in some natural formulations currently on the market and which are available to naturopaths.) This was the standard treatment before l-T_4 was available commercially, but reproducible results were difficult, if not impossible, to obtain due to the variability of thyroid hormone content in these preparations.[22]

In younger people diagnosed with hypothyroidism, treatment with T_4 should be instigated at the highest calculated dose, whereas in older people the dose should be conservative and slowly titrated up to avoid complications, particularly in those people with coronary artery disease. However, long-term treatment above the optimal dose can lead to osteoporosis and atrial fibrillation and should therefore be avoided.[22,45] In autoimmune hypothyroid women planning pregnancy, TSH levels should be kept below 2.5 μU/L, with a 30% increase in l-T_4 dosage once pregnancy has been confirmed.[22]

Table 17.4 lists the treatments currently employed to treat hypo- and hyperthyroidism.

Table 17.4 Conventional treatment for hyper- and hypothyroidism

CONDITION	DRUG	ACTION
Hyperthyroidism	Propylthiouracil Carbamidazole (active metabolite: methimazole)	Antithyroid drugs: inhibit formation of thyroid hormone; immunosuppressive
	Propranolol	Beta-blocker: ↓ sympathetic nervous system activity ↓ peripheral T_4 to T_3 conversion
	Radioactive Iodine	Radiation destroys part or all of thyroid gland (could lead to hypothyroidism)
	Surgery	Partial or total thyroidectomy (could lead to hypothyroidism)
Hypothyroidism	Oroxine (thyroxine) (l-T_4)	Replacement of thyroid hormone (T_4)
	In some cases, liothyronine (l-T_3) has been added to T_4.	Replacement of thyroid hormones (T_3 and T_4)
	Desiccated extract of beef or pork thyroid	Replacement of thyroid hormones (T_3 and T_4)

KEY TREATMENT PROTOCOLS

Diagnostic aids

Temperature regulation

Accurate diagnosis is vital for an effective treatment protocol. In the early stages of thyroid disorders the symptoms can be quite general (such as loose stools or constipation, and changes in energy) and part of a multitude of disease entities. When the prominent signs and symptoms of hyper- or hypothyroidism appear the disease is quite advanced. It is therefore imperative to find early markers so intervention can be started to prevent the manifestation of advanced disease states.

One such marker is body temperature. Ideally, a temperature reading needs to be taken at the same time each day in the morning, straight after waking and before getting out of bed. The reason for taking the temperature in the morning is the influence melatonin exerts on thyroid hormones.[48] The thermometer should be placed under the tongue until it beeps (for digital thermometers) or for a minimum of 5 minutes (if using a mercury one). Ear thermometers or taking the temperature under arm is too inaccurate for this purpose (although the latter has been advocated for decades). This should be repeated for 4 consecutive days and an average taken of the readings. For a woman of childbearing age, the temperature should be taken in the first half of her cycle, ideally the days straight after menses, as there is a natural rise in temperature at ovulation and throughout the second half of the cycle.

> **NATUROPATHIC TREATMENT AIMS**
>
> - Reduce stress.
> - Support stressed systems with adaptogens and anxiolytics (if indicated).
> - Enhance optimal thyroid function.
> - Increase quality of life.
> - Hyperthyroidism:
>   - Support overactive metabolic pathways, organs and systems through nutrient-dense foods, antioxidants, energy-production cofactors and other specific nutrients as indicated.
>   - Slow down thyroid function using phytotherapy.
> - Hypothyroidism:
>   - Ensure precursors (tyrosine, iodine) and cofactors (selenium, zinc) for thyroid hormone production are replete.
>   - Stimulate thyroid function using phytotherapy.

A normal reading is between 36.5 and 37.0°C. Low readings have been linked to thyroid underfunction, and values above this range to hyperthyroidism. Research in elderly hospitalised patients revealed a link between low core (rectal) temperature, low T_3 and high rT_3, and mortality. Further, low serum albumin and weight loss (as indicators of malnutrition) have also been linked to hypothermia (defined as a core temperature between 35.0 and 36.5°C). Interestingly, TSH did not make a significant difference in these patients.[49] However, when healthy males were subjected to different sleep temperatures a significant increase was found in plasma cortisol and TSH with lowered body temperature.[50] Likewise, a rise in TSH and drop in T_3 and T_4 were noted in cold climates and winter months, especially in people above the age of 40 years.[51] In some subjects with fever, rT_3 was found to be directly correlated whereas T_3 was inversely correlated to body temperature, at 40°C reducing to levels seen only in severe hypothyroidism.[52] It seems that the thyroid gland is very sensitive to either heat or cold stress as a result of the hypothalamus–pituitary–thyroid axis dysregulation, and reacts by reducing its hormone production.[48,51]

A number of factors can interfere with the accuracy of the temperature method. Late nights, lack of sleep, infections and acute illnesses will alter the readings. Antidepressant medication has also been linked to lower body temperature. A significant rise in TSH and a drop in T_3 and T_4 have been noted after administration of antidepressants such as tricyclics and selective serotonin reuptake inhibitors (SSRIs), but also after lithium and electroshock treatment. In some patients a blunted TSH response to TRH has been found.[53] This begs the question whether these treatments interfere with negative feedback loops (such as between T_3 and TSH or TSH and TRH) or whether tyrosine was needed preferentially to produce adrenalin?

A low morning temperature may be the first indicator of suboptimal thyroid function. If this is the case it should be followed by a blood test. However, with no prior thyroid pathology it is unlikely that a medical practitioner will order anything other than TSH. Yet it is obvious from the above research that a TSH reading alone will not always reflect the actual functioning of the thyroid. If there is suspicion of thyroid pathology despite a low-normal TSH, T_3, T_4, thyroid antibodies and ideally rT_3 should be assessed. Currently, rT_3 is an out-of-pocket expense to the patient but worth doing if there is good clinical indication for this.

Physical and pathology tests

Since goitre is one of the earliest symptoms of iodine deficiency, the thyroid gland should be palpated to check for enlargement.[40] Further tests that are recommended are a 24-hour urinary iodine excretion,[40] and red blood cell (solidus and/or 24-hour urinary excretion of) selenium and zinc. If any of these are low, appropriate supplementation should be instigated. These tests will confirm or deny the results of a dietary analysis with regard to these elements. Protein status should be evaluated by investigating dietary protein intake and digestive capacity, and possibly by body composition analysis. If protein is found to be low, then it is likely that tyrosine will also be low. If stress is suspected to play a major part in the aetiology of the thyroid disorder then it would be prudent to also assess cortisol.

Addressing underlying pathology

Treatment depends on the findings as a result of case taking, dietary analysis and pathology tests. If stress is a major contributor, **adaptogens** (for example, *Withania somnifera, Rhodiola rosea, Panax ginseng* and *Glycyrrhiza glabra*) or anxiolytics (for example, *Piper methysticum, Valeriana spp., Passiflora incanata*) could be of use.[54-57] If autoimmunity is present **anti-inflammatory** (for example *bioflavonoids,*[58] *enzymes*[58] and *Curcuma longa)*[54] and **immunosuppressant** (for example, *Tylophora indica* and *Hemidesmus indicus*)[54] agents may be indicated.

Hyperthyroidism
Managing increased metabolic rate

In hyperthyroidism, metabolic rate and, with this, energy production are increased. The overactive metabolism needs to be supported through nutrient-dense foods with ample amounts of fruit and vegetables for **antioxidant support**. Further, supplementation with Krebs cycle and oxidative phosphorylation nutrients, notably B vitamins, magnesium, coenzyme Q10 and carnitine (Table 17.5), is highly advisable.[1,4]

An increased metabolic rate brings with it increases in inflammation and oxidative stress, particularly if autoimmunity is also present.[59] The best cellular defence includes broad-spectrum antioxidants (including the vitamins A, C and E, the minerals zinc and selenium, and the bioactive substances α-lipoic acid, N-acetyl cysteine and coenzyme Q10),

Table 17.5 Treatments for hyperthyroidism

SUPPLEMENT	AMOUNT	RATIONALE
B complex	1 b.i.d.	High quality, high dose, preferably in their activated (phosphorylated) forms, for ready use in energy production in the Krebs cycle
Coenzyme Q10	100 mg/day	Essential for energy production in the electron transport chain
Magnesium	100–400 mg/day	Needed in Krebs cycle and for any ATP-dependent reactions
Antioxidants	1 b.i.d.	Broad-spectrum, high dose, to dampen the oxidative damage occurring through the higher metabolic rate and autoimmunity (if present).[60]
Vitamin C	1000 mg/day	Shown to benefit hyperthyroidism. Best taken in small frequent doses.[61]
Leonurus cardiaca	15–40 mL/wk	To reduce iodine metabolism and thyroid hormone production[54,56]
Lycopus virginicus	15–25 mL/wk	Adjuvant therapy for thyroid hyperfunction. Inhibition of peripheral deiodination of T_4 to T_3.[54,56]

as well as intracellular antioxidant support (notably glutathione and superoxide dismutase).[60] **Essential fatty acids** are also needed. **Vitamin C** at 1000 mg per day has shown beneficial effects in hyperthyroidism.[61]

Herbal and nutritional treatment

In order to dampen thyroid hormone production herbs such as ***Lycopus virginicus*** and ***Leonurus cardiaca*** are useful.[54,56] In a rat model, oral administration of *L. virginicus* has reduced T_3 levels; this is thought to be the result of decreased peripheral T_4 conversion to T_3.[65] *L. cardiaca* is used for nervous cardiac disorders such as palpitations,[56] and since these symptoms also occur in hyperthyroidism this herb has been used as an adjuvant for this condition.[54] Other herbs with thyroid-blocking action include *Melissa officinalis* and *Lithospermum* spp.[66,67]

Dietary goitrogens[39,40] (see the box below) or smoking can have an inhibitory effect on thyroid function by interfering with iodine uptake and thyroid hormone production. Paradoxically, excess iodine intake can also impede thyroid hormone production.[39,40]

GOITROGENS[39,40,62–64]

- Regular intake of any substance containing thiocyanate, such as:
  - raw brassica (coleslaw or cassava)
  - tobacco
- Others:
  - millet
  - soy

Table 17.6 Treatment protocol for hypothyroidism

NUTRIENT	AMOUNT	RATIONALE
Iodine[39,40,74]	150 µg/day	Constituent of thyroid hormone
Tyrosine[74]	1000–3000 mg/day	Constituent of thyroid hormone. Needs to be taken between meals.
Selenium[39,74]	100–200 µg/day	Facilitates the conversion from T_4 to the active form T_3.
Zinc[5,6]	25 mg 1–2/day	Supports thyroid hormone regulation
Withania somnifera[72,73]*	5–13 mL/day 1:2 extract	Increasing T_3 and T_4
Bacopa monnieri[71]	5–13 mL/day 1:2 extract	Increasing T_4
Fucus vesiculosus[54]	4.5–8.5 mL/day 1:1 extract	Contains iodine
Desiccated thyroid extract[22]		Contains T_3 and T_4

*Research done in mice

However, this is not recommended as a treatment as increased production of thyroid hormones could be the result, at least initially, thus contributing to the problem.

Hypothyroidism
Cofactors for hormone production
For hypothyroidism, hormone precursors and cofactors, such as combinations of **tyrosine**, **iodine**, **selenium** and **zinc**, are recommended to support the thyroid (Table 17.6). However, hyperthyroidism can develop as a result of recent supplementation with iodine to correct a hypothyroid state. Commonly, nodules develop on the thyroid gland, secreting thyroid hormones that are not regulated by TSH. If this should occur iodine supplementation needs to cease and treatment as for hyperthyroidism instigated.[40]

Iodine
Nutritionally, goitrogens (see above) in large amounts, particularly raw, should be avoided, especially if iodine status is already compromised.[39,40] Food rich in iodine includes seaweed products, seafood, eggs and products where iodine has been added to the feed. In the past, iodine has been used to sterilise milking equipment, resulting in iodine-rich milk. But in recent years iodine has been replaced by other methods of sterilisation (notably chlorine), so dairy is not a good source of iodine any longer.[35] In certain parts of the world, such as Australia and New Zealand where goitre used to be prevalent, iodine has been added to table salt.[39] However, the decreasing use of salt has further contributed to lowered iodine status.[35]

Available iodine supplements include potassium iodide and potassium iodate, iodised vegetable oil, nascent (atomic) iodine and Lugol's solution. When treating iodine deficiency it was noted that simultaneously correcting other nutrient deficiencies, notably iron and vitamin A, produced significantly better results.[4,40]

In pregnancy the requirement for thyroid hormone increases; this needs to be met by adequate iodine status. Therefore, additional iodine at about 125 μg/day should be supplied to allow for the increase in metabolic demand.[68–70]

Herbal and nutritional treatment

Certain herbs, such as *Withania somnifera*, *Bacopa monnieri* and *Fucus vesiculosus*, may be beneficial in hypothyroidism.[54,71–73] *W. somnifera* has also been shown to cause a decrease in hepatic lipid peroxidation and may thus be useful in concomitant heart and liver disease.[73]

CAM EVIDENCE IN THYROID DISORDERS

It should be noted that currently there is a scarcity of evidence from robust human studies for the use of nutritional and herbal interventions to treat thyroid disorders. More studies are required to firmly endorse these interventions.

Comprehensive diagnosing

In both hyper- and hypothyroidism, despite the best treatment measures, symptoms can persist, leading to compromised quality of life. It would therefore be prudent to not only assess thyroid function through laboratory testing and temperature readings, but also through a comprehensive interview or questionnaire that takes the patient's symptoms and overall health status into account.[75]

INTEGRATIVE MEDICAL CONSIDERATIONS

In mild cases of hypo- or hyperthyroidism diet and lifestyle changes, and nutritional and herbal supplements, may be sufficient. If TSH or thyroid hormones show severe disturbances or do not normalise (or at least show a trend towards normal) with natural treatment within 3 to 6 months, medication should be considered. A careful balance needs to be reached where medication and supplements enhance each other without causing imbalances in the opposite direction. This needs to be done in conjunction with the patient's GP.

Since the HPA axis is often involved in thyroid disorders other hormones, such as cortisol and insulin, and imbalanced physiological processes could be at the root of the condition. It may therefore be prudent to test for these hormones as well and treat any resultant imbalances.

Any therapies that help reduce stress are of value, such as bodywork, mind therapies and relaxation techniques. Homoeopathy and traditional Chinese medicine can help balance body energies, thus setting the stage for healing to take place. The homoeopathic remedy Thyroidinum has been given in cases of thyroid dysfunction,[76] however individualisation of remedies may yield better results long-term.

Case Study

A 48-year-old female presented with weight loss of 5 kg over a period of 6 months, despite eating normally. **Her BMI at the time of the consultation was 17.** There were no other syptoms. She had experienced a number of stressors in the previous 2 years, including losing her husband (whom she had nursed) to cancer and completing university studies while still working full-time. **A blood test revealed a TSH of 0.1 (0.3–5), T_3 of 6.8 (3.5–6.5) and T_4 of 23 (10–20). This was treated** (see the protocol below), and a follow-up **blood test 6 months later revealed normal thyroid function.** The patient's weight had returned to normal.

However, **3 years later the patient returned.** She was still eating the same (healthy) diet but had **noticed that her weight had steadily increased** over the past few months. She also felt sore and stiff most of the time, and her bowels tended towards constipation. Her **morning temperature was 36.1°C.** A thyroid test showed **TSH at 5.9 with T_3 and T_4 both at the low end of normal. Thyroid antibodies were elevated,** with **peroxidase AB at 81 (0–12)** and **thyroglobulin AB at 45 (0–34). Urinary iodine was low at 62** μg/L, indicative of mild to moderate deficiency. **ESR was 8 (1–30),** suggestive of low-grade inflammation. **Cortisol was low-normal** at 183 (160–650). She was **diagnosed with Hashimoto's thyroiditis.**

SUGGESTIVE SYMPTOMS[1,3,10,11]

Hyperthyroidism

- Weight loss
- Heat intolerance
- Increased appetite

- Irritability
- Tremor
- Increased pulse

Hypothyroidism

- Goitre
- Weight gain or difficulty losing it
- Cold intolerance
- Tiredness
- Constipation
- Mental slowness

- Depression
- Slow pulse
- Dry hair and skin
- Menstrual disorders in women
- Decreased body temperature

Example treatment

Hyperthyroidism

In the first consultation, the diagnosis of hyperactive thyroid was made on the basis of the laboratory results and her symptom of weight loss (confirmed by medical diagnosis). Her diet was reviewed and she was encouraged to eat nutrient-dense food and to avoid refined carbohydrates and processed food in order to provide the best nutrition to her overactive metabolism. Iodine in the form of iodised salt and sea-

Herbal prescription (hyperthyroidism)

Rhodiola rosea 1:1	30 mL
Lycopus virginicus 1:2	40 mL
Leonurus cardiaca 1:2	30 mL
7 mL b.d.	100 mL

Nutritional prescription

Activated vitamin B complex	1 tablet b.d.
Coenzyme Q10	100 mg/day
Magnesium citrate	300 mg/day
Broad-spectrum antioxidant	1 tablet b.d.

weed products were best avoided, too, so that the thyroid was deprived of one of the materials from which to make thyroid hormones. Raw brassica, such as coleslaw, was advised to increase iodine binding for elimination.

To dampen thyroid function and increase resilience, she was prescribed a herbal formula containing *Rhodiola rosea* to counteract stress and to improve stamina, and

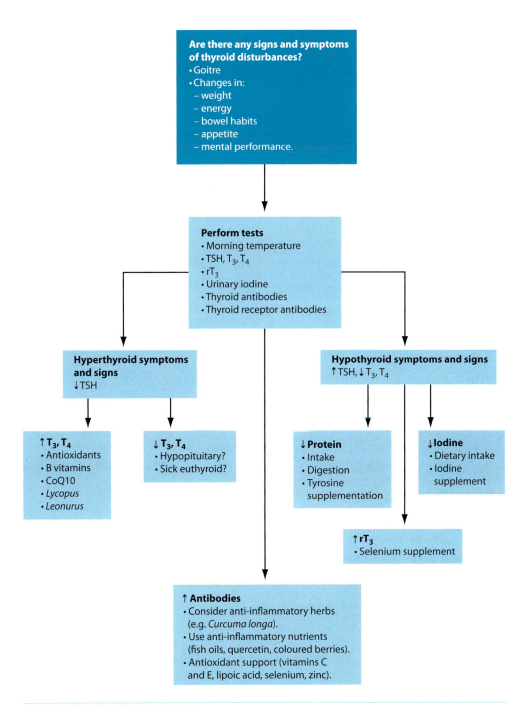

Figure 17.4 Naturopathic treatment decision tree—thyroid abnormalities

Lycopus virginicus and *Leonurus cardiaca* to dampen thyroid hyperactivity. She was also treated with nutritional supplements to support her increased metabolism: activated vitamin B complex to provide cofactors for the Krebs cycle in their coenzyme form, coenzyme Q_{10} to support energy production in the electron transport chain, magnesium citrate to support Krebs cycle function and ATP-dependent reactions, and a broad-spectrum antioxidant to minimise oxidative damage due to an overactive metabolism.

Further, she was advised to practise a relaxation technique such as guided imagery or meditation. This patient needed time for herself after years of emotional and physical stress. Informal counselling was used as part of the therapeutic relationship. Intensive exercise (other than hatha yoga, a gentle walk or swim) was discouraged to prevent further weight loss.

Three months later, the patient had been very compliant. Her weight had increased by 2 kg. A recent blood test showed that her thyroid hormones had returned to near normal. She was advised to stay on the supplements at half dose for a further 6 weeks and to have thyroid hormones retested in another 3 months' time (by which time they had normalised).

Hypothyroidism (3 years later)

At a follow-up consultation 3 years later, the patient complained of unexplained weight gain, fatigue, dry skin and cold hands. She was referred to her GP for a blood test; she was diagnosed with Hashimoto's disease. Her medical practitioner wanted to treat her with thyroxine, which she was trying to avoid.

Her diet was changed by removing raw brassica such as coleslaw, and the use of iodised salt and seaweed products was encouraged. Spices (such as ginger for its warming and anti-inflammatory properties and turmeric for its anti-inflammatory and antioxidant properties) were advised, to be used on a daily basis. According to the patient's wish no liquid herbal formula was prescribed. *Rhodiola rosea* was suggested for physical and mental stamina, and *Curcuma longa* for anti-inflammatory and antioxidant support. A thyroid and adrenal support formula containing tyrosine, potassium iodide, selenium, *Withania somnifera* and nutritional cofactors to provide precursors and cofactors for thyroid hormone formation was also prescribed. For anti-inflammatory support, a bioflavonoid formula containing quercetin, rutin and vitamin C was given, as well as fish oils in high strength.

> **Herbal prescription (hypothyroidism)**
>
> | | |
> |---|---|
> | *Rhodiola rosea* 1 g | 1 capsule b.d. |
> | *Curcuma longa* 2 g | 1 tablet/day |
> | *Fucus vesiculosus* 1 g | 1 tablet/day |
>
> **Nutritional prescription**
>
> | | |
> |---|---|
> | Thyroid and adrenal support nutrients | 2 capsules b.d. |
> | Bioflavonoid formula | 1 tablet b.d. |
> | Omega-3 fish oils | 3 g t.d.s. |
> | Digestive support | 1 with each meal |

Expected outcomes and follow-up protocols

After 3 months, the patient is expected to report improvement regarding hypothyroidism symptoms, in addition to balancing her weight. This should reflect on her blood test with antibodies and TSH readings normalising. If no beneficial effect occurs after 4–6 weeks of treatment, the prescription should be altered to address a potential underlying autoimmune pathology (see Chapter 28 on autoimmunity for treatment details). If after 3 months of treatment no change had occurred on follow-up blood tests (and symptoms), she would be advised to start thyroxine at 50 µg/day. The prescription can still be repeated and use adjuvantly, with the exception of the thyroid and adrenal support formula, which can be reduced to 1 capsule b.d. Regular blood tests are advised and the prescription modified for the patient's current health status. After the thyroid parameters have normalised, she can be advised to consider slowly reducing thyroxine (with medical support), while continuing with her herbal and nutriceutical prescription. Some patients may have the hyperthyroidism return, and thereby may need to titrate up the dose of thyroxine; however, others may find that they stay euthyroid. The key factor for practioners to note in treating thyroid conditions is that

Table 17.7 Review of the major evidence

INTERVENTION	METHODOLOGY	RESULT	COMMENT
Iodine[36]	Cross-sectional study of school children in Melbourne Urine sample for iodine assay ($n = 577$, aged 11–18 years)	76% had abnormal results. 27% had moderate-severe deficiency. Girls had significantly lower values than boys.	Similar results were found in Sydney and Tasmania, indicative of a widespread mild iodine deficiency in Australia.
Iodine[33]	Cross-sectional study of school children in Tasmania Urine sample for iodine assay ($n = 225$, aged 7–17 years)	Median urinary iodine excretion was 84 μg/L, indicative of mild iodine deficiency. 20% had less than 50 μg/L (indicative of moderate to severe iodine deficiency).	The research on iodine shows that deficiency is more prevalent than suspected.
Iodine[32]	Cross-sectional study of school children in central coast NSW Urine sample for iodine assay ($n = 324$, aged 5–13 years)	Median urinary iodine excretion was 82 μg/L, indicative of mild iodine deficiency. 14% had less than 50 μg/L (indicative of moderate to severe iodine deficiency). No goitre was detected in any of the children.	Yet another study corroborating the results of other studies and confirming the widespread iodine deficiency in Australia.
Selenium[39]	Prospective RCT Critically ill patients with multiple injuries ($n = 31$, aged 42 ± 16 years) 500 μg/day selenium or placebo for 5 days after injury	Faster and higher increase in T_3 and T_4, rT_3 rising less in active group and earlier normalisation	Not only selenium levels but also inflammatory cytokines, present in critically ill patients, interfere with thyroid hormone synthesis.
Selenium[42]	Comparative study Children with congenital hypothyroidism (CH) ($n = 18$, aged 0.5–15.4 years compared to euthyroid controls) 20–60 μg/day selenomethionine for 3 months	TSH difference abolished between CH and controls. Significant decrease in thyroglobulin.	Selenium not only increases conversion of T_4 to T_3 and therefore negative feedback to TSH, it also reduces antibody production. This effect does not seem to be mediated by glutathione peroxidase.
Mercury[44]	Cross-sectional study of chloralkali workers exposed to mercury vapour for a mean 13.3 years ($n = 47$) Control group matched for age ($n = 47$)	Significantly increased rT_3. Free T_4:free T_3 ratio was higher in the subgroup with highest exposure to mercury. Lowest urinary iodine in exposed workers correlated to the highest rT3.	Low iodine status seems to be an additional risk factor for the toxic effects of mercury exposure.
Soy and seaweed[63]	RCT cross-over 5 g/day of seaweed (= 475 mg iodine) for 7 weeks Last week: addition of soy protein isolate (2 mg/day isoflavones) ($n = 25$, postmenopausal women)	Significant urinary iodine and serum TSH increase with seaweed. No change with soy protein isolate.	It is surprising that TSH rose with iodine supplementation as the opposite was expected. It could be that other constituents of soy are responsible for their goitrogenic action.

in some instances people may alternate from hyperthyroidism to hypothyroidism and vice versa. Due to this, regular monitoring of signs and symptoms and blood tests is advised.

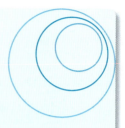

KEY POINTS

- Stress may induce both hyper- and hypothyroidism.
- Both hyper- and hypothyroidism can be the result of autoimmunity.
- In hyperthyroidism the increased metabolic activity needs to be supported through nutrient-dense diet and supplements, notably B vitamins and antioxidants.
- Nutritional deficiencies, particularly iodine and selenium, are indicated in hypothyroidism.
- Subclinical hypothyroidism is often underdiagnosed and therefore not treated.

Further reading

Danzi S, Klein I. Recent considerations in the treatment of hypothyroidism. Curr Opin Investig Drugs. 2008;9(4):357–362.

Vaidya B, Pearce SHS. Management of hypothyroidism in adults. BMJ 2008;337(7664):284–289.

Woolever DR, Beutler AI. Hypothyroidism: a review of the evaluation and management. Family Practice Recertification 2007;29(4):45–52.

References

1. Lord RS, Alexander BJ. Laboratory evaluations for integrative and functional medicine. 2nd edn. Duluth: Georgia: Metametrix Institute, 2008.
2. Thibodeau G, Patton K. Anatomy and physiology. 5th edn. St. Louis: CV Mosby, 2003.
3. Woolever DR, Beutler AI. Hypothyroidism: a review of the evaluation and management. Family Practice Recertification 2007;29(4):45–52.
4. Gropper S, et al. Advanced nutrition and human metabolism. 5th edn. Australia: Wadsworth, Cengage Learning, 2009.
5. Ganapathy S, Volpe SL. Zinc, exercise, and thyroid hormone function. Crit Rev Food Sci Nutr 1999;39(4):369–390.
6. Maxwell C, Volpe SL. Effect of zinc supplementation on thyroid hormone function. A case study of two college females. Ann Nutr Metab 2007;51(2):188–194.
7. Tierney LM, et al. Medical diagnosis and treatment. 44th edn. New York: McGraw-Hill, 2005.
8. Brown KM, Arthur JR. Selenium, selenoproteins and human health: a review. Public Health Nutr 2001;4(2B):593–599.
9. Leonard JL. Non-genomic actions of thyroid hormone in brain development. Steroids 2008;73(9–10):1008–1012.
10. Crowley LV. An introduction to human disease: pathology and pathophysiology correlations. 6th edn. Sudbury: Jones and Bartlett Publishers, 2004.
11. Kumar P, Clark M. Clinical medicine. 5th edn. London: W. B. Saunders, 2002.
12. Kosovskiĭ MI, et al. [Glucose tolerance disorders in patients with hypothyroidism]. Probl Endokrinol 1992;38(2):26–29.
13. Clausen N, et al. Counterregulation of insulin-induced hypoglycaemia in primary hypothyroidism. Acta Endocrinol 1986;111(4):516–521.
14. Stanická S, et al. Insulin sensitivity and counter-regulatory hormones in hypothyroidism and during thyroid hormone replacement therapy. Clin Chem Lab Med 2005;43(7):715–720.
15. Fommei E, Lervasi G. The role of thyroid hormone in blood pressure homeostasis: evidence from short-term hypothyroidism in humans. J Clin Endocrinol Metab 2002;87(5):1996–2000.
16. Chopra IJ. Nonthyroidal illness syndrome or euthyroid sick syndrome? Endocr Pract 1996;2(1):45–52.
17. Douyon L, Schteingart DE. Effect of obesity and starvation on thyroid hormone, growth hormone, and cortisol secretion. Endocrinol Metab Clin North Am 2002;31(1):173–189.
18. Ochi Y, Kajita Y. [Determination of thyroid hormone]. Nippon Rinsho 1999;57(8):1794–1799.
19. Dickey RA, et al. Optimal thyrotropin level: normal ranges and reference intervals are not equivalent. Thyroid 2005;15(9):1035–1039.
20. Wartofsky L, Dickey RA. The evidence for a narrower thyrotropin reference range is compelling. J Clin Endocrinol Metab 2005;90(9):5483–5488.
21. Brown B. Moving towards balance—hypothyroidism. Online. Available: http://www.moving-towards-balance.com.au/MTB_Hypothyroidism.html. Accessed 19 April 2009.
22. Danzi S, Klein I. Recent considerations in the treatment of hypothyroidism. Curr Opin Investig Drugs 2008;9(4):357–362.
23. Vaidya B, Pearce SHS. Management of hypothyroidism in adults. Br Med J 2008;337(7664):284–289.
24. Krysiak R, et al. [Subclinical hypothyroidism]. Wiad Lek 2008;61(4–6):139–145.
25. Papi G, et al. Subclinical hypothyroidism. Curr Opin Endocrinol Diabetes Obes 2007;14(3):197–208.
26. Villar H, et al. Thyroid hormone replacement for subclinical hypothyroidism. Cochrane Database Systemat Rev 2007;(3):CD003419.
27. Gharib H. Commentary: review: Available evidence does not support a benefit for thyroid hormone replacement in adult with subclinical hypothyroidism. ACP J Club 2008:Sect. 6.
28. Tchong L, et al. Hypothyroidism: management across the continuum. J Clin Outcomes Manag 2009;16(5):231–235.

29. Arrigo T, et al. Subclinical hypothyroidism: the state of the art. J Endocrinol Invest 2008;31(1):79–84.
30. Tsigos C, Chrousos GP. Hypothalamic-pituitary-adrenal axis, neuroendocrine factors and stress. J Psychosom Res 2002;53(4):865–871.
31. Taniyama M, et al. Urinary cortisol metabolites in the assessment of peripheral thyroid hormone action: application for diagnosis of resistance to thyroid hormone. Thyroid 1993;3(3):229–233.
32. Guttikonda K, et al. Iodine deficiency in urban primary school children: a cross-sectional analysis. Med J Aust 2003;179(7):346–348.
33. Guttikonda K, et al. Recurrent iodine deficiency in Tasmania, Australia: a salutary lesson in sustainable iodine prophylaxis and its monitoring. J Clin Endocrinol Metab 2002;87(6):2809–2815.
34. Gunton JE, et al. Iodine deficiency in ambulatory participants at a Sydney teaching hospital: is Australia truly iodine replete? [see comment]. Med J Aust 1999;171(9):467–470.
35. Li M, et al. Re-emergence of iodine deficiency in Australia. Asia Pac J Clin Nutr 2001;10(3):200–203.
36. McDonnell CM, et al. Iodine deficiency and goitre in schoolchildren in Melbourne. Med J Aust 2003;178(4):159–162.
37. Mann JI, Aitken E. The re-emergence of iodine deficiency in New Zealand? N Z Med J 2003;116(1170):U351.
38. Thomson CD. Selenium and iodine intakes and status in New Zealand and Australia. Br J Nut 2004;91(5):661–672.
39. Higdon J. An evidence-based approach to vitamins and minerals. New York: Thieme, 2003.
40. Shils ME, et al. Modern nutrition in health and disease. Philadelphia: Lippincott Williams & Wilkins, 2006.
41. Berger MM, et al. Influence of selenium supplements on the post-traumatic alterations of the thyroid axis: a placebo-controlled trial. Intensive Care Med 2001;27(1):91–100.
42. Chanoine JP, et al. Selenium decreases thyroglobulin concentrations but does not affect the increased thyroxine-to-triiodothyronine ratio in children with congenital hypothyroidism. J Clin Endocrinol Metab 2001;86(3):1160–1163.
43. Gärtner R. Selenium and thyroid hormone axis in critical ill states: an overview of conflicting view points. J Trace Elem Med Biol 2009;23(2):71–74.
44. Ellingsen DG, et al. Effects of low mercury vapour exposure on the thyroid function in chloralkali workers. J Appl Toxicol 2000;20(6):483–489.
45. Clarke N, Kabadi UM. Optimizing treatment of hypothyroidism. Treat Endocrinol 2004;3(4):217–221.
46. Paoletti J. Differentiation and treatment of hypothyroidism, functional hypothyroidism, and functional metabolism. International Journal of Pharmaceutical Compounding 2008;12(6):489–487.
47. Joffe RT, et al. Treatment of clinical hypothyroidism with thyroxine and triiodothyronine: a literature review and metaanalysis. Psychosomatics 2007;48(5):379–384.
48. Mazzoccoli G, et al. The hypothalamic-pituitary-thyroid axis and melatonin in humans: possible interactions in the control of body temperature. Neuro Endocrinol Lett 2004;25(5):368–372.
49. Nogues R, et al. Influence of nutrition, thyroid hormones, and rectal temperature on in-hospital mortality of elderly patients with acute illness. Am J Clin Nutr 1995;61(3):597–602.
50. Beck U, et al. Temperature and endocrine activity during sleep in man. Activation of cortisol and thyroid-stimulating hormone, inhibition of human growth hormone secretion by raised or decreased ambient and body temperatures. Arch Psychiatr Nervenkr 1976;222(2–3):245–256.
51. Reed HL. Circannual changes in thyroid hormone physiology: the role of cold environmental temperatures. Arctic Med Res 1995;54(Suppl 2):9–15.
52. Ljunggren JG, et al. The effect of body temperature on thyroid hormone levels in patients with non-thyroidal illness. Acta Med Scand 1977;202(6):459–462.
53. Höflich G, et al. Thyroid hormones, body temperature, and antidepressant treatment. Biol Psychiatry 1992;31(8):859–862.
54. Bone K. A clinical guide to blending liquid herbs. USA: Elsevier, 2003.
55. Blumenthal M. The ABC clinical guide to herbs. Austin: American Botanical Council, 2003.
56. Blumenthal M. The complete German Commission E monographs—therapeutic guide to herbal medicines [CD-ROM]. Austin: American Botanical Council, 1999.
57. Mills S, Bone K. Principles and practice of phytotherapy. Sydney: Churchill Livingstone, 2000.
58. Pizzorno J, Murray M. Textbook of natural medicine. 3rd edn USA: Churchill Livingstone, 2006.
59. Gershwin M, et al. Handbook of nutrition and immunity. Totowa, New Jersey: Humana Press, 2004.
60. Ma A, et al. Antioxidant therapy for prevention of inflammation, ischemic reperfusion injuries and allograft rejection. Cardiovasc Hematol Agents Med Chem 2008;6(1):20–43.
61. Seven A, et al. Biochemical evaluation of oxidative stress in propylthiouracil treated hyperthyroid patients. Effects of vitamin C supplementation. Clin Chem Lab Med 1998;36(10):767–770.
62. Doerge DR, Sheehan DM. Goitrogenic and estrogenic activity of soy isoflavones. Environ Health Perspect 2002;3:349–353.
63. Teas J, et al. Seaweed and soy: companion foods in Asian cuisine and their effects on thyroid function in American women. J Med Food 2007;10(1):90–100.
64. Messina M, Redmond G. Effects of soy protein and soybean isoflavones on thyroid function in healthy adults and hypothyroid patients: a review of the relevant literature. Thyroid 2006;16(3):249–258.
65. Winterhoff H, et al. Endocrine effects of Lycopus europaeus L. following oral application. Arzneimittelforschung 1994;44(1):41–45.
66. Yarnell E, Abascal K. Botanical medicine for thyroid regulation. Alternative and Complementary Therapies 2006;12(3):107.
67. Auf'mkolk M, et al. Extracts and auto-oxidized constituents of certain plants inhibit the receptor-binding and the biological activity of Graves' immunoglobulins. Endocrinology 1985;116(5):1687–1693.
68. Glinoer D. Feto-maternal repercussions of iodine deficiency during pregnancy. An update. Ann Endocrinol 2003;64(1):37–44.
69. Glinoer D. Pregnancy and iodine. Thyroid 2001;11(5):471–481.
70. Glinoer D. What happens to the normal thyroid during pregnancy? Thyroid 1999;9(7):631–635.
71. Kar A, et al. Relative efficacy of three medicinal plant extracts in the alteration of thyroid hormone concentrations in male mice. J Ethnopharmacol 2002;81(2):281.
72. Panda S, Kar A. Changes in thyroid hormone concentrations after administration of ashwagandha root extract to adult male mice. J Pharm Pharmacol 1998;50(9):1065–1068.
73. Panda S, Kar A. Withania somnifera and Bauhinia purpurea in the regulation of circulating thyroid hormone concentrations in female mice. J Ethnopharmacol 1999;67(2):233–239.
74. Braun L, Cohen M. Herbs and natural supplements. 2nd edn. Sydney: Churchill Livingstone, 2007.
75. Razvi S, et al. Instruments used in measuring symptoms, health status and quality of life in hypothyroidism: a systematic qualitative review. Clin Endocrinol 2005;63(6):617–624.
76. Tarkas PI. Thyroidinum. Indian Journal of Homoeopathic Medicine 1989;24(1):67.

Section 6 Female reproductive system

Unlike the male reproductive system, the female reproductive system is located entirely within the pelvic region. This system is controlled by a complex series of feedback loops, for example the hypothalamic–pituitary–ovarian (HPO) axis, that regulate, monitor and control the release of various sex hormones such as testosterone, oestrogen and progesterone. The levels of each of these hormones fluctuate at various stages of the cycle under this control, and each has a specific role—for example, oestrogen promotes growth of the endometrial tissue lining the uterus for eventual embryo implantation or shedding at menses. The developments, maturation, release and (if fertilised) implantation of the embryo is also dependent on appropriate regulation of this process. However, other body processes can also affect this regulation; for example, the hypothalamic–pituitary–adrenal axis or high levels of insulin may affect HPO regulation of sex hormones.

Naturopathic medicine lends itself to the treatment of female reproductive complaints specifically because of this complexity. However, this complexity has meant that the female reproductive system is in many respects an enigma to conventional medicine, and most medical therapeutic options therefore tend to focus on specific reproductive tissue or hormonal activity. Although these are undeniably important, many female reproductive disorders are the result of a complex milieu of which these form only a part. For example, exogenous endometrial tissue implantation may be encouraged by increased levels of inflammation (perhaps from increased intestinal permeability or from other, non-reproductive sources); and naturopaths understood and treated the link between hyperinsulinaemia and anovulation long before it became accepted in conventional gynaecological and endocrinology practice. Naturopathic medicine has also long appreciated the significant relationship between emotional and psychological wellbeing and reproductive symptoms, as both a side effect and a causative factor. Moreover, naturopathic medicine has appreciated that a normal reproductive cycle is just that—normal—and that deviations such as dysmenorrhoea reflect a disharmony. Women are not meant to undergo traumatic experiences for significant periods each month and the cessation of menses with age is recognised as a normal stage of life—one that needs to be supported, not medicated.

Naturopathy has traditional roots in the treatment of female reproductive disorders, which was often the realm of 'wise women' who often employed various herbal medicines to treat common reproductive system conditions and to aid healthy childbirth. Various traditional herbal 'spasmolytics' and 'uterine tonics' are still used today by modern clinicians (although more evidence is now required to elucidate the mechanisms behind these effects). Naturopathic treatment commonly focuses on restoring the reproductive system to optimal function—with a regular cycle with minimal discomfort. In addition to appropriate biological interventions, naturopaths should encourage female patients to be more self-aware of their bodies and their reproductive cycles.

This particular section does not deal with fertility; rather this is discussed in detail in Chapter 31 on fertility, preconception care and pregnancy. Instead this section focuses on conditions associated with the reproductive system that can be experienced by women of reproductive age and that are commonly expected to be seen in clinical practice; however, the complexity of the female reproductive system is such that many of the principles discussed herein may be relevant to other female reproductive cases, even if they do not share the same medical diagnosis.

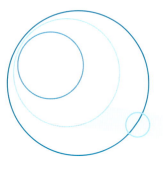

Dysmenorrhoea and menstrual complaints

Jon Wardle
ND, MPH

AETIOLOGY AND CLASSIFICATION

Menstrual complaints are often broadly—and sometimes incorrectly—categorised under the broad moniter of premenstrual syndrome (PMS). PMS is defined as a recurrent set of physical and behavioural symptoms occurring cyclically 7–14 days before menstruation (the luteal phase) and are troublesome enough to interfere with some aspects of the female's life.[1] In common clinical usage this has also extended to symptoms (such as dysmenorrhoea) that occur during menstruation and cease by the end of the full flow of menses. Despite its high prevalence PMS remains poorly understood and often not prioritised in medical treatment.[1] Multiple aetiologies have been proposed, most prominently those in Table 18.1. In reality a number of these may be responsible for underlying imbalances, even in the same patient. The numerous proposed aetiologies for PMS mean that more than 150 individual symptoms have been associated with the condition. The most common are listed in Table 18.2.[1]

Although diagnosis is difficult given the broad range of possible aetiologies and symptoms, premenstrual dysphoric disorder (PMDD), a more severe form of PMS, is a recent addition to the *Diagnostic and Statistical Manual of Mental Disorders IV.*[2] To be diagnosed with PMDD a woman must have at least five of the following symptoms occurring cyclically at a level serious enough to interfere with normal daily activities:

1. feelings of sadness or hopelessness, possible suicidal thoughts
2. feelings of tension or anxiety
3. mood swings marked by periods of teariness
4. persistent irritability or anger
5. disinterest in daily activities and relationships

Table 18.1 Proposed aetiologies of premenstrual syndrome[1]

CATEGORY	EXAMPLE
Fluid and electrolyte balance	• Aldosterone excess • High sodium:potassium ratio • Rennin/angiotensin abnormalities
Hereditary factors	• Genetic risk
Hormonal factors	• Oestrogen deficiency • Oestrogen excess • High oestrogen:progesterone ratio • Progesterone deficiency • High prolactin
Inflammatory mediators	• Prostaglandin excess • Prostaglandin deficiency
Psychological factors	• Poor coping skills • Poor self-esteem • Beliefs about menstrual cycle
Social factors	• Current and former marital and sexual relationships • Stress • Cultural and societal attitudes about PMS • Poor social networks
Biochemical factors	• Various vitamin and mineral deficiencies • Dopamine deficiency

Table 18.2 The most common symptoms of premenstrual syndrome

Abdominal bloating	Depression	Lethargy
Anxiety	Dizziness	Low self-esteem
Back pain	Fatigue	Mood swings
Breast tenderness	Headache	Nervousness
Change in appetite	Insomnia	Social isolation
Clumsiness	Irritability	Sugar cravings
Constipation	Joint pain	Water retention

6. trouble concentrating
7. fatigue or low energy
8. food cravings or bingeing behaviour
9. sleep disturbances
10. feeling out of control
11. physical symptoms such as bloating, breast tenderness, headaches and joint or muscle pain.

Patients fulfilling the diagnositic criteria for PMDD also fulfil medical diagnostic criteria for PMS, but not necessarily vice versa. However, it may be viewed as disturbing that behavioural aspects form the focus of diagnosis in PMDD, when in clinical practice a vast array of hormonal and physiological interactions take place within a woman's body around the time of menstruation, resulting in a variety of broader symptoms and forming a more complex basis of underlying aetiology.

Dysmenorrhoea

While PMS is often used as an all-encompassing moniker for menstrual complaints, menstrual symptoms do not occur only prior to menstruation. Dysmenorrhoea is painful menstruation and is the most common menstrual complaint, as well as having the most potential to substantially interfere with patients' lives. In fact, dysmenorrhoea is the most frequent gynaecological problem in adolescent girls (the prevalence is 80 to 90%). Daily activities are frequently affected and it is the most common cause of regular absenteeism in young women.

Primary dysmenorrhoea classically presents as a cramping lower abdominal pain that usually begins during the day before menstruation. The pain gradually eases after the start of menstruation and is sometimes gone by the end of the first day of bleeding. Primary dysmenorrhoea occurs in a high percentage of young women only in ovulatory cycles and the pain is normally limited to the first 48 to 72 hours of menstruation.[1]

Secondary dysmenorrhoea may occur during other parts of the menstrual cycle and can be either relieved or worsened by menstruation. Pain from secondary dysmenorrhoea is often described as a dull and aching rather than being spasmodic or cramping in nature. It can occur before menstruation (up to 1 week) or get worse once menstruation starts.

Hormonal and biochemical influences

Endocrine studies have suggested that PMS is not the result of a simple excess or deficiency in certain hormone levels.[3] Low progesterone,[4] excessive oestrogen[5] or normal levels of both[6] have not been associated with increasing incidence of PMS. Though prolactin levels have been associated with several symptoms of PMS there has been little hard evidence to suggest that elevated prolactin levels are present in women with PMS.[6,7] Similarly while aldosterone is thought to be at least partly responsible for the congestive symptoms of PMS there have been no reports of significant differences between women with and without PMS.[5] It has been postulated that PMS is not associated with abnormal hormone levels, but rather an abnormal response to sex hormones[8] which may be exacerbated during episodes of stress.[9] High blood flow is also associated with an increased instance of dysmenorrhoea.[10]

It is thought that deviations from normal ovarian function—rather than hormone levels per se—are associated with changes to other body systems (such as neurotransmitters) seen in PMS.[11] Serotonin is thought to be particularly affected by changes in hormone levels and responsible for many mood change symptoms associated with PMS.[12]

It has also been hypothesised that women with PMS may have lower levels of circulating endogenous opiates (or serotonin) or a more sudden withdrawal after the postovulation surge, leaving them more susceptible to depression and more sensitive to pain in the luteal phase.[13–15] Prostaglandins are also associated with the PMS symptoms of breast pain, fluid retention, abdominal cramping, headaches, irritability and depression.[16] The high levels of the leukotrienes that increase uterine muscle spasm (C4 and D4) in the menstrual blood of women with dysmenorrhoea also support the hypothesis that prostaglandins are an important part of the aetiology.[17] Anti-inflammatory prostaglandins may also be associated with reducing the exaggerated effects of prolactin.[18]

Psychosocial factors can also influence the menstrual cycle. Emotional and physical stressors such as travel, illness, stress, weather changes and other environmental factors can influence the length of the menstrual cycle, ovulation and severity of

PMS.[19] One study found that 75% of women receiving care for PMS had another diagnosis that could account for their symptom complex—predominantly depression and other mood disorders.[20]

RISK FACTORS

Epidemiological data observe a strong relationship between smoking or exposure to tobacco products and a higher incidence of dysmenorrhoea.[21–23] Obesity is also a risk factor for menstrual disturbances, with women who have a body mass index (BMI) over 30 incurring a threefold risk of developing them.[24] Approximately three-quarters of women have a separate diagnosis—particularly mood disorders or other hormone-mediated diagnoses—that contribute significantly to their symptoms.[25] High levels of caffeine may be associated with increased prevalence and severity of PMS symptoms,[26,27] though this may be due to an additive relationship of sugar with caffeine.[28] Many women medicate themselves with caffeine during PMS symptoms, which may exacerbate their symptoms.[29]

CONVENTIONAL TREATMENT

The basic aim of treatment of menstrual disorders in conventional treatment focuses on symptomatic relief and coping strategies in line with the hormonal dysfunction rather than reliance on medication. Conventional treatment of primary dysmenorrhoea is usually associated with pain management (such as ibuprofen) or a combined oral contraceptive pill. Secondary dysmenorrhoea is more complex and may be associated with other conditions such as pelvic infection or endometriosis. Common symptomatic relief for dysmenorrhoea with analgesics such as paracetamol or ibuprofen or antiprostaglandin agents such as indomethacin or mefenamic acid may also be recommended. In cases of secondary dysmenorrhoea the conventional treatment is to identify and treat the cause.

Various pharmaceutical agents are used in conventional treatment, including diuretics (such as spironolactone—particularly with fluid retention), vitamins (such as B6), SSRI agents or danazol (particularly with severe mastalgia).[30] Hormone therapy is also common, and consists of hormonal agents such as oral contraceptive pill (OCP), progestogens or implants. However, these have little evidence of efficacy in PMS.[31] Progesterone treatment is increasingly popular, particularly amongst integrative medical practitioners; however, the evidence for effective treatment with progesterone alone is unclear.[32]

KEY TREATMENT PROTOCOLS

Although various diagnoses can often present in menstrual disorders, naturopathic treatment focuses not on treatment of particular disorders, but rather the restoration of a normal menstrual cycle. Other chapters in the reproductive section focus on various aspects of hormone normalisation, so this chapter focuses on specific symptoms associated with PMS, particularly dysmenorrhoea as it is often the most encountered

NATUROPATHIC TREATMENT AIMS

- Remove risk factors.
- Regulate HPO axis function and normalise hormones.
- Reduce inflammation and inflammatory mediators.
- Treat menstrual pain symptomatically.
- Address psychological factors (causations and clinical manifestations).

symptom in clinical practice. A normal menstrual cycle should be free of the discomfort associated with pathological conditions such as PMS, PMDD or dysmenorrhoea. This return to normalcy can be sought through a number of mechanisms, most commonly hormonal regulation via the hypothalamic–pituitary–ovarian (HPO) axis.

HPO-axis regulation

As opposed to conditions specifically linked to certain hormone excesses such as endometriosis (oestrogen) and PCOS (androgen), treatment of broader menstrual disorders focuses on hormone normalisation, often through modulation of the HPO axis. In this sense naturopathic treatments are not necessarily associated with specific actions on hormones, but rather work to restore the appropriate function of the body's own natural processes that regulate these hormones. For example, while ***Vitex agnus-castus*** was initially thought to work on increasing progesterone levels or decreasing prolactin, research is suggesting it has a role even further upstream on the HPO due to its dopaminergic action.

In addition to prescriptive naturopathic medicines, many of which are explored in more detail in other reproductive chapters, a number of different lifestyle factors, discussed below, can disrupt the functioning of the HPO axis.

Dietary factors

Dietary factors may also play a significant role. Women with PMS typically consume more dairy products, refined sugar and high sodium foods than women without PMS.[33] Fish, eggs and fruit have been associated with less dysmenorrhoea while wine is associated with more.[36] Women following a low-fat, vegetarian diet also had lower incidence

ABRAHAM'S CLASSIFICATIONS

In 1983 Dr Guy Abraham publicised a system for the classification of PMS into four distinct subgroups.[33–35] These subtypes have since had a major influence on naturopathic practice. However, while they may be somewhat clinically useful in a broad sense they should be treated as guidelines only as they have not been confirmed by research and patients rarely fit neatly into one group. The subtypes are discussed below.

PMS-A (anxiety)
This is thought to be related to high levels of oestrogen and a deficiency of progesterone. Its symptom complex is irritability, anxiety and emotional lability.

PMS-C (carbohydrate craving)
This is thought to be caused by enhanced intracellular binding of insulin though its exact mechanism is unclear. The symptom complex of this category is increased appetite, carbohydrate craving, headache and heart palpitations.

PMS-D (depression)
This is thought to be due to low levels of oestrogen leading to excessive breakdown of neurotransmitters and could be due to symptoms related to enhanced androgen or progesterone production.

PMS-H (hyperhydration)
This is thought to be caused by elevations of aldosterone due to excessive oestrogen, sodium consumption, adrenal stress or magnesium deficiency. The symptom complex of this subtype is weight gain, breast tenderness and fullness, peripheral swelling and abdominal bloating.

of dysmenorrhoea.[22,23,37] This was theorised to be due to increased sex-hormone binding globulin (which was measured in the study) and its effects on oestrogen or arachidonic acid. A diet high in oily fish and avoidance of foods with significant arachidonic acid content reduces the severity of dysmenorrhoea, possibly through improving the synthesis of anti-inflammatory prostaglandins and leukotrienes. Higher amounts of fibre have been associated with lower levels of menstrual pain.[38] High intakes of total and saturated fats and low unrefined carbohydrate and fibre consumption were also associated with dysmenorrhoea.[39]

Regulating blood sugar levels may be important in modulating hormonal status. It has been observed that PMS symptoms are worse in women with abnormal glucose tolerance.[40] The body appears more sensitive to insulin during the luteal phase; this has led some researchers to theorise that hypoglycaemia may account for some premenstrual symptoms. Consumption of foods high in sugar content—particularly chocolate—may also increase the severity of menstrual symptoms.[28] Regulating eating patterns may therefore help to improve dysmenorrhoea—eating breakfast was associated with a lower incidence of dysmenorrhoea[41] as was a history of calorie-restrictive dieting.[42] This relationship was also observed irrespective of BMI.[43]

Other lifestyle factors

Increased or regular exercise is associated with lower incidence of dysmenorrhoea and most other premenstrual symptoms.[44–49] This may be due in part to the apparent hormone normalisation role of exercise or increased physical activity,[50] or its effects on stress reduction in women with dysmenorrhoea.[51] More detailed information on the effects of stress on reproductive function can be found in Chapter 20 on polycystic ovarian syndrome and Chapter 31 on fertility, preconception care and pregnancy.

A study of 380 women found that those with higher levels of stress were twice as likely to experience dysmenorrhoea in their cycle.[52] Relaxation therapy through various meditative or relaxation techniques has been demonstrated to improve premenstrual symptoms and dysmenorrhoea.[53,54]

PMS supplements
Herbal medicines

Vitex agnus-castus has had demonstrated effect in the treatment of a variety premenstrual symptoms.[55–58] *V. agnus-castus* reduces prolactin through its action on dopamine receptors.[57–62] However, other studies have suggested a dose-dependent effect, as lower doses (120 mg) were found to increase secretion while higher doses (204–480 mg) were found to decrease secretion.[63] It may also have effects on progesterone levels; one study has shown it can normalise progesterone levels in women with hyperprolactinaemia within 3 months[61] while another has suggested it can stimulate progesterone receptor expression.[64] Recent research has suggested that *V. agnus-castus* may exert activity in the opiate system, and the activation of mood regulatory and analgesic pathways via this system may be at least partly responsible for its efficacy in menstrual disorders.[65]

Cimicifuga racemosa is thought to modulate oestrogen levels by reducing LH secretion.[66,67] Although no clinical studies are available it has a strong tradition of use in dysmenorrhoea and menstrual disorders and has been approved by Commission E for use in these conditions.[34,35,68]

Tea from the leaves of *Rosa gallica* has also been demonstrated to mildly improve dysmenorrhoea and other menstrual symptoms in women.[69] *Psidii guajavae folium* (guava) has been demonstrated to be effective in dysmenorrhoea.[70] *Matricaria recutita* has been commonly used for treatment of dysmenorrhoea.[71] Uterine tonic herbs may also be used in PMS treatment (see Chapter 31).

Hypericum perforatum may be useful in women displaying irritability or depression in PMS, and one small pilot trial has demonstrated a significant reduction in PMS symptom scores.[72] Other **nervine herbs** such as *Valeriana officinalis, Piper methysticum, Passiflora incarnata* and *Melissa officinalis* have also been traditionally used in PMS for similar circumstances.[34,35,68] *Ginkgo biloba* has also demonstrated improvement in psychosocial aspects of PMS, though it is most effective at reducing congestive symptoms such as breast pain, tenderness and fluid retention.[73]

Nutritional medicines

Calcium supplementation has been shown to reduce PMS symptoms.[74,75] Women who had 1000–1200 mg calcium reported that their menstrual pain reduced by half.[74] **Magnesium** has also been shown to reduce PMS mood and fluid retention symptoms.[76,77] Although serum magnesium levels are often normal in women with PMS, they can have lower red blood cell magnesium levels than women without and levels are known to fluctuate throughout the cycle.[78–80] **Vitamin E** can be useful for breast symptoms, tension, irritability and lack of co-ordination in PMS.[81–83] **Vitamin A** also has a long history of use in PMS treatment.[84] **Zinc** levels have also been demonstrated to be low in women with PMS.[85]

Symptomatic pain relief

Topical application of warmth

There may be an element of clinical truth in the traditional habit of curling up with a **hot water bottle**. Application of heat to the abdomen has also been demonstrated to be at least as effective as ibuprofen or paracetamol in clinical studies.[86,87] **Massage** with liniments or warming salves (for example ginger) or moxibustion may also offer relief.

Herbal smooth muscle relaxants

Herbs with demonstrated ability to relax smooth muscle, such as *Valeriana officinalis* (though in animal studies only),[88] *Lavendula angustifolia*,[89] *Matricaria recutita*[90] and *Foeniculum vulgare*[91] may be used in the treatment of dysmenorrhoea, usually beginning a few days before menstruation and continuing until bleeding stops. *Zingiber officinale* has been shown to be equally effective as the NSAIDs ibuprofen and mefenamic acid in the symptomatic treatment of menstrual pain.[92] This may be particularly useful in women who experience nausea in conjunction with menstrual pain. It can be taken as an infusion or several preparations—often sold for travel sickness or nausea—are available. *F. vulgare* was found to reduce the severity of dysmenorrhoea when taken (20 drops of liquid tincture five times per day) during the first 3 days of menses and is thought to be as effective as commonly used conventional analgesics.[93]

Viburnum opulus and *V. prunifolium* both have a strong tradition of use as uterine relaxants[34,35,68] in addition to many early case reports,[94,95] though they are yet to be clinically studied. While these are not symptomatic in the sense that they immediately resolve symptoms, they are effective only in treating the symptoms of dysmenorrhoea and do not address the underlying cause.

Endocrine interactions

In addition to high blood sugar or cortisol, low thyroid function may exacerbate PMS symptoms and low thyroid function has been found in women with PMS.[96–98] The menstrual cycle appears to have an effect on thyroid function, with rT3 concentrations found to be higher in the luteal as opposed to follicular phase.[97] Given the complex interactions that exist between hormonal systems this is not unusual. Thyroid treatment is expanded in Chapter 17 on thyroid abnormalities.

OTHER THERAPEUTIC CONSIDERATIONS

Although naturopathic philosophy dictates finding the underlying cause for dysmenorrhoea, there is little likelihood of patient compliance (and therefore ultimately clinical success) without addressing symptomatic complaints. This may necessitate either an integrated approach to treatment with conventional medications or a separate prescription for purely symptomatic naturopathic medications.

TRADITIONAL HERBAL REPRODUCTIVE MEDICINE[34,35,68]

Naturopathy has a rich history in treating disorders of the female reproductive system and it would be remiss from a historical and clinical context to ignore this component. Herbal medicine in particular has a long tradition. Some herbs, such as *Vitex agnus-castus, Paeonia lactiflora* and *Cimicifuga racemosa*, have been used as generalist reproductive herbs, and are thought to work predominantly as hormonal regulators rather than having specific activity (it is now thought that they act directly on HPO regulation).

Fluid retention
Diuretics such as *Taraxacum officinale* have traditionally been used for symptoms of fluid retention.

Oestrogen support
Some herbs have been traditionally considered 'oestrogenic' in nature, in that they support oestrogen function in the body, though they may not be intrinsically oestrogenic themselves. Some examples are *Chamaelirium luteum* and *Dioscorea villosa*.

Spasmolytic herbs
Spasmolytic herbs have been used traditionally for menstrual cramping. These include *Angelica sinensis, Viburnum* spp., *Ligistium wallichii* and *Rubus idaeus*. *Achillea millefolium* is specifically used as a spasmolytic that also reduces bleeding.

Antihaemorrhagic
Antihaemorrhagics include *Achillea millefolium, Equisetum arvense, Alchemillia vulgaris, Lamium album, Panax notoginseng* and uterine antihaemorrhagics such as *Capsella bursa-pastoris* and *Trillium erectum*.

Anodyne
Corydalis ambigua, Piscidia erythrina, Tanacetum parthenium and *Anemone pulsatilla* have been traditionally used for pain management in reproductive disorders.

Uterine tonics
Uterine tonics are herbs that have traditionally been used for their normalising effect on the uterus and assisting with normal uterine function. They include *Rubus idaeus, Angelica sinensis, Chamaelirium luteum, Aletris farinose, Caulophyllum thalictroides* and more recently *Tribulus terrestris*.

TRADITIONAL HERBAL REPRODUCTIVE MEDICINE[34,35,68] *(Continued)*

Emmenagogues

Emmenagogues—or uterine stimulants—are traditionally used when there is a desire to increase the strength of uterine contractions. They are traditionally prescribed to initiate menstruation caused by hormonal irregularities or when the period is slow or delayed. Due to their action they are also contraindicated in pregnancy. Examples are *Ruta graveolens*, *Artemesia vulgaris*, *Salvia officinalis* and *Mentha pulegium*. Emmenagogues have also been prescribed for certain conditions associated with heavy bleeding due to 'poor uterine tone', usually indicated by heavy flow, little pain and significant clotting. They are also used in combination with uterine tonics after miscarriage to adequately expel tissue and promote healing and regeneration.

Circulatory stimulants

Another concept often discussed in various humoral medicines (including traditional Chinese medicine, traditional naturopathy and Ayurvedic medicine) is the concept of warming herbs being used in reproductive conditions that are cold or stagnant in nature. They are used to promote circulation and blood flow and to remove obstruction. Examples are *Zingiber officinale* and *Cinnamomum zeylanicum*. Pain is often related to blood or Qi stagnation in traditional Chinese medicine and equivalent ancient naturopathic humoral tradition.

In practice naturopathy is a holistic modality, and also makes use of other various herbal action—nervines, adaptogens and so on—as deemed appropriate for the individual patient. Treatment very rarely makes use of reproductive herbs alone.

The patient should also be counselled on appropriate or sensible dressing to cope with breast tenderness or abdominal bloating (such as loose-fitting clothes around the abdomen or a firm-fitting bra to wear during episodes of PMS).

INTEGRATIVE MEDICAL CONSIDERATIONS

Oral contraceptive use

Vitamin B6 supplementation can restore biochemical values and treat PMS symptoms in women taking oral contraception.[99] Hormone supplementation is also commonly used in conventional medicine to treat menstrual symptoms and may affect levels of vitamins A, B2, B3, B5, B12 and folate. OCP use may also reduce the action of *Vitex agnus-castus*.[100]

Acupressure

Acupressure has been demonstrated to be an effective treatment for dysmenorrhoea.[101,102]

Traditional Chinese medicine

Traditional Chinese herbal medicine was found to be more effective than acupuncture in the treatment of dysmenorrhoea[103] and a variety of effective herbal treatments are available.[104] As prescription is usually determined by a physical state diagnosis based on a classical Chinese understanding of the human body, a comprehensive knowledge of traditional Chinese medicine theory is required to appropriately prescribe many of these herbal formulations.[105] Acupuncture has also been found to be moderately effective in the treatment of dysmenorrhoea. This was best seen in patients who committed to weekly treatments and was most effective when combined with herbal and dietary treatments.

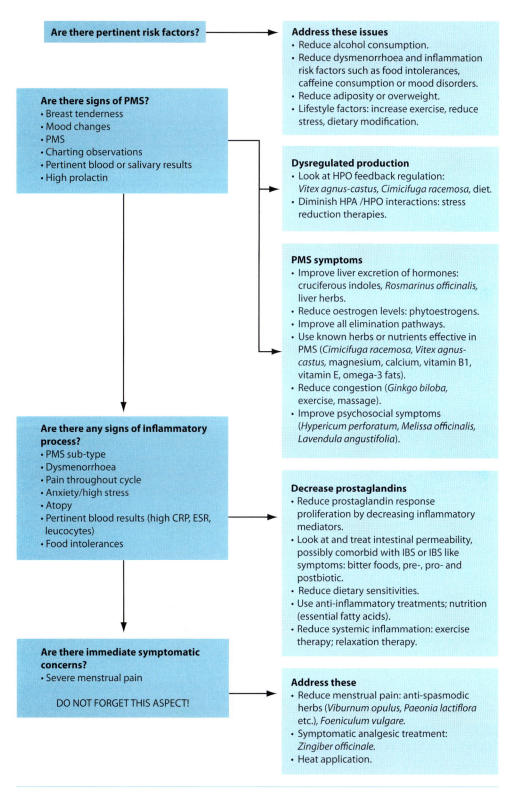

Figure 18.1 Naturopathic treatment decision tree—dysmenorrhoea and menstrual complaints

Chiropractic

A Cochrane review of spinal manipulation in dysmenorrhoea found spinal manipulation to be no better than sham manipulation, though did suggest it was more effective than no treatment.[106]

Qi gong

Chinese exercise therapy or Qi gong has also had documented encouraging success in alleviating various premenstrual symptoms.[107,108]

Homoeopathy

A small preliminary pilot study has demonstrated a positive effect of individualised homoeopathic treatment on premenstrual symptoms, with at least 30% improvement in symptoms observed in 90% of patients receiving homoeopathy versus 37.5% of those who were not.[109]

TENS

Transcutaneous electrical nerve stimulation (TENS) has been demonstrated as a non-invasive, clinically significant intervention for dysmenorrhoea.[110] TENS may also reduce cortisol and prolactin levels through the opioid-modulating analgesia system.[111]

Aromatherapy

Topical application of a 2:1:1 mixture of the aromatherapy oils *Lavandula officinalis*, *Salvia sclarea* and *Rosa centifolia* was demonstrated to be effective in symptomatic treatment of dysmenorrhoea in one small study.[112] Other aromatherapy treatments may also be suitable.

Massage

Regular massage may be a useful adjunct therapy in severe perimenstrual disorders. One small trial has demonstrated positive effects on pain and water retention in the longer term but only short-term benefit for mood and anxiety.[113] Another small trial of abdominal massage using TCM meridian theory has also shown benefit in regard to perimenstrual symptoms such as pain and bloating.[114]

Case Study

A 24-year-old woman comes into the clinic presenting with **severe menstrual cramping** each cycle. The pain is described as 'acute and stabbing'. Her periods have **not become heavier** but the pain is getting worse. They are **relieved after the first few days.** She also gets **anxious** and **'moody'** before her cycle begins.

SUGGESTIVE SYMPTOMS

- Uterine cramping
- Behavioural or mood changes or swings
- Abdominal bloating
- Appetite changes
- Breast tenderness

Example treatment

The patient was given a herbal tablet of *Vitex agnus-castus* to help modulate HPO activity. A combination herbal tablet as in the 'Herbal formula' box was also given to provide symptomatic relief. Its rationale is anti-spasmodic, anti-inflammatory and analgesic. The patient was also prescribed 6000 mg of fish oil daily to provide anti-inflammatory action and address nutritional deficiencies.

The patient was given dietary advice: she was told to initially avoid foods that were commonly associated with inflammatory mediators (wheat and bovine dairy); she was told to increase consumption of foods rich in anti-inflammatory fatty acids such as fish (tuna particularly), avocado and nuts; and was told to increase fibre in her diet, including the addition of legumes and whole grains. Her diet was amended to increase the variety of foods.

> **Herbal formula (tablets)**
>
> *Vitex agnus-castus* taken once   1000 mg
> 1 tablet daily or once daily
> *Viburnum* combination tablet
> combining:
> * *Corydalis ambigua*   600 mg
> * *Zingiber officinale*   400 mg
> * *Viburnum opulus*   400 mg
> Taken 3–4 times daily 2 days before period until 2 days after
>
> **Nutritional prescription**
>
> Omega-3 fish oil 6000 mg daily

The patient had adhered to all prescriptive medicines but had found it difficult to completely remove dairy and wheat. However, her symptoms had still dramatically improved. She was told to continue the *V. agnus-castus* and try not to take the *Viburnum* combination for the next cycle, but instead to take a *Z. officinale* supplement for symptomatic relief. She was told to continue the dietary and lifestyle recommendations and was now free to use dairy and wheat; however, she was counselled on the importance of consuming these as part of a varied diet and taught to focus on wholegrain wheat products and fermented or cultured dairy products.

The patient returned periodically for health visits. After 6 months she was confident enough to cease the *V. agnus-castus*. Her menstrual cramping does not usually return but can flare up occasionally—during which time she takes the *Z. officinale* supplement symptomatically. The patient is now often aware of the situations causing these flare-ups and is able to alter diet and lifestyle accordingly.

Expected outcomes and follow-up protocols

Pain reduction in dysmenorrhoea is the most commonly sought treatment in PMS. Many of the other symptoms of PMS are related to the same underlying issue. A symptomatic treatment for menstrual cramping (such as the *Viburnum* mix) should be given in line with this request; however, eventual HPO modulation or menstrual cycle correction should remain the ultimate goal. Smooth muscle relaxants or uterine tonics alone should never constitute the entirety of treatment. Noticeable improvement should occur within the first cycle and continue throughout the cycles. After a few cycles of noticeably less pain the symptomatic treatments should be ceased and the prescription should focus on HPO modulation and its effectors only.

Table 18.3 Review of the major evidence

STUDIES	METHODOLOGY	RESULT	COMMENT
Thiamine Gokhale 1996[115]	3-month RCT ($n = 556$) crossover design with women with moderate to severe spasmodic dysmenorrhoea. 100 mg thiamine vs placebo	Thiamine significantly increased the proportion of women with no pain before crossover after 60 days compared with placebo (51% vs 0%). After completion of the RCT, 87% of all women experienced no pain.	No analysis was made to determine differences between levels of dysmenorrhoea.

Table 18.3 Review of the major evidence *(Continued)*

STUDIES	METHODOLOGY	RESULT	COMMENT
Vitamin E Butler & McKnight 1955,[116] Ziaei et al. 2005[117]	4 menstrual cycle RCT ($n = 278$) with women aged 15–17 years with primary dysmenorrhoea. 400 IU vitamin E vs placebo	Vitamin E group had lower VAS pain scores at 2 months (3 vs 5; $p \leq 0.001$) and 4 months (0.5 vs 6; $p \leq 0.001$); shorter pain duration at 2 months (4.2 hours vs 15 hours; $p \leq 0.001$) and four months (1.6 hours vs 17 hours; $p \leq 0.001$); and lower blood loss at 2 months (54 vs 70; $p \leq 0.001$) and 4 months (46 vs 70; $p \leq 0.001$) than placebo group.	The form of vitamin E was not made known. Blood loss was also self-measured using a 'staining score' of menstrual pads.
Omega-3 fats Harel et al. 1996[118] Deutch 1995[119]	4-month RCT ($n = 42$). Crossover design with adolescents with dysmenorrhoea. Fish oil (1080 mg EPA; 720 mg DHA) 1.5 mg vitamin E vs placebo	Reduction in Cox Menstrual Symptom Scale Score of 69.9 to 44.0 ($p \leq 0.001$) for fish oil group vs placebo	Omega-3 containing oils have encouraging evidence for reducing menstrual symptoms.
Magnesium Wilson & Murphy 2001[120]	Cochrane systematic review found 7 randomised trials.	Magnesium was more effective than placebo for pain relief and resulted in less extra medication being required.	Trials included in review were: • Seifert et al. 1989[122] (RCT, $n = 50$—magnesium more effective than placebo at pain relief after 6 months and reduction in prostaglandins after 2 months (PGF2 at 45% of baseline levels in magnesium group vs 90% in placebo) • Fontana-Kleiber & Hogg 1990[123] (RCT, $n = 21$. Magnesium more effective than placebo for pain relief on three-point scale after 5 months).
Benassi et al. 1992[121]	Open 6 menstrual cycle trial ($n = 30$). Women with dysmenorrhoea. 4.5 mg magnesium picolanate vs placebo	VAS pain scores reduced significantly ($p \leq 0.05$) on first day of cycle throughout intervention.	Pain scores reduced significantly for first day of cycle, but changes were not significant for second or third days of cycle.
Psidii guajavae folium extract Doubova et al. 2007[70]	4-month RCT ($n = 197$). Women with dysmenorrhoea were assigned to one of four groups: 3 mg guava extract; 6 mg guava extract; 1200 mg ibuprofen; or placebo.	Reduction in VAS pain score consistently over three cycles ($p \leq 0.001$) though was slightly less than ibuprofen group.	Although study showed reduction in pain scores from baseline in all groups, results were inconsistent over three cycles except for 6 mg and ibuprofen groups.

(Continued)

Table 18.3 Review of the major evidence *(Continued)*

STUDIES	METHODOLOGY	RESULT	COMMENT
Zingiber officinale Ozgoli et al. 2009[92]	RCT (*n* = 150) in women with dysmenorrhoea assigned to take one of three interventions four times daily: 250 mg powdered ginger; 250 mg mefenamic acid or 400 mg ibuprofen.	Significant reduction in pain scores across all groups ($p \leq 0.05$).	No significant difference occurred between interventions ($p \leq 0.05$)
Foeniculum vulgare Modaress & Asidipour 2006[93]	2 cycle RCT (n =110) in adolescent women with dysmenorrhoea assigned to take either 250 mg mefenamic acid every 6 hours or 30 drops of *Foeniculum* extract every 6 hours	80% of girls in the fennel group and 73% of girls in the mefenamic acid group showed complete pain relief or pain decrease, while 80% in the fennel group and 62% in the mefenamic acid group no longer needed to rest.	No significant difference in pain relief between the two groups
Namovar et al. 2003[124]	(*n* = 30). Adolescent women with moderate to severe dysmenorrhoea were given no treatment in first cycle, 250 mg mefenamic acid every 6 hours in second cycle, and 25 drops fennel extract in third cycle.	Both mefenamic acid and fennel extract reduced menstrual pain ($p \leq 0.001$). No significant difference was observed during first day though mefenamic acid was significantly superior on second and third days. There was no significant difference in time taken to enact effect between mefenamic acid and fennel extract.	Study design and methodological flaws may reduce validity.
French maritime bark Kohama et al. 2004[125]	3 cycle open CT (n = 47) in women with dysmenorrhoea assigned to take 60 mg FMB per dysmenorrhoeal day	Abdominal pain was reduced in first cycle ($p \leq 0.05$) and further in second cycle ($p \leq 0.01$).	No significant reduction in back pain nor days experiencing pain

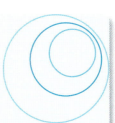

KEY POINTS

- Menstrual problems are not associated with simple hormone excess or deficiency, but rather a complex interconnection of factors that interfere with the HPO axis.
- PMS symptoms are often treated successfully through amelioration of underlying causes with dietary and lifestyle modification—women were not designed to 'malfunction' once a month.
- Symptomatic treatment is very important. However, smooth muscle relaxants or analgesics should be considered only a temporary solution and treatment of the underlying factors should be prioritised.
- Treatment of primary dysmenorrhoea should see positive results within the first one or two cycles. Secondary dysmenorrhoea requires treatment of its causative aetiology and is often more complex (see Chapter 19 on endometriosis).

Further reading

Altman G, et al. Increased symptoms in female IBS patients with dysmenorrhea and PMS. Gastroenterol Nurs 2006;29(1):4–11.

Girman A, et al. An integrative medicine approach to premenstrual syndrome. Am J Obstet Gynecol 2003;188(5 Suppl):S56–S65.

Hudson T. Women's encyclopedia of natural medicine. New York: McGraw-Hill, 2008.

Ozgoli G, et al. Comparison of effects of ginger, mefenamic acid, and ibuprofen on pain in women with primary dysmenorrhea. J Altern Complement Med 2009;15:129–132.

Proctor M, et al. Diagnosis and management of dysmenorrhoea. BMJ 2006;332(7550):1134–1138.

Trickey R. Women, hormones and the menstrual cycle: herbal and medical solutions from adolescence to menopause. Sydney: Allen & Unwin, 2003.

References

1. Edmonds K, ed. Obstetrics and gynaecology. London: Blackwell, 2007.
2. American Psychiatric Association. Diagnostic and statistical manual of mental disorders. 4th edn. Arlington: American Psychiatric Association, 2000.
3. Roca C, et al. Implications of endocrine studies of premenstrual syndrome. Psychiat Ann 1996;26:576–580.
4. Backstrom T, Carstensen H. Estrogen and progesterone in plasma in relation to premenstrual tension. J Steroid Biochem 1974;5:257–260.
5. Munday M, et al. Correlations between progesterone, estradiol and aldosterone levels in the premenstrual syndrome. Clin Endocrinol 1981;14(1):1–9.
6. Rubinow D, et al. Changes in plasma hormones across the menstrual cycle in patients with menstrually related mood disorder and in control subjects. Am J Obstet Gynecol 1988;158:5–11.
7. O'Brien P, Symonds E. Prolactin levels and the premenstrual syndrome. Br J Obstet Gynecol 1982;89:306–308.
8. Dalton K. The aetiology of premenstrual syndrome is with the progesterone receptors. Med Hypotheses 1990;31:323–327.
9. Nock B. Noradrenergic regulation of progestin receptors: new findings. Ann N Y Acad Sci 1986;474:415–422.
10. Sundell G, et al. Factors influencing the prevalence and severity of dysmenorrhoea in young women. Br J Obstet Gynecol 1990;97:588–594.
11. Rubinow D, Schmidt C. The treatment of premenstrual syndrome—forward into the past. New Engl J Med 1995;332:1574–1575.
12. Kessel B. Premenstrual syndrome: advances in diagnosis and treatment. Obstet Gynecol Clin North Am 2000;27(3):625–639.
13. Chuong C, et al. Neuropeptide levels in the premenstrual syndrome. Fertil Steril 1985;44:760–765.
14. Rapkin A. The role of serotonin in the premenstrual syndrome. Clin Obstet Gynecol 1992;35(3):629–636.
15. Steiner M, Pearlstein T. Premenstrual dysphoria and the serotonin system: pathophysiology and treatment J Clin Psychiatry 2000;61(12):S17–S21.
16. Budoff P. The use of prostaglandin inhibitors for the premenstrual syndrome. J Reprod Med 1983;28:465–468.
17. Nigam S, et al. Increased concentrations of eiconasoids and platelet-activating factor in menstrual blood from women with primary dysmenorrhoea. Eicosanoids 1991;4(3):137–141.
18. Horrobin D. The role of essential fatty acids and prostaglandins in the premenstrual syndrome. J Reprod Med 1983;28(7):465–468.
19. Hamilton J, et al. Premenstrual mood changes: a guide to evaluation and treatment. Psychiat Ann 1984;30:474–482.
20. DeJong R, et al. Premenstrual mood disorder and psychiatric illness. Am J Psychiat 1985;142:1359–1361.
21. Chen C, et al. Prospective study of exposure to environmental tobacco smoke and dysmenorrhea. Environ Health Perspect 2000;108(11):1019–1022.
22. Hornsby P, et al. Cigarette smoking and disturbance of menstrual function. Epidemiology 1998;9(2):193–198.
23. Parazzini F, et al. Cigarette smoking, alcohol consumption, and risk of primary dysmenorrhea. Epidemiology 1994;5(4):469–472.
24. Masho S, et al. Obesity as a risk factor for premenstrual syndrome. J Psychosom Obstet Gynecol 2005;26(1):33–39.
25. DeJong R, et al. Premenstrual mood disorder and psychiatric illness. Am J Psychiatry 1985;142:1359–1361.
26. Rossignol A, Bonnlander H. Caffeine-containing beverages, total fluid consumption, and premenstrual syndrome. Am J Public Health 1990;80(9):1106–1110.
27. Rossignol A, et al. Tea and premenstrual syndrome in the People's Republic of China. Am J Public Health 1989;79(1):67–69.
28. Rossignol A, Bonnlander H. Prevalence and severity of the premenstrual syndrome. Effects of foods and beverages that are sweet or high in sugar content. J Reprod Med 1991;36:131–136.
29. Rossignol A, et al. Do women with premenstrual symptoms self-medicate with caffeine? Epidemiology 1991;2(6):403–408.
30. Murtagh J. General practice. Sydney: McGraw-Hill, 2007.
31. Wyatt K. Premenstrual syndrome. Clin Evid 2000;9: 2125–2144.
32. Ford O, et al. Progesterone for premenstrual syndrome. Cochrane Database Syst Rev 2006(4):CD003415.
33. Abraham G. Nutritional factors in the etiology of the premenstrual syndrome. J Reprod Med 1983;28:446–464.
34. Mills S, Bone K. Principles and practice of phytotherapy. Edinburgh: Churchill Livingstone, 2000.
35. Blumenthal M, et al., eds. Herbal medicine: expanded Commission E monographs (English translation). Austin: Integrative Medicine Communications, 2000.
36. Balbi C, et al. Influence of menstrual factors and dietary habits on menstrual pain in adolescence age. Eur J Obstet Gynecol Reprod Biol 2000;91(2):143–148.
37. Barnard N, et al. Diet and sex-hormone binding globulin, dysmenorrhea, and premenstrual symptoms. Obstet Gynecol 2000;95(2):245–250.
38. Nagata C, et al. Associations of menstrual pain with intakes of soy, fat and dietary fiber in Japanese women. Eur J Clin Nutr 2005;59(1):88–92.
39. Nagata C, et al. Soy, fat and other dietary factors in relation to premenstrual symptoms in Japanese women. BJOG 2004;111(6):594–599.
40. Roy S, et al. Changes in glucose oral tolerance during normal menstrual cycle. J Indian Med Assoc 1971;57(6): 201–204.

41. Fujiwara T. Skipping breakfast is associated with dysmenorrhoea in young women in Japan. Int J Food Sci Nutr 2003;54(6):505–509.

42. Fujiwara T. Diet during adolescence is a trigger for subsequent development of dysmenorrhoea in young women. Int J Food Sci Nutr 2007;58(6):437–444.

43. Montero P, et al. Influence of body mass index and slimming habits on menstrual pain and cycle irregularity. J Biosoc Sci 1996;28(3):315–323.

44. Golomb L, et al. Primary dysmenorrhea and physical activity. Med Sci Sports Exerc 1998;30(6):906–909.

45. Pullon S, et al. Treatment of premenstrual symptoms in Wellington women. N Z Med J 1989;102(862):72–74.

46. Jahromi M, et al. Influence of a physical fitness course on menstrual cycle characteristics. Gynecol Endocrinol 2008;24(11):659–662.

47. Aganoff J, Boyle G. Aerobic exercise, mood states and menstrual cycle symptoms. J Psychosom Res 1994;38:183–192.

48. Choi P, Salmon P. Symptom changes across the menstrual cycle in competitive sportswomen, exercisers and sedentary women. Br J Clin Pschol 1995;34(3):447–460.

49. Prior J, Vigna Y. Conditioning exercise and premenstrual symptoms. Reprod Med 1987;32:423–428.

50. Stoddard J, et al. Exercise training effects on premenstrual distress and ovarian steroid hormones. Eur J Appl Physiol 2007;99(1):27–37.

51. Lustyk M, et al. Stress, quality of life and physical activity in women with varying degrees of premenstrual symptomatology. Women Health 2004;39(3):35–44.

52. Wang L, et al. Stress and dysmenorrhoea: a population based prospective study. Occup Environ Med 2004;61(12):1021–1026.

53. Goodale I, et al. Alleviation of premenstrual syndrome with the relaxation response. Obstet Gynecol 1990;75(4):649–655.

54. Arias A, et al. Systematic review of the efficacy of meditation techniques as treatments for medical illness. J Altern Complement Med 2008;12(8):817–823.

55. Schellenberg R. Treatment for the premenstrual syndrome with agnus castus fruit extract: prospective, randomised, placebo controlled study. BMJ 2001;322(7279):134–137.

56. Loch E, et al. Treatment of premenstrual syndrome with a phytopharmaceutical formulation containing Vitex agnus castus. J Womens Health Gend Based Med 2000;9(3):315–320.

57. Wuttke W, et al. Chaste tree (Vitex agnus-castus)—pharmacology and clinical indications. Phytomed 2003;10(4):348–57.

58. Berger D, et al. Efficacy of Vitex agnus-castus L. Extract Ze 440 in patients with pre-menstrual syndrome (PMS). Arch Gynecol Obstet 2000;264(3):150–153.

59. Jarry H, et al. In vitro prolactin but not LH and FSH release is inhibited by compounds in extracts of Agnus castus: direct evidence for a dopaminergic principle by the dopamine receptor assay. Exp Clin Endocrinol 1994;102(6):448–454.

60. Sliutz G, et al. Agnus castus extracts inhibit prolactin secretion of rat pituitary cells. Horm Metab Res 1993;25(5):253–255.

61. Milewicz A, et al. [Vitex agnus-castus extract in the treatment of luteal phase defects due to latent hyperprolactinemia. Results of a randomized placebo-controlled double-blind study] [in German]. Arzneimittelforschung 1993;43(7):752–756.

62. Meier B, et al. Pharmacological activities of Vitex agnus-castus extracts in vitro. Phytomedicine 2000;7(5):373–381.

63. Merz P, et al. The effects of a special Agnus castus extract (BP1095E1) on prolactin secretion in healthy male subjects. Exp Clin Endocrinol Diabetes 1996;104(6):447–453.

64. Liu J. Evaluation of estrogenic activity of plant extracts for the potential treatment of menopausal symptoms. J Agricult Food Chem 2001;49(5):2472–2479.

65. Webster D, et al. Activation of the mu-opiate receptor by Vitex agnus-castus methanol extracts: implication for its use in PMS. J Ethnopharmacol 2006;106(2):216–221.

66. Duker E, et al. Effects of extracts from Cimicifuga racemosa on gonadotrophin release in menopausal women and ovariectomized rats. Planta Med 1991;57(5):420–424.

67. Seidlova-Wuttke, et al. Evidence for selective estrogen receptor modulator activity in a black cohosh (Cimicifuga racemosa) extract: comparison with estradiol-17 beta. Eur J Endocrinol 2003;149:351–362.

68. Scientific Committee of the British Herbal Medical Association. British herbal pharmacopoeia. 1st edn. Bournemouth: British Herbal Medicine Association, 1983.

69. Tseng Y, et al. Rose tea for relief of primary dysmenorrhea in adolescents: a randomized controlled trial in Taiwan. J Midwifery Womens Health 2005;50(5):e51–57.

70. Doubova S, et al. Effect of a Psidii guajavae folium extract in the treatment of primary dysmenorrhea: a randomized clinical trial. J Ethnopharmacol 2007;110(2):305–310.

71. Banikarim C, et al. Prevalence and impact of dysmenorrhea on Hispanic female adolescents. Arch Pediatr Adolesc Med 2000;154:1226–1229.

72. Stevinson C, Ernst E. A pilot study of Hypericum perforatum for the treatment of premenstrual syndrome. BJOG 2000;107(7):870–876.

73. Tamborini A, Taurelle R. [Value of standardized Ginkgo biloba extract (EGb 761) in the management of congestive symptoms of premenstrual syndrome]. Rev Fr Gynecol Obstet 1993;88(7–9):447–457.

74. Thys-Jacobs S, et al. Calcium carbonate and the premenstrual syndrome: effects on premenstrual and menstrual symptoms. Am J Obstet Gynecol 1998;179(2):444–452.

75. Thys-Jacobs S, et al. Calcium supplementation in premenstrual syndrome. J Gen Intern Med 1989;4:183–189.

76. Facchinetti F, et al. Oral magnesium successfully relieves premenstrual mood changes. Obstet Gynecol 1991;78:177–181.

77. Walker A, et al. Magnesium supplementation alleviates premenstrual symptoms of fluid retention. J Womens Health 1998;7:1157–1165.

78. Abraham G, Lubran M. Serum red cell magnesium levels in patients with PMT. Am J Clin Nutr 1981;34:2364–2366.

79. Sherwood R, et al. Magnesium and the premenstrual syndrome. Ann Clin Biochem 1986;23:667–670.

80. Facchinetti F, et al. Premenstrual increase of intracellular magnesium levels in women with ovulatory, asymptomatic menstrual cycles. Gynecol Endocrinol 1988;2:249–256.

81. London R, et al. Evaluation and treatment of breast symptoms in women with the premenstrual syndrome. J Reprod Med 1981;28:503–508.

82. London R, et al. The effect of alpha-tocopherol on premenstrual symptomatology: a double-blind study. J Am Coll Nutr 1983;2(2):115–122.

83. London R, et al. Efficacy of alpha-tocopherol in the treatment of the premenstrual syndrome. J Reprod Med 1987;32(6):400–404.

84. Argonz J, Abinzano C. Premenstrual tension treated with vitamin A. J Clin Endocrinol Metab 1950;10(12):1579–1590.

85. Chuong C, Dawson E. Zinc and copper levels in premenstrual syndrome. Fertil Steril 1994;62:313–320.

86. Akin M, et al. Continuous, low-level, topical heat wrap therapy as compared to acetaminophen for primary dysmenorrhea. J Reprod Med 2004;49(9):739–745.

87. Akin M, et al. Continuous low-level topical heat in the treatment of dysmenorrhea. Obstet Gynecol 2001;97(3):343–349.

88. Hazelhoff B, et al. Antispasmodic effects of Valeriana compounds: an in-vivo and in-vitro study on the guinea pig ileum. Arch Int Pharmacdyn Ther 1982;257:274–287.

89. Lis-Belchin M, Hart S. Studies on the mode of action of the essential oil of lavender (*Lavandula angustifolia*). Phytother Res 1999;13(6):540–542.

90. Achterrath-Tuckermann U, et al. Pharmacological investigations with compounds of chamomile. V. Investigations on the spasmolytic effect of compounds of chamomile and Kamillosan on the isolated guinea pig ileum. Planta Med 1980;39(1):38–50.

91. Ostad S, et al. The effect of fennel essential oil on uterine contraction as a model for dysmenorrhea, pharmacology and toxicology study. J Ethnopharmacol 2001;76(3):299–304.

92. Ozgoli G, et al. Comparison of effects of ginger, mefenamic acid, and ibuprofen on pain in women with primary dysmenorrhea. J Altern Complement Med 2009.[Epub ahead of print].

93. Modaress Nejad V, Asadipour M. Comparison of the effectiveness of fennel and mefenamic acid on pain intensity in dysmenorrhoea. East Mediterr Health J 2006;12(3–4):423–427.

94. Munch J, Pratt H. The uterine-sedative action of authentic Viburnum. XI. Bioassay methods. Pharmaceut Arch 1941;12:88–91.

95. Jarboe C, et al. Uterine relaxant properties of Viburnum. Nature 1966;212:837.

96. Brayshaw N, Brayshaw D. Thyroid hypofunction in premenstrual syndrome. N Engl J Med 1986;315:1486–1487.

97. Girdler S, et al. Thyroid axis function during the menstrual cycle in women with premenstrual syndrome. Psychoneuroendocrinology 1995;20(4):395–403.

98. Schmidt P, et al. Thyroid function in women with premenstrual syndrome. J Clin Endocrinol Metab 1993;76(3):671–674.

99. Bermond P. Therapy of side effects of oral contraceptive agents with vitamin B6. Acta Vitaminol Enzymol 1982;4(1–2):45–54.

100. Braun L, Cohen M. Herbs and natural supplements: an evidence based guide. Sydney: Churchill Livingstone, 2007.

101. Taylor D, et al. A randomized clinical trial of the effectiveness of an acupressure device (relief brief) for managing symptoms of dysmenorrhea. J Altern Complement Med 2002;8:357–370.

102. Pouresmail Z, Ibrahimzadeh R. Effects of acupressure and ibuprofen on the severity of primary dysmenorrhea. J Trad Chin Med 2002;22:205–210.

103. Zhu X, et al. Chinese herbal medicine for primary dysmenorrhoea. Cochrane Database Syst Rev 2008;(2):CD005288.

104. Jia W, et al. Common traditional Chinese medicinal herbs for dysmenorrhea. Phytother Res 2006;20(10):819–824.

105. Maciocia G. Obstetrics and gynecology in Chinese medicine. Edinburgh: Churchill Livingstone, 1997.

106. Proctor M, et al. Spinal manipulation for primary and secondary dysmenorrhoea. Cochrane Database Syst Rev 2006;(3):CD002119.

107. Jang H, Lee M. Effects of qi therapy (external qigong) on premenstrual syndrome: a randomized placebo controlled study. J Altern Complement Med 2004;10:456–462.

108. Jang H, et al. Effects of qi-therapy on premenstrual syndrome. Int J Neurosci 2004;114:909–921.

109. Yakir M, et al. Effects of homeopathic treatment in women with premenstrual syndrome: a pilot study. Br Homeopath J 2001;90:148–153.

110. Proctor M, et al. Transcutaneous electrical nerve stimulation and acupuncture for primary dysmenorrhoea. Cochrane Database Syst Rev 2002;(1):CD002123.

111. Akinbo S, et al. Effect of transcutaneous electric nerve stimulation (TENS) on hormones profile in subjects with primary dysmenorrhoea—a preliminary study. South African Journal of Physiotherapy 2007;63(3):45–48.

112. Han S, et al. Effect of aromatherapy on symptoms of dysmenorrhea in college students: a randomized placebo-controlled clinical trial. J Altern Complement Med 2006;12(6):535–541.

113. Hernandez-Reif M, et al. Premenstrual symptoms are relieved by massage therapy. J Psychosom Obstet Gynaecol 2000;21(1):9–15.

114. Kim J, et al. [The effects of abdominal meridian massage on menstrual cramps and dysmenorrhea in full-time employed women]. Taehan Kanho Hakhoe Chi 2005;35(7):1325–1332.

115. Gokhale L. Curative treatment of primary (spasmodic) dysmenorrhoea. Indian J Med Res 1996;103:227–231.

116. Butler E, McKnight E. Vitamin E in the treatment of primary dysmenorrhoea. Lancet 1955;268(6869):844–847.

117. Ziaei S, et al. A randomised controlled trial of vitamin E in the treatment of primary dysmenorrhoea. BJOG 2005;112(4):466–469.

118. Harel Z, et al. Supplementation with omega-3 polyunsaturated fatty acids in the management of dysmenorrhea in adolescents. Am J Obstet Gynecol 1996;174(4):1335–1338.

119. Deutch B. Menstrual pain in Danish women correlated with low n-3 polyunsaturated fatty acid intake. Eur J Clin Nutr 1995;49(7):508–516.

120. Wilson M, Murphy P. Herbal and dietary therapies for primary and secondary dysmenorrhoea. Cochrane Database Syst Rev 2001;(3):CD002124.

121. Benassi L, et al. Effectiveness of magnesium pidolate in the prophylactic treatment of primary dysmenorrhoea. Clin Experimental Obstet Gynecol 1992;19(3):176–179.

122. Seifert B, et al. [Magnesium—a new therapeutic alternative in primary dysmenorrhea]. Zentralbl Gynakol 1989;111(11):755–760.

123. Fontana-Klaiber H, Hogg B. [Therapeutic effects of magnesium in dysmenorrhea]. Schweiz Rundsch Med Prax 1990;79(16):491–494.

124. Namavar Jahromi B, et al. Comparison of fennel and mefenamic acid for the treatment of primary dysmenorrhea. Int J Gynaecol Obstet 2003;80(2):153–157.

125. Kohama T, et al. Analgesic efficacy of French maritime pine bark extract in dysmenorrhea: an open clinical trial. J Reprod Med 2004;49(10):828–832.

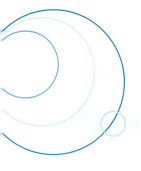

19
Endometriosis

Jon Wardle
ND, MPH

OVERVIEW AND AETIOLOGY

Endometriosis is the abnormal growth of endometrial tissue in areas other than the wall of the uterus.[1] The exact cause of endometriosis is unknown although a number of theories do exist. It is one of the more common causes of infertility in Western societies. However, sufferers may experience combinations of many underlying causes and no person is identical in their symptoms or causes. Theories in naturopathic medicine include the following (see Figure 19.1):

- Excessive oestrogens may promote the proliferation of endometrial tissue. Oestrogen levels may be higher for a number of reasons, including increased production or decreased excretion, or may be dominated by oestrogen metabolites that are more proliferative, inflammatory and genotoxic.[2,3]
- Environmental toxins may mimic hormones in the body, exacerbating endometriosis symptoms.[4]
- Although retrograde menstruation is present in most cycling women, not all these women have endometriosis. It is thought inflammatory mediators may cause endometrial tissue to adhere to other tissues;[5] an autoimmune component has also been linked to endometriosis.[6]
- There may be a genetic component. Endometriosis has been linked to dysfunctions in embryonic development.
- Other theories suggest that endometriosis does not represent transplanted endometrial tissue but starts de novo from local stem cells. This process has been referred to as *coelomic metaplasia*. Various triggers, such as excessive oestrogen levels, menses, toxins or immune factors, may be necessary to start this process. This would explain the rare instances of endometriosis in men.[7,8]

RISK FACTORS

Several risk factors need to be addressed in the patient with endometriosis. Although often hormonal or inflammatory in nature, removal of these risk factors may be enough to significantly reduce symptoms. Lack of exercise can increase levels of oestrogen and inflammatory mediators and reduce oestrogen excretion.[9] However, strenuous physical activity during menstruation may increase risk. Epidemiological data also suggest that positive correlations of symptoms and occurrence are

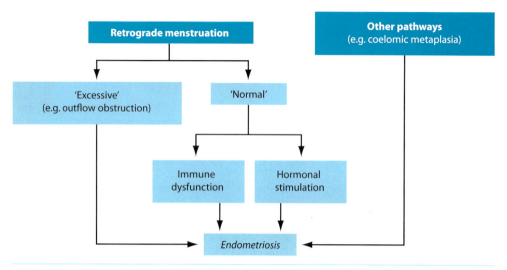

Figure 19.1 Postulated theories for the development of endometriosis

seen with increased cigarette smoking; increased carbohydrate, alcohol and coffee intake; stress; and low body mass index.[10] Aromatase found in adipose tissue may also increase the formation of oestrogen.[11] Therefore weight loss may be indicated in some patients.

CONVENTIONAL TREATMENT

Conventional medical treatment aims to reduce the symptoms of endometriosis and improve fertility. This can be done surgically (most often laparoscopic to remove tissue, although occasionally hysterectomy is required) or medically. Medical interventions focus predominantly on reduction of excessive oestrogen levels. These include those androgenic in nature, such as danazol or progesterone supplementation; inducing hypo-oestrogenic states by decreasing FSH and LH through the use of gonadotrophin-releasing hormone agonists (GnRH agonists); continuous hormonal contraception to stop bleeding; or aromatase inhibitors to block the formation of oestrogens, particularly in adipose tissue.[1]

KEY TREATMENT PROTOCOLS

In naturopathic treatment, endometriosis is most often theorised as a disorder of inflammation or hormonal imbalance and may have a number of underlying factors.

Oestrogen modulation

Hypothalamic–pituitary–ovarian axis modulation

Oestrogen levels in the body may be affected by disruptions of the hypothalamic–pituitary–ovarian (HPO) axis. The anterior pituitary releases FSH (follicle stimulating hormone) and LH (luteinising

NATUROPATHIC TREATMENT AIMS
- Address risk and exacerbating factors.
- Modulate oestrogen levels.
- Decrease inflammation.
- Address secondary aims and symptoms.
- Address dietary and lifestyle issues affecting the condition.

AROMATASE

Aromatase is an enzyme of the cytochrome P450 superfamily the function of which is to aromatise androgens, thereby producing oestrogens. Normally, it is found in the ovaries, and to a much lesser extent in the skin and fat. Aromatase is not present in the normal endometrium but is expressed aberrantly in endometriosis.[2,12–14]

Prostaglandin E2 (PGE_2) was found to be the most potent known inducer of aromatase activity in endometrial cells.[15,16] Inflammation may not only increase aromatase, but also make endometrial tissue more sensitive to its effects.[17] Factors known to increase aromatase activity are hyperinsulinaemia, increased adiposity, obesity and ageing.[18]

Aromatase activity may be decreased by increased consumption of dietary phytoestrogens[19] in addition to reduction in adiposity and inflammation.

hormone), which encourages oestrogen release from growing ovarian follicles. Ordinarily feedback loops regulate hormone release from the HPO axis, but in some reproductive disorders this may be disrupted. Herbal medicines such as ***Vitex agnus-castus***[20] and ***Cimicifuga racemosa***[21] may help restore proper functioning of the HPO axis through direct and indirect means. Exercise has been shown to both reduce oestrogen production and increase oestrogen excretion[10] (see Chapter 18 on premenstrual syndrome and dysmenorrhoea).

Oestrogen-like compounds and oestrogen receptor activity

Many compounds—both natural and synthetic—may mimic endogenous sex hormones.[4,22,23] Several chemicals in current industrial use may interfere with the body's hormone responses. Compounds such as dioxins, polychlorinated biphenyls (PCBs) and bisphenols (found in pesticides, petrochemicals and plastics) may bind to and activate endogenous oestrogen receptor sites. However, unlike natural hormones these xenoestrogens (literally 'foreign oestrogens') may exert effects many times more potent than endogenous oestrogens.[24] **Phytoestrogens** (literally 'plant oestrogens') also bind to and activate these oestrogen receptor sites although they are often much less powerful than regular oestrogen and therefore act as oestrogen modulators by preventing the more powerful compounds—endogenous hormones and the xenoestrogens—binding in excess oestrogen conditions but binding to empty sites in oestrogen-deficient conditions.[25] A compound exhibiting this activity is known as a selective oestrogen receptor modulator (SORM)—similar in effect to the pharmaceutical compound tamoxifen. The isoflavones (such as genistein and dadzein) from soy products, lignans from lentils and flaxseed, coumestans from ***Trifolium pratense*** and flavonoids found in a variety of sources are examples of phytoestrogens. Sources of phytoestrogens are listed in Table 19.1. Although most research has focused on phytoestrogenic compounds from soy products, most dietary consumption of these compounds in Western diets occurs from lignans.[26] Different soy products may also vary in their phytoestrogenic content: soybeans, tofu and tempeh are good sources while soy milk is generally not. Studies suggest that ***Cimicifuga racemosa*** may contain negligible amounts of phytoestrogenic compounds while still exerting strong oestrogen modulating ability.[13] This is thought to be related more to its effects on luteinising hormone. *V. agnus-castus* has also shown significant competitive binding to oestrogen receptors in vitro.[27]

The generalisation that all phytoestrogens are inherently weaker than endogenous oestrogen is not correct. The herbs *T. pratense* and *Humulus lupulus* actually exert stronger activity in the body than endogenous oestrogen. This may make them therapeutically useful in oestrogen-deficient conditions—those associated with menopause, for example—but may potentially exacerbate symptoms of oestrogen-dependent disorders and render their use inappropriate in high doses in conditions such as endometriosis.[28,29] It is also prudent to avoid herbs known to promote oestrogenic symptoms, such as *Chamaelirium luteum* and *Dioscorea villosa*. Studies suggest that long-term treatment with high-dose phytoestrogenic compounds (in excess of 150 mg of soy isoflavones daily for 5 years) can lead to endometrial hyperplasia.[30] This suggests a role for lower doses associated with modified dietary intake for long-term management. **Cruciferous indoles**, in addition to their activity on oestrogen excretion and conversion, may also directly inhibit stimulation of oestrogen receptors by oestrogen or oestrogen-like compounds[31,32] though the particular mechanism is unknown at this time.

Oestrogen excretion

Inadequate oestrogen excretion may result in excess circulating oestrogens. The main route of elimination of excess oestrogens is the liver. The major pathways of elimination are the phase II liver pathways glucoronidation, sulphation and methylation.[35] These pathways bind the used hormones with a water-soluble substance, which can then be eliminated through bile and eventually faeces.

If toxins overload the system, these pathways can become congested. **Cruciferous indoles**, such as indole-3-carbinol (I3C) and di-indolyl-methane (DIM), found in brussels sprouts, broccoli, cabbage, garlic and other 'sulfurous' vegetables,[36] are

Table 19.1 Relative phytoestrogenic content (μg/100 g) of commonly used therapeutic supplements[2,14,15,33,34]

Trifolium pratense	1,767,000
Flaxseed (crushed)	546,000
Soybeans	103,920
Tofu	27,150
Sesame seed	8,008
Flax bread	7,540
Multigrain bread	4,798
Pumpkin	3,870
Chickpeas	3,600
Lentils	3,370
Soy milk	2,457

particularly useful for the oestrogen-specific pathways as they induce enzyme reactions that assist with detoxification and conversion of 17β-estradiol to less active forms (2-hydroxyestrone as opposed to 16α-hydroxyestrone).[37–43] While these trials are largely based on direct supplementation (of 300–400 mg/day of I3C or 100 mg/day of DIM) studies suggest food supplementation may also be effective.[36,39,44] Herbs such as ***Silybum marianum*** and ***Bupleurum falcatum*** can also improve liver enzyme activity in regards to oestrogen clearance.[45] Figure 19.2 shows examples of supplements, foods and herbs useful in improving liver function. ***Rosmarinus officinalis*** has been found to directly increase hepatic metabolism of oestrogens and reduce their uterotropic action in animal studies.[46] Vitamin B complexes may increase the inactivation of oestrone in the body.[47] Other useful treatment tools are listed in Table 19.2.

Phase I liver detoxification processes convert oestrogens to either 2-hydroxyoestrone (2OH oestrone), 16- or 4-hydroxyoestrone. 2OH oestrone is a 'cancer-protective' metabolite (oestrogen antagonist) and the latter two are 'pro-carcinogenic' (oestrogen agonists).[48] Each of the enzymes involved are subject to genetic polymorphisms that are measurable in more complex cases. Other factors can also affect this oestrogen conversion (see Figure 19.3).[48]

The liver is not the only organ associated with oestrogen excretion. The entero-hepatic circulatory system will recycle sex hormones if intestinal transit time is sufficiently slow. If there is not enough fibre in the diet, the oestrogens will be recirculated before they are excreted. Increased fibre consumption has been associated with lower oestrogen metabolites.[34] Fibre is also required to increase dioxin, PCB and other oestrogen-like molecules from the body in animal models.[49,50]

Supporting liver function

Healthy detoxification consists of both appropriate phase I and phase II detoxification. Phase I is a stage in which lipid soluble substances are transformed into intermediate substances via the cytochrome P450 set of enzymes.[33] In many instances this may render substances even more toxic or otherwise reactive than previously.[33] Therefore appropriate

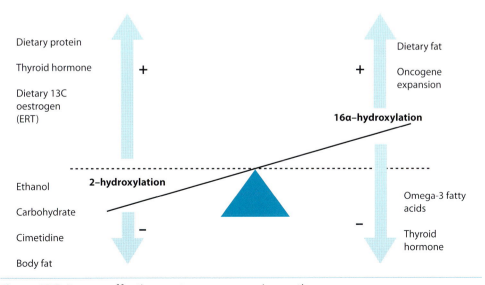

Figure 19.2 Factors affecting oestrogen conversion pathways

Table 19.2 Detoxification enzyme reactions involving common naturopathic medicines

PHASE	INDUCE	INHIBIT
I*	Cruciferous vegetables[51]	Legumes[52]
	Garlic[53]	Grapefruit juice[54]
	Smoking[55]	Starfruit juice[56]
	Thymus vulgare[57]	Taraxacum officinale[58]
	Adhatoda vasica[59]	Mentha pieperita[58]
	Charcoaled meat products	Matricaria recutita[58]
	Niacin	Humulus lupulus[60]
	High protein diets	Glycyrrhiza glabra[61,62]
	Hypericum perforatum[63]	Rosmarinus officinalis[64]
		Withania somnifera[65]
		Echinacea spp.[66]
		Chlorophyll[36]
		Berberine-containing herbs[67,68]
		Schisandra chinensis[69]
II*	Curcumin[70,71]	Low protein status
	Vaccinum spp.[72]	Zinc deficiency
	Green tea[73,74]	B12 deficiency
	Cruciferous vegetables[75–77]	Folic acid deficiency
	Taraxacum officinale[58]	
	Humulus lupulus[60,78]	
	Glycyrrhiza glabra[61]	
	Rosmarinus officinalis[64,79]	
	Thymus vulgare[57]	
	Adhatoda vasica[59]	
	Withania somnifera[65]	
	Flavonoids[36]	
	Schisandra chinensis[80]	

*For simplification purposes, phases I and II have not been split into their components.

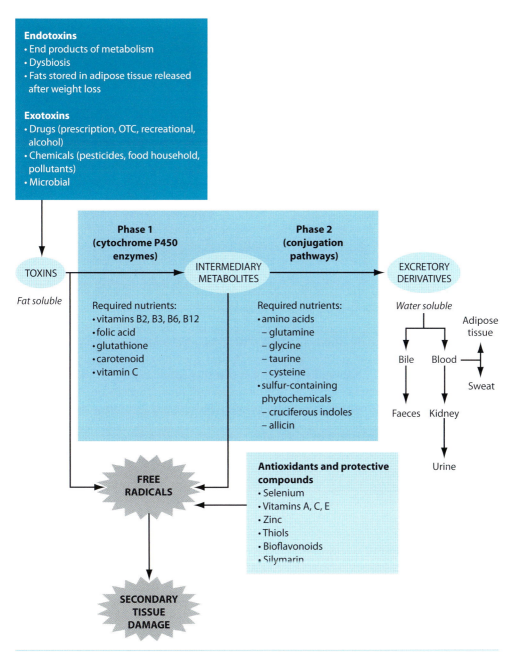

Figure 19.3 Biochemical and nutritional factors affecting oestrogen conversion and metabolism

phase II detoxification processes need to be supported. Phase II processes make the intermediate substances from phase I detoxification water-soluble by conjugating them with amino acids like glucoronic acid, glutathione and glycine or undergoing processes such as methylation, sulphation, acetylation and sulphoxidation.[33] These substances can then be excreted through the stool, sweat or urine (and to lesser extent lungs)—elimination pathways, which also need to be appropriately encouraged in detoxification.

THE LIVER IN GYNAECOLOGY

The reproductive section of the book may seem a strange place to discuss liver pathology, but the liver has long played a key role in gynaecology diagnosis and treatment in traditional medicine. In Western humoral theory most gynaecological complaints were caused by an excess of yellow bile (hot womb—fiery and red menstrual loss) or a deficiency resulted in too little menses and a feeling of coldness or heaviness on the area ('damp'). In traditional Chinese medicine the liver has long been associated with common gynaecological complaints such as PMS, irregular menses, amenorrhoea, infertility and dysmenorrhoea. Both systems related the mental symptoms often associated with PMS to liver disharmony. These broader concepts have had a great influence on contemporary naturopathic practice. Detoxification of hormones is still a key treatment aim in gynaecological disorders such as PMS, dysmenorrhoea, fibroids and endometriosis.

Phase I (p450) enzymes are relatively resistant to depletion due to nutritional considerations; however, Phase II enzymes are particularly dependent on nutritional substrates required for conjugation. Pathological factors, such as cardiovascular, liver and kidney disease, can also affect the liver's detoxification mechanisms. Like many medications, naturopathic medicines have the ability to interact with detoxification pathways in the liver.

Many studies are either in vitro or animal in vivo and therefore clinical significance often remains unknown. It should also be noted that there often exists a lack of in vivo–in vitro correlation with respect to studies on interaction of phase I interactions. For example, while **Silybum marianum** has documented in vitro evidence of induction of cytochrome p450 enzymes, in vivo evidence does not seem to suggest a significant effect.[81–83] Further studies have also demonstrated that co-administration of *S. marianum* with other medications does not reduce levels of that medication, again suggesting no clinically significant interaction.[84–87] The induction of CYP enzymes by *H. perforatum* also seems to bear little clinical significance when compared to in vitro results.[88,89] However, quality issues need to be considered as evidence suggests that specific compounds in naturopathic medicines that vary from product to product may be responsible for this induction—for example, levels of hyperforin may be responsible for induction in *H. perforatum* products and these levels can differ significantly in different products.[88,90] However, a number of factors can belie in vitro pharmacokinetic suggestion in human physiology, including not just individual differences in people themselves, but also significant differences in different versions of the 'same' naturopathic products. Therefore caution should still be observed. It should also be noted that in a clinical setting induction or inhibition of phase I or phase II enzymes, and by extension possible interaction with other medications, does not necessarily preclude use of these naturopathic medicines. Rather it implies that these factors should be taken into appropriate consideration when prescribing them and that the patient's use of concomitant medicines should be routinely monitored (see the drug–CAM interactions table in Appendix 1).

In some instances dietary inclusion may be more beneficial than supplementation. Glutathione—a key nutrient in phase II metabolism of toxins—is best obtained from food sources, as many supplements may have limited bioavailability.[36] Diets low in protein may predispose patients to lowered liver detoxification, as key amino acids are involved in these liver processes.[91] Increasing crude protein intake will also help to improve availability of amino acid precursors to conjugation.

POLYPHARMACY

Although most attention is paid to the effects that naturopathic medicines can have on the efficacy of conventional medicines, conventional medicines can affect the efficacy of naturopathic medicines. In a polypharmacy patient various interactions could significantly affect the effectiveness of the desired prescription. Nor is polypharmacy limited only to conventional medicines. Too many naturopathic medicines could present the same difficulties. These effects need to be taken into consideration when formulating a treatment plan.

Detoxification

Inhibiting phase I reactions is generally thought of as cancer protective, as it reduces the production of potentially toxic intermediates. However, supporting phase II reactions will also reduce exposure to these intermediates. Antioxidants are also an essential part of detoxification protocol. The liver-supportive naturopathic medicines **glutathione** and ***Silybum marianum*** work largely through their antioxidant activity, sequestering these potentially dangerous or mutagenic intermediate compounds.

Improving liver function, with respect to supporting and implementing balance between phase I and phase II reactions, remains the primary treatment aim in supporting detoxification. However, this process can be supported in other ways.

Modulation of intestinal microflora with **probiotics** and **synbiotics** (including dietary intervention with yoghurt) has also been demonstrated to improve the liver's general function and detoxification ability in humans, most probably through the reduction of endotoxin load or ammonia production and resorption in the intestine.[92–95]

Exercise will also promote hepatic biotransformation processes.[96,97] Fasting is also known to enhance the detoxification process,[98] in part because the main source of energy is hydrolysed fatty acid tissue from adipose tissue stores, where many toxins are stored.[99] However, due prudence needs to be displayed, as fasting may liberate toxins faster than they can be eliminated (because in part the adequate substrates from phase II detoxification may be missing or compromised) and may potentially endanger the patient.

Hydrotherapy is thought to increase filtration through the liver by encouraging blood circulation, in addition to aiding excretion through sweating.[100] Sauna therapy has also been used to encourage elimination through the skin, with substantial elimination and significant clinical improvement thought possible through this mechanism.[101,102] **Sauna** exposure of 5–15 minutes per day is safe and effective in enhancing detoxification, though caution is advised in patients with recent myocardial infarction or other serious cardiovascular complications, and patients need to be advised that eliminating toxins through the skin may initially irritate (though ultimately improve) conditions such as atopic dermatitis.[103] Many nutrients—particularly trace elements such as zinc, copper, iron and chromium as well as electrolytes—may be lost through sweating and may need monitoring or replacement.

An **Ayurvedic herbal formula** consisting of *Capparis spinosa*, *Cichorium intybus*, *Solanum nigrum*, *Terminalia arjuna*, *Cassia occidentalis*, *Achillea millefolium* and *Tamarix gallica* has been found to stimulate liver detoxification in addition to exerting hepatoprotective properties.[104]

Some herbs have a history of use for detoxification and are used in traditional herbal medicine for their role in supporting liver function. Herbs traditionally labelled **hepatics** or 'liver' herbs (including *S. marianum*, *Cynara scolymus*, *Bupleurum falcatum*, *Schisandra* *chinensis, Peamus boldo* and *Taraxacum officinale*) have also been used to detoxify wastes, including excessive hormones, and may also be considered.[105–107]

Detoxification may be of assistance to people with chronic, though not life-threatening, diseases. One study investigated the use of a nutrient supplement specifically targeted at supporting phase I and phase II detoxification mechanisms in 84 patients for 10 weeks, and found significant improvement in symptoms in the intervention group.[108] The same product exhibited similar results in another trial as well as a 23% increase in liver detoxification as measured by caffeine-clearance tests.[109] Other small or uncontrolled trials have also demonstrated improvement in nutritional and psychological symptoms, as well as excretion of toxic markers such as PCBs, following a **detoxification regimen** using high dose niacin, individualised vitamin and mineral supplementation and poly-unsaturated oils combined with physical exercise and sauna therapy.[110–112] Other more generalised integrative detoxification (that have not relied purely on high-level supple-mentation) programs have also shown improvements.[113]

While initially promising, in reality the area is very underexplored and many claims are based on extrapolations of existing data of varying quality or from programs focusing on drug and alcohol detoxification.

Detoxification is also an area in which unproven and often ineffective remedies are aggressively marketed, both to practitioners and to patients, implying careful consid-eration before their use in clinical practice.[114] Therefore, while detoxification regimens may provide a clinically valuable adjuvant to treatment, naturopathic practitioners should be sure to focus on more relevant primary treatment aims in the clinical setting. More extreme detoxification methods can be every dangerous and should be avoided. While it is true that many traditional methods may fall into this category, it should also be acknowledged that these traditions were borne of a time when environmental toxic burdens were far lower and would have resulted in fewer side effects and lower risk.

Inflammation
Inflammatory cytokines
Endometriosis is a chronic inflammatory disease, characterised by altered function of immune-related cells, an increased number of activated macrophages and their secreted products, such as growth factors, cytokines and angiogenic factors in the peritoneal environment.[6,118–125] The presence of inflammatory mediators may actually encourage endometrial tissue ordinarily found in retrograde menstruation to adhere to tissue.[5]

ENDOMETRIOSIS AND IBS

Endometriosis and irritable bowel syndrome exhibit markedly similar symptoms and one is, in fact, quite commonly misdiagnosed for the other.[115,17] IBS is often associated with marked increases in inflammatory mediated cytokines IL-6, IL-10 and TNF-α. These inflammatory mediators are associated with altered bowel bacteria.[116] These same cytokines are implicated in encouraging endometrial tissue to adhere to other tissue when in excess amounts in the peritoneal fluid. This is thought to be in some part due to the migration from these cells in dysbiosis (see the 'leaky gut' theory in Chapter 3 on irritable bowel syndrome). Positive correlations have been observed between dysbiosis and endometriosis in rhesus monkeys,[117] and successful treatment of IBS with probiotics has been demonstrated to improve endometriosis outcomes.[17]

IL-6, IL-8 and TNF-α appear to be most associated with this phenomenon though others may also play a role. These specific cytokines are also linked to irritable bowel syndrome (IBS) and intestinal dysbiosis (see the box above). One theory is that these cytokines migrate to nearby areas, and in this case encourage endometrial tissue to adhere. High oestrogen levels may exacerbate this role by modulating immune response on macrophages and monocytes through their functional receptors.[126] Higher oestrogen levels have also been associated with increased intestinal permeability and promotion of gram-negative intestinal bacteria.[127] Probiotics, increasing fibre (and in particular the immune regulating fibres such as FOS), anti-inflammatory foods such as fish oils, garlic and ginger, and herbs such as *Viburnum opulus* and *Boswellia serrata* can also reduce inflammation in endometriosis.[128] Even subclinical inflammation has been associated with progression of endometriosis indicating that even mild anti-inflammatory approaches may prove clinically useful.[129]

Angiogenesis and apoptosis

Excessive endometrial angiogenesis is proposed as an important mechanism in the pathogenesis of endometriosis and is thought to play an underlying role in the proliferation seen in the condition.[130] Nuclear factor-kappa B (NF-κB) is thought to play an integral role in this increased proliferation. In endometriosis cells NF-κB appears to be continuously activated, and suppression of NF-κB activity by NF-κB inhibitors or proteasome inhibitors suppresses proliferation of endometrial cells in vitro.[131] Various inflammatory mediators, growth factors and oxidative stress are thought to be responsible for this activation. **Curcumin** has been demonstrated to reduce angiogenesis and proliferation and induce apoptosis in endometrial cells in vitro and inactivates NF-κB.[36,132] Other therapeutic agents specifically indicated to reduce angiogenesis and proliferation—although they have not been specifically studied in endometriosis—include **vitamin D** and foods rich in **flavonoids**, **cruciferous indoles** and **resveratrol** (see the box below).[36,128] Correction of exacerbating factors, particularly inflammatory mediators, may also reduce proliferation.

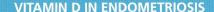

VITAMIN D IN ENDOMETRIOSIS

Vitamin D analogues, such as danazol, have long been used in the treatment of endometriosis. However, vitamin D itself, and the vitamin D system, is thought to play a role in the immune complex changes observed in endometriosis.[136] The active D3 form has been described as a potent regulator of cell growth and differentiation in endometriosis.[137] Variations in vitamin D binding protein (DBP) have also been found in patients with endometriosis.[138] It is thought that DBP may influence inflammatory mediators in the body. Only 5% of DBP is actually bound to vitamin D and its metabolites. The remainder has several important functions, including conversion to a powerful macrophage activating factor involved in increasing inflammatory processes in the body. Vitamin D is also associated with increased HDL cholesterol levels,[139] which are associated with reductions in symptoms of endometriosis.[140]

An experimental treatment protocol using aromatase inhibitors given concomitantly with supplemental vitamin D has achieved promising results in the treatment of endometriosis.[141] Research has also demonstrated reduced lesion weight in endometriosis cells with vitamin D.[142]

Some evidence suggests that endometriotic tissue may not have enhanced proliferative abilities, but rather reduced apoptosis.[133–135] Therapeutic interventions that may increase apoptosis, such as *Curcuma longa*, *Scutellaria baicalensis*, **zinc**, selenium and foods rich in a broad range of various phytochemicals (including **flavonoids**, **cruciferous indoles** and **isothiocynates**) may be useful in the treatment of endometriosis.[36,128]

Prostaglandin regulation

Oestrogen is also reported to increase PGE2 formation by stimulating cyclooxygenase type 2 (COX-2) enzymes in endometrial stromal cells,[143,144] thereby producing a positive feedback loop for continuous local production of oestrogen and prostaglandins; this favours the proliferative and inflammatory characteristics of endometriosis.

The prostaglandins series 1 and 3 have anti-inflammatory effects that may help patients with endometriosis.

Animal studies have found reduced production levels of inflammatory prostaglandins PGE_2 and $PGF_{2\alpha}$, and decreased endometrial implant diameter in those animals treated with eicosapentaenoic acid (EPA) and docosahexaenoic acid (DHA) of marine origin.[145] In vitro studies have also found that **omega-3 fatty acids** found in fish oils reduced survival rates of endometrial cells when compared to omega-6 (n-6), mixed polyunsaturated fats (PUFA) or control groups.[146] Epidemiological data of fish oil consumption in women with endometriosis have shown reduced symptoms with increased consumption.[147] Increased consumption of other inflammatory polyunsaturated fats, particularly of the omega-6 series, was also linked with an increase in symptoms.[148] Exercise, increasing water consumption and eliminating food allergies will also reduce inflammatory mediators.

Endometrial tissue damage

Adhesions

Adhesions increase when women have endometriosis. Vitamin E has been specifically demonstrated to reduce adhesion formation.[149–151] This action is thought to be primarily through reduction of series 2 prostaglandins and better removal of pelvic debris by white blood cells.[152] Although unpublished, Italian research has demonstrated a reduction in adhesion weight when treated with **vitamin D** compounds.[144,153] **Zinc**, *Calendula officinalis* and **vitamin C** are also traditionally used.

Surgery

It is accepted that in specific patients endometriosis can spread directly. The risk of endometrial implantation is increased by surgery, particularly surgery to remove endometrial tissue.[3] This is due to the increase of inflammatory mediators to the area.[6] Reducing inflammation and encouraging appropriate healing responses can reduce the risk of recurring endometrial growths after surgery.

INTEGRATIVE MEDICAL CONSIDERATIONS

Traditional Chinese medicine

Acupuncture has documented success in relieving the pain of dysmenorrhoea. In traditional Chinese medicine endometriosis is seen as a disorder of Qi, Blood and Liver stagnation, an approach that has had documented success in the literature.[154,155] **Gui Zhi Fu Ling Wan** is indicated to move blood, transform stagnation and remove masses—particularly in lower abdominal areas. Its modern integrated naturopathic application extends to

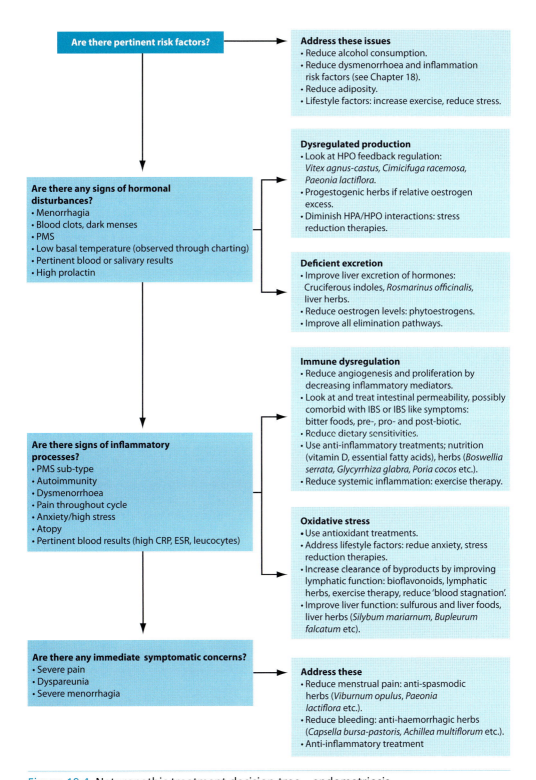

Figure 19.4 Naturopathic treatment decision tree—endometriosis

dysmenorrhoea, endometriosis and fibroids (see Chapter 18 on dysmenorrhoea), in particular the emperor herbs *Cinnamomum zeylanicum*, *Poria cocos* and *Paeonia lactiflora*.[156] Chinese exercise therapy (qi gong) referral may also be appropriate in this condition.

Oral contraceptive pills

Hormone supplementation is commonly used in conventional medicine to reduce endometriosis symptoms. Women taking contraceptive agents therapeutically may become deficient in vitamins B2, B3, B5, B12 and folate and may experience raised levels of vitamin A.[128] Hormone use may reduce the effects of *Vitex agnus-castus* and increase the hypertensive side effects associated with *Glycyrrhiza glabra*. Any treatment that aims to increase liver function will reduce the effectiveness of the hormonal drugs.[128]

Case Study

A 24-year-old female patient presents to the clinic complaining of intensely **painful periods**, which she has experienced since menarche. The **pain is more noticeable towards the end of the period** and she also experiences pain in the middle of the cycle, albeit in differing areas (she points to upper and lower abdominal areas). **Her bleeding is heavy**, and she is often required to take an 'emergency bag' of sanitary products whenever she leaves her house during her period. She experiences daily **nausea, indigestion** and **flatulence.** She and her partner have been **trying unsuccessfully to fall pregnant** for the past 9 months.

Example treatment

The patient was advised to stop trying to get pregnant for 4 months while herbal treatment was undertaken. She was prescribed the liquid herbal formula in the table displayed taken at a dose of 5 mL three times daily. The treatment rationale was anti-spasmodic (*Achillea millefolium* and *Viburnum opulus*), antihaemorrhagic (*Achillea millefolium*), anti-inflammatory (*Glycyrrhiza glabra*) and the reproductive herbs *Vitex agnus-castus* and *Cimicifuga racemosa* to modulate hormone levels through their various mechanisms.

She was also given dietary advice including increasing the consumption of onions, garlic, Chinese cabbage or other cruciferous vegetables to at least once per day to promote liver metabolism of hormones; and including lentils, chickpeas and ground flaxseed meal at least four times per week. Her refined carbohydrates and dairy consumption were reduced. She was prescribed 1 tablespoon *Ulmus fulva* with 1 teaspoon of raw honey in warm water at night to encourage healthy intestinal bacterial populations, settle digestive dysfunction and reduce constipation. She was referred to a local qi gong class. She was also required to do 30 minutes of moderately strenuous exercise at least every second day except during her period. She was also prescribed cod liver oil at a dose of 600 IU of vitamin D equivalent to reduce inflammation, provide fatty acids and reduce lesions. These were to be reviewed after 1 month.

At the second consultation the patient had adhered to the dietary changes and followed all recommendations. She had begun qi gong classes and started walking 20 minutes every day. She had no further

Herbal formula	
Vitex agnus-castus 1:2	10 mL
Cimicifuga racemosa 1:2	20 mL
Achillea millefolium 1:2	20 mL
Viburnum opulus 1:2	30 mL
Glycyrrhiza glabra 1:2	20 mL
Nutritional formula	
Vitamin D 600 IU daily to be taken via cod liver oil	
Ulmus fulva powder 10 g once per day	

Table 19.3 Review of the major evidence

INTERVENTION	STUDIES	METHODOLOGY	OUTCOME MEASURES	RESULTS
Diet	Parazzini et al. 2004[44]	RCT ($n = 504$)	Weekly consumption of selected dietary items Symptom scores	A reduction in risk for high intake of green vegetable and an increased risk for intake of ham, beef and other red meat. No association with intake of coffee, alcohol, fish and milk
Diet	Britton et al. 2000[148]	RCT ($n = 673$) only 280 with endometriosis	Yearly consumption of food items and symptom scores	Vegetable and polyunsaturated fats increase symptoms.
Fish oil	Covens et al. 1988[145]	RCT, animal (rabbits, $n = 38$)	PGE_2 concentration and implant size	Peritoneal PGE_2 concentrations and endometrial implant diameter were significantly lower in intervention group.
Genistein	Cotroneo & Lamartiniere 2001[158]	RCT, animal (rats, $n = 92$)	Endometrial implant growth Uterine growth	High doses of injected genistein supported growth of endometrial tissue while dietary genistein reduced tissue size. No association between genistein and uterine growth
French maritime bark (60 mg daily)	Kohama et al. 2007[159]	RCT, human ($n = 58$)	Endometriosis symptom scores, CA-125 and oestrogen (E2) levels	French maritime bark extract reduced symptom scores more slowly than conventional GnRHa although recurrence occurred after 28 weeks in GnRHa group. CA-125 was reduced though no change was observed in E2 levels.

abdominal pain or digestive discomfort. Her bleeding had reduced noticeably since the previous cycle. She was advised to continue dietary and lifestyle prescriptions, along with the herbal formula until review in 1 month.

At the third consult, the patient had slipped a little on her diet, but to her surprise this had led to only minor symptoms returning. At this stage it was suggested that the patient move towards a tablet form of *Vitex agnus-castus*—to be continued for a period of 4 months before review at a dose of two 500 mg tablets, twice daily (at which stage it was discontinued). The patient at this time had vastly improved menstrual symptoms though she still had significant dark clotting in her menses and occasional stabbing pain—though to nowhere near the extent previously experienced. A Chinese herbal formula for blood stasis was prescribed: cinnamon and hoelen formula (containing *Poria cocos*, *Cinnamomum zeylanicum* and *Paeonia lactiflora*) at a dose of 10 g per day. The patient returned after 3 months with a 'normal' menstrual cycle. Nervous support and preconception care were the new foci of her treatment.

Expected outcomes and follow-up protocols

Pain reduction is often the most commonly sought treatment. This is thought to be due to underlying excessive cytokine levels[157] and will be addressed in due course, though immediate symptomatic relief for dysmenorrhoea (through, for example, the supplementation of *Viburnum opulus* in the 3 days before the period) and menorrhagia (through supplementation of *Capsella bursa-pastoris* or *Achillea millefolium*) can occur in the first cycle after treatment. Concomitant with these symptomatic treatments, longer-term aims of normalising underlying menstrual function should be undertaken. Noticeable improvement in general should occur by the second cycle, providing dietary and lifestyle changes are also addressed. This should be especially noticeable in terms of abdominal pain, bloating and concomitant gastrointestinal symptoms. Women with larger or more ingrained endometrial growths will require oestrogen modulating and anti-inflammatory treatment for some months to reduce and remove well-established endometrial growths, particularly those in 'enclosed' or 'removed' areas—such as those in areas not commonly associated with menstrual flow (for example, the intestines and kidneys). Patients should be notified that this could take up to 12 months in difficult cases, and that results are extremely variable between patients.

KEY POINTS

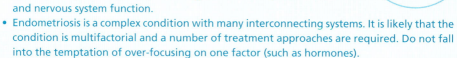

- Endometriosis shares many properties with autoimmune conditions. Examine the inflammatory status of the patient and do not rely on hormonal modulation alone.
- Endometriosis is an oestrogen-dependent condition. Look at the factors that may influence this, including liver function, HPO function and nervous system function.
- Endometriosis is a complex condition with many interconnecting systems. It is likely that the condition is multifactorial and a number of treatment approaches are required. Do not fall into the temptation of over-focusing on one factor (such as hormones).
- Many of these factors have underlying nutritional or lifestyle aetiologies. Do not overcomplicate things. Studies suggest that sometimes simple dietary modifications may be enough to significantly improve outcomes.

Further reading

Fjerbaek A, Knudsen UB. Endometriosis, dysmenorrhea and diet—what is the evidence? Eur J Obstet Gynecol Reprod Biol 2007;132(2):140–147.

Guidice LC, Kao LC. Endometriosis. Lancet 2004;364(9447):1789–1799.

Halis G, Arici A. Endometriosis and inflammation in infertility. Ann N Y Acad Sci 2004;1034:300–315.

Hudson T. Women's encyclopedia of natural medicine. New York: McGraw-Hill, 2008.

Trickey R. Women, hormones and the menstrual cycle. Sydney: Allen & Unwin, 2003.

References

1. Edmonds K, ed. Obstetrics and gynaecology. London: Blackwell, 2007.
2. Mazur W, Adlercreutz H. Naturally occurring estrogens in food. Pure Applied Chem 1998;70:1759–1776.
3. Guidice L, Kao L. Endometriosis. Lancet 2004;364 (9447):1789–1799.
4. Rier S. The potential role of exposure to environmental toxicants in the pathophysiology of endometriosis. Ann N Y Acad Sci 2002;955:201–212.
5. Halme J, et al. Peritoneal macrophages from patients with endometriosis release growth factor activity in vitro. J Clin Endocrinol Metab 1988;66:1044–1049.
6. Leibovic D, et al. Immunobiology of endometriosis. Fertil Steril 2001;75:1–10.
7. Schrodt G, et al. Endometriosis of the male urinary system: a case report. J Urol 1980;124(5):722–723.
8. Martin J, Hauck A. Endometriosis in the male American surgeon. Am Surg 1985;51(7):426–430.
9. Westerlind K, Williams N. Effect of energy deficiency on estrogen metabolism in premenopausal women. Med Sci Sports Exerc 2007;39(7):1090–1097.
10. Missmer S, et al. Incidence of laparoscopically confirmed endometriosis by demographic, anthropometric and lifestyle factors. Am J Epidemiol 2004;160(8):784–796.
11. Wake D, et al. Increased aromatase expression in human subcutaneous adipose tissue in obesity. Endocrine Abstracts 2004;7:60.
12. Adlercreutz H. Epidemiology of phytoestrogens. Ballieres Clin Endocrin Metabol 1998;12:605–623.
13. Petterson H, Kiessling K. Liquid chromatographic determination of the plant estrogens coumestrol and isoflavones in animal feed. J Assoc Off Anal Chem 1984;67(3):503–506.
14. Bulun S, et al. Role of aromatase in endometrial disease. J Steroid Biochem Mol Biol 2001;79:19–25.
15. Lea R, Whorwell P. Irritable bowel syndrome or endometriosis or both? Eur J Gastroenterol Hepatol 2003;15(10):1131–1133.
16. Noble L, et al. Prostaglandin E2 stimulates aromatase expression in endometriosis-derived stromal cells. J Clin Endocrinol Metab 1997;82:600–606.
17. Bukulmez O, et al. Inflammatory status influences aromatase and steroid receptor expression in endometriosis. Endocrinology 2008;149(3):1190–1204.
18. Simpson E, et al. Aromatase—a brief overview. Annu Rev Physiol 2002;64:93–127.
19. Brooks J, Thompson L. Mammalian lignans and genistein decrease the activities of aromatase and 17beta-hydroxysteroid dehydrogenase in MCF-7 cells. J Steroid Biochem Mol Biol 2005;94(5):461–467.
20. Wuttke W, et al. Chaste tree (Vitex agnus-castus) pharmacology and clinical indications. Phytomedicine 2003; 10(4):348–357.
21. Seidlova-Wuttke D. Evidence for selective estrogen receptor modulator activity in a black cohosh (Cimicifuga racemosa) extract: comparison with estradiol-17 beta. Eur J Endocrinol 2003;149:351–362.
22. Birnbaum L, Cummings A. Dioxins and endometriosis: a plausible hypothesis. Environ Health Perspect 2002;110(1):15–21.
23. Foster W, Agarwal S. Environmental contaminants and dietary factors in endometriosis. Ann N Y Acad Sci 2002;955:213–229.
24. Tsutsumi O. Assessment of human contamination of estrogenic endocrine-disrupting chemicals and their risk for human reproduction. J Steroid Biochem Mol Biol 2005;93(2–5):325–330.
25. Wang L. Mammalian phytoestrogens: enterodiol and enterolactone. J Chromatogr B Analyt Technol Biomed Life Sci 2002;777(1–2):289–309.
26. Valsta L, et al. Phyto-oestrogen database of foods and average intake in Finland. Br J Nutr 2003;89:S31–S38.
27. Liu J. Evaluation of estrogenic activity of plant extracts for the potential treatment of menopausal symptoms. J Agric Food Chem 2001;49(5):2472–2479.
28. Beck V, et al. Comparison of hormonal activity (estrogen, androgen and progestin) of standardized plant extracts for large scale use in hormone replacement therapy. J Steroid Biochem Mol Biol 2003;84(2–3):259–268.
29. Zava D, et al. Estrogen and progestin bioactivity of foods, herbs, and spices. Proc Soc Exp Biol Med 1998;217(3):369–378.
30. Unfer V, et al. Endometrial effects of long-term treatment with phytoestrogens: a randomized, double-blind, placebo-controlled study. Fertil Steril 2004;82:145–148.
31. Ashok B, et al. Abrogation of oestrogen-mediated cellular and biochemical effects by indole-3-carbinol. Nutr Cancer 2001;41(1–2):180–187.
32. Meng Q, et al. Indole-3-carbinol is a negative regulator of estrogen receptor-alpha signalling in human tumour cells. J Nutr 2000;130(12):2927–2931.
33. Sowers M, et al. Selected diet and lifestyle factors are associated with estrogen metabolites in a multiracial/ethnic population of women. J Nutr 2006;136(6):1588–1595.
34. Thompson L, et al. Phytoestrogen content of foods consumed in Canada, including isoflavones, lignans and coumestan. Nutr Cancer 2006;54(2):184–201.
35. Voet D. Biochemistry. 3rd edn. New York: Wiley & Sons, 2004.
36. Higdon J. An evidence-based approach to dietary phytochemicals. Stuttgart: Thieme, 2007.
37. Bradlow H, et al. Long-term responses of women to indole-3-carbinol or a high fibre diet. Cancer Epidemiol Biomarkers Prev 1994;3(7):591–595.
38. Dalessandri K, et al. Pilot study: effect of 3,3'-diindolylmethane supplements on urinary hormone metabolites in postmenopausal women with a history of early stage breast cancer. Nutr Cancer 2004;50(2):161–167.
39. McAlindon T, et al. Indole-3-carbinol in women with SLE: effect on estrogen metabolism and disease activity. Lupus 2001;10(11):779–783.
40. Michnovicz J, Bradlow H. Altered oestrogen metabolism and excretion in humans following consumption of indole-3-carbinol. Nutr Cancer 1991;16:59–66.
41. Michnovicz J, et al. Changes in levels of urinary estrogen metabolites after oral indole-3-carbinol treatment in humans. J Natl Cancer Inst 1997;89(10):718–723.
42. Michnovicz J. Increased estrogen 2-hydroxylation in obese women using oral indole-3-carbinol. Int J Obes Relat Metab Disord 1998;22(3):227–229.
43. Wong G, et al. Dose-ranging study of indole-3-carbinol for breast cancer prevention. J Cell Biochem Suppl 1997;(28–29)Supp 1:S111–S116.
44. Parazzini F, et al. Selected food intake and risk of endometriosis. Human Reprod 2004;19(8):1755–1759.
45. Morazzoni P, Bombardelli E. Silybum marianum (Carduus Marianus). Fitoterapia 1995;66:3–42.
46. Zhu B, et al. Dietary administration of an extract from rosemary leaves enhances the liver microsomal metabolism of endogenous estrogens and decreases their uterotropic action in CD-1 mice. Carcinogenesis 1998;19(10): 1821–1827.
47. Zondek B, Finkerlstein M. Effect of vitamin B complex on inactivation of estrone in vivo and in vitro. Science 1947;105(2723):259–260.
48. Sepkovic D, Bradlow H. Estrogen hydroxylation—the good and the bad. Ann N Y Acad Sci 2009;1155:57–67.
49. Aozasa O, et al. Enhancement in fecal excretion of dioxin isomer in mice by several dietary fibers. Chemosphere 2001;45(2):195–200.
50. Kimura Y, et al. Some dietary fibers increase elimination of orally administered polychlorinated biphenyls but not that of retinol in mice. J Nutr 2004;134:135–142.

51. Wattenberg L. Studies on polycyclic hydrocarbon hydroxylases of the intestine possibly related to cancer: effects of diet on benzpyrene hydroxylase activity. Cancer 1971;28:99–102.

52. Cardador-Martínez A, et al. Relationship among antimutagenic, antioxidant and enzymatic activities of methanolic extract from common beans (*Phaseolus vulgaris* L). Plant Foods Hum Nutr 2006;61(4):161–168.

53. Brady J, et al. Modulation of rat hepatic microsomal monooxygenase activities and cytotoxicity by diallyl sulfide. Toxicol Appl Pharmacol 1991;108:342–354.

54. Uno T, Yasui-Furukori N. Effect of grapefruit juice in relation to human pharmacokinetic study. Curr Clin Pharmacol 2006;1(2):157–161.

55. Kroon L. Drug interactions with smoking. Am J Health Syst Pharm 2007;64(18):1917–1921.

56. Zhang J, et al. Inhibition of human liver cytochrome P450 by star fruit juice. J Pharm Pharm Sci 2007;10(4):496–503.

57. Sasaki K, et al. Thyme (*Thymus vulgaris L.*) leaves and its constituents increase the activities of xenobiotic-metabolizing enzymes in mouse liver. J Med Food 2005;8(2):184–189.

58. Maliakal P, Wanwimolruk S. Effect of herbal teas on hepatic drug metabolizing enzymes in rats. J Pharm Pharmacol 2001;53(10):1323–1329.

59. Singh R, et al. Modulatory influence of *Adhatoda vesica* (*Justicia adhatoda*) leaf extract on the enzymes of xenobiotic metabolism, antioxidant status and lipid peroxidation in mice. Mol Cell Biochem 2000;213(1–2):99–109.

60. Stevens J, Page J. Xanthohumol and related prenylflavonoids from hops and beer: to your good health! Phytochemistry 2004;65(10):1317–1330.

61. Chan H, et al. Inhibition of glycyrrhizic acid on aflatoxin B1-induced cytotoxicity in hepatoma cells. Toxicoloy 2003;188(2–3):211–217.

62. Jeong H, et al. Hepatoprotective effects of 18beta-glycyrrhetinic acid on carbon tetrachloride-induced liver injury: inhibition of cytochrome P450 2E1 expression. Pharmacol Res 2002;46(3):221–227.

63. Whitten D, et al. The effect of St John's wort extracts on CYP3A: a systematic review of prospective clinical trials. Br J Clin Pharmacol 2006;62(5):512–516.

64. Offord E, et al. Mechanisms involved in the chemoprotective effects of rosemary extract studied in human liver and bronchial cells. Cancer Lett 1997;114(1–2):275–281.

65. Padmavathi B, et al. Roots of *Withania somnifera* inhibit forestomach and skin carcinogenesis in mice. Evid Based Complement Alternat Med 2005;2(1):99–105.

66. Raner G, et al. Effects of herbal products and their constituents on human cytochrome P450(2E1) activity. Food Chem Toxicol 2007;45(12):2359–2365.

67. Xin H, et al. The effects of berberine on the pharmacokinetics of cyclosporin A in healthy volunteers. Methods Find Exp Clin Pharmacol 2006;28(1):25–29.

68. Imanshahidi M, Hosseinzadeh H. Pharmacological and therapeutic effects of *Berberis vulgaris* and its active constituent, berberine. Phytother Res 2008;22(8):999–1012.

69. Iwata H, et al. Identification and characterization of potent CYP3A4 inhibitors in *Schisandra* fruit extract. Drug Metab Dispos 2004;32(12):1351–1358.

70. Dinkova-Kostova A, Talalay P. Relation of structure of curcumin analogs to their potencies as inducers of phase 2 detoxification enzymes. Carcinogenesis 1999;20:911–914.

71. Iqbal M, et al. Dietary supplementation of curcumin enhances antioxidant and phase II metabolizing enzymes in ddY male mice: possible role in protection against chemical carcinogenesis and toxicity. Pharmacol Toxicol 2003;92(1):33–38.

72. Bomser J, et al. In vitro anticancer activity of fruit extracts from Vaccinium species. Planta Med 1996;62:212–216.

73. Khan S, et al. Enhancement of antioxidant and phase II enzymes by oral feeding of green tea polyphenols in drinking water to SKH-1 hairless mice: possible role in cancer chemoprevention. Cancer Res 1992;52:4050–4052.

74. Stoner G, Mukhtar H. Polyphenols as cancer chemopreventive agents. J Cell Biochem 1995;22(Suppl):169–180.

75. Zhang Y, et al. A major inducer of anticarcinogenic protective enzymes from broccoli: isolation and elucidation of structure. Proc Natl Acad Sci U S A 1992;89:2399–2403.

76. Uda Y, et al. Induction of the anticarcinogenic marker enzyme, quinone reductase, in murine hepatoma cells in vitro by flavonoids. Cancer Lett 1997;120:213–216.

77. Nho C, Jeffery E. The synergistic upregulation of phase II detoxification enzymes by glucosinolate breakdown products in cruciferous vegetables. Toxicol Appl Pharmacol 2001;174(2):146–152.

78. Dietz B, et al. Xanthohumol isolated from *Humulus lupulus* inhibits menadione-induced DNA damage through induction of quinone reductase. Chem Res Toxicol 2005;18(8):1296–1305.

79. Sotelo-Félix J, et al. Evaluation of the effectiveness of *Rosmarinus officinalis* (Lamiaceae) in the alleviation of carbon tetrachloride-induced acute hepatotoxicity in the rat. J Ethnopharmacol 2002;81(2):145–154.

80. Lee S, et al. Induction of the phase II detoxification enzyme NQO1 in hepatocarcinoma cells by lignans from the fruit of schisandra chinensis through nuclear accumulation of Nrf2. Planta Med 2009. In press.

81. Gurley B, et al. In vivo assessment of botanical supplementation on human cytochrome P450 phenotypes: *Citrus aurantium, Echinacea purpurea,* milk thistle, and saw palmetto. Clin Pharmacol Ther 2004;76(5):428–440.

82. Gurley B, et al. Clinical assessment of CYP2D6-mediated herb-drug interactions in humans: effects of milk thistle, black cohosh, goldenseal, kava kava, St John's wort, and echinacea. Mol Nutr Food Res 2008;52(7):755–763.

83. Gurley B, et al. Effect of milk thistle (*Silybum marianum*) and black cohosh (*Cimicifuga racemosa*) supplementation on digoxin pharmacokinetics in humans. Drug Metab Dispos 2006;34(1):69–74.

84. DiCenzo R, et al. Coadministration of milk thistle and indinavir in healthy subjects. Pharmacotherapy 2003;23(7):866–870.

85. Piscitelli S, et al. Effect of milk thistle on the pharmacokinetics of indinavir in healthy volunteers. Pharmacotherapy 2002;22(5):551–556.

86. Mills E, et al. Milk thistle and indinavir: a randomized controlled pharmacokinetics study and meta-analysis. Eur J Clin Pharmacol 2005;61(1):1–7.

87. Doehmer J, et al. Assessment of drug-drug interaction for silymarin. Toxicol In Vitro 2008;22(3):610–617.

88. Mueller S, et al. No clinically relevant CYP3A induction after St John's wort with low hyperforin content in healthy volunteers. Eur J Clin Pharmacol 2009;65(1):81–87.

89. Will-Shahab L, et al. St John's wort extract (Ze 117) does not alter the pharmacokinetics of a low-dose oral contraceptive. Eur J Clin Pharmacol 2009;65(3):287–294.

90. Mueller S, et al. The extent of induction of CYP3A by St. John's wort varies among products and is linked to hyperforin dose. Eur J Clin Pharmacol 2006;62(1):29–36.

91. Soeters P, et al. Amino acid adequacy in pathophysiological states. J Nutr 2004;134(6 Suppl):1575S–1582S.

92. Liu Q, et al. Synbiotic modulation of gut flora: effect on minimal hepatic encephalopathy in patients with cirrhosis. Hepatology 2004;39(5):1441–1449.

93. Bajaj J, et al. Probiotic yogurt for the treatment of minimal hepatic encephalopathy. Am J Gastroenterol 2008;103(7):1707–1715.

94. Sharma P, et al. An open-label randomized controlled trial of lactulose and probiotics in the treatment of minimal hepatic encephalopathy. Eur J Gastroenterol Hepatol 2008;20(6):506–511.

95. Sheth A, Garcia-Tsao G. Probiotics and liver disease. J Clin Gastroenterol 2008;42(Supp 2):80–84.
96. Duncan K, et al. Running exercise may reduce risk for lung and liver cancer by inducing activity of antioxidant and phase II enzymes. Cancer Lett 1997;116(2):151–158.
97. Yiamouyiannis C, et al. Chronic physical activity: hepatic hypertrophy and increased total biotransformation enzyme activity. Biochem Pharmacol 1992;44(1):121–127.
98. Imamura M, Tung T. A trial of fasting cure for PCB-poisoned patients in Taiwan. Prog Clin Biol Res 1984;137:147–153.
99. Müllerová D, Kopecký J. White adipose tissue: storage and effector site for environmental pollutants. Physiol Res 2007;56(4):375–381.
100. Stiefelhagen P. Functional disorders call for total therapy—Kneipp's hydrotherapy instead of psychopharmaceuticals. MMW Fortschr Med 2005;147(18):4–8.
101. Krop J. Chemical sensitivity after intoxication at work with solvents: response to sauna therapy. J Altern Complement Med 1998;4(1):77–86.
102. Chambaz A, et al. Urinary caffeine after coffee consumption and heat dehydration. Int J Sports Med 2001;22(5):366–372.
103. Hannuksela M, Ellahham S. Benefits and risks of sauna bathing. Am J Med 2001;110(2):118–126.
104. Huseini H, et al. The efficacy of Liv-52 on liver cirrhotic patients: a randomized, double-blind, placebo-controlled first approach. Phytomedicine 2005;12(9):619–624.
105. Scientific Committee of the British Herbal Medical Association. British herbal pharmacopoeia. 1st edn. Bournemouth: British Herbal Medicine Association, 1983.
106. Blumenthal M, et al., eds. Herbal medicine: expanded Commission E monographs (English translation). Austin: Integrative Medicine Communications, 2000.
107. Mills S, Bone K. Principles and practice of phytotherapy. Edinburgh: Churchill Livingstone, 2000.
108. Bland J, et al. A medical food-supplemented detoxification program in the management of chronic health problems. Altern Ther Health Med 1995;1(5):62–71.
109. MacIntosh A, Ball K. The effects of a short program of detoxification in disease-free individuals. Altern Ther Health Med 2000;6(4):70–75.
110. Schnare D, et al. Evaluation of a detoxification regimen for fat stored xenobiotics. Med Hypotheses 1982;9(3):265–282.
111. Tretjak Z, et al. PCB reduction and clinical improvement by detoxification: an unexploited approach? Hum Exp Toxicol 1990;9(4):235–244.
112. Kilburn K, et al. Neurobehavioral dysfunction in firemen exposed to polychlorinated biphenyls (PCBs): possible improvement after detoxification. Arch Environ Health 1989;44(6):345–350.
113. Rea W, et al. Reduction of chemical sensitivity by means of heat depuration, physical therapy and nutritional supplementation in a controlled environment. J Nutr Environ Med 1996;6:141–148.
114. Cohen M. Detox: science or sales pitch? Aust Fam Physician 2007;30(12):1009–1010.
115. Kumar D. Irritable bowel syndrome, chronic pelvic inflammatory disease and endometriosis. Eur J Gastroenterol Hepatol 2004;16(12):1251–1252.
116. Tamboli C, et al. Dysbiosis in inflammatory bowel disease. Gut 2004;53(1):1–4.
117. Bailey M, Coe C. Endometriosis is associated with an altered profile of intestinal microflora in female rhesus monkeys. Human Reprod 2002;17(7):1704–1708.
118. Braun D, et al. Spontaneous and induced synthesis of cytokines by peripheral blood monocytes in patients with endometriosis. Fertil Steril 1996;65:1125–1129.
119. Bullimore D. Endometriosis is sustained by tumour necrosis factor-alpha. Med Hypotheses 2003;60:84–88.
120. Gurgan T, et al. Serum and peritoneal fluid levels of IGF I and II and insulinlike growth binding protein-3 in endometriosis. J Repro Med 1999;44:450–454.
121. Kim J, et al. Insulin-like growth factors (IGFs), IGF-binding proteins (IGFBPs), and IGFBP-3 protease activity in the peritoneal fluid of patients with and without endometriosis. Fertil Steril 2000;73:996–1000.
122. Koninckx P, et al. Endometriotic disease: the role of peritoneal fluid. Hum Reprod Update 1998;4:741–751.
123. Punnonen J, et al. Increased levels of interleukin-6 and interleukin-10 in the peritoneal fluid of patients with endometriosis. Am J Obstetr Gynecol 1996;174:1522–1526.
124. Rana N, et al. Basal and stimulated secretion of cytokines by peritoneal macrophages in women with endometriosis. Fertil Steril 1996;65:925–930.
125. Richter O, et al. TNF-alpha secretion by peritoneal macrophages in endometriosis. Zentralbl Gynakol 1998;120:332–336.
126. Capellino S, et al. Role of estrogens in inflammatory response: expression of estrogen receptors in peritoneal fluid macrophages from endometriosis. Ann N Y Acad Sci 2006;1069:263–267.
127. Enomoto N, et al. Role of Kuppfer cells and gut-derived endotoxins in alcoholic liver injury. J Gastroenterol Hepatol 2000;15(Suppl):D20–D25.
128. Braun L, Cohen M. Herbs and natural supplements: an evidence based guide. Sydney: Churchill Livingstone, 2007.
129. Agic A, et al. Is endometriosis associated with systemic subclinical inflammation? Gynecol Obstet Invest 2006;62:139–147.
130. Healy DL, et al. Angiogenesis: a new theory for endometriosis. Human Reproduction Update 1998;4(5):736–740.
131. Guo S. Nuclear factor-κB (NF-κB): an unsuspected major culprit in the pathogenesis of endometriosis that is still at large? Gynecol Obstet Inv 2007;63(2):71–97.
132. Wieser F, et al. Curcumin suppresses angiogenesis, cell proliferation and induces apoptosis in an in vitro model of endometriosis [Poster]. Fertil Steril 2007;88:S204–S205.
133. Beliard A, et al. Reduction of apoptosis and proliferation in endometriosis. Fertil Steril 2004;82:80–85.
134. Gebel H, et al. Spontaneous apoptosis of endometrial tissue is impaired in women with endometriosis. Fertil Steril 1998;69:1042–1047.
135. Scotti S, et al. Reduced proliferation and cell adhesion in endometriosis. Mol Hum Reprod 2000;6:610–617.
136. Vigano P, et al. Cycling and early pregnant endometrium as a site of regulated expression of the vitamin D system. J Mol Endocrinol 2006;36:415–424.
137. Agic A, et al. Relative expression of 1,25-dihydroxyvitamin D3 receptor, vitamin D 1 alpha-hydroxylase, vitamin D 24-hydroxylase, and vitamin D 25-hydroxylase in endometriosis and gynecologic cancers. Reprod Sci 2007;14(5):486–497.
138. Ferroro S, et al. Vitamin D binding protein in endometriosis. J Soc Gynecol Investig 2005;12(4):272–277.
139. Moyad M. The potential benefits of dietary and/or supplemental calcium and vitamin D. Urol Oncol 2003;21(5):384–391.
140. Choktanasiri W, et al. Long-acting triptorelin for the treatment of endometriosis. Int J Gynecol Obstet 1996;54(3):237–243.
141. Ailawadi R, et al. Treatment of endometriosis and chronic pelvic pain with letrozole and norethindrone acetate: a pilot study. Fertil Steril 2004;81(2):290–296.
142. Panina P. Use of vitamin D compounds to treat endometriosis. Bioxil SpA. Italy 2006.
143. Tamura M, et al. Estrogen up-regulates cyclooxygenase-2 via estrogen receptor in human uterine microvascular endothelial cells. Fertil Steril 2004;81(5):1351–1356.

144. Kluft C, et al. Pro-inflammatory effects of oestrogens during use of oral contraceptives and hormone replacement treatment. Vascul Pharmacol 2002;39(3):149–154.

145. Covens A, et al. The effect of dietary supplementation with fish oil fatty acids on surgically induced endometriosis in the rabbits. Fertil Steril 1988;49(4):698–703.

146. Gazvani M, et al. High n-3:n-6 fatty acids rations in culture medium reduce endometrial-cell survival in combined endometrial gland and stromal cell cultures from women with and without endometriosis. Fertil Steril 2001;76(4):717–722.

147. Fjerbaek A, Knudsen U. Endometriosis, dysmenorrhea and diet—what is the evidence? Eur J Obstet Gynecol Reprod Biol 2007;132(2):140–147.

148. Britton J, et al. Diet and benign ovarian tumours (United States). Cancer Causes Control 2000;11(5):389–401.

149. Hemedah O, et al. Prevention of peritoneal adhesions by administration of sodium carboxymethyl cellulose and oral vitamin E. Surgery 1993;114(5):907–910.

150. Kalferentzos F, et al. Prevention of peritoneal adhesion formation in mice by vitamin E. J R Coll Surg Edinb 1987;32(5):288–290.

151. Kagoma P, et al. The effect of vitamin E on experimentally induced peritoneal adhesions in mice. Arch Surg 1985;120(8):949–951.

152. Meydani M. Vitamin E. Lancet 1995;345(8943):170–175.

153. Perez-Fernandez R, et al. Vitamin D, Pit-1, GH, and PRL: possible roles in breast cancer development. Curr Med Chem 2007;14(29):3051–3058.

154. Li J, et al. [Clinical observation on treatment of endometriosis by tonifying qi and promoting blood circulation to remove stasis and purgation principle] [in Chinese]. Zhongguo Zhong Xi Yi Jie He Za Zhi 1999;19(9):533–535.

155. Wang R, Zhou L. [Clinical observation on treatment of endometriosis with principle of activating blood circulation to remove stasis]. [in Chinese]. Zhongguo Zhong Xi Yi Jie He Za Zhi 2004;24(3):258–259.

156. Maciocia G. Obstetrics and gynecology in Chinese medicine. Edinburgh: Churchill Livingstone, 1997.

157. Thomson J, Redwine D. Chronic pelvic pain associated with autoimmunity and systemic and peritoneal inflammation and treatment with immune modification. J Reprod Med 2005;50:745–758.

158. Cotroneo M, Lamartiniere S. Pharmacologic, but not dietary genistein supports endometriosis in a rat model. Toxicol Sci 2001;61(1):68–75.

159. Kohama T, et al. Effect of French maritime pine bark extract on endometriosis as compared with leuprorelin acetate. J Reprod Med 2007;52(8):703–708.

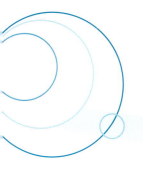

20
Polycystic ovarian syndrome

Jon Wardle
ND, MPH

CLASSIFICATION AND AETIOLOGY

Polycystic ovarian syndrome (PCOS) is a term to describe a constellation of clinical and biochemical features. For many of these the aetiology remains poorly understood. Several factors also preclude difficulties in diagnosis of PCOS, including a heterogeneous range of symptoms that can change over time and the lack of a precise and uniform consensus on diagnosis. In 2003 a consensus workshop indicated PCOS to be present if two out of three criteria are met: oligoovulation and/or anovulation, excess androgen activity (as determined by elevated free androgen index) and polycystic ovaries (by gynaecological ultrasound); and other endocrine disorders such as hyperprolactinaemia are excluded.[1] Elevated fasting insulin or high insulin levels in glucose tolerance tests may also be used to suggest diagnosis. Other blood tests may be suggestive but not diagnostic, for example if the LH:FSH ratio is greater than 1:1, or if there are low levels of sex hormone binding globulin. The presence of ovarian cysts does not automatically imply a diagnosis of PCOS. The prevalence of PCOS is thought to be between 5 and 10% of women and is one of the main causes of infertility in Western women.[2,3]

The symptoms of PCOS usually appear upon menarche, and are associated with early puberty brought about by early secretion of androgens.[4] This may also be associated with low birth weight. However, the condition can develop a considerable time after menarche in the presence of other environmental factors such as weight gain and subsequent insulin resistance.

Increased ovarian androgen biosynthesis in the polycystic ovary syndrome results from abnormalities at all levels of the hypothalamic–pituitary–ovarian (HPO) axis. Androgen excess in women with PCOS may be of either ovarian or adrenal origin. It is also postulated that insulin may induce overactivity of 11β-hydroxysteroid dehydrogenase, resulting in excessive adrenal androgen production.[5] Androgens may be converted to oestrone in fatty tissue, causing blood oestrone and ultimately stimulating LH production, which triggers ovarian androgen production. Increased frequency of luteinising hormone (LH) pulses in PCOS may result from an increased frequency of hypothalamic gonadotrophin-releasing hormone (GnRH) pulses, resulting in higher production of LH compared with follicle-stimulating hormone (FSH). The increase in pituitary secretion of LH can lead to an increase in androgen production by ovarian theca cells. Increased efficiency in the conversion of androgenic precursors in theca cells leads to enhanced production of androstenedione, which can then be converted by 17β-hydroxysteroid dehydrogenase (17βOHSD) to form testosterone or aromatised by the aromatase enzyme to form oestrone, which can be further converted to oestradiol by 17βOHSD (see Figure 20.1).[5]

Insulin acts synergistically with LH to enhance androgen production. Insulin also inhibits hepatic synthesis of sex hormone-binding globulin (which ordinarily binds to testosterone) and therefore increases the proportion of testosterone that is biologically available. Testosterone inhibits and oestrogen stimulates hepatic synthesis of sex hormone-binding globulin.[5]

Polycystic ovaries in PCOS develop when the ovaries are stimulated to produce excessive amounts of androgens—particularly testosterone—through the release of excessive luteinising hormone (LH) by the anterior pituitary gland or through high levels of insulin in the blood.[6] This causes the follicle to begin maturation but the lack of LH surge results in anovulation, meaning the ovum does not release, and ultimately a cyst is formed (see Figure 20.2).

RISK FACTORS

A majority of, though not all, patients in Western settings with PCOS have insulin resistance and are often overweight.[7] Elevated insulin levels contribute to or cause the abnormalities seen in the hypothalamic–pituitary–ovarian (HPO) axis that lead to PCOS. Hyperinsulinaemia may increase GnRH pulse frequency, LH dominance over FSH, increased ovarian androgen production, decreased follicular maturation, and decreased SHBG binding—all of which can lead to the development of PCOS.[5]

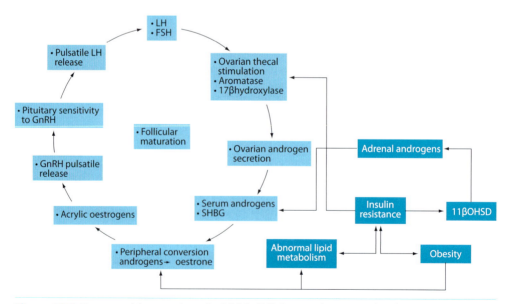

Figure 20.1 Hormonal interactions in PCOS. SHBG = sex-hormone binding globulin, LH = luteinising hormone, FSH = follicle-stimulating hormone, GnRH = gonadotrophin-releasing hormone, 11βOHSD = 11β-hydroxysteroid dehydrogenase

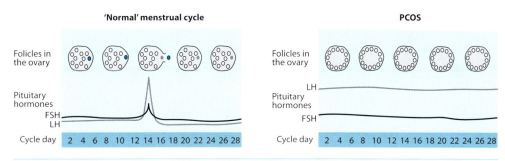

Figure 20.2 Hormonal and reproductive changes in PCOS compared to normal menstruation. FSH = follicle-stimulating hormone, LH = luteinising hormone

Insulin resistance is a common finding among patients of normal weight as well as overweight patients.

It is easy to view the typical PCOS patient with insulin hypersensitivity as the conventional overweight type. However, insulin resistance is also common in lean women with PCOS.[8] It is also easy to view PCOS as a primarily androgen-dependent disorder; however, oestrogen dominance is also commonly present in women with PCOS. Although weight loss is generally associated with good clinical effect and being overweight is common in women with PCOS, it should never be assumed that women with PCOS will always be overweight. This trend should be noted to prevent the misdiagnosis of the condition in women who are not overweight.

Thyroid problems may make PCOS symptoms worse[9] and women with PCOS also have a high prevalence of autoimmune thyroid conditions.[10] Thyroid function should therefore also be checked in patients with PCOS (see Chapter 17 on thyroid abnormalities).

Liver support may also be required in women with PCOS. Approximately 30% of women with PCOS have raised liver enzymes, and diabetes and insulin resistance also increase the risk of non-alcoholic liver disease.[11,12] Hyperinsulinaemia may inhibit the production of SHBG in the liver.

CONVENTIONAL TREATMENT

Due to the functional nature of diagnosis, conventional treatment in PCOS is generally focused on a number of goals. These may include reducing hyperinsulinaemia; restoring normal menstruation, reproductive function and fertility; and reducing associated symptoms such as hirsutism.[13]

Weight reduction and exercise are generally seen as first-line treatments in the management of PCOS. Primary treatment of insulin resistance with metformin or thiazolidenediones is used if the former interventions have had little success.

Anovulation can be treated with ovulation-induction drugs such as clomiphene, bromocriptine, gonadotrophin or GnRH. This treatment has a relatively high risk profile and most often reserved to force ovulation when the patient is trying to conceive. When

EXCLUDE PREGNANCY

It is always important to exclude pregnancy in women of any age presenting with amenorrhoea. It is not unknown in clinical practice to see a patient who has unknowingly become pregnant, despite denying the possibility.

conception is still not achieved assisted reproductive techniques such as in vitro fertilisation are commonly recommended.

The treatment of hirsutism and acne in PCOS generally focuses on reducing androgen levels. Electrolysis, as well as more temporary measures such as waxing and bleaching, is recommended for hirsutism.

If pregnancy is desired, assisted reproductive techniques, including radical drug therapy with clomiphene or a similar agent, or in vitro fertilisation techniques, are also commonly prescribed (see Chapter 31 on fertility, preconception care and pregnancy).[13]

NATUROPATHIC DIAGNOSIS TECHNIQUES
Charting
Due to the often significant timeframes encountered when treating patients with PCOS, tools such as charting may be employed to observe hormonal status changes over time. Menstrual cycle charting based on basal body temperature (BBT) has been traditionally used in naturopathic practice to ascertain changes in levels of hormone levels in reproductive females (see Figure 20.3). It is thought to reflect the menstrual cycle in two ways: (1) within 1–2 days before LH surge there should be a low point in BBT; and (2) following ovulation women should generally see a sustained increase in BBT of between 0.2 and 0.5°C.[14] This rise is most likely due to the thermogenic effect of a metabolite of progesterone.

There has been some contention as to the effectiveness of BBT charting in pregnancy outcomes; however, its use in naturopathy has been extended more broadly to the menstrual cycle in general.

It should be noted that focusing on individual components of charting is very often inadequate.[14] However, when integrated they can form a useful clinical tool that provides a broad overview of reproductive function and actively involves patients in their treatment. Despite the fact that more specific and accurate investigations currently exist, charting may still have a role to play in clinical practice as it is inexpensive, non-invasive and generally reliable. It also actively involves the patient in the therapeutic and diagnostic process. However, interpretation can be subjective and difficult and in more complex cases other investigative techniques may be more appropriate.

Temperature should be taken (sublingually) immediately upon rising. Several factors—including alcohol consumption the night before, restless sleep, variations in waking time and illness—may affect temperature and should be noted on the chart.

Sustained temperature rise shows the most likely day of ovulation (the actual rise begins 12 hours before ovulation during the LH surge).

Consistently low temperature (under 36.5°C) may indicate a hypothyroid condition, which may play a role in poor reproductive function (see Chapter 17 on thyroid abnormalities).

Progesterone
Adequate progesterone levels will result in a sustained, noticeable and prompt rise in BBT. A small or unsustained rise with dips in temperature will be indicative of poor progesterone levels. However, temperature levels alone do not confirm appropriate levels of progesterone. The luteal phase needs to be at least 11 days to indicate adequate progesterone levels. Progesterone levels need to peak approximately 7 days after ovulation to ensure adequate uterine lining for implantation.

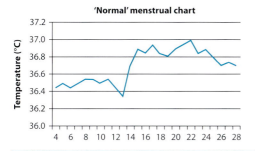
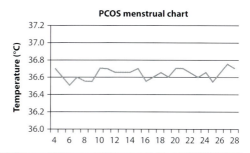

Figure 20.3 The 'normal' chart (left) shows a concordance in temperature with expected levels of progesterone and an immediate strong rise in temperature, giving a strong indication of ovulation. The PCOS chart (right) shows an anovular cycle with no pattern differentiating follicular and luteal phases. Mucus changes may be evident in this case and may represent follicular activity and surges in oestrogen that do not result in ovulation.

Follicular phase length

Long or short follicular phase length (less than 11 days) is indicative of oestrogen imbalances. In short follicular phases this may be further compounded by effects on the corpus luteum, resulting in inadequate progesterone production.

Mucus

Ovarian follicular activity combined with surges in oestrogen that do not result in ovulation are a common occurrence in PCOS. Mucus changes may be evident in these women.

KEY TREATMENT PROTOCOLS

Follicle stimulating hormone and luteinising hormone regulation

Some herbal medicines may affect levels of FSH and LH and may therefore proffer some benefit in the treatment of PCOS. Despite its status as a phytoestrogen, *Cimicifuga racemosa* does not seem to affect the release of prolactin and FSH, though it does reduce LH, in the limited research currently conducted.[15] This central effect is thought to be due to its role on dopaminergic regulation of reproductive hormones rather than its effects on oestrogen receptors.[16,17] The *British Herbal Pharmacopeia* lists *C. racemosa's* main actions as being useful in ovarian dysfunction and ovarian insufficiency.[18]

> **NATUROPATHIC TREATMENT AIMS**
> - Reduce underlying issues such as overweight or insulin resistance.
> - Reduce androgen excess.
> - Regulate and balance hormones more generally.
> - Promote ovulation.
> - Encourage lifestyle changes.

Vitex agnus-castus has had conflicting results, with some studies showing no change in FSH or LH, and another suggesting increased LH release.[19–21] *V. agnus-castus* is thought to have antiandrogenic properties. *Humulus lupulus* also reduces LH with continued use and may therefore be useful to reduce androgens in PCOS.[22] A review of **soy** studies suggests that soy consumption has no effects on FSH or TSH.[23]

Unpublished (though publicly available) data suggest that supplementation with the herb *Tribulus terrestris* for 3 months may normalise ovulation and result in pregnancy in women with endocrine infertility.[24] *Mentha spicata* (via tea therapy—2 cups per day for 5 days) use has been associated with increases in LH, FSH and oestrogen levels in women with PCOS.[25]

Glycyrrhiza glabra is a commonly used herb in the treatment of PCOS. Though trials for its stand-alone treatment in PCOS are lacking, there exists a theoretical basis behind its use. *G. glabra* has been demonstrated to reduce testosterone levels in healthy women.[26] Various forms of *Glycyrrhiza* have been used in a combination product (as the key ingredient with *Paeonia lactiflora*) in the treatment of PCOS in some small trials that showed reduction in FSH:LH ratio, ovarian testosterone production and improvements in ovulation.[27,28] However, the situation in the combination product has been confused further by the fact that while this research has focused on *G. uralensis* clinical application is still dominated by *G. glabra*. The clinical effects of these minor differences are unknown. *G.racemoza* may also exert further potent phytoestrogenic activity independent of these effects.[29] *Glycyrrhiza glabra* is also demonstrated to reduce body fat mass in normal weight subjects.[30] A *Paeonia lactiflora* and *Glycyrrhiza glabra* combination has been found to have numerous effects on PCOS, including regulating FSH:LH ratios (possibly through stimulation of pituitary dopamine receptors),[27] lowering testosterone levels and improving oestradiol to testosterone ratios.[28,31]

Exogenous **melatonin** has been demonstrated to enhance LH secretion, LH pulse amplitude and LH sensitivity to GnRH.[32–34] This was thought to be the result of melatonin supplementation mimicking the effects of PCOS—possibly due to the effects of melatonin on increasing cortisol levels. This effect is known to increase in hypo-oestrogenic states.[35] However, while most studies have been in postmenopausal or older women, melatonin supplementation in younger women has been associated with return to menstrual regularity, as well as the reduction of LH levels in younger women with high baseline levels, in clinical settings.[36,37] This has led to calls for a possible role of melatonin in the treatment of PCOS and, despite its popularity in some streams of naturopathic medicine, it remains unclear at this stage what role it may play; further research is required.[38] Other factors known to affect melatonin levels should also be considered (see Chapter 14 on insomnia).

Other factors may also affect LH levels. Various human studies have suggested that inadequate nutrition or short periods of fasting reduces LH pulsing, though not always LH levels.[39–41] This is thought to be due to relative increases in cortisol caused by these states.[42] Animal studies seem to suggest that increased endotoxin load can reduce plasma LH levels.[43]

HPO and hypothalamic–pituitary–adrenal (HPA) axis interaction

It is well known that women with PCOS exhibit abnormalities in cortisol metabolism as well as higher levels than controls.[44] It is also known that a return to states of normal cortisol from high cortisol level in women with amenorrhoea or menstrual disturbances often precedes the resumption of normal ovarian activity.[45] These findings further support the role for stress reduction in regulating LH and FSH function in the treatment of reproductive disorders such as PCOS.

The reproductive axis is inhibited at all levels by various components of the HPA axis. Corticotrophin-releasing hormone (CRH) can either directly or indirectly (through β-endorphin) suppress gonadotrophin-releasing hormone. Glucocorticoids may also exert inhibitory effects by rendering target tissues resistant to reproductive hormones, inhibiting GnRH and LH secretion and inhibiting ovarian oestrogen and progesterone biosynthesis.[5] The effects of the HPA axis interaction with the female reproductive system can result in idiopathic or hypothalamic amenorrhoea (for example, that associated with stress, depression, anxiety or eating disorders) in its own right, or result in the hypogonadism associated with Cushing's syndrome,[5] though it may also result in further indirect complication of other disorders of hormonal dysregulation like PCOS.

However, these interactions can also be bidirectional. Corticotrophin-releasing hormone, for example, is regulated to some extent in reproductive tissue by oestrogen. Corticotrophin-releasing hormone is responsible for a number of functions in reproductive tissue (see Table 20.1), and disorders or events (such as chronic stress adaptation) that affect these levels may also have clinically relevant effects on reproductive function. Due to this bidirectional activity, a multifaceted approach to disorders, focusing on regulation of both reproductive and adrenal hormones, may be more successful in conditions such as PCOS rather than targeting one system alone, particularly considering PCOS may often be a disorder of oestrogen excess (via adipose tissue) as well as androgen excess. For this reason, generalised hormone-balancing protocols may also be beneficial in PCOS. Further information on balancing reproductive hormones can be found in Chapter 19 on endometriosis.

Weight management

Although not all people presenting with PCOS are overweight, in those that are, weight loss is an essential part of PCOS treatment. Not only can realistic weight loss result in dramatic improvement in the condition, but being overweight can also make treatment

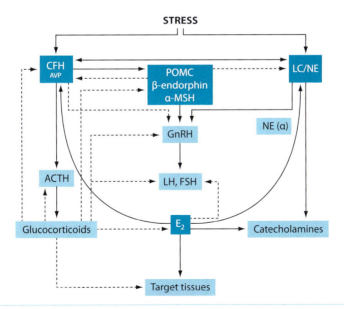

Figure 20.4 Interactions of the HPO and HPA axes.
CRH = corticotrophin-releasing hormone, GnRH = gonadotropin-releasing hormone, LH = luteinising hormone, E_2 = ovarian estradiol, α-MSH = melanocyte-stimulating hormone, ACTH = adrenocorticotropic hormone, AVP = arginine-vasopressin, FSH = follicle-stimulating hormone, NE (α) = norepinephrine stimulation via α-noradrenergic receptors, POMC = proopiomelanocortin, solid line = stimulation, broken line = inhibition

Table 20.1 Reproductive corticotrophin-releasing hormone, potential physiological roles and potential pathogenic effects[46]

REPRODUCTIVE CRH	POTENTIAL PHYSIOLOGICAL ROLES	POTENTIAL PATHOGENIC EFFECTS
Ovarian CRH	Follicular maturation Ovulation Luteolysis Suppression of female sex steriod production	Premature ovarian failure (↑ secretion) Anovulation(↓ secretion) Corpus luteum dysfunction (↓ secretion) Ovarian dysfunction (↓ secretion)
Uterine CRH	Decidualisation	Infertility (↓ secretion)
	Blastocyst implantation	Recurrent spontaneous abortion (↓ secretion)
	Early maternal tolerance	
Placental CRH	Labour	Premature labour (↑ secretion)
	Maternal hypercortisolism Fetoplacental circulation Fetal adrenal steroidogenesis	Delayed labour (↓ secretion) Preeclampsia and eclampsia (↑ secretion)

less effective.[47,48] Weight loss also proffers more effectiveness than current medication for insulin resistance and related disorders.[49] Specific individual pharmacotherapy of any kind—including that of dietary and herbal supplements—is generally clinically ineffective in weight loss in the insulin-resistant individual[50] and therefore therapy should focus on an integrated approach to weight management.

As little as 2–5% reduction in weight can be enough to improve metabolic and reproductive indices in women with PCOS.[51] This modest improvement can restore ovulatory function and improve insulin sensitivity by over 70%.[52] A 5–10% reduction in weight can reduce central fat stores by 30% and weight loss also increases SHBG concentration, reduces testosterone concentration and androgenic stimulation of the skin (resulting in reduction in hirsutism), improves menstrual function and conception rates and reduces miscarriage rates in women with PCOS.[53–59]

High protein diets are typically associated with excellent weight loss results in insulin-resistant and PCOS women.[60,61] Although higher-protein or lower-carbohydrate diets are often successful in weight loss in women with PCOS, this weight loss may not automatically equate to improvements in insulin parameters or ovarian function.[62] However, Mediterranean-style diets have been associated with both weight loss and improved insulin parameters in both generic insulin resistant and PCOS patients.[63,64]

An Israeli study comparing three common **diets—low-fat, low-carbohydrate and Mediterranean**—found that all diets were effective.[65] However, the low-carbohydrate and Mediterranean diets appeared to be more effective than the low-fat diet over 2 years. This suggests that dietary interventions may best be individualised to patient needs rather than protocol-driven.

Long-term modest weight loss is far more important in PCOS than acute weight loss. In fact drastic weight loss in women with PCOS may have negative effects on reproductive function.[66] Patient compliance may be improved in low-carbohydrate or higher-protein diets compared to low-fat diets. This is evidenced by a systematic review of

FATNESS OR FITNESS?

It is easy to assume that all that is required to treat PCOS is to reduce the weight of the patient. However, improving physical fitness may often be more effective than crude weight loss in PCOS management. Similarly, an assumption should not be made that leanness equates to fitness (endometriosis, for example, is far more common in lean women). It may be prudent to aim for goals that more accurately reflect fitness levels (stamina in daily tasks and energy levels) rather than crude measurements. Weight management should focus on achieving a healthy weight and not some arbitrary number. Some women will never acquire an 'athletic' body type even at peak fitness. Holistic treatment may in these cases extend to reducing the psychological effect of body issues as well as physical considerations, and encouraging the patient to be comfortable with their healthy body. This may require referral to non-clinical resources (for example, advice on flattering clothing choices) as much as clinical ones.

dietary interventions that suggested that participant attrition was higher in low-fat diet clinical trials.[67] Patients who have consistent eating habits were more likely to maintain their desired weight than those who follow stricter, but variable, protocols or gave themselves more flexibility during holidays.[68]

Diets higher in mono-unsaturated and polyunsaturated fats did not result in higher weight regain after crash dieting than low-fat diets and also resulted in significantly better lipid and insulin profiles.[69] Studies of low-carbohydrate diets in patients with blood sugar dysregulation have also routinely demonstrated improvements in blood sugar and insulin profiles.[70–74] There appears to be no negative long-term consequences in insulin sensitivity in these diets.[75] However, composition of diets may be important, whereas saturated fats can induce insulin resistance, and mono-unsaturated fats can improve insulin sensitivity.[75]

Although short-term trials do not seem to indicate macronutrient composition is as important as caloric restriction in short-term weight loss in women with PCOS,[62,76] the improved longer-term outcomes and compliance suggest a role for Mediterranean-style or high-protein dietary changes. However, rather than advocating drastic low-carbohydrate measures in diet, a more prudent approach is to increase protein, which can improve satiety and reduce carbohydrate intake by default.

However, it is not just a reduction in carbohydrate that is required. Changes in the types of carbohydrate consumed—shifting towards complex rather than simple carbohydrates—can also improve outcomes in weight management,[77] as can increasing fibre and separation of carbohydrate intake from protein intake.[78,79] Eating breakfast was also associated with successful weight maintenance.[68,80]

Care needs to be particularly taken with many foods advertised as 'low fat' or similar as these may often be high in sugar or other carbohydrates to compensate for lost taste advantage. Patients need to be adequately counselled on how to identify appropriate dietary additions. Care also needs to be taken when advising particular supplements for weight loss for patients with PCOS. Very few supplements have demonstrated success in weight loss despite many manufacturers making unsubstantiated claims. **5-hydroxy-tryptophan** supplementation, for example, has normalised eating patterns in obese patients by reducing their intake of fat, energy and carbohydrate even when diets during the studies were unrestricted.[81–84] There is also some evidence to suggest that **green tea** (from *Camellia sinensis*) can raise metabolic rates, increase thermogenesis, speed up fat oxidation and improve insulin sensitivity and glucose tolerance.[85–88] Its effects on insulin sensitivity and weight loss may be related to the combination of catechins and caffeine,[89] though there is speculation that its association with weight management is thought to be related to its caffeine content alone.[90] Milk can reduce the glucose tolerance actions of tea by up to 90%.[91] However, these should not be relied upon as primary treatments and rather should be adjuncts to a diet and lifestyle modification prescription.

Dietary counselling and exercise may result in a trend towards normalisation of hormone levels (as observed by LH:FSH ratio) in PCOS patients, even in the absence of weight loss.[92] In overweight, infertile women with amenorrhoea or anovulation, 12 weeks of exercise and diet therapy were also associated with development of menstrual regularity and normalisation of E1:E2 ratio (see Chapter 19 on endometriosis).[93]

The role of leptin

Leptin is a hormone secreted by adipocytes and regulates body weight via its effects on metabolism and satiety. However, levels of this hormone appear to be related to the overweight status of the patient. Leptin levels are higher in overweight women with and without PCOS.[94,95] Leptin also acts directly on ovarian function through specific receptors.[96–99] Generally, leptin inhibits the hypothalamic–pituitary–adrenal axis and stimulates the reproductive system, which may result in ovarian over-production of androgens.

Impaired postprandial cholecystokinin (CCK) secretion, possibly associated with increased levels of testosterone, may also play a role in the greater frequency of binge eating and being overweight in women with PCOS.[100] The hormone ghrelin—implicated in appetite regulation—was found to be lower in PCOS women than in controls, indicating alterations in satiety.[101] In overweight women with PCOS a dysfunctional leptin resistance may be observed and this may be one reason weight loss is a successful intervention in PCOS.[102,103]

Insulin resistance

The treatment of insulin resistance is covered in more depth in Chapter 16 on diabetes type 2, though some advances have been made specifically in relation to PCOS. Inositol has the ability to increase ovulation and reduce hyperandrogenism in women with PCOS, including those without weight issues, as well as improving insulin parameters.[104–107] **Bitters** are traditionally used by naturopaths to both improve digestive function and regulate blood sugar levels.[108] Vinegar (for example, apple cider vinegar) may be particularly helpful to reduce postprandial blood glucose levels and improve insulin sensitivity.[109–112]

Galega officinales is traditionally used to treat insulin resistance and contains chromium salts as well as guanidines.[113,114] Early research established hypoglycaemic activity in these guanidine compounds.[18,115] The drug metformin, used successfully in conventional treatment of PCOS, is a synthetic guanidine derivative. Other herbs that may show promise in the treatment of insulin resistance more generally include *Momordica indica*, *Gymnema sylvestre* and *Aloe vera*.[116] Interventions useful in insulin resistance are covered in more depth in Chapter 16 on diabetes type 2.

Chromium was found to improve insulin resistance parameters, though not ovulation, in women with PCOS.[117,118] Insulin resistance may be associated with higher aromatase activity.[119] This is explored further in Chapter 19 on endometriosis.

Hirsutism

Hirsutism is common in women with PCOS and often weight loss alone has been associated with reducing the effects of hirsutism.[53,57,58] An infusion of ***Mentha spicata*** was found to lower free testosterone, while not lowering total testosterone or DHEA, in a small study of women with PCOS and hirsutism.[25,120] ***Serenoa repens*** has also been found to reduce the severity of androgenic dermatological conditions (alopecia) in both men and women and may therefore be useful in PCOS.[121,122] **Zinc** may also be of some value in reducing androgenic activity in skin.[123] Hormonal modulation more generally will also assist with skin conditions associated with excess androgens, and is discussed in more detail in Chapter 24 on acne.

INTEGRATIVE MEDICAL CONSIDERATIONS

Acupuncture

Women with PCOS treated with acupuncture have shown improvements in hormone levels, ovulation and basal body temperature.[124] This is thought to be particularly related to the effects of acupuncture on the sympathetic nervous system in PCOS.

Asian herbal medicine

There has been much discussion surrounding the successful treatment of PCOS with the herbs *P. lactiflora* and *G. glabra*. This is based on successful treatment of PCOS in a series of small uncontrolled studies in a combination herbal product of which these two herbs were only two components of many.[27,28] A Japanese combination (*unkei-to*) has also demonstrated some effect in women with PCOS,[125,126] as have a variety of other combination herbal products.[127,128]

These remedies have a strong tradition of use in PCOS which is being reinforced through modern research; however, they need to be properly prescribed in accordance with traditional Chinese medicine or *kampo* principles. It should also be remembered that, due to the difficulties in developing a uniform diagnosis of PCOS, these formulations may not be applicable to all populations with or manifestations of PCOS. It is known, for example, that the metabolic characteristics and responses to treatment of Asian women with PCOS may be significantly different to those seen in Western populations.[127] Their use in contemporary naturopathic practice needs to take these principles into consideration.

Homoeopathy

A case series has found that individualised homoeopathic treatment may be successful at restoring ovulation in women with amenorrhoea.[129]

Psychotherapeutic options

Some women with PCOS fail to fall within social norms regarding outer appearance and may feel stigmatised and feel a loss of feminine identity—this may affect mood, sexual function and quality of life more generally.[130] Appropriate counselling and psychotherapeutic options may help lessen the impact on quality of life in PCOS patients.

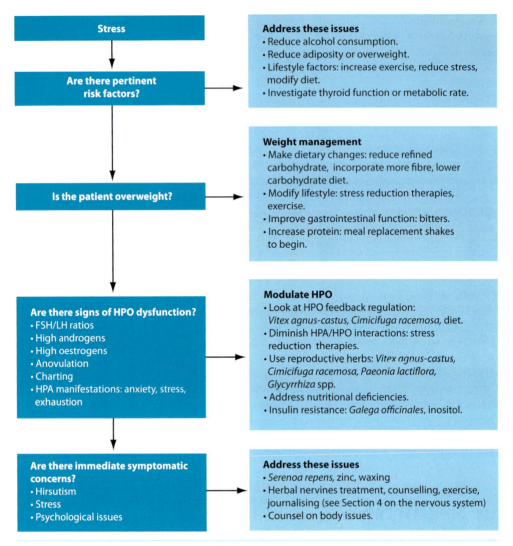

Figure 20.5 Naturopathic treatment decision tree

Case Study

A 26-year-old woman presents with **irregular periods** with **heavy cramping**. She has successfully lost weight previously, but has since put it back on over the last 2 years and is currently slightly **overweight**, with a BMI of 27. She finds it difficult to maintain weight loss, despite eating well and exercising. She has **hair growth** on her abdomen and upper lip.

SUGGESTIVE SYMPTOMS

- Oligomenorrhoea or irregular menstruation
- Overweight
- Hirsutism or acne
- Insulin resistance
- Infertility or failure to conceive
- Ovarian cysts

Example treatment

Prescription

The patient was prescribed the liquid herbal formula in the box below. The treatment rationale was to encourage ovulation, reduce FSH and androgen levels. Zinc was given to assist with hirsutism.

Herbal formula		
Cimicifuga racemosa	2:1	15 mL
Glycyrrhiza glabra	2:1	35 mL
Paeonia lactiflora	2:1	30 mL
Serenoa repens	2:1	20 mL
5 mL t.d.s.		100 mL
Nutritional prescription		
Zinc (amino acid chelate)	15 mg	

The patient was also advised to begin a higher-protein diet and to reduce her refined carbohydrates. She was given the name of several recipe books to help her in this endeavour. She was given recipes to help her incorporate foods such as legumes that she had had little experience with. She was told to increase her consumption of vegetables, particularly cruciferous, and told to keep a diet diary for next visit.

The patient was also recommended a protein powder to take as a morning tea supplement. She was recommended to take either apple cider vinegar or bitters before meals. After discussion it was decided the exercise most suited to her was walking. She was instructed to purchase an mp3 player and a public transport card. She was to walk for one album each day (enough to break into a sweat) and walk to the nearest available public transport instead of driving to work. (It was ascertained that this would result in similar or reduced commuting times.)

After the first consultation the patient had had difficulty with compliance of the herbal mixture due to the taste of *Serenoa*. It was recommended instead that she move to a tablet containing equal proportions of *Cimicifuga racemosa*, *Paeonia lactiflora* and *Glycyrrhiza glabra* (but no *S. repens*) to the liquid tincture instead. It had been 4 weeks; she had lost 4.5 kg and is enthusiastic about her new diet. She enquired about other possible exercises and was recommended qi gong, swimming or bike riding as activities that may fit into her lifestyle. Her hirsutism remained and she still not had a period.

At the third consultation the patient is continuing with weight loss—12 kg since the initial visit 3 months ago. She has experienced her first period, which lasted for seven days and was quite heavy. She was told to continue with the formula, though a *Vitex agnus-castus* tablet was added to help her cycle become regular. She has noticed more energy. Her hirsutism is still present, but reducing slowly. The patient is counselled that it is still early and, while results are positive, full amelioration of symptoms may take some time.

Expected outcomes and follow-up protocols

Many patients ignore PCOS until they unsuccessfully attempt to conceive. Even once PCOS has been resolved these patients may require further preconception care on a more individual basis. Referral to a fertility program or specialist may be warranted.

Treatment needs to be looked at long term. It may be months before the initial menstrual bleeding (which may seem 'excessive' in both volume and timeframe by normal standards once it does finally arrive). Patients need to be counselled on this before embarking on treatment to ensure they know what to expect and to ensure they do not get disheartened by the lack of immediate results. Charting can be a useful tool to indicate changes in hormone levels that are getting closer to those required for ovulation, even when menstrual changes are not apparent. Patients with amenorrhoea may also require a change in their prescription at the point of their first menstrual bleed to assist their cycle to become regular.

Table 20.2 Review of the major evidence

STUDIES	METHODOLOGY	RESULT	COMMENT
Camellia sinensis Chan et al. 2006[86]	3-month 2-arm RCT ($n = 34$) 2% weight/volume Lung Chen green tea powder standardised to 540 mg epigallocatechin gallate (equivalent to 1.5 cups of tea) vs placebo	Non-significant reduction of 2.4% of BMI in green tea group while control group BMI increased significantly during trial.	Sample size was small and therefore statistical power low. While not an effective agent in reducing BMI, green tea may play a role in weight maintenance and reducing further weight gain in PCOS. Larger studies are needed to confirm the result.
Whey protein Kasim-Karakas et al. 2007[131]	RCT ($n = 28$) measuring changes in hormone levels of women with PCOS after acute glucose (oral 5 hour glucose challenge test) and acute protein intakes (with whey protein). Protein suppressed ghrelin significantly more than glucose and had more satietogenic effect.	Glucose ingestion caused significantly more hyperinsulinaemia and stimulated cortisol and DHEA more than protein.	Study represents short-term effects only, though provides some mechanistic support for increasing protein and decreasing simple sugars in PCOS treatment.
Inositol Nestler et al. 1998[104]	6–8 week RCT of 44 obese women with PCOS given either 1200 mg d-chiro-inositol or placebo	19/22 women in inositol group ovulated vs 6/22 in placebo group ($p \leq 0.001$). Serum triglycerides, insulin, free testosterone and blood pressure all increased significantly when compared to placebo (at least $p \leq 0.007$).	D-chiro-inositol increases the action of insulin in patients with the polycystic ovary syndrome, thereby improving ovulatory function and decreasing serum androgen concentrations, blood pressure and plasma triglyceride concentrations.
Iuorno et al. 2002[105]	6–8 week RCT of 20 lean women with PCOS given 600 mg inositol once daily or placebo	Serum triglycerides, insulin, free testosterone and blood pressure all increased significantly when compared to placebo (at least $p \leq 0.03$).	
Mentha spicata Akdoğan et al. 2007[25]	21 women with hirsutism were given one cup of *Mentha spicata* infusion b.d. for 5 days.	There was a significant decrease in free testosterone and increase in luteinising hormone, follicle-stimulating hormone and oestradiol. No significant decreases in total testosterone or dehydroepiandrostenedione sulfate levels were observed.	*Mentha spicata* may have anti-androgenic effects in PCOS.
Peony and liquorice combination[27,28]	24 week RCT of 34 women with PCOS given 7.5 g of TJ-68 (herbal medicine containing peony and liquorice).	Significant reductions in FSH:LH ratio, ovarian testosterone production and improvements in ovulation.	These small trials used a combination herbal medicine prescribed according to traditional Chinese medicine or *kampo* principles. Their use in naturopathic prescription may not mirror this.

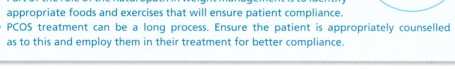

KEY POINTS

- Use dietary and lifestyle modification first—it is more effective than medication.
- Address the other risk factors that are associated with PCOS (cardiovascular, etc.).
- Part of the role of the naturopath in weight management is to identify appropriate foods and exercises that will ensure patient compliance.
- PCOS treatment can be a long process. Ensure the patient is appropriately counselled as to this and employ them in their treatment for better compliance.

Reduction of hirsutism is also a long-term treatment. Hair follicles will often take at least 3–6 months (their life cycle) before effects are observed in women with PCOS. It may be prudent to counsel them to make cosmetic adjustments until then if this is a big concern, in addition to counselling them on the long timeframe of treatment.

Further reading

Kalantaridou S, et al. Stress and the female reproductive system. J Reprod Immunol 2004;62(1–2):61–68.

Giallauria F, et al. Androgens in polycystic ovary syndrome: the role of exercise and diet. Semin Reprod Med 2009;27(4):306–315.

Huang S, Chen A. Traditional Chinese medicine and infertility. Curr Opin Obstet Gynecol 2008;20(3): 211–215.

Trickey R. Women, hormones and the menstrual cycle: herbal and medical solutions from adolescence to menopause. Sydney: Allen & Unwin, 2003.

Wilkes S, Murdoch A. Obesity and female fertility: a primary care perspective. J Fam Plann Reprod Health Care 2009;35(3):181–185.

Revised 2003 consensus on diagnostic criteria and long-term health risks related to polycystic ovary syndrome (PCOS). Hum Reprod 2004;19(1):41–47.

References

1. Revised 2003 consensus on diagnostic criteria and long-term health risks related to polycystic ovary syndrome (PCOS). Hum Reprod 2004;19:41–47.
2. Asuncion M, et al. A prospective study of the prevalence of the polycystic ovary syndrome in unselected Caucasian women from Spain. J Clin Endocrinol Metab 2000;85:2434–2438.
3. Knochenhauer E, et al. Prevalence of the polycystic ovary syndrome in unselected black and white women of the southeastern United States: a prospective study. J Clin Endocrinol Metab 1998;83:3078–3082.
4. Ibanez L, et al. Polycystic ovary syndrome after precocious pubarche: ontogeny of the low-birthweight effect. Clin Endocrinol (Oxf) 2001;55:667–672.
5. Speroff L, Fritz M. Clinical gynecologic endocrinology and infertility. 7th edn. Philadelphia: Lippincott Williams & Wilkins, 2005.
6. Kovacs, G, Norman, R, eds. Polycystic ovarian syndrome. Cambridge: Cambridge University Press, 2008.
7. Wilkes S, Murdoch A. Obesity and female fertility: a primary care perspective. J Fam Plann Reprod Health Care 2009;35(3):181–185.
8. Altuntas Y, et al. Reactive hypoglycemia in lean young women with PCOS and correlations with insulin sensitivity and with beta cell function. Eur J Obstet Gynecol Reprod Biol 2005;119(2):198–205.
9. Ghosh S, et al. Subclinical hypothyroidism: a determinant of polycystic ovary syndrome. Horm Res 1993;39:61–66.
10. Jannsen O, et al. High prevalence of autoimmune thyroiditis in patients with polycystic ovary syndrome. Eur J Endocrinol 2004;150:363–369.
11. Schwimmer J, et al. Abnormal aminotransferase activity in women with polycystic ovary syndrome. Fertil Steril 2005;83:494–497.
12. El-Serag H, et al. Diabetes increases the risk of chronic liver disease and hepatocellular carcinoma. Gastroenterology 2004;126:460–468.
13. Edmonds K, ed. Obstetrics and gynaecology. London: Blackwell, 2007.
14. Martinez A, et al. The reliability, acceptability and applications of basal body-temperature (BBT) records in the diagnosis and treatment of infertility. Eur J Obstet Gynecol Reprod Biol 1992;47:121–127.
15. Duker E, et al. Effects of extracts from *Cimicifuga racemosa* on gonadotropin release in menopausal women and ovariectomized rats. Planta Med 1991;57:420–424.
16. Borrelli F, et al. Pharmacological effects of *Cimicifuga racemosa*. Life Sci 2003;73:1215–1229.
17. Jarry H, et al. In vitro effects of the *Cimicifuga racemosa* extract BNO 1055. Maturitas 2003;44:S31–S38.
18. Scientific Committee of the British Herbal Medical Association. British herbal pharmacopoeia. 1st edn. Bournemouth: British Herbal Medicine Association, 1983.

19. Laurintzen C, et al. Treatment of premenstrual tension with *Vitex agnus-castus*: controlled, double blind study versus pyroxidin. Phytomedicine 1997;4:183–189.
20. Milewicz A, et al. [*Vitex agnus-castus* extract in the treatment of luteal phase defects due to latent hyperprolactinemia. Results of a randomized placebo-controlled double-blind study] [in German]. Arzneimittelforschung 1993;43(7):752–756.
21. Jarry H, et al. In vitro prolactin but not LH and FSH release is inhibited by compounds in extracts of Agnus castus: direct evidence for a dopaminergic principle by the dopamine receptor assay. Exp Clin Endocrinol 1994;102(6):448–454.
22. Okamato R, Kumai A. Antigonadotrophic activity of hop extract. Acta Endocrinol 1992;127(4):371–377.
23. Balk E, et al. Effects of soy on health outcomes. Evid Rep Technol Assess (Summ) 2005;126:1–8.
24. Tabakova P, et al. Clinical study of Tribestan® in females with endocrine sterility. Sofia: Bulgarian Pharmacology Group, 2000.
25. Akdoğan M, et al. Effect of spearmint (*Mentha spicata Labiatae*) teas on androgen levels in women with hirsutism. Phytother Res 2007;21(5):444–447.
26. Armanini D, et al. Licorice reduces serum testosterone in healthy women. Steroids 2004;69(11–12):763–766.
27. Takahashi K, Kitao M. Effects of TJ-68 (shakuyaku-kanzo-to) on polycystic ovarian disease. Int J Fertil Menopausal Stud 1994;39(2):69–76.
28. Takahashi K, et al. Effects of traditional medicine (Shakuyaku-kanzo-to) on testosterone secretion in patients with polycystic ovary syndrome detected by ultrasound. Nippon Sanka Fujinka Gakkai Zasshi 1988;40(6):789–796.
29. Setchell K, Cassidy A. Dietary isoflavones: biological effects and relevance to human health. J Nutr 1999;129:758S–767S.
30. Armanini D, et al. Effect of licorice on the reduction of body fat mass in healthy subjects. J Endocrinol Invest 2003;26(7):646–650.
31. Yaginuma T, et al. Effect of traditional herbal medicine on serum testosterone levels and its induction of regular ovulation in hyperandrogenic and oligomenorrheic women. Nippon Sanka Fujinka Gakkai Zasshi 1998;34(7):939–944.
32. Cagnacci A, et al. Exogenous melatonin enhances luteinizing hormone levels of women in the follicular but not in the luteal menstrual phase. Fertil Steril 1995;63:996–999.
33. Cagnacci A, et al. Melatonin enhances the luteinizing hormone and follicle-stimulating hormone responses to gonadotropin-releasing hormone in the follicular, but not in the luteal, menstrual phase. J Clin Endocrinol Metab 1995;80:1095–1099.
34. Cagnacci A, et al. Influence of melatonin administration on glucose tolerance and insulin sensitivity of postmenopausal women. Clin Endocrinol (Oxf) 2001;54:339–346.
35. Cagnacci A, et al. Melatonin enhances cortisol levels in aged women: reversible by estrogens. J Pineal Res 1997;22(2):81–85.
36. Bellipanni G, et al. Effects of melatonin in perimenopausal and menopausal women: a randomized and placebo controlled study. Exp Gerontol 2001;36(2):297–310.
37. Bellipanni G, et al. Effects of melatonin in perimenopausal and menopausal women: our personal experience. Ann N Y Acad Sci 2005;1057:393–402.
38. Cagnacci A, Volpe A. A role for melatonin in PCOS? Fertil Steril 2002;77(5):1089.
39. Loucks A, Heath E. Dietary restriction reduces luteinizing hormone (LH) pulse frequency during waking hours and increases LH pulse amplitude during sleep in young menstruating women. J Clin Endocrinol Metab 1994;78:910–915.
40. Olson B, et al. Short-term fasting affects luteinizing hormone secretory dynamics but not reproductive function in normal-weight sedentary women. J Clin Endocrinol Metab 1995;80:1187–1193.
41. Alvero R, et al. Effects of fasting on neuroendocrine function and follicle development in lean women. J Clin Endocrinol Metab 1998;83:76–80.
42. Bergendahl M, et al. Short-term fasting suppresses leptin and (conversely) activates disorderly growth hormone secretion in midluteal phase women—a clinical research center study. J Clin Endocrinol Metab 1999;84(3):883–894.
43. Daniel JA, et al. Regulation of the growth hormone and luteinizing hormone response to endotoxin in sheep. Domest Anim Endocrinol 2002;23(1–2):361–370.
44. Yildiz B, Azziz R. Adrenocortical dysfunction in polycystic ovary syndrome. In: Kovacs G, Norman R, eds. Polycystic ovary syndrome. 2nd edn. Cambridge: Cambridge University Press, 2007.
45. Kondoh Y, et al. A longitudinal study of disturbances of the hypothalamic-pituitary-adrenal axis in women with progestin-negative functional hypothalamic amenorrhea. Fertil Steril 2001;76(4):748–752.
46. Kalantaridou S, et al. Stress and the female reproductive system. J Reprod Immunol 2004;62(1–2):61–68.
47. Dale O, et al. The impact of insulin resistance on the outcome of ovulation induction with low-dose follicle stimulating hormone in women with polycystic ovarian syndrome. Hum Reprod 1998;13:567–570.
48. Homburg R. Adverse effect of luteinizing hormone on fertility: fact or fantasy. Bailleres Clin Obstet Gynecol 1998;12:555–563.
49. Knowler W, et al. Reduction in the incidence of type 2 diabetes with lifestyle intervention or metformin. N Engl J Med 2002;346:393–403.
50. Norris S, et al. Efficacy of pharmacotherapy for weight loss in adults with type 2 diabetes mellitus: a meta-analysis. Arch Intern Med 2004;164(13):1395–1404.
51. Moran L, et al. Effects of lifestyle modification in polycystic ovarian syndrome. Reprod Biomed Online 2006;12:569–578.
52. Huber-Buchholz M, et al. Restoration of reproductive potential by lifestyle modification in obese polycystic ovary syndrome: role of insulin sensitivity and luteinizing hormone. J Clin Endocrinol Metab 1999;84:1470–1474.
53. Kiddy D, et al. Improvement in endocrine and ovarian function during dietary treatment of obese women with polycystic ovary syndrome. Clin Endocrinol (Oxf) 1992;36:105–111.
54. Pasquali R, et al. Effect of long-term treatment with metformin added to hypocaloric diet on body composition, fat distribution, and androgen and insulin levels in abdominally obese women with and without the polycystic ovary syndrome. J Clin Endocrinol Metab 2000;85:2767–2774.
55. Crosignani P, et al. Overweight and obese anovulatory patients with polycystic ovaries: parallel improvements in anthropometric indices, ovarian physiology and fertility rate induced by diet. Hum Reprod 2003;18:1928–1932.
56. Moran L, et al. Dietary composition in restoring reproductive and metabolic physiology in overweight women with polycystic ovary syndrome. J Clin Endocrinol Metab 2003;88:812–819.
57. Piacquadio D, et al. Obesity and female androgenic alopecia: cause and effect? J Am Acad Dermatol 1994;30:1028–1030.
58. Ruutiainen K, et al. Influence of body mass index and age on the grade of hair growth and hormonal parameters of hirsute women. Int J Gynecol Obstet 1988;24:361–368.
59. Clark A, et al. Weight loss results in significant improvement in pregnancy ovulation and outcome rates in anovulatory obese women. Hum Reprod 1995;10:2705–2712.

60. Mathers J, Daly M. Dietary carbohydrates and insulin sensitivity. Curr Opin Clin Nutr Metab Care 1998;1: 553–557.
61. Skov A, et al. Randomized trial on protein vs. carbohydrate in ad libitum fat reduced diet for the treatment of obesity. Int J Obes Relat Metab Disord 1999;23: 528–536.
62. Stamets K, et al. A randomized trial of the effects of two types of short term hypocaloric diets on weight loss in women with polycystic ovary syndrome. Fertil Steril 2004;81:630–637.
63. Carmina E, et al. Difference in body weight between American and Italian women with polycystic ovary syndrome: influence of diet. Hum Reprod 2003;18: 2289–2293.
64. Esposito K, et al. Effect of a mediterranean-style diet on endothelial dysfuntion and markers of vascular inflammation in the metabolic syndrome: a randomized trial. JAMA 2004;292:1440–1446.
65. Shai I, et al. Weight loss with a low-carbohydrate, Mediterranean, or low-fat diet. N Engl J Med 2008;359(3):229–241.
66. Tsagareli V, et al. Effect of a very-low-calorie diet on in vitro fertilization outcomes. Fertil Steril 2006;86: 227–229.
67. Hession MR, et al. Systematic review of randomized controlled trials of low-carbohydrate vs. low-fat/low-calorie diets in the management of obesity and its comorbidities. Obes Rev 2009;10(1):36–50.
68. Wing R, Phelan S. Long-term weight loss maintenance. Am J Clin Nutr 2005;82(Supp 1):222S–225S.
69. Due A, et al. Comparison of 3 ad libitum diets for weight-loss maintenance, risk of cardiovascular disease, and diabetes: a 6-mo randomized, controlled trial. Am J Clin Nutr 2008;88:1232–1241.
70. Brinkworth GD, et al. Long-term effects of a high-protein, low-carbohydrate diet on weight control and cardiovascular risk markers in obese hyperinsulinemic subjects. Int J Obes Relat Metab Disord 2004;28(5):661–670.
71. Sharman MJ, et al. A ketogenic diet favorably affects serum biomarkers for cardiovascular disease in normal-weight men. J Nutr 2002;132(7):1879–1885.
72. Wolever TM, Mehling C. Long-term effect of varying the source or amount of dietary carbohydrate on postprandial plasma glucose, insulin, triacylglycerol, and free fatty acid concentrations in subjects with impaired glucose tolerance. Am J Clin Nutr 2003;77(3):612–621.
73. Volek JS, et al. Fasting lipoprotein and postprandial triacylglycerol responses to a low-carbohydrate diet supplemented with n-3 fatty acids. J Am Coll Nutr 2000;19(3):383–391.
74. Gannon MC, Nuttall FQ. Effect of a high-protein, low-carbohydrate diet on blood glucose control in people with type 2 diabetes. Diabetes 2004;53:2375–2382.
75. Lara-Castro C, Garvey WT. Diet, insulin resistance, and obesity: zoning in on data for Atkins dieters living in South Beach. J Clin Endocrinol Metab 2004;89(9):4197–4205.
76. Moran L, et al. Short-term meal replacements followed by dietary macronutrient restriction enhance weight loss in polycystic ovary syndrome. Am J Clin Nutr 2006;84(1):77–87.
77. Hung T, et al. Fat versus carbohydrate in insulin resistance, obesity, diabetes and cardiovascular disease. Curr Opin Clin Nutr Metab Care 2003;6:165–176.
78. Landin K, et al. Guar gum improves insulin sensitivity, blood lipids, blood pressure, and fibrinolysis in healthy men. Am J Clin Nutr 1992;56:1061–1065.
79. Vuksan V, et al. Beneficial effects of viscous dietary fiber from Konjac-mannan in subjects with the insulin resistance syndrome: results of a controlled metabolic trial. Diabetes Care 2000;23(1):9–14.
80. Wyatt H, et al. Long-term weight loss and breakfast in subjects in the National Weight Control Registry. Obes Res 2002;10:78–82.
81. Ceci F, et al. The effects of oral 5-hydroxytryptophan administration on feeding behavior in obese adult female subjects. J Neural Transm 1989;76(2):109–117.
82. Cangiano C, et al. Effects of oral 5-hydroxy-tryptophan on energy intake and macronutrient selection in non-insulin dependent diabetic patients. Int J Obes Relat Metab Disord 1998;22(7):648–654.
83. Cangiano C, et al. Eating behavior and adherence to dietary prescriptions in obese adult subjects treated with 5-hydroxytryptophan. Am J Clin Nutr 1992;56(5): 863–867.
84. Cangiano C, et al. Effects of 5-hydroxytryptophan on eating behavior and adherence to dietary prescriptions in obese adult subjects. Adv Exp Med Biol 1991;294: 591–593.
85. Venables M, et al. Green tea extract ingestion, fat oxidation, and glucose tolerance in healthy humans. Am J Clin Nutr 2008;87(3):778–784.
86. Chan C, et al. Effects of Chinese green tea on weight, and hormonal and biochemical profiles in obese patients with polycystic ovary syndrome—a randomized placebo-controlled trial. J Soc Gynecol Investig 2006;13(1):63–68.
87. Dulloo A, et al. Efficacy of a green tea extract rich in catechin polyphenols and caffeine in increasing 24-h energy expenditure and fat oxidation in humans. Am J Clin Nutr 1999;70(6):1040–1045.
88. Chantre P, Lairon D. Recent findings of green tea extract AR25 (Exolise) and its activity for the treatment of obesity. Phytomedicine 2002;9(1):3–8.
89. Dulloo A, et al. Green tea and thermogenesis: interactions between catechin-polyphenols, caffeine and sympathetic activity. Int J Obes Relat Metab Disord 2000;24: 252–258.
90. Kovacs E, et al. Effects of green tea on weight maintenance after body-weight loss. Br J Nutr 2004;91: 431–437.
91. Anderson R, Polansky M. Tea enhances insulin activity. J Agric Food Chem 2002;50:7182–7186.
92. Bruner B, et al. Effects of exercise and nutritional counseling in women with polycystic ovary syndrome. Appl Physiol Nutr Metab 2006;31(4):384–391.
93. Miller P, et al. Effect of short-term diet and exercise on hormone levels and menses in obese, infertile women. J Reprod Med 2008;53(5):315–319.
94. Telli M, et al. Serum leptin levels in patients with polycystic ovary syndrome. Fertil Steril 2002;77(5):932–935.
95. Takeuchi T, Tsutsumi O. Basal leptin concentrations in women with normal and dysfunctional ovarian conditions. Int J Gynecol Obstet 2000;69(2):127–133.
96. Mitchell M, et al. Adipokines: implications for female fertility and obesity. Reproduction 2005;130(5):583–597.
97. Finn P, et al. The stimulatory effect of leptin on the neuroendocrine reproductive axis of the monkey. Endocrinology 1998;139(11):4652–4662.
98. Cioffi J, et al. The expression of leptin and its receptors in pre-ovulatory human follicles. Mol Hum Reprod 1997;3(6):467–472.
99. Brannian J, Hansen K. Leptin and ovarian folliculogenesis: implications for ovulation induction and ART outcomes. Semin Reprod Med 2002;20(2):103–112.
100. Hirschberg A, et al. Impaired cholecystokinin secretion and disturbed appetite regulation in women with polycystic ovary syndrome. Gynecol Endocrinol 2004;19(2): 79–87.
101. Moran L, et al. Ghrelin and measures of satiety are altered in polycystic ovary syndrome but not differentially affected by diet composition. J Clin Endocrinol Metab 2004;89:3337–3344.
102. Spritzer P, et al. Leptin concentrations in hirsute women with polycystic ovary syndrome or idiopathic hirsutism: influence on LH and relationship with hormonal, metabolic, and anthropometric measurements. Hum Reprod 2001;16(7):1340–1346.

103. Moschos S, et al. Leptin and reproduction: a review. Fertil Steril 2002;77(3):433–444.
104. Nestler J, et al. Ovulatory and metabolic effects of D-chiro-inositol in the polycystic ovary syndrome. N Engl J Med 1999;340(17):1314–1320.
105. Iuorno M, et al. Effects of D-chiro-inositol in lean women with the polycystic ovary syndrome. Endocr Pract 2002;8(6):417–423.
106. Nestler J, et al. Role of inositolphosphoglycan mediators of insulin action in the polycystic ovary syndrome. J Pediatr Endocrinol Metab 2000;13(Suppl 5):1295–1298.
107. Gerli S, et al. Effects of inositol on ovarian function and metabolic factors in women with PCOS: a randomized double-blind placebo controlled trial. Eur Rev Med Pharmacol Sci 2003;7:151–159.
108. Mills S, Bone K. Principles and practice of phytotherapy. Edinburgh: Churchill Livingstone, 2000.
109. Brighenti F, et al. Effect of neutralized and native vinegar on blood glucose and acetate responses to a mixed meal in healthy subjects. Eur J Clin Nutr 1995;49(5):242–247.
110. Ostman E, et al. Vinegar supplementation lowers glucose and insulin responses and increases satiety after a bread meal in healthy subjects. Eur J Clin Nutr 2005;59(9):983–988.
111. Johnston C, et al. Vinegar improves insulin sensitivity to a high-carbohydrate meal in subjects with insulin resistance or type 2 diabetes. Diabetes Care 2004;27(1):281–282.
112. Liljeberg H, Björck I. Delayed gastric emptying rate may explain improved glycaemia in healthy subjects to a starchy meal with added vinegar. Eur J Clin Nutr 1998;52(5):368–371.
113. Neef H, et al. Hypoglycaemic activity of selected European plants. Phytother Res 1995;6(2):45–48.
114. Neef H, et al. Inhibitory effects of Galega officinalis on glucose transport across monolayers of human intestinal epithelial cells (Caco-2). Pharm Pharmacol Lett 1996;6(2):86–89.
115. Muller H, Reinwein H. Pharmacology of galegin. Arch Expll Path Pharm 1927;125:212–228.
116. Yeh G, et al. Systematic review of herbs and dietary supplements for glycemic control in diabetes. Diabetes Care 2003;26:1277–1294.
117. Lucidi R, et al. Effect of chromium supplementation on insulin resistance and ovarian and menstrual cyclicity in women with polycystic ovary syndrome. Fertil Steril 2005;84(6):1755–1777.
118. Lydic M, et al. Chromium picolinate improves insulin sensitivity in obese subjects with polycystic ovary syndrome. Fertil Steril 2006;86(1):243–246.
119. la Marca A, et al. Insulin-lowering treatment reduces aromatase activity in response to follicle-stimulating hormone in women with polycystic ovary syndrome. Fertil Steril 2002;78(6):1234–1239.
120. Grant P. A randomised clinical trial of the effects of spearmint herbal tea on hirsutism in females with polycystic ovarian syndrome. Endoce Abst 2008;15:P282.
121. Prager N, et al. A randomized, double-blind, placebo-controlled trial to determine the effectiveness of botanically derived inhibitors of 5-alpha-reductase in the treatment of androgenetic alopecia. J Altern Complement Med 2002;8(2):143–152.
122. Morganti P, et al. Effect of gelatine-cystine and Serenoa repens extract on free radical levels and hair growth. J Appl Cosmetol 1998;16:57–64.
123. Stamatiadis D, et al. Inhibition of 5 alpha-reductase activity in human skin by zinc and azelaic acid. Br J Dermatol 1988;119:627–632.
124. Stener-Victorin E, et al. Acupuncture in polycystic ovary syndrome: current experimental and clinical evidence. J Neuroendocrinol 2008;20(3):290–298.
125. Ushiroyama T, et al. Effects of switching to wen-jing-tang (unkei-to) from preceding herbal preparations selected by eight-principle pattern identification on endocrinological status and ovulatory induction in women with polycystic ovary syndrome. Am J Chin Med 2006;34(2):177–187.
126. Ushiroyama T, et al. Effects of unkei-to, an herbal medicine, on endocrine function and ovulation in women with high basal levels of luteinizing hormone secretion. J Reprod Med 2001;46(5):451–456.
127. Yu Ng E, Ho P. Polycystic ovary syndrome in Asian women. Semin Reprod Med 2008;26(1):14–21.
128. Huang S, Chen A. Traditional Chinese medicine and infertility. Curr Opin Obstet Gynecol 2008;20(3):211–215.
129. Cardigno P. Homoeopathy for the treatment of menstrual irregularities: a case series. Homeopathy 2009;98(2):97–106.
130. Janssen O, et al. Mood and sexual function in polycystic ovary syndrome. Semin Reprod Med 2008;26(1):45–52.
131. Kasim-Karakas S, et al. Relation of nutrients and hormones in polycystic ovary syndrome. Am J Clin Nutr 2007;85(3):688–694.

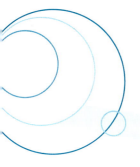

21
Menopause

Jon Wardle
ND, MPH

OVERVIEW

Menopause represents the natural transition from fertility to age-related non-fertility. The term 'menopause' specifically means the cessation of menstruation, and most often occurs between the ages of 45 and 55 years, with the average age for the last period being 51 years.

All healthy women will transition from a reproductive (premenopausal) period—marked by regular ovulation and cyclic menstrual bleeding—to a postmenopausal period marked by amenorrhoea. The onset of the menopausal transition is marked by changes in the menstrual cycle and in the duration or amount of menstrual flow (see Table 21.1). Subsequently, cycles are missed, but the pattern is often erratic early in the menopausal transition. Therefore the menopause is defined retrospectively after 12 months of continued amenorrhoea.

The term 'perimenopause' is most often used to describe the time leading up to and directly following menopause.[2] During perimenopause, hormone levels fluctuate and women may experience a variety of symptoms including vasomotor symptoms (hot flushes and night sweats), vulvovaginal atrophy, emotional fluctuations and cognitive decline (memory problems). Some women experience very little in the way of these symptoms; for others this time is particularly debilitating. Low oestrogen levels postmenopause also increase the risk of a number of other physical conditions including osteoporosis and cardiovascular disease. The various symptoms of the menopausal transition are associated with a variety of physiological changes and the responses to these changes. Figure 21.1 shows the symptoms associated with changes in hormone levels.

In the postmenopausal phase FSH rise to levels 10–15 times the level that can be expected during the follicular phase of a reproductive cycle, while LH levels increase to around three times that experienced during menstruation. The ovaries do continue to excrete minimal amounts of oestrogens, and continue to excrete significant amounts of androgens.[2]

It should also be noted that individual women will experience the menopausal transition differently. The prevalence rates of the main symptoms can vary greatly across the different stages of menopause (see Figure 21.2).[4]

Table 21.1 The stages of menopause

STAGES	−5	−4	−3	−2	−1	0		1
Terminology	Reproductive			Menopausal transition		Postmenopausal		
	Early	Peak	Late	Early	Late	Early		Late
				Perimenopause				
Duration	Variable			Variable		A	B	Until demise
						1 year	4 years	
Menstrual cycles	Variable to regular	Regular		Variable cycle length (> 7 days different from normal)	≥ 2 skipped cycles and an interval of amenorrhoea (> 60 days)	Amenorrhoea for 12 months	None	
Endocrine	Normal FSH	↑FSH		↑FSH		↑FSH		

Source: Adapted from Soules et al.[1]

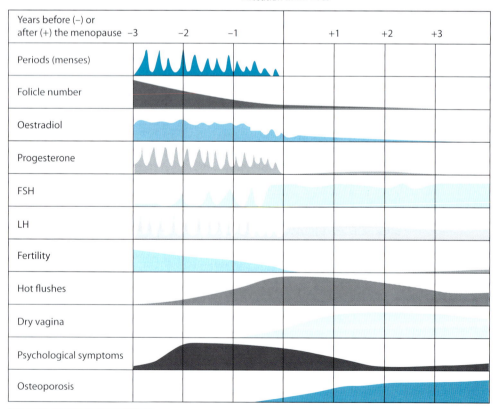

Figure 21.1 Menopausal symptom and hormone changes over time[3]

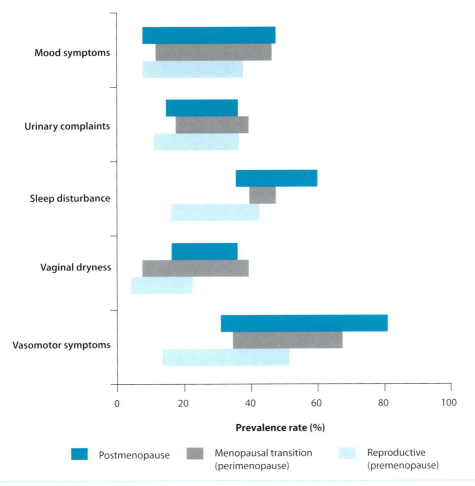

Figure 21.2 Prevalence rates of the main symptoms of menopause[4]

CONVENTIONAL TREATMENT

Conventional practitioners tend to underestimate the effects of perimenopausal symptoms on their patients.[5] However, fewer than 25% of women experience a (relatively) symptom-free menopause and over 25% of women experience debilitating symptoms.[6] Many women turn to conventional practitioners for explanation and reassurance rather than treatment.[3]

Much controversy has raged during recent years over what is termed the 'medicalisation' of naturally occurring life stages, of which the most publicised is menopause. Conventional practice has often viewed menopause as a condition of oestrogen deficiency, and treatment is based on the use of supplemental hormones, commonly referred to as hormone therapy (HT).

There is much conjecture and controversy surrounding the use of HT in menopause. There are definite benefits to using HT. HT is effective for vasomotor symptoms, vulvovaginal atrophy symptoms, osteoporosis-related fracture prevention, and benefits cardiovascular and central nervous systems.[7] However, continued use of HT can increase the risk for venous thromboembolism and increases the risk of developing breast cancer.[7]

BIOIDENTICAL HORMONE THERAPY: SAFER, MORE EFFECTIVE?

Most of the data suggesting risks associated with hormone therapy have been conducted using equine or synthetic hormones, and there is little evidence of the safety or efficacy of bioidentical or natural hormones. Theoretically they are suggested to proffer advantage in that they are more closely aligned with the innate hormones seen in the body and can be individually tailored (when compounded), but they should not automatically be considered the safer option. Both the Therapeutic Goods Administration of Australia and the Federal Drug Administration in the United States of America consider the adverse effects of HT as reported to be a 'class effect'—that is, that bioidentical hormones can be considered to have the same risks and benefits as conventional HT. In fact most conventional HT used in Australia already uses oestradiol and other forms considered to be bioidentical. However, progestin is known to have very different, often contradictory, physiological actions to natural progesterone in many women. Regardless, focusing solely on direct hormone replacement does not address the underlying causes of the symptoms experienced by perimenopausal women and therefore when used alone may not be reflective of naturopathic or holistic best practice. While HT use is ultimately a matter for discussion between physician and patient, it should form only part of the treatment strategy in the naturopathic management of menopause.

HT may be recommended in certain circumstances—specifically, distressing symptoms or significant osteoporosis.[7] Longer-term use of HT is generally considered a matter for discussion between the physician and the patient, with risks taken into account in addition to potential benefit to bone health and quality of life. Generally, long-term use is discouraged and physicians are encouraged to use lower therapeutic doses.

Various forms of oestrogen have been used for many years as a hormonal supplement to treat menopausal symptoms and are generally thought to be the most effective treatment for vasomotor symptoms. Oestrogen is therefore no longer recommended for prevention of chronic conditions, although it is effective and approved for osteoporosis prevention.[4] Women with an intact uterus are usually prescribed the 'opposed' regimen (when oestrogen is combined with a progestin to avoid the development of endometrial hyperplasia and endometrial cancer). Testosterone may also be given to women. Examples of commonly used HT in Australia are listed in Tables 21.2 and 21.3.

However, much conventional medical treatment of menopause is comprised of educational and lifestyle management of symptoms. Several other classes of prescription medications are also used in the treatment of menopausal symptoms, including antihypertensive medications such as clonidine for hot flushes and various antidepressants or anxiolytics for psychological symptoms. Much of this research has come from the treatment of menopausal women with breast cancer, in whom hormone therapy is contraindicated.

RISK FACTORS

Although much focus tends to be drawn towards the effect that HT can have on increasing breast cancer risk, other modifiable lifestyle factors such as little exercise, smoking, postmenopausal weight gain and high alcohol consumption may increase the risk of not only breast cancer but other menopausal symptoms as well.[8]

Table 21.2 Oestrogens often used in menopause[3]

GENERIC NAME	PROPRIETARY NAME/S (EXAMPLES)	DAILY DOSE RANGE	USUAL DAILY PROTECTIVE DOSE
Oral			
Conjugated equine oestrogen	Premarin	0.3–2.5 mg	0.625 mg
Oestradiol valerate	Progynova	1.0–4.0 mg	2.0 mg
Oestriol	Ovestin	1.0–4.0 mg	2.0 mg
Piperazine oestrone sulphate	Ogen	0.625–5 mg	1.25 mg
Implants			
Oestradiol	Oestradiol implants	20–100 mg	50 mg
Skin patch			
Oestradiol	Various	25–100 µg every 3½ to 7 days	50 µg
Topical gel			
Oestradiol 0.1%	Sandrena	0.5–1.5 mg	1 mg
Nasal spray			
Oestradiol	Aerodiol	150–600 µg	300 µg
Vaginal preparations			
Creams			
Oestriol 1 mg/g	Ovestin	0.5 g	0.5 g
Pessaries			
Oestradiol	Vagifem	25 µg	1 pessary (25 µg)
Oestriol	Ovestin ovula	0.5 mg	0.5 mg

Note: Vaginal therapy is usually given continuously for 2 weeks, then twice weekly.

Table 21.3 Progestogens often used in menopause

GENERIC NAME	DAILY DOSE RANGE	USUAL DAILY PROTECTIVE DOSE
Dydrogesterone	10–20 mg	10 mg
Medroxyprogesterone acetate	2.5–20 mg	10 mg
Norethisterone	1.25–5 mg	2.5 mg

Risk factors for severity of symptoms during perimenopause include genetics (symptoms experienced by the mother may give a guide), body mass index (BMI)—women with a higher BMI may experience a lower level of perimenopause symptoms due to the production of oestrogen by aromatase in adipose tissue (see Chapter 19 on endometriosis).

The duration of symptoms appears independent of HT but is less in those groups with higher physical activity.[9] Other lifestyle factors, such as increased alcohol and caffeine use and smoking, are also associated with worsened menopausal symptoms.[10]

KEY TREATMENT PROTOCOLS

Perimenopause is a natural stage of life and not a disease or a disorder. Therefore it does not automatically require any kind of medical intervention or treatment. However, this natural transition is not always a smooth one and in certain cases the physical, mental and emotional effects associated with perimenopause can be quite severe and may significantly disrupt the lives of women experiencing them. Naturopathic treatment therefore focuses on reducing these effects and ensuring quality of life throughout this transition. Various lifestyle

NATUROPATHIC TREATMENT AIMS
- Improve quality of life.
- Reduce symptoms (hot flushes, psychological symptoms and fatigue).
- Maintain ideal weight and health parameters (for cardiovascular and bone health).
- Manage stress.
- Address sexual health.
- Modify diet to improve symptoms and to reduce osteoporosis and cardiovascular risk.

and dietary habits can have significant effects on the severity of menopausal symptoms, so treatment should otherwise focus on ensuring optimal health.

Naturopathic treatment focuses on general improvement in physiology as opposed to correction or counteracting the effects of menopause with oestrogen supplementation. Many clinicians make the assumption that only climacteric symptoms are of concern in menopausal patients. As naturopathic treatment of a perimenopausal patient is focused on supportive care throughout the process, rather than correction of an aetiological or pathological condition, a broader clinical enquiry that extends beyond symptoms relating to oestrogen deficiency needs to be undertaken. Enquiries need to be made about mental state—anger and irritability, depression, moodiness, loss of self-esteem and sleeping difficulties. Sexual function and urinary function also need to be explored in depth.

Women undergoing the menopause transition turn to complementary medicines not only to seek effective treatment but also to gain greater control over their symptoms.[17] It is therefore essential that a strong participatory relationship is encouraged during treatment and that the naturopath does not fall into the habit of product-prescribing only.

When looking at the literature there seems to be little relation to gross product sales (the most commonly sold complementary therapies for menopause) and specific clinical effectiveness. However, these therapies may be working on broader improvements or act on a psychosomatic level by offering the patients the opportunity to take control of their condition. For example, while acupuncture does not seem to have specific effects on menopausal symptoms such as hot flushes[18] it does seem to offer improvements to quality of life scores in perimenopausal women overall.[19]

For example, treatment with a combination *Hypericum perforatum* and *Cimicifuga racemosa* product for 16 weeks resulted in a 50% reduction in Menopause Rating Scale (MRS) scores, with a 41.8% reduction in the Hamilton Depression Rating Scale.[20]

OESTROGEN-LIKE COMPOUNDS AND OESTROGEN RECEPTOR ACTIVITY

Many compounds—both natural and synthetic—may mimic endogenous sex hormones.[11–13] *Phytoestrogens* may bind to and activate these oestrogen receptor sites. Given the use of hormone replacement therapy in conventional treatment, these compounds are gaining popularity amongst both the public and practitioners for relieving menopausal symptoms.

For example, the phytoestrogenic isoflavones found in *Trifolium pratense* and soy are thought to have beneficial effects on cognitive abilities, bone mineral density and plasma lipid concentrations in menopausal women.[14] Phytoestrogenic activity may also be utilised in traditional Chinese medicine. *Astragalus membranaceus* and *Scutellaria baicalensis* are traditionally used in the treatment of menopausal symptoms in traditional Chinese medicine and exert oestrogenic activity in vivo.[15]

Dietary intake of phytoestrogens and an increased consumption of whole-grain foods may also be associated with a reduction in vasomotor symptoms.[16]

Many compounds exerting oestrogenic activity will be discussed in relation to symptoms. Many have not actually been studied extensively for menopausal symptoms, but phytoestrogens are discussed in more detail in Chapter 19 on endometriosis.

Although *C. racemosa* was effective in treating neurovegetative symptoms of depression in menopausal women, combination treatment was more effective than *C. racemosa* treatment alone.[21] These changes seem more significant than the effects on vasomotor symptoms alone. And while *H. perforatum* does not seem to exert a significant effect on hot flush symptoms, it does proffer significant improvement on quality of life scales due to its effect on other symptoms associated with menopause and should therefore also be considered.[22] *C. racemosa* also has positive effects on overall quality of life scales and other broader menopause rating scales when used alone in addition to its effects on individual symptoms.[23] Several relaxation therapies have also proven to be effective in alleviating or reducing a number of perimenopausal symptoms, rather than having specific outcomes.

Major symptoms
Hot flushes
Exercise
Because exercise has demonstrated effects on sex steroids, it may moderate at least the severity, if not the frequency, of hot flushes.[9,24–26] One epidemiological study found that women who belonged to a gymnasium club reported lower incidence of hot flushes than those who were not, although their individual exercise regimens were unreported.[27] However, studies on exercise, while generally demonstrating reduced severity and incidence of hot flushes, suggest it has had the greatest effect on quality of life scores.

Herbal medicine
A 2007 systematic review of 17 trials of which 11 could be included showed a demonstrated effect of **Trifolium pratense** in reducing hot flush symptoms in menopause.[34] A 2005 review of trials found 12 clinical trials of **C. racemosa** in vasomotor symptoms,

BLACK COHOSH SAFETY

Although concerns relating to the hepatotoxicity of *Cimicifuga racemosa* have been raised, systematic reviews have suggested it can be generally thought to be a safe medicine, with the main side effects being mild and reversible, and no direct causal link to *Cimicifuga* was found in cases of severe hepatotoxicity.[28–31] In the most recent trial, long-term supplementation of *Cimicifuga* for a period of 1 year was found to have no effects on hepatic blood flow or liver function.[32] However, an association does exist as hepatotoxicity has occurred in several people taking supplements containing *Cimicifuga*. This is thought to be related to issues of product quality, concomitant medications or individual genetic susceptibility. Although the specific mechanism relating to hepatotoxicity associated with *Cimicifuga* use is unknown, one theory gaining credence is an immunologic reaction to triterpene glycosides in the plant in susceptible individuals, rather than the direct result of inherent toxicity.[33] Therefore these issues should be considered when advising or treating patients using these therapies, as they should for any other pharmacological intervention.

all but one of which demonstrated benefit,[35] and a later non-specific review found significant benefit also.[36]

C. racemosa may act through a number of pathways independent of its activity as a phytoestrogen. Recent evidence suggests that it may have an effect on opiate receptors.[37] *Cimicifuga* extract has also been demonstrated to exert dopaminergic activity in vitro.[38] This may in part also explain the effects of *Cimicifuga* in menopause as dopaminergic drugs are often used to treat menopausal symptoms such as hot flushes. Some studies have suggested that *Cimicifuga* has an equipotent effect to oestrogen[39] although this does not seem reflective of the entirety of the data.[40,41] It should be noted, however, that significant heterogeneity exists in the results for differing formulations, suggesting that quality issues need to be considered before prescribing.

Angelica sinensis and ***Matricaria recutita*** in combination has been demonstrated to reduce hot flushes and improve sleep in menopausal women,[42] but other trials have failed to demonstrate these results when *Angelica sinensis* was used alone.[43,44]

Humulus lupulus supplementation over 12 weeks was found to reduce discomforting symptoms of menopause, particularly hot flushes, even at low doses.[45] This is thought to be due to the oestrogenic nature of *H. lupulus*.[46] *Salvia officinalis* was also demonstrated to improve symptoms of hot flushes and nights sweats in perimenopausal women.[47]

Psychosocial interventions

Several trials have shown that relaxation training can have positive effects on hot flush symptoms.[48–51] These include biofeedback, breathing exercises and meditation. Yoga may also be beneficial in reducing menopausal symptoms exacerbated by mental stress.[52,53]

Psychological interventions

Panax ginseng has been demonstrated to improve psychological symptoms, particularly fatigue, insomnia and depression, in menopausal women.[54]

In menopausal women with psychological and psychosomatic symptoms, sole therapy using ***Hypericum perforatum*** demonstrated significant improvement

(76.4% self-evaluation and 79.2% physician evaluation), including improved sexual wellbeing.[55]

Piper methysticum as an adjuvant treatment has been demonstrated to reduce anxiety in perimenopausal women.[56] It may also be useful in treating sleep disorders not associated with vasomotor symptoms that are often experienced by perimenopausal women (see Chapter 14 on insomnia).

Sexual function and libido

Women undergoing the perimenopausal transition often experience changes in libido or dyspareunia which can be influenced by a number of physiological or psychosocial ways. Hormone changes may influence sexual function in a number of ways. Low levels of oestrogens and androgens seem to be directly related to libido, as do low levels of testosterone.[57] Physical changes enacted by alterations in hormone levels—for example, vaginal dryness associated with lower levels of oestrogen—will have a significant negative effect on sexual response. Lack of lubrication can result in soreness and tenderness, and ultimately less enjoyment during sexual encounters for these reasons. Anticipation of painful sex due to lack of lubrication after a negative experience may further decrease desire. Patients need to be counselled adequately on the practical implications of the menopausal transition as many women may not have previously needed to apply measures such as endogenous lubrication. Oestrogens also have a vasodilatory effect that can result in increased blood flow in vaginal, clitoral and urethral areas; this may reduce during menopause, and loss of oestrogen is also associated with relaxation of vaginal tissue and muscle tone in genital areas. Encouraging circulation and tone in these areas—for example, through **pelvic floor exercises** or more general regimens such as exercise, yoga or tai chi—may also be useful.

Physical changes alone are not solely responsible for the negative effects of the perimenopausal transition on sexual function and libido. Psychological changes such as depression, anxiety and low self-esteem can all affect sexual desire and enjoyment, as can many of the medicines prescribed for these conditions. Conversely, the effects of menopausal changes on a woman's sex life can also precipitate psychological changes. The social construct of menopause in modern society can also have a deleterious effect in this regard. Menopause in Western societies is often viewed negatively, particularly in relation to the loss of femininity. This is in stark contrast to many traditional cultures, who often view the transition as a positive one that affords them respect as elders and relief from child-bearing. Patients need to be counselled appropriately throughout this period, encouraged to explore their femininity and sexual selves and reminded that these aspects of themselves need not diminish once menstruation ceases. One study has shown that while yoga therapy did not increase general self-esteem, it was significant in improving esteem relating to perceived sexual attractiveness.[58]

Many **herbal medicines** have been used to increase libido. *Asparagus racemosus* is colloquially referred to as 'she with one thousand husbands' in the Ayurvedic tradition in reference to its effects on sexual function and has demonstrated positive results in animal studies, but is yet to be tested through human trials.[59] This situation is also true of other traditionally used aphrodisiac herbs such as *Turnera diffusa* and *Tribulus terrestris*. A product containing *Panax ginseng*, *Turnera diffusa*, *Ginkgo biloba* and l-arginine has been found to significantly increase libido in women at all stages of the menopausal transition compared to placebo in two small trials.[60,61]

Treating the psychological symptoms associated with menopause may also improve libido. *Hypericum perforatum*—a herb commonly used to treat the psychosocial problems associated with menopause—was found to improve libido when used to treat seasonal affective disorder[62] and improved sexual wellbeing in 80% of perimenopausal women when prescribed for psychosocial symptoms.[55] *Trigonella foenum-graecum* has been used for postmenopausal vaginal dryness in the North American naturopathic tradition.[63]

Vaginal atrophy and incontinence

After menopause the vaginal lining may thin due to lower oestrogen levels. This may result in painful intercourse and a greater susceptibility to vaginal infections. Regular intercourse may be beneficial as it increases blood flow to the genitalia, but adequate lubrication is required—natural or supplemental. Naturopathic treatment options for recurrent bladder infections are covered in Chapter 27.

Vitamin D may have a role in reducing vaginal atrophy. Supplementation with vitamin D has reduced vaginal atrophy in one small trial.[64]

Incontinence incidence may increase in postmenopausal women. Many women may resign themselves to this being a normal part of the ageing process, but there are several therapeutic options available. **Pelvic floor exercises** may reduce the incidence of incontinence in postmenopausal women and improve quality of life.[65] Increased **physical exercise** more generally may also be beneficial in reducing the incidence or severity of urinary incontinence.[66]

Urinary tract infections

Approximately 15% of menopausal women will experience frequent bladder infections.[2] General recommendations for urinary tract infections are discussed in Chapter 27 on urinary tract infection, but there are several factors to take into consideration when treating urinary tract infections in perimenopausal women, such as decreased acidity of the urine and loss of bladder elasticity, due to lower oestrogen levels and the fact that urinary tract infections are often symptomless during the menopause.

Long-term considerations

Although much focus tends to be drawn towards the association between hormone therapy and increasing breast cancer, other modifiable lifestyle factors such as little exercise, smoking, postmenopausal weight gain and high alcohol consumption have similar rates of increased risk of breast cancer.[8] And although fat intake alone is not associated with

CAM AND OSTEOPOROSIS

Diet and lifestyle advice
- Diet high in calcium-rich foods, leafy vegetables, some phytoestrogens, low in refined carbohydrates, reduced acidic foods
- Adequate sunshine
- Weight-bearing exercise
- Avoidance of smoking
- Reduction of alcohol

Possible prescription
- Calcium and magnesium
- Vitamins K and D
- Omega-3 fats
- Trace elements: silica, boron
- Bioflavonoids
- Folate, B6, B12

increased risk of breast cancer, attention to this lifestyle factor can help to improve the cardiovascular outcomes usually associated with the menopausal transition.[67] Attention needs to be paid to the long-term consequences of the menopausal transition as well as short-term symptomatic treatment.

Dietary modification is an essential part of treating the perimenopausal patient. Not only are long-term risks such as osteoporosis and cardiovascular health significantly affected by dietary intakes, but dietary factors also have important effects on symptom severity during the menopausal transition. No consultation is complete without investigation of the dietary component.

Osteoporosis

In a clinical setting osteoporosis is often addressed in the context of menopausal treatment because it is found in postmenopausal women and can be largely prevented by correcting oestrogen deficiency. Approximately 30% of postmenopausal women are estimated to have osteoporosis.[68] The hypo-oestrogenic state leads to loss of bone density in postmenopausal women by activation of the bone remodelling units with an excess of bone resorption compared to bone formation.[69]

Adequate dietary intakes are necessary for prevention and treatment of osteoporosis.

Another dietary intervention that may be beneficial for osteoporosis in postmenopausal women is **omega-3 fatty acids**. Several human and animal studies have shown significant decreases in bone resorption and a protective effect on bone with omega-3 fatty acids.[70–72]

Adequate **calcium** and **vitamin D** consumption are essential in the treatment of osteoporosis. It is generally recommended that 1500 mg of calcium and 800 IU per day of vitamin D are recommended for postmenopausal women.[7] Dietary sources of calcium are listed in Table 21.4. However, dietary intake of calcium alone may not be sufficient, particularly in women who have undergone early menopause.[73] Sunlight exposure of 5–10 minutes per day may be required, particularly considering that older people may synthesise vitamin D less well over time. Supplementation of both calcium and vitamin D may be necessary. However, large studies such as the Women's Health Initiative have shown that reliance on supplementation can be fraught, as compliance can be low—only 59% of women were taking more than 80% of their recommended supplementation towards the study's end.[74] Dietary modification should therefore form the basis of treatment. More dietary recommendations for bone health can be found in Chapter 22 on osteoarthritis.

Phytoestrogenic therapy may offer a limited protective role.[75] Considering that HT and SORM therapy are both used to prevent the effects of osteoporosis, this is worth exploring. Increased soy consumption may inhibit bone resorption and stimulate bone formation[76,77] and population studies indicate that the incidence of osteoporosis is lower in countries with higher soy consumption.[14]

Regular exercise can increase bone density in postmenopausal women.[68] However, high impact exercise may be counterproductive as more severe forms of exercise may result in micro-damage, increasing the risk of fracture.[78] Regular tai chi exercise may improve bone density scores and offer protection against fracture in postmenopausal women.[79] Further benefits of specific exercises are discussed in Chapter 22 on osteoarthritis.

Cardiovascular health

Women are offered a higher degree of protection against cardiovascular disease before the menopause due to higher oestrogen levels. However, reductions in oestrogen levels postmenopause result in women having the same incidence of cardiovascular disease

Table 21.4 Calcium content of foods[4]

FOOD	AMOUNT	CALCIUM CONTENT (MG)
Yoghurt	200 g (1 small tub)	520
Calcium-enriched milk	250 mL (1 cup)	475
Skim milk	250 mL (1 cup)	400
Tahini	20 g	310
Full fat milk	250 mL (1 cup)	300
Calcium-enriched soy milk	250 mL (1 cup)	290
Sardines	5 whole	286
Cheddar cheese	30 g (1 slice)	232
Parmesan cheese	20 g	230
Salmon (tinned)	½ cup with bones	220
Prawns	1 cup	132
Mussels	6 whole	120
Dried figs	3	108
Tofu	80 g	96
Ice-cream	60 g (2 scoops)	90
Soy beans, chickpeas or kidney beans	½ cup	70
Dried apricots	10 halves	42
Silverbeet or spinach	½ cup	38
Oranges	1 whole	35
Broccoli	1 cup	25

as men by the age of 70 years.[80] Despite this protective mechanism it is still estimated that 94% of adverse cardiovascular risk in women is associated with modifiable risk factors such as type II diabetes, hypertension, diet, stress, smoking and obesity.[81] Therefore women who have previously not had to consider cardiovascular health implications may need to investigate this issue in more depth (see the section on the cardiovascular system).

Exercise
As well as the benefits of regular exercise in treating specific menopausal symptoms such as hot flushes previously outlined, exercise confers a number of other benefits in the peri-menopausal patient. These benefits include decreased bone loss, improved circulation,

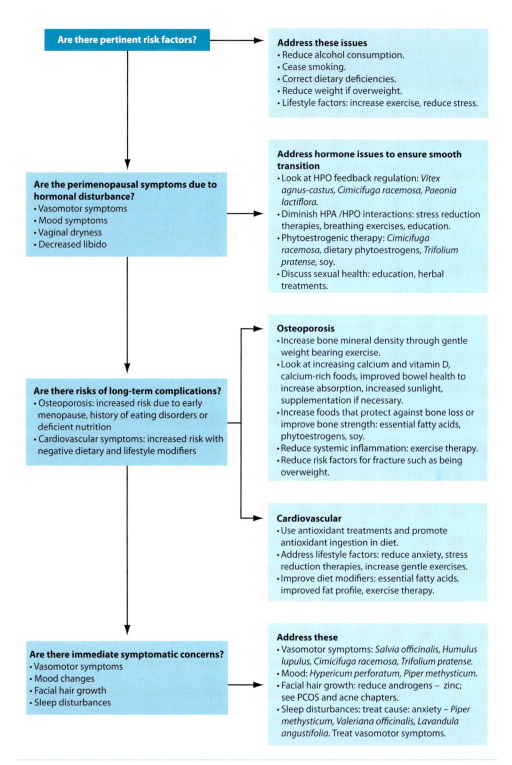

Are there pertinent risk factors?

Address these issues
- Reduce alcohol consumption.
- Cease smoking.
- Correct dietary deficiencies.
- Reduce weight if overweight.
- Lifestyle factors: increase exercise, reduce stress.

Are the perimenopausal symptoms due to hormonal disturbance?
- Vasomotor symptoms
- Mood symptoms
- Vaginal dryness
- Decreased libido

Address hormone issues to ensure smooth transition
- Look at HPO feedback regulation: *Vitex agnus-castus, Cimicifuga racemosa, Paeonia lactiflora.*
- Diminish HPA /HPO interactions: stress reduction therapies, breathing exercises, education.
- Phytoestrogenic therapy: *Cimicifuga racemosa*, dietary phytoestrogens, *Trifolium pratense,* soy.
- Discuss sexual health: education, herbal treatments.

Osteoporosis
- Increase bone mineral density through gentle weight bearing exercise.
- Look at increasing calcium and vitamin D, calcium-rich foods, improved bowel health to increase absorption, increased sunlight, supplementation if necessary.
- Increase foods that protect against bone loss or improve bone strength: essential fatty acids, phytoestrogens, soy.
- Reduce systemic inflammation: exercise therapy.
- Reduce risk factors for fracture such as being overweight.

Are there risks of long-term complications?
- Osteoporosis: increased risk due to early menopause, history of eating disorders or deficient nutrition
- Cardiovascular symptoms: increased risk with negative dietary and lifestyle modifiers

Cardiovascular
- Use antioxidant treatments and promote antioxidant ingestion in diet.
- Address lifestyle factors: reduce anxiety, stress reduction therapies, increase gentle exercises.
- Improve diet modifiers: essential fatty acids, improved fat profile, exercise therapy.

Are there immediate symptomatic concerns?
- Vasomotor symptoms
- Mood changes
- Facial hair growth
- Sleep disturbances

Address these
- Vasomotor symptoms: *Salvia officinalis, Humulus lupulus, Cimicifuga racemosa, Trifolium pratense.*
- Mood: *Hypericum perforatum, Piper methysticum.*
- Facial hair growth: reduce androgens – zinc; see PCOS and acne chapters.
- Sleep disturbances: treat cause: anxiety – *Piper methysticum, Valeriana officinalis, Lavandula angustifolia.* Treat vasomotor symptoms.

Figure 21.3 Naturopathic treatment decision tree—menopause

cardiovascular function and risk profile, improved mental wellbeing and stress reduction and increased endurance and energy. Perimenopausal patients usually comprise an older demographic than the typical patient, and encouraging healthy behaviours can ensure healthy ageing and protection against many age-related conditions.

As menopause is not a defined medical condition but rather a collection of symptoms associated with a transitional stage through life, many of the treatments are covered in other relevant chapters. Table 21.5 focuses on vasomotor symptoms.

INTEGRATIVE MEDICAL CONSIDERATIONS

Acupuncture

Acupuncture does offer specific effects on menopausal symptoms such as hot flushes,[24,82] but demonstrates significantly greater improvements to quality of life scores in perimenopausal women more broadly.[19] Traditional Chinese medicine has a long history of treating menopausal symptoms and, typically, acupuncture would not be used alone.[83] However, to be effective these treatments need to be prescribed according to traditional Chinese medicine theory.

Homoeopathy

Homoeopathic treatment has shown encouraging results, but requires further research. Homoeopathy has been successful in treating oestrogen withdrawal symptoms in women with breast cancer.[84] As the symptoms treated in menopausal patients can vary substantially, individualised treatment is advised.

Osteopathy

One small trial of osteopathic manipulations has demonstrated improvements in menopausal symptoms.[85]

Case Study

A 51-year-old female patient presents to your clinic with **night sweats, mild hot flushing** during the day, **abdominal bloating** and **emotional swings**. Her menstrual cycle was previously 28 days with mild cramping and light flow. In the last 12 months her **menstrual flow has slowly become heavier with clotting and cramping**, and her **cycle has slowly shortened** to approximately 19–21 days. She is **irritable** and **tired**. Her **sleep is poor** as she wakes frequently during the night due to the intense sweating.

SUGGESTIVE SYMPTOMS

- Night sweats and hot flushing
- Mood swings
- Insomnia
- Irregular cycles

Example treatment

Prescription

She was prescribed the herbal tablet in the box on the right to be taken one tablet, once daily.

She was told to take three kava tablets half an hour before bed, and two tablets during periods of extreme irritability. She

Herbal prescription

- *Cimicifuga racemosa* tablet: equiv. to 42.25 mg rhizome 1 tablet 2 times per day
- *Piper methysticum* tablet: aqueous extract equiv. to 50 mg kava lactones 2 tablet 2 times per day

Table 21.5 Review of the major evidence

INTERVENTION	KEY LITERATURE	SUMMARY OF RESULTS	COMMENT
Cimicifuga racemosa	Geller & Studee 2005[35]	A 2005 review of trials found 12 clinical trials of *Cimicifuga racemosa* in vasomotor symptoms, all but one of which demonstrated benefit.	Although *Cimicifuga racemosa* has been demonstrated to improve vasomotor symptoms and menopause and quality of life scores, there are marked differences between various formulations, suggesting quality issues need to be appropriately explored when prescribing.
Trifolium pratense	Coon, Pittler & Ernst 2007[34]	A 2007 systematic review of 17 trials of which 11 could be included showed a demonstrated effect of *Trifolium pratense* in reducing hot flush symptoms in menopause.	Systematic review
Phytoestrogen diet	Murkies et al. 2008[16]	6-week RCT (*n* = 58). Groups randomised to diets supplemented with soy or whole-grain wheat flour. Significant reduction in vasomotor symptoms in soy (↓ 40%) and wheat groups (↓ 25%) (*p* ≤ 0.001). Significant reductions also observed in menopause scores and FSH levels.	More rapid reduction observed in soy group.
Acupuncture	Borud et al. 2009[82]	12-week RCT (*n* = 267). Groups randomised to receive either 10 acupuncture sessions and self-care advice or self-care advice only. Hot flush frequency was significantly reduced in acupuncture (↓ 5.8 per 24 hours) versus control group (↓ 3.7 per 24 hours—difference of 2.1). Hot flush intensity ↓ 3.2 in acupuncture group vs ↓ 1.8 in control group. Both results *p* ≤ 0.001.	Pragmatic trial which may be more reflective of clinical practice.
Humulus lupulus	Heyerick 2006[45]	12-week RCT (*n* = 67). Groups received either 100 mg or 250 mg *Humulus lupulus* extract. Hot flush frequency was significantly decreased at 6 weeks (*p* ≤ 0.023) but not 12 weeks (*p* ≤ 0.086). Results were not dose dependent, with lower dose achieving better results at both 6 and 12 weeks.	Although promising, this trial is hampered by its small study size. Given that it affirms traditional use, further studies are warranted.

(Continued)

Table 21.5 Review of the major evidence *(Continued)*

INTERVENTION	KEY LITERATURE	SUMMARY OF RESULTS	COMMENT
Salvia officinalis and *Medicago sativa*	De Leo et al. 1998[47]	Open trial (*n* = 30). 20 women had vasomotor symptoms completely disappear, 4 women significantly reduced symptoms and 6 women showed some reduction in symptom scores.	While affirming traditional use, this study suffers from poor design and further trials are necessary.

was counselled on sleep hygiene issues. She was also prescribed 1 tablespoon *Ulmus fulva* with 1 teaspoon of raw honey in warm water at night to encourage healthy intestinal bacterial populations, settle digestive dysfunction and reduce abdominal discomfort.

She was also given dietary advice, including increasing the consumption of lentils, chickpeas and ground flaxseed meal at least four times per week, and her bread was changed to a heavier soy and linseed from white bread. Her refined carbohydrates and dairy consumption were reduced. She was referred to a local tai chi class for relaxation and exercise. She was also required to do 30 minutes of moderately strenuous exercise at least every second day. These arrangements were to be reviewed after 1 month.

Most importantly, she was counselled about the process and given appropriate literature regarding the changes she could expect, and was reassured that she was undergoing a natural process.

Follow-up treatment

The patient had adhered to the dietary changes and followed all recommendations. She had begun tai chi classes and started walking 20 minutes every day. She was still experiencing symptoms, though they were reducing in intensity. She also indicated that she was no longer feeling fatigued. She was advised to continue dietary and lifestyle advice, along with the herbal formula until review in 1 month. She was also told to begin keeping a journal of symptoms—to enable her to understand the condition better and act as a stress outlet.

At the third treatment the patient had vastly improved menopausal symptoms though she was still experiencing variability. She was less irritable and depressed. The new focus of her treatment was aimed at general health improvement. She continued taking the herbal formula for a year after her initial treatment, after which time she felt she no longer needed it and stopped.

Expected outcomes and follow-up protocols

Perimenopause is a natural part of the lifecycle and therefore symptoms are not necessarily indicative of pathology. The changes will result in symptoms and these can be expected to continue for some time (1 year or more). Naturopathic treatments will not be instantaneous; for example, *C. racemosa* treatment will require 2 weeks to observe its effect and 3 months before optimal benefit can be observed.[59] Patients should be moved towards a general health program as soon as possible as this will ultimately improve their symptoms and lessen their duration.

KEY POINTS

- Menopause is a natural process and needs to be supported, not treated.
- Improving health parameters more generally will improve symptoms.
- Menopause is experienced differently by each woman; what works in many of your patients may not work in your current patient. Particular care in this regard needs to be undertaken when developing a herbal or nutritional prescription.
- Much of the distress of perimenopause is associated with stigma or confusion. Remind your patients that this is not 'the end' of anything and provide reassurance.
- Involve patients in treatment processes—encourage a shift towards self-care modalities.

Further reading

Coon J, et al. *Trifolium pratense* isoflavones in the treatment of menopausal hot flushes: a systematic review and meta-analysis. Phytomedicine 2007;14(2–3):153–159.

Geller S, Studee L. Botanical and dietary supplements for menopausal symptoms: what works, what does not. J Womens Health (Larchmt) 2005;14(7):634–649.

Hudson T. Women's encyclopedia of natural medicine. New York: McGraw-Hill, 2008.

Society of Obstetricians and Gynaecologists of Canada. Canada, menopause and osteoporosis update. J Obstet Gynaecol Can 2009;31(1):S27–S30.

References

1. Soules M, et al. Executive summary: Stages of Reproductive Aging Workshop (STRAW). Fertil Steril 2001;76:874–878.
2. Edmonds K, ed. Obstetrics and gynaecology. London: Blackwell, 2007.
3. Murtagh J. General practice. Sydney: McGraw-Hill, 2007.
4. Nelson H. Menopause. Lancet 2008;371(9614):760–770.
5. Ghali W, et al. Menopausal hormone therapy: physician awareness of patient attitudes. Am J Med 1997;(103):3–10.
6. Porter M, et al. A population based survey of women's experience of the menopause. Br J Obstet Gynaecol 2002;103:1025–1028.
7. Society of Obstetricians and Gynaecologists of Canada. Menopause and osteoporosis update. J Obstet Gynaecol Can 2009;31(1 Suppl 1):S27–S30.
8. Reeves G, et al. Million Women Study Collaboration. Cancer incidence and mortality in relation to body mass index in the Million Women Study: cohort study. BMJ 2007;335:1134.
9. Col N, et al. Duration of vasomotor symptoms in middle-aged women: a longitudinal study. Menopause 2009;16(3):453–457.
10. Greendale G, Gold E. Lifestyle factors: are they related to vasomotor symptoms and do they modify the effectiveness or side effects of hormone therapy? Am J Med 2005;118(12):148–154.
11. Rier S. The potential role of exposure to environmental toxicants in the pathophysiology of endometriosis. Ann N Y Acad Sci 2002;955:201–212.
12. Birnbaum L, Cummings A. Dioxins and endometriosis: a plausible hypothesis. Environ Health Persp 2002;110(1):15–21.
13. Foster W, Agarwhal S. Environmental contaminants and dietary factors in endometriosis. Ann N Y Acad Sci 2002;955:213–229.
14. Geller S, Studee L. Soy and red clover for mid-life and aging. Climacteric 2006;9(4):245–263.
15. Zhang C, et al. In vitro estrogenic activities of Chinese medicinal plants traditionally used for the management of menopausal symptoms. J Ethnopharmacol 2005;98(3):295–300.
16. Murkies A, et al. Dietary flour supplementation decreases post-menopausal hot flushes: effect of soy and wheat. Maturitas 2008;61(1–2):27–33.
17. Gollschewski S, et al. Women's perceptions and beliefs about the use of complementary and alternative medicines during menopause. Complement Ther Med 2008;16(3):163–168.
18. Lee M, et al. Acupuncture for treating menopausal hot flushes: a systematic review. Climacteric 2009;12(1):16–25.
19. Ailfhaily F, Ewies A. Acupuncture in managing menopausal symptoms: hope or mirage? Climacteric 2007;10(5):371–380.
20. Uebelhack R, et al. Black cohosh and St John's wort for climacteric complaints: a randomized trial. Obstet Gynecol 2006;107(2.1):247–255.
21. Briese V, et al. Black cohosh with or without St John's wort for symptom-specific climacteric treatment—results of a large-scale, controlled, observational study. Maturitas 2007;57(4):405–414.
22. Al-Akoum M, et al. Effects of *Hypericum perforatum* (St John's wort) on hot flashes and quality of life in perimenopausal women: a randomized pilot trial. Menopause 2009;16(2):307–314.
23. Mollá M, et al. *Cimicifuga racemosa* treatment and health related quality of life in post-menopausal Spanish women. Gynecol Endocrinol 2009;25(1):21–26.
24. Lindh-Astrand L, et al. Vasomotor symptoms and quality of life in previously sedentary postmenopausal women randomised to physical activity or estrogen therapy. Maturitas 2004;48(2):97–105.
25. Ivarsson T, et al. Physical exercise and vasomotor symptoms in postmenopausal women. Maturitas 1998;29(2):139–146.

26. Thurston R, et al. Physical activity and risk of vasomotor symptoms in women with and without a history of depression: results from the Harvard Study of Moods and Cycles. Menopause 2006;13:553–560.

27. Hammar M, et al. Does physical exercise influence the frequency of postmenopausal hot flushes? Acta Obstet Gynecol Scand 1990;69(5):409–412.

28. Huntley A, Ernst E. A systematic review of the safety of black cohosh. Menopause 2003;10(1):58–64.

29. Teschke R, Schwarzenboeck A. Suspected hepatotoxicity by *Cimicifugae racemosae* rhizoma (black cohosh, root): critical analysis and structured causality assessment. Phytomedicine 2009;16(1):72–84.

30. Firenzuoli F, et al. Black cohosh hepatic safety: follow-up of 107 patients consuming a special Cimicifuga racemosa rhizome herbal extract and review of literature. Evidence Based Complement Altern Med 2008: doi:10.1093/ecam/nen009.

31. Borrelli F, Ernst E. Black cohosh (*Cimicifuga racemosa*): a systematic review of adverse events. Am J Obstet Gynecol 2008;199(5):455–466.

32. Nasr A, Nafeh H. Influence of black cohosh (*Cimicifuga racemosa*) use by postmenopausal women on total hepatic perfusion and liver functions. Fertil Steril 2009; 92(5):1780–1782.

33. Chitturi S, Farrell G. Hepatotoxic slimming aids and other herbal hepatotoxins. J Gastrolenterol Hepatol 2008;23:366–373.

34. Coon J, et al. Trifolium pratense isoflavones in the treatment of menopausal hot flushes: a systematic review and meta-analysis. Phytomedicine 2007;14(2–3):153–159.

35. Geller S, Studee L. Botanical and dietary supplements for menopausal symptoms: what works, what does not. J Womens Health (Larchmt) 2005;14(7):634–649.

36. Cheema D, et al. Non-hormonal therapy of postmenopausal vasomotor symptoms: a structured evidence-based review. Arch Gynecol Obstet 2007;276(5):463–469.

37. Reame N, et al. Black cohosh has central opioid activity in postmenopausal women: evidence from naloxone blockade and positron emission tomography neuroimaging. Menopause 2008;15(5):832–840.

38. Jarry H, et al. In vitro effects of the *Cimicifuga racemosa* extract BNO 1055. Maturitas 2003;44 Supp 1:31–38.

39. Wuttke W, et al. The *Cimicifuga* preparation BNO 1055 vs. conjugated estrogens in a double-blind placebo-controlled study: effects on menopause symptoms and bone markers. Maturitas 2003;44(Suppl):S67–S77.

40. Borrelli F, Ernst E. Black cohosh (*Cimicifuga racemosa*) for menopausal symptoms: a systematic review of its efficacy. Pharmacol Res 2008;58(1):8–14.

41. Low Dog T. Menopause: a review of botanical dietary supplements. Am J Med 2005;118(Suppl 12B):98–108.

42. Kupfersztain C, et al. The immediate effect of natural plant extract, *Angelica sinensis* and *Matricaria chamomilla* (Climex) for the treatment of hot flushes during menopause. A preliminary report. Clin Exp Obstet Gynecol 2003;30(4):203–206.

43. Hirata J, et al. Does dong quai have estrogenic effects in postmenopausal women? A double-blind, placebo-controlled trial. Fertil Steril 1997;68(6):981–986.

44. Haines C, et al. A randomized, double-blind, placebo-controlled study of the effect of a Chinese herbal medicine preparation (dang gui buxue tang) on menopausal symptoms in Hong Kong Chinese women. Climacteric 2008;11(5):439–440.

45. Heyerick A, et al. A first prospective, randomized, double-blind, placebo-controlled study on the use of a standardized hop extract to alleviate menopausal discomforts. Maturitas 2006;54(2):164–175.

46. Chadwick L, et al. The pharmacognosy of *Humulus lupulus* L. (hops) with an emphasis on estrogenic properties. Phytomedicine 2006;13(1–2):119–131.

47. De Leo V, et al. Treatment of neurovegetative menopausal symptoms with a phytotherapeutic agent. Minrva Ginecol 1998;50(5):207–211.

48. Freedman R, Woodward S. Behavioral treatment of menopausal hot flushes: evaluation by ambulatory monitoring. Am J Obstet Gynecol 1992;167(2):436–439.

49. Irvin J, et al. The effects of relaxation response training on menopausal symptoms. J Psychosom Obstet Gynaecol 1996;17(4):202–207.

50. Nedstrand E, et al. Applied relaxation and oral estradiol treatment of vasomotor symptoms in postmenopausal women. Maturitas 2005;51(2):154–162.

51. Carmody J, et al. A pilot study of mindfulness-based stress reduction for hot flashes. Menopause 2006;13(5):760–769.

52. Booth-LaForce C, et al. A pilot study of a hatha yoga treatment for menopausal symptoms. Maturitas 2007;57(3):286–295.

53. Chattha R, et al. Treating the climacteric symptoms in Indian women with an integrated approach to yoga therapy: a randomized control study. Menopause 2008;15(5):862–870.

54. Tode T, et al. Effect of Korean red ginseng on psychological functions in patients with severe climacteric syndromes. Int J Gynaecol Obstet 1999;67(3):169–174.

55. Grube B, et al. St John's Wort extract: efficacy for menopausal symptoms of psychological origin. Adv Ther 1999;16(4):177–186.

56. De Leo V, et al. Evaluation of combining kava extract with hormone replacement therapy in the treatment of postmenopausal anxiety. Maturitas 2001;39(2):185–188.

57. Gracia C, et al. Predictors of decreased libido in women during the late reproductive years. Menopause 2004;11(2):144–150.

58. Elavsky S, McAuley E. Exercise and self-esteem in menopausal women: a randomized controlled trial involving walking and yoga. Am J Health Promot 2007;22(2):83–92.

59. Mills S, Bone K. Principles and practice of phytotherapy. Edinburgh: Churchill Livingstone, 2000.

60. Ito T, et al. The enhancement of female sexual function with ArginMax, a nutritional supplement, among women differing in menopausal status. J Sex Marital Ther 2006;32(5):369–378.

61. Ito T, et al. A double-blind placebo-controlled study of ArginMax, a nutritional supplement for enhancement of female sexual function. J Sex Marital Ther 2001;27(5):541–549.

62. Wheatley D. Hypericum in seasonal affective disorder (SAD). Curr Med Res Opin 1999;15(1):33–37.

63. Braun L, Cohen M. Herbs and natural supplements: an evidence-based guide. Sydney: Elsevier, 2007.

64. Yildirim B, et al. The effects of postmenopausal vitamin D treatment on vaginal atrophy. Maturitas 2004;49(4):334–337.

65. Borello-France D, et al. Continence and quality-of-life outcomes 6 months following an intensive pelvic-floor muscle exercise program for female stress urinary incontinence: a randomized trial comparing low- and high-frequency maintenance exercise. Phys Ther 2008;88(12):1545–1553.

66. Peterson J. Minimize urinary incontinence: maximize physical activity in women. Urol Nurs 2008;28(5):351–356.

67. Prentice R, et al. Low-fat dietary pattern and risk of invasive breast cancer: the Women's Health Initiative Randomized Controlled Dietary Modification Trial. JAMA 2006;295:629–642.

68. Bonaiuti D, et al. Exercise for preventing and treating osteoporosis in postmenopausal women. Cochrane Database Syst Rev 2002;(3):CD000333.

69. Bjarnason N. Postmenopausal bone remodelling and hormone replacement. Climacteric 1998;1(1):72–79.

70. Griel A, et al. An increase in dietary n-3 fatty acids decreases a marker of bone resorption in humans. Nutr J 2007;6:2.

71. Sun D, et al. Dietary n-3 fatty acids decrease osteoclas-togenesis and loss of bone mass in ovariectomized mice. J Bone Miner Res 2003;18(7):1206–1216.
72. Fernandes G, et al. Protective role of n-3 lipids and soy protein in osteoporosis. Prostaglandins Leukot Essent Fatty Acids 2003;68(6):361–372.
73. Bischoff-Ferrari H, et al. Fracture prevention with vitamin D supplementation: a meta-analysis of randomized controlled trials. JAMA 2005;293:2257–2264.
74. Jackson R, et al. Women's Health Initiative Investigators. Calcium plus vitamin D supplementation and the risk of fractures. N Engl J Med 2006;354:669–683.
75. Potter S, et al. Soy protein and isoflavones: their effects on blood lipids and bone density in postmenopausal women. Am J Clin Nutr 1998;83 Supp:1375S–1379S.
76. Ma D, et al. Soy isoflavone intake increases bone mineral density in the spine of menopausal women: meta-analysis of randomized controlled trials. Clin Nutr 2008;27(1):57–64.
77. Ma D, et al. Soy isoflavone intake inhibits bone resorption and stimulates bone formation in menopausal women: meta-analysis of randomized controlled trials. Eur J Clin Nutr 2008;62(2):155–161.
78. Rittweger J. Can exercise prevent osteoporosis? J Musculo-skelet Neuronal Interact 2006;6(2):162–166.
79. Wayne P, et al. The effects of tai chi on bone mineral density in postmenopausal women: a systematic review. Arch Phys Med Rehabil 2007;88(5):673–680.
80. Tunstall-Pedoe H. Myth and paradox of coronary risk and menopause. Lancet 1998;351(9113):1425–1427.
81. Yusuf S, et al. INTERHEART Study Investigators. Effect of potentially modifiable risk factors associated with myocardial infarction in 52 countries (the INTERHEART study): case-control study. Lancet 2004;364:937–952.
82. Borud E, et al. The Acupuncture on Hot Flushes Among Menopausal Women (ACUFLASH) study, a randomized controlled trial. Menopause 2009;16(3):484–493.
83. Maciocia G. Obstetrics and gynecology in Chinese medicine. Edinburgh: Churchill Livingstone, 1997.
84. Thompson E, Reilly D. The homoeopathic approach to the treatment of symptoms of oestrogen withdrawal in breast cancer patients. A prospective observational study. Homoeopathic 2003;92(3):131–134.
85. Cleary C, Fox J. Menopausal symptoms: an osteopathic investigation. Complement Ther Med 1994;2:181–186.

Section 7 Musculoskeletal system

The musculoskeletal system is the mechanical structure that provides form, stability and movement to the human body. Although the broader muscle and skeletal systems are quite different, they are connected via a complex array of bone, muscle, cartilage, joints, tendons, ligaments and other connective tissue. The musculoskeletal system is responsible not just for locomotion, but also for the protection of vital organs from physical damage. The musculoskeletal system is also biochemically active—the skeleton is the main storage repository for calcium and phosphorus and has a critical role in blood cell production.

The musculoskeletal system is the mechanical workhorse of the human body and lends itself to disorders of degeneration. This degeneration may come from a number of underlying reasons, from physical wear and tear to the consequences of increased systemic inflammation. Conditions commonly encountered in naturopathic practice in this system include various forms of arthritis (such as rheumatoid, osteo- or viral arthritis), fibromyalgia and gout. Other commonly encountered disorders in this system include those of a more acute nature—for example, promoting the repair for healing of physical sports or trauma injuries through specific and non-specific support, and long-term management of long-standing joint diseases. These conditions may present with pain and discomfort that affect activities of daily living such as sleep and psychological wellbeing, which in turn may negatively affect other health disorders. Because of this the clinician, in treating the many chronic musculoskeletal system conditions, should focus on the endgame of 'improving quality of life'.

Musculoskeletal system conditions form a significant therapeutic challenge, representing approximately a quarter of the workload of a primary care practitioner. Many common locomotor problems will be short-lived or self-limiting, or may be ameliorated with analgesia and physical therapy such as osteopathy or appropriate exercise therapy. However, appropriate early treatment of musculoskeletal system disorders is vital, as this can reduce the incidence of further architectural damage, the development of chronic pain disorders and various comorbidities that may ensue. Many musculoskeletal system conditions can also be managed effectively by the patient, providing good symptom-control education has been part of the consultative process.

Naturopaths treating musculoskeletal system disorders also have to school themselves in a broad array of therapeutic modalities. Herbal and nutritional medicines are potentially beneficial in treating patients with these disorders, as are various lifestyle modifications. However, musculoskeletal system treatment is particularly well served by many therapies underutilised or under-referred in contemporary naturopathic practice. These include hydrotherapy, various forms of physical and exercise therapy, dry needling or acupuncture and various counselling techniques.

Naturopathic protocols used to treat musculoskeletal system disorders commonly involve attenuating the inflammatory cascade, reducing pain and improving circulation and relaxation of the fascia. In conditions such as arthritis or musculoskeletal system injuries, remedial programs may be of assistance in improving outcomes. Herbal medicines that effect anti-inflammatory, antispasmodic and analgesic activity may be of benefit. Musculoskeletal system conditions are generally amenable to topical preparations that effect rubefacient and anti-inflammatory actions. Nutrients that are commonly prescribed may enhance the repair of soft tissue or joint architecture, and reduce inflammation.

This section gives an overview of the treatment of important conditions in this system, looking at both physical and systemic interactions in the naturopathic treatment of simple and complex conditions. This section focuses on the two main musculoskeletal system conditions—osteoarthritis and fibromyalgia—and details other symptomatic aspects such as general muscle pain. For further information on managing pain in osteoarthritis, consult Chapter 37 on polypharmacy and pain management.

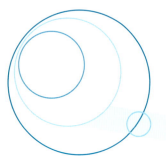

22
Osteoarthritis

Paul J. Orrock

ND, RN, MAppSc, DO

DEFINITION AND AETIOLOGY

Osteoarthritis, also called degenerative joint disease, is primarily a disease of ageing, as 90% of all people have radiographic features of it in the weight-bearing joints by the age of 40 years.[1,2,3] It is defined by degeneration of the cartilage and subsequent hypertrophy of the bone surrounding the articulations. There are no systemic signs of disease with this condition. Typically the pain is localised to joints in a non-symmetrical pattern, and is usually relieved by rest and gentle motion. There are hereditary and mechanical risk factors involved in this condition, with obesity and repetitive mechanical loading especially provocative in the lower limb articulations. Degeneration in a joint can be primary by 'wear and tear' or secondary to an articular injury, for example a fracture, or metabolic diseases like hyperparathyroidism.[2,3]

Incidence and cost

In Australia, arthritis and musculoskeletal conditions are large contributors to illness, pain and disability.[4] Accounting for more than 4% of the overall disease burden, measured in terms of disability-adjusted life years (DALY), these conditions account for a significant proportion of healthy years of life lost. More than 6.1 million Australians are reported to have arthritis or a musculoskeletal condition. Most commonly reported conditions are back pain and various forms of arthritis. Further, over 1 million Australians are reported to have disability associated with arthritis and related disorders, with mobility limitation the major feature. These conditions are the second most common reason for presentation to a general practitioner,[3,5] and the third leading cause of health expenditure.[6] In view of this large disease burden—the number of people affected and the high disability impact—arthritis and musculoskeletal conditions were declared a National Health Priority Area (NHPA) in July 2002. 1.3 million Australians (almost 7% of the population) have diagnosed osteoarthritis and females (8%) are more likely than males (5%) to have the disease.[3]

RISK FACTORS

The risk factors for osteoarthritis have been categorised into a succinct list of modifiable and unmodifiable factors.[7]

Modifiable

The first and most obvious factor is injury to a joint complex, and this is especially true in men. Trauma to the meniscus and cruciate ligament tears are particularly provocative in the development of osteoarthritis, and this relationship remains despite surgical repair.[2,3,7]

Obesity is a major risk factor in both the development of weight-bearing joint osteoarthritis and its severity and subsequent disability.[3,6–8] Women are particularly susceptible in this factor, and obesity appears to be predisposing to osteoarthritis, and not just secondary to becoming sedentary because of it.

The link between occupational overuse and the development of osteoarthritis has been shown in many different work activities, particularly when the knee is involved in repeated bending, kneeling, squatting or climbing,[3,7] and this effect is exacerbated by the addition of heavy-load lifting.[9]

Unmodifiable

The prevalence of osteoarthritis has an interesting age and gender relationship. Men more commonly have the radiological signs of the condition before the age of 50 years, and conversely women have it after that age. Women are more likely to have bilateral knee osteoarthritis as well as hand osteoarthritis. The disease increases in incidence and severity with age.[7]

In terms of family history, there is an inherited tendency towards osteoarthritis, with the heritability component estimated in twin studies at 60–65% for hip and hand osteoarthritis, and 40–50% for knee osteoarthritis, although there has been no single gene defect identified.[10] There is also evidence that race is involved as a risk factor. For example, there is evidence that Chinese subjects have a lower incidence of hand and hip osteoarthritis.[11] These risk factors can compound, as in obesity with occupational bending and twisting. There is some evidence that recreational overuse is a risk, specifically in elite sports.[7]

DIAGNOSIS

A joint can be defined or diagnosed to have osteoarthritis by symptoms, structural changes, or both (see Figure 22.1). The symptoms of osteoarthritis include:
- pain
- stiffness
- tenderness
- limitation of movement
- crepitus, and occasionally
- swelling.[3]

Radiological changes on X-ray are useful to identify some of the key signs of the osteoarthritic joint: the narrowing of the joint space, marginal osteophyte formation, subchondral sclerosis and the hypertrophy of the periarticular bones. However, radiological changes are not always observed in people with joint symptoms, and people with radiological changes do not always have symptoms. Cartilage is not seen on X-ray as it is not radio-opaque, so ultrasound and magnetic resonance imaging (MRI) and visualisation under arthroscopy might be necessary to clarify the joint changes.[2,3]

In clinical research studies, the diagnosis and severity of osteoarthritis is commonly measured using the Western Ontario and McMaster Universities Osteoarthritis Index (WOMAC). The WOMAC evaluates three clinical domains including pain, stiffness

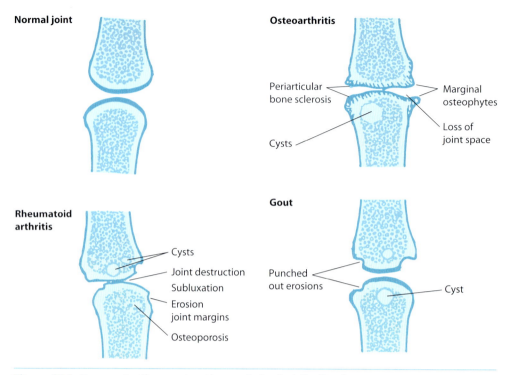

Figure 22.1 Demonstrating contrasting radiological finding between common arthritides

and physical function in people with osteoarthritis of the hip and knee, and assesses change in symptoms of patients who have received therapeutic intervention. Ordinal Likert scales are used to grade the severity of each domain, and the instrument has been extensively evaluated for validity.[12,13]

The differential diagnosis of osteoarthritis from other forms of arthritide, like rheumatoid arthritis and gout, should include a consideration of the pattern of joint involvement and whether signs of inflammation are present (see Table 22.1 and Figure 22.2). If the patient has a recent history of infection or fever, is less than 40 years old or presents with abnormal routine blood tests, other forms of arthritis (such as rheumatoid or septic) should be considered (see Chapter 28 on autoimmunity). Laboratory tests (for example, ESR, rheumatoid factor and synovial fluid analysis) may be used to rule out alternative diagnoses.[2,3,14]

CONVENTIONAL TREATMENT

The foundations of conventional treatment can be summarised as:[2,3,15,16]

- supervised exercise program
- weight loss
- non-steroidal anti-inflammatory drug (NSAID) medication
- intraarticular injection with steroids
- total joint replacement.

The exercise program and weight-loss strategies are elements of the self-help management plan that all health practitioners would support—see the discussion below regarding the evidence.

Table 22.1 Differential diagnosis of joint patterns

CHARACTERISTIC	STATUS	DISEASE
Inflammation	Present	Rheumatoid arthritis, systemic lupus erythematosus, gout
	Absent	Osteoarthritis
Number of involved joints	Monoarticular	Gout, trauma, septic arthritis, Lyme disease, osteoarthritis
	Oligoarticular (2–4 joints)	Reiter's disease, psoriatic arthritis, inflammatory bowel disease
	Polyarticular (5 or more)	Rheumatoid arthritis, systemic lupus erythematosus
Site of joint involvement	Distal interphalangeal	Osteoarthritis, psoriatic arthritis (not rheumatoid arthritis)
	Metacarpophalangeal, wrists	Rheumatoid arthritis, systemic lupus erythematosus (not osteoarthritis)
	First metatarsophalangeal	Gout, osteoarthritis

Source: Adapted from 2009 Current Medical Diagnosis and Treatment.[2]

Prescription of NSAIDs is included as the first choice for pain and inflammation control, with the addition of analgesics where necessary. The prescription should be accompanied by an assessment of the presence of risk factors for NSAIDs including age, hypertension, upper gastrointestinal events and cardiovascular, renal or liver disease. Other issues to be considered are aspirin allergy and polypharmacy (for example, concurrent use of diuretics, ACEI and/or anticoagulants).[2,3,15,16]

In Australia, the percentage of people with osteoarthritis using the common medications are: 8.0% use celecoxib (NSAID), 6.6% paracetamol, 5.3% meloxicam (NSAID), 3.9% diclofenac sodium (NSAID).[3]

NATUROPATHIC TREATMENT AIMS
- Remove obstacles to health:
  - obesity
  - sedentary lifestyle
  - pro-inflammatory diet.
- Support healing:
  - nutrient support for joint complexes
  - physical medicine for circulation and drainage.
- Reduce pain:
  - improve sleep
  - reduce medication intake.
- Improve functional capabilities:
  - range of motion
  - activities of daily living.
- Limit progression of degeneration.
- Address comorbidities of chronic pain:
  - depression.
- Improve daily functioning.
- Encourage lifestyle changes.

KEY TREATMENT PROTOCOLS
The goals in the naturopathic treatment of people with osteoarthritis are to:
- modify inflammation and reduce pain
- enhance joint integrity and repair damage in order to maintain mobility and flexibility
- slow the progression of the disease.

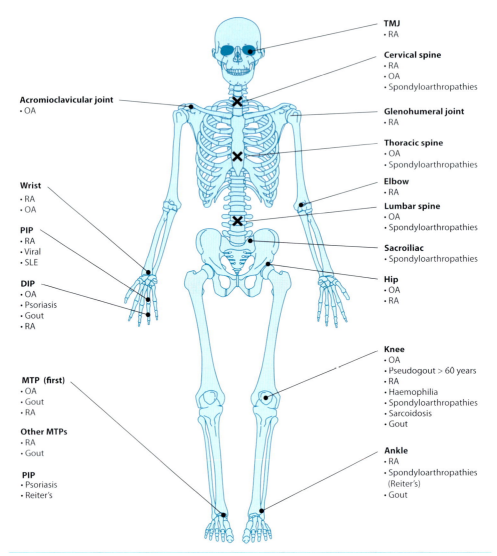

TMJ
• RA

Cervical spine
• RA
• OA
• Spondyloarthropathies

Glenohumeral joint
• RA

Thoracic spine
• OA
• Spondyloarthropathies

Elbow
• RA

Lumbar spine
• OA
• Spondyloarthropathies

Sacroiliac
• Spondyloarthropathies

Hip
• OA
• RA

Knee
• OA
• Pseudogout > 60 years
• RA
• Haemophilia
• Spondyloarthropathies
• Sarcoidosis
• Gout

Ankle
• RA
• Spondyloarthropathies
 (Reiter's)
• Gout

Acromioclavicular joint
• OA

Wrist
• RA
• OA

PIP
• RA
• Viral
• SLE

DIP
• OA
• Psoriasis
• Gout
• RA

MTP (first)
• OA
• Gout
• RA

Other MTPs
• RA
• Gout

PIP
• Psoriasis
• Reiter's

Figure 22.2 Differential diagnosis in arthritis based on patterns of regional joint presentations

This schedule of therapeutic aims has a large number of individualised permutations based on the many pieces of information that are gleaned from the personal history and lifestyle analysis of each person with osteoarthritis. In naturopathic medicine, this is a vital component of the management of a multifactorial condition such as osteoarthritis. As in any naturopathic approach to case reasoning, the therapeutic order is useful to prioritise management, and to ensure the naturopathic principles are followed.[19] The following is a summary of modalities that may be used within naturopathic medicine that have been investigated for this condition.

The naturopathic approach to the management of this condition reflects the evidence-based guidelines of a number of mainstream groups. The Osteoarthritis Research Society International (OARSI) has published practice guidelines for managing hip and knee osteoarthritis.[20] The guidelines state that the optimal management requires

TREAT THE WHOLE PATIENT

Although clinical treatment will inevitability focus on amelioration of pain, degeneration and inflammation in arthritis patients, it is also important to consider how this affects their day-to-day lives.

Qualitative studies of patients with rheumatoid arthritis suggested that fatigue, not pain, was the factor associated with their condition that affected their life the most.[17] Similar findings have since been observed in osteoarthritis patients as well.[18] Fatigue may be associated with pain, pain medication, poor sleeping patterns or any number of factors. Arthritis may also affect the patient's ability to perform daily tasks and interact socially or with their partner, and has other psychosocial or emotional ramifications, all of which need to be appropriately addressed in the naturopathic treatment of arthritis.

a combination of non-pharmacological and pharmacological approaches. The first priority is education of the patient about the condition and the importance of changes in lifestyle, exercise and weight reduction in order to unload the damaged joints. The initial focus should be on self-help and patient-driven treatments rather than on passive therapies delivered by health professionals.[21] The focus on self-help in obesity and exercise management is also a key element of the guidelines from both the Royal Australian College of General Practitioners[22] and the National Arthritis and Musculoskeletal Conditions Advisory Group.[14]

The approach in naturopathic medicine to 'address weakened or dysfunctioning systems or organs' coincides with the clinical approach of looking for the existence of comorbidities that may be linked to the primary problem (see Figure 22.3). This is clear in the management of osteoarthritis, where assessment and treatment may be necessary in the (among others):

- nutritional/dietary domain—especially with regard to obesity and weight control
- cardiovascular system—limiting the ability to exercise
- psycho-emotional aspect—the effects of chronic pain and disability
- gastrointestinal system—absorption of nutrients, food sensitivities and reactions to conventional medications.[21,23]

Attenuate inflammation

The process of inflammation plays a central role in many disorders, especially those in the musculoskeletal system. Like many processes in the body, there can be positive outcomes from a resolution or there can be uncontrolled and damaging results. The activators of inflammation can include injury, radiation, infection, oxidative stress and certain foods. Tissue injury stimulates the release of inflammatory signalling molecules such as bradykinin, and the release of inflammatory cytokines such as IL-1, TNF and IL-6. Cells that respond to infection or injury include macrophages and mast cells.[24] Macrophages and other immune cells secrete chemokines that recruit leukocytes from the circulation to the site of inflammation. Mast cells release histamine, prostaglandins and leukotrienes that act as chemokines, increase vascular permeability and act on the vascular endothelium to increase tissue recruitment of leukocytes.[24] Cyclooxygenase (COX) is an enzyme that is responsible for the formation of pro-inflammatory prostaglandins, prostacyclins and thromboxanes from the omega-6 arachidonic acid (see Chapter 28 on autoimmunity for further detail).

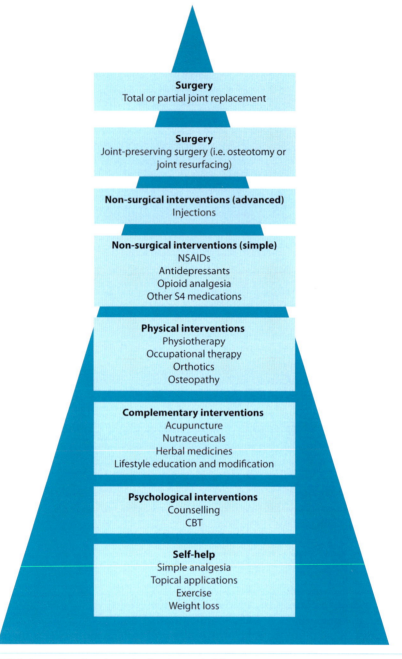

Figure 22.3 Integrative treatment of osteoarthritis
Source: Adapted from Dieppe PA, Lohmander LS. Pathogenesis and management of pain in osteoarthritis. Lancet 2005;365(9463):965–973.

Omega-3 essential fatty acids compete with the omega-6, thereby moderating the inflammatory effect. There is evidence that omega-3 oils containing eicosapentaenoic acid (EPA) and docosahexaenoic acid (DHA) have anti-inflammatory actions,[25,26] but clinical data are lacking with regard to the treatment of osteoarthritis.[25,27] The most widely available sources of EPA and DHA are cold water oily fish such as salmon, herring, mackerel, anchovies and sardines.

Harpagophytum procumbens, a South African herb, has been reviewed for efficacy and safety in the treatment of osteoarthritis with favourable results, especially in the reduction of pain.[28,26] The mechanism of action has not been established, but is thought to be the anti-inflammatory activity of harpagoside.[29] An 8-week, single-group, open clinical trial demonstrated statistically significant improvements in patient assessment of global pain, stiffness and function. There were also statistically significant reductions in mean pain scores for hand, wrist, elbow, shoulder, hip, knee and back pain. Quality of life measurements (using the SF-12 health survey) were significantly increased from baseline and 60% of patients either reduced or stopped concomitant pain medication. Adverse effects have been described as no different to placebo.[27,30]

A proprietary blend of *Solidago virgaurea*, *Populus tremula* and *Fraxinus excelsior* has been demonstrated to be effective in reducing pain and inflammation

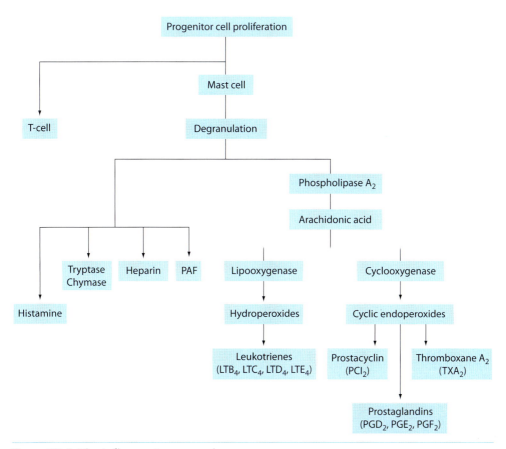

Figure 22.4 The inflammatory cascade
Source: Pearlman DS. Pathophysiology of the inflammatory response. J Allergy Clin Immunol 1999;104:S132–S137.

in arthritis via a variety of mechanisms. While most of the 43 studies justifying the formulation's use have focused on pain measures, many have also uncovered various anti-inflammatory mechanisms, with efficacy often comparable to conventional anti-inflammatory medication.[31,32]

The gum resin extracted from the herb ***Boswellia serrata*** has some evidence as a potent anti-inflammatory, anti-arthritic and analgesic agent.[33] A recent double-blind, randomised placebo-controlled trial of 75 subjects with osteoarthritis demonstrated that an extract of *B. serrata* (5-Loxin®) conferred clinically and statistically significant improvements in pain scores and physical function scores, and these changes were recorded in the treatment group as early as 7 days after the start of treatment.[34]

Salix* spp.** through the active constituent salicin, has anti-inflammatory and analgesic activity. Standardised preparations of the bark have shown positive effects in a number of trials in musculoskeletal conditions, with an analgesic effect dominant in low back pain.[26,35] In a recent non-blinded trial of 131 subjects with arthrosis of the hip and knee, willow bark had equivalent effect to NSAIDs, with fewer side effects.[36] A recent review found that, for treating mild or fairly severe cases of gonarthrosis and coxarthrosis, the effect of willow bark extract was comparable to that of standard therapies.[36] ***Uncaria* spp.** is known to have anti-inflammatory activity in vitro, possibly by inhibiting the production of the pro-inflammatory cytokine, TNF-α,[26] but clinical trials have been inconclusive.[27] ***Zingiber officinale has been found to have anti-inflammatory actions.[26,37] In a double-blind, randomised controlled trial of 261 subjects with knee osteoarthritis, ginger was found to significantly reduce symptoms and had mild adverse effects.[38]

An interesting pilot study using a real practice model showed that **herbal medicine formulas** prescribed for the individual by a herbal practitioner resulted in improvement of symptoms of osteoarthritis of the knee.[39] Twenty adults, previously diagnosed with osteoarthritis of the knee, were recruited into this randomised, double-blind, placebo-controlled, pilot study carried out in a primary-care setting. All subjects were seen in consultation three times by a herbal practitioner who was blinded to the randomisation coding. Each subject was prescribed treatment and given lifestyle advice according to usual practice: continuation of conventional medication where applicable, healthy-eating advice and nutrient supplementation. Individualised herbal medicine was prescribed for each patient, but only dispensed for those randomised to active treatment—the remainder were supplied with a placebo. At baseline and outcome (after 10 weeks of treatment), subjects completed a food frequency questionnaire and the Western Ontario and McMaster Universities Osteoarthritis Index (WOMAC) knee health and Measure Yourself Outcome Profile (MYMOP) wellbeing questionnaires. There was significant improvement in the active group ($n = 9$) for the mean WOMAC stiffness subscore at week 5 and week 10, but not in the placebo group ($n = 5$). Also the mean WOMAC total and subscores all showed clinically significant improvement (20%) in knee symptoms at weeks 5 and 10 compared with baseline. Moreover, the mean MYMOP symptom 2 subscore, mostly relating to osteoarthritis, showed significant improvement at week 5 and week 10 compared with baseline for the active, but not for the placebo, group. This pilot study showed that herbal medicine prescribed for the individual by a herbal practitioner resulted in improvement of symptoms of osteoarthritis of the knee. This methodology mirrors normal clinical procedures, and should encourage similar larger clinical trials that have more relevance to naturopathic practice.

Enhance joint integrity and repair damage

Primary and secondary prevention are the main foci of naturopathic medicine, and maintaining and repairing articular and periarticular tissue is a foundation for the management of osteoarthritis. Developing, maintaining and repairing collagen-based connective tissue requires optimal tissue levels of the essential amino acids, as well as vitamin C and iron as cofactors. Bone and cartilage are built on a matrix of minerals, mainly calcium and phosphorus, and an extracellular ground substance of proteoglycans (see Figure 22.5). Proteoglycans are glycoproteins that have a core protein with glycosaminoglycan (GAG) chains.

Glucosamine and **chondroitin** are both natural components of proteoglycans, the building blocks of cartilage, and are thought to increase its synthesis when taken orally. Glucosamine is manufactured from oyster and crab shells, and chondroitin from bovine or shark cartilage. There are conflicting results in the research findings for both symptom relief and limiting the progression of the disease.

The large Glucosamine/Chondroitin Arthritis Intervention Trial (GAIT) trials[40,41] have found varying positive and negative results in both domains of clinical effect, and one study[27] puts forward a list of concerns that may explain why the body of evidence remains equivocal, including:

- the tendency of industry-sponsored trials to have positive results
- poor supplement quality
- varying dosing methods
- trials too brief to allow slow therapeutic effect
- underpowered trails.[27]

A recent randomised, double-blind, placebo-controlled trial of chondroitin sulfate given to 622 patients with knee osteoarthritis for 2 years found that the structure-modifying and symptom-modifying effects of chondroitin sulfate over the long-term suggest that it could be a disease-modifying agent.[42]

Methylsulfonylmethane (**MSM**) has been used as a sulfur-based nutritional supplement in conditions with joint pain, but a recent systematic review of clinical trials was

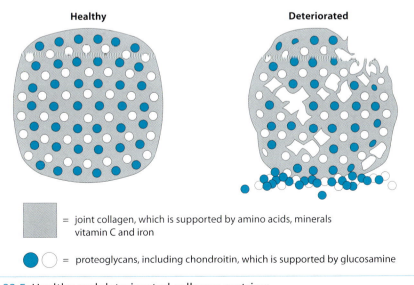

Healthy **Deteriorated**

= joint collagen, which is supported by amino acids, minerals vitamin C and iron

= proteoglycans, including chondroitin, which is supported by glucosamine

Figure 22.5 Healthy and deteriorated collagen matrices

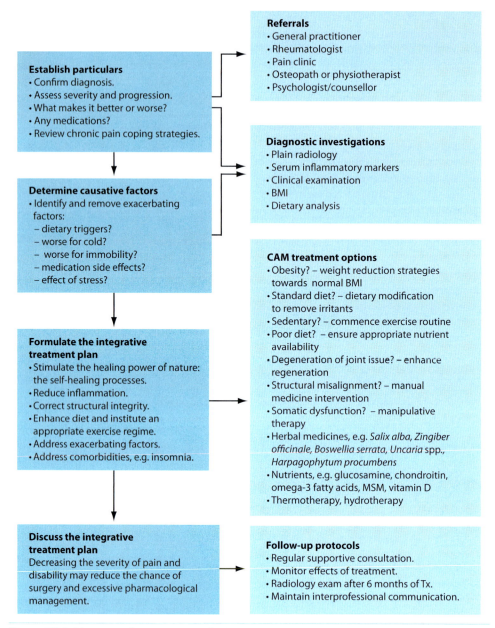

Establish particulars
• Confirm diagnosis.
• Assess severity and progression.
• What makes it better or worse?
• Any medications?
• Review chronic pain coping strategies.

Determine causative factors
• Identify and remove exacerbating factors:
  – dietary triggers?
  – worse for cold?
  – worse for immobility?
  – medication side effects?
  – effect of stress?

Formulate the integrative treatment plan
• Stimulate the healing power of nature: the self-healing processes.
• Reduce inflammation.
• Correct structural integrity.
• Enhance diet and institute an appropriate exercise regime.
• Address exacerbating factors.
• Address comorbidities, e.g. insomnia.

Discuss the integrative treatment plan
Decreasing the severity of pain and disability may reduce the chance of surgery and excessive pharmacological management.

Referrals
• General practitioner
• Rheumatologist
• Pain clinic
• Osteopath or physiotherapist
• Psychologist/counsellor

Diagnostic investigations
• Plain radiology
• Serum inflammatory markers
• Clinical examination
• BMI
• Dietary analysis

CAM treatment options
• Obesity? – weight reduction strategies towards normal BMI
• Standard diet? – dietary modification to remove irritants
• Sedentary? – commence exercise routine
• Poor diet? – ensure appropriate nutrient availability
• Degeneration of joint issue? – enhance regeneration
• Structural misalignment? – manual medicine intervention
• Somatic dysfunction? – manipulative therapy
• Herbal medicines, e.g. *Salix alba, Zingiber officinale, Boswellia serrata, Uncaria* spp., *Harpagophytum procumbens*
• Nutrients, e.g. glucosamine, chondroitin, omega-3 fatty acids, MSM, vitamin D
• Thermotherapy, hydrotherapy

Follow-up protocols
• Regular supportive consultation.
• Monitor effects of treatment.
• Radiology exam after 6 months of Tx.
• Maintain interprofessional communication.

Figure 22.6 Naturopathy treatment decision tree—osteoarthritis

unable to reach a firm conclusion on its usefulness, because of methodological flaws and despite a number of positive trial findings.[43–45]

Improving joint mobility

The result of inflammation and fibrosis in osteoarthritis is limited joint motion, and this interferes with activities of daily living and has the global effect of reducing fitness and compliance to exercise therapy.

Massage and physical therapy provide viable options for managing osteoarthritis. There have been some trials using massage for osteoarthritis, but methodological quality is lacking, particularly with regard to the difficulties of blinding and control. A randomised controlled trial of 68 adults with radiologically confirmed osteoarthritis of the knee demonstrated significant improvements from standard Swedish massage in the WOMAC global scores, pain, stiffness and physical function domains.[48] The subjects also had improvement in the visual analogue scale of pain assessment, range of motion in degrees and time to walk 50 feet (15.24 metres).

Evidence of efficacy in treating osteoarthritis may exist for the addition of physical therapy modalities. The term 'multimodal therapy' generally includes range of motion exercise, soft tissue mobilisation and muscle strengthening and stretching—all within the scope of the naturopath inclined to physical medicine.[49] Studies suggest that patients with osteoarthritis receive moderate short-term (up to 8 weeks) clinical impact measured on WOMAC global and pain scores.

Adding therapeutic oils to the massage appears to have potential as an alternative method for short-term knee pain relief. In a double-blind, placebo-controlled trial of 59 older people, the intervention group had ginger and orange **essential oils** added to the massage oil, and the improvements of WOMAC-measured physical function and pain were superior in the intervention group compared with both the placebo and the control group at post 1-week time but not sustained at post 4 weeks.[50]

Reduce pain

Pain management is a vital component of chronic disease therapy in general, and non-pharmacological approaches should be considered in patients with osteoarthritis (see Chapter 37 on polypharmacy and pain management for more detail of pain management in osteoarthritis).

Thermotherapy may reduce the pain associated with osteoarthritis. It involves the application of heat or cold (such as a heat or ice pack and ice massage) to treat symptoms of osteoarthritis. This could be applied by a massage therapist, physical therapist or naturopath in an integrated setting. The application of cold is known to have an effect by reducing swelling and inflammation, numbing pain and blocking nerve impulses and muscle spasms to the joint.

QUALITY MATTERS

As with many complementary medicines, quality and dosing variances can affect the therapeutic application and efficacy of treatment in trials. Glucosamine comes in a variety of forms which, though they theoretically can be hydrolysed in the stomach into equivalent forms, may have effects on therapeutic dosing requirements. Additionally, quality issues may also arise. Some formulations are demonstrated to be consistently more effective than placebo or other formulations in clinical trials.[46,1] Although concerns have been raised that these positive results may be related to industry sponsorship, it has been deemed equally likely that these results may also be due to the stricter quality controls of some formulations.[47] In clinical practice recommending any generic complementary medicine can be fraught; it is recommended that practitioners make specific recommendations for products they know to have high standards of quality and efficacy.

A Cochrane systematic review[51] found that it is most effective in an acute stage of osteoarthritis when minor joint inflammation is present and is administered through the application of an ice pack wrapped in a towel for 20 minutes, 5 days a week for 2 weeks.

Vitamin D deficiency appears to be prevalent in people with chronic musculoskeletal pain.[52–54] The mechanism appears to be related to a decrease in calcium absorption leading to dysfunctional collagen deposition in the periosteum, which generates painful stimuli. Oral supplementation with vitamin D in deficient subjects leads to a reduction in pain.[55]

The Framingham study data[56] link vitamin D deficiency to osteoarthritis. In a study of 556 subjects, dietary and supplement intake of vitamin D and serum levels of 25-hydroxyvitaminD were evaluated. Osteoarthritis was measured using knee radiographs. The authors concluded that low intake and low serum levels of vitamin D each appeared to be associated with an increased risk for progression of osteoarthritis of the knee.[56] These conclusions have been supported in a more recent review.[57]

Address oxidation

When inflammation is present, the breakdown of cells and tissues creates a burden of products of oxidation. The process of oxidation (producing reactive oxygen species) is a key factor in conditions of ageing, and the extracellular space depends on trace elements for **antioxidation**.

The Framingham study demonstrated that in an open trial of 640 subjects vitamin C 150–500 mg/day and beta-carotene 6000–10,000 IU/day in the diet was found to reduce risk of cartilage loss and knee pain over 8 years, with possible effects from vitamin E 8–10 mg/day in patients with knee osteoarthritis.[58]

This early promise has not been supported in trials since, with two systematic reviews finding very limited evidence for vitamin C or E.[45,59]

Remove metabolic waste products

A traditional naturopathic protocol used to treat osteoarthritis involves stimulation of the body's detoxification pathways to clear metabolic waste. While this philosophy has not yet been scientifically tested via rigorous studies, traditional evidence does support this practice.[60,61] The traditional use of **herbal 'alteratives'** and **'diuretics'** such as celery seed or dandelion leaf, or nettles to treat rheumatism, appears to be predicated upon these herbs' abilities to stimulate the removal of metabolic waste by increasing diuresis and potentially reducing blood composition of metabolic byproducts. This protocol may be potentially beneficial in treating gout (see the box on gout below).

INTEGRATIVE MEDICAL CONSIDERATIONS

Self-management

Self-management education programs have an important role to play in the management of chronic conditions such as osteoarthritis, and suit an integrative model of shared care between conventional and complementary medicine practitioners. Self-management education programs are interventions designed to educate the patient in self-care activities that promote health and the management of chronic diseases, increasing their motivation and decreasing the negative effects the condition has on their daily function.[63] The National Health Priority Action Council states that, by taking the behavioural approach to the management of the psychosocial aspects of chronic disease, patients have outcomes of decreased pain and improved quality of life.[63] This approach matches the holistic underpinning of naturopathic medicine.

GOUT[62]

Overview
- Acute onset of pain, usually in the evening
- Primarily male population
- Usually presents as monoarticular joint pain in the metatarsophalangeal joint
- High serum uric acid, urate crystals in the joint
- Genetic causations, triggered by increased alcohol and poor diet

Protocols
- Modify diet (reduce/avoid alcohol, high-purine foods, excess refined carbohydrates, saturated fats)
- Encourage hydration: 2.5 L per day keeps uric acid in solution and promotes excretion. Reversing dehydration also important.
- Reduce weight and exercise in moderation.
- Remove/reduce uric acid (via herbal diuretics and aquaretics, folic acid).
- Reduce inflammation via botanical and nutrient prescription.

CAM interventions
- Dietary advice (low purines and alcohol, healthy carbs/protein/fats balance, increase anthocyanidin-rich fruits such as cherries, blueberries)
- Folic acid has a similar mechanism of action to conventional gout medications such as allopuronol (it reduces xanthine oxidase) but requires large doses—over 5 mg—to be therapeutically effective. A trial of 10–20 mg daily should be considered.
- Lifestyle advice (exercise, reduced weight if required)
- Anti-inflammatories (such as bromelain, quercetin, omega-3, *Glycyrrhiza glabra*, *Harpagophytum procumbems*, *Boswellia serrata*)
- Diuretics/aquaretics (such as *Taraxacum officinale*, *Urtica dioica*, *Apium graveolens*)

Weight loss

Obesity is clearly a risk factor for developing osteoarthritis, particularly for women. There is very strong evidence that people who are obese (with a body mass index (BMI) of over 30) are at higher risk of their osteoarthritis being symptomatic and progressing than those with a BMI less than 30. The relationship between obesity and osteoarthritis is thought to be because of the increased stress on articular surfaces in the weight-bearing joints.[2,3,8,64] Reducing obesity in the patient with osteoarthritis should be considered as both a primary and a secondary prevention strategy. The condition is multifactorial, and is best managed in a multidisciplinary team including naturopaths.

The Arthritis, Diet, and Activity Promotion Trial (ADAPT) was a randomised, single-blind controlled clinical trial that demonstrated that weight loss was central to the improvement in WOMAC physical function, pain and stiffness scores; these results were enhanced when combined with a moderate exercise program.[64]

Exercise

Exercise guidance is a foundation of a naturopathic approach to wellness, and in the management of osteoarthritis coincides with the mainstream evidence-based guidelines. Exercise is important both as a treatment of symptoms and to prevent the development of osteoarthritis. Increasing physical activity improves general physical health and assists in the management of obesity, both vital risk factors for osteoarthritis, as mentioned.

Enhancing muscular strength is an outcome of exercise programs, and muscular weakness and dysfunction can cause joint instability and subsequent injury. To prevent this injury and resultant degeneration, and to prevent further injury in the degenerative joint, exercise programs must be a central component of the management plan in osteoarthritis.

Physical exercise of a light-to-moderate intensity increases muscle strength as well as range of motion, aerobic capacity and endurance that contributes to improved physical functioning and pain reduction. Various programs (see Table 22.2) offer different benefits and no specific type of exercise regimen has been shown to be superior.[2,3,20,22] A number of Cochrane reviews support the application of therapeutic exercise in the management of osteoarthritis,[65] with evidence for moderate intensity[66] and aquatic programs.[67]

An interesting systematic review looked at tai chi, a traditional Chinese martial art style, which has been one of the most researched therapeutic exercises. The authors report that there is evidence suggesting that tai chi may be effective for pain control in patients with knee osteoarthritis, but the evidence is not as convincing for pain reduction or improvement of physical function.[68]

Acupuncture

Acupuncture is commonly used in an integrated clinical setting by acupuncturists, medical practitioners, physiotherapists and naturopaths, and has been assessed for efficacy in the treatment of osteoarthritis. In a randomised, controlled, single-blind trial of 88 subjects, acupuncture plus diclofenac was more effective than placebo acupuncture plus diclofenac for the symptomatic treatment of osteoarthritis of the knee.[73] A recent meta-analysis regarding acupuncture for knee osteoarthritis was inconclusive, concluding that sham-controlled trials show clinically irrelevant short-term benefits of acupuncture for treating knee osteoarthritis.[74] This study reveals the difficulties of control with research into therapies like acupuncture, where the placebo is not inert but has some effect, in many cases equal to the active intervention.

 Case Study

A 72-year-old widow presents with **osteoarthritis** at **multiple painful sites**—both knees, right hip and her fingers. These have had a **gradual onset of 10 years** and are slowly progressing. She **complains of sleeplessness** and is **very stiff in the morning**, which has limited her voluntary work. Her BMI is 32, and her diet is random, as she cooks for herself, but is very busy with social activities. These activities and her normal beach walk have been **adversely affected by her pain and limited mobility**.

SUGGESTIVE SYMPTOMS

- Widespread musculoskeletal pain
- Pain in joints—insidious onset, typically hip, knee and fingers
- Pain is relieved by rest
- Brief morning stiffness, relieved by gentle motion
- Fatigue
- Weakness in activities of daily living

Differential diagnosis[2]

- Osteoarthritis
- Rheumatoid arthritis
- Other autoimmune disorders
- Anaemia
- Depression
- Malignancy

Table 22.2 Exercise interventions in osteoarthritis

NAME	DESCRIPTION	INDICATIONS	CAUTIONS/CON-TRAINDICATIONS	COMMENTS
ROM exercise	Active movement within range	Maintain joint ROM, ↑ joint nutrition, prevent soft tissue shortening[69]	Painful ROM	Foundation of rehabilitation for painful musculoskeletal conditions
Myofascial stretching	Static loading or proprioceptive neuromuscular facilitation (PNF—use of contract and release)	↑ muscle length and flexibility —optimise ROM[69]	Patient incomprehension	Good evidence basis[69]
Yoga asanas	Full ROM postures with adjunctive breathing exercises	General ROM maintenance and optimisation; strengthening; painful musculoskeletal conditions, balance and coordination, anxiety, depression[70]	Articular instability, poor instruction	Evidence is inconclusive—large number of low-quality RCTs
Resistance training	Repetitive weight resisted motion within ROM	↑ muscle strength and endurance; ↑ BMR, ↑ muscle mass; ↑ BMD; improved glucose metabolism[69]	Soft tissue injury/inflammation	Exercise professional required to set form and progression
Aerobic conditioning	Varied exercise aiming to increase oxygen demand and use	Obesity, general conditioning to prevent disease, depression[69]	Cardiac/respiratory disease, painful weight-bearing conditions	Requires careful grading in intensity, excellent evidence profile
Tai chi	Chinese system of slow movements	Painful musculoskeletal conditions[71]	Nil known	Traditional use in aged population group
Aquatic	Variety of exercises in water	↑ coordination, flexibility and strength,[69,67] for painful conditions	Wounds/infection	Decreases load on weight bearing tissues
Pilates	Resisted movement system with apparatus and floor exercises	↑ muscle strength and control—trunk/lumbo/pelvic.[72] Injury rehabilitation	None known	Requires careful guidance to establish muscle control.

Abbreviations: ROM = range of motion; BMR = basal metabolic rate; BMD = Bone mineral density

OSTEOARTHRITIS: COMORBID DEPRESSION AND PAIN

Patients with chronic diseases such as osteoarthritis have a higher rate of depression and anxiety than the general population.[14] Osteoarthritis also has a feature of chronic pain, which can result in feelings of lowered self-worth, anxiety and depression.[23] The practitioner needs to be educated about the effect these psychosocial aspects have on the condition and its progression. Osteoarthritis can also affect relationships and community and social activities,[23,14] which are all addressed in the naturopathic assessment of the individual.

A recent study of depression in 1021 patients with osteoarthritis[75] revealed that subjects who had concomitant depression had more contacts to general practitioners and to providers of complementary alternative medicine, resulting in increased health-service use. The authors conclude that appropriate treatment of depression would increase quality-of-life measures and also lower costs by decreasing health-service use, and that depression aggravates the burden of osteoarthritis significantly.[75] See Chapter 37 on polypharmacy and pain management for further consideration of pain management in naturopathic medicine.

Physical examination
- Musculoskeletal
- Observe for asymmetry/oedema.
- Palpate for signs of inflammation and joint complex disorder.
- Range of motion—active and passive

Diagnostic imaging
- Plain X-rays of affected joints

Laboratory
- Rheumatoid factor
- Erythrocyte sedimentation rate
- Antinuclear antibodies
- C-reactive protein

Example treatment
Herbal and nutritional prescription
The herbal prescription is designed to exert anti-inflammatory, analgesic and circulatory stimulatory actions. The nutritional supplements are prescribed to assist in reducing joint pain and enhancing mobility via anti-inflammatory activity and structural modification.

Physical medicine
- Therapeutic massage with ginger oil once a week for 1 month, including range of motion and then maintenance—consider referral to a manual medicine practitioner.
- Symptomatic cold packs on affected regions.

Herbal formula

Salix alba 1:1	25 mL
Harpagophytum procumbens 2:1	35 mL
Uncaria guanensis 1:2	30 mL
Zingiber officinale 1:2	10 mL
5 mL t.d.s.	100 mL
Boswellia serrata tablets 4 g b.d.	

Nutritional prescription

Glucosamine sulfate 500 mg t.d.s.
MSM 3 g powder b.d.
Vitamin D 1000 IU/day

Table 22.3 Review of the major evidence

INTERVENTION	KEY LITERATURE	SUMMARY OF RESULTS	COMMENT
Omega-3 EPA, DHA	Setty et al. 2005[26]	Inconclusive in vivo evidence in osteoarthritis	Review article.
Harpagophytum procumbens	Brien et al. 2006[26] Warnock et al. 2007[30]	Two high quality RCTs; n = 211; osteoarthritis multiple sites; ↓ pain. Single group open study; n = 259; ↓ pain, stiffness, function (p < 0.0001); ↑ QOL SF-12; 60% patients ↓ medications.	Systematic review.
Boswellia serrata	Ernst 2009[33]	n = 171 (3 RCTs); osteoarthritis knee; ↓ pain, WOMAC scores	Systematic review, individual trials small sample sizes.
Salix spp.	Chrubasik et al. 2001[35] Beer et al. 2008[36]	Open randomised; n = 93; low back pain; ↓ pain; equal effect to NSAID group. Open observational; n =128; knee and hip osteoarthritis; ↓ clinical symptoms and WOMAC scores.	Encouraging evidence to support a botanical with strong traditional use
Zingiber officinale	Altman 2001[38]	RCT; n = 247; osteoarthritis knee pain on standing; ↓ pain (p < 0.043)	Traditionally combines well with *Salix* spp.
Glucosamine and Chondroitin	Sawitzke et al. 2008[41] Kahan et al. 2009[42]	RCT; knee osteoarthritis; n = 572; joint space width not different to control. RCT; knee osteoarthritis; ↓ joint space width (p < 0.0001)	Glucosamine and chondroitin sulfate combined Chondroitin sulfate alone
MSM	Brien et al. 2008[43]	Mild/moderate osteoarthritis knee; n = 168; ↓ pain (p value not reported)	Systematic review of RCTs' 'methodological flaws'
Antioxidants	McAlindon et al. 2005[58]	Framingham cohort; n = 640; VC, beta-carotene and VE ↓ knee osteoarthritis progression and cartilage loss	No effect on primary prevention
Massage and physical therapy	Perlman et al. 2006[48]	n = 68; osteoarthritis knee; Swedish massage for 8 weeks; WOMAC pain, stiffness (p < 0.001), ROM (p = 0.03)	RCT, underpowered, not full blinding of assessors
Thermotherapy	Brosseau et al. 2003[66]	3 RCTs, knee osteoarthritis; improved function and knee strength, decreased swelling.	Systematic review
Acupuncture	Manheimer et al. 2007[74]	9 RCTs; knee osteoarthritis; pain, function compared to usual care.	Meta-analysis; sham controlled have variation in design.

Dietary and lifestyle advice
- Education about condition—arthritis support group
- Weight loss program to reduce BMI
- Dietary change to ensure regular quality meals, ensuring EFAs and antioxidants
- Guided exercise program:
  - aquarobics once per week
  - muscular strengthening in local gym once per week.

Expected outcomes and follow-up protocols

The early management plan could be organised around 4–6 weeks of gradual symptomatic improvement with weekly consultations and settling in of the lifestyle changes. The patient's GP and exercise physiologist would receive a letter outlining the naturopathic management plan, and setting realistic goals for pain reduction, increased flexibility and reducing the BMI.

Chronic disease management requires a well-established therapeutic relationship and supportive team, so consultations every 6–8 weeks for 12 months would be important to monitor and maintain compliance to the exercise and dietary changes. Aggravations are expected as the patient increases activities towards her expectations, and these would be managed by physical therapy, acupuncture and short-term pain- and inflammation-based herbal medicines, in conjunction with her conventional medications.

Acknowledgment

The author would like to acknowledge Justin Sinclair for his assistance with integrative approaches to osteeoarthritis.

Further reading

Chaitow L, ed. Naturopathic physical medicine. Edinburgh: Elsevier, 2008.

Brosseau LY, et al. Thermotherapy for treatment of osteoarthritis. Cochrane Database Syst Rev 2003;4:CD002826.

Towheed T, et al. Glucosamine therapy for treating osteoarthritis. Cochrane Database Syst Rev 2006;2:CD002946.

References

1. Reginster J, et al. Current role of glucosamine in the treatment of osteoarthritis. Rheumatology (Oxford) 2007;46(5):731–735.
2. 2009 Current medical diagnosis and treatment. 48th edn. New York: McGraw Hill Medical, 2009.
3. Australian Institute of Health and Welfare. A picture of osteoarthritis in Australia. Canberra: Australian Institute of Health and Welfare, 2007.
4. Australian Institute of Health and Welfare. Arthritis and musculoskeletal conditions in Australia, 2005. Canberra: Australian Institute of Health and Welfare, 2005.
5. Australian Institute of Health and Welfare. General practice activity in Australia 2000-01. Canberra: Australian Institute of Health and Welfare, 2001.
6. Australian Institute of Health and Welfare. Health system expenditure on disease and injury in Australia, 2000-01. Canberra: Australian Institute of Health and Welfare, 2005.
7. March LB, Bagga H. Epidemiology of osteoarthritis in Australia. Med J Aust 2004;180(5 Suppl):SS6–SS10.
8. Hart DS, Spector TD. The relationship of obesity, fat distribution and osteoarthritis in women in the general population: the Chingford study. J Rheumatol 1993;20:331–335.
9. Coggon DC, et al. Occupational activity and osteoarthritis of the knee. Arthritis Rheum 2000;43:1443–1449.
10. Spector TC, et al. Genetic influences on osteoarthritis in women: a twin study. BMJ 1996;312:940–943.
11. Zhang YX, et al. Lower prevalence of hand osteoarthritis among Chinese subjects in Beijing compared with white subjects in the United States: the Beijing Osteoarthritis study. Arthritis Rheum 2003;48:1034–1040.
12. Bellamy NB, et al. Validation study of WOMAC: a health status instrument for measuring clinically important patient relevant outcomes to anti-rheumatic drug therapy in patients with osteoarthritis of the hip or knee. J Rheumatol 1988;15:1833–1840.
13. Auw Yang KR, et al. Validation of the short-form WOMAC function scale for the evaluation of osteoarthritis of the knee. J Bone Joint Surg 2007;89-B(1): 50–56.
14. National Arthritis and Musculoskeletal Conditions Advisory Group. Evidence to support the national action plan for osteoarthritis, rheumatoid arthritis and osteoporosis: opportunities to improve health-related quality of life and reduce the burden of disease and disability. Canberra: Department of Health and Ageing, 2004.

15. American College of Rheumatology. American College of Rheumatology Subcommittee on Osteoarthritis guidelines. Recommendations for the medical management of osteoarthritis of the hip and knee: 2000 update. Arthritis Rheum 2000;43:1905–1915.
16. Jordan KA, et al. EULAR Recommendations 2003: an evidence based approach to the management of knee osteoarthritis: Report of a Task Force of the Standing Committee for International Clinical Studies Including Therapeutic Trials (ESCISIT). Ann Rheum Dis 2003;62(12):1145–1155.
17. Hewlett S, et al. Patients' perceptions of fatigue in rheumatoid arthritis: overwhelming, uncontrollable, ignored. Arthritis Rheum 2005;53(5):697–702.
18. Power J, et al. Fatigue in osteoarthritis: a qualitative study. BMC Musculoskelet Disord 2008;1(9):63.
19. Zeff J, et al. A hierarchy of healing: the therapeutic order. The unifying theory of naturopathic medicine. In: Pizzorno JE, Murray MT, eds. Textbook of natural medicine. 3rd edn. Edinburgh: Churchill Livingstone, 2006.
20. Zhang WM, et al. OARSI recommendations for the management of hip and knee osteoarthritis, part II: OARSI evidence-based, expert consensus guidelines. Osteoarthritis Cartilage 2008;16(2):137e–162e.
21. Hart J. Osteoarthritis and complementary therapies. Alternative and Complementary Therapies 2008;14(3):116–120.
22. Royal Australian College of General Practitioners. Osteoarthritis Working Group: Guideline for the non-surgical management of hip and knee osteoarthritis. 2009. Online. Available: http://www.nhmrc.gov.au/PUBLICATIONS/synopses/_files/cp117-hip-knee-osteoarthritis.pdf.
23. Kelly A. Managing osteoarthritis pain. Nursing 2006;36(11):20–21.
24. Laufer S, et al., eds. Inflammation and rheumatic diseases: the molecular basis of novel therapies. Stuttgart: Thieme, 2008.
25. Calder P. Dietary modification of inflammation with lipids. Proc Nutr Soc 2002;61:345–358.
26. Setty AS, L.H. Herbal medications commonly used in the practice of rheumatology: mechanisms of action, efficacy, and side effects. Semin Arthritis Rheum 2005;34(6):773–784.
27. Tancred J. Joint care. Journal of Complementary Medicine 2009;8(2):12–19.
28. Brien SL, et al. Devil's claw (*Harpagophytum procumbens*) as a treatment for osteoarthritis: a review of efficacy and safety. J Altern Complement Med 2006;12(10):981–993.
29. Braun L, Cohen M. Herbs and natural supplements. An evidence-based guide. Sydney: Elsevier, 2005.
30. Warnock MM, et al. Effectiveness and safety of devil's claw tablets in patients with general rheumatic disorders. Phytother Res 2007;21(12):1228–1233.
31. Ernst E. The efficacy of Phytodolor® for the treatment of musculoskeletal pain—a systematic review of randomized clinical trials. Nat Med J 1999;2(1):14–16.
32. Gundermann K, Müller J. Phytodolor—effects and efficacy of a herbal medicine. Wien Med Wochenschr 2007;157(13–14):343–347.
33. Ernst E. Frankincense: a systematic review. BMJ 2009;337:a2813.
34. Sengupta KA, et al. A double blind, randomized, placebo controlled study of the efficacy and safety of 5-Loxin® for treatment of osteoarthritis of the knee. Arthritis Res Ther 2008;10(4):R85.
35. Chrubasik SK, et al. Treatment of low-back pain with a herbal or synthetic anti-rheumatic: a randomized controlled study. Willow bark extract for low-back pain. Rheumatology (Oxford) 2001;40:1388–1393.
36. Beer A-M, Wegener T. Willow bark extract (*Salicis cortex*) for gonarthrosis and coxarthrosis—results of a cohort study with a control group. Phytomedicine 2008;15:907–913.
37. Tjendraputra ET, et al. Effect of ginger constituents and synthetic analogues on cyclooxygenase-2 enzyme in intact cells. Bioorg Chem 2001;29(3):156–163.
38. Altman RM, Marcussen KC. Effects of a ginger extract on knee pain in patients with osteoarthritis. Arthritis Rheum 2001;44(11):2531–2538.
39. Hamblin LL, et al. Improved arthritic knee health in a pilot RCT of phytotherapy. J R Soc Promot Health 2008;128(5):255–262.
40. Clegg DR, et al. Glucosamine, chondroitin sulfate, and the two in combination for painful knee osteoarthritis. N Engl J Med 2006;354(8):795–808.
41. Sawitzke AS, et al. The effect of glucosamine and/or chondroitin sulfate on the progression of knee osteoarthritis: a report from the glucosamine/chondroitin arthritis intervention trial. Arthritis Rheu 2008;58(10):3183–3191.
42. Kahan AU, et al. Long-term effects of chondroitins 4 and 6 sulfate on knee osteoarthritis: the study on osteoarthritis progression prevention, a two-year, randomized, double-blind, placebo-controlled trial. Arthritis Rheum 2009;60(2):524–533.
43. Brien SP, et al. Systematic review of the nutritional supplements dimethyl sulfoxide (DMSO) and methylsulfonylmethane (MSM) in the treatment of osteoarthritis. Osteoarthritis Cartilage 2008;16(11):1277–1288.
44. Kim LA, et al. Efficacy of methylsulfonylmethane (MSM) in osteoarthritis pain of the knee: a pilot clinical trial. Osteoarthritis Cartilage 2006;14(3):286–294.
45. Ameye LG, Chee WS. Osteoarthritis and nutrition: from nutraceuticals to functional foods: a systematic review of the scientific evidence. Arthritis Res Ther 2006;8(4):R127.
46. Towheed T, et al. Glucosamine therapy for treating osteoarthritis. Cochrane Database Syst Rev 2006;(2):CD002946.
47. Vlad SL, et al. Glucosamine for pain in osteoarthritis: why do trial results differ? Arthritis Rheum 2007;56(7):2267–2277.
48. Perlman AS, et al. Massage therapy for osteoarthritis of the knee: a randomized controlled trial. Arch Intern Med 2006;166(22):2533–2538.
49. Orrock P. Naturopathic physical medicine. In: Chaitow L, ed. Naturopathic physical medicine. Edinburgh: Elsevier, 2008.
50. Yip YB, Tam ACY. An experimental study on the effectiveness of massage with aromatic ginger and orange essential oil for moderate-to-severe knee pain among the elderly in Hong Kong. Complement Ther Med 2008;16(13):131–138.
51. Brosseau LY, et al. Thermotherapy for treatment of osteoarthritis. Cochrane Database Syst Rev 2003;(4):CD004259.
52. Thomas ML-J, et al. Hypovitaminosis D in medical inpatients. N Engl J Med 1998;338(12):///–/83.
53. Nesby-O'Dell SS, et al. Hypovitaminosis D prevalence and determinants among African American and white women of reproductive age: third National Health and Nutrition Examination Survey, 1988–1994. Am J Clin Nutr 2002;79:187–192.
54. Plotnikoff GA, Quigley JM. Prevalence of severe hypovitaminosis D in patients with persistent, nonspecific musculoskeletal pain. Mayo Clin Proc 2003;78(12):1463–1470.
55. Holick M. Vitamin D deficiency: what a pain it is. Mayo Clin Proc 2003;78(12):1457–1459.
56. McAlindon TF, et al. Relation of dietary intake and serum levels of vitamin D to progression of osteoarthritis of the knee among participants in the Framingham Study. Ann Intern Med 1996;125(5):353–359.
57. Holick M. Vitamin D deficiency: medical progress. N Engl J Med 2007;357(3):266.
58. McAlindon TJ, et al. Do antioxidant micronutrients protect against the development and progression of knee osteoarthritis? Arthritis Rheum 2005;39(4):648–656.
59. Wang YP, et al. The effect of nutritional supplements on osteoarthritis. Altern Med Rev 2004;9(3):275–296.

60. Chaitow L, ed. Naturopathic physical medicine. Edinburgh: Elsevier, 2008.
61. Mills S, Bone K. Principles and practice of phytotherapy. Edinburgh: Churchill Livingstone, 2000.
62. Demio P. Gout. In: Rakel D, ed. Integrative medicine. 2nd edn. Philadelphia: Saunders Elsevier, 2008.
63. National Health Priority Action Council. National service improvement framework for ostearthritis, rheumatoid arthritis and osteoporosis. Canberra: Department of Health and Ageing, 2006.
64. Messier SL, et al. Exercise and dietary weight loss in overweight and obese older adults with knee osteoarthritis. Arthritis Rheum 2004;50(5):1501–1510.
65. Fransen MM, et al. Exercise for osteoarthritis of the hip or knee. Cochrane Database Syst Rev 2003;(3):CD004376.
66. Brosseau LM, et al. Intensity of exercise for the treatment of osteoarthritis. Cochrane Database Syst Rev 2003;(3):CD004376.
67. Bartels EL, et al. Aquatic exercise for the treatment of knee and hip osteoarthritis. Cochrane Database Syst Rev 2007;(4):CD005523.
68. Soo Lee MP, et al. Tai chi for osteoarthritis: a systematic review. Clin Rheumatol 2008;27(2):211–218.
69. Bandy WD, Sanders B. Therapeutic exercise: techniques for intervention. 1st edn. Philadelphia: Lippincott Williams and Wilkins, 2001.
70. Lipton L. Using yoga to treat disease: an evidence based review. JAAPA 2008;21(2):34–41.
71. Lee M, et al. Tai chi for osteoarthritis: a systematic review. Clinical Rheumatology 2008;27(2):211–218.
72. Bernardo L. The effectiveness of Pilates training in healthy adults: an appraisal of the research literature. J Bodyw Mov Ther 2007;11:106–110.
73. Vas JM, et al. Acupuncture as a complementary therapy to the pharmacological treatment of osteoarthritis of the knee: randomised controlled trial. BMJ 2004;329:1216.
74. Manheimer EL, et al. Meta-analysis: acupuncture for osteoarthritis of the knee. Ann Intern Med 2007;146(12): 868–877.
75. Rosemann TG, et al. The impact of concomitant depression on quality of life and health service utilisation in patients with osteoarthritis. Rheumatol Int 2007;27(9):859–863.

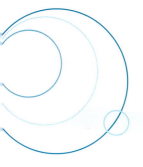

23
Fibromyalgia

Leslie Axelrod

ND, LAc

AETIOLOGY, EPIDEMIOLOGY AND CLASSIFICATION

The American College of Rheumatology (ACR) definition of fibromyalgia (FM) has been based on generalised pain as the primary symptom; however, many of these patients present with a wide variety of complaints including, but not limited to, increased frequency of fatigue, non-restorative sleep, IBS, headache and impaired cognition and mood.[1] It is more prevalent in women, ages 20–50 years, but has also been seen in paediatric and geriatric populations. It affects 0.5% to 5.8% of the population in North America and Europe.[2] The diagnosis has been based primarily on subjective reporting of widespread pain, with the absence of objective findings or a known aetiology. Research has identified biochemical and metabolic abnormalities that are common to this particular group. Presently, there is a movement to redefine this disorder to include its multisystem effect and find objective, measurable biomarkers.[3]

The 1990 American College of Rheumatology criteria for classification of fibromyalgia[1] are widespread pain for at least 3 months, defined as the presence of all of the following:
- pain on the right and left sides of the body
- pain above and below the waist (including shoulder and buttock pain)
- pain in the axial skeleton (cervical, thoracic or lumbar spine, or anterior chest)
- pain in 11 of 18 tender point sites on digital palpation.

Pain, on digital palpation, must be present in at least 11 of the following 18 tender point sites (see Figure 23.1). All sites are bilateral:
- occiput—at the suboccipital muscle insertions (trapezius, sternocleidomastoid, semi-spinalis capitus, splenius capitus)
- low cervical—at the anterior aspects of the intertransverse spaces at C5–C7
- trapezius—at the midpoint of the upper border
- supraspinatus—at origins, above the scapula spine near the medial border
- second rib—upper lateral to the second costochondral junction
- lateral epicondyle—2 cm distal to the epicondyles
- gluteal—in upper outer quadrants of buttocks in anterior fold of muscle
- greater trochanter—posterior to the trochanteric prominence
- knee—at the medial fat pad proximal to the joint line.

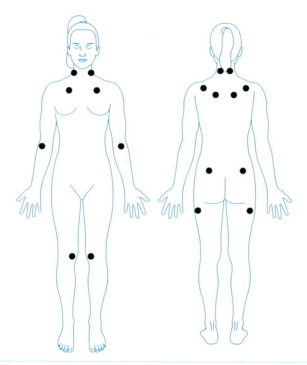

Figure 23.1 Fibromyalgia: diagnostic tender points

Digital palpation should be performed with an approximate force of 4 kg, enough pressure for the examiner's nail bed to blanch. A tender point has to be painful at palpation, not just 'tender'.

The aetiology of fibromyalgia is not fully understood, but ongoing research has been elucidating some possible mechanisms for this syndrome. Biochemical, metabolic and cellular changes have been demonstrated in multiple systems including mitochondrial dysfunction with aberrations in ATP synthesis and use, central nervous system (CNS) changes affecting cerebral blood flow, neurotransmitter synthesis and function and increased pain perception.[4] HPA axis function is affected, resulting in a hyporesponsiveness of the adrenals and circadian rhythm abnormalities.[5] Somatic and visceral alterations have also been demonstrated in the literature.[6] The result of these changes contributes to the high incidence of comorbidities associated with this syndrome.

RISK FACTORS

There are a variety of risk factors associated with FM patients, including genetics, and comorbidities with other rheumatological conditions and chronic fatigue syndrome (see Chapter 35 on chronic fatigue syndrome). One of the most consistent findings is that the prevalence among females compared to males is as high as 9:1,[2] which is also common to these comorbid conditions. Previous history of domestic violence, abuse and emotional trauma appear to be factors as evidenced by the epidemiological data.[7] The presence of poverty, poor support and lower educational status may be a predisposing factor associated with the high incidence of mood disorders and decreased pain threshold.[8] These triggers, when combined with the prevalence of non-restorative sleep,

Table 23.1 Predictive risks factors for developing fibromyalgia[7,8]

AGE 20–50 YEARS	FEMALE > MALE (9:1)
Lower education level and socioeconomic status	Non-restorative sleep
Increased incidence of anxiety, depression and somatisation	Comorbidity with other rheumatic diseases, such as rheumatoid arthritis and lupus
History of physical, sexual, emotional abuse or trauma	Comorbidity with chronic fatigue syndrome
Poor social support system	High prevalence of gastrointestinal dysfunction and dysbiosis
Abnormal stress response	Other family members with symptoms of fibromyalgia and common enzyme defect

predispose the FM patient to irregularities in the HPA axis that are common in this cohort.[9] This spectrum of systemic changes along with aberrations in the health of the gastrointestinal tract contribute to this cascade via alterations in serotonin synthesis and use, nutritional deficiencies and immune dysfunction and must be differentiated from other disease patterns presenting with myalgias.[3]

CONVENTIONAL TREATMENT

A variety of allopathic medications have been used in the treatment of FM, including muscle relaxants, antidepressants, anticonvulsants and other CNS agents. The antidepressants typically prescribed are tricyclic antidepressants (TCAs), selective serotonin reuptake inhibitors (SSRIs), serotonin and noradrenaline reuptake inhibitors (SNRIs) and monoamine oxidase inhibitors (MAOIs).[10] NSAIDs and steroids alone have not been shown to be effective.[10] Review of a meta-analysis on patients using the muscle relaxant cyclobenzaprine revealed a reduction in pain initially and improvement in sleep, but no change in tender points or fatigue.[11] A recent meta-analysis representing the efficacy of different antidepressant classes on the parameters associated with fibromyalgia revealed amitriptyline and duloxetine as having the most overall effectiveness. The author's conclusion of the meta-analysis was that, based on the data, these two medications can justifiably be recommended, in the short term, for pain and sleep disturbances.[12]

Table 23.2 Medication overall effect using p value*: meta-analysis of 18 randomised controlled trials (RCTs)[12]

SYMPTOM	SSRIs (FLUOXETINE AND PAROXETINE)	SNRIs (DULOXETINE, MILNACIPRAN)	MAOs (MOCLOBEMIDE, PIRLINDOLE)	TCAs (AMITRIPTYLINE)
Pain	**0.04**	**< 0.001**	**0.03**	**< 0.001**
Fatigue	0.25	0.23	0.66	**0.003**
Sleep	0.18	**< 0.001**	0.19	**< 0.001**
Depressed mood	**0.02**	**0.001**	0.88	0.76

*$p < 0.05$ significant (bold)

TREATMENT OF GENERAL MUSCLE TENSION AND PAIN

- Lifestyle education:
  - sleep
  - exercise
  - diet
  - rest
  - sunshine
- Physical and manipulative modalities:
  - adjustment
  - soft tissue manipulation
  - myofascial release
  - massage
  - physical therapy
  - stretching
  - yoga
- Dietary and nutritional factors:
  - anti-inflammatory diet
  - anti-allergic diet
  - gluten free
  - correct nutritional deficiencies and biochemical imbalances
- Mind/body techniques:
  - meditation
  - biofeedback
  - hypnosis
  - eye movement desensitisation and reprocessing (EMDR)
  - cognitive behavioural therapy
- Pain management:
  - botanical
  - homoeopathy
  - hydrotherapy
  - acupuncture
  - therapeutic injections
  - medication
- Address underlying issues:
  - neuroendocrine
  - hypothalamic–pituitary–adrenal axis
  - toxicity
  - gastrointestinal dysbiosis and permeability.

Due to the increased side effects of the TCAs, low doses are typically prescribed; this may account for the lack of improvement in depression. The median duration for the RCTs was 8 weeks (4 to 28 weeks). The long-term effect of the medications and posttreatment improvement has not been elucidated in-depth in the literature. Median drop-out rates did not differ between the placebo and antidepressant groups due to adverse effects. Because of the possibility of suicidal thinking, in the United States of America most medications approved for fibromyalgia carry a black box warning from the Food and Drug Administration (FDA); these include duloxetine (SNRI), milnacipran (SNRI) and pregabalin, a GABA analogue typically used to treat neuropathic pain and seizures.[13,14]

KEY TREATMENT PROTOCOLS

Mitochondrial and cellular changes

Metabolic changes occur at the cellular level, causing functional aberrations in FM patients. These include changes in glycolysis and isoenzyme production and reduction of energy reserves. Increased lactate production and decreased lactate dehydrogenase isoenzymes were present in the muscle tissue of FM patients.[15] A small study using magnetic resonance spectroscopy revealed decreased phosphocreatine, an essential muscle energy storage form, and reduced ATP levels in the quadriceps of FM patients

NATUROPATHIC TREATMENT AIMS
- Reduce pain.
- Improve sleep.
- Address mood and cognitive changes.
- Address any digestive dysfunction.
- Improve daily functioning.

compared to controls during rest.[16] Total oxidative capacity and phosphorylation potential was also reduced during rest and exercise.[16] Another study found decreased platelet ATP, along with higher calcium and magnesium levels, implying irregularities in the calcium magnesium pump mechanisms at the cellular level.[17] These biochemical aberrations contribute to the fatigue, weakness and exercise intolerance associated with FM.

The role of **magnesium** includes glycolysis and mitochondrial function.[18] ATP biosynthesis and metabolism in FM patients are affected by a disturbance in its use.[19] Inconsistencies in the levels of magnesium are evident in the various blood components. Increased platelet magnesium and calcium levels have been found, and low serum and RBC magnesium levels are noted.[20,21] Reduced serum magnesium levels appear to correlate with fatigue, but not to the number of tender points.[22] In a small placebo controlled trial, **malic acid**, a precursor to malate (an intermediary in the citric acid cycle), was combined with magnesium. The effects of a 4-week course of magnesium/malic acid 300/1200 mg were compared to those of a 600/2400 mg dosage. Significant reductions in pain and tenderness measures were seen at higher dosages given for at least 2 months.[21,23] A randomised, double blind, placebo controlled 8-week study using an IV micronutrient therapy (IVMT), **Myers' cocktail** (which contains magnesium), thiamine, vitamin C, calcium and B vitamins demonstrated statistically significant improvement in tender points, pain, depression and quality of life in the IVMT group at 8 weeks, while the placebo group of IV lactated Ringer's solution showed statistically significant improvement in tender points. The dramatic response of the placebo group negated a statistical significance between the groups. The response persisted for 4 weeks posttreatment for both groups.[24] An 8-week uncontrolled case study of seven previously non-responsive patients by Massey revealed a 60% decrease in pain and 80% reduction in fatigue.[25]

The irregularities of the calcium–magnesium pump mechanism as suggested by Bazzichi may play a role in the muscle pain attributed to fibromyalgia.[16] Other aberrations in calcium absorption and use may exist in the patient presenting with widespread pain. **Vitamin D** in the form of 1 alpha, 25-(OH)2-vitamin D3 promotes the calcium-dependent exocytotic activities of the cell when coupled with ATP, potentiating the bone anabolic effects of this nutrient.[26,27] A deficiency of vitamin D may masquerade as a generalised non-specific pain, depression and poor fibromyalgia assessment scores.[28] One author proposes that the widespread pain associated with low levels of vitamin D is secondary to reduced calcium absorption, which increases PTH levels.[29] Elevated PTH causes increased urinary excretion of phosphorus, resulting in low levels of circulating calcium phosphate, ultimately leading to a poorly mineralised collagen matrix. Endosteal and periosteal swelling may occur secondary to the affected collagen on the surfaces, triggering bone and muscle pain.

In multiple studies of patients presenting with persistent non-specific muscle pain as well as fibromyalgia, 25-OH vitamin D levels were frequently depressed.[29,30] Supplementation of vitamin D2, 50,000 IU weekly for 8 weeks, yielded significant clinical improvement in mild to moderately (10–25 ng/mL) deficient patients, but not severely deficient patients.[28] However, this regimen of supplementation has not consistently yielded pain reduction in moderately deficient patients, even after 3 months.[31] Vitamin D deficiency has also been associated with decreased cognitive performance and mood disorders, especially anxiety and depression.[32,33] Evaluation of 25-OH vitamin D levels and correction of low serum levels are warranted in all patients presenting with widespread pain. In addition to the possible benefit to FM, depressed levels of vitamin D have been associated with increased risk of breast cancer and osteoporosis in this primarily female population.[34] The optimal level of 25-OH vitamin D remains a controversial topic and one study recommended a minimum of ≥ 40 ng/mL for breast cancer prevention.[34] The optimal level for fibromyalgia patients still remains unclear.[34]

Phosphorylated **D-ribose** is a component of ATP and NADH as D-ribose-5-phosphate, and may be helpful to FM patients. A small uncontrolled trial of 41 patients with FM and/or chronic fatigue syndrome, given 5 g of ribose three times daily, revealed significant improvement in energy and wellbeing according to a visual analogue scale.[35] Due to the limitations and positive results of the study, further investigation of D-ribose would be valuable.

Neurotransmitter effects

The concept of 'somatisation' has been associated with fibromyalgia secondary to the increased reporting of hypersensitivity to pain, cognitive dysfunction, depression, anxiety, social isolation and insomnia.[36] There is an increased incidence of adverse life events and psychological distress common to this primarily female cohort.[7] In addition to psychosocial stressors, the biochemical changes associated with neurotransmitter synthesis and use have been implicated and may contribute to the mental and emotional state of these patients (see Section 4 on the nervous system).

There is a genetic correlation of FM in families secondary to a defect in neurotransmitter metabolism. This polymorphic rate defect displays itself in catecholamine turnover secondary to catecholamine-O-methyl transferase enzyme and is linked to dopaminergic, adrenergic/non-adrenergic neurotransmission and the mu-opioid system.[37] This aberration has been associated with increased nociceptive response to painful stimuli. In addition to dopamine and epinephrine metabolism, reduced levels of serotonin and its precursors, **tryptophan** and **5-hydroxytryptophan** (5-HTP), are seen.[38,39] Low levels of plasma and serum serotonin (5-HT) have been highlighted in the literature and pharmacological treatment has focused on the use of antidepressants, most recently SSRIs and SNRIs, for treatment of pain, sleep and mood disturbances.[40] In FM patients, low levels of serotonin in combination with elevated levels of substance P, a neurotransmitter that has been associated with enhanced pain perception secondary to normal stimuli, has been considered to be a precipitating factor for the increased pain hypersensitivity found in fibromyalgia.[41]

The conversion of tryptophan to serotonin involves the intermediary, 5-hydroxytryptophan (5-HTP). This biochemical pathway may be inhibited by stress, insulin resistance, tetrahydrobiopterin, pyridoxal 5-phosphate and magnesium deficiency.[42] Supplementation with 5-HTP alone has shown significant improvement in the number of tender points, anxiety, fatigue, pain intensity and quality of sleep during a 90-day trial of patients with primary fibromyalgia syndrome. Mild transient side effects were reported in 30% of the patients.[42,43]

Another metabolic pathway is the use of **S-adenosyl methionine (SAMe)** in the conversion of 5-HT to melatonin. It acts as a coenzyme and a methyl donor, and has been shown to be an effective antidepressant in psychiatric populations.[44] In FM patients there is a correlation with depression and the number of trigger points. When patients were treated with 200 mg of injectable SAMe, both depression and the number of trigger points significantly improved.[45] A 6-week trial of oral SAMe revealed improvement in fatigue, mood and morning stiffness.[46] Reduction in pain, but not tender point count, occurred during week 6 of the trial and may warrant a longer investigation to realise the potential benefits.

The use of botanicals specifically for the treatment of FM has not been well documented in the scientific literature. Since combination formulas are the traditional mode of botanical dispensing, a balanced combination of botanicals would most likely best address the complex nature of a FM patient. However, single botanicals addressing the separate components of this syndrome will be presented, allowing the naturopathic practitioner to develop an individualised compound to best suit the needs of their patients (see Table 23.3).

The botanical **Rhodiola rosea** was found to increase 5-HT levels in the hippocampus of depressive rats to normal levels using 1.5 g/kg, 3 g/kg and 6 g/kg dosages.[49] A randomised placebo controlled double-blind study of **Hypericum perforatum** in the treatment of depressive patients with somatic complaints including depression, fatigue and disturbed sleep resulted in 70% of the patients being symptom-free after 4 weeks.[50] *H. perforatum* administration in the unstressed rat population revealed a decrease in tryptophan, an increase in corticosterone and lower 5-HT in the hippocampus and amygdala under stressful physical conditions. Serum 5-HT levels increased more than 110%, 163% and 172% in the hypothalamus, amygdala and hippocampus respectively ($p < 0.01$), demonstrating an adaptive response to stress. Tryptophan and corticosterone levels did not change significantly.[51] In addition, a meta-analysis, including the Cochrane database, comparing HP to key SSRIs revealed that there was a similar efficacy between the medications, but fewer side effects with the HP.[52,53] The botanical **Scutellaria baicalensis**, which has traditionally been used as a 'nervine', contains a metabolite similar to hyperforin, which is found in *H. perforatum* and would demonstrate similar actions.[54]

Table 23.3 Fibromyalgia: herbal medicine actions and examples[47,48]

1. Adaptogens/tonics
Withania somnifera, Panax ginseng, Rhodiola rosea, Eleutherococcus senticosus
2. Antispasmodics
Viburnum opulus, Piper methysticum, Piscidia erythrina, Scutellaria lateriflora
3. Nervines
Scutellaria lateriflora, Passiflora incarnata, Matricaria recutita, Melissa officinalis
4. Thymoleptics
Hypericum perforatum, Avena sativum, Lavandula angustifolia, Turnera diffusa
5. Hypnotics
Humulus lupulus, Passiflora incarnata, Valeriana spp.
6. Analgesics
Corydalis ambigua, Eschscholtzia californica
7. Digestives (aromatics, bitters, mucilages)
Zingiber officinale, Taraxacum officinale, Ulmus fulva
8. Circulatory stimulants
Zingiber officinale, Ginkgo biloba, Cinnamomum zeylanicum, Zanthoxylum spp.

The circadian rhythm

Dysregulated circadian rhythms, manifesting as poor sleep patterns, non-restorative sleep and chronic fatigue, have been reported in fibromyalgia patients.[55] Elevation of late evening cortisol and alterations in melatonin levels may contribute to the poor sleep patterns seen in this cohort.[56] Normal basal circadian rhythm is typically evidenced by a sharp rise in serotonin synthesis and a release of 5-HT in the early evening, preceding an elevation in melatonin production. There are conflicting data regarding melatonin secretion in FM patients. Decreased urinary melatonin secretion levels were found between the hours of 11 p.m. and 7 a.m.[57–59] Meanwhile, in another study, plasma melatonin levels were elevated in FM patients between the hours of 11 p.m. and 6:50 a.m. compared to controls, but secretory patterns remained similar.[5] This discrepancy between urinary and plasma melatonin levels was not demonstrated in normal non-depressed patients.[60] Despite the discrepancy and different methods of evaluation, it was found that administration of 3 mg of **melatonin** at bedtime in a small uncontrolled study revealed significant improvement in tender point count, pain severity and sleep after 30 days.[59]

HPA-axis modulation

Another contributing factor to the non-restorative sleep, low energy and heightened pain perception may be associated with abnormalities in the hypothalamic–pituitary–adrenal (HPA) axis.[61] Dexamethasone suppression tests in FM patients show statistically significant increased release of ACTH with no resulting change in cortisol, indicating a hyporesponsiveness of the adrenal function to stimuli.[61] The increased ACTH/cortisol ratios, compared to controls, correlate to increased stress and anxiety measures. Also, the percentage of cortisol suppression is related to pain and fatigue as reported by patients.[62] Corticoid response to acute exercise is also impaired in fibromyalgia patients.[63] In addition to lower basal plasma and urinary cortisol levels, there is a decreased expression of corticosteroid receptors, all of these contributing to the abnormal glucocorticoid response.[64] The combined dysfunction associated with the HPA axis and the adrenal response contributes to the aetiopathology and symptomology of fibromyalgia.

A combination of **Eleutherococcus senticocus**, **Schisandra chinensis** and **Rhodiola rosea** revealed improved exercise endurance and tolerance to stress.[65,66] In addition, a single administration of **Panax ginseng** up-regulated the release of ACTH and corticosteroid initially, but did not maintain this effect after 7 days of ginseng administration. However, ginseng was shown to modulate the effect of hydrocortisone administration on the pituitary adrenocortical system even after 7 days.[67]

Digestive dysbiosis

It is estimated that 30–70% of patients with FM have irritable bowel syndrome (IBS) concurrently.[68,69] In addition to altered visceral and somatic perception, both patient subsets have decreased serotonin synthesis and use, which may contribute to increased sensitivity to abdominal pain.[6,70] In addition, the low levels of serotonin may alter motor and secretory function that may result in diarrhoea or constipation, both manifestations of IBS.[70] Increased intestinal and gastroduodenal permeability is associated with FM. In addition increased incidence of dysbiotic changes, as evidenced by the lactulose hydrogen breath test, implicates the prevalence of small intestinal bowel overgrowth (SIBO) in both these groups. The proximal small intestine typically has low levels of colonic type bacteria, but issues such as dysmotility and lack of gastric acid may exacerbate SIBO. The intensity of abdominal pain in FM patients with SIBO appears to correlate to the degree of bacterial overgrowth found in the small intestine.[71] In a double-blind randomised placebo controlled trial, FM patients identified with SIBO were treated to achieve full eradication of the pathogenic flora compared to a non-eradicated group. The group that achieved complete eradication of dysbiotic flora had a significant improvement in pain and depression, in comparison to the non-eradicated group.[72] Eradication with antibiotics is standard treatment for SIBO, but recurrence rate is high, especially in populations using proton pump inhibitors, which decrease gastric secretions.[73] There have been a limited number of small studies and case reports showing improvement in SIBO via natural therapeutics.

Studies using **glutamine** and **fibre** in animal studies demonstrated a reduction of bacterial translocation into lymph nodes, along with improvement in gut barrier function secondary to glutamine.[74–76] A nutrient solution of **L-arginine** alone at levels of 300 and 600 mg or in combination with nucleotides and omega-3 fatty acids showed a reduction in bacterial translocation.[77] In addition the **omega-3 fatty acids** may improve the outcome of fibromyalgia patients over time by modulating inflammatory cytokines[78] (see Chapter 28 on autoimmunity). Consideration should also be given to ensuring motility and normal gastric secretions, since their reduction may perpetuate SIBO. The modification of SIBO and bacterial translocation may decrease the inflammatory response that appears to develop with long-standing fibromyalgia.

Immune alterations

Immune activation was apparent in dermal biopsies of fibromyalgia patients that revealed significantly elevated levels of IgG deposits in the dermis. In addition there was higher mean number of mast cells and an association between degranulated mast cells and the individual IgG immunofluorescence scores.[79] This IgG correlation may account, in part, for the prevalence of rhinitis in this cohort (70%) in the absence of positive skin allergy tests in 50–65% of this population.[80] Both IBS and migraines, common manifestations associated with FM, also demonstrate elevated IgG levels.[81,82] In a study of IBS patients, food antigen specific IgE antibodies were not significantly different between FM patients and controls. IgG4 antibodies were significantly elevated in one study, but did not significantly correlate with the severity of symptoms.[83]

IBS and migraines may both benefit by eliminating IgG positive foods, and reduction of circulating IgG may be beneficial in the treatment of fibromyalgia patients. In addition to the role of IgG in functional bowel disturbances, IBS and migraines, it is possible that dermal IgG may contribute to sensory alterations and widespread pain. It appears that IgG plays a more significant role than IgE in the pathogenesis of a variety of co-existing complaints and that standard scratch testing and IgE titres are not the most accurate method of testing for this cohort. Also, since the severity of symptoms does not always correlate with the antibody titres, it is important to eliminate all reactive foods, even low scoring ones.[83] ELISA testing of food antigens and subsequent trial elimination would be justified in this population.

Circulatory disturbances

It has been hypothesised that circulatory changes may be partially responsible for the pain, presence of tender points, exercise intolerance, Raynaud's phenomenon and cognitive changes present in FM.[84] Alterations in microcirculation and temperature were at the level of tender points, resulting in lower skin temperature. A lack of blood flow was implicated by decreased erythrocyte velocity and increased concentration of erythrocytes at tender points.[84] Muscle biopsy revealed increased dialysate lactate secondary to alterations in nitric oxide pathways; this may contribute to the reported exercise intolerance and exertion fatigue reported during aerobic exercise in these patients.[85] Impaired cerebral perfusion flow is also evident by brain single photon emission computed tomography (SPECT) and clinically correlated with the severity and associated disability of the small group evaluated.[86]

The correlation between circulatory and oxygenation disturbances with FM may explain the beneficial effect of **CoQ10** and ***Ginkgo biloba***. A small, uncontrolled study of 200 mg daily of both coenzyme Q10 (CoQ10) and *G. biloba* showed promise for improving quality of life measures.[87] Increased tissue perfusion was demonstrated by both substances. CoQ10 is present primarily in the mitochondria and assists in the generation of ATP via cellular respiration, but also has been shown to be protective against lipid peroxidation secondary to cerebral hypo/hyperperfusion in rats.[88,89] CoQ10 is also effective in the treatment of fatigue and migraines.[88,90] *G. biloba* increased blood flow velocity cerebrally, as well as having an effect on promoting vasculogenesis capacity, via endothelial progenitor cells stimulation, in the peripheral blood, resulting in improved perfusion of the peripheral tissues.[91,92]

INTEGRATIVE MEDICAL CONSIDERATIONS

The fibromyalgia patient is complex with irregularities in a multitude of processes including, but not limited to, cellular, neuroendocrine, digestive, vascular and emotional alterations. The ubiquitous nature of this condition would benefit by a combination of energetic medicine, lifestyle and mind/body interventions.

Homoeopathy

A double-blind, randomised, parallel-group, placebo controlled study using individualised homoeopathic medicine with daily LM potency over a 3-month period was been shown to be effective in treating fibromyalgia. The number of tender points, pain on palpation and quality of health all improved significantly.[93] Another study using individualised homoeopathic prescriptions revealed more significant improvement on fatigue and function with less effect on pain.[94]

Acupuncture

Acupuncture diagnosis commonly assesses pain as 'Blood and Qi [energy] Stagnation' and focuses on movement of these vital substances.[95] One study demonstrated an elevated number of erythrocytes in conjunction with a decrease in regional blood flow at the level of tender points of FM patients; this correlates to the Chinese theory of Blood Stagnation.[84] Lower skin temperature was also found.[84] A follow-up study measured these indices pre- and post-acupuncture treatment. The therapeutic effect of acupuncture revealed a significant increase in blood flow and temperature at the level of the tender points posttreatment.[96] Acupuncture has been shown to increase serotonin levels in rats with the insertion of a bilateral acupoint, urinary bladder 23. Elevated levels began after 20 minutes and maintained for 60 minutes posttreatment.[97] Substance P levels were reduced using electroacupuncture of local and distal points in a rat model.[98]

Acupuncture may have an adaptogenic response on cortisol levels. Animal studies on horses and rabbits using electroacupuncture showed an increase in cortisol levels post treatment.[99–101] The inconsistencies of positive results with acupuncture, specifically on fibromyalgia patients, may be based in part on the techniques used. In a meta-analysis of

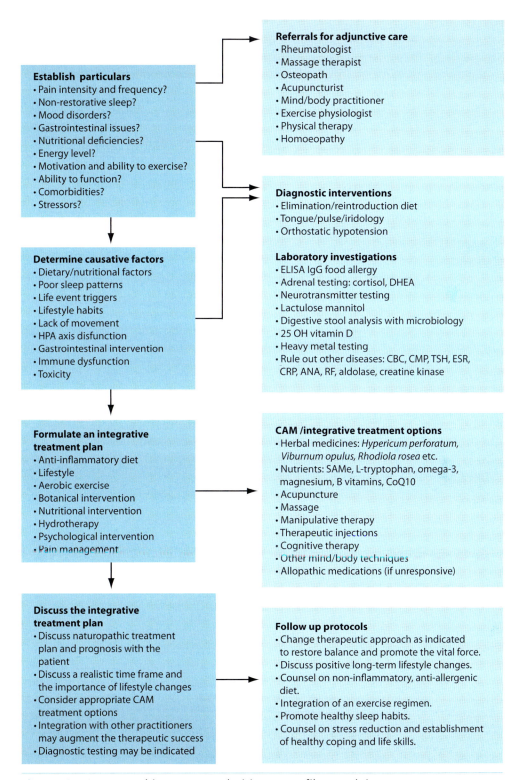

Establish particulars
- Pain intensity and frequency?
- Non-restorative sleep?
- Mood disorders?
- Gastrointestinal issues?
- Nutritional deficiencies?
- Energy level?
- Motivation and ability to exercise?
- Ability to function?
- Comorbidities?
- Stressors?

Referrals for adjunctive care
- Rheumatologist
- Massage therapist
- Osteopath
- Acupuncturist
- Mind/body practitioner
- Exercise physiologist
- Physical therapy
- Homoeopathy

Determine causative factors
- Dietary/nutritional factors
- Poor sleep patterns
- Life event triggers
- Lifestyle habits
- Lack of movement
- HPA axis disfunction
- Gastrointestinal intervention
- Immune dysfunction
- Toxicity

Diagnostic interventions
- Elimination/reintroduction diet
- Tongue/pulse/iridology
- Orthostatic hypotension

Laboratory investigations
- ELISA IgG food allergy
- Adrenal testing: cortisol, DHEA
- Neurotransmitter testing
- Lactulose mannitol
- Digestive stool analysis with microbiology
- 25 OH vitamin D
- Heavy metal testing
- Rule out other diseases: CBC, CMP, TSH, ESR, CRP, ANA, RF, aldolase, creatine kinase

Formulate an integrative treatment plan
- Anti-inflammatory diet
- Lifestyle
- Aerobic exercise
- Botanical intervention
- Nutritional intervention
- Hydrotherapy
- Psychological intervention
- Pain management

CAM /integrative treatment options
- Herbal medicines: *Hypericum perforatum, Viburnum opulus, Rhodiola rosea* etc.
- Nutrients: SAMe, L-tryptophan, omega-3, magnesium, B vitamins, CoQ10
- Acupuncture
- Massage
- Manipulative therapy
- Therapeutic injections
- Cognitive therapy
- Other mind/body techniques
- Allopathic medications (if unresponsive)

Discuss the integrative treatment plan
- Discuss naturopathic treatment plan and prognosis with the patient
- Discuss a realistic time frame and the importance of lifestyle changes
- Consider appropriate CAM treatment options
- Integration with other practitioners may augment the therapeutic success
- Diagnostic testing may be indicated

Follow up protocols
- Change therapeutic approach as indicated to restore balance and promote the vital force.
- Discuss positive long-term lifestyle changes.
- Counsel on non-inflammatory, anti-allergenic diet.
- Integration of an exercise regimen.
- Promote healthy sleep habits.
- Counsel on stress reduction and establishment of healthy coping and life skills.

Figure 23.2 Naturopathic treatment decision tree—fibromyalgia

five randomised controlled studies, out of 11 evaluated, results were based on variables including reduction of pain, number of tender points and improvement in quality of life and sleep. The studies involving electroacupuncture overall achieved the best results. In addition, most of the positive studies used individualised treatments.[100] The negative studies used manual therapy, which may not have had sufficient stimulation to 'obtain Qi' in a population that has sensory perception alterations.

Cupping and moxibustion techniques, which were not addressed in the meta-analysis, may also have beneficial effects when included in the acupuncture treatment.[102] The validity of sham acupuncture continues to be controversial, especially in a population with widespread pain. In acupuncture, insertion of needles into a painful point, termed an 'ashi' point, which is not otherwise considered a standard acupuncture point, is considered to be an effective treatment strategy for pain reduction. Meanwhile, the US National Institutes of Health consensus stance is that acupuncture is a sufficient adjuvant therapy to treat FM patients.[103]

Exercise and manual therapy

Exercise intolerance is a common manifestation in fibromyalgia patients. Multiple studies, including a meta-analysis of eight studies, showed that aerobic-only exercise training programs revealed significant improvement in outcome measures, including physical function and global wellbeing while reducing pain, tender points and fibromyalgia impact scores. Stretching and relaxation exercises did not yield the same effect. Improvement was seen as early as 6 weeks and maintained with exercise up to 12 months in some studies.[104–105] A review of pool exercise studies yielded improvement in mood and sleep as well as physical function and pain. The improvements, as reviewed in follow-up studies, showed a positive response for up to 2 years.[107]

Muscle stimulation may also be achieved with manual therapies. A small study of FM patients receiving twice weekly 30-minute massage treatments showed a decrease of substance P, reduction in pain and anxiety, in addition to improvement in quality and number of sleep hours.[108]

Mind/body therapy

The psychological component of FM in this primarily female population has been explored. Violence against women is epidemic as demonstrated in a cross-sectional, self-administered, anonymous survey of 1952 female patients. Physical, sexual and alcohol abuse and emotional status were all investigated among a diverse community-based population. The results of the survey indicated that one in 20 women had experienced domestic violence in the past year, one in five in their adult life and one in three as either a child or an adult. Participants that had experienced abuse within the past year were more likely to have depression, anxiety and somatisation.[109] Findings of another large case-controlled study of 574 women revealed an increased prevalence of abuse among FM patients over controls. There was a significant correlation between frequency of abuse and FM.[7] A Spanish epidemiological and quality of life study revealed low educational level, low social class and self-reported depression are much more prevalent in this FM population.[110] Depression co-existing with FM appears to decrease the pain threshold in these patients.[111] Effective treatment of FM must address the psychological impact as well as the biochemical changes to effect a long-standing improvement.

The prognosis for FM patients is partially dependent on social support and self-efficacy, which has been shown to predict positive lifestyle changes in FM patients.[112]

A randomised controlled study of 91 patients with fibromyalgia using mindfulness training during eight weekly session of 2.5 hours revealed alleviation of depressive symptoms, as assessed by the Beck Depression Inventory.[113] The effect of a 6-week guided imagery program was to improve functional status and self-efficacy in the management of pain. Actual pain level did not change significantly.[114]

Case Study

A 52-year-old female presents with **generalised aching pain** in her extremities and back for the past 6 months. She takes trazadone and cyclopenzaprine for sleep, but still **wakes unrefreshed**. She reports **anxiety**, **poor concentration** and a constant sensation of her body vibrating. She is extremely **fatigued**. She has a long history of irritable bowel syndrome.
PE: 11/18 Positive tender points
CBC, CMP, ESR, CRP normal
Low 25-OH vitamin D

SUGGESTIVE SYMPTOMS

- Widespread musculoskeletal pain
- Presence of tender points
- All four quadrants involved
- Non-restorative sleep, insomnia
- Fatigue

- Mood disorders: anxiety and depression
- Gastrointestinal: IBS, visceral and somatic changes
- Neurological: cognitive changes, headaches and migraines

Example treatment

The formula is designed to reduce pain, and improve sleep, cognition and mood. Chronic pain and lack of sleep create a vicious cycle, which contributes to the anxiety, cognitive changes and fatigue associated with this condition. This is due, in part, to a disruption in the hypothalamic–pituitary–adrenal axis.[115] Reduction of pain and promotion of a restorative sleep are essential to daily functioning of this patient.

The presence of irritable bowel syndrome may indicate food intolerances and should be investigated. In addition, dysbiosis, which is common to this cohort, may exacerbate the condition and should be treated according to the presenting organisms and imbalances in the normal flora. To improve physical function, a graduated aerobic exercise program (water- or land-based) improves fibromyalgia scores, pain, cognition, anxiety and sleep. Manual therapies (massage, manual lymph drainage) have been helpful in pain, fatigue and anxiety.[108,116]

Herbal formula

Rhodiola rosea 1:1	20 mL
Schisandra chinensis 1:1	25 mL
Viburnum opulus 1:2	15 mL
Hypericum perforatum 1:2	20 mL
Melissa officinalis 1:2	20 mL
5 mL t.d.s.	100 mL
Ginkgo biloba tablets 1 g t.d.s.	

Nutritional prescription

5-HTP 100 mg b.d.
Magnesium malate 600/2400 q.d.
Vitamin D3 5000 IU q.d.
Glutamine 1000 mg t.d.
Micronutrient IV once weekly for 4 weeks
Consider melatonin 3 mg p.r.n. sleep

Nutritional intervention

- 5-HTP enhances serotonin levels that will reduce her anxiety and improve sleep. A decrease in pain perception has also been associated with 5-HTP supplementation.
- Magnesium malate decreases the tender point index.

- Vitamin D supplementation—correction of her low levels is indicated since deficiency has been implicated in cases of widespread pain as well as anxiety.[117] Daily sunlight therapy without sunscreen for approximately 10–15 minutes may be recommended.[8]
- Micronutrient IV once weekly for 4 weeks is indicated to supplement possible deficiencies secondary to malabsorption and gastrointestinal dysfunction. The nutrients included would assist in ATP and mitochondrial function, musculoskeletal function and many other biochemical reactions.
- Consider melatonin if her current regimen is not sufficient for sleep.[59]

Herbal intervention

- *Rhodiola rosea* is an adaptogen that improves serotonin levels, fatigue, sleep patterns and mental performance,[118–119] and positively affects neurotransmitters with normalisation of stress-induced elevation of serotonin, corticosterone, norepinephrine and dopamine.[120]
- *Ginkgo biloba* increases cerebral circulation, cognition and perfusion of peripheral tissues.[121,122] In combination with CoQ10, it also has analgesic properties and improves quality of life measures in FM patients.[123]
- *Schisandra chinensis* acts as adaptogen. It has a sedative effect that would be helpful for sleep.[124,125] In addition it increases work capacity, improves tissue respiration, acts as an antioxidant and improves phase II detoxification of the liver.[126]
- *Viburnum opulus* acts as an analgesic and increases gastroduodenal mucosal protective activity.[127,128]
- *Hypericum perforatum* has analgesic properties, modulates serotonin and acts as an antioxidant.[129]
- *Melissa officinalis* has calming and analgesic properties, and positively affects mood, anxiety and sleep. It has an antinociceptive action on pain receptors.[130–132] *M. officinalis* also acts as an antispasmodic on smooth muscle and the gastrointestinal tract, and would be helpful for IBS.[133]

Expected outcomes and follow-up protocols

In the case above, it is essential to correct sleep patterns to promote rejuvenation and strengthening of the vital force. Pain reduction is imperative for the patient to be able to function, as well as heal. Nutraceutical and botanical supplementation, physical modalities (myofascial release and massage) as well as acupuncture have been shown to be effective. Pain-relieving pharmaceuticals may be considered as part of the plan in severe non-responsive cases. Lifestyle changes are an integral part of the program. Exercise will improve oxygenation of the tissues and regulation of mood, sleep and other factors. Fatigue and exercise intolerance may be a challenge for the patient to initiate and follow through. In these instances a trained professional may be indicated for the success of the program.

The digestion must be addressed to improve barrier function and absorption. Dietary changes should be the focus, with botanical and nutraceuticals intervention as an adjunct. Dysbiotic changes are common to this cohort and re-establishment of normal gut flora should be promoted. Correction of nutritional deficiencies, especially vitamin D, may yield beneficial results and should be implemented. If insomnia, anxiety and fatigue continue, salivary cortisol may be valuable to assess aberrations in the HPA axis. Fibromyalgia affects patients on a profound level and modalities such as homoeopathy, acupuncture and mind/body techniques can provide a deep level of healing on the physical, mental, emotional and spiritual levels.

Table 23.4 Review of the major evidence

INTERVENTION	KEY LITERATURE	SUMMARY OF RESULTS	COMMENT
5-HTP	Caruso et al. 1990[42]	$n = 50$ with improvement in all parameters of the study	Positive results were found in the majority of parameters. Particularly indicated with co-existing sleep and mood disturbances.
	Sarzi et al. 1992[43]	$n = 50$, 90-day study. 50% had 'good' to 'fair' improvement. 30% reported side effects.	
SAMe	Tavoni et al. 1987[45]	$n = 17$ with injectable form. Reduction of painful trigger sites ($p < 0.02$). Improvement in depression ($p < 0.05$)	Especially useful with co-existing depression.
	Jacobsen et al. 1991[45]	$n = 44$ with oral form revealed improvement in clinical disease activity ($p = 0.04$), pain ($p = 0.002$), fatigue ($p = 0.02$), morning stiffness ($p = 0.03$), and mood by face scale ($p = 0.006$)	Study length was only 6 weeks with more significant improvement in tender points at the end of the trial.
Magnesium/ malic acid	Abraham 1992[21]	$n = 15$. Tender point index score of 19.6 ± 2.1 before and 8 ± 1.1 and 6.5 ± 0.74 after ($p < 0.001$). Placebo controlled.	Small studies. It appears to be dose-dependent with better results at 2 months.
	Russell et al. 1995[23]	$n = 24$. Super malic found to be safe and effective.	
Micronutrient IV	Ali et al. 2009[24]	$n = 31$. Randomised, placebo controlled. Relief of symptoms for most patients compared to base line. Both IVMT and placebo had statistically significant results, but not compared to each other.	Lactated Ringer's solution was the placebo providing rehydration and electrolytes, which may be responsible for the improvement in the placebo group; this contributed to the absence of statistical significance of the study.
	Massey et al. 2007[25]	$n = 7$ uncontrolled, no placebo	
D-ribose	Teitelbaum et al. 2006[35]	$n = 41$. Significantly reduced symptoms of FMS in uncontrolled study.	Many of the patients studied had co-existing chronic fatigue syndrome, which may affect results.
CoQ10/ginkgo	Lister 2002[87]	$n = 25$. Progressive improvement of quality of life. 64% claimed to be better. 9% claimed to be worse in small uncontrolled study using non-specific overall rating questionnaire.	The single study had limitations, but CoQ10 and ginkgo show promise for helping cognition, migraines and fatigue.

(Continued)

Table 23.4 Review of the major evidence *(Continued)*

INTERVENTION	KEY LITERATURE	SUMMARY OF RESULTS	COMMENT
Vitamin D	Arvold et al. 2009[28]	Short-term improvement of overall fibromyalgia score, but did not significantly improve musculoskeletal symptoms.	May be valuable for patients with widespread pain and should be supplemented if they have low serum levels, but no consistent improvement with FM patients.
Homoeopathy	Bell et al. 2004[93] Relton et al. 2009[94]	Individualised homoeopathy significantly better than placebo.	This therapy is dependent on the skill of the practitioner.
Acupuncture	Mayhew & Ernst 2007[134]	Meta-analysis of five RCTs revealed mixed results.	Improvement in FM may be more dependent on the technique used, with overall significantly better results using electroacupuncture.
	Li et al. 2006[102]	$n = 66$. Therapeutic group better than control group ($p \leq 0.01$). Acupuncture with cupping therapy is effective.	
Exercise	Busch et al. 2008[104]	Aerobic only training may improve FM symptoms.	Aerobic exercise was consistently more effective than stretching and relaxation exercises.
	Gowans et al. 2007[107]	Pool exercise may be an effective intervention for FMS.	
	Richards & Scott 2002[107]	Simple, cheap, effective and potentially widely available treatment.	

KEY POINTS

- Fibromyalgia is a multi-system disease and is a debilitating chronic condition.
- Management must address the sleep and persistent pain issues.
- Restoration of normal HPA axis and neurotransmitter function is required.
- The gastrointestinal tract must be addressed to increase nutrient absorption, preventing immune alterations due to dysbiosis and increased intestinal permeability.
- A comprehensive integrative approach including nutrition, botanicals, lifestyle, mind/body and energetic therapeutics would be of great benefit to this population.

Further reading

Busch AJ, et al. Exercise for fibromyalgia: a systematic review. J Rheumatol 2008;35(6):1130–1144.

Dadabhoy D, et al. Biology and therapy of fibromyalgia. Evidence-based biomarkers for fibromyalgia syndrome. Arthritis Res Ther 2008;10(4):211.

Gran JT. The epidemiology of chronic generalized musculoskeletal pain. Best Pract Res Clin Rheumatol 2003;17(4):547–561.

References

1. Wolfe F, et al. The American College of Rheumatology 1990 criteria for the classification of fibromyalgia. Report of the Multicenter Criteria Committee. Arthritis Rheum 1990;33(2):160–172.
2. Gran JT. The epidemiology of chronic generalized musculoskeletal pain. Best Pract Res Clin Rheumatol 2003;17(4):547–561.
3. Dadabhoy D, et al. Biology and therapy of fibromyalgia. Evidence-based biomarkers for fibromyalgia syndrome. Arthritis Res Ther 2008;10(4):211.
4. Sprott H, et al. Increased DNA fragmentation and ultra-structural changes in fibromyalgic muscle fibres. Ann Rheum Dis 2004;63(3):245–251.
5. Korszun A, et al. Melatonin levels in women with fibromyalgia and chronic fatigue syndrome. J Rheumatol 1999;26(12):2675–2680.
6. Mayer EA, Raybould HE. Role of visceral afferent mechanisms in functional bowel disorders. Gastroenterology 1990;99(6):1688–1704.
7. Ruiz-Perez I, et al. Risk factors for fibromyalgia: the role of violence against women. Clin Rheumatol 2009;28(7):777–786.
8. Holick MF. The influence of vitamin D on bone health across the life cycle. J Nutr 2005;135(11):2726S–2727S.
9. Gur A, Oktayoglu P. Central nervous system abnormalities in fibromyalgia and chronic fatigue syndrome: new concepts in treatment. Curr Pharm Des 2008;14(13):1274–1294.
10. Lautenschlager J. Present state of medication therapy in fibromyalgia syndrome. Scand J Rheumatol Suppl 2000;113:32–36.
11. Tofferi JK, et al. Treatment of fibromyalgia with cyclobenzaprine: A meta-analysis. Arthritis Rheum 2004;51(1):9–13.
12. Hauser W, et al. Treatment of fibromyalgia syndrome with antidepressants: a meta-analysis. JAMA 2009;301(2):198–209.
13. Russell IJ, et al. The effects of pregabalin on sleep disturbance symptoms among individuals with fibromyalgia syndrome. Sleep Med 2009;10(6):604–610.
14. Food and Drug Administration News. FDA proposes new warnings about suicidal thinking, behavior in young adults who take antidepressant medications, in P07–77. May 2, 2007.
15. Is fibromyalgia caused by a glycolysis impairment? Nutr Rev 1994;52(7):248–250.
16. Park JH, et al. Use of P-31 magnetic resonance spectroscopy to detect metabolic abnormalities in muscles of patients with fibromyalgia. Arthritis Rheum 1998;41(3):406–413.
17. Bazzichi L, et al. ATP, calcium and magnesium levels in platelets of patients with primary fibromyalgia. Clin Biochem 2008;41(13):1084–1090.
18. Werbach M. Nutritional influences on illness. 2nd edn. Tarzana: Third Line Press, 1996.
19. Eisinger J. Metabolic abnormalities in fibromyalgia. Clinical Bulletin of Myofascial Therapy 1998;3(1):3–21.
20. Eisinger J, et al. Selenium and magnesium status in fibromyalgia. Magnes Res 1994;7(3–4):285–288.
21. Abraham GE. Management of fibromyalgia: rationale for the use of magnesium and malic acid. Journal of Nutritional Medicine 1992;3:49–59.
22. Sendur OF, et al. The relationship between serum trace element levels and clinical parameters in patients with fibromyalgia. Rheumatol Int 2008;28(11):1117–1121.
23. Russell IJ, et al. Treatment of fibromyalgia syndrome with Super Malic: a randomized, double blind, placebo controlled, crossover pilot study. J Rheumatol 1995;22(5):953–958.
24. Ali A, et al. Intravenous micronutrient therapy (Myers' Cocktail) for fibromyalgia: a placebo-controlled pilot study. J Altern Complement Med 2009;15(3):247–257.
25. Massey PB. Reduction of fibromyalgia symptoms through intravenous nutrient therapy: Results of a pilot clinical trial. Altern Ther Health Med 2007;13(3):32–34.
26. Xiaoyu Z, et al. 1alpha,25(OH)2-vitamin D3 membrane-initiated calcium signaling modulates exocytosis and cell survival. J Steroid Biochem Mol Biol 2007;103(3-5):457–461.
27. Biswas P, Zanello LP. 1alpha,25(OH)(2) vitamin D(3) induction of ATP secretion in osteoblasts. J Bone Miner Res 2009;24(8):1450–1460.
28. Arvold DS, et al. Correlation of symptoms with vitamin D deficiency and symptom response to cholecalciferol treatment: a randomized controlled trial. Endocr Pract 2009;15(3):203–212.
29. Plotnikoff GA, Quigley JM. Prevalence of severe hypovitaminosis D in patients with persistent, non-specific musculoskeletal pain. Mayo Clin Proc 2003;78(12):1463–1470.
30. Badsha H, et al. Myalgias or non-specific muscle pain in Arab or Indo-Pakistani patients may indicate vitamin D deficiency. Clin Rheumatol 2009;28(8):971–973.
31. Warner AE, Arnspiger SA. Diffuse musculoskeletal pain is not associated with low vitamin D levels or improved by treatment with vitamin D. J Clin Rheumatol 2008;14(1):12–16.
32. Wilkins CH, et al. Vitamin D deficiency is associated with worse cognitive performance and lower bone density in older African Americans. J Natl Med Assoc 2009;101(4):349–354.
33. Armstrong DJ, et al. Vitamin D deficiency is associated with anxiety and depression in fibromyalgia. Clin Rheumatol 2007;26(4):551–554.
34. Crew KD, et al. Association between plasma 25-hydroxyvitamin D and breast cancer risk. Cancer Prev Res (Phila Pa) 2009;2(6):598–604.
35. Teitelbaum JE, et al. The use of D-ribose in chronic fatigue syndrome and fibromyalgia: a pilot study. J Altern Complement Med 2006;12(9):857–862.
36. Schochat T, Raspe H. Elements of fibromyalgia in an open population. Rheumatology (Oxford) 2003;42(7):829–835.
37. Zubieta JK, et al. COMT val158met genotype affects mu-opioid neurotransmitter responses to a pain stressor. Science 2003;299(5610):1240–1243.
38. Russell IJ, et al. Serum amino acids in fibrositis/fibromyalgia syndrome. J Rheumatol Suppl 1989;19:158–163.
39. Yunus MB, et al. Plasma tryptophan and other amino acids in primary fibromyalgia: a controlled study. J Rheumatol 1992;19(1):90–94.
40. Wolfe F, et al. Serotonin levels, pain threshold, and fibromyalgia symptoms in the general population. J Rheumatol 1997;24(3):555–559.
41. Russell IJ, et al. Elevated cerebrospinal fluid levels of substance P in patients with the fibromyalgia syndrome. Arthritis Rheum 1994;37(11):1593–1601.
42. Caruso I, et al. Double-blind study of 5-hydroxytryptophan versus placebo in the treatment of primary fibromyalgia syndrome. J Int Med Res 1990;18(3):201–209.
43. Sarzi Puttini P, Caruso I. Primary fibromyalgia syndrome and 5-hydroxy-L-tryptophan: a 90-day open study. J Int Med Res 1992;20(2):182–189.
44. Kagan BL, et al. Oral S-adenosylmethionine in depression: a randomized, double-blind, placebo-controlled trial. Am J Psychiatry 1990;147(5):591–595.
45. Tavoni A, et al. Evaluation of S-adenosylmethionine in primary fibromyalgia. A double-blind crossover study. Am J Med 1987;83(5A):107–110.
46. Jacobsen S, Danneskiold-Samsoe B, Andersen RB. Oral S-adenosylmethionine in primary fibromyalgia. Double-blind clinical evaluation. Scand J Rheumatol 1991;20(4):294–302.
47. Bone K. A clinical guide to blending liquid herbs: herbal formulations for the individual patient. St Louis: Churchill Livingstone, 2003.

48. Grieves B. A modern herbal. Chatham: Jonathan Cape Ltd 1973:(1931).

49. Chen QG, et al. The effects of *Rhodiola rosea* extract on 5-HT level, cell proliferation and quantity of neurons at cerebral hippocampus of depressive rats. Phytomedicine 2009;16(9):830–838.

50. Hubner WD, et al. *Hypericum* treatment of mild depressions with somatic symptoms. J Geriatr Psychiatry Neurol 1994;7(Suppl 1):S12–S14.

51. Ara I, Bano S. St. John's Wort modulates brain regional serotonin metabolism in swim stressed rats. Pak J Pharm Sci 2009;22(1):94–101.

52. Rahimi R, et al. Efficacy and tolerability of *Hypericum perforatum* in major depressive disorder in comparison with selective serotonin reuptake inhibitors: a meta-analysis. Prog Neuropsychopharmacol Biol Psychiatry 2009;33(1):118–127.

53. Linde K, et al. St John's wort for major depression. Cochrane Database Syst Rev 2008;(4):CD000448.

54. Dygai AM, et al. [The modulating effects of preparations of Baikal skullcap (*Scutellaria baicalensis*) on erythron reactions under conditions of neurotic exposures]. Eksp Klin Farmakol 1998;61(1):37–39.

55. Korszun A. Sleep and circadian rhythm disorders in fibromyalgia. Curr Rheumatol Rep 2000;2(2):124–130.

56. Crofford LJ, et al. Basal circadian and pulsatile ACTH and cortisol secretion in patients with fibromyalgia and/or chronic fatigue syndrome. Brain Behav Immun 2004;18(4):314–325.

56. Klein DC, et al. The melatonin rhythm-generating enzyme: molecular regulation of serotonin N-acetyltransferase in the pineal gland. Recent Prog Horm Res 1997;52:307–357; discussion 357–358.

58. Wikner J, et al. Fibromyalgia—a syndrome associated with decreased nocturnal melatonin secretion. Clin Endocrinol (Oxf) 1998;49(2):179–183.

59. Citera G, et al. The effect of melatonin in patients with fibromyalgia: a pilot study. Clin Rheumatol 2000;19(1):9–13.

60. Matthews CD, et al. Human plasma melatonin and urinary 6-sulphatoxy melatonin: studies in natural annual photoperiod and in extended darkness. Clin Endocrinol (Oxf) 1991;35(1):21–27.

61. Griep EN, et al. Altered reactivity of the hypothalamic-pituitary-adrenal axis in the primary fibromyalgia syndrome. J Rheumatol 1993;20(3):469–474.

62. Wingenfeld K, et al. The low-dose dexamethasone suppression test in fibromyalgia. J Psychosom Res 2007;62(1):85–91.

63. Paiva ES, et al. Impaired growth hormone secretion in fibromyalgia patients: evidence for augmented hypothalamic somatostatin tone. Arthritis Rheum 2002;46(5):1344–1350.

64. Macedo JA, et al. Glucocorticoid sensitivity in fibromyalgia patients: decreased expression of corticosteroid receptors and glucocorticoid-induced leucine zipper. Psychoneuroendocrinology 2008;33(6):799–809.

65. Sun LJ, et al. [Effects of schisandra on the function of the pituitary-adrenal cortex, gonadal axes and carbohydrate metabolism in rats undergoing experimental chronic psychological stress, navigation and strenuous exercise]. Zhonghua Nan Ke Xue 2009;15(2):126–129.

66. Panossian A, et al. Adaptogens exert a stress-protective effect by modulation of expression of molecular chaperones. Phytomedicine 2009;16(6–7):617–622.

67. Filaretov AA, et al. Role of pituitary-adrenocortical system in body adaptation abilities. Exp Clin Endocrinol 1988;92(2):129–136.

68. Almansa C, et al. Prevalence of functional gastrointestinal disorders in patients with fibromyalgia and the role of psychologic distress. Clin Gastroenterol Hepatol 2009;7(4):438–445.

69. Wallace DJ, Hallegua DS. Fibromyalgia: the gastrointestinal link. Curr Pain Headache Rep 2004;8(5):364–368.

70. Crowell MD. Role of serotonin in the pathophysiology of the irritable bowel syndrome. Br J Pharmacol 2004;141(8):1285–1293.

71. Goebel A, et al. Altered intestinal permeability in patients with primary fibromyalgia and in patients with complex regional pain syndrome. Rheumatology (Oxford) 2008;47(8):1223–1227.

72. Pimentel M, et al. Eradication of small intestinal bacterial overgrowth reduces symptoms of irritable bowel syndrome. Am J Gastroenterol 2000;95(12):3503–3506.

73. Lauritano EC, et al. Small intestinal bacterial overgrowth recurrence after antibiotic therapy. Am J Gastroenterol 2008;103(8):2031–2205.

74. Spaeth G, et al. Fibre is an essential ingredient of enteral diets to limit bacterial translocation in rats. Eur J Surg 1995;161(7):513–518.

75. Evans MA, Shronts EP. Intestinal fuels: glutamine, short-chain fatty acids, and dietary fiber. J Am Diet Assoc 1992;92(10):1239–1246,1249.

76. Xu D, et al. Elemental diet-induced bacterial translocation associated with systemic and intestinal immune suppression. J Parenter Enteral Nutr 1998;22(1):37–41.

77. Aydogan A, et al. Effects of various enteral nutrition solutions on bacterial translocation and intestinal morphology during the postoperative period. Adv Ther 2007;24(1):41–49.

78. Kang JX, Weylandt KH. Modulation of inflammatory cytokines by omega-3 fatty acids. Subcell Biochem 2008;49:133–143.

79. Enestrom S, et al. Dermal IgG deposits and increase of mast cells in patients with fibromyalgia—relevant findings or epiphenomena? Scand J Rheumatol 1997;26(4):308–313.

80. Baraniuk JN, et al. Nasal secretion analysis in allergic rhinitis, cystic fibrosis, and nonallergic fibromyalgia/chronic fatigue syndrome subjects. Am J Rhinol 1998;12(6):435–440.

81. Zuo XL, et al. Alterations of food antigen-specific serum immunoglobulins G and E antibodies in patients with irritable bowel syndrome and functional dyspepsia. Clin Exp Allergy 2007;37(6):823–830.

82. Arroyave Hernandez CM, et al. Food allergy mediated by IgG antibodies associated with migraine in adults. Rev Alerg Mex 2007;54(5):162–168.

83. Zar S, et al. Food-specific IgG4 antibody-guided exclusion diet improves symptoms and rectal compliance in irritable bowel syndrome. Scand J Gastroenterol 2005;40(7):800–807.

84. Jeschonneck M, et al. Abnormal microcirculation and temperature in skin above tender points in patients with fibromyalgia. Rheumatology (Oxford) 2000;39(8):917–921.

85. McIver KL, et al. NO-mediated alterations in skeletal muscle nutritive blood flow and lactate metabolism in fibromyalgia. Pain 2006;120(1–2):161–169.

86. Guedj E, et al. Clinical correlate of brain SPECT perfusion abnormalities in fibromyalgia. J Nucl Med 2008;49(11):1798–1803.

87. Lister RE. An open, pilot study to evaluate the potential benefits of coenzyme Q10 combined with *Ginkgo biloba* extract in fibromyalgia syndrome. J Int Med Res 2002;30(2):195–199.

88. Mizuno K, et al. Antifatigue effects of coenzyme Q10 during physical fatigue. Nutrition 2008;24(4):293–299.

89. Tsukahara Y, et al. Antioxidant role of endogenous coenzyme Q against the ischemia and reperfusion-induced lipid peroxidation in fetal rat brain. Acta Obstet Gynecol Scand 1999;78(8):669–674.

90. Sandor PS, et al. Efficacy of coenzyme Q10 in migraine prophylaxis: a randomized controlled trial. Neurology 2005;64(4):713–715.

91. Zhang J, et al. The therapeutic effect of *Ginkgo biloba* extract in SHR rats and its possible mechanisms based on cerebral microvascular flow and vasomotion. Clin Hemorheol Microcirc 2000;23(2–4):133–138.

92. Chen J, et al. Effects of *Ginkgo biloba* extract on number and activity of endothelial progenitor cells from peripheral blood. J Cardiovasc Pharmacol 2004;43(3):347–352.

93. Bell IR, et al. Improved clinical status in fibromyalgia patients treated with individualized homeopathic remedies versus placebo. Rheumatology (Oxford) 2004;43(5):577–582.

94. Relton C, et al. Healthcare provided by a homeopath as an adjunct to usual care for fibromyalgia (FMS): results of a pilot randomised controlled trial. Homeopathy 2009;98(2):77–82.

95. Maciocia G. The practice of Chinese medicine: the treatment of diseases with acupuncture and Chinese herbs. London: Churchill Livingstone, 1994.

96. Sprott H, et al. [Microcirculatory changes over the tender points in fibromyalgia patients after acupuncture therapy (measured with laser-Doppler flowmetry)]. Wien Klin Wochenschr 2000;112(13):580–586.

97. Yoshimoto K, et al. Acupuncture stimulates the release of serotonin, but not dopamine, in the rat nucleus accumbens. Tohoku J Exp Med 2006;208(4):321–326.

98. Tu WZ, et al. [Effect of electroacupuncture of local plus distal acupoints in the same segments of spinal cord on spinal substance P expression in rats with chronic radicular pain]. Zhen Ci Yan Jiu 2008;33(1):7–12.

99. Schneider A, et al. Neuroendocrinological effects of acupuncture treatment in patients with irritable bowel syndrome. Complement Ther Med 2007;15(4):255–263.

100. Cheng R, et al. Electroacupuncture elevates blood cortisol levels in naive horses; sham treatment has no effect. Int J Neurosci 1980;10(2–3):95–97.

101. Liao YY, et al. Effect of acupuncture on adrenocortical hormone production: I. Variation in the ability for adrenocortical hormone production in relation to the duration of acupuncture stimulation. Am J Chin Med 1979;7(4):362–371.

102. Li CD, et al. [Clinical study on combination of acupuncture, cupping and medicine for treatment of fibromyalgia syndrome]. Zhongguo Zhen Jiu 2006;26(1):8–10.

103. Acupuncture. NIH consensus statement online 1997 Nov 3-5;15(5):1–34.

104. Busch AJ, et al. Exercise for fibromyalgia: a systematic review. J Rheumatol 2008;35(6):1130–1144.

105. Richards SC, Scott DL. Prescribed exercise in people with fibromyalgia: parallel group randomised controlled trial. BMJ 2002;325(7357):185.

106. Valim V, et al. Aerobic fitness effects in fibromyalgia. J Rheumatol 2003;30(5):1060–1109.

107. Gowans SE, deHueck A. Pool exercise for individuals with fibromyalgia. Curr Opin Rheumatol 2007;19(2):168–173.

108. Field T, et al. Fibromyalgia pain and substance P decrease and sleep improves after massage therapy. J Clin Rheumatol 2002;8(2):72–76.

109. McCauley J, et al. The 'battering syndrome': prevalence and clinical characteristics of domestic violence in primary care internal medicine practices. Ann Intern Med 1995;123(10):737–746.

110. Mas AJ, et al. Prevalence and impact of fibromyalgia on function and quality of life in individuals from the general population: results from a nationwide study in Spain. Clin Exp Rheumatol 2008;26(4):519–526.

111. de Souza JB, et al. The deficit of pain inhibition in fibromyalgia is more pronounced in patients with comorbid depressive symptoms. Clin J Pain 2009;25(2):123–127.

112. Beal CC, Stuifbergen AK, Brown A. Predictors of a health promoting lifestyle in women with fibromyalgia syndrome. Psychol Health Med 2009;14(3):343–353.

113. Sephton SE, et al. Mindfulness meditation alleviates depressive symptoms in women with fibromyalgia: results of a randomized clinical trial. Arthritis Rheum 2007;57(1):77–85.

114. Menzies V, et al. Effects of guided imagery on outcomes of pain, functional status, and self-efficacy in persons diagnosed with fibromyalgia. J Altern Complement Med 2006;12(1):23–30.

115. Novati A, et al. Chronically restricted sleep leads to depression-like changes in neurotransmitter receptor sensitivity and neuroendocrine stress reactivity in rats. Sleep 2008;31(11):1579–1585.

116. Ekici G, et al. Comparison of manual lymph drainage therapy and connective tissue massage in women with fibromyalgia: a randomized controlled trial. J Manipulative Physiol Ther 2009;32(2):127–133.

117. Kaluff AV, et al. Increased anxiety in mice lacking vitamin D receptor gene. Neuroreport 2004;15(8):1271–1274.

118. Kelly GS, *Rhodiola rosea*: a possible plant adaptogen. Altern Med Rev 2001;6(3):293–302.

119. Fintelmann V, Gruenwald J. Efficacy and tolerability of a *Rhodiola rosea* extract in adults with physical and cognitive deficiencies. Adv Ther 2007;24(4):929–939.

120. Spasov AA, et al. A double-blind, placebo-controlled pilot study of the stimulating and adaptogenic effect of *Rhodiola rosea* SHR-5 extract on the fatigue of students caused by stress during an examination period with a repeated low-dose regimen. Phytomedicine 2000;7(2):85–89.

121. Birks J, Grimley Evans J. *Ginkgo biloba* for cognitive impairment and dementia. Cochrane Database Syst Rev 2009;(1):CD003120.

122. Shah ZA, et al. *Ginkgo biloba* normalises stress-elevated alterations in brain catecholamines, serotonin and plasma corticosterone levels. Eur Neuropsychopharmacol 2003;13(5):321–325.

123. Biddlestone L, et al. Oral administration of *Ginkgo biloba* extract, EGb-761 inhibits thermal hyperalgesia in rodent models of inflammatory and post-surgical pain. Br J Pharmacol 2007;151(2):285–291.

124. Huang F, et al. Sedative and hypnotic activities of the ethanol fraction from *Fructus schisandrae* in mice and rats. J Ethnopharmacol 2007;110(3):471–475

125. Panossian A, Wikman G. Pharmacology of *Schisandra chinensis* Bail: an overview of Russian research and uses in medicine. J Ethnopharmacol 2008;118(2):183–212.

126. Lee SB, et al. Induction of the phase II detoxification enzyme NQO1 in hepatocarcinoma cells by lignans from the fruit of *Schisandra chinensis* through nuclear accumulation of Nrf2. Planta Med 2009: In press.

127. Calle J, et al. Antinociceptive and uterine relaxant activities of *Viburnum toronis* alive (Caprifoliaceae). J Ethnopharmacol 1999;66(1):71–73.

128. Zayachkivska OS, et al. Influence of *Viburnum opulus* proanthocyanidins on stress-induced gastrointestinal mucosal damage. J Physiol Pharmacol 2006;57(Suppl 5):155–167.

129. Uchida S, et al. Antinociceptive effects of St. John's wort, *Harpagophytum procumbens* extract and grape seed proanthocyanidins extract in mice. Biol Pharm Bull 2008;31(2):240–245.

130. Guginski G, et al. Mechanisms involved in the antinociception caused by ethanolic extract obtained from the leaves of *Melissa officinalis* (lemon balm) in mice. Pharmacol Biochem Behav 2009;93(1):10–16.

131. Awad R, et al. Bioassay-guided fractionation of lemon balm (*Melissa officinalis* L.) using an in vitro measure of GABA transaminase activity. Phytother Res 2009;23(8):1075–1081.

132. Soulimani R, et al. Neurotropic action of the hydroalcoholic extract of *Melissa officinalis* in the mouse. Planta Med 1991;57(2):105–109.

133. Sadraei H, et al. Relaxant effect of essential oil of *Melissa officinalis* and citral on rat ileum contractions. Fitoterapia 2003;74(5):445–452.

134. Mayhew E, Ernst E. Acupuncture for fibromyalgia—a systematic review of randomized clinical trials. Rheumatology (Oxford) 2007;46(5):801–804.

Section 8 Integumentary system

The integumentary system is comprised of the epidermis, dermis, hairs and nails, and surface glands, in addition to lymph and blood systems that nourish the tissue and remove metabolic waste. The skin is the largest organ of the human body, and is responsible for many functions including barrier protection, immunological defence, insulation and temperature regulation. Beyond the superficial layer of the skin, there are other tissues such as blood and lymphatic vessels. Treatment of skin conditions must take into consideration the entire integumentary system.

Naturopathy and traditional herbal medicine have long had a custom of preparing various external therapeutic applications that possess specific physical and pharmacological properties for the treatment of skin conditions. In modern times this tradition has continued. For example, the healing properties of honey are now being rediscovered in many hospitals; ti tree oil was placed in the ration packs of Australian soldiers during World War II to combat infectious skin diseases; and lavender and valerian formed an integral part of some rehabilitation treatments after World War I. Many of these treatments are being 'newly discovered' not only by modern dermatology, but also by contemporary naturopathic practice.

The skin has a complex interplay with the immune, haematological and nervous systems. Many skin conditions are not necessarily caused by a topical microbial infection and reaction, but are related to immunological or other pathological issues by systemic or underlying disorders. These processes themselves may occur for a variety of reasons, including environmental or dietary influence, psychological or emotional factors or an underlying and possible diagnosable pathology. From a naturopathic perspective, the management of skin conditions requires an investigative approach to identify the underlying issue that is causing the physiological imbalance; this may be a dietary intolerance or a psychological factor. Understanding the pathophysiology of the diagnosed condition, although important, provides only a superficial view of many skin conditions. Hence a thorough case history and an understanding of the interrelationship of many physiological systems—especially the nervous and digestive/hepatobiliary systems—are important.

The skin in naturopathic medicine is also traditionally viewed as the 'third elimination organ', a dynamic entity that can both eliminate and absorb toxins or other pharmacologically active agents. Managing these processes has always been a core tenet of the naturopathic treatment of skin disease and other conditions that require the elimination of pathogens or metabolic waste. Common interventions used in naturopathic practice to support the skin include herbal 'alteratives' and 'depuratives' (for example, *Echinacea* spp. or *Arctium lappa*) and 'hepatics' (for example, *Taraxacum officinale*), as the liver is seen as playing a crucial role in many skin conditions. 'Skin nutrients', including vitamin A, essential fatty acids, biotin, zinc, vitamin C, niacin and protein, are also commonly prescribed. These interventions may address the underlying toxicity that may contribute to skin conditions as well as providing key precursors and cofactors required for the repair and maintenance of integumentary tissue.

This section outlines some of the more common skin conditions seen in contemporary naturopathic practice. Many of these principles can be extended to many other skin conditions that are not covered. Furthermore, the principle of 'encouraging and supporting the channels of elimination', covered throughout this section, will be applicable to many other conditions, such as arthritis.

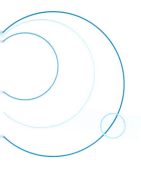

24
Acne vulgaris

Amie Steel
ND, MPH

AETIOLOGY

Acne vulgaris is a condition typified by inflammation of the pilosebaceous follicles in the skin.[1] It is characterised by a variety of lesions including nodules, papules, pustules and open and closed comedones. However, the sequence of the pathophysiological development of these lesions is still unclear. The dominant hypothesis at this stage focuses on increased circulating androgens stimulating sebaceous gland activity, and the resulting sebum production triggering hyperkeratosis. This process blocks the follicle and results in dilation and the ultimate formation of a comedone.[1] The transition from a comedone to a lesion such as a pustule, papule or nodule is believed to be due to a bacterium, called *Propionibacterium acnes*, colonising the follicle and triggering an inflammatory response within the follicle wall.[2] This cascade involves T helper cells (CD4+), most likely subtype T helper 1, and macrophages, which infiltrate the local area, possibly as a result of antigenic stimulation. The antigen identified as the most likely initiator of inflammation is *Propionibacterium acnes* (see the box below). This trigger is believed to develop due to weakness in the follicular basement membranes, associated with reduced linoleic acid levels in the follicular wall. This has been explained through increased sebum production depleting local fatty acid stores. Once an inflammatory cascade has begun, hyperproliferation of follicles can occur. As keratinised cells and sebum compact within the follicular lumen, a 'horny plug' forms. This process ultimately results in the development of a comedone and is referred to as 'comedonegenesis'.[2]

RISK FACTORS

Predisposing and exacerbating factors relating to the development of acne vulgaris include hereditary predisposition, premenstrual hormonal fluctuations, increased androgen levels, heavy or irritating clothing, backpacks or helmets, the application of oily creams, the use of certain drugs and exposure to increased heat and humidity.[5] Some dietary factors, such as dairy intake[6] or glycaemic load,[7] may also increase the risk of acne; however, specific attributable risk in this area remains unclear until further research is done.

PROPIONIBACTERIUM ACNES

Propionibacterium acnes was initially considered the cause of acne vulgaris following its identification in acne lesions in 1896. This has been supported by evidence of a failure of antibiotic treatment of acne due to erythromycin-resistant strains of *P. acnes*. However, more recent research has determined that *P. acnes* may trigger or exacerbate acne vulgaris, but it is not the only factor. In fact, some acne lesions do not have any sign of bacterial infection. It is now considered that *P. acnes* is not the primary cause of acne, although it is still considered a significant contributor to the inflammation.[3,4] *P. acnes* is more commonly connected with the appearance of pustules, rather than the least severe comedones. This occurs due to the bacteria breaking down sebum into specific fatty acids, which trigger an inflammatory response. The inflammation weakens the dermal layer and opportunistic staphylococcal organisms invade, forming a pustule.[5]

CONVENTIONAL TREATMENT

Treatment of acne vulgaris focuses on the bacterial and hormonal aetiology of the condition. The hormonal mainstays of medical intervention include oral contraceptives and antiandrogen medication (spironolactone, cyproterone acetate or flutamide).[8] Approaching acne management through hormonal regulation is justified through the presence of androgen receptors in the basal layer of sebaceous glands and in the outer root sheath keratinocytes in the hair follicle. Oral contraceptives interfere with the stimulation of these receptors by reducing ovarian production of androgens, while the other antiandrogen medications act as receptor blockers.[8] Topical management through the use of peeling agents (benzoyl peroxide, tretinoin or isotretinoin) and antibacterial agents (tetracycline) are also commonly used to control lesions.[5]

The most common drug used in severe, chronic acne vulgaris is isotretinoin. Isotretinoin affects epidermis health through a number of mechanisms, including promotion of epidermal cell differentiation, stimulation of keratinocyte proliferation and reduction of sebaceous gland size (by suppressing the proliferation of basal sebocytes and sebum production). Immunomodulatory and anti-inflammatory properties have also been identified. Isotretinoin is usually prescribed on average for 20 weeks, with a starting dose of between 0.5 and 1 mg/kg/day and concomitant prescription of oral antibiotics for the first 4 weeks of treatment.[9]

Naturopathic management of patients taking this medication needs to be approached carefully due to potential side effects of oral retinoid therapy (see the box below). Individuals who have been prescribed isotretinoin should avoid pregnancy, due to potential congenital malformations associated with the drug. There is also a risk of psychiatric conditions such as depression, psychoses and suicidal thoughts. It is also worth noting that, however rare, liver conditions such as acute hepatitis can be triggered through isotretinoin therapy and, because of this, hepatoprotective interventions may be worth considering. At the very least ethanol extracts of herbs may need to be modified to reduce potentially compounding the impact upon liver health. Most commonly, however, isotretinoin affects mucous membranes and can cause cheilitis, dry eyes, dry mouth, dry skin and desquamation of lips.[10] Furthermore, recent research has also identified elevated serum homocysteine levels in patients with cystic acne undergoing isotretinoin therapy,[11] as well as decreased plasma folate concentrations.[12] The health implications of these results are discussed in more detail

POTENTIAL SIDE EFFECTS OF ISOTRETINOIN THERAPY

The side effects of isotretinoin therapy are essentially the same as vitamin A toxicity (hypervitaminosis A syndrome) and include the following:[9]
- hepatoxicity
- musculoskeletal disorders
- transient hyperlipidaemia
- cheilitis
- teratogenicity
- pseudotumor cerebri (benign intracranial hypertension)
- psychiatric effects.

in Section 3 on the cardiovascular system. Some possible complementary prescriptions that may support individuals taking isotretinoin include zinc, methionine, arginine, vitamin E, soy protein, fish oil and L-carnitine. However, any inclusion of these interventions in the treatment plan would require careful and close monitoring as research in this area is still preliminary.[10]

KEY TREATMENT PROTOCOLS

The understanding of acne vulgaris from a naturopathic perspective focuses on the factors that can contribute to androgen excess and inflammatory responses. As there are a number of underlying factors that can be involved, depending on the individual, the treatment will centre on those that have been identified to be relevant to the patient. However, more general management of inflammation and androgen excess is also an important component of the naturopathic approach to treatment.

NATUROPATHIC TREATMENT AIMS
- Increase detoxification through all channels of elimination.
- Reduce oxidative load and improve antioxidant status.
- Regulate blood sugar levels.
- Reduce production of inflammatory compounds.
- Regulate sympathetic and parasympathetic nervous system activity.
- Reduce serum androgen levels.
- Reduce sebum production and sebocyte proliferation.

Hormone modulation

The sebaceous glands, and the skin in general, are sites for androgen synthesis within the human body. In fact, prior to puberty, the sebaceous glands, particularly in the face and scalp, are the primary sites of androgen conversion from adrenal precursor hormones such as DHEA-S. All key enzymes required to convert cholesterol to androgens, particularly testosterone, are locally present within the sebaceous gland. Androgens, specifically dihydrotestosterone, are understood to be involved in both the regulation of cell proliferation and lipogenesis. In contrast, oestrogens are understood to inhibit excessive sebaceous gland activity, possibly by increasing androgen binding to its binding globulin.[3,13]

Management of acne focusing specifically on the elevated androgen levels includes the application of herbs such as **Serenoa repens**. *Serenoa repens* acts to reduce the conversion of testosterone to dihydrotestosterone through inhibition of the enzyme responsible, 5-α-reductase. Although no research is apparently specifically related to acne vulgaris, successful outcomes have been found when using this herb in a range of other androgen-dominant conditions.[14–16] A different approach to the herbal management of hormone modulation often considered in acne vulgaris is ***Vitex agnus-castus***.[17] *V. agnus-castus* has been traditionally used for the regulation of hormonal conditions particularly focusing on sexual and reproductive functions,[18] and this has been supported through more recent research identifying dopaminergic and oestrogenic compounds extracted from the herb.[19] Another herbal intervention to be considered is a *kampo* (traditional Japanese medicine) combination formula of ***Paeonia* spp.** and ***Glycyrrhiza* spp.**, which has been found to reduce testosterone and improve oestrogen/testosterone ratio in women with polycystic ovarian syndrome.[20] Although the exact mechanism is unclear, it has been argued that this occurs due to an increased aromatase activity, thereby converting testosterone to 17β-oestradiol, and/or central nervous system activity resulting in an increase in pituitary secretion of follicle-stimulating hormone and luteinising hormone.[20]

Similarly, other natural substances may be used in the management of acne vulgaris, although not yet specifically investigated for the condition, based upon their known activity within the body. For example, enterolactone, a phytoestrogenic compound derived from flaxseed, has been found to reduce the Free Androgen Index.[21] However, this substance is activated from precursors found in flaxseed by the microflora found in the human colonic intestinal tract; this microflora may be affected by the use of oral antibiotics.[22]

FREE ANDROGEN INDEX (FAI)

The Free Androgen Index (sometimes called the Testosterone Free Index, or TFI) is determined by calculating the ratio of the total testosterone concentration to the concentration of sex hormone binding globulin. It often increases in severe acne, hirsutism, polycystic ovarian syndrome and male androgenic alopecia (male-pattern baldness).[34]

Androgens and the stress response

Research has found that the symptoms of acne vulgaris are worse in times of psychological stress. Physiological adaptation to stress may also be a contributing factor to acne vulgaris due to the hormonal cascade this produces. In particular, increased physiological stress results in hypothalamic secretion of noradrenalin and thereby corticotrophic-releasing hormone (CRH). CRH then stimulates release of adrenocorticotrophic hormone (ACTH) from the anterior pituitary. The primary target of ACTH is the adrenal cortex through which it affects adrenal androgen secretion.[23] Furthermore, CRH also inhibits secretion of gonadotrophic releasing hormone, resulting in lower gonadic hormones, thereby further exacerbating the androgen:oestrogen imbalance often seen in acne vulgaris.[23] For this reason, herbs that have adaptogenic activity may be considered (see Chapter 8 on respiratory disorders), including ***Rhodiola rosea***,[24] ***Panax ginseng*** and ***Withania somnifera***.[25]

Androgen metabolism and clearance

Naturopathically, the skin has been referred to as 'the third kidney'. The rationale behind this statement is the role the skin plays in detoxification of the system. Both phase I and phase II detoxification enzymes are found in human skin. The phase I enzymes are mostly represented by alcohol dehydrogenase; however, CYP450 enzymes are also present although at much lower levels.[26] The subtypes of CYP450 found in

ALTERATIVES AND DEPURATIVES

Historically, naturopaths have emphasised the importance of detoxification to manage a number of conditions including renal, urinary, hepatic, endocrine and skin disease.[32] It is explained by Benedict Lust in his seminal text that 'the origin of all is again to be readily explained by accumulations of foreign matter; and here we have especially to do with the accumulations affecting the normal function of those organs so important for the secretion of waste matter from the body: the kidneys and the skin'.[32] This is the foundation upon which the herbal medicine management of skin disorders was originally based: the use of alteratives and depuratives. An alterative or depurative has been defined as a herb that 'improves detoxification and aids elimination to reduce the accumulation of metabolic waste products within the body'.[28] Herbs that are traditionally considered to have this action include (but are by no means limited to) *Iris versicolor*, *Arctium lappa*, *Galium aparine*, *Echinacea* spp., *Chionanthus virginicus*, *Berberis aquifolium*, *Smilax ornata* and *Rumex crispus*. However, it is interesting to note that no current research validating the empirical use of these herbs has been found. This is an important area within naturopathic management of skin diseases, and such research would provide great benefit to evidence-based naturopathic practice.

the skin are generally involved in hydroxylation of a number of compounds, including retinoids, prostanoids, inflammatory mediators, arachidonic acid and cholesterol. In contrast, the phase II enzymes are expressed in high concentrations. These include glutathione-*S*-transferase, catechol-O-methyltransferase and steroid sulfotransferase.[26] Likewise, aromatase has been found in high concentrations in sebaceous glands and may act to clear excess androgens.[27] This implies that the skin does have an important role in detoxification, particularly through phase II enzymes. It also suggests that compromised or stressed liver detoxification may place further burden on the skin, thereby aggravating dermal conditions such as acne vulgaris. With this in mind, it may be more accurate to refer to the skin as the 'second liver' rather than the third kidney.

Clearance of excess hormones and other aggravating substances has historically been managed naturopathically using **depurative herbs.** These herbs are associated with improved detoxification and elimination of metabolic wastes.[28] There are a number of herbs which have been traditionally used for chronic skin disorders, including *Iris versicolor*, *Arctium lappa*, *Galium aparine*, *Berberis aquifolium* and *Smilax ornata* (see the box on alteratives and depuratives for more information). However, very little modern research has been undertaken investigating the benefits of these herbs in acne vulgaris.[17] More recently, naturopaths have been using an extract from cruciferous vegetables, known as indole-3-carbinol, to stimulate hepatic metabolism of excess steroidal hormones, including androgens.[29] Like the depurative herbs, however, there is no specific research linking this compound with acne vulgaris, but understanding its mechanism of action does suggest some potential clinical benefit.

In contrast to these beneficial interventions, cigarette smoking and tobacco-related products have been found to inhibit aromatase activity,[30] and as such may exacerbate acne vulgaris, but this has not yet been supported through epidemiological research.[31]

Androgens and diet

A potential confounding factor within hormone imbalances related to acne may come from the diet.[6] For example, milk intake as a teenager has been associated with an increased incidence of acne. The researchers found that these results were not linked to saturated fat intake as skim milk consumption had a higher association. The researchers hypothesised that the hormonal content of the milk may be a contributing factor, particularly for adolescent females, but this requires further investigation.

Likewise, a diet with a high glycaemic load can result in increased plasma levels of glucose, insulin and insulin-like growth factor-1 (IGF-1), all of which have been associated with an increased Free Androgen Index[13] (see the box above). By following a low-glycaemic load and high protein diet, researchers have found reduced lesion count, reduced FAI and increased IGF binding protein-1.[7] However, research in this area is still inconclusive due to conflicting results.[33]

Inflammation, infection and topical management

Immune modulation to reduce inflammation and bacterial infection of the acne lesions is another important component of the naturopathic management of acne vulgaris. This is often achieved through minimising oxidation, decreasing physiological stress and reducing inflammatory triggers such as elevated blood glucose levels and bacterial infection of the lesion. However, more direct anti-inflammatory approaches may also be included in the treatment of acne vulgaris. One such option is **quercetin**, a compound synthesised by plants, with a known anti-inflammatory effect through inhibition of TNF-α, NFκB, IL-2 and IFNγ.[35] Another commonly used compound is **bromelain**, derived from pineapples. Bromelain is an enzyme complex that acts to reduce inflammation, although the exact mechanism requires further clarification.[36]

Oxidative stress and inflammatory mediators

Oxidative stress has been found to be increased in patients with acne vulgaris; however, it is unclear whether this is a cause or symptom.[37] However, as oxidative stress has been linked to inflammatory responses, it is an important factor to address when managing this condition.

Dietary intake of *trans*-fatty acids, found in margarines, spreads, frying and cooking oils,[38] has been associated with increased inflammatory markers such as C-reactive protein,[39] TNF receptor-1 and TNF receptor-2.[40] For this reason, it is recommended that dietary intake of processed and deep-fried foods be reduced in individuals with acne vulgaris.

Furthermore, compromised levels of dietary antioxidants have been linked with acne vulgaris. One study identified a strong relationship between low levels of vitamin A and vitamin E and acne. In fact, it was found that levels in the lower quintile were associated with the severity of the condition.[41] The link between oxidative stress and acne vulgaris also suggests that **medicinal herbs** with known antioxidant activity, such as *Rosmarinus officinalis*,[42] *Camellia sinensis*[42] and *Curcuma longa* may be beneficial.[43] However, it must be noted that no known clinical research has been undertaken investigating the oral use of these herbs in acne vulgaris.

Nutrients such as selenium[44] and zinc[45] also have known antioxidant activity and may be beneficial in reducing oxidative stress in acne vulgaris. Selenium has undergone preliminary clinical trials for patients with acne vulgaris, particularly focusing on improving erythrocyte glutathione peroxidase (an endogenous antioxidant enzyme that

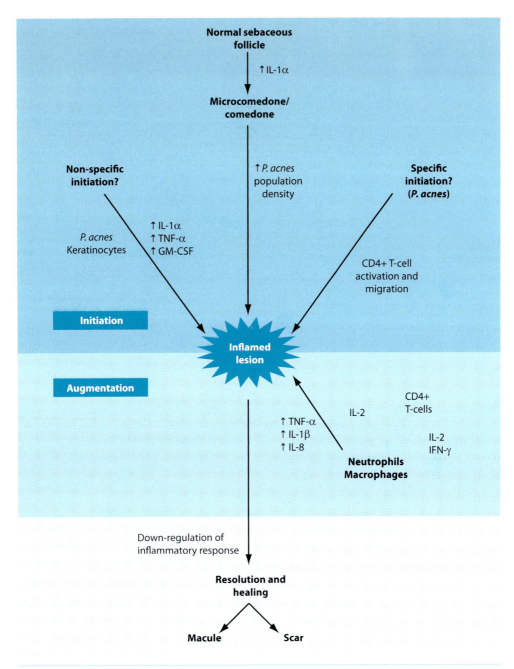

Figure 24.1 Events in the evolution of an inflammatory acne lesion
Source: Farrar MD, Ingham E. Ache: inflammation. Clinics in Dermatology 2004;22:380–384.

relies on selenium as a cofactor) activity.[46] The clinical significance of this research is not yet clear, although it is known that lower glutathione peroxidase levels are found in patients with acne compared with controls.[47] Clinical research for oral zinc supplements in acne vulgaris has also been undertaken, and found to result in mild but statistically significant improvements.[48,49]

Stress and the inflammatory response

Cutaneous tissue is the site of a complex system of autocrine and paracrine functions that are stimulated by prostaglandins. Increased inflammatory response stimulates a cascade of stress hormone release, which begins with corticotrophic-releasing hormone and culminates in the release of cortisol, thereby generating an anti-inflammatory response. However, the expression of CRH receptors is modulated by hormones such as testosterone and oestrogen.[3] This process is supported by the well-accepted evidence that acne vulgaris is aggravated by mental stress. This may be explained by stimulation of the HPA axis under stress, causing an increase in adrenal secretion of cortisol and androgens.[50] This further supports the potential benefits associated with the adaptogenic herbs mentioned above, and also suggests that herbs with both anti-inflammatory and adrenal tonic activity such as *Glycyrrhiza glabra*[28] may be beneficial.

Topical treatments and antimicrobial activity

Medical management of acne vulgaris usually incorporates an aspect of antibacterial and topical treatments, and naturopathic approaches are no different. Essential oils are often used topically on acne lesions with the main focus of such treatments being antimicrobial activity. Such an example is *Cymbopogon nardus*, which has been identified through an in vitro study to exert antimicrobial activity on *Propionibacterium acnes*.[51] Another study compared *Melaleuca alternifolia* essential oil with benzoyl peroxide, a common topical antibacterial treatment.[52] This study found both treatments to be effective, although the *M. alternifolia* had a slower response rate and fewer side effects. In fact, in vitro research[53] has found that *P. acnes* is susceptible to *M. alternifolia* at concentrations as low as 0.25%.

Topical application of *Camellia sinensis* has also been investigated in relation to sebum production. A recent animal study[54] found that a number of green tea catechins (including epigallocatechin-3-gallate) reduced sebocyte proliferation, and other compounds such as kaempferol reduce sebocyte lipogenesis. This potential treatment has been further explored using patients with acne vulgaris and a 2% 'tea lotion';[55] however, the exact formula of the tea lotion was not defined and as such the clinical relevance is unclear.

Preliminary research has identified a polysaccharide found in *Camellia sinensis* extracts that reduces *Propionibacterium acnes* adhesion to human cutaneous tissue.[56] This research needs to be expanded further to explore the application of green tea extract on topical acne lesions, but the implications are promising. In contrast, a small human study investigating the effect of topical application of *Curcuma longa* in reducing acne inflammation found no benefit.[57]

INTEGRATIVE MEDICAL CONSIDERATIONS

Beyond the naturopathic treatments already considered, there are a number of other therapies which may be considered when developing an integrative medical treatment plan.

Psychotherapy

One such consideration is psychotherapy. Given the physiological impact of stress on the pathogenesis of acne and the importance of emotional health to overall wellbeing, it is important to consider counselling as an important therapy adjunctive to acne

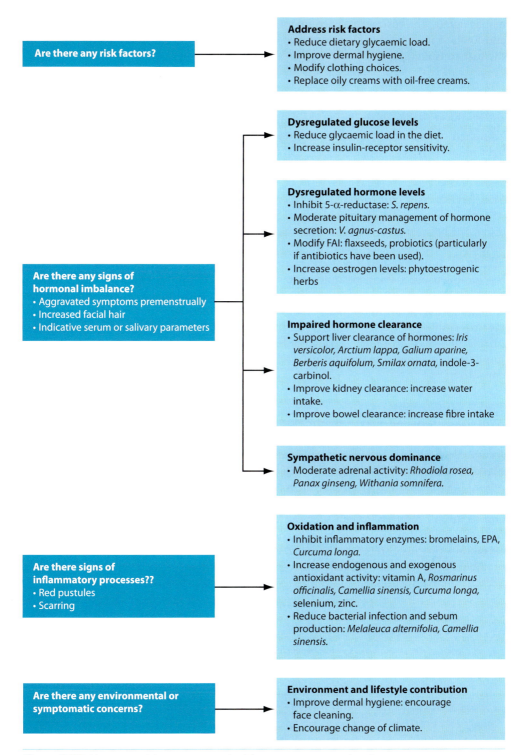

Figure 24.2 Naturopathic treatment decision tree—acne vulgaris

management. The basic acknowledgment of emotional responses such as embarrassment and low self-image is an important part of this process and can be implemented from the first consultation.[58]

Phototherapy

Phototherapy is another method of treatment to be considered. Blue light phototherapy has been trialled recently for acne management,[59] and was found to reduce lesions (although not to affect *P. acnes* colonies). A similar result has also been found for red light phototherapy.[60]

Hygiene considerations

Skin hygiene is a controversial consideration within a treatment regimen associated with the management of acne vulgaris. Some preliminary research has found that the difference between showering immediately after exercise-induced sweating and waiting 4 hours before showering made no statistically significant difference to the symptoms of acne.[61] Similar research was conducted regarding face-washing and acne, comparing groups using a standard mild cleanser and washing once, twice and four times a day for 6 weeks.[62] The group washing twice per day had improvements in both open comedones and non-inflammatory lesions; however, there appeared to be no real advantage to washing more frequently than this. Hygiene considerations more generally—such as higher environmental bacterial levels on floors, bedding and so on—have been implicated in other skin conditions such as atopic dermatitis and therefore could be considered.[63]

Ayurvedic medicine

Ayurvedic medicine may also provide some support in the management of acne vulgaris. An in vitro study was undertaken to explore the effect of a number of Ayurvedic herbs on inflammatory mediators associated with *P. acnes* infection and the pathogenesis of acne vulgaris.[64] Of the herbs studied, *Rubia cordifolia*, *Curcuma longa*, *Hemidesmus indicus*, *Azadirachta indica* and *Sphaeranthus indicus* were found to reduce the inflammatory mediators interleukin-8 and tumour necrosis factor-α, and to inhibit reactive oxygen species (free radicals). *Curcuma longa* and *Hemidesmus indicus* are often used in Western herbal medicine, but it is worth noting that the extraction process for the herbs used was reflective of practices used in Ayurvedic medicine and may not directly correspond with ethanol-based extracts as used in Western herbal medicine.

Case Study

A 21-year-old female presents to the clinic with **inflamed acne comedones** and **pustules** on her cheeks and chin. Her skin has been a problem for the past 4 or 5 years, but the problem has increased in severity over the last 2 months. She is a student, and she finds managing work and study **quite stressful**. She has not noticed any connection between her acne and her menstrual cycle. She **reports a strong hunger signal**, and craves both hot chips and sweet foods. This is reflected in her **diet which contains refined carbohydrates and fried fatty foods**.

SUGGESTIVE SYMPTOMS

- Comedones (blackheads or whiteheads)
- Pustules (raised red mass containing purulent exudate)

Example treatment

Prescription

In this example case, the approach to treatment is to improve metabolite clearance and reduce the effect of exacerbating factors, while providing agents to reduce inflammation and promote connective tissue healing. The herbal formula as shown in the treatment box includes herbs selected due to their vulnerary (*C. officinalis*, *C. asiatica* and *H. perforatum*), anti-inflammatory (*C. asiatica* and *C. officinalis*), depurative (*C. asiatica*), adaptogenic (*C. asiatica* and *S. chinensis*), anti-depressant (*H. perforatum* and *S. chinensis*) and nervine tonic (*H. perforatum*, *S. chinensis* and *C. asiatica*) activity.[28,65] Further support of the internal herbal formula is provided through the topical wash consisting of *C. officinalis*, *C. sinensis* and *M. alternifolia*.

The treatment aims are also supported through the use of a nutritional formula containing selenium, vitamin A, vitamin E, bromelains, quercetin and zinc to assist in reducing inflammation and oxidation, while promoting connective tissue repair.[36,66,67] However, it is vital that this is combined with dietary recommendations to reduce sugar and refined carbohydrate intake, and increase consumption of unprocessed grains and whole foods. Finally, it is also important to encourage more lifestyle balance, particularly by increasing the amount of time spent on enjoyable activities, to assist in the reduction of stress response.

Herbal formula

Calendula officinalis 1:2	20 mL
Centella asiatica 1:2	30 mL
Hypericum perforatum 1:2	25 mL
Schisandra chinensis 1:2	25 mL
5 mL b.d.	100 mL

Nutritional prescription

Quercetin 400 mg b.d.
Bromelains 100 mg b.d.
Zinc (gluconate) 4 mg b.d.
Selenium 13 μg b.d.
Vitamin A 2500 IU b.d.
Vitamin E 242 IU b.d.

Topical wash

1 cup infusion of:
Calendula officinalis (5 g)
Camellia sinensis (5 g)
and
Melaleuca alternifolia (100% essential oil) (5 drops)
Apply topically using a clean cloth or cotton wool daily.

Expected outcomes and follow-up protocols

In the above case, it is expected that within 1 month there should be a noticeable improvement in symptoms, although all lesions may not have cleared. However, concomitant improvements such as reduction in food cravings, improved sleep and better mood can be expected. With these changes, the herbal formula can be modified to focus more on lymphatic clearance rather than nervous system support. This can be achieved through the replacement of *Schisandra chinensis* with an *Echinacea angustifolia/purpurea* blend, while maintaining her nutritional supplement and dietary changes. Within 1 more month, new lesions can be expected to cease, and ongoing treatment can then focus on regulation of the HPA axis through adaptogenic herbs such as *Turnera diffusa* and *Glycyrrhiza glabra*.

Given that the patient in the example case is young and living away from home for the first time on a student's income, it is important to develop her prescription carefully, taking in to account her cooking skills, time commitments and budget. As such, her supplements have been restricted to one herbal and one nutritional formula at a time, thereby minimising the financial pressure. The dietary recommendations proposed also take her life skills into consideration. The first consultation provides some gentle recommendations that work within her current diet and do not involve very expensive food or

Table 24.1 Review of the major evidence

INTERVENTION	METHODOLOGY	RESULT	COMMENT
Low glycaemic-load diet[70]	12-week RCT ($n = 43$), male 15–25 years Low glycaemic load diet (25% protein, 45% low GI carbohydrates) vs placebo (carbohydrate dense with no reference to GI)	Significant reduction in total lesion counts compared to placebo: −23.5 to −12.0. Weight, BMI and insulin sensitivity also improved in the intervention group.	This was not compared with a high GI diet, or even a moderate GI diet. The placebo was essentially uncontrolled; this may not be a realistic comparative base.
Topical tea tree oil water-based gel[52]	RCT ($n = 124$) 5% tea tree oil water-based gel vs 5% benzoyl peroxide lotion	Both reduced number of inflamed and non-inflamed lesions. Onset was slower with tea tree oil gel.	No placebo group was included in this study, and blinding was difficult due to the distinctive odour of tea tree oil.
Topical vitamin C and vitamin A[71]	8-week RCT ($n = 45$) 5% sodium ascorbyl phosphate (SAP) lotion or 0.2% retinol lotion or both	5% SAP lotion reduced acne lesions by 48.82%, retinol lotion reduced lesions by 49.5% and the combination therapy reduced lesions by 63.1%.	The researchers noted that excessive application of the retinol lotion resulted in skin irritation and enhanced sun burn. No placebo group was used. Not common forms as used in naturopathy.

Note: RCT = randomised controlled trial

a lot of meal preparation. This can then be modified when she returns, has experienced some successes and is keen to take on further changes.

It may take 2 to 3 months of consistent treatment before results are noticed with acne vulgaris. In fact, it may be beneficial in a condition such as this to have less frequent consultations. Rather than seeing a patient fortnightly, this may need to spread out to 4 to 8 weeks. This is particularly important if hormonal imbalance is a strong contributing factor for the individual. If blood sugar irregularities become evident through case taking, and basic dietary changes are not addressing them, further investigation may be necessary. Specifically, a glucose tolerance test (with insulin) may identify subacute glucose intolerance or pancreatic insufficiency. If this is the case the treatment regimen will need to be modified to incorporate a stronger focus in this area. Particularly useful treatment options here include *Gymnema sylvestre*[68] and magnesium[69] (see Section 5 on the endocrine system for more information).

KEY POINTS

- Hormonal imbalance, particular androgen excess, plays a large role in the pathophysiology of acne vulgaris.
- Inflammation is a key consideration in the management of acne vulgaris and can be affected by bacterial infection, dietary choices, stress response or hormonal imbalance.
- Managing acne vulgaris can be achieved with little steps, but it is always important to address dietary and lifestyle factors, however slowly.

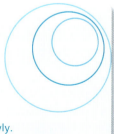

Further reading

Cordain L. Implications for the role of diet in acne. Seminars in Cutaneous Medicine and Surgery 2005;24:84–91.

Desai A, et al. Systemic retinoid therapy: a status report on optimal use and safety of long-term therapy. Drug Actions, Reactions, and Interactions 2007;25(2):185–193.

Farrar MD, Ingham E. Acne: inflammation. Clinics in Dermatology 2004;22:380–384.

Jaffer SN, Qureshi AA. Dermatology quick glance. USA: McGraw-Hill Professional, 2003.

References

1. Olutunmbi Y, et al. Adolescent female acne: etiology and management 2008;21(4):171–176.
2. Holland DB, Jeremy AHT. The role of inflammation in the pathogenesis of acne and acne scarring. Seminars in Cutaneous Medicine and Surgery 2005;24:79–83.
3. Zouboulis CC. Acne and sebaceous gland function. Clinics in Dermatology 2004;22:360–366.
4. Farrar MD, Ingham E. Acne: inflammation. Clinics in Dermatology 2004;22:380–384.
5. Gould BE. Pathophysiology for the health professional. 3rd edn. Philadelphia: Saunders Elsevier, 2006.
6. Adebamowo CA, et al. High school dietary dairy intake and teenage acne. J Am Acad Dermatol 2005;52:207–214.
7. Smith RN, et al. The effect of a high-protein, low glycemic-load diet versus a conventional, high glycemic-load diet on biochemical parameters associated with acne vulgaris: a randomized, investigator-masked, controlled trial. J Am Acad Dermatol 2007;57:247–256.
8. George R, et al. Hormonal therapy for acne. Seminars in Cutaneous Medicine and Surgery 2008;27:188–196.
9. Desai A, et al. Systemic retinoid therapy: a status report on optimal use and safety of long-term therapy. Dermatologic Clinics 2007;25(2):185–193.
10. Hanson N, Leachman S. Safety issues in isotretinoin therapy. Seminars in Cutaneous Medicine and Surgery 2001;20(3):166–183.
11. Polat M, et al. Plasma homocysteine level is elevated in patients on isotretinoin therapy for cystic acne: a prospective controlled study. J Dermatol Treat 2008;19(4):229–232.
12. Chanson A, et al. Decreased plasma folate concentration in young and elderly healthy subjects after a short-term supplementation with isotretinoin. J Eur Acad Dermatol Venereol 2008;22(1):94–100.
13. Danby FW. Diet and acne. Clinics in Dermatology 2008;26:93–96.
14. Prager N, et al. A randomized, double-blind, placebo-controlled trial to determine the effectiveness of botanically derived inhibitors of 5-alpha-reductase in the treatment of androgenetic alopecia. Journal of Alternative and Complementary Medicine 2002;8(2):143–152.
15. Talpur N, et al. Comparison of saw palmetto (extract and whole berry) and cernitin on prostate growth in rats. Molecular and Cellular Biochemistry 2003;250(1–2):21–26.
16. Wadsworth TL, et al. Effects of dietary saw palmetto on the prostate of transgenic adenocarcinoma of the mouse prostate model (TRAMP). Prostate 2007;67(6):661–673.
17. Yarnell E, Abascal K. Herbal medicine for acne vulgaris. Alternative and Complementary Therapies 2006;12(6):303–309.
18. Felter HW, Lloyd JU. King's American dispensary. 18th edn. Portland: Eclectic Medical Publications, 1905, reprinted 1983.
19. Jarry H, et al. In vitro assays for bioactivity-guided isolation of endocrine active compounds in Vitex agnus-castus. Maturitas 2006;55(Suppl 1):S26–S36.
20. Takahashi K, Kitao M. Effect of TJ-68 (shakuyaku-kanzo-to) on polycystic ovarian disease. International Journal of Fertility 1994;39(2):69–76.
21. Demark-Wahnefried W, et al. Pilot study of dietary fat restriction and flaxseed supplementation in men with prostate cancer before surgery: exploring the effects on hormonal levels, prostate-specific antigen, and histopathologic features. Urology 2001;58(1):47–52.
22. Kilkkinen A, et al. Use of oral antimicrobials decreases serum enterolactone concentration. American Journal of Epidemiology 2002;155(5):472–477.
23. Charmandari E, et al. Endocrinology of the stress response 1. Annual Review of Physiology 2005;67(1):259–284.
24. Spasov AA, et al. A double-blind, placebo-controlled pilot study of the stimulating and adaptogenic effect of Rhodiola rosea SHR-5 extract on the fatigue of students caused by stress during an examination period with a repeated low-dose regimen. Phytomedicine 2000;7(2):85–89.
25. Bhattacharya SK, Muruganandam AV. Adaptogenic activity of *Withania somnifera*: an experimental study using a rat model of chronic stress. Pharmacology, biochemistry and behaviour 2003;75(3):547–555.
26. Luu-The V, et al. Analysis of phases 1 and 2 metabolism enzymes in human skin suggests important role of phase 2 enzymes in the detoxification. Toxicology Letters 2008;180S:s121.
27. Chen W, et al. Cutaneous androgen metabolism: basic research and clinical perspectives. Journal of Investigative Dermatology 2002;119(5):992–1007.
28. Bone K. A clinical guide to blending liquid herbs. Missouri: Churchill Livingstone, 2003.
29. Jellinck PH, et al. Distinct forms of hepatic androgen 6β-hydroxylase induced in the rat by indole-3-carbinol and pregnenolone carbonitrile. Journal of Steroid Biochemistry and Molecular Biology 1994;51(3–4):219–225.
30. Osawa Y, et al. Aromatase inhibitors in cigarette smoke, tobacco leaves and other plants. Journal of Enzyme Inhibition and Medicinal Chemistry 1990;4(2):187–200.
31. Firooz A, et al. Acne and smoking: is there a relationship? BMC Dermatology 2005;5(1):2.
32. Lust B. Universal buyer's guide naturopathic encyclopaedia directory and yearbook for drugless therapy 1918–1919. New York: Lust and Butler, 1918.
33. Kaymak Y, et al. Dietary glycemic index and glucose, insulin, insulin-like growth factor-I, insulin-like growth factor binding protein 3, and leptin levels in patients with acne. J Am Acad Dermatol 2007;57:819–823.
34. Vankrieken L. Testosterone and the free androgen index. www.diagnostics.siemens.com: Siemens Diagnostic, 2000.
35. Sun Yu E, et al. Regulatory mechanisms of IL-2 and IFN[gamma] suppression by quercetin in T helper cells. Biochemical Pharmacology 2008;76(1):70–78.
36. Taussig SJ, Batkin S. Bromelain, the enzyme complex of pineapple (*Ananas comosus*) and its clinical application. An update. Journal of Ethnopharmacology 1988;22(2):191–203.
37. Arican O, et al. Oxidative stress in patients with acne vulgaris. Mediators of Inflammation 2005;6(2005):380–384.
38. Hulshof KFAM, et al. Intake of fatty acids in Western Europe with emphasis on trans fatty acids: the TRANSFAIR study. European Journal of Clinical Nutrition 1999;53(2):143–157.

39. Lopez-Garcia E, et al. Consumption of trans fatty acids is related to plasma biomarkers of inflammation and endothelial dysfunction. J Nutr 2005 March 1, 2005;135(3):562–566.

40. Mozaffarian D, et al. Dietary intake of trans fatty acids and systemic inflammation in women. American Journal of Clinical Nutrition 2004;79(4):606–612.

41. El-akawi Z, et al. Does the plasma level of vitamins A and E affect acne condition? Clinical and Experimental Dermatology 2006;31(3):430–434.

42. Chen H-Y, et al. Evaluation of antioxidant activity of aqueous extract of some selected nutraceutical herbs. Food Chemistry 2007;104(4):1418–1424.

43. Kumar GS, et al. Free and bound phenolic antioxidants in amla (*Emblica officinalis*) and turmeric (*Curcuma longa*). Journal of Food Composition and Analysis 2006;19(5):446–452.

44. Elango N, et al. Enzymatic and non-enzymatic antioxidant status in stage (III) human oral squamous cell carcinoma and treated with radical radio therapy: Influence of selenium supplementation. Clinica Chimica Acta 2006;373(1–2):92–98.

45. Mariani E, et al. Effects of zinc supplementation on antioxidant enzyme activities in healthy old subjects. Experimental Gerontology 2008;43(5):445–451.

46. Michaelsson G, Edqvist LE. Erythrocyte glutathione peroxidase activity in acne vulgaris and the effect of selenium and vitamin E treatment. Acta Derm Venereol 1984;64(1):9–14.

47. Aybey B, et al. Glutathione peroxidase (GSH-Px) enzyme levels of patients with acne vulgaris. Journal of the European Academy of Dermatology and Venereology 2005;19(6):766–767.

48. Goransson K, et al. Oral zinc in acne vulgaris: a clinical and methodological study. Acta Derm Venereol 1978;58(5):443–448.

49. Dreno B, et al. Low doses of zinc gluconate for inflammatory acne. Acta Derm Venereol 1989;69(6):541–543.

50. Tanida N, et al. Relation between mental stress-induced activity and skin conditions: a near-infrared spectroscopy study. Brain Research 2007;1184:210–216.

51. Lertsatitthanakorna P, et al. In vitro bioactivities of essential oils used for acne control. International Journal of Aromatherapy 2006;16(1):43–49.

52. Bassett IB, et al. A comparative study of tea-tree oil versus benzoylperoxide in the treatment of acne. Medical Journal of Australia 1990;153(8):455–458.

53. Carson CF, Riley TV. Susceptibility of *Propionibacterium acnes* to the essential oil of *Melaleuca alternifolia*. Letters in Applied Microbiology 1994;19(1):24–25.

54. Kim JK, et al. Evaluation of skin sebosuppression by components of total green tea (*Camellia sinensis*) extracts. Food Science and Biotechnology 2008;17(3):464–469.

55. Sharquie KE, et al. Topical therapy of acne vulgaris using 2% tea lotion in comparison with 5% zinc sulphate solution. Saudi Med J 2008;29(12):1757–1761.

56. Lee J-H, et al. Inhibition of pathogenic bacterial adhesion by acidic polysaccharide from green tea (*Camellia sinensis*). Journal of Agricultural and Food Chemistry 2006;54:8717–8723.

57. Shaffrathul JH, et al. Turmeric: role in hypertrichosis and acne. Indian Journal of Dermatology 2007;52(2):116.

58. Panconesi E, Hautmann G. Psychotherapeutic approach in acne treatment. Dermatology 1998;196(1):116.

59. Ammad S, et al. An assessment of the efficacy of blue light phototherapy in the treatment of acne vulgaris. J Cosmet Dermatol 2008;7(3):180–188.

60. Na JI, Suh DH. Red light phototherapy alone is effective for acne vulgaris: randomized, single-blinded clinical trial. Dermatol Surg 2007;33(10):1228–1233.

61. Short RW, et al. A single-blinded, randomized pilot study to evaluate the effect of exercise-induced sweat on truncal acne. Pediatr Dermatol 2008;25(1):126–128.

62. Choi JM, et al. A single-blinded, randomized, controlled clinical trial evaluating the effect of face washing on acne vulgaris. Pediatr Dermatol 2006;23(5):421–427.

63. Leung A, et al. Severe atopic dermatitis is associated with a high burden of environmental *Staphylococcus aureus*. Clin Exp Allergy 2008;38(5):789–793.

64. Jain A, Basal E. Inhibition of *Propionibacterium acnes*-induced mediators of inflammation by Indian herbs. Phytomedicine 2003;10:34–38.

65. British Herbal Medicine Association. British herbal pharmacopoeia. London: British Herbal Medicine Association, 1996.

66. Kohlmeier M. Nutrient metabolism. San Diego: Academic Press, 2003.

67. Gropper SS, et al. Advanced nutrition and human metabolism. 5th edn. Belmont: Wadsworth, 2009.

68. Sugihara Y, et al. Antihyperglycemic effects of gymnemic acid IV, a compound derived from *Gymnema sylvestre* leaves in streptozotocin-diabetic mice. Journal of Asian Natural Products Research 2000;2(4):321–327.

69. Paolisso G, et al. Magnesium and glucose homeostasis. Diabetologia 1990;33(9):511–514.

70. Smith RN, et al. A low-glycemic-load diet improves symptoms in acne vulgaris patients: a randomized controlled trial. Am J Clin Nutr 2007;86(1):107–115.

71. Ruamrak C, et al. Comparison of clinical efficacies of sodium ascorbyl phosphate, retinol and their combination in acne treatment. International Journal of Cosmetic Science 2009;31(1):41–46.

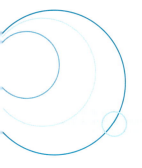

Inflammatory skin disorders— atopic eczema and psoriasis

Amie Steel
ND, MPH

AETIOLOGY

Atopic dermatitis (eczema) is most frequently diagnosed in infancy, but may continue through the adult years.[1] It involves an inherited tendency towards type 1 hypersensitivity reactions, and as such it is common to also see eczema or other allergic conditions (such as allergic rhinitis and asthma) in an individual's family history.[1] The physiological response to the allergen causes chronic inflammation and requires pathology testing for conclusive diagnosis. In particular, a full blood count to identify elevated eosinophil levels and a serum IgE test are both important, and emphasise the allergenic basis of the disease.[1] The presentation of atopic dermatitis may vary depending on the life stage of the individual. Infantile eczema tends to involve lesions that are moist, red, vesicular and covered with crusts. They will tend to occur on the face, neck, buttocks and extensor surfaces of the arms and legs.[1] Adults may also present with some moist, red lesions; however, these will mainly be concentrated in flexor regions of the arms and legs. More commonly, adults will present with dry, scaling lesions and with lichenification (thick, leathery patches) in the other areas. Pruritus (itching) is a commonly reported symptom irrelevant of the age.[1] Over time affected regions may become more sensitive to irritants such as soaps, fabrics and changes in climate (temperature and humidity).[1] These irritants impair skin barrier function by damaging the stratum corneum intercellular bilayers, through either the lipid organisation or removing the lipids overall.[2] Interestingly, a recent worldwide prospective cohort study ($n = 490,102$) found the prevalence of eczema in children in countries such as United Kingdom, New Zealand and Australia is increasing by more than 14% per year.[3]

In contrast, psoriasis is more likely to present in adolescence, although it also has an as yet undefined familial link. The pathophysiology of psoriasis is generally considered to be unknown.[4] It has been mostly linked with increased cellular proliferation and hyperkeratinisation of the dermal layer, and has been described as 'an autoimmune disease with systemic features',[4] due to the presence of T-cells that remain activated and cause the skin to constantly regenerate.[4] Like eczema, psoriasis also begins with small red papules, but lesions eventually develop a silvery plaque (although the basal layer remains red and inflamed). Most commonly, psoriatic lesions are seen on the face, scalp, elbow and knees.[1] The key inflammatory markers involved in the development of psoriasis is tumour necrosis factor and interferon-γ.[5] Another important intracellular compound is cyclic-AMP (cAMP), which is understood to regulate cellular proliferation, although the precise mechanism and resulting effect on psoriasis are still unclear.[6]

Another observation that may, over time, assist in the understanding of psoriasis pathophysiology is the comorbidity of psoriasis with other conditions such as obesity, diabetes, heart disease and bowel disorders. It has been hypothesised, based on the known aetiology of the former conditions, that diet and lifestyle may therefore play a role in the development of psoriasis. Furthermore, it has been argued that the connection between bowel disorders and skin may be due to autointoxication through intestinal absorption of microbial antigens.[4] However, these hypotheses are still unproven and as such the cause and development of psoriasis require further exploration.

A key consideration in the clinical management of psoriasis and eczema is the potential similarity in presentation and sometimes treatment principles of the two conditions, contrasted by the very different pathophysiological nature. Eczema is an atopic, allergic condition, while psoriasis has autoimmune features. With this in mind, it is important to confirm the accuracy of the diagnosis before initiating a treatment plan (see the box on testing for atopy). Generic autoimmune considerations can be found in Chapter 28 on autoimmunity.

RISK FACTORS

The most important identified risk factor associated with both eczema and psoriasis is heredity; this link is much stronger in atopic eczema. The potential to develop an atopic condition of any kind is much more likely if it is already present within the family.[1] Further contributing factors worth considering in eczema rely on the identification of irritants. Common examples include strong detergents, wool, specific allergenic foods

COMMON FOOD ALLERGENS IN ATOPY

Foods commonly identified as allergens in atopic dermatitis include:[7]
- cow's milk
- egg white
- peanut
- wheat
- nuts
- fish.

(eggs, dairy, fish and nuts), psychological stress and scratching.[1,2] Change in climate can also be an ongoing aggravating factor in eczema.[2] Psoriasis has more lifestyle risk factors such as smoking, alcohol consumption, stress and obesity.[8]

CONVENTIONAL TREATMENT

Conventional management of eczema ideally involves identification of the allergens, and perhaps also any aggravating factors. Beyond this, pharmaceutical treatment relies heavily upon topical glucocorticoids to reduce chronic inflammation, and antihistamine to reduce pruritis.[1]

Management of psoriasis mostly focuses on interventions to reduce cellular proliferation, including glucocorticoids, tar preparations and ultraviolet light. Severe cases may result in the use of methotrexate.[1]

KEY TREATMENT PROTOCOLS

Gastrointestinal support

The gastrointestinal system is considered to be an important consideration in the management of skin disorders such as atopic eczema and psoriasis. The principle behind this connection focuses on intestinal hyperpermeability as an important factor in pathogenesis. It is proposed that weakness in gap junctions between enterocytes in the jejunum and lower duodenum allows toxins to migrate

GALT AND THE HYGIENE HYPOTHESIS

The gut-associated lymphoid tissue (GALT) consists of Peyer's patches, lymphoid nodules and the appendix. To induce an allergenic response from a food-based antigen, such as casein in cow's milk, the compound must be transported into Peyer's patches from the intestinal lumen. However, a healthy intestinal cell is lined with epithelial cells constituting a thick layer of glycoproteins. In addition to this, further protection is provided by mucins, digestive enzymes and secretory IgA (sIgA). The process of developing immune reactivity to specific antigens is quite complex and involves many types of immune cells within the GALT, and is explained in more detail in Chapter 28 on autoimmunity. However, it has been suggested that larger particles being processed in the B-cells within the Peyer's patches may result in the development of T helper 2 cell dominance, while immune response to microbes will stimulate T helper 1 cells (see Figure 25.1).[10] If this occurs at an early age, it exacerbates the T helper 2 dominance that naturally occurs during gestation as a way of protecting the developing fetus from maternal immunity, and may contribute to the development of atopy.[11] It is upon this understanding that the foundations for the hygiene hypothesis are laid. Initially, the rationale behind the hygiene hypothesis was linked to the epidemiological evidence that individuals in developed countries with improved sanitary practices had higher prevalence of atopic conditions. It was argued that this was due to a lack of provocation of the GALT, resulting in a maintenance of T helper 2 dominance.[11] However, more recent researchers now suggest that, although this may be true, the same benefit can be achieved by ensuring exposure to commensal gut microbiota, rather than relying on pathogenic infections to stimulate T helper 1 cells and redress the balance.[12]

into the circulation from the intestinal lumen. As these are processed and excreted through the skin they contribute to the dermal physiological changes associated with skin conditions.[9] For this reason, a focus of naturopathic treatment in eczema and psoriasis is gastrointestinal support to promote healthy permeability, and reduce the absorption of undigested peptides and food antigens.

Dysbiosis and immune function

Dysbiosis, or imbalance in the gastrointestinal bacterial population, has been associated with the development of atopic disease. It is suggested that an incorrect balance of bacteria results in inflammatory damage and reduced mucous membrane function throughout the digestive tract, thereby contributing to the pathogenesis of the condition.

For example, a recent randomised controlled trial (RCT) has indicated that maternal supplementation with ***Lactobacillus rhamnosus*** in the final weeks of gestation and up to 6 months postnatally if breastfeeding, concomitant with ongoing supplementation for the infant up to 2 years old, results in a decreased prevalence of eczema in individuals with a strong family history.[13] This may be explained by other research, which found that a similar dose of *L. rhamnosus* also resulted in a decrease in eczema symptoms.[14] The difference in this study was the measurement of objective pathology markers such as C-reactive protein (CRP) and interleukin-6. Interestingly, the levels of CRP were markedly higher in the group given *L. rhamnosus* than the placebo group. From this, it is suggested that the probiotic bacteria result in an inflammatory

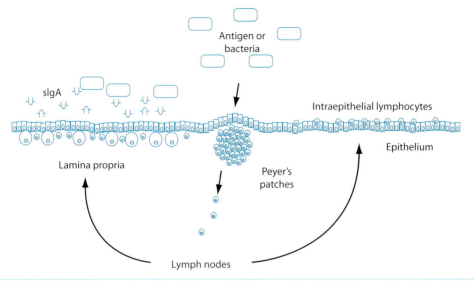

Figure 25.1 Overview of intestinal immune responses[10]

response being generated from within the intestinal epithelial cells, contributing to the healing of eczema. As CRP inhibits the production of a range of inflammatory cytokines and chemokines, this may contribute to the explanation. Furthermore, interleukin-6 (also increased in the intervention group) stimulates mucosal protein synthesis and IgA production, thereby reducing intestinal permeability and counteracting elevated IgE levels.[14] The rationale behind using probiotics to prevent atopy has been reviewed through a meta-analysis focusing on infants and was found to suggest promising results, although further research is needed.[15] However, a recent meta-analysis of the use of probiotics to treat eczema did not yield such positive results and as such the relevance of using probiotics to manage an already established atopic condition may be questioned.[16]

In conjunction with possible probiotics use, some medicinal herbs may be useful, due to their anti-microbial properties; however, research into this approach for the management of eczema has not been undertaken. In particular, using herbs such as **Ocimum basilicum**,[17] **Allium sativum**[18] and **Hydrastis canadensis**[19] may help to reduce the growth of pathogenic organisms prior to reinoculation with beneficial flora via probiotic supplementation.

Intestinal permeability

Intestinal permeability has been proposed to be an important component within the underlying pathophysiology of atopic conditions such as eczema. The concept of intestinal permeability is structured upon the tight junctions that exist between intestinal cells. These tight junctions are built from a number of membrane proteins. A number of factors proposed to increase intestinal permeability such as oxidative stress and inflammatory cytokines are also linked with atopy. This suggests that the relationship between intestinal permeability and eczema may be bilateral. Similarly, psoriasis has been described as a non-specific manifestation of bowel pathology in which undigested peptides and antigens from food and microbes are absorbed into the intestinal portal system and are eventually transported to the skin for elimination.[9] This viewpoint is congruent with the traditional naturopathic approach for skin conditions (see the box on alteratives and depuratives in the previous chapter). For more information on the pathophysiology of intestinal permeability and poor food digestion, see Chapter 5 on food allergy and intolerance.

Probiotics are the most validated approach to managing intestinal permeability in eczema. For example, a probiotic mix (*L. rhamnosus* 19070-2 and *L. reuteri* DSM-12246) was found to reduce intestinal hyperpermeability.[20] However, the same study also found that there was a direct correlation between the lactulose:mannitol ratio (a measure of intestinal permeability) and the severity of eczema (see the box on birth, breastfeeding and atopy). Another probiotic organism, *Saccharomyces boulardii*, has also been found to reduce intestinal hyperpermeability.[21] However, neither of these treatments has been evaluated for the management of psoriasis.

Another important consideration when addressing intestinal permeability is to ensure the adequate digestion of food and therefore prevent large undigested food particles being absorbed. With this in mind, herbs containing **bitter principles** are often used to provide vagal stimulation of gastric acid. Such herbs include *Gentiana lutea, Andrographis paniculata, Taraxacum officinale* and *Cynara scolymus*.[22] A similar effect has also been traditionally achieved through diet, by the ingestion of foods such as dandelion leaves, and **lemon juice in warm water**. An example of a nutrient which may be useful in this situation is **zinc** due to its role as a cofactor to carbonic anhydrase.[23]

Immune modulation

Modulating immune response is inevitably involved in the management of inflammatory conditions such as atopic dermatitis and psoriasis. This can occur on two levels. Superficial management, such as reducing histamine release, can still provide some

BIRTH, BREASTFEEDING AND ATOPY

Breastfeeding is promoted by the World Health Organization (WHO) as an important factor in infant health.[24] WHO recommends exclusive breastfeeding up to 6 months, and nutritionally sound complementary feeding starting from 6 months and continuing up to 2 years old and later if appropriate. One rationale behind this stance is the potential risk associated with feeding infants products other than breast milk in developing atopic conditions, amongst other acute and chronic health risks. Breast milk contains a number of physiological factors that benefit the infant, beyond its nutrient composition, and may be important in preventing atopy. These include a range of immune factors designed to reduce the likelihood of bacterial infection, and epidermal growth factor, which assists in the development of the intestinal lining, thereby improving nutrient absorption and reducing sensitisation to foreign particles.[24] Colostrum is also provided to breastfeeding infants in the first few days of life, and provides an immune protection to the infant while it becomes accustomed to the newly developing colony of gut microbiota.[24] Inoculation with the strains of microbes that constitute the colony is achieved at birth through vaginal delivery. In contrast, infants birthed through caesarean section have a different profile of microbiota, and an increased risk of atopy, suggesting the composition of flora is vital to healthy immune induction.[25] Furthermore, preventative supplementation with probiotics given to women in late stages of pregnancy only benefited infants born through caesarean section.[26]

beneficial results. This can be achieved through the use of **antiallergy** herbs such as *Albizzia lebbeck*,[27] or **nutrients** such as vitamin C,[28] magnesium,[29] zinc, copper and vitamin B6.[30] On a deeper level, regulating T-cell activity and reducing oxidative stress may also be important.

Inflammation

Inflammation is a key feature of the pathogenesis of atopic dermatitis.[31] This has been linked to an overproduction of IgE antibodies, which is linked to an inherited sensitivity and dysregulation of T- and B-cells. Furthermore, through its effects on eicosanoid production, the arachidonic acid cascade is considered to be a potential trigger to the onset of atopic dermatitis, and to be involved in the ongoing modification of symptoms.[31] For example, it is understood that histamine contributes to itching, but it has been suggested that the itching threshold is lowered by products of the arachidonic acid cascade such as PGE_1, PGE_2 and PGH_2.[31] Considering the role that essential fatty acids such as gamma-linoleic acid and docosohexaenoic acid play in regulating this cascade, it is unsurprising that research has found a strong connection between essential fatty acid deficiency, essential fatty acid supplementation and eczema management (see the box on EFA deficiency and eczema). Other anti-inflammatory interventions as proposed in Chapter 24 on acne vulgaris may also be indicated in eczema. Although a small clinical trial without placebo was undertaken to investigate the benefit of oral curcuminoids (from ***Curcuma longa***) in patients with psoriasis with inconclusive results,[32] larger and better designed studies are still needed in this area.

Current understanding of immune function indicates that T helper 2 cells promote IgE production.[37] An imbalance between T helper 1, which is induced by infection, and T helper 2 cells, associated with allergic reactions, is evident in atopic eczema.[38] This knowledge has led to the development of the 'hygiene hypothesis' as an explanation of

EFA DEFICIENCY AND ECZEMA

The most abundant fatty acid in the skin is linoleic acid (omega-6).[33] Gamma-linolenic acid is known to be converted to arachidonic acid through a series of enzymatic reactions. However, the enzyme required to convert the GLA metabolite, dihomo γ linolenic acid (DGLA), to arachidonic acid, delta-5-desaturase, is not present in skin epidermis (see Figure 25.2). Furthermore, the enzymes 15-lipoxygenase and cyclo-oxygenase are both still active, and act upon DGLA to form the anti-inflammatory compound 15-hydroxyeicosatrenoic acid (15-HETrE). In fact, 15-HETrE may have a more potently anti-inflammatory effect than similar metabolites of 15-lipoxygenase activity from omega-3 fats such as DHA and EPA.[33]

However, GLA supplementation does not seem to prevent the development of eczema; rather its benefits appear to focus on ameliorating the symptoms.[34] A pilot study found that supplementation with DHA (5.4 g/day) still reduced the symptoms of atopic dermatitis.[35]

In both eczema and psoriasis, leukotriene B4 and 15-HETrE, byproducts of arachidonic acid metabolism, are elevated. Furthermore, it has been suggested that individuals with atopic dermatitis may have a defect in the conversion of linoleic acid to γ-linolenic acid (via delta-6 desaturase). This may also explain why no therapeutic benefit has been associated with flaxseed oil supplementation, as it has with fish oil.[36]

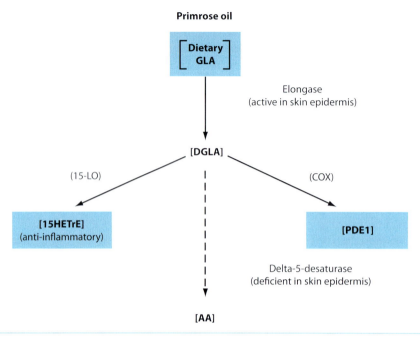

Figure 25.2 The anti-inflammatory role of evening primrose oil in skin tissue[33]

the aetiology of atopy (see the box on GALT and the hygiene hypothesis above). More recently, however, molecular research has identified the association between genetic predisposition to the development of atopy with polymorphisms in receptors to bacterial endotoxins, thereby reducing an individual's T helper 1 response. This does not necessarily mean the 'hygiene hypothesis' is untrue, but it may indicate that the underlying process is somewhat complex.[39] As such, herbs that have been traditionally defined as immunomodulatory, such as ***Withania somnifera, Echinacea angustifolia*** and ***Eleutherococcus senticosus***,[22] are often used. Recent in vitro research has also found that the equivalent of 10 mg of zinc per day increases levels of interferon-γ, which is primarily associated with T helper 1 activity; however, the clinical significance of this activity is still unclear.

An interesting contrast to atopic eczema in the T helper story is psoriasis. Psoriatic conditions are generally associated with elevated T helper 1 levels. The T helper 1 response that occurs in psoriasis is most commonly associated with a previous streptococcal or staphylococcal throat infection. The sensitised T helper 1 cells that result from this infection then migrate to the dermal layer, and produce cytokines such as interferon-γ. These cytokines contribute to hyperproliferation, a key feature of psoriasis.[40] A substantial amount of evidence suggests that a key intervention in managing T helper 1 dominant conditions such as psoriasis is **vitamin D**, which acts by promoting T helper 2 responses while blocking T helper 1. Similarly, retinoic acid (**vitamin A**) has also been found to reduce T helper 1 cell cytokines, while increasing T helper 2 transcription.[41] Although this implies that both vitamins A and D may be beneficial in psoriasis, and are to be avoided in atopic dermatitis, this may not be the case. Vitamin A deficiency still appears to increase the severity of atopic conditions. It has been suggested that this is due to an important link between vitamin A and atopy, encompassing its role in the maintenance and repair of the lamina propria, and the resulting gut-associated lymphoid tissue function.[41]

Oxidation

As atopic dermatitis is an inflammatory condition, oxidative stress is a potential side effect to be considered. Although at this stage it is not considered to be a causative factor, oxidative load may be placing a further burden on immunity and contributing to later problems. In support of this, impaired nitrogen and oxygen radical quenching has been suggested in preliminary research.[42] Similarly, psoriatic patients have also been linked with increased oxidative stress.[43] With this in mind, antioxidant nutrients such as **vitamin C**, selenium and zinc may be indicated,[23] although no known research focused on eczema has been conducted in this area. Antioxidant herbs, although they have not yet been researched for eczema specifically, may also be beneficial.

Stress

Stress has been found to enhance humoral immunity, at the expense of cell-mediated immunity, resulting in T helper 2 cell dominance and thereby favouring the production of IgE and creating a predisposition to allergy.[38] In support of this, increased activity of the hypothalamus-pituitary-adrenal (HPA) axis and consequent inflammatory reactions have been associated with individuals with diagnosed atopic dermatitis, including changes in eosinophil counts and serum IgE levels.[37] This may be explained by the effect of glucocorticoids in suppressing T helper 1 and promoting T helper 2 activity. Further evidence of this is seen in patients undergoing corticosteroid therapy resulting in increased serum IgE levels.[38] As such, it has been suggested that stress hormones in early life may generate Th2 cell predominance.[37] Stress may also affect the pathophysiology of atopic dermatitis by contributing to intestinal dysbiosis (as discussed above). This may occur through increased bacterial adherence and decreased luminal lactobacilli.[37]

Based upon this knowledge, herbal interventions that have immune and HPA-modulating activity, such as ***Eleutherococcus senticosus*** and ***Rhodiola rosea***, are recommended.[46] Similarly, nutrients that support parasympathetic nervous system activity,

ASTHMA AND ECZEMA

One of the most common examples used to explain the naturopathic principle *tolle causum*, or 'treat the cause', is the link between eczema and asthma, known medically as the atopic march. A systematic review on this topic found that one in three children who developed atopic dermatitis in the first 4 years of life would develop asthma.[44] Further research has also identified the persistence of this risk through to adult life.[45] The rationale behind this, from a naturopathic perspective, is that the dysfunctional physiological process that contributes to the development of atopic dermatitis is not addressed at its roots by conventional therapy such as topical emollients, topical steroid creams and antihistamines. Instead, the immune dysfunction such as T helper 2 predominance develops into cellular memory,[45] and may result in other compounds, such as inhaled antigens, becoming allergenic, thereby resulting in atopic rhinitis or asthma.

such as **choline**, **magnesium**, **vitamin B1** and **vitamin B5**, [23] may also be indicated (see Section 4 on the nervous system for more information).

Connective tissue function
Dermal barrier function
Maintaining dermal barrier function is an important component in minimising the damage caused by atopic dermatitis. It is generally understood that most of the issues surrounding disturbed barrier function are due to disturbed lipid composition in the stratum corneum layer of the epidermis.[2] It was upon this knowledge that the rationale for essential fatty acid supplementation in atopic dermatitis was initially based. It was identified that low levels of long-chain fatty acids were found in the serum and the cell membranes of individuals with atopic dermatitis, and that this state contributed to increased inflammation and transepidermal water loss.[36] Following on from this, a range of studies have investigated the effect of essential fatty acids status and the consequent benefit of supplementation in atopic dermatitis; however, the outcomes of these studies have been mixed.[47–49] Although this area has not been particularly well researched, nutrients that support collagen synthesis, such as **vitamin C**, **lysine**, **proline**, **copper** and **iron**, may also be considered.[23] Likewise, herbs that promote collagen synthesis, such as *Centella asiatica*,[50] could be beneficial, and has been shown to have potential benefit in psoriatic conditions.[51]

INTEGRATIVE MEDICAL CONSIDERATIONS
Homoeopathy
Homoeopathy may be used in the management of atopic dermatitis; however, as is the nature of classical homoeopathy, it is difficult to identify a specific remedy as it is very focused on the individual. An interesting study[52] that used a comparative cohort design to review the efficacy of homoeopathic treatment of eczema compared with conventional treatment was conducted. Although there were some flaws in the study, it identified an equal benefit for younger children taking the homoeopathic remedy compared with conventional treatment.

Psychotherapeutic treatment
Psychotherapeutic treatment may also provide support when managing patients with atopic dermatitis.[53] The rationale behind this may be multifaceted. It has been suggested that, as atopic dermatitis is known to be exacerbated during circumstances of perceived stress, relaxation techniques and cognitive behavioural exercises may assist the individual in managing their response, and as such reduce its physiological impact. Furthermore, behavioural interventions can reduce the habit of scratching displayed by individuals with atopic dermatitis, and as such have a favourable effect on the itch–scratch cycle. There are a number of interventions which have been investigated, and the overall outcome seems promising.[53]

Environment
Climatic change may also be a beneficial intervention to consider in the management of atopic dermatitis. In particular, moving to subtropical climates from subarctic or temperate climates, even for a period of 4 weeks, can incur benefits to patients for up to 3 years. The benefit may be due to a number of reasons, including exposure to sea water and increased ultraviolet A and B radiation.[54] Climatotherapy and

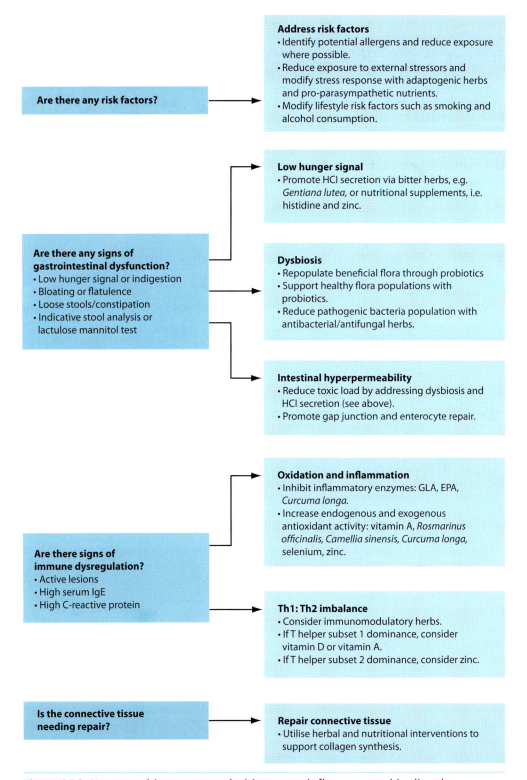

Figure 25.3 Naturopathic treatment decision tree—inflammatory skin disorders

balneotherapy—whereby patients with skin conditions such as psoriasis and atopic dermatitis attend spas, exposing themselves to mineral waters and sun for periods of a few weeks—can also offer improvement in these conditions, particularly for those that have responded poorly to treatment.[55,56]

Adjuvant topical treatments

One small trial has shown improvement in psoriasis using topically applied caffeine.[57] This is thought to be due to the actions of caffeine on increasing intracellular cAMP. Caffeine cream can be quite easily prepared by crushing caffeine tablets available from pharmacies together with a cream base. A small study of patients with mild psoriasis also found improvement in symptoms with *Aloe vera*, though care needs to be taken in case the patient is sensitive to this treatment.[58] Glycyrrhetinic acid, found in *Glycyrrhiza glabra*, may potentiate the action of hydrocortisone in skin by inhibiting the enzyme 11β-hydroxysteroid dehydrogenase.[59]

Traditional Chinese medicine

A Cochrane review of Chinese herbal medicine for atopic eczema suggested that it may be an effective treatment option for atopic eczema.[60] A later trial has suggested that acupuncture combined with Chinese herbal medicine is more effective in the treatment of atopic dermatitis than herbal medicine alone.[61]

Case Study

A 32-year-old female presents to the clinic with previously diagnosed eczema. She has **dry, scaly patches** around her **mouth**, **fingers** and on the **inside of her elbows**. They are very **red, itchy** and **papular** and are only relieved by using low-perfume moisturisers and steroidal creams. They appear to be **aggravated by stress** and the **change of seasons**. She was initially diagnosed with eczema at 5 years old; this has persisted for most of her life. This patient **does not report feeling any hunger signal**, and finds that she **craves sweets**. Her **flatus is 'offensive'** and worse when she eats meat products. She moves her bowels every 1 or 2 days, but her motions are small and unformed.

SUGGESTIVE SYMPTOMS

- Pruritis
- Eosinophilia
- Increased serum IgE levels
- Moist, red vesicular lesions (in infants)
- Dry, scaling lesions (in adults)
- More prevalent in the flexor surfaces of arms and legs, hands and feet

Example treatment

The initial prescription for this case is quite simple, as it is important to not prescribe strong antihistamine or immune-modulating interventions prior to allergy testing because this may skew the results. As such, 3000 mg of fish oil in the morning and mixed probiotics including strains of *Lactobacillus rhamnosus* and *Lactobacillus plantarum* are a safe and evidence-based protocol while she undergoes specific IgE testing to identify the allergens in her diet

Nutritional prescription

Omega-3 fish oil 3 × 1000 mg capsules with breakfast
Probiotic complex ½ tsp (equivalent to 10 × 10⁹ organisms)

Investigations

Specific IgE test

and/or environment that may be contributing to her condition. It may be useful to provide general dietary recommendations to reduce common allergens such as cow's milk and wheat (see the box on common food allergens in atopy at the beginning of the chapter) after she has been tested and results are pending.

Expected outcomes and follow-up protocols

Upon receipt of her IgE allergy profile results, dietary modifications can be undertaken to reduce intake of allergenic foods. Beyond this, modifying her prescription to focus on addressing possible intestinal hyperpermeability may be indicated. This can include *Saccharomyces boulardii* and a prebiotic formula, containing glutamine (an important energy substrate for enterocytes[23]) as well as *Ulmus rubra* and pectin. Further digestive support to stimulate gastric acid and support protein digestion, such as *Gentiana lutea*, may also be useful at this stage. If preferred, antihistamine herbs (such as *Albizzia lebbeck*) may be included in the treatment. Alternatively, it may be worth waiting to see if the antihistamine activity is necessary once the allergens have been removed from the diet.

After 4–8 weeks of intestinal repair, it is beneficial to revisit previous triggers such as stress and provide HPA support (such as *Glycyrrhiza glabra* and *Rehmannia glutinosa*) to ameliorate the effect this has on the immune system.

It is possible to have initiated this case with immune modulating herbs such as *Hemidesmus indicus, Albizzia lebbeck* or *Echinacea angustifolia*, but as the patient was undertaking allergy testing these therapies were not used initially. Any testing that is being undertaken to determine baseline physiological activity must not be masked by potent therapeutic interventions such as herbal or high-dose nutritional supplementation. Also, given the weight of evidence that suggests the potential benefit of probiotics in the management of this condition, it is proposed that using these interventions initially allows for a clear measure of their efficacy in the individual case. It then allows the practitioner to consider other interventions to address other contributing aspects of the patient's health rather than as a focus of treatment. This is important to remember that, as an individual can only take on so many prescribed products at any one time, ensuring that the prescription is most effective in the long run is important.

Table 25.1 Review of the major evidence

INTERVENTION	METHODOLOGY	RESULT	COMMENT
Evening primrose seed oil (Efamol)[47]	12-week 2-arm RCT ($n = 99$) Moderate to severe diagnosis of atopic dermatitis Evening primrose oil 500 mg (360 mg linoleic acid and 45 mg of GLA) vs placebo (500 mg paraffin) 3 dose regimens: 2 capsules twice daily; 4 capsules twice daily; 6 capsules twice daily	The higher dose groups showed significantly evening primrose oil was significantly superior to placebo with regard to itch ($p < 0.003$), scaling ($p < 0.002$), and general impression of severity ($p < 0.01$).	All participants were using concomitant mild topical steroids, emollients and systemic antihistamines. No objective measurements were used. All measurements were subjective. A more robust approach would be to include serum IgE, eosinophil or other markers.

(Continued)

Table 25.1 Review of the major evidence *(Continued)*

INTERVENTION	METHODOLOGY	RESULT	COMMENT
Lactobacillus rhamnosus[13]	2-year 3-arm *RCT (n = 474) Lactobacillus rhamnosus* HN001 (6 × 10^9 CFU) vs *Bifidobacterium animalis* subsp. *lactis* HN019 (9 × 10^9 CFU) vs placebo. *Pregnant women*: taken from 35 weeks' gestation until 6 months if breastfeeding *Infants*: taken from birth to 2 years	High-risk infants receiving *L. rhamnosus* had a reduced risk of eczema (*p* = 0.01) compared with placebo. It did not seem to have the same effect on atopy overall. No significant effect was noted for *B. animalis* spp. *lactis*.	Participants were unable to continue if they gave birth before 37 weeks' gestation, and/or had not begun the intervention for ≥ 2 weeks before birth. This effectively limited the understanding of this type of intervention on premature births. While this is an important control for the study, it would be interesting to have this aspect explored in future studies. High risk was defined as a primary family history.
Lactobacillus rhamnosus GG[62]	4 weeks 2-arm RCT (*n* = 230) Infants with suspected cow's milk allergy, in conjunction with skin treatment (emollients and 1% hydrocortisone cream) and elimination diet were given *Lactobacillus rhamnosus* GG (5 × 10^9 CFU) vs mix of probiotics (*L. rhamnosus* GG, *L. rhamnosus* LC705, *Bifidobacterium breve* Bbi99 and *Propionibacterium freudenreichii* spp. *Shermanii* JS) vs placebo.	The whole group showed a reduction in symptoms of 65%. In the IgE-sensitive group, *L. rhamnosus* GG showed a greater reduction in symptoms compared with placebo.	Although the researchers did find that exclusion of infants who took antibiotics during the course of the study further amplified the effect of *L. rhamnosus* GG on symptoms, they did not control for previous use of antibiotics in infants or maternally while breastfeeding. This may have further confounded the results.
Borage oil[48]	12 weeks 4-arm RCT (*n* = 140) *Adults*: 4 × capsules (equiv. 920 mg GLA) twice daily vs placebo *Children*: 2 × capsules (equiv. 460 mg GLA) twice daily vs placebo	SASSAD score indicated a stronger effect in the placebo compared with the intervention group.	The study did not investigate the essential fatty acid status of participants at base line, nor the previous dietary intake. Furthermore, the placebo used for the children arm was olive oil, which may have contributed to the therapeutic effect.
Glycyrrhiza glabra topical gel[63]	2 weeks 3-arm RCT (*n* = 108) 2% topical gel vs 1% topical gel vs placebo applied three times daily	Symptoms were reduced by 60–84% in the 2% topical gel and 35–56% in the 1% topical gel.	The researchers did not use any standardised measurements tools, only a Likert scale. Also, the placebo was not described. However, a high level of detail pertaining to the sourcing and processing of the herbal extract and gel preparation was included.

Table 25.1 Review of the major evidence *(Continued)*

INTERVENTION	METHODOLOGY	RESULT	COMMENT
Probiotic mix (*Lactobacillus rhamnosus* 19070-2 and *L. reuterii* DSM 12246)[20]	6-week 2-arm RCT (*n* = 41) Probiotics (10 × 10^10 CFU) twice daily vs placebo	39% reduction in gastrointestinal symptoms. Probiotic treatment lowered the lactulose to mannitol ratio.	Placebo consisted of skim milk powder, which is a common allergen for atopic dermatitis.
Narrow band ultraviolet B phototherapy[64]	12 weeks 3-arm RCT (*n* = 73) UV-B vs UV-A vs fluorescent twice daily	Mean reductions in total disease activity and extent of disease were significant compared with visible light.	Difficult to maintain true placebo as fluorescent light has some visibility so technicians would have known it was placebo.
Probiotics[15]	Meta-analysis 6 studies (*n* = 1549) Probiotics vs control *or* probiotics strain vs different probiotics strain *or* probiotics and prebiotic vs control	There was an overall reduction in clinical eczema in infants, but there was too much heterogeneity between studies for the results to be conclusive.	6 other studies identified but were not included in the analysis because they did not use allergy or food sensitivity as a measured outcome.
Psychological Intervention[53]	Meta-analysis 8 studies (mean *n* = 96.8) Heterogenous interventions including behavioural therapy, autogenic training, cognitive behavioural therapy, educational program and aromatherapy.	Overall showed a positive result, but due to the heterogeneity the studies a true meta-analysis was not possible.	The inclusion of aromatherapy failed to consider the potential physiological effect of the essential oils. This is particularly an issue as the aromatherapy study used counselling and massage on the controls, and as such was investigating the physiological effects of the oils.

KEY POINTS

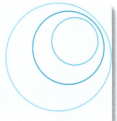

- Ensure that, where possible, any allergenic triggers are removed as a primary step in management.
- Pay close attention to any signs of dysbiosis and treat accordingly.
- Provide lifestyle support to reduce stress response.
- Avoid using any immune modulating interventions prior to testing for antigens as this may mask results.

Further reading

Jaffer SN, Qureshi AA. Dermatology quick glance. USA: McGraw-Hill Professional, 2003.

Krutmann J. Pre- and probiotics for human skin. Journal of Dermatological Science 2009;54(1):1–5.

McMillin DL, et al. Systemic aspects of psoriasis: an integrative model based on intestinal etiology. Integrative Medicine 1999;2:105–113.

Wright RJ, et al. The impact of stress on the development and expression of atopy. Current Opinion in Allergy and Clinical Immunology 2005;5:23–29.

References

1. Gould BE. Pathophysiology for the health professional. 3rd edn. Philadelphia: Saunders Elsevier, 2006.

2. Proksch E, et al. Skin barrier function, epidermal proliferation and differentiation in eczema. Journal of Dermatological Science 2006;43:159–169.

3. Williams H, et al. Is eczema really on the increase worldwide? Journal of Allergy and Clinical Immunology 2008;121:947–954.

4. McMillin DL, et al. Systemic aspects of psoriasis: an integrative model based on intestinal etiology. Integrative Medicine 2000;2:105–113.

5. Arican O, et al. Serum levels of TNF-alpha, IFN-gamma, IL-6, IL-8, IL-12, IL-17, and IL-18 in patients with active psoriasis and correlation with disease severity. Mediatus Inflamm 2005;5:273–279.

6. Takahashi H, et al. Cyclic AMP differentially regulates cell proliferation of normal human keratinocytes through ERK activation depending on the expression pattern of B-Raf. Archives of Dermatological Research 2004;296(2):74–82.

7. Host A, Halken S. Practical aspects of allergy-testing. Paedicatric Respiratory Reviews 2003;4(4):312–318.

8. Neimann AL, et al. The epidemiology of psoriasis. Expert Rev Dermatol 2006;1:63–75.

9. McMillin DL, et al. Systemic aspects of psoriasis: an integrative model based on intestinal etiology. Integrative Medicine 1999;2:105–113.

10. Simecka JW. Mucosal immunity of the gastrointestinal tract and oral tolerance. Advanced Drug Delivery Reviews 1998;34:235–259.

11. Rautava S, et al. New therapeutic strategy for combating increasing burden of allergic disease: probiotics—a Nutrition, Allergy, Mucosal Immunology and Intestinal Microbiota (NAMI) Research Group report. Journal of Allergy and Clinical Immunology 2005;116:31–37.

12. Adlerberth I, et al. Gut microbiota and development of atopic eczema in 3 European birth cohorts. Journal of Allergy and Clinical Immunology 2007;120:343–350.

13. Wickens K, et al. A differential effect of 2 probiotics in the prevention of eczema and atopy: a double-blind, randomized, placebo-controlled trial. Journal of Allergy and Clinical Immunology 2008;122:788–794.

14. Viljanen M, et al. Induction of inflammation as a possible mechanism of probiotic effect in atopic eczema-dermatitis syndrome. Journal of Allergy and Clinical Immunology 2005;115:1254–1259.

15. Osborn DA, Sinn JKH. Probiotics in infants for prevention of allergic disease and food hypersensitivity. Cochrane Database of Systemic Reviews 2009;(4):CD006475.

16. Boyle RJ, et al. Probiotics for treating eczema (review). Cochrane Database of Systemic Reviews 2008;(1):CD006135.

17. Suppakul P, et al. Antimicrobial properties of basi and its possible application in food packaging. Journal of Agricultural and Food Chemistry 2003;51(11):3197–3207.

18. Iciek M, et al. Biological properties of garlic and garlic-derived organosulfur compounds. Environmental and Molecular Mutagenesis 2009;50(3):247–265.

19. Hwang BY, et al. Antimicrobial constituents from goldenseal (the rhizomes of Hydrastis canadensis) against selected oral pathogens. Planta Medica 2003;69(7):623–627.

20. Rosenfeldt V, et al. Effect of probiotics on gastrointestinal symptoms and small intestinal permeability in children with atopic dermatitis. Journal of Pediatrics 2004;145:612–616.

21. Vilela GE, et al. Influence of Saccharomyces boulardii on the intestinal permeability of patients with Crohn's disease in remission. Scandanavian Journal of Gastroenterology 2008;43(7):842–848.

22. British Herbal Medicine Association. British herbal pharmacopoeia. London: British Herbal Medicine Association, 1996.

23. Gropper SS, et al. Advanced nutrition and human metabolism. 5th edn. Belmont: Wadsworth, 2009.

24. World Health Organization. Infant and young child feeding: model chapter for textbooks for medical students and allied health professionals. World Health Organization, 2009:1–99.

25. Bager P, et al. Caesarean delivery and risk of atopy and allergic disease: meta-analyses. Epidemiology of Allergic Disease 2008;38:634–642.

26. Kuitunen M, et al. Probiotics prevent IgE-associated allergy until 5 years in caesarean-delivered children but not in the total cohort. Journal of Allergy and Clinical Immunology 2009;123:335–341.

27. Tripathi RM, et al. Studies on the mechanism of action of Albizzia lebbeck, an Indian indigenous drug used in the treatment of atopic allergy. Journal of Ethnopharmacology 1979;1(4):385–396.

28. Clemetson CAB. Histamine and ascorbic acid in human blood. J Nutr 1980;110(4):662–668.

29. Bois P, et al. Histamine-liberating effect of magnesium deficiency in the rat. Nature 1963;197(4866):501–502.

30. Maintz L, et al. Evidence for a reduced histamine degradation capacity in a subgroup of patients with atopic eczema. Journal of Allergy and Clinical Immunology 2006;117(5):1106–1112.

31. Ikai K, Imamura S. Role of eicosanoids in the pathogenesis of atopic dermatitis. Prostaglandins, Leukotrienes and Essential Fatty Acids 1993;48:409–416.

32. Kurd SK, et al. Oral curcumin in the treatment of moderate to severe psoriasis vulgaris. A prospective clinical trial. J Am Acad Dermatol 2008;58:625–631.

33. Ziboh VA, et al. Significance of lipoxygenase-derived fatty acids in cutaneous biology. Prostaglandins and Other Lipid Mediators 2000;63:3 13.

34. Kitz R, et al. Impact of early dietary gamma-linolenic acid supplementation on atopic eczema in infancy. Pediatric Allergy and Immunology 2006;17:112–117.

35. Koch C, et al. Docosahexaenoic acid (DHA) supplementation in atopic eczema: a randomised, double-blind, controlled trial. British Journal of Dermatology 2008;158:786–792.

36. Wright S. Essential fatty acids and the skin. Prostaglandins, Leukotrienes and Essential Fatty Acids 1989;38:229–236.

37. Wright RJ, et al. The impact of stress on the development and expression of atopy. Current Opinion in Allergy and Clinical Immunology 2005;5:23–29.

38. Marshall GD, Roy SR. Stress and allergic diseases. In: Ader R, ed. Psychoneuroimmunology. Elsevier: Academic Press, 2007.

39. Prescott SL, Dunstan JA. Immune dysregulation in allergic respiratory disease: the role of T regulatory cells. Pulmonary Pharmacology and Therapeutics 2005;18:217–228.

40. Baker BS, et al. A major aetiological factor for psoriasis. Trends in Immunology 2006;27(12):545–552.

41. Mora JR, et al. Vitamin effects on the immune system: vitamins A and D take centre stage. Nature Reviews: Immunology 2008;8:685–698.

42. Omata N, et al. Increased oxidative stress in childhood atopic dermatitis. Life Sciences 2001;69:223–228.

43. Kokcam I, Naziroglu M. Antioxidants and lipid peroxidation status in the blood of patients with psoriasis. Clinica Chimica Acta 1999;289:23–31.

44. van der Hulst AE, et al. Risk of developing asthma in young children with atopic eczema: a systematic review. Journal of Allergy and Clinical Immunology 2007;120:565–569.

45. Burgess JA, et al. Childhood eczema and asthma incidence and persistence: a cohort study from childhood to middle age. Journal of Allergy and Clinical Immunology 2008;122(2):280–285.

46. Safonova GM, et al. Protective effects of plant polyphenols on the immune system in acute stress. Doklady Biological Sciences 2001;378(1–6):223–235.

47. Wright S. Oral evening primrose seed oil improves atopic eczema. Lancet 1982;2(8308):1120–1122.
48. Takwale A, et al. Efficacy and tolerability of borage oil in adults and children with atopic eczema: randomised, double blind, placebo controlled parallel group trial. British Medical Journal 2003;327:1–4.
49. Newson RB, et al. Umbilical cord and maternal blood red cell fatty acids and early childhood wheezing and eczema. Journal of Allergy and Clinical Immunology 2004;114:531–537.
50. Shukla A, et al. In vitro and in vivo wound healing activity of asiaticode isolated from *Centella asiatica*. Journal of Ethnopharmacology 1999;65(1):1–11.
51. Sampson JH, et al. In vitro keratinocyte antiproliferant effect of *Centella asiatica* extract and triterpenoid saponins. Phytomedicine 2001;8(3):230–235.
52. Keil T, et al. Homoeopathic versus conventional treatment of children with eczema: a comparative cohort study. Complementary Therapies in Medicine 2008;16:15–21.
53. Chida Y, et al. The effects of psychological intervention on atopic dermatitis. International Archives of Allergy and Immunology 2007;144:1–9.
54. Byremo G, et al. Effect of climatic change in children with atopic eczema. Allergy 2006;61:1403–1410.
55. Kazandjieva J, et al. Climatotherapy of psoriasis. Clin Dermatol 2008;26(5):477–485.
56. Matz H, et al. Balneotherapy in dermatology. Dermatol Ther 2003;16(2):132–140.
57. Vali A, et al. Evaluation of the efficacy of topical caffeine in the treatment of psoriasis vulgaris. J Dermatolog Treat 2005;16(4):234–237.
58. Paulsen E, et al. A double-blind, placebo-controlled study of a commercial *Aloe vera* gel in the treatment of slight to moderate psoriasis vulgaris. J Eur Acad Dermatol Venereol 2005;19(3):326–331.
59. Teelucksingh S, et al. Potentiation of hydrocortisone activity in skin by glycyrrhetinic acid. Lancet 1990;335(8697):1060–1063.
60. Zhang W, et al. Chinese herbal medicine for atopic eczema. Cochrane Database Syst Rev 2005;(2):CD002291.
61. Salameh F, et al. The effectiveness of combined Chinese herbal medicine and acupuncture in the treatment of atopic dermatitis. J Altern Complement Med 2008;14(8):1043–1048.
62. Viljanen M, et al. Probiotics in the treatment of atopic eczema/dermatitis syndrome in infants: a double-blind placebo-controlled trial. Allergy 2005;60:494–500.
63. Saeedi M, et al. The treatment of atopic dermatitis with licorice gel. Journal of Dermatological Treatment 2003;14:153–157.
64. Reynolds NJ, et al. Narrow-band ultraviolet B and broad-band ultraviolet A phototherapy in adult atopic eczema: a randomised controlled trial. Lancet 2001;357:2012–2016.

Section 9 Urogenital system

The urogenital system consists of the urinary tract (including the renal system), and in males the sexual reproductive organs. The urinary tract is primarily responsible for cleaning and filtering excess fluid and waste material from the blood (via the kidneys, ureters, bladder and urethra). In addition, the kidneys have further hormonal and blood pressure monitoring functions. Urogenital system disorders are likely to become more pronounced in the future with an ageing Western population. As people age the kidneys may lose some of their ability to remove wastes from the blood and bladder, while the pelvic muscle and penile tissue lose tone and strength. Increased rates of incontinence occur in the elderly, as the sphincter muscles in the pelvis lose strength. In most men the prostate will get larger as they grow older; this phenomenon is responsible for benign prostatic hyperplasia. In addition, functional disorders such as erectile dysfunction may also occur. So elderly patients need to be screened for urogenital system conditions more often than their younger counterparts.

Systemic symptoms, including headaches, fatigue and nocturia, may result from genitourinary pathology. Urogenital health in both men and women is linked to environmental, immune, hormonal and sexual health. While genetic and environmental factors have a pronounced effect on urogenital system conditions, psychological factors should also be considered, especially in matters relating to sexuality (function and performance). While physical symptoms may be limited to this system more than others, conditions such as erectile dysfunction or incontinence may have significant emotional or psychological effects. Self-esteem issues need careful consideration, and emotional and psychological support and therapy are important therapeutic adjuncts.

Naturopathic medicine has long had an association with the treatment of urogenital disorders. The original Hippocratic Oath contains an admonition on the dangers of operating for 'stones', and the diuretic properties of plants have been documented for the treatment of 'stones' since the time of Pliny the Elder. Common urogenital conditions treated by naturopaths include benign prostatic hypertrophy, urinary tract infections, erectile dysfunction and, to a lesser extent, urinary calculi. Kidney infection or disease is a more serious medical condition, and medical intervention is required (though CAM therapies may provide adjuvant support).

Naturopathic medicine has an array of therapeutic options to address both symptomatic and underlying urogenital system conditions. Dietary advice provides a cornerstone of treating many urogenital system disorders, for example essential fatty acids in benign prostatic hyperplasia, increased water and alkalinity in urinary tract infections, mineral balance or low oxalates in urinary calculi. Herbal medicines may also be of assistance in providing anti-inflammatory, antiseptic, diuretic and other specific actions that are required in many urogenital system disorders.

This section focuses on some of the complexities in three of the most commonly seen urogenital system conditions: benign prostatic hypertrophy, erectile dysfunction and urinary tract infections.

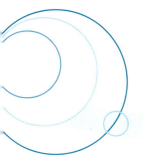

26
Benign prostatic hypertrophy

Kieran Cooley
ND, MSc

AETIOLOGY AND EPIDEMIOLOGY

While benign prostatic hypertrophy of the prostate (BPH) (or more accurately benign prostatic *hyperplasia*) and erectile dysfunction (ED) are typically seen in the *ageing* male, these can occur at any age. Current understanding of the disease involves imbalanced states of androgens (particularly dihydrotestosterone [DHT]), oestrogens, insulin and insulin-like growth factor (IGF), and detrusor dysfunction of the bladder neck.[1] The chief complaint of patients with BPH is urinary frequency, urgency, nocturia, decreased and intermittent force of stream and the sensation of incomplete emptying of the bladder, although these symptoms are neither specific or necessary for the diagnosis of BPH and do not correlate with the extent or degree of hypertrophy of the prostate.[1] One study suggests that 20% of men in their 40s and 90% of men in their 70s have varying degrees of BPH,[2] although incidence rates for age groups vary depending on population demographics (some suggest 50% of men older than 60, and 80% of men over 80 years).[3] Increasing age is the predominant factor associated with prevalence of BPH. Likewise, the incidence and prevalence of ED are also linked to age, with United States of America data suggesting a tripling of the incidence occurring between the ages of 40 and 70 years, and up to 66% of men having suffered from some erectile dysfunction (mild to complete) by the age of 70 years.[4] Worldwide estimates suggest up to 330 million men could be affected by this disorder,[5] although criticism exists pertaining to the over-medicalisation and resulting prescription rates for drugs providing only symptomatic relief for some age-associated disorders like ED.[6] Conversely, both ED and BPH may suffer from under-diagnosis due to the symptomatic nature and psychological stigma associated with each of these diseases.[7]

Previously, diagnosis of BPH was thought to involve solely lower urinary tract symptoms (LUTS) syndrome;[1] however, recent evidence suggests that LUTS is often due to anatomical disorders (detrusor muscle dysfunction)[8,9] and that symptoms of BPH do not correlate well with prostate size. However, an enlarged prostate could contribute to detrusor dysfunction and urinary retention, often termed 'LUTS-BPH'. Clinicians should note that not all men with BPH have LUT symptoms and LUTS is not specific or exclusive to BPH.

There is little certainty surrounding the exact pathogenesis of BPH. It is characterised by periurethral prostate tissue proliferation, which is indicated by an increase in the number (not size) of epithelial and stromal cells.[10] This has been posited to be a relatively normal (or at least highly pervasive) process of ageing, often linked to the prostate tissue response to increase in androgens (dihydrotestosterone [DHT]) that occurs in the ageing male. Environmental exposure to hormone disruptors like xenoestrogens may result in a cascade of events that influence the development of dysfunctional regulation of testosterone, 17β-oestradiol and DHT (see Figure 26.1).[10] The enzymes aromatase and 5-alpha reductase are involved in hormone regulation and these are often targets of both conventional as well as naturopathic treatment. Other evidence suggests that increased exposure to growth factors (insulin and insulin-like growth factor (IGF)) initiates the onset of hyperproliferation, ultimately leading to decreased urinary and vascular flow and an increased risk for ED, LUTS, prostatitis and prostate cancer, all of which can be associated disorders.[1] As the prostate enlarges, it causes discomfort in the groin and increased pressure on the bladder, leading to variable urine flow rates, frequent urination, nocturia and a sense of incomplete voiding. With chronicity or severity of enlargement, blockage of the urethra can occur, increasing the risk for urinary tract infections, bladder stones and possible kidney damage.

In 2001 a landmark paper suggested a link between ED, BPH, cardiovascular disease and depression in the ageing male,[11] supporting earlier suggestions linking some of these disorders to vascular function.[12] Since then, further evidence has confirmed a strong correlation among these disorders, with significantly higher prevalence rates of any of the listed conditions when a comorbidity from any of the other disorders exists. The correlation is particularly strong between BPH and ED, possibly due to a shared vasculogenic pathophysiology, revolving around atherosclerosis and endothelial dysfunction or injury, in production of nitric oxide (NO).[13] Other factors associated with cardiovascular disease and/or depression (such as central obesity, increased circulating levels of insulin, diabetes, decreased physical activity, hypertension and increased oxidative stress) are also implicated in the state that promotes the hyperproliferation

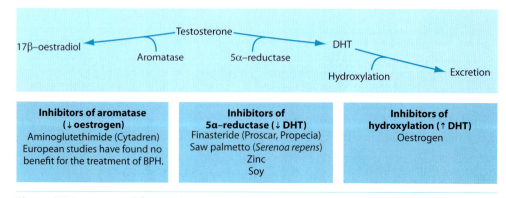

Figure 26.1 Hormonal factors in BPH
Source: Rakel D, ed. Integrative medicine. 2nd edn. Philadelphia: Saunders, 2007.

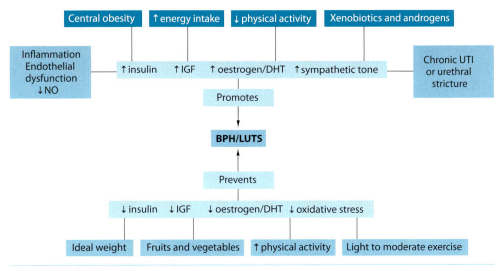

Figure 26.2 Factors affecting BPH or LUTS

of prostatic tissue and decreased functioning of circuitry relating to achieving an erection.[14,15]

RISK FACTORS[1,3,16]

Several factors may promote BPH/LUTS, whereas other influences may have a protective effect (see Figure 26.2). The following is a list of potential risk factors and indicators of BPH:

- Urethral structure as a result of recurrent urinary tract infection, bladder infection or trauma or bladder neck contractions (congenital or acquired) can induce LUTS and stimulate the onset of hyperproliferation.
- Comorbid conditions such as cardiovascular disease, erectile dysfunction and depression are also implicated in increased incidence or potential for earlier onset of BPH.
- Increased serum prostate-specific antigen (PSA) can be indicative of BPH, but it is neither sensitive nor specific to BPH although monitoring change in this marker over time gives some small clinically relevant indication of prostate status or change. Suggested PSA levels that may indicate a hyperproliferative prostate are > 1.6 ng/mL for men in their 50s, > 2.0 ng/mL for men in their 60s and > 2.3 ng/mL for men in their 70s.
- A positive digital rectal exam is the strongest indicator of BPH and regular screening is recommended in men over 50 years old or those exhibiting symptoms.

CONVENTIONAL TREATMENT

Conventional treatment of BPH varies often begins with 'watchful waiting' if the symptoms are mild. Alpha-blockers (alfuzosin and tamsulosin) are often selected for decreasing sympathetic tone with minimal change in blood pressure to give LUT symptom relief and are often employed in those without significantly raised levels of PSA.[1,16] 5-alpha reductase inhibitors (finasteride or dutasteride) inhibit the conversion of testosterone to DHT and are the most frequently prescribed treatment, sometimes in conjunction with alpha-blockers with greater success. If symptoms are severe, there is a long history of smoking or risk factors for cancer, or PSA levels are relatively high, surgical removal of the prostate (transurethral resection of the prostate or TURP) may be indicated.

KEY TREATMENT PROTOCOLS

A comprehensive strategy addressing cardiovascular risk and reduction of inflammation is required to address the underlying vascular cause. Additional strategies to provide symptomatic relief from LUTS are necessary for short-term management of this debilitating disorder. The initial approach in treating this disorder is always to assess the lifestyle of the patient and recommend judicious and achievable adjustments when required.

> ### NATUROPATHIC TREATMENT AIMS
> - Address risk factors including achievement of healthy weight and increased physical activity.
> - Regulate hormones, particularly through aromatase and 5-alpha reductase as well as environmental sources of hormones.
> - Address symptom relief and quality-of-life issues.
> - Protect endothelial function through decreasing inflammation, improving NO production.
> - Address latent, recurrent or chronic infection and sources of oxidative stress.

Lifestyle and exercise modification

As mentioned above, lifestyle modification is an important protocol in treating BPH and ED. Observational studies indicate that there is a positive association between abdominal obesity and BPH,[17,18] and an inverse association between physical activity and BPH.[19,20] Diets high in fats or in calories may encourage abdominal obesity and sympathetic nervous system activity, both of which can increase the risk of BPH. Sympathetic nervous system activation (which is the 'fight or flight' arm of the autonomic nervous system) may cause the prostate smooth muscle to contract, resulting in a worsening of lower urinary tract symptoms. Studies suggest that there is no increased risk of BPH with higher caloric intake when accompanied by increased physical activity.[18] With respect to ED, weight loss, physical activity, smoking cessation and decreased sympathetic activity (relaxation) have also been suggested as beneficial treatments.[21] Dietary sources of caffeine and other diuretics should be reduced, and fluid intake monitored to reduce nocturia and urinary output to the bladder from the kidneys.

Three potential mechanisms for physical activity and decreased risk for BPH and ED may be proposed:
1. It may increase blood flow to the area, allowing the body to remove wastes efficiently.
2. It may decrease sympathetic stress responses, thus relaxing prostatic tissue.
3. It may reduce excess abdominal weight, increasing overall lower body pressure, thus relaxing the prostate and rectal region and improving blood flow into and out of the area.

Nutritional hormonal modulation (5-alpha reductase, aromatase, dihydrotestosterone and oestrogen)

Clinicians should consider dietary strategies to modulate hormones, hydroxylation of DHT and maintain healthy cholesterol and cardiovascular states; these strategies include avoiding sources of pesticides,[22] increasing fruit consumption, increasing the intake of zinc and essential fatty acid, decreasing butter consumption, avoiding margarine,[23] decreasing coffee consumption[24] and keeping cholesterol levels below 200 mg/dL.[25]

Inconclusive evidence exists regarding protein intake and BPH. Some research demonstrates that a **high-protein diet** (total calories made up of 44% protein, 35% carbohydrate and 21% fat) can inhibit 5-alpha reductase, while a low-protein diet (10% protein, 70% carbohydrate and 20% fat) may stimulate the enzyme.[26] Contrary to this evidence, a large 8-year observational study of 3523 men with BPH suggests that total protein intake is positively associated with BPH, with the association being slightly stronger for animal protein intake than for vegetable protein intake.[18] A second epidemiological study based in China also revealed a correlation between higher animal intake and the incidence of BPH (91.1% in those eating high animal diets as opposed to 11.8% in those not eating animal protein).[27]

Authors of these studies suggest that a high protein intake may result in a greater osmolar load, which may be one possible mechanism for its detrimental effects on symptoms of BPH. This will increase urinary output and thus impose undue extra burden on an already partially obstructed or strained elimination system.[18] Consistent with an anti-inflammatory approach, a diet high in quality, plant-derived and coldwater fish-based protein sources in moderate amounts seems prudent, given the current evidence.

Zinc supplementation has reduced the size of the prostate (confirmed by rectal palpation, radiography and endoscopy) and reduced overall symptomatology in the majority of patients with BPH in studies conducted in the 1970s as well as recently.[28] The clinical efficacy of zinc is probably due to its critical involvement in many aspects of androgen metabolism. High amounts of oestrogen can inhibit intestinal uptake of zinc, whereas elevated androgens increase absorption. Because oestrogen levels are increased in men with BPH, zinc uptake may be low, suggesting a higher functional need for this nutrient and begging the need for additional supplementation.[29,30] However, one case-control study suggested a positive association between zinc levels and BPH.[31] This deviation from other research may be partially explained by dietary confounding factors.

The relationship between zinc levels and 5-alpha reductase activity in hyperplastic prostates is inconsistent; however, zinc has been shown to inhibit the activity of 5-alpha reductase, and decreases the conversion of testosterone to DHT.[32-35] Zinc can also inhibit specific binding of androgens to the cytosol and nuclear androgen receptors present in high amounts in prostatic tissue.[32] These mechanisms suggest that zinc has more of a preventative role by maintaining a nutritional status that discourages prostate hypertrophy. No interventional studies investigating the use of zinc for BPH exist, although observational studies suggest it has a safe and effective role in diminishing the size of the prostate, particularly for prostate cancer, although one study suggests it can increase urinary symptoms.[36-40]

Zinc is also involved in the regulation of prolactin secretion, leading to increased uptake of testosterone and subsequent rise in DHT in the prostate.[41-43] Natural (from beer, stress and tryptophan)[44,45] and pharmaceutical prolactin antagonists (bromocriptine)[46] have been shown to reduce many of the symptoms of prostatic hyperplasia. However, this strategy can have severe side effects, particularly pertaining to cardiovascular and neurological systems, including severe changes in mood.[47,46]

A 100 g serving of soybeans or **soy** products contains 90 mg of **beta-sitosterol**, which has been shown to decrease cholesterol; this is a potential mechanism for soy's effect on BPH. The cholesterol-lowering effects of phytosterols are well documented,[48,49] while also showing an effect on treating BPH.[9] One double-blind study[50] in 200 men using beta-sitosterol (20 mg) or placebo three times daily demonstrated an increase in the maximum urine flow rate from a baseline of 9.9 mL/s to 15.2 mL/s and a decrease in mean residual urinary volume of 30.4 mL from 65.8 mL in the beta-sitosterol group. No changes were observed in the placebo group. An increased consumption of soy and soy foods is associated with a decrease in the risk of prostate cancer,[51,52] which is associated with the incidence of BPH. Phytoestrogens in soy (isoflavonoids, genistein and daidzein), as well as *Trifolium pratense* are implicated due to their effect on oestrogen receptors[51,53] and inhibition of 5-alpha reductase.[54] Other sources of beta-sitosterols such as *Hypoxis hemerocallidea* may also be of benefit, although many of these studies are lacking in the rigour of reporting including dose and method of extraction as well as adverse-event reporting.[55] Clinical use of these substances may be most appropriate for men with BPH in the 'watchful waiting' stage of the condition[56] with clinically effecting doses of beta-sitosterol ranging from 60–130 mg daily.[57,58]

One study[59] suggested that 60 mg twice daily of the dried, ground flowers of *Opuntia* spp. over 2 to 6 months was effective at reducing urinary urgency and the sensation of a full bladder, although this remains to be repeated in other studies and stands as preliminary evidence.

The diet should be as free as possible from environmental toxins such as pesticides and other contaminants because many of these compounds (such as dioxin, polyhalogenated biphenyls, hexachlorobenzene and dibenzofurans) increase 5-alpha reduction of steroids.[26] Diethylstilbestrol produces changes in rat prostates histologically similar to BPH.[60] While cadmium is a known antagonist of zinc and can influence testosterone levels through effects on the activity of 5-alpha reductase, its concentration in, and effects on, the prostate are unclear. Several studies have produced conflicting results.[61,62]

Herbal hormonal modulation (5-alpha reductase, aromatase, dihydrotestosterone and oestrogen)

During the 1990s, botanical medicine in Germany and Australia were considered 'first-line' treatments for BPH and accounted for greater than 90% of all drugs in the medical management of BPH.[63] In Italy, plant extracts accounted for roughly 50% of all medications prescribed for BPH, while alpha-blockers and 5-alpha reductase inhibitors account for only 5.1% and 4.8%, respectively.[64]

Clinical success with any of the botanical treatments of BPH may be determined by the degree of obstruction as indicated by the residual urine content.[1,22] For mild LUTS symptoms and residual urine levels less than 50 mL, the results are usually excellent. For levels between 50 and 100 mL, the results are usually quite good. Residual urine levels greater than 100 mL will be more difficult to produce significant improvements in the customary 4- to 6-week period without co-management using other therapies including pharmaceuticals, and with botanical medicine adding little to the overall reduction in symptoms within a 4–6 week period. One small (n = 40) but well-designed clinic-based research study investigating the open use of phytotherapy for LUTS/BPH demonstrated a statistically significant superiority of phytotherapy use (as both adjuvant to pharmacological treatment or as a stand-alone) over use of alpha-blockers to reduce urinary retention, and improve erectile and ejaculatory dysfunction.[65] Adulteration and/or contamination in herbal products for erectile dysfunction is relatively widespread[66,67] particularly in 'commercial' natural health products in some countries. As with usual prescriptions, clinicians should ensure that patients are accessing high quality products.

The liposterolic extract of the fruit of *Serenoa repens*, native to Florida in the USA, has been shown to significantly improve the signs and symptoms of BPH in numerous clinical studies. The mechanism of action is postulated to be related to inhibition of DHT binding to both the cytosolic and the nuclear androgen receptors, inhibition of 5-alpha reductase, interference with intraprostatic oestrogen receptors and an anti-inflammatory effect.[10] As a result of this multitude of effects, positive results have been produced in numerous double-blind clinical studies. However, different extracts of *S. repens* (permixon) may have more of an anti-inflammatory mechanism of action in modulating BPH;[63,66–70] clinicians should be mindful of these differences in therapeutic action from the myriad of extraction methods used in natural health products and the multifaceted effects of herbal medicines, particularly *S. repens*.[68]

Synthesis research, including systematic reviews of clinical trials, has previously reported excellent results using *S. repens*.[71,72] One examination of 21 randomised, controlled trials involving a total of 3139 men (including 18 double-blind trials) demonstrated that men treated with *S. repens* experienced decreased urinary tract symptom scores, less nocturia, better urinary tract symptom self-rating scores and peak urine flow improvements compared with men receiving placebo.[71] This analysis also showed that, matched up with men receiving the DHT inhibitor finasteride (Proscar), men treated with *S. repens* had similar improvements in urinary tract symptom scores and peak urine. A related review also reported that adverse effects due to *S. repens* were mild and infrequent with erectile dysfunction appearing more frequently with finasteride (4.9%) than with *S. repens* (1.1%).[72] However, a recent update to this Cochrane review, which included nine new studies comparing *S. repens* to either placebo or finasteride, demonstrated no significant benefit for treating any symptoms of BPH except nocturia.[73] The large variability in patient population, severity of disease and extraction or source of *S. repens*, as demonstrated by a lack of heterogeneity between studies and wide confidence intervals for outcomes, highlights some of the challenges in herbal medicine research when applying research results to individuals. At the same time, these results indicate that clinical success in using serenoa for BPH is variable, with the greatest likelihood for improvement occurring in men with mild to moderate symptoms receiving treatment within the first 4–6 weeks of onset.

Overall, it can be stated that some men with mild to moderate BPH experience some improvement in symptoms during the first 4 to 6 weeks of therapy using *S. repens*. All major symptoms of BPH are improved, especially nocturia. And despite an efficacy profile similar to finasteride for mild to moderate severity, serenoa has a lower risk profile and is less expensive.[74] The most common side effect is gastrointestinal distress, and this is easily remedied by taking *S. repens* with food.

Cernilton®, a proprietary combination of water-soluble and acetone-soluble extract of *Secale cereale*, has been used to treat prostatitis and BPH for years in Europe.[75,76] Several short clinical studies and one systematic review suggest it to be beneficial in the treatment of BPH,[77–83] with patients reporting moderate improvement. Patients who respond typically have reductions of nocturia and diurnal frequency of around 70%, as well as significant reductions in residual urine volume. The extract has been shown to exert some anti-inflammatory action and produce a contractile effect on the bladder while simultaneously relaxing the urethra.[84]

In one study, the clinical efficacy of Cernilton® in the treatment of symptomatic BPH was examined over a 1-year period.[76] Seventy-nine males of an average age of 68 years (range 62 to 89), with a mean baseline prostatic volume of 33.2 cm^2, were administered 63 mg Cernilton® pollen extract twice daily for 12 weeks. Average urine maximum flow rate increased from 5.1 to 6 mL/s. Average flow rate increased from 9.3 to 11 mL/s. Residual urine volume decreased from 54.2 mL to less than 30 mL. Urgency and discomfort improved by 76.9% with dysuria, incomplete emptying, intermittency, delayed or prolonged voiding all having 60–70% improvement. Nocturia improved by 56.8%. Overall, 85% of the test subjects experienced benefit, 11% reporting 'excellent', 39% reporting 'good', 35% reporting 'satisfactory' and 15% reporting 'poor' as a description of their outcome.

A systematic review conducted in 2000 compiling two placebo-controlled studies, two comparative trials (both lasting 12 to 24 weeks) and three double-blind studies of 444 men showed that, although Cernilton® did not improve urinary flow rates, residual volume or prostate size compared with placebo or the comparative study agents, it did improve self-rated urinary symptom scores and reduced nocturia compared with placebo.[81] Again, this review highlights some of the variability in evidence for the use of this herbal extract with the chances of clinical success in using this as a stand-alone treatment remaining unclear.

Extracts from the bark of ***Pygeum africanum*** used in research studies are fat-soluble sterols and fatty acids. Virtually all of the research on pygeum has featured a pygeum extract standardised to contain 14% triterpenes including beta-sitosterol and 0.5% *n*-docosanol. The suggested therapeutic action has been suggested to be due, in part, to the inhibition of growth factors EGF, bFGF and IGF-I, which are responsible for the prostatic overgrowth.[85,86]

Clinical trials totalling more than 600 patients have demonstrated pygeum extract to be effective in reducing the symptoms and clinical signs of BPH, especially in early cases.[86,87] The research studies suggest pygeum having a superiority in objective parameters, especially urine flow rate and residual urine content, over saw palmetto. However, as the two extracts have somewhat overlapping mechanisms of actions, they can be used in combination.

Lepidium meyenii (**maca**) is a root belonging to the brassica family traditionally known for its aphrodisiac properties in both men and women.[88] A recent randomised, double-blind placebo-controlled trial demonstrated a subjective improvement on the International Index of Erectile Function (IIEF-5) and Satisfaction Profile (SAT-P) using 2400 mg/day of dry extract of maca compared to placebo.[89] Although both groups improved significantly from baseline self-rated psychological performance scores, there was a statistically significant superiority in the maca group in physical and social performance. This represents a small but statistically significant clinical effect from using this dose of maca in men with mild erectile dysfunction. Two other randomised, placebo-controlled studies with limited information suggest that 1.5 and 3 g/day dose of maca can improve erectile dysfunction without altering testosterone levels in men with this disorder.[90,91] Further research is necessary to better determine the mechanism of action, the clinical relevance and optimal dose and constituents in maca for use in erectile dysfunction. No clinical evidence exists for the use of maca for treating BPH.

Extracts of ***Urtica dioica*** have also been shown to be effective in the treatment of BPH, although less research evidence exists compared to other botanical medicines. A number of long-term, double-blind studies have shown it to be more effective than a placebo, with no adverse effects reported.[92,93] A randomised, multicentre, double-blind study in 431 patients using extracts of both *S. repens* and *U. dioica* found clinical benefit equal to that of finasteride,[94] with a larger, second study lasting 24 weeks confirming its benefit in reducing residual urine and improving peak flow.[92] A similar therapeutic action between urtica and serenoa extracts appears to exist in that each interact with binding of DHT to cytosolic and nuclear receptors.[95] Other in vitro studies also show that lignans found in *U. dioica* may modulate hormonal effects due to their affinity for sex hormone-binding globulin.[96]

In vitro studies of ***Epilobium*** **spp.** suggest steroid receptor and aromatase inhibition activity as well as potent cyclo-oxygenase-2 (COX-2) and antioxidant potential, so this herb could theoretically be used in BPH.[97,98] Other cell-line research supports this and elucidates the antihyperplastic and potential anticancer action of *Epilobium parviflorum* extract (oenothein B) as a potent inhibitor of DNA synthesis in a human prostate cell line. Aqueous extracts have also demonstrated plausible COX-2 action,[99] although ethanolic extracts appear to have the most potential inhibitory action on this enzyme linked to inflammatory pathways.[100] These results have yet to be duplicated in clinical trials.

Inflammation

While limited, some studies suggest that the inflammatory process including the production of cytokines (interleukin 1 and 6, and tissue necrosis factor alpha) increases prostatic tissue proliferation.[63,75] Other research links the presence of platelet-derived growth factor (PDGF) (produced during the inflammatory processes) and androgens with the incidence of BPH and hyperproliferation of prostate cells.[101,102] In these studies, DHT failed to produce a mitogenic response in prostate cells without the presence of PDGF.

In a large, Italian, case-control study **essential fatty acids** (**EFA**) consisting of linoleic, linolenic and arachidonic acids have resulted in significant improvement for many BPH patients.[103] All 19 subjects in an uncontrolled study showed diminution of residual urine, with 12 of the 19 having no residual urine by the end of several weeks of treatment. Prostatic and seminal lipid levels and ratios are often abnormal,[104] and supplementation may be addressing an underlying EFA deficiency. Cell-line research suggests differences in essential fatty acid composition in hyperplastic or cancerous prostate cells.[105,106] Because of concern regarding increased oxidation of unsaturated acids,[18] a basic antioxidant regimen should be employed when taking EFAs.

The role of tomatoes, tomato sauce and **lycopene** in BPH is not clear; however, epidemiological and population-based studies suggest that their consumption is linked to decreased incidence of BPH,[106] a reduction in PSA levels,[107] and decreased progression of BPH to prostate cancer.[109] The therapeutic action of lycopene in this disorder may be due to its potent antioxidant properties.

Sympathetic nervous system hyperactivity

Reduction of urethral stricture and relaxation of smooth muscles is aided by parasympathetic stimulation or parasympathetic mimetic agents.[110] Reduction in sympathetic nervous activity and/or parasympathetic stimulation may aid in LUTS symptom relief, as evidenced by some studies suggesting that a combination of **glycine**, **alanine** and **glutamic acid** (in the form of two 6-grain capsules administered three times daily for 2 weeks and one capsule three times daily thereafter) relieved many BPH symptoms. Nocturia was relieved or reduced in 95%, urgency reduced in 81%, frequency reduced in 73% and delayed micturition alleviated in 70% in one study[111] with similar results reported in other controlled studies.[112] The mechanism of action is unknown. These amino acids may act as inhibitory neurotransmitters, providing symptom relief and reducing the feelings of a full bladder, or providing an overall nervine function that can positively affect urine flow in men suffering from BPH.[113]

While no clinical evidence supports the use of hops (*Humulus lupulus*), the antiproliferative effects of flavonoids on prostate cancer cell lines, as well as its nervine and parasympathetic action, may warrant further research and clinical benefit.[68,114] Other **nervine** and **antispasmodic** botanical medicines may have a potential supportive role in managing BPH; examples are *Scutellaria lateriflora* and *Passiflora incarnata*. However, no studies have presently been conducted to assess this potential.

Vascular functioning

Chronic ischaemia can result in thickening of the prostate and growth of tissue in response to an altered endothelial growth factor resulting from the diminished blood supply.[115] Atherosclerosis and diminished blood supply appear to be potential root causes in BPH and ED. Improving vascular function via herbal and nutrient interventions (discussed in the ED section), managing cholesterol and moderating alcohol consumption, in addition to dietary strategies to address cardiovascular risk, will possibly prove beneficial (see Section 3 on the cardiovascular system).

In addition to epidemiological studies suggesting a relationship between higher cholesterol levels and cardiovascular disease with higher incidence of BPH and ED, the breakdown products of cholesterol itself can also be cytotoxic and carcinogenic and have been shown to accumulate in hyperplastic or cancerous prostate tissue.[104]

Hypocholesterolaemic (statin) drugs have been shown to have a favourable influence on BPH possibly by limiting subsequent formation of epoxycholesterols (metabolic by-products of cholesterol).[116] As discussed above, the regulation of cardiovascular risk factors (such as elevated LDL and total cholesterol) and decreased HDL may help in the holistic prevention and treatment of BPH.

Although only beer has been associated with increasing prolactin levels, higher overall alcohol intake may be associated with BPH. In a large Hawaiian study involving 6581 men, an alcohol intake of at least 740 mL/month was directly correlated with the diagnosis of BPH,[31] with a stronger association for beer, wine and sake compared with distilled spirits. While this indicates a relationship in incidence, a smaller study suggested that men waiting for TURP surgery were more likely to avoid the surgical procedure (having remission of symptoms) with higher consumption of alcohol.[24] This study also described the correlation of higher rates of BPH in men with coronary disease. Although these studies are apparently contradictory in relationship to alcohol, it is possible that in men at higher risk for coronary artery disease due to higher levels of low-density lipoproteins, alcohol may play an overall protective role by reducing these lipoproteins.

INTEGRATIVE MEDICAL CONSIDERATIONS

The severity of the symptoms will dictate whether surgery or catheterisation is necessary for acute urinary obstruction. Counselling may be necessary to address the psychological issues of sexual dysfunction. Progression of BPH to prostate cancer is of concern and should be monitored appropriately using regular DRE with possible PSA testing. Acupuncture and moxibustion can increase blood flow, and some studies have provided evidence that it may be considered as a viable adjunctive treatment,[133–135] particularly when combined with hypnotherapy.[136] Numerous studies on the effect of acupuncture on urinary frequency have been conducted; however, no studies exist on the use of acupuncture for BPH specifically, and many of these studies involve ageing women.[137–141] Other studies suggest trigger point release therapy and relaxation as being beneficial for addressing ED and BPH, particularly if chronic pelvic pain is involved.[142] Counselling and psychiatry may be beneficial for addressing the psychological roots or manifestations of ED and the symptoms of BPH. Pelvic floor (kegal) exercises have been shown to be beneficial in up to 35% of ED patients[143,144] with some potential shown for their ability to improve urinary function.[145]

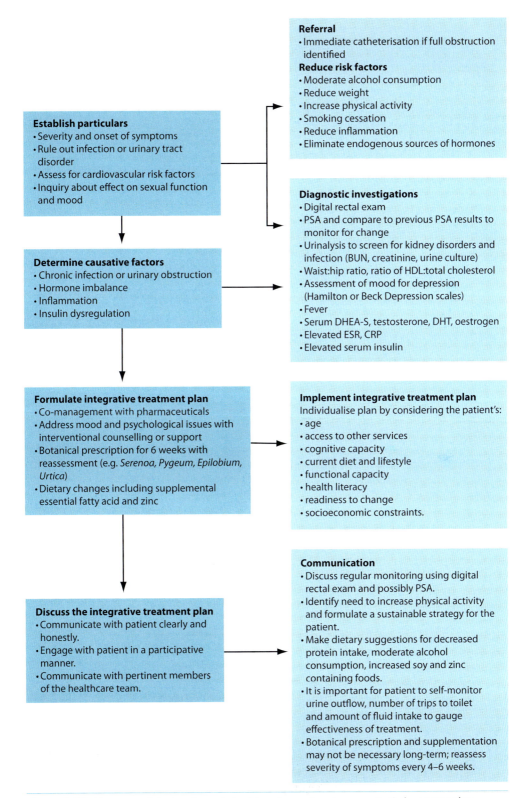

Establish particulars
- Severity and onset of symptoms
- Rule out infection or urinary tract disorder
- Assess for cardiovascular risk factors
- Inquiry about effect on sexual function and mood

Determine causative factors
- Chronic infection or urinary obstruction
- Hormone imbalance
- Inflammation
- Insulin dysregulation

Formulate integrative treatment plan
- Co-management with pharmaceuticals
- Address mood and psychological issues with interventional counselling or support
- Botanical prescription for 6 weeks with reassessment (e.g. *Serenoa, Pygeum, Epilobium, Urtica*)
- Dietary changes including supplemental essential fatty acid and zinc

Discuss the integrative treatment plan
- Communicate with patient clearly and honestly.
- Engage with patient in a participative manner.
- Communicate with pertinent members of the healthcare team.

Referral
- Immediate catheterisation if full obstruction identified

Reduce risk factors
- Moderate alcohol consumption
- Reduce weight
- Increase physical activity
- Smoking cessation
- Reduce inflammation
- Eliminate endogenous sources of hormones

Diagnostic investigations
- Digital rectal exam
- PSA and compare to previous PSA results to monitor for change
- Urinalysis to screen for kidney disorders and infection (BUN, creatinine, urine culture)
- Waist:hip ratio, ratio of HDL:total cholesterol
- Assessment of mood for depression (Hamilton or Beck Depression scales)
- Fever
- Serum DHEA-S, testosterone, DHT, oestrogen
- Elevated ESR, CRP
- Elevated serum insulin

Implement integrative treatment plan
Individualise plan by considering the patient's:
- age
- access to other services
- cognitive capacity
- current diet and lifestyle
- functional capacity
- health literacy
- readiness to change
- socioeconomic constraints.

Communication
- Discuss regular monitoring using digital rectal exam and possibly PSA.
- Identify need to increase physical activity and formulate a sustainable strategy for the patient.
- Make dietary suggestions for decreased protein intake, moderate alcohol consumption, increased soy and zinc containing foods.
- It is important for patient to self-monitor urine outflow, number of trips to toilet and amount of fluid intake to gauge effectiveness of treatment.
- Botanical prescription and supplementation may not be necessary long-term; reassess severity of symptoms every 4–6 weeks.

Figure 26.3 Naturopathic treatment decision tree—benign prostatic hypertrophy

ERECTILE DYSFUNCTION

Overview
- Erectile dysfunction is classified as organic (circulatory or a side effect of medication, particularly anti-depressant or neurogenic) or psychological.[117]
- Significant psychosomatic or mind/body connections affect this disorder.[118]
- Normal erectile function involves a balance between excitatory and inhibitory psychological, vascular and neural responses,[12,119] involves release of nitric oxide (NO) gas into the endothelial cells of the penis and causes the subsequent relaxation of smooth muscle cells lining the corpus cavernosum so that there is increased blood to flow into the organ and retention of blood in the spongy erectile tissue.
- Parasympathethic nervous activity and conversion of guanosine triphosphate (GTP) into cyclic guanosine monophosphate (cGMP) by the enzyme guanylate cyclase.[8] An erection subsides when cGMP is hydrolysed by phosphodiesterase type 5 enzymes (PDE5), causing smooth muscle contraction and emptying of the corpus cavernosum.
- Screening and diagnostic evaluation should include a complete patient history to identify the presence of comorbid conditions, particularly diabetes, dyslipidaemia and hypertension[119] as well as assessment of any neurological or circulatory obstacles to proper innervation of the pelvic area.

Conventional treatments
Conventional treatments focus on providing symptomatic relief through pharmacological substances (phosphodiesterase type-5 (PDE-5) inhibitors such as sildenafil or tadalafil) as first-line therapy, removing causative agents (the side effects of beta-adrenergic blockers, antidepressants or spironolactone), and counselling.[13,121]

CAM treatments
Arginine
Three small, pilot, randomised, controlled studies provided relative support for the clinical effectiveness of L-arginine in doses ranging from 1500 mg—5 g/day used over a 2–6-week period for ED.[122–124] While the study[123] using 1500 mg/day for 2 weeks did not demonstrate a significant benefit over placebo, the other two studies demonstrated a 20–40% self-reported improvement in symptoms of ED. It is unclear whether foods rich in L-arginine such as legumes, whole grains and nuts consumed in moderate-to-large amounts would have a similar effect. Other studies using L-arginine in combination with other natural substances such as pycnogenol[125] or yohimbine[126] generally supported the notion that L-arginine can have some positive effect on the symptoms of erectile dysfunction; however, further research is necessary.

Herbs
Panax ginseng has the most promising evidence for safe and effective treatment of ED, with 900 mg/day for 8 weeks showing clinical and physiological effectiveness in up to 60% of men with ED.[8,127] Yohimbine (5.4 mg t.i.d. for 8 weeks) also shows promising results, although significant side effects associated with its therapeutic action as an alpha-2-adrenergic receptor make it a less desirable treatment option.[128] Based on vasodilatory actions, *Ginkgo biloba* may benefit some men where penile blood flow is impaired (however, the clinical evidence is mixed).[129,130] *Tribulus terrestris* may be a viable option to treat ED, via increasing the release of nitric oxide from the endothelium and nitrergic nerve endings in penile tissue (clinical studies have not yet, however, confirmed its efficacy).[131,132]

Case Study

A 55-year-old male presents with **frequent difficult urination**. Over the past few months he has noticed **inability to maintain an erection**. This has been **diagnosed as occurring due to BPH**. His BMI is 26.5 and his waist:hip ratio is 1.2. His diet is low in vegetables and relatively high in red meat. In his early 40s he suffered from **obstructive uropathy** over a period of 2 years; this was due to renal calculi and treated using ultrasound.

SUGGESTIVE SYMPTOMS

- Weak, painful or incomplete micturition
- Acute or chronic retention of urine
- Urinary urgency, particularly nocturnal
- Inability to achieve or maintain a full erection (male)
- Increased abdominal mass and other cardiovascular risk factors
- Potential co-occurring mood and libido changes

Example treatment

Urinalysis was performed to rule out urinary tract infection and patient was advised that the urogenital health of his partner is necessary for a healthy sexual relationship. Patient was advised to increase physical activity, including a mix of aerobic and anaerobic activity for at least 30 minutes three times per week to address mood, weight loss, blood flow and cardiovascular risk. The treatment rationale was aimed at regulating androgens and addressing inflammation using an aggressive dose of *Serenoa repens*, Cernilton®, *Pygeum africanum* and zinc, address urinary tract symptoms using

Herbal prescription

Urtica dioica (radix) 1:2	35 mL
Epilobium spp. 1:2	35 mL
Pygeum africanum 1:2	30 mL
5 mL t.d.s.	100 mL
Serenoa repens tablets 160 mg b.d.	
Flower pollen extract (e.g. Cernilton®) 63 mg two or three times/day	

Nutritional prescription

Flaxseed oil 1 tbsp two times/day
Zinc amino acid chelate 50 mg/day
High-fibre diet including 100 g of soy products each day

stinging nettle, and 1 tablespoon of flaxseed oil two times/day to address inflammation and cardiovascular risk markers. Dietary advice was given, including consumption of a diet high in soluble fibre to help address cardiovascular risk and regulate weight, consume 100 g of soy products (soybeans or tofu) each day to assist hormone regulation, and increase fruit consumption to facilitate hydroxylation and elimination of DHT. Other prescriptive options include increased consumption of pumpkin seeds, which are sources of essential fatty acids and zinc. Limit alcohol consumption, particularly beer. Regulation of androgens and hormones may take up to 2 months and patients may need additional or integrative support to manage symptoms while addressing the root cause. Acute catheterisation if urine outflow is sufficiently obstructed, or co-management using alpha-blockers to address symptoms that significantly affect quality of life (nocturia and urinary frequency), may be necessary.

Expected outcomes and follow-up protocols

If PSA levels are used as one means of monitoring prostate health, this test should be done once every 6 months (especially if there is a significantly enlarged prostate on digital rectal exam). Reassessment of symptoms of BPH should occur every 6 weeks if moderate, and at least every 4 weeks if severe. Patients should keep a diary of daily trips

Table 26.1 Review of the major evidence

INTERVENTION	KEY LITERATURE	SUMMARY OF RESULTS	COMMENT
Serenoa repens	Meta-analyses Wilt et al. 2002[71] Tacklind et al. 2009[73] (update of Wilt 2002)	Initial review[71] indicated significant improvements in urinary symptoms compared to placebo or pharmaceutical treatment amongst 21 trials, However, an updated review incorporating nine newer studies suggested weighted mean difference in nocturia significantly better than placebo, not significant for other urinary symptoms.[73] RR compared to tamsulosin: 0.91 (not significant superiority) [73]	Significant heterogeneity amongst the 30 RCTs in most recent analyses, particularly with respect to dose and extract of serenoa as well as length of study (range 4–26 weeks)
Beta-sitosterol	Systematic review Wilt et al. 1999[58]	A total of 4 studies of varied extracts/doses over a 4–26 week period showed significant improvements in peak urine flow, with two studies showing a 4.9 decrease in International Prostate Symptom Scores (IPSS) (95% CI = –6.3 to –3.5, $p < 0.05$) with no observed reduction in prostate size on palpation.	Longer-term studies with sufficient reporting of safety are required, although amongst these studies only 8% of participants experienced any adverse reactions.
Zinc	Cell or animal research Sinquin 1984[62] Fahim 1993[28]	Metabolites of testosterone produced via 5-alpha reductase were significantly increased in prostate cells with addition of zinc. Significant ($p < 0.05$) reduction in prostate weight and 5-alpha reductase activity following intraprostatic zinc injections compared to sham and placebo in rat model	Mechanism of action for altering testosterone/androgen profile using zinc is established. Based on this and epidemiological data on zinc in men with BPH, human clinical studies are warranted.
Acupuncture	Systematic review Lee et al. 2009[133]	Randomised studies suggested significant improvement using 4–10 weeks 1–2×/week of acupuncture or electroacupuncture (up to 63% responder rate); however, not statistically superior to sham acupuncture in one study. Non-significant RR: 2.73 (95% CI 0.42–17.78, $p = 0.29$) favouring acupuncture vs sham acupuncture. Large heterogeneity between studies	A total of 4 studies evaluating acupuncture for erectile dysfunction were included for review; however, 25 case reports/series as well as studies combining acupuncture and herbs or moxibustion were also identified. Studies suffered from small sample size and poor design, including control groups, randomisation and blinding. Large response to sham acupuncture (43%). Further research is warranted.

(Continued)

Table 26.1 Review of the major evidence *(Continued)*

INTERVENTION	KEY LITERATURE	SUMMARY OF RESULTS	COMMENT
Diet	Epidemiological studies Kristal et al. 2008[107] Rohrmann et al. 2007[146] Meyer et al. 2005[38]	Hazard ratios (HR) for BPH increased for daily consumption of red meat (1.38) and lower for vegetable consumption > 3 servings/day) (0.68) and consumption of > 2 servings alcohol/day (0.68). 31% increased HR for highest consumers of total fat ($p < 0.05$). Vegetable consumption was inversely associated with BPH (fifth compared with first quintile OR 0.89; 95% CI = 0.80–0.99; p for trend = 0.03), whereas fruit intake was not. Consumption of fruit and vegetables rich in beta-carotene (p for trend = 0.004), lutein (p for trend = 0.0004), or vitamin C (p for trend = 0.05) was inversely related to BPH. Population-based study confirms consuming supplements containing zinc, vitamin E, vitamin C, selenium and beta-carotene over 8-year period had no significant effect on PSA or IGF levels ($p > 0.05$).	Although not as strong, HR for > 33.3 mg/day zinc (0.68 95% CI 0.54–87, $p = 0.026$ for trend), > 12,589 µg/day lycopene (0.82 95% CI = 0.65–1.03, $p = 0.056$) and > 15.6 µg/ day vitamin D (0.82 95% CI = 0.66–1.03, $p = 0.032$) demonstrate possible links to the incidence of BPH. With increasing vitamin C intake from foods, men were less likely to have BPH (p for trend = 0.0009). Neither alpha- nor gamma-tocopherol intake from foods was associated with BPH (p for trend = 0.05 and 0.84, respectively). Supplementation with antioxidants did significantly reduce the hazard ratio of developing prostate cancer in men with normal PSA at baseline (HR 0.52; 95% CI = 0.29–0.92).
Lifestyle	Epidemiological studies Platz et al. 1998[19] Rohrmann et al. 2005[147] Shiels et al. 2009[148]	Physical activity was inversely related with total BPH (extreme quintiles: OR 0.75, 95% CI = 0.67–0.85, p for trend < 0.001), surgery for BPH (OR 0.76, 95% CI = 0.64–0.90, p for trend < 0.001), and symptomatic BPH (OR 0.75, 95% CI = 0.64–0.87, p for trend < 0.001) Former heavy smokers (≥ 50 pack-years) had a higher odds of LUTS than never smokers (OR 2.01, 95% CI = 1.04–3.89). Men who drank alcohol daily had a lower chance of LUTS than non-drinkers (OR 0.59, 95% CI = 0.37–0.95, p trend = 0.07). All levels of moderate and vigorous activity were statistically significantly inversely associated with LUTS (p trend = 0.06), whereas men who reported no leisure-time physical activity had a greater odds of LUTS (OR 2.06, 95% CI =1.26–3.39). Men currently smoking had higher serum testosterone, free testosterone and oestradiol levels ($p < 0.05$ for all measures).	Walking, the most prevalent activity, was inversely related to BPH risk; men who walked 2 to 3 hours/ week had a 25% lower risk of total BPH. Confirmation across multiple epidemiological studies amongst varied populations of men that smoking is linked to hormone levels and incidence of BPH and that physical activity is inversely associated with LUTS.

to the toilet, fluid intake and attempts to collect urine output, as a means of assessing the effectiveness of treatment as well as whether adjunctive or emergency care is warranted.

Improvements to ED may take time, particularly if there is a strong psychological component, and a discussion with the patient that encourages realistic expectations for changes but that adds no undue pressure should take place. Individual or couples counselling may be warranted. If the root cause of BPH and ED is likely to be vascular in origin, and there are no signs or diagnostic tests indicating hypertension, infection, hormone abnormalities or inflammation, 3 g/day of L-arginine could improve ED as well as circulation. If no improvements occur within 3 months, other therapeutic options include removal of the potential sources of inflammation in the diet, supplementation using glycine, alanine and glutamic acid (6 g/day), and the use of herbal medicines such as *Epilobium* spp. for BPH and *Ginkgo biloba* or *Tribulus terrestris* for ED.

KEY POINTS

- BPH shares many properties with cardiovascular, erectile dysfunction, depression and urinary tract infection disorders.
- The holistic treatment approach should look beyond hormonal regulation and include therapies to reduce inflammation, reduce oxidative stress and improve nitric oxide production.
- BPH is predominantly an androgen-mediated disorder. Factors that decrease the production of dihydrotestosterone should be included in most treatment protocols.
- Counselling to address issues of ageing, mood and sexual health may be important in moderating quality of life and the mental/emotional aspects of these diseases.

Further reading

Edwards, JL. Diagnosis and management of benign prostatic hyperplasia. Am Fam Physician 2008;77(10):1403–1410.

Mantzoros CS, et al. Insulin-like growth factor 1 in relation to prostate cancer and benign prostatic hyperplasia. Br J Canc 1997;76(9):1115–1118.

Moyad MA, et al. Prevention and treatment of erectile dysfunction using lifestyle changes and dietary supplements: what works and what is worthless, parts 1 and 2. Uro Clin N Am 2004;31:249–273.

Rosenberg MT. Diagnosis and management of erectile dysfunction in the primary care setting. Int J Clin Prac 2007;61(7):1198–1208.

Zakaria L, et al. Common conditions of the aging male: erectile dysfunction, benign prostatic hyperplasia, cardiovascular disease and depression. Int Urol Nephrol 2001;33(2):283–292.

Zhu YS, Imperato-McGinley JL. 5 alpha-reductase isozymes and androgen actions in the prostate. Ann N Y Acad Sci 2009;1155:43–56.

References

1. Edwards JL. Diagnosis and management of benign prostatic hyperplasia. Am Fam Physician 2008;77(10): 1403–1410.
2. Arrighi HM, et al. Natural history of benign prostatic hyperplasia and risk of prostatectomy. The Baltimore Longitudinal Study of Aging. Urology 1991;38(1 Suppl):4–8.
3. Dull P, et al. Managing benign prostatic hyperplasia. Am Fam Physician 2002;66(1):77–84.
4. Feldman HA, et al. Impotence and its medical and psychosocial correlates: results of the Massachusetts Male Aging Study. J Urol 1994;151(1):54–61.
5. Goldstein I. Male sexual circuitry. Working Group for the Study of Central Mechanisms in Erectile Dysfunction. Sci Am 2000;283(2):70–75.
6. Shankar PR, Subish P. Disease mongering. Singapore Med J 2007;48(4):275–280.
7. Nehra A, Kulaksizoglu H. Global perspectives and controversies in the epidemiology of male erectile dysfunction. Curr Opin Urol 2002;12(6):493–496.
8. McKay D. Nutrients and botanicals for erectile dysfunction: examining the evidence. Altern Med Rev 2004;9(1):4–16.
9. Thomas JA. Diet, micronutrients, and the prostate gland. Nutr Rev 1999;57(4):95–103.

10. Comhaire F, Mahmoud A. Preventing diseases of the prostate in the elderly using hormones and nutriceuticals. Aging Male 2004;7(2):155–169.
11. Zakaria L, et al. Common conditions of the aging male: erectile dysfunction, benign prostatic hyperplasia, cardiovascular disease and depression. Int Urol Nephrol 2001;33(2):283–292.
12. Sullivan ME, et al. Nitric oxide and penile erection: is erectile dysfunction another manifestation of vascular disease? Cardiovasc Res 1999;43(3):658–665.
13. Rosenberg MT. Diagnosis and management of erectile dysfunction in the primary care setting. Int J Clin Pract 2007;61(7):1198–1208.
14. Jacobsen SJ. Risk factors for benign prostatic hyperplasia. Curr Urol Rep 2007;8(4):281–288.
15. Moyad MA. Lifestyle changes to prevent BPH: heart healthy = prostate healthy. Urol Nurs 2003;23(6):439–441.
16. Engl T, et al. Uropharmacology: current and future strategies in the treatment of erectile dysfunction and benign prostate hyperplasia. Int J Clin Pharmacol Ther 2004;42(10):527–533.
17. Soygur T, et al. Effect of obesity on prostatic hyperplasia: its relation to sex steroid levels. Int Urol Nephrol 1996;28(1):55–59.
18. Suzuki S, et al. Intakes of energy and macronutrients and the risk of benign prostatic hyperplasia. Am J Clin Nutr 2002;75(4):689–697.
19. Platz EA, et al. Physical activity and benign prostatic hyperplasia. Arch Intern Med 1998;158(21):2349–2356.
20. Platz EA, et al. Interrelation of energy intake, body size, and physical activity with prostate cancer in a large prospective cohort study. Cancer Res 2003;63(23):8542–8548.
21. Wisard M. [Erectile dysfunction: physical exercise, losing weight, stop smoking, reducing alcohol, relaxing, it could also work!]. Rev Med Suisse 2007;3(136):2773–2774, 2776, 2778.
22. Morrison AS. Epidemiology and environmental factors in urologic cancer. Cancer 1987;60(3 Suppl):632–634.
23. Lagiou P, et al. Diet and benign prostatic hyperplasia: a study in Greece. Urology 1999;54(2):284–290.
24. Gass R. Benign prostatic hyperplasia: the opposite effects of alcohol and coffee intake. BJU Int 2002;90(7):649–654.
25. Demark-Wahnefried W, et al. Pilot study to explore effects of low-fat, flaxseed-supplemented diet on proliferation of benign prostatic epithelium and prostate-specific antigen. Urology 2004;63(5):900–904.
26. Kappas A, et al. Nutrition-endocrine interactions: induction of reciprocal changes in the delta 4-5 alpha-reduction of testosterone and the cytochrome P-450-dependent oxidation of estradiol by dietary macronutrients in man. Proc Natl Acad Sci U S A 1983;80(24):7646–7649.
27. Zhang SX, et al. [Comparison of incidence of BPH and related factors between urban and rural inhabitants in district of Wannan]. Zhonghua Nan Ke Xue 2003;9(1):45–47.
28. Fahim MS, et al. Zinc arginine, a 5 alpha-reductase inhibitor, reduces rat ventral prostate weight and DNA without affecting testicular function. Andrologia 1993;25(6):369–375.
29. Leake A, et al. The effect of zinc on the 5 alpha-reduction of testosterone by the hyperplastic human prostate gland. J Steroid Biochem 1984;20(2):651–655.
30. Leake A, et al. Subcellular distribution of zinc in the benign and malignant human prostate: evidence for a direct zinc androgen interaction. Acta Endocrinol (Copenh) 1984;105(2):281–288.
31. Chyou PH, et al. A prospective study of alcohol, diet, and other lifestyle factors in relation to obstructive uropathy. Prostate 1993;22(3):253–264.
32. Zaichick V, et al. Zinc in the human prostate gland: normal, hyperplastic and cancerous. Int Urol Nephrol 1997;29(5):565–574.
33. Leake A, et al. The effect of zinc on the 5 alpha-reduction of testosterone by the hyperplastic human prostate gland. J Steroid Biochem 1984;20(2):651–655.
34. Leake A, et al. Subcellular distribution of zinc in the benign and malignant human prostate: evidence for a direct zinc androgen interaction. Acta Endocrinol (Copenh) 1984;105(2):281–288.
35. Wallace AM, Grant JK. Effect of zinc on androgen metabolism in the human hyperplastic prostate. Biochem Soc Trans 1975;3(4):540–542.
36. Johnson AR, et al. High dose zinc increases hospital admissions due to genitourinary complications. J Urol 2007;177(2):639–643.
37. Silk R, LeFante C. Safety of zinc gluconate glycine (Cold-Eeze) in a geriatric population: a randomized, placebo-controlled, double-blind trial. Am J Ther 2005;12(6):612–617.
38. Meyer F, et al. Antioxidant vitamin and mineral supplementation and prostate cancer prevention in the SU.VI. MAX trial. Int J Cancer 2005;116(2):182–186.
39. Neuhouser ML, et al. Dietary supplement use in the Prostate Cancer Prevention Trial: implications for prevention trials. Nutr Cancer 2001;39(1):12–18.
40. Patterson RE, et al. Vitamin supplements and cancer risk: the epidemiologic evidence. Cancer Causes Control 1997;8(5):786–802.
41. Judd AM, et al. Zinc acutely, selectively and reversibly inhibits pituitary prolactin secretion. Brain Res 1984;294(1):190–192.
42. Login IS, et al. Zinc may have a physiological role in regulating pituitary prolactin secretion. Neuroendocrinology 1983;37(5):317–320.
43. Farnsworth WE, et al. Interaction of prolactin and testosterone in the human prostate. Urol Res 1981;9(2):79–88.
44. De Rosa G, et al. Prolactin secretion after beer. Lancet 1981;2(8252):934.
45. Corenblum B, Whitaker M. Inhibition of stress-induced hyperprolactinaemia. Br Med J 1977;2(6098):1328.
46. Farrar DJ, Osborne JL. The use of bromocriptine in the treatment of the unstable bladder. Br J Urol 1976;48(2):235–238.
47. Boyd A. Bromocriptine and psychosis: a literature review. Psychiatr Q 1995;66(1):87–95.
48. Miettinen TA, et al. Serum plant sterols and cholesterol precursors reflect cholesterol absorption and synthesis in volunteers of a randomly selected male population. Am J Epidemiol 1990;131(1):20–31.
49. Tilvis RS, Miettinen TA. Serum plant sterols and their relation to cholesterol absorption. Am J Clin Nutr 1986;43(1):92–97.
50. Berges RR, et al. Randomised, placebo-controlled, double-blind clinical trial of beta-sitosterol in patients with benign prostatic hyperplasia. Beta-sitosterol Study Group. Lancet 1995;345(8964):1529–1532.
51. Denis L, et al. Diet and its preventive role in prostatic disease. Eur Urol 1999;35(5–6):377–387.
52. Engelhardt PF, Riedl CR. Effects of one-year treatment with isoflavone extract from red clover on prostate, liver function, sexual function, and quality of life in men with elevated PSA levels and negative prostate biopsy findings. Urology 2008;71(2):185–190:discussion 190.
53. Messina MJ. Emerging evidence on the role of soy in reducing prostate cancer risk. Nutr Rev 2003;61(4):117–131.
54. Jarred RA, et al. Anti-androgenic action by red clover-derived dietary isoflavones reduces non-malignant prostate enlargement in aromatase knockout (ArKo) mice. Prostate 2003;56(1):54–64.

55. Drewes SE, et al. Hypoxis hemerocallidea—not merely a cure for benign prostate hyperplasia. J Ethnopharmacol 2008;119(3):593–598.

56. Katz AE. Flavonoid and botanical approaches to prostate health. J Altern Complement Med 2002;8(6):813–821.

57. Wilt T, et al. Beta-sitosterols for benign prostatic hyperplasia. Cochrane Database Syst Rev 2000;(2):CD001043.

58. Wilt TJ, et al. Beta-sitosterol for the treatment of benign prostatic hyperplasia: a systematic review. BJU Int 1999;83(9):976–983.

59. Gerber GS. Phytotherapy for benign prostatic hyperplasia. Curr Urol Rep 2002;3(4):285–291.

60. Yamashita A, et al. Influence of diethylstilbestrol, Leuprolelin (a luteinizing hormone-releasing hormone analog), Finasteride (a 5 alpha-reductase inhibitor), and castration on the lobar subdivisions of the rat prostate. Prostate 1996;29(1):1–14.

61. Lahtonen R. Zinc and cadmium concentrations in whole tissue and in separated epithelium and stroma from human benign prostatic hypertrophic glands. Prostate 1985;6(2):177–183.

62. Sinquin G, et al. Testosterone metabolism by homogenates of human prostates with benign hyperplasia: effects of zinc, cadmium and other bivalent cations. J Steroid Biochem 1984;20(3):773–780.

63. Sivkov AV, et al. [Morphological changes in prostatic tissue of patients with benign prostatic hyperplasia treated with permixon]. Urologiia 2004;(5):10–16.

64. Buck AC. Phytotherapy for the prostate. Br J Urol 1996;78(3):325–336.

65. Dedhia RC, et al. Impact of phytotherapy on utility scores for 5 benign prostatic hyperplasia/lower urinary tract symptoms health states. J Urol 2008;179(1):220–225.

66. Fleshner N, et al. Evidence for contamination of herbal erectile dysfunction products with phosphodiesterase type 5 inhibitors. J Urol 2005;174(2):636–641:discussion 641; quiz 801.

67. Gryniewicz CM, et al. Detection of undeclared erectile dysfunction drugs and analogues in dietary supplements by ion mobility spectrometry. J Pharm Biomed Anal 2009;49(3):601–606.

68. Buck AC. Is there a scientific basis for the therapeutic effects of serenoa repens in benign prostatic hyperplasia? Mechanisms of action. J Urol 2004;172(5 Pt 1):1792–1799.

69. Magri V, et al. Activity of Serenoa repens, lycopene and selenium on prostatic disease: evidences and hypotheses. Arch Ital Urol Androl 2008;80(2):65–78.

70. Vela Navarrete R, et al. BPH and inflammation: pharmacological effects of Permixon on histological and molecular inflammatory markers. Results of a double blind pilot clinical assay. Eur Urol 2003;44(5):549–555.

71. Wilt T, et al. *Serenoa repens* for benign prostatic hyperplasia. Cochrane Database Syst Rev 2002;(3):CD001423.

72. Wilt TJ, et al. Phytotherapy for benign prostatic hyperplasia. Public Health Nutr 2000;3(4A):459–472.

73. Tacklind J, et al. Serenoa repens for benign prostatic hyperplasia. Cochrane Database Syst Rev 2009;(2):CD001423.

74. Gordon AE, Shaughnessy AF. Saw palmetto for prostate disorders. Am Fam Physician 2003;67(6):1281–1283.

75. Asakawa K, et al. [Effects of cernitin pollen-extract (Cernilton) on inflammatory cytokines in sex-hormone-induced nonbacterial prostatitis rats]. Hinyokika Kiyo 2001;47(7):459–465.

76. Yasumoto R, et al. Clinical evaluation of long-term treatment using Cernilton pollen extract in patients with benign prostatic hyperplasia. Clin Ther 1995;17(1):82–87.

77. Buck AC, et al. Treatment of outflow tract obstruction due to benign prostatic hyperplasia with the pollen extract, Cernilton. A double-blind, placebo-controlled study. Br J Urol 1990;66(4):398–404.

78. Dutkiewicz S. Usefulness of Cernilton in the treatment of benign prostatic hyperplasia. Int Urol Nephrol 1996;28(1):49–53.

79. Hayashi J, et al. [Clinical evaluation of Cernilton in benign prostatic hypertrophy]. Hinyokika Kiyo 1986;32(1):135–141.

80. Horii A, et al. [Clinical evaluation of Cernilton in the treatment of the benign prostatic hypertrophy]. Hinyokika Kiyo 1985;31(4):739–746.

81. MacDonald R, et al. A systematic review of Cernilton for the treatment of benign prostatic hyperplasia. BJU Int 2000;85(7):836–841.

82. Maekawa M, et al. [Clinical evaluation of Cernilton on benign prostatic hypertrophy–a multiple center double-blind study with Paraprost]. Hinyokika Kiyo 1990;36(4):495–516.

83. Ueda K, et al. [Clinical evaluation of Cernilton on benign prostatic hyperplasia]. Hinyokika Kiyo 1985;31(1):187–191.

84. Habib FK, et al. Identification of a prostate inhibitory substance in a pollen extract. Prostate 1995;26(3):133–139.

85. Yablonsky F, et al. Antiproliferative effect of *Pygeum africanum* extract on rat prostatic fibroblasts. J Urol 1997;157(6):2381–2387.

86. Boulbes D, et al. *Pygeum africanum* extract inhibits proliferation of human cultured prostatic fibroblasts and myofibroblasts. BJU Int 2006;98(5):1106–1113.

87. Edgar AD, et al. A critical review of the pharmacology of the plant extract of *Pygeum africanum* in the treatment of LUTS. Neurourol Urodyn 2007;26(4):458–463:discussion 464.

88. Kamatenesi-Mugisha M, Oryem-Origa H. Traditional herbal remedies used in the management of sexual impotence and erectile dysfunction in western Uganda. Afr Health Sci 2005;5(1):40–49.

89. Zenico T, et al. Subjective effects of *Lepidium meyenii* (maca) extract on well-being and sexual performances in patients with mild erectile dysfunction: a randomised, double-blind clinical trial. Andrologia 2009;41(2):95–99.

90. Gonzales GF, et al. Effect of *Lepidium meyenii* (maca), a root with aphrodisiac and fertility-enhancing properties, on serum reproductive hormone levels in adult healthy men. J Endocrinol 2003;176(1):163–168.

91. Gonzales GF, et al. Effect of *Lepidium meyenii* (maca) on sexual desire and its absent relationship with serum testosterone levels in adult healthy men. Andrologia 2002;34(6):367–372.

92. Lopatkin N, et al. Efficacy and safety of a combination of sabal and urtica extract in lower urinary tract symptoms–long-term follow-up of a placebo-controlled, double-blind, multicenter trial. Int Urol Nephrol 2007;39(4):1137–1146.

93. Safarinejad MR. *Urtica dioica* for treatment of benign prostatic hyperplasia: a prospective, randomized, double-blind, placebo-controlled, crossover study. J Herb Pharmacother 2005;5(4):1–11.

94. Sokeland J. Combined sabal and urtica extract compared with finasteride in men with benign prostatic hyperplasia: analysis of prostate volume and therapeutic outcome. BJU Int 2000;86(4):439–442.

95. Wagner H, et al. [Biologically active compounds from the aqueous extract of *Urtica dioica*]. Planta Med 1989;55(5):452–454.

96. Schottner M, et al. Lignans from the roots of *Urtica dioica* and their metabolites bind to human sex hormone binding globulin (SHBG). Planta Med 1997;63(6):529–532.

97. Ducrey B, et al. Inhibition of 5 alpha-reductase and aromatase by the ellagitannins oenothein A and oenothein B from Epilobium species. Planta Med 1997;63(2):111–114.

98. Hevesi Toth B, Kery A. [Epilobium parviflorum—in vitro study of biological action]. Acta Pharm Hung 2009;79(1):3–9.

99. Hevesi BT, et al. Antioxidant and antiinflammatory effect of *Epilobium parviflorum* Schreb. Phytother Res 2009;23(5):719–724.

100. Steenkamp V, et al. Studies on antibacterial, anti-inflammatory and antioxidant activity of herbal remedies used in the treatment of benign prostatic hyperplasia and prostatitis. J Ethnopharmacol 2006;103(1):71–75.

101. Vlahos CJ, et al. Platelet-derived growth factor induces proliferation of hyperplastic human prostatic stromal cells. J Cell Biochem 1993;52(4):404–413.

102. Gleason PE, et al. Platelet derived growth factor (PDGF), androgens and inflammation: possible etiologic factors in the development of prostatic hyperplasia. J Urol 1993;149(6):1586–1592.

103. Bravi F, et al. Macronutrients, fatty acids, cholesterol, and risk of benign prostatic hyperplasia. Urology 2006;67(6):1205–1211.

104. Boyd E, Berry N. Prostatic hypertrophy as part of generalized metabolic disease. J Urol 1939;41:406–411.

105. Chaudry AA, et al. Arachidonic acid metabolism in benign and malignant prostatic tissue in vitro: effects of fatty acids and cyclooxygenase inhibitors. Int J Cancer 1994;57(2):176–180.

106. Narayan P, Dahiya R. Alterations in sphingomyelin and fatty acids in human benign prostatic hyperplasia and prostatic cancer. Biomed Biochim Acta 1991;50(9):1099–1108.

107. Kristal AR, et al. Dietary patterns, supplement use, and the risk of symptomatic benign prostatic hyperplasia: results from the prostate cancer prevention trial. Am J Epidemiol 2008;167(8):925–934.

108. Edinger MS, Koff WJ. Effect of the consumption of tomato paste on plasma prostate-specific antigen levels in patients with benign prostate hyperplasia. Braz J Med Biol Res 2006;39(8):1115–1119.

109. Schwarz S, et al. Lycopene inhibits disease progression in patients with benign prostate hyperplasia. J Nutr 2008;138(1):49–53.

110. Bullock TL, Andriole Jnr GL. Emerging drug therapies for benign prostatic hyperplasia. Expert Opin Emerg Drugs 2006;11(1):111–123.

111. Damrau F. Benign prostatic hypertrophy: amino acid therapy for symptomatic relief. J Am Geriatr Soc 1962;10:426–430.

112. Feinblatt HM, Gant JC. Palliative treatment of benign prostatic hypertrophy; value of glycine-alanine-glutamic acid combination. J Maine Med Assoc 1958;49(3):99–101 passim.

113. Thor PJ, et al. [The autonomic nervous system function in benign prostatic hyperplasia]. Folia Med Cracov 2006;47(1–4):79–86.

114. Delmulle L, et al. Anti-proliferative properties of prenylated flavonoids from hops (Humulus lupulus L.) in human prostate cancer cell lines. Phytomedicine 2006;13(9–10):732–734.

115. Kozlowski R, et al. Chronic ischemia alters prostate structure and reactivity in rabbits. J Urol 2001;165(3):1019–1026.

116. Hinman, F, ed. Benign prostatic hypertrophy. New York: Springer-Verlag, 1983.

117. Baldwin DS. Sexual dysfunction associated with antidepressant drugs. Expert Opin Drug Saf 2004;3(5):457–470.

118. Sachs BD. The false organic-psychogenic distinction and related problems in the classification of erectile dysfunction. Int J Impot Res 2003;15(1):72–78.

119. Price D, Hackett G. Management of erectile dysfunction in diabetes: an update for 2008. Curr Diab Rep 2008;8(6):437–443.

120. Mikhail N. Management of erectile dysfunction by the primary care physician. Cleve Clin J Med 2005;72(4):293–294, 296–297, 301–305 passim.

121. Guay AT, et al. American Association of Clinical Endocrinologists medical guidelines for clinical practice for the evaluation and treatment of male sexual dysfunction: a couple's problem—2003 update. Endocr Pract 2003;9(1):77–95.

122. Chen J, et al. Effect of oral administration of high-dose nitric oxide donor L-arginine in men with organic erectile dysfunction: results of a double-blind, randomized, placebo-controlled study. BJU Int 1999;83(3):269–273.

123. Klotz T, et al. Effectiveness of oral L-arginine in first-line treatment of erectile dysfunction in a controlled crossover study. Urol Int 1999;63(4):220–223.

124. Zorgniotti AW, Lizza EF. Effect of large doses of the nitric oxide precursor, L-arginine, on erectile dysfunction. Int J Impot Res 1994;6(1):33–35;discussion 36.

125. Stanislavov R, Nikolova V. Treatment of erectile dysfunction with pycnogenol and L-arginine. J Sex Marital Ther 2003;29(3):207–213.

126. Kernohan AF, et al. An oral yohimbine/L-arginine combination (NMI 861) for the treatment of male erectile dysfunction: a pharmacokinetic, pharmacodynamic and interaction study with intravenous nitroglycerine in healthy male subjects. Br J Clin Pharmacol 2005;59(1):85–93.

127. Rowland DL, Tai W. A review of plant-derived and herbal approaches to the treatment of sexual dysfunctions. J Sex Marital Ther 2003;29(3):185–205.

128. Ernst E, Pittler MH. Yohimbine for erectile dysfunction: a systematic review and meta-analysis of randomized clinical trials. J Urol 1998;159(2):433–436.

129. Wheatley D, Triple-blind placebo-controlled trial of Ginkgo biloba in sexual dysfunction due to antidepressant drugs. Hum Psychopharmacol 2004;19(8):545–548.

130. Cohen AJ, Bartlik B. Ginkgo biloba for antidepressant-induced sexual dysfunction. J Sex Marital Ther 1998;24(2):139–143.

131. Adimoelja A. Phytochemicals and the breakthrough of traditional herbs in the management of sexual dysfunctions. Int J Androl 2000;23(Suppl 2):82–84.

132. Adaikan PG, et al. Proerectile pharmacological effects of Tribulus terrestris extract on the rabbit corpus cavernosum. Ann Acad Med Singapore 2000;29(1):22–26.

133. Lee MS, et al. Acupuncture for treating erectile dysfunction: a systematic review. BJU Int 2009;104(3):366–370.

134. Yang YK, et al. [Effects of moxibustion on erectile function and NO-cGMP pathway in diabetic rats with erectile dysfunction]. Zhongguo Zhen Jiu 2007;27(5):353–356.

134. Zhao L. Clinical observation on the therapeutic effects of heavy moxibustion plus point-injection in treatment of impotence. J Tradit Chin Med 2004;24(2):126–127.

136. Rowland DL, Slob AK. Understanding and diagnosing sexual dysfunction: recent progress through psychophysiological and psychophysical methods. Neurosci Biobehav Rev 1995;19(2):201–209.

137. Kim JH, et al. Randomized control trial of hand acupuncture for female stress urinary incontinence. Acupunct Electrother Res 2008;33(3–4):179–192.

138. Tian FS, et al. [Study on acupuncture treatment of diabetic neurogenic bladder]. Zhongguo Zhen Jiu 2007;27(7):485–487.

139. Emmons SL, Otto L. Acupuncture for overactive bladder: a randomized controlled trial. Obstet Gynecol 2005;106(1):138–143.

140. Katz AR. Urinary tract infections and acupuncture. Am J Public Health 2003;93(5):702;author reply 702–703.

141. Alraek T, et al. Acupuncture treatment in the prevention of uncomplicated recurrent lower urinary tract infections in adult women. Am J Public Health 2002;92(10):1609–1611.

142. Anderson RU, et al. Sexual dysfunction in men with chronic prostatitis/chronic pelvic pain syndrome: improvement after trigger point release and paradoxical relaxation training. J Urol 2006;176(4 Pt 1):1534–1538;discussion 1538–1539.

143. Dorey G, et al. Pelvic floor exercises for treating postmicturition dribble in men with erectile dysfunction: a randomized controlled trial. Urol Nurs 2004;24(6):490–497,512.

144. Dorey G, et al. Pelvic floor exercises for erectile dysfunction. BJU Int 2005;96(4):595–597.

145. Vasconcelos M, et al. Voiding dysfunction in children. Pelvic-floor exercises or biofeedback therapy: a randomized study. Pediatr Nephrol 2006;21(12): 1858–1864.

146. Rohrmann S, et al. Meat and dairy consumption and subsequent risk of prostate cancer in a US cohort study. Cancer Causes Control 2007;18(1):41–50.

147. Rohrmann S, et al. Association of cigarette smoking, alcohol consumption and physical activity with lower urinary tract symptoms in older American men: findings from the third National Health And Nutrition Examination Survey. BJU Int 2005;96(1):77–82.

148. Shiels MS, et al. Association of cigarette smoking, alcohol consumption, and physical activity with sex steroid hormone levels in US men. Cancer Causes Control 2009;20(6):877–886.

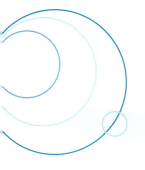

Recurrent urinary tract infection

Michelle Boyd
ND

AETIOLOGY AND EPIDEMIOLOGY

A urinary tract infection (UTI) is by simplest definition an infection that affects any part of the urinary tract, including the kidneys, ureters, bladder and urethra. Most infections will involve the lower tract, which includes the urethra and the bladder. UTIs are most commonly caused by the organism *Escherichia coli*.[1] Infections typically develop when bacteria or viruses enter the urinary system through the urethra. Once inside the bladder, the bacteria begin multiplying until their numbers are large enough to cause infectious symptoms (usually more than 100,000 organisms per mL in a mid-stream urine sample). Infections may cause swelling of the urethra (urethritis), bladder (cystitis), epididymis (epididymitis) or one or both testicles (orchitis).[1] Females are far more likely to present with UTIs than males, as the female urethra is closer to the anus (and its bacterial load) than the male urethra. Most UTIs are classified as 'uncomplicated', being caused by a transient infection of a single strain of proliferative bacteria.[2] Other cases, however, are classed as 'complicated' and are caused by urinary tract dysfunction or disease, or via an overarching medical condition such as diabetes. In the latter case concern exists in regard to potential renal damage; medical referral is advised.

Common symptoms associated with UTI include urgency to urinate, a burning sensation during micturition, haematuria, cloudy or foul (or otherwise abnormal) smelling urine, and frequently passing small amounts of urine.[1,3] Symptoms suggestive of urethritis include a burning sensation during micturition and, in men, penile discharge. Symptoms suggestive of cystitis may include pelvic pressure, lower abdominal pain and painful and frequent urination.[1,3] Symptoms suggestive of epididymitis in men include scrotal pain; tenderness in the testes and groin; painful intercourse, ejaculation and urination; and orchitis.[1,3]

Screening of asymptomatic women has shown that approximately 5% will have some form of UTI, 11% of women will experience UTI in any given year and 50% of women will experience symptoms of cystitis at some stage in their life.[4,5] All males who present with a UTI should be referred for investigation to exclude any underlying abnormality such as prostatitis. The differential diagnoses of vaginitis or vulvovaginal infections (such as *Candida* spp.) are also often associated with vaginal discharge.[1]

RISK FACTORS

Sexual intercourse frequency is the strongest risk factor for UTIs in younger populations.[1] Exposure to spermicide and new sexual partners are additive risk factors.[6] Diabetes is also a risk factor for UTIs, particularly for complicated UTIs, and women who require medical management for this condition will run roughly twice the risk of developing a UTI than non-diabetic women.[7] Low levels of oestrogen can dramatically change the microflora from one dominated by *Lactobacillus* to one dominated by *E. coli*, therefore increasing the risk of UTI (it should be noted that this may be of clinical relevance only in postmenopausal women).[8]

CONVENTIONAL TREATMENT

Conventional treatment of UTIs relies on antibiotic therapy, and in most cases of uncomplicated infection can be managed easily, with antibiotic treatment expected to cure 80–90% of uncomplicated UTIs.[5] Optimal treatment also includes adjuvant recommendations such as increasing fluid intake, encouraging complete bladder emptying and urinary alkalinisation for severe dysuria.[5] Simple analgesics such as paracetamol are recommended for pain. Recurrent UTIs are usually defined as three or more UTIs in a 12-month period, and in these women a larger focus on preventive treatment is advised, even as far as prophylactic antibiotic use after sexual intercourse.[5]

KEY TREATMENT PROTOCOLS

The primary naturopathic treatment goals for UTIs are to initially combat the urinary pathogen and ameliorate symptoms such as pain and fever. Long-term treatment protocols are to enhance the patient's immune function to appropriately remove and resist infection, remove possible irritants, restore urinary tract microflora, prevent bacteria from adhering to the mucosal wall of the bladder, and promote preventive behaviours.

> **NATUROPATHIC TREATMENT AIMS**
> - Educate the patient with lifestyle advice to aid in UTI prevention.
> - Target UTI with antimicrobials and increase water intake.
> - Remove aggravating factors such as a highly acidic diet.
> - Promote appropriate immune function.
> - Restore urinary tract microflora balance.

Herbal medicine has a strong tradition of use in genitourinary conditions (see Table 27.1), although many herbal medicines' mechanisms of action and clinical efficacy have yet to be validated.

Antimicrobial activity

Encouraging healthy bacterial balance may be achieved by preventing dysbiosis and promoting healthy gastrointestinal bacteria populations. As most infections are the result of *E. coli* from the digestive tract, promoting a diet that favours healthy microflora ratios may be beneficial in reducing the incidence of UTI. A Finnish study, for example, found that women who consumed fermented dairy products containing probiotic strains had a reduced risk of developing UTI.[11] The consumption of fresh juices, particularly berry

Table 27.1 Traditional herbal actions in urinary tract infection*

HERB	ANTI-ADHERENT	ANTI-INFLAMMATORY	ANTILITHIC	ANTISEPTIC (URINARY)	ASTRINGENT	BLADDER TONIC	DIURETIC	DEMULCENT (URINARY)	IMMUNE MODULATING	SPASMOLYTIC
Andrographis		✓							✓	
Buchu		✓		✓			✓	✓		
Corn silk		✓	✓				✓	✓		
Couch grass							✓	✓		
Cramp bark					✓					✓
Cranberry	✓			✓						
Crataeva nurvala		✓	✓			✓				
Goldenrod		✓		✓			✓			
Horsetail			✓		✓	✓	✓			
Hydrangea		✓					✓			
Liquorice		✓						✓	✓	
Marshmallow		✓						✓		
Nettle		✓					✓			
Parsley		✓					✓			
Arctostaphylos uva-ursi		✓		✓	✓					

*Adapted from Commission E and British Herbal Pharmacopoeia monographs[9,10]

juices, was also associated with decreased risk of developing UTI. Clinical investigation of women who are predisposed to recurrent UTI has also uncovered reduced beneficial microflora populations even during times of non-infection.[12,13]

Although it is known that pathogenic urogenital flora proliferate at the time of infection, attempts to restore balance with **probiotic supplements** to reduce UTI show mixed results.[14] Specific strains of probiotics can be beneficial for preventing recurrent UTIs in women and generally have a good safety profile. *Lactobacillus rhamnosus* and *L. reuteri* either intravaginally or orally are most effective, while *L. casei shirota* and *L. crispatus* showed efficacy in some studies; *L. rhamnosus* does not seem as effective.[15,16] Controversy still surrounds the use of probiotics for UTI prophylaxis due to limited and mixed evidence. As with all instances in using specific probiotic strains for specific therapeutic effects, care needs to be taken to identify the appropriate strain (see Chapter 3 on irritable bowel syndrome for more discussion on suitable probiotic strains for specific conditions).

The isoquinoline alkaloid **berberine** from *Hydrastis canadensis*, *Coptis chinensis* and *Berberis vulgaris* has a strong effect in treating UTIs due to bacteriostatic activity.[17] Its effects have been confirmed against a number of bacteria including *Staphylococcus* spp., *E. coli* and *Streptococcus* spp.[18] ***Arctostaphylos uva-ursi***, rich in the phenolic constituent arbutin, also provides strong antimicrobial activity and has preliminary clinical evidence.[19] Clinical studies using these botanicals are now required to confirm this activity in humans.

Inhibition of bacteria adhering to bladder wall

A key protocol in treating UTIs is to reduce bacterial proliferation in the bladder and their adherence to the bladder wall. In addition to increasing diuresis and providing an antimicrobial and bacteriostatic action, interventions that interfere with bacterial adherence will be of benefit. A key lifestyle measure in reducing bacterial colonisation and adherence on bladder tissue is complete urination after sexual intercourse. The main phytotherapy studied for this action is ***Vaccinium macrocarpon*** (**cranberry**), and its cousins **blueberry** and **bilberry**. In vitro and animal studies have demonstrated that cranberry consumption inhibits the binding of bacterial strains such as *E. coli* to uroepithelial cells.[17,19] It appears that the anthocyanidins are responsible for this activity. A Cochrane review and meta-analysis revealed that cranberry or cranberry and lingonberry significantly reduced people's chances of developing UTIs over a 12-month period.[20] It was concluded that cranberry juice or tablets may preferentially benefit women with chronic recurring UTIs compared with elderly men or people with bladder infections due to catheterisation.

A botanical with traditional use in UTIs is ***Juniperus* spp.** This medicinal plant may provide an anti-UTI effect via bacteriostatic, diuretic and anti-adhesion effects, but to date no human clinical trials substantiate this.[19] It should be noted that a common misconception exists about *Juniperus* spp. and nephrotoxicity. Close evaluation of the literature reveals that a review of the evidence does not support this effect, and that previous case studies may be based on adulteration of the juniper oil.[19] As mentioned previously, the isoquinoline alkaloid **berberine** has a potential effect in treating UTIs due to bacteriostatic action; this constituent also has demonstrated anti-adhesion activity against a number of bacteria including *Staphylococcus* spp., *E. coli* and *Streptococcus* spp.[18,17] The nutrient **D-mannose** may also provide anti-adhesion activity against bacteria such as *E. coli*. This simple sugar has been shown to bind to uroepithelial cells to which bacteria normally adhere, thereby interfering with colonisation.[17] While a promising intervention it should noted that current evidence is based on in vitro and animal studies.

Enhancement of diuresis

The most obvious way to increase diuresis is by use of aquaretics: agents that increase water excretion via effects on glomerular filtration as opposed to affecting electrolyte control with diuretics.[19] Water and herbal teas related to treatment are the preferable methods of increasing liquid intake. Although most botanicals used for this effect are regarded as being aquaretic, there have been some studies on the diuretic effects of certain herbs that are noted to be potentially beneficial in conditions like oedema and hypertension.[19] Reference is particularly made in this instance to the herb ***Taraxacum officinale*** where the leaf especially has demonstrated diuretic affects due in part to potassium content.[21] An added benefit for use of *T. officinale* in diuresis is that potassium levels are compensated for the loss of this mineral in urine output.[22] The first human study to evaluate the diuretic effects of this herb showed promise for its use as a diuretic.[23] The pilot study used fresh leaf hydroethanolic extract of *T. officinale* (8 mL t.d.s.) in 17 participants to investigate whether an increased urinary frequency and volume would result (compared to prerecorded baseline measurements). Results revealed a significant increase in the frequency of urination in the 5-hour period after the first dose. There was also a significant increase in the excretion ratio in the 5-hour period after the second dose of extract. The third dose, however, failed to significantly alter any of the measured parameters. For more detail on the use of *T. officinale* as a diuretic, refer to Chapter 10 on hypertension.

Reduction of inflammation and pain

Symptomatic relief of pain and inflammation is also important in treating UTIs. The use of **herbal anti-inflammatories** and **demulcents** are specifically indicated and are highly recommended (see the detailed lists in Tables 27.1 and 27.4). Further details on treating pain and inflammation may be found in Chapter 28 on autoimmunity, Chapter 22 on osteoarthritis and Chapter 37 on pain management.

Preventive measures

Clinicians are advised to provide lifestyle advice to assist in UTI prevention (see Table 27.2). A key consideration is to advise that the patient communicate to their sexual partner/s about the potential influence their sexual hygiene may have on the genesis of a UTI. To effectively prevent UTIs, the sexual partner is advised to adopt the same lifestyle advice as the patient being treated (especially males) as they may be the prime source of recurrent infection. Although studies on fluid intake and susceptibility to UTI appear inconclusive, adequate hydration is important and may improve the results of interventional treatment.[25] Supporting healthy immune function is also an important preventive measure. One small trial has found that 100 mg of **vitamin C** reduced the incidence of UTI in pregnant women.[26] A recent meta-analysis noted, however, that vitamin C may be of little use as an acidifying agent lowering urinary pH.[27] The

REMOVE BLADDER IRRITANTS[24]

Some substances may have an irritant effect on bladder epithelial tissue, predisposing patients to infection and delaying treatment effects. These are caffeine, refined sugars, dietary allergens, nicotine, alcohol and certain medications.

Table 27.2 Lifestyle factors useful in the prevention of UTIs[28,29,11]

Hydration and urination

- Drink at least eight glasses of water per day.
- Urinate often as retaining urine in the bladder may promote bacterial growth.
- Completely empty the bladder when urinating.

Urogenital area hygiene

- Good hygiene and urination should be observed (by both sexual partners) before and after sexual activity.
- Any potential irritants that are vaginally inserted should be avoided where possible in women with recurrent infections—these may include diaphragms or tampons that contain potentially irritating chemicals.
- Always cleanse the urogenital and anal areas from front to back.

Clothing

- Wear appropriate clothing—avoid tight-fitting underwear and wear breathable natural fibres like cotton for underwear and stockings.

Sensitivities and allergies

- Allergens and sensitivity by-products may cause irritation of the bladder wall so avoidance is recommended.
- UTIs after sexual activity may also result from latex or spermicidal allergies. Therefore reviewing birth control methods may be advised.

preventive action for the use of vitamin C in the case of UTIs may be by way of its indirect rather than direct effects.

Medicinal teas

One potentially beneficial CAM intervention in the treatment of UTIs is the use of **medicinal teas**, which, in addition to providing antimicrobial, anti-inflammatory, demulcent or diuretic activity, also increase the amount of water consumed. As Reinard Ludewig (1989)[40] espoused, 'persons who prefer their daily coffee, cocoa, or tea to caffeine tablets are unknowingly accepting and enjoying the pleasure of gentle-acting phytomedicines'. Traditional herbal pharmacopoeias advocate the use of medicinal herbal teas (infusions and decoctions) for the treatment of UTIs, to promote diuresis, disinfect the urine and prevent the formation of renal gravel and stones (see Table 27.3).[40]

Writings in *The American Eclectic Materia Medica and Therapeutics* (1863) reflected the practice of the day, declaring without doubt that 'infusion and decoction are the most eligible forms of administering such vegetable remedies' as they 'yield either a part or all of their virtues to water infusion'. They reiterated that, although much 'tea' was laughed at, 'this practice has proven eminently successful' and the added advantage was 'that the patient will receive sufficient [liquid], a matter that is of the first importance in the treatment of many diseases'.[41]

Teas, as aqueous preparations, are efficient in extracting water-soluble plant chemicals, in particular essential oils, and the presence of saponins enhances the bioavailability of other, less-soluble compounds.[38] Furthermore, therapeutic infusions have added benefits not gleaned from herbal liquid extracts and solid dose forms. The ritual of preparing a herbal tea, savouring the aroma and slowly sipping, to ultimately experience the

Table 27.3 Teas commonly used in UTIs[9,10]

HERB DETAILS			MONOGRAPH INDICATIONS					
BOTANICAL AND COMMON NAMES	PLANT PART	DOSAGE AND ADMINISTRATION	GERMAN COMMISSION E	WHO	ESCOP	GERMAN STANDARD LICENCE	BRITISH HERBAL COMPENDIUM	BRITISH HERBAL PHARMACOPOEIA
Agathosma betulina	Leaf	1–2 g by infusion t.d.s.					Mild UTI	Cystitis, urethritis. Specific: acute catarrhal cystitis
Agropyron repens	Rhizome	4–8 g in decoction t.d.s.						Cystitis, urethritis, lithuria. Specific: cystitis with irritation or inflammation of urinary tract
Althaea officinalis	Leaf	Leaf: 2–5 g by infusion t.d.s.						Leaf: cystitis, urethritis, urinary gravel or calculus
Arctostaphylos uva-ursi	Leaf	Steep 3 g in 150 mL boiled water 15 mins up to q.i.d.	Inflammatory disorders of efferent UT		Uncomplicated UTIs, cystitis	Support therapy for bladder and kidney catarrh		Cystitis, urethritis, dysuria, pyelitis and lithuria. Specific: acute catarrhal cystitis with dysuria and highly acid urine
Armoracia rusticana	Root	Steep 2 g in 150 mL boiled water for 5 mins	Supportive therapy for UTIs				Inflammation or mild infections of genitourinary tract	
Echinacea spp.	Root	Steep 2 g in 150 mL boiled water for 5 mins		Supportive therapy for UTIs				
Equisetum arvense	Green stems	Steep 2 g in 150 mL boiled water 10 – 15 mins t.d.s.	Lower UTIs and inflammation and renal gravel			Lower UTIs and inflammation and renal gravel		

(Continued)

Table 27.3 Teas commonly used in UTIs[9,10] (Continued)

	HERB DETAILS			MONOGRAPH INDICATIONS					
BOTANICAL AND COMMON NAMES	PLANT PART	DOSAGE AND ADMINISTRATION	GERMAN COMMISSION E	WHO	ESCOP	GERMAN STANDARD LICENCE	BRITISH HERBAL COMPENDIUM	BRITISH HERBAL PHARMACOPOEIA	
Juniperus communis	Berry	Dried ripe fruits infusion 1:20 in boiling water dosed 100 mL t.d.s.						Acute or chronic cystitis. Specific: cystitis, in absence of renal inflammation	
Petroselinum crispum	Herb and root	Steep 2 g in 150 mL water t.d.s.	Diuresis and prevent and treat kidney gravel						
Solidago virgaurea	Aerial (above ground)	Steep 3 g in 150 mL boiled water for 10 to 15 mins, 2 to 4 times daily between meals	Diuresis for inflammatory lower UTIs, prevent and treat urinary calculi and kidney gravel		Diuresis for inflammatory urinary tract and renal gravel, adjuvant bacterial UTIs	Diuresis in inflammation of kidneys and bladder	Mild infections of UT	Cystitis	
Urtica dioica	Leaf	Steep 2–5 g in 150 mL boiled water for 10 to 15 mins, t.d.s.	Diuresis for inflammatory lower urinary tract, prevent and treat kidney gravel		Irrigation therapy in inflammatory conditions of lower urinary tract	Increase urine volume and treat urine associated complaints			
Zea mays	Styles and stigmas	4–8 g by infusion t.d.s.						Cystitis, urethritis and nocturnal enuresis. Specific: acute or chronic inflammation of urinary system	

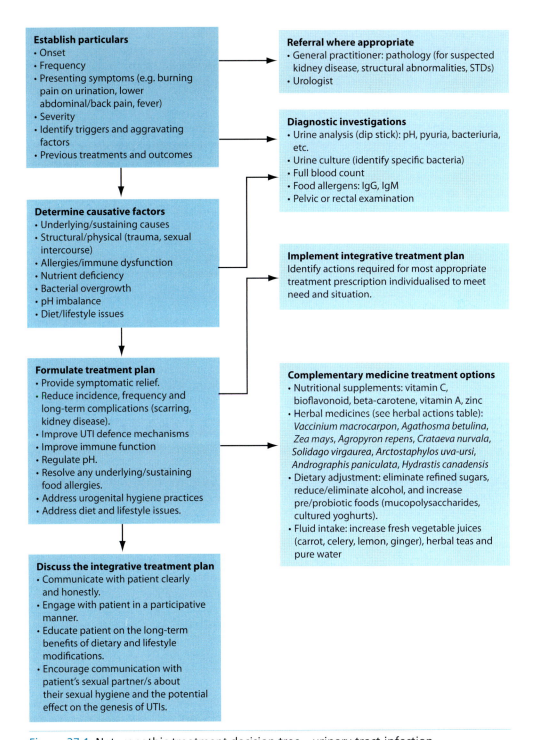

Figure 27.1 Naturopathic treatment decision tree—urinary tract infection

soothing, warm sensation that, at some level, brings relaxation to an otherwise stressed individual, has added therapeutic value.

There are important considerations in the selection of herbs to create a balanced blend that is both therapeutic and palatable. Weiss instructs that every formulation requires three components: (1) the basic remedy (the *remedium cardinal*), (2) an adjuvant to enhance or complement the action of the basic remedy, and (3) a 'corrigent' to improve palatability and compliance.[42] Preparation instructions also need to be communicated well as the method used has the potential to impede or potentiate the therapeutic benefits of an herbal tea. Herbal parts containing volatile oils (for example, in delicate leaves and seeds) should be gently infused in hot water in an enclosed vessel (teapot) so as not to damage or lose these therapeutic plant compounds. Chemical compounds contained in harder bark or root components may need to be 'drawn out' in boiling water for 10 to 15 minutes. Furthermore, dosage instructions will potentiate the curative properties attributed to both the preparation and the ingestion practices of taking tea. Unless otherwise indicated, 1 or 2 teaspoons of tea are used per cup (150 mL) of hot water, of which 2 to 3 cups are to be taken daily on an empty stomach to aid absorption, preferably drunk on rising, mid-afternoon and before bed.[42]

INTEGRATIVE MEDICAL CONSIDERATIONS

There are important medical implications associated with UTIs. UTIs elevate the risk of pyelonephritis and are associated with impaired renal function and end-stage renal disease.[1] It is therefore imperative that anyone presenting with an UTI with suspected kidney disease should be referred to a general practitioner for assessment with possible further referral to an urologist (see Table 27.4 for other common urinary conditions).[30]

Conventional treatment of UTIs with antibiotics along with a high recurrence rate of UTIs, especially among young women, has led to issues of antibiotic resistance. Various authors have reported on antibiotic resistance and its implications for the long-term use of antibiotics for the effective management of urinary tract and kidney infections.[31,32,33,34] One case-control study concluded that exposure to antibiotics is a strong risk factor for a resistant *E. coli* UTI.[35] An integrative approach using various herbal and nutritional therapeutics to support and resolve UTIs may provide promise. A Norwegian study found that acupuncture reduced the UTI rate by around half in women who had a history of recurrent UTIs.[36] However, treatment needs to be individualised based on the diagnosis and prescription of trained practitioners. Acupuncture also seems to result in improved quality of life of women with recurrent UTIs.[37]

Case Study

A 33-year-old female presents with chronic, **recurrent UTIs** that have affected her all her adult life. They have been previously treated but not resolved with antibiotic treatment. She currently reports of **extreme pain and discomfort upon urination**. No blood appears in her urine. She mentions that it seems to get **worse after she has sex with her partner**.

SUGGESTIVE SIGNS AND SYMPTOMS

- Urogenital pain
- Lower back pain
- Fever, chills
- Haematuria

- Dysuria
- Frequency, nocturia and urgency
- Foul-smelling urine
- Fatigue

Table 27.4 Treatment of other urogenital conditions[3,38,39,17,19]

UROGENITAL DISORDER	TREATMENT PROTOCOL	CAM INTERVENTIONS	COMMENT
Kidney stones	• Reduce inflammation. • Assist breakdown of urinary gravel. • Increase diuresis. • Provide analgesia.	• Low oxalate diet • Low purine diet • Increase water intake • Antilithic, anti-inflammatory botanicals • Vitamin B6, magnesium	• Monitor closely for referral for medical help if condition worsens, e.g. increased pain or blood in urine. • Address pain with analgesic medicines. • Evidence of antilithic activity is currently based only on traditional evidence. • Ultrasound may assist.
Pyelonephritis/ kidney infection	• Refer immediately for medical help (antibiotics are usually prescribed). • Support adjuvantly. • Reduce inflammation. • Provide analgesia. • Tonify kidneys (traditional protocol).	• Antimicrobial, anti-inflammatory, demulcent, diuretic botanicals • Increase water (with adequate electrolytes) • Urogenital hygiene • Low renal-irritant diet	• Chronic recurring kidney infections and nephritis may be unresponsive to repeated antibiotics. • Anti-microbial herbs, e.g. *Arcostaphytes uva-ursi, Hydrastis canadensis, Echinacea* spp. may assist in this case.
Vaginal thrush	• Anti-fungal action • Recolonise tissue with appropriate microflora. • Reduce itching. • Support immune and nervous systems.	• Anti-fungal/microbial pessary or douche containing tea tree oil, *Hydrastis canadensis*, probiotics. • Low yeast diet • Immune tonics • Nervines	• Screen for trigger, e.g. stress, diet change or antibiotic use. • Considered in traditional Chinese medicine as a 'damp' condition—avoid 'damp' diets and exposure to wet environments.

Example treatment

The treatment protocol is designed to promote symptomatic relief and reduce the incidence, frequency and long-term complications (scarring and kidney disease) of recurrent UTIs.

Prescription

The herbal treatment is designed to promote UTI defence mechanisms by:

- improving the flow and volume of urine to reduce stagnation and adherence and facilitate 'flushing out' of infective bacteria by (1) increasing urine volume (using diuretic teas and increase water intake), (2) promoting ease (painless) urination (using urinary demulcents, anti-inflammatories) and (3) facilitating complete bladder emptying and improving bladder tone (using a spasmolytic to reduce lower bladder sphincter resistance, and a bladder tonic) and (4) reducing bacterial adherence to the bladder wall.
- improving immune function (immune modulation).

Vaccinium macrocarpon, Echinacea angustifolia and *Hydrastis canadensis* provide anti-adhesive (bacterial), immune-enhancing and antimicrobial activity, respectively. The use of the botanical as a medicinal tea (detailed below) will not only increase urine volume and diuresis, but it will also provide soothing demulcent effects and further enhance the anti-inflammatory and antiseptic actions of the herbal prescription. The herbal tea is advised to be taken at a different time to the *Hydrastis canadensis* tablets as the tannins from peppermint and bearberry may bind with the berberine alkaloids. Although peppermint is spasmolytic and antimicrobial in action,[9] the main purpose for it being included in the tea blend is to enhance flavour (taste).

The combination of peppermint and buchu creates a delightful aromatic experience. The additional use of traditional Ayurvedic herb *C. nurvala* may also provide a 'bladder tonic' activity although this is based on traditional evidence.

Herbal prescription

Vaccinium macrocarpon tablets 3 g
Dose: 2 tablets t.d.s.
Echinacea angustifolia (standardised for alkylamides) tablets 1 g
Dose: 2 tablets t.d.s.
Hydrastis canadensis (standardised for berberine) tablets 1 g
Dose: 1 tablet t.d.s.
Herbal tea: buchu, corn silk, goldenrod, bearberry, marshmallow, peppermint
1 cup t.d.s. on empty stomach on rising, mid-afternoon and before bed (prepare in teapot fresh each morning for use throughout the day). See the herb tea blend preparation box below for further instructions.

Probiotics

See the list in the text.
2 capsules each night 1 hour before dinner

Probiotics are prescribed to rebalance the microflora in the bladder containing more than 20 billion organisms in a blend of *Lactobacillus acidophilus*, *L. casei*, *L. plantarum*, *L. rhamnosus*, *L. gasseri*, *L. delbruecki* spp. *bulgaricus*, *Streptococcus thermophilus*, *Bifidobacterium longum*, *B. breve* and *B. lactis*.

Dietary and lifestyle advice

Recommendations are made (as in Table 27.2) to further reduce susceptibility to and incidence of UTIs and to promote general wellbeing and healthy immune function. Dietary advice may include reducing or eliminating intake of refined sugar and alcohol, and increase pre- and probiotic foods (mucopolysaccharides and cultured yoghurts).

HERBAL TEA BLEND

Herb/herb part	g per week
Buchu leaves	20
Corn silk styles and stigmas	20
Goldenrod aerial parts	10
Bearberry leaves	15
Marshmallow root	15
Peppermint leaves	20
Total	100 g

Dose: 5 g per cup of tea, infused in covered vessel (teapot) for 15 minutes. 1 cup t.d.s. on empty stomach on rising, mid -afternoon and before bed.

Herbs are combined and mixed in a blender to reduce particle size. This improves the extraction of the therapeutic compounds from the infusion process.

Table 27.5 Review of the major evidence

INTERVENTION	METHODOLOGY	RESULT	COMMENT
Probiotics: *L. rhamnosus* and *L. reuteri* or placebo; vaginal suppository[43] *L. rhamnosus* and *L. reuteri* or *Lactobacillus* growth factor; vaginal suppository[44]	RCT (*n* = 41) RCT (*n* = 55)	21% recurrence in probiotic group versus 47% recurrence in placebo group 73% reduction in both groups over previous year	Intervention given post-successful acute treatment with antibiotics No significant difference between groups although both exhibited significant reductions over the year of the study
Vaccinium macrocarpon (cranberry)[20]	Cochrane review 10 studies (*n* = 1049) Cranberry tablets or juice versus placebo control	Cranberry significantly reduced the incidence of UTIs at 12 months. RR 0.65, 95% CI: 0.46–0.90	Trials appear to benefit women preferentially over elderly men or people with catheterisation using cranberry for UTI prevention. Optimum dose or method (juice or tablet) needs clarification

Increased fluid intake, using fresh vegetable juices (for example, a blend of celery, carrot, lemon and ginger), herbal teas and pure water, is also advised. Urogenital hygiene practices—pre- and postcoital hygiene and increased urination—are also recommended.

Expected outcomes and follow-up protocols

It would be expected that within a few days of starting the prescription (likely in less than 1 day) there would be relief of symptoms. Reduced UTI recurrence can be promoted by increasing immune resistance and improved balance of bowel and urogenital flora. Furthermore, a reduced UTI recurrence rate may be effected if diet and lifestyle advice is adhered to. Herbal prescription should be continued a couple of days after the symptoms have resolved to completely address the pathogen. Preventive measures should be continued. A prophylactic prescription can be provided to enhance immune function, maintain bowel and urogenital flora, improve mucous membrane integrity and urinary tract function, and to address any contributing factors such as stress. The use of the herbal tea prescribed and cranberry tablets can be continued long-term, and is advised in people with chronic recurrent UTIs.

KEY POINTS

- UTIs are common, especially in young women, and recurrence rate is high.
- UTIs elevate the risk of pyelonephritis and are associated with impaired renal function and end-stage renal disease, so UTIs should be treated assertively and comprehensively.
- Conventional treatment of UTIs with antibiotics may lead to patterns of antibiotic resistance, so judicious use is advised.
- Various CAM therapeutics (herbal and nutritional) have value in the treatment and prevention of UTIs and can be considered as stand-alone interventions or adjuvants with antibiotics.
- Implementation of lifestyle advice (for example, sexual hygiene) is advised to assist the prevention of recurrence.

Further reading

Barrons R, Tassone D. Use of *Lactobacillus* probiotics for bacterial genitourinary infections in women: a review. Clin Ther 2008;30:453–468.

Head K. Natural approaches to prevention and treatment of infections of the lower urinary tract. Altern Med Rev 2008;13:227–244.

Jepson R, Craig J. Cranberries for preventing urinary tract infections. Cochrane Database Syst Rev 2008;(23):CD001321.

Yarnell E. Botanical medicines for the urinary tract. World J Urol 2002;20:285–293.

References

1. Wein AJ, et al. Campbell-Walsh Urology. 9th edn. Philadelphia: Saunders Elsevier, 2007.
2. Boon, et al. Davidson's principles and practice of medicine. 20th edn. Edinburgh: Churchill Livingstone, 2006.
3. Kumar P, Clark M. Clinical medicine. 5th edn. London: W.B. Saunders, 2002.
4. Foxman B, et al. Urinary tract infection: self reported incidence and associated costs. Ann Epidemiol 2000;10:509–515.
5. Murtagh J. General practice. Sydney: McGraw-Hill, 2007.
6. Scholes D, et al. Risk factors for recurrent urinary tract infection in young women. J Infect Dis 2000;182:1177–1182.
7. Boyko E, et al. Diabetes and the risk of acute urinary tract infection among postmenopausal women. Diabetes Care 2002;25:1778–1783.
8. Stamm W. Estrogens and urinary-tract infection. J Infect Dis 2007;195:623–624.
9. Blumenthal M, et al. Herbal medicine expanded Commission E monographs. Newton: Integrative Medicine Communications, 2000.
10. British Herbal Medicine Association Scientific Committee. British herbal pharmacopoeia. Bournemouth: British Herbal Medicine Association, 1983.
11. Kontiokari T, et al. Dietary factors protecting women from urinary tract infection. Am J Clin Nutr 2003;77:600–604.
12. Gupta K, et al. Inverse association of H_2O_2-producing lactobacilli and vaginal *Escherichia coli* colonization in women with recurrent urinary tract infections. J Infect Dis 1998;178:446–450.
13. Kirjavainen P, et al. Abnormal immunological profile and vaginal microbiota in women prone to urinary tract infections. Clin Vaccine Immunol 2009;16:29–36.
14. Reid G. Probiotic agents to protect the urogenital tract against infection. Am J Clin Nutr 2001;73:437S–443S.
15. Barrons R, Tassone D. Use of *Lactobacillus* probiotics for bacterial genitourinary infections in women: a review. Clin Ther 2008;30:453–468.
16. Reid G. Probiotic lactobacilli for urogenital health in women. J Clin Gastroenterol 2008;42:S234–S236.
17. Head K. Natural approaches to prevention and treatment of infections of the lower urinary tract. Altern Med Rev 2008;13:227–244.
18. Scazzocchio F, et al. Antibacterial activity of *Hydrastis canadensis* extract and its major isolated alkaloids. Planta Med 2001;67:561–564.
19. Yarnell E. Botanical medicines for the urinary tract. World J Urol 2002;20:285–293.
20. Jepson RG, et al. Cranberries for preventing urinary tract infections. Cochrane Database Syst Rev 2004;(2):CD001321.
21. Hook I, et al. Evaluation of dandelion for diuretic activity and variation of potassium content. Int J Pharmacog 1993;31(1):29–34.
22. Schütz K, et al. *Taraxacum*—a review on its phytochemical and pharmacological profile. J Ethnopharmacol 2006;107:313–323.
23. Clare BA, et al. The diuretic effect in human subjects of an extract of *Taraxacum officinale* folium over a single day. J Altern Complement Med 2009;15(8):929–934.
24. Wyman JF, et al. Practical aspects of lifestyle modifications and behavioural interventions in the treatment of overactive bladder and urgency urinary incontinence. Int J Clin Pract 2009;63(8):1177–1191.
25. Beetz R. Mild dehydration: a risk factor of urinary tract infection. Eur J Clin Nutr 2003;57:S52–S58.
26. Ochoa-Brust G, et al. Daily intake of 100 mg ascorbic acid as urinary tract infection prophylactic agent during pregnancy. Acta Obstet Gynecol Scand 2007;86:783–787.
27. Masson P, et al. Meta-analyses in prevention and treatment of urinary tract infections. Infect Dis Clin North Am 2009;23:355–385.
28. Foxman B, Frerichs R. Epidemiology of urinary tract infection: II. Diet, clothing, and urination habits. Am J Public Health 1985;75(11):1314–1317.
29. Foxman B, Chi J. Health behavior and urinary tract infection in college-aged women. J Clin Epidemiol 1990;43(4):329–337.
30. Foxman B. Epidemiology of urinary tract infections: incidence, morbidity, and economic costs. Dis Mon 2003;49:53–70.
31. Foxman B, et al. Antibiotic resistance and pyelonephritis. Clin Infect Dis 2007;45:281–283.
32. Karlowsky JA, et al. Fluoroquinolone-resistant urinary isolate of *Escherichia coli* from outpatients are frequently multidrug resistant: results from the North American Urinary Tract Infection Collaborative Alliance-Quinolone Resistance Study. Antimicrob Agents Chemother 2006;50(6):2251–2254.
33. McNulty CAM, et al. Clinical relevance of laboratory-reported antibiotic resistance in acute uncomplicated urinary tract infection in primary care. J Antimicrob Chemother 2006;58:1000–1008.
34. Mazzulli T. Resistance trends in urinary tract pathogens and impact on management. J Urol 2002;168:1720–1722.
35. Hillier S, et al. Prior antibiotics and risk of antibiotic-resistant community-acquired urinary tract infection: a case-control study. J Antimicrob Chemother 2007;60:92–99.
36. Alraek T, et al. Acupuncture treatment in the prevention of uncomplicated recurrent lower urinary tract infections in adult women. Am J Public Health 2002;92:1609–1611.
37. Alraek T, Baerheim A. An empty and happy feeling in the bladder … : health changes experienced by women after acupuncture for recurrent cystitis. Complement Ther Med 2001;9:219–223.
38. Mills S, Bone K. Principles and practice of phytotherapy. Edinburgh: Churchill Livingstone, 2000.
39. Grases F, et al. Urolithiasis and phytotherapy. Int Urol Nephrol 1994;26:507–511.
40. Cited in Schulz V, et al. Rational phytotherapy a physicians' guide to herbal medicine. Berlin: Springer, 2001.
41. Bergner P. Tinctures vs teas. Medical Herbalism 2001;10(4):3.
42. Weiss R. Herbal medicine. Gothenburg: Ab Arcanum and Beaconsfield: Beaconsfield Publishers, 1985.
43. Reid G, et al. Influence of three day antimicrobial therapy and *Lactobacillus* vaginal suppositories on recurrence of urinary tract infections. Clin Ther 1992;14:11–16.
44. Reid G, et al. Installation of *Lactobacillus* and stimulation of indigenous organisms to prevent recurrence of urinary tract infections. Microecol Ther 1995;23:32–45.

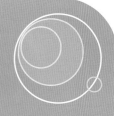

PART C
Specialised clinical conditions

In contemporary naturopathic treatment, some conditions cannot be categorised by the systems they affect. Instead, they share common aetiology that can affect a variety of systems. This focus on aetiology requires a more complex understanding and analysis of naturopathic treatment and its effects on biochemical processes. For example, autoimmunity refers not to a pathology limited to a specific site or system, but rather to a dysfunctional process whereby the body's immune system fails to recognise 'self'. Cancer also is not limited to specific systems but instead represents uncontrolled growth, invasion or metastasis of cells in any location. Many of the broad principles will remain the same for this process in any bodily location. These specialised conditions also share a complexity that necessitates a more detailed investigation.

The 'cancer journey' in particular is a long and varied one, and cannot be limited to aetiological considerations alone. There is a plethora of strategies for prevention, a multitude of treatment options, and palliative care considerations for those who fail to go into remission. These range from biological agents that can directly affect the biochemistry of cancer (in a positive or negative manner) to addressing the various general physical and psychological consequences that arise from cancer and its treatment. The complexity is further augmented by the many varied and complex pharmaceutical medicine regimens that are encountered in naturopathic oncology practice. Considerations pertinent to the successful integration of naturopathic and conventional oncology practice are discussed in Chapter 29 on cancer.

In some instances the principles discussed in detail also have relevance for other sections of the book. For example, while the detailed investigation of naturopathic treatment on various inflammatory pathways has obvious relevance in autoimmunity, it also has direct relevance for the underlying causes of many other conditions covered in this text. Chapter 28 on autoimmunity in particular reveals a thorough review of the pathogenesis of autoimmune conditions, in addition to a variety of traditional and evidence-based CAM interventions used to address these disorders.

In summary, this section outlines the extensive principles behind the treatment of these specialised conditions. These principles can be applied to a broad range of autoimmune diseases and cancers respectively. In Chapter 29 on cancer, however, the treatment of specific cancers are outlined as individual case examples as this reflects the clinical focus required.

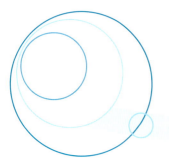

28

Autoimmunity

Joanne Bradbury

ND, BNat (Hons)

OVERVIEW

Autoimmunity is a normal event, while autoimmune diseases result from an aberration of this normal phenomenon.[1] Autoimmune diseases are characterised by chronic inflammation with a loss of tolerance to 'self' or 'auto' antigens. The causes for the loss of tolerance, the shift from normal immune function to autoimmune pathology, are poorly understood but are generally agreed to be multifactorial, involving a combination of genetic, environmental, hormonal and immune factors.[1,2] Probable key factors include abnormal cytokine biology and the direct activation of larger than normal quantities of auto- or self-reactive CD4 positive T-cells. Conventionally, autoimmune disorders are diagnosed and treated by physicians specialising in the particular system involved, as shown in Table 28.1. A new paradigm is emerging that groups the pathogeneses of the wide spectrum of autoimmune diseases by their common underlying mechanism: immune system dysregulation, mediated by an imbalance of pro-inflammatory and regulatory cytokines.[3]

AETIOLOGY

Genetic factors

In the immune system, cell surface protein molecules called human leukocyte antigens (HLA) recognise self from non-self. These antigens are unique for each individual and are encoded by a group of genes on the sixth chromosome called the major histocompatibility complex (MHC).[5] On exposure to a foreign antigen, MHC antigens present a component of the invading antigen to circulating T-cells. MHC class I interact with cytotoxic T (CD8+) cells, which track down and kill specific cells, and MHC class II interact with helper T (CD4+) cells which, in the presence of pro-inflammatory cytokines, activate a full immune response (discussed further below under 'T-cells').[6]

Certain MHC class II genotypes are associated with increased susceptibility to autoimmune diseases. This susceptibility may be clustered within specific populations; for instance, increased risk of rheumatoid arthritis is associated with HLA-DR1 (in Asians, Spanish and Jewish Israeli nationals) and HLA-DR4 (in Caucasians).[6]

Table 28.1 Major autoimmune disorders[4]

AUTOIMMUNE DISEASE	SYSTEM AFFECTED	MAIN ORGANS AFFECTED
Systemic lupus erythematosus (SLE)	Systemic	Skin, joints, kidneys, lungs, heart, brain and blood cells
Rheumatoid arthritis	Systemic; muscular skeletal	Connective tissue in joints
Dermatitis herpetiformis	Integumentary	Skin, particularly elbows, knees, back and back of neck
Multiple sclerosis	Nervous	Myelin sheath in neurons of brain and spinal chord
Myasthenia gravis	Nervous; neuromuscular junction	Muscles , particularly the muscles around the eyes
Pernicious anaemia	Blood (haematologic); gastrointestinal	Parietal cells in stomach
Goodpasture's disease	Renal; respiratory	Kidney and lungs
Graves' disease (hyperthyroidism)	Endocrine	Thyroid gland
Hashimoto's thyroiditis	Endocrine	Thyroid gland
Type I diabetes mellitus	Endocrine	Pancreatic beta cells
Coeliac disease	Gastrointestinal	Villi in small intestine
Ulcerative colitis (inflammatory bowel disease)	Gastrointestinal	Mucosa of colon, particularly large colon
Crohn's disease	Gastrointestinal	Can affect entire colon wall, most commonly the lower ileum

Some autoimmune diseases are associated with a single mutation, such as autoimmune lymphoproliferative syndrome. Importantly, not everyone that has the mutant gene manifests the disease. Of those that do, there is a wide variation in the progression and severity of the disease. This implies that there are other factors controlling and regulating the pathogenesis of autoimmune disease.[7]

Most autoimmune diseases involve a combination of several genetic mutations. The net effect of a combination of mutations may manifest as a pathological phenotype (that is, the way a genotype actually manifests in an individual), depending on the presence or absence of protective factors, both genetic and non-genetic.[7]

Certain HLA alleles are protective against autoimmune disease. Protective genes and susceptibility genes may both be present in an individual. The net effect of protective and susceptibility genes determine an individual's genetic susceptibility to autoimmune diseases.[8]

Specific gene-environment interactions are increasingly being discovered as research into the human genome progresses.[9] It is estimated that there may be as many as 20 mutations associated with autoimmune diseases; these mutations are expected to be fully elucidated over the next few years as a result of work on the human genome project.[10] However, it is important to note that not all individuals bearing susceptibility genes actually manifest the disease conditions. Gene–gene and gene–environment interactions that may help our understanding of the pathogenesis of autoimmune disease are gradually being discovered.

Environmental factors such as diet and lifestyle may interact with genes to trigger, delay or prevent autoimmune diseases. While it is not possible to avoid our genotype, our phenotype is more malleable. How our genotype actually manifests takes account of environmental factors and how these factors interact with our genes. Environmental triggers and an individual's reaction to these triggers may offer effective therapeutic intervention points for the prevention, delay or mitigation of autoimmune disease in genetically susceptible individuals.

Environmental factors

Viral and bacterial infections, certain chemicals and drugs and mechanical injury have been implicated as potential triggers of autoimmune diseases in susceptible humans and animals.[7,10,11] Two mechanisms that are widely accepted explanations of how an infection may cause autoimmunity are known as *molecular mimicry* and *bystander activation*.

'Molecular mimicry' is the term given to the process of activation of autoreactive helper T (Th or CD4+) cells through cross-reactivity between foreign antigens and self antigens. The foreign antigen may so closely resemble a self antigen that the immune system, having reacted successfully to this foreign antigen, starts reacting to the self antigen as well.[5] 'Bystander activation' refers to the spontaneous activation of local autoreactive Th cells as part of a coordinated inflammatory response, which may occur as a result of any threat to homeostasis (such as infection).[12]

Recent research has identified another potential mechanism whereby bacteria may elicit autoimmune pathology. A group of bacteria called *superantigens*, which includes *streptococcal* and *staphylococcal* exotoxins, seem to short-cut the usual immune mechanisms of presentation and directly trigger CD4 cells to launch a full inflammatory response. The result is an enormous release of pro-inflammatory cytokines from T-cells, especially tumour necrosis factor-alpha (TNF-α) and IL-2. Exposure to superantigens has been shown to drive the intense inflammatory responses that result in acute toxic shock or chronic inflammatory disease, such as rheumatic fever.[5]

Antigen triggers need not come from the external environment—they may be endogenous proteins. Endogenous proteins that have been implicated in the pathogenesis of rheumatoid arthritis include human cartilage glycoprotein 39, citrullinated protein and heavy-chain binding protein.[13]

Dietary antigens have also been implicated in the pathogenesis of autoimmune pathology, especially the gastrointestinal autoimmune diseases.[14] For instance, cereal grains are known inducers of two autoimmune diseases (coeliac disease and dermatitis herpetiformis); removal of gluten from the diet ameliorates symptoms in these conditions. A process of molecular mimicry is strongly suspected in the pathophysiology of these conditions.[15] An inflammatory environment in the intestine (from dietary antigens) is associated with increased permeability and increased frequency of potentially

AUTOIMMUNE GENOTYPE

While it is not possible to avoid our genotype, our phenotype (how our genotype actually manifests in an individual) is more malleable, as it takes account of environment and lifestyle factors.

pathogenic antigens crossing the intestinal epithelium and entering the internal environment ('leaky gut syndrome'). This is mediated by IFN-γ and TNF-α, both altering the tight junctions between cells, while IFN-γ increases the uptake of proteins for transportation into the mucosal cells.[16]

Recent in vitro work has postulated a role for certain internal environmental conditions that may favour the recognition and binding of large numbers of autoantigens by antibodies. After transient exposure to protein destabilising (but not denaturing) conditions, such as low or high pH, high-salt environments and redox-reactive agents, a small percentage of autoantibodies become extremely autoreactive.[17] High salt and its sequelae, widespread low-level metabolic acidity, are hallmarks of the Western diet and are suspected as having an involvement in many so-called modern lifestyle diseases.[18]

Whatever the environmental trigger, the process of antibody autoreactivity is mediated by cytokines, which turn on and off the signals for T-cells specific for self antigens.[19] Thus, in the pathogenesis of autoimmunity, cytokine biology may provide the weakest link in the chain of events that result in pathology.[11]

Inflammatory mechanisms
Cytokines
Cytokines are chemical messengers that coordinate the whole immune system.[19] They include interleukins (IL), interferons (IFN), tumour necrosis factors (TNF), colony stimulating factors (CSF) and transforming growth factors (TGF). These messenger molecules are actually secreted by and communicate with most, and probably all, bodily systems including the brain. Consequently, they may well be a vital link in the 'mind–body connection'. In this section the discussion of cytokine function will be limited to the immune system and how altered cytokine biology appears to play a critical role in the mediation of autoimmune pathology.

Cytokines are found in tissues and in the blood and act as in autocrine, paracrine and endocrine ways. At their target cells cytokines bind to membrane receptors that use second messenger systems. The ensuing enzymatic cascade then results in stimulation or inhibition of cell functions. They can regulate the expression of membrane proteins, including cytokine receptors, and they can stimulate the expression and secretion of their own and other kinds of cytokines.[20] In the immune system, cytokines are mainly secreted from activated macrophages and helper T lymphocytes (CD4+ cells). T helper (Th) cells are central to the regulation of the adaptive immune system, both the humoral and cellular arms.[21] T helper cells are primarily regulated by T regulatory (Treg) cells (once known as suppressor T lymphocytes). An important role of Treg cells is the inhibition of B lymphocytes from differentiating into plasma cells, the precursors of antibodies. Altered regulatory T-cell functioning has been associated with autoimmune disease.[22]

T-cells
T-cells are lymphocytes that have T-cell receptors (TCRs) on the surface membrane. These cells differ from B cells in that they do not respond to soluble antigen but respond to an antigen only when presented bound to MHC molecules, which distinguish self from non-self antigens. Ligands that bind to MCH class I proteins alert T-cells to intracellular infections, resulting in cloning of cytotoxic T (CD8) cells specific for the antigen infection.

Antigen-specific cytotoxic T-cells hunt down and destroy the infected cells. Ligands that bind to MCH class II proteins alert T-cells to a threat that requires a coordinated immune system response, to be mediated by the cloning of antigen-specific helper T (CD4) cells.[23]

Depending on the nature of the antigen, T helper cells differentiate into distinct subsets, which tailor the adaptive immune system to suit the threat at hand. For instance, bacteria and viruses typically activate the cellular arm whereas helminths activate the humoral arm of adaptive immunity.[24]

CD4+ and CD8+ T-cells

MHC classes I and II antigens are recognised by two distinct subsets of T-cells. These T-cell subsets are distinguished by their respective cell surface proteins.[25] Cell surface molecules have been designated as CD or 'cluster of differentiation', as they were identified using statistical cluster analysis to identify the specific cells that differentiated after being stimulated by certain antigens.

A numeric system was designated to CD cells as they were identified.[26] The T-cell subsets that express CD4 molecules (CD4+ T-cells) may belong to either the helper or regulatory T-cell subsets, where those T-cells that express CD8 molecules (CD8+ T-cells) are cytotoxic T-cells.[23] The CD4 and CD8 proteins function as co-receptors in that they cooperate with the T-cell receptor (TCR) to recognise and respond to an antigen bound to MHC classes II and I, respectively.

A portion of the CD4 and CD8 receptor sits outside the cell and directly interacts with the MHC on the antigen-presenting cell. The combination of the TCR and CD4 or CD8 binding to MHC is the first signal required for T-cell activation.[27]

T helper 1/T helper 2 hypothesis

For 20 years the study of immunology has used the Th1:Th2 hypothesis paradigm, which depicts many disease states to be characterised by the relationship or balance of T helper type 1 (CD4+Th1 or simply Th1) cells and T helper type 2 (CD4+Th2 or Th2) cells.[28]

During Th1 differentiation, activated antigen-presenting cells such as macrophages and dendritic cells (DCs) produce IL-12. IL-12 signals CD4+ cells to differentiate into Th1 cells, which secrete IL-2, a pro-inflammatory mediator. Interleukin-12 in the presence of IL-18 signals natural killer (NK) cells to secrete IFN-γ,[28] another potent pro-inflammatory mediator.

Th1 cells augment a predominately cellular immune response by stimulating T-cytotoxic activity and NK cells, activating macrophages and stimulating the production of other key inflammatory mediators such as nitric oxide (NO).[28] Th1 differentiation mediates a potent inflammatory response and an ongoing predominance of Th1 cytokines drives chronic inflammatory activity.[3]

During Th2 differentiation IL-4 induces naive T helper cells to differentiate into T helper type 2 (Th2) cells. Th2 cells secrete the cytokines IL-4, IL-5, IL-6, IL-10 and IL-13. This subset of cells activates and coordinates a predominately humoral immune response by stimulating the activity of oesinophils, mast cells and B-cell differentiation into plasma cells, which secrete antibodies.[28]

Cytokines derived from Th1 and Th2 have been shown to regulate each other by antagonistic and mutually inhibitive activity.[29] For instance, IL-10 inhibits IL-12 secretion from antigen-presenting cells, but even after IL-12 has been induced in vivo, IL-10 down-regulates its receptors, thereby limiting the effectiveness of IL-12.[30] Th2 cytokines are known to suppress the activation of macrophages, the proliferation of T-cells and the production of pro-inflammatory cytokines.[28] The Th2 cytokines, IL-4 and IL-10, are considered the major anti-inflammatory cytokines. Within this Th1:Th2 paradigm, most autoimmune diseases have been viewed as Th1-driven disorders.[28,31] The typical cytokine profile in Th1-mediated autoimmune diseases, such as rheumatoid arthritis, multiple sclerosis, autoimmune thyroid disease, type 1 diabetes and Crohn's disease, is an overproduction of IL-12, IFN-γ, TNF-α and under-expression of the immunoregulatory Th2 cytokine, IL-10.[28]

Most researchers recognise the oversimplicity and rigidity of the Th1:Th2 phenotypes paradigm, but as a simplistic model it is exceedingly useful and has rejuvenated enormous clinical interest and research in the field of helper T-cell immunology. However, the story continues to unfold as new and exciting research suggests much more plasticity and diversity in CD4+Tcell subsets in vivo, previously underestimated as it was not easily demonstrated in vitro.[32]

The emerging paradigm in understanding T helper cell subsets

The recent discovery of Th-17 cells uncovers a whole new arm of adaptive immunity, specific for inflammation and autoimmunity as illustrated in Figure 28.1.[24] A potent pro-inflammatory cytokine, IL-17, stimulates the production of TNF-α, IL-1β, IL-6, IL-8 and G-CSF (the colony-stimulating factor that increases neutrophils).[27]

Increased levels of Th17 cells have been found to be associated with both animal and human autoimmune diseases.[32–36] Many cytokines, such as IL-1, IL-6, IL-21, TNF-α, IL-23 and TGF-β, are known to stimulate IL-17 production from naive CD4+ T-cells in the presence of inflammatory stimuli such as toll-like receptors.[32]

Low levels of TGF-β in the presence of IL-6 and IL-21, IL-1 and IL-23 appear to stimulate IL-17 while high levels of TGF-β suppress IL-17. IL-17 is regulated by TGF-β and IL-10 both directly and indirectly via conversion of naive T-cells into Treg cells.

Toll-like receptors are pattern-recognition receptors that have evolved to recognise specific bacteria and are found on many antigen-presenting cells, such as dendritic cells, in the innate immune system. When activated, toll-like receptors induce inflammation via activation of inflammatory transcription factors such as NF-κB, which up-regulate the production of pro-inflammatory cytokines, such as IL-17 from Th17 cells and IFG-γ from Th1 cells, as shown in Figure 28.2.

Cytokines as the third signal

Recently, a 'third signal', provided by pro-inflammatory cytokines, has been postulated as a necessary requirement for full T-cell activation.[37] For instance, a soluble antigen injected into mice resulted in an increase in antigen-specific CD4+T-cells in lymph nodes and follicles. However, CD4+ cells activated in this way simply died off and did not react when re-exposed to the antigen. Although the CD4+ cells differentiated into antigen-specific T-cells in the first instance, when they received no further signal within a week after exposure to the antigen, they became hypo-responsive to the antigen on re-exposure.[37,38]

While the T-cells may differentiate they do not necessarily make the transition into a long-term, sustained adaptive immune response, as characterised not only by the proliferation of antigen-specific T-cells, but by the transition to the cloning of specific helper T-cell subsets and memory cells, which in turn influence B cells to generate antigen-specific antibodies. If, on the other hand, bacteria are present during activation, there is a sustained increase in antigen-specific T-cell cloning, along with migration of T-cells to lymph regions rich in B cells, resulting in the stimulation of antigen-specific antibodies.

An important observation was made during these studies. It was noted that the effect of the bacteria was mediated by the secretion of the cytokine, IFN-γ, from T-cells.[39]

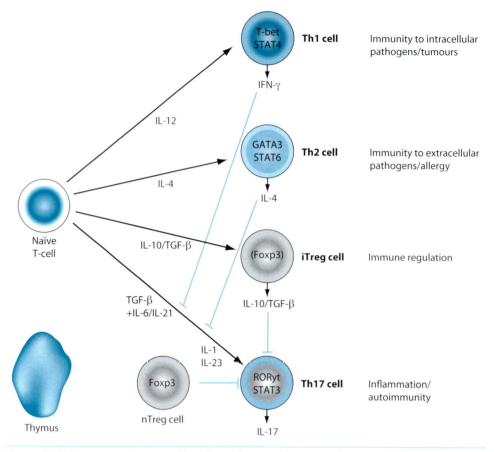

Figure 28.1 The emerging paradigm in understanding CD4+ (T helper) cell subsets, showing their respective differentiation and function.
Source: Mills 2008[32]

More importantly, the enhanced effect on T-cell activation by the bacteria was replicated when the bacteria were altogether replaced by the pro-inflammatory cytokines, tumour necrosis factors and IL-1. In addition, the bacterial-induced IFN-γ was replicated by IL-12. Thus, successful activation of T-cells in vivo after exposure to an antigen requires the presence of certain pro-inflammatory cytokines even in the absence of bacteria or other infecting agent.[39]

This 'three-signal model' has been further developed to specify IL-1 as the actual third signal for the antigen-induced activation of naive CD4+ T-cells, and IL-12 as that for CD8+ T-cells.[37] It has been proposed that the first two signals are adequate for a transient, localised response but that a long-term, sustained response depends on the presence of certain pro-inflammatory cytokines. IL-1 and TNF-α appear to have significant roles in the cytokine-driven longevity of antigen-specific memory T-cell populations.[38]

Autoreactive CD4+ T-cells
Low levels of auto-reactive (or self-reactive) CD4+ T-cells naturally circulate in the blood of healthy people and are regulated by regulatory CD4+ T (Treg) cells.[40] Naturally occurring regulatory T-cells such as CD4+CD25+ suppress the proliferation of auto-reactive T-cells and are therefore critical in the maintenance of peripheral tolerance.[41]

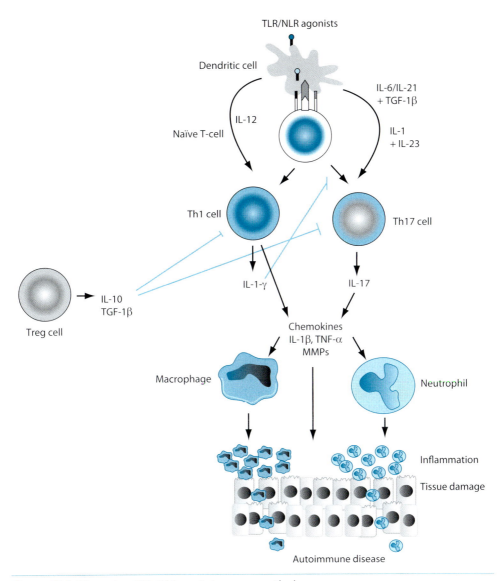

Figure 28.2 The role of Th17 in autoimmune pathology
Source: Mills 2008[32]

The regulatory cytokines IL-4, IL-10 and TFB-β are believed to be involved in the suppression of activated autoreactive T helper cells by regulatory T-cells.[42] Activation of autoreactive T helper cells and their subsequent differentiation into autoantigen-specific pro-inflammatory Th1 subsets is a pivotal step in the pathogenesis and progression of autoimmune diseases, such as multiple sclerosis.[12]

Cytokines are the signalling molecules that activate and deactivate autoreactive T-cells.[19] However, pro-inflammatory cytokines such as TNF-α, which have been heavily implicated in the pathogenesis of autoimmune diseases, have also been shown to have immunoregulatory activity. It may be that in the short term TNF-α is pro-inflammatory, but chronic exposure leads to down-regulation of the immune response.[43]

One known mechanism is via pituitary-stimulated secretion of glucocorticoids (see Section 5 on the endocrine system for discussion of the HPA axis), which may constitute a homeostatic role for TNF-α in inflammation. It may also be that other cytokines more specific to autoimmune pathology, such as IL-17, are more critical to the long-term sustained activation of the immune system as observed in autoimmune diseases.[44]

Pro-inflammatory cytokines activate local autoreactive T-cells as a normal part of the coordinated response to a threat to homeostasis, such as infection or cell damage. In some cases, however, autoreactive T-cells may induce IL-12 secretion from antigen-presenting cells in the absence of infection or other threats to homeostasis, launching an unnecessary inflammatory response and enhancing susceptibility to autoimmune disease.[30] This appears to be mediated by abnormal cytokine biology.

This approach is reflected by the new range of biological agents increasingly used in the medical treatment of autoimmune diseases (as discussed later under 'Conventional treatments') that manipulate cytokine biology. Natural approaches also utilise this strategy, as environmental factors such as the manipulation of dietary fatty acids are increasingly understood to influence cytokine biology (see a full discussion in the later section, 'Key treatment protocols').

RISK FACTORS

As work on the human genome continues, so does our knowledge of how multiple susceptibility and protective genes combine to contribute towards an autoimmune-prone phenotype.[45] However, the presence of a genetic susceptibility does not necessarily mean it will manifest as an autoimmune disease. Environmental factors may interact with genetic susceptibility to alter immunity to result in the production of autoantibodies.

Once genetically susceptible individuals have been identified, disease may be prevented, delayed or mitigated by avoiding or minimising exposure to known triggers.[46] In a large Danish cohort study involving 37,338 twins, genetic factors were found to be less important than environmental factors.[47] Environmental factors include exposure to infections and environmental chemicals but also include the internal environment, such as sex and stress hormones, and immune dysfunction.

Altered immune function

Ageing of the immune system has been associated with a decline of its ability to recognise self from non-self, thereby increasing the risk of the development of autoimmune diseases.[48] People with autoimmune diseases have immune systems that resemble those in the elderly, such as involution of the thymus, and premature ageing has been postulated as a risk factor for autoimmune disease.[49] On the other hand, young age is a risk factor for multiple sclerosis, with 70% of people with multiple sclerosis aged between 20 and 40 years.[50]

Viruses have been shown in animal models to be potent triggers of autoimmunity through molecular mimicry and promoters of pathogenic responses through bystander activation. Humans with rheumatoid arthritis and SLE have an altered virus-specific response to the Epstein-Barr virus, for example. Of particular note, the virus-specific T-cells that drive autoimmune pathology appear to be directed by cytokines rather than by the virus itself.[51] In genetically susceptible individuals, a combination of a latent Epstein-Barr viral load and altered immune regulation, for instance a functional deficit of Epstein-Barr virus-specific T-cells, may trigger rheumatoid arthritis and SLE.[52] The occurrence of chronic recurrent infections is a known risk factor for rheumatoid arthritis.[53] A partial or complete deficiency in the complement proteins is a risk factor for SLE.[54,55] Immunodeficiency, for any reason (congenital or iatrogenic), increases the risk of non-Hodgkin lymphoma. Inflammatory diseases also increase the risk of non-Hodgkin lymphoma, with more severe inflammation increasing risk further.[56] Interestingly, a prospective cohort of 27,290 postmenopausal women found that NSAID use was associated with an increased risk of non-Hodgkin lymphoma.[57] It is likely that the NSAID use indicates an unresolved underlying inflammation, which is the actual risk factor for non-Hodgkin lymphoma.

Exposure to chemicals

There is conclusive evidence that smoking is a risk factor for rheumatoid arthritis.[58] There is also evidence that mercury from dental amalgam may increase the production of autoantibodies in mercury-sensitive patients with autoimmune thyroiditis.[59] Occupational and environmental exposure to asbestos and silica, respectively, increases the risk of developing an autoimmune disease.[60,61] Occupational exposure to mineral oil increased the risk of autoimmunity by 30%.[58] Epidemiological studies that have looked at vaccinations and exposure to environmental toxins have failed to show them as strong risk factors for autoimmunity, but because there is evidence for an association in animal and case-controlled studies there has been a call for more research in this area.[62,63]

Diet and lifestyle

Many dietary and lifestyle factors may exacerbate autoimmune diseases. Early exposure to cow's milk has been associated with increased risk of autoimmune diseases, especially type I diabetes.[64] Antigens from milk, grains and legumes have also been found to contain peptides that mimic those found in the joints of people with rheumatoid arthritis.[15] Vitamin D deficiency is a risk factor for SLE and multiple sclerosis.[65] Dietary fatty acids is a possible risk factor in multiple sclerosis.[66] Sleep deprivation was shown to be a risk factor for disease in mice with a genetic susceptibility to develop SLE.[67] Ultraviolet radiation and geographic location are known risk factors for multiple sclerosis.[66]

Hormones

Sex is a risk factor for autoimmune diseases. The prevalence of many autoimmune diseases, such as multiple sclerosis, rheumatoid arthritis and SLE, are higher in women than men. For instance, 90% of SLE cases occur in women.[68] On average, women experience their first symptoms of rheumatoid arthritis during menopause, around the time of the decline of ovarian oestrogens.[69] In a randomised controlled trial of hormone replacement therapy (HRT) in rheumatoid arthritis of 200 women, those that responded well to the HRT (they had significantly increased serum oestrogen levels) demonstrated improvements in disease symptoms and progression compared with controls.[70]

Oestrogen appears to have a dual role in immune function, suppressing inflammation while stimulating antibody production.[71] Oestrogen receptors have been found on cells from many different systems, including immune cells. In a mouse model of rheumatoid arthritis, when oestrogen receptors were blocked there was an earlier onset of the disease.[72]

Phytoestrogens are very interesting compounds from plants and can produce mild oestrogenic activity in humans. One such example is quercetin from soybeans. It was demonstrated that quercetin could block antigen-specific Th 1 differentiation in neurons and ameliorate clinical severity and duration of disease in a mouse model of multiple sclerosis by binding to oestrogen receptors.[73] This suggests a potentially promising role for phytoestrogens in autoimmune disease.

Stress

Stress is a risk factor for many autoimmune diseases.[53,74,75] Stress is also known to worsen symptoms in many autoimmune diseases, particularly rheumatoid arthritis and multiple sclerosis.[76,77] Animal and human studies have linked defective neuroendocrine function with enhanced susceptibility of autoimmune diseases, such as rheumatoid arthritis, SLE, type 1 diabetes and Sjögren's syndrome.[78–81] In animal models of autoimmune disease, the onset of the disease is associated with a lack of HPA axis responsiveness (see Section 5 on the endocrine system for discussion) to IL-1, where resistance to autoimmune pathology was maintained by normal HPA axis–immune system responsiveness.[82]

CONVENTIONAL TREATMENTS

Conventional treatments focus on suppressing and managing the symptoms. Treatment will depend on the type and severity of the autoimmune disease. The conventional treatments for three major autoimmune diseases are given in Table 28.2.

Research into new drugs for autoimmune diseases are primarily focused on biological agents in inflammatory pathways.[83] In order to suppress inflammation and prevent damage, the inhibition of pro-inflammatory cytokines, especially TNF-α and IL-1, would appear to be the most useful approach.[84] However, these are new and expensive drugs, and need to be monitored for potential adverse effects.[85]

In a review of the literature comparing clinical trial outcomes to clinical practice[86] anti-TNF-α therapies were shown to produce remarkable improvements in clinical trials, reducing clinical symptoms and slowing disease progression; however, in clinical practice these improvements were found to be much more modest. It should be noted that while anti-TNF-α therapy has enjoyed spectacular success in clinical trials and modest success in clinical practice, it has also been associated with some serious side effects such as the induction of a reversible syndrome very similar to lupus (SLE is associated with the under-expression of TNF-α).[7]

Side effects from other therapeutic agents also exist; for example, long-term use of corticosteroids is associated with thinning of the skin and loss of bone mineral density. The immunosuppressant drugs (chemotherapies) are associated with highly toxic side effects, such as fatigue, nausea and vomiting, mouth ulcers and hair loss.

KEY TREATMENT PROTOCOLS

Naturopathic approaches to autoimmune conditions should aim to correct the underlying imbalance in cytokine biology in order to reduce the effect of chronic inflammation and associated tissue damage. Factors that are known to influence cytokine biology should be explored in individuals with autoimmune conditions on a case-by-case basis. In organ-specific and systemic autoimmune conditions, the tissues and organs affected should also be supported according to the details given in the relevant chapters in this book. Two key nutritional factors known to influence cytokine biology in a beneficial way are (1) **omega-3 fatty acids**, and (2) **antioxidants**. The Western diet is losing the protective antioxidants and omega-3 fatty acids, as they have been gradually processed out of the food supply over time. The loss of these protective factors, together with a gain of dietary precursors to inflammatory and pro-oxidant agents, has led to a chronic imbalance in our diet. The Western diet has effectively become a pro-inflammatory diet.

It is essential that the imbalances of the background diet be fully understood and corrected as a priority in dealing with chronic inflammation. Correcting dietary imbalances has been shown to augment medical interventions, and may reduce reliance upon them.[89,90] Dietary modifications that favour balanced immune function should, for the most part, be sustained throughout life.

Lifestyle factors must also be explored thoroughly for potential pro-inflammatory and protective influences. Pro-inflammatory influences need to be identified and minimised. Psychological stress induces an inflammatory state in the immune system by generating the production of pro-inflammatory cytokines.[91] Chronic stress results in a chronically imbalanced and under-functioning immune system (see Section 5 on the endocrine system).

The perception of stress is the net result of the perceptions of the actual stressor minus available coping resources. Potential stressors need to be identified and reduced, and available coping resources need to be increased. This may require referral for psychological counselling, meditation or relaxation training, relationship counselling, or other integrative health-care stress and mood management interventions.

Table 28.2 Conventional treatment for common autoimmune diseases[81,82,84,87]

AUTOIMMUNE CONDITION	THERAPEUTIC AGENTS	METHOD OF ACTION
Rheumatoid arthritis	Simple analgesics such as paracetamol and aspirin, and non-steroidal anti-inflammatory drugs (NSAIDs) are given in the first instance for symptomatic relief. Corticosteroids, systemic such as prednisolone Corticosteroids, local injections into single joints Disease-modifying anti-rheumatic drugs (hydroxychloroquine, gold compounds, d-penicillamine and sulfasalazine) Immunosuppressive drugs (methotrexate, leflunomide, azathioprine and cyclosporine) Cytotoxic chemotherapies, such as cyclophosphamide Biological agents, anti-cytokine therapies such as etanercept and infliximab	NSAIDs have their action by inhibition of the enzyme cyclooxygenase (COX), which releases arachidonic acid from cell phospholipids and metabolises it into prostaglandins and leukotrienes. Widespread systemic anti-inflammatory effects by binding to glucocorticoids receptors, which down-regulates inflammatory processes. Local administration of prednisolone reduces the side effects of systemic intake. Unknown mode of action but believed to slow disease progression by modifying immune system. Slow-acting drugs. Suppress immune system in various ways. Methotrexate suppresses folic acid metabolism, inhibiting the proliferation of white blood cells. Very potent immunosuppressants, as used as chemotherapies in neoplastic diseases. Block pro-inflammatory cytokine production and secretion, particularly tumour necrosis factors.
SLE	Non-steroidal anti-inflammatory drugs (NSAIDs) are given in the first instance for symptomatic relief. Antimalarials, such as hydroxychloroquine, chloroquine and quinacrine Dehydroepiandrosterone (DHEA) Immunosuppressive drugs, such as azathioprine, methotrexate, cyclosporin A, tacrolimus	COX inhibitors Interfere with the antigen-presenting ability of macrophages, down-regulating the CD4+ response to autoantigens.[88] An adrenal steroid hormone often suppressed by prednisolone; may counter some of the side effects of corticosteroids Suppress immune system in various ways. Azathioprine suppresses purine metabolism, inhibiting the proliferation of white blood cells.
Crohn's disease	Cytotoxic chemotherapies, such as cyclophosphamide	Very potent immunosuppressants, used as chemotherapies in neoplastic diseases.

(Continued)

Table 28.2 Conventional treatment for three autoimmune diseases[81,82,84,87] (*Continued*)

AUTOIMMUNE CONDITION	THERAPEUTIC AGENTS	METHOD OF ACTION
Crohn's disease (*continued*)	Anticholinergics, for symptomatic relief of cramps	Muscle relaxants; neuromuscular blocking agents
	Antidiarrhoeals, such as diphenoxylate and loperamide, for symptomatic relief of diarrhoea	Comprehensive control of diarrhoea Increase stool firmness
	Hydrophilic muciloids, such as psyllium husks and slippery elm powder	Local anti-inflammatory drugs in the colon, probably by inhibiting cyclooxygenase and lipoxygenase
	Pro-drugs, such as sufasalazine and mesalomine, which are broken down by gut flora into locally acting anti-inflammatory drugs	Anti-inflammatory effects, which reduce pain, fever and cramping.
	Corticosteroids, systemic, during acute stages Corticosteroids, locally acting, such as budesonide	Act locally in colon as anti-inflammatory, reducing side effects of systemic corticosteroid treatment.
	Broad-spectrum antibiotics, such as metronidazole (Flagyl), mainly used if there is an infected fistula or abscess Immunosuppressants, such as azathioprine, methotrexate and cyclosporine	Effective against anaerobic bacterial pathogens. Suppress immune system in various ways. Cyclosporine inhibits the release of interleukins.
	Biological agents, anti-cytokine therapies, such as the monoclonal antibody tumour necrosis factor inhibitor infliximab Surgery	IL-1 blockers, IL-12 antibodies, anti-CD4 antibodies, adhesion molecule inhibitors, anti-inflammatory cytokines, monoclonal antibody tumour necrosis factor inhibitor Bowel resection is necessary for intestinal obstruction or persistent fistula or abscesses, but does not cure the disease.

NATUROPATHIC TREATMENT AIMS

- Regulate cytokine biology:
  - reduce production of proinflammatory cytokines (TNF-α, IL-1β, IL-6, IFN-γ, IL-8, IL-17)
  - increase production of regulatory cytokines (IL-10, IL-4, TGF-β).
- Reduce oxidative stress.
- Reduce and prevent chronic infection.
- Support the affected organ or tissue (see the relevant chapters).
- Reduce low-grade systemic metabolic acidosis.
- Support HPA axis resiliency (see Section 5 on the endocrine system).
- Reduce and manage psychological, emotional and physical stress (see the sections on the nervous and endocrine systems).
- Increase capacity of cellular detoxification pathways.
- Instigate a program of moderate physical exercise.

Protective lifestyle factors need to be instigated and sustained throughout life in all individuals interested in balancing immune function, and especially those with chronic inflammation. For instance, physical exercise has a protective influence on the immune system through several known mechanisms. Interestingly, moderate physical activity actually provides an essential nutrient, glutamine, for immune cells that is stored in skeletal muscles and released through muscle contractions. Glutamine is the precursor for an essential intracellular antioxidant, glutathione, which protects the cell from damage and subsequent inflammation. Exercise also has a favourable effect on cytokine biology, inducing anti-inflammatory factors.

Research into the newly established field of psychoneuroimmunology has greatly advanced the understanding of the psychological and emotional factors that influence immune function. It is known that negative and stressful emotions directly stimulate the production of pro-inflammatory cytokines that mediate and intensify disease.[92] The idea that emotions affect health outcomes is not new and can be dated as far back as Hippocrates. What is new is that, through psychoneuroimmunology, science is providing evidence to support the 'mind–body' link.[93] Laughter,[94] meditation,[95,96] spiritual beliefs,[97] positive thinking[98] and even choir singing and listening[99] have all been shown to beneficially influence immune parameters. For more detail on this exceedingly interesting field of research, see the discussion in Chapter 6 on respiratory infections and immune insufficiency.

Dietary modulation to reduce inflammation

In human evolution, there have been two major changes that have resulted in an increased consumption of grain (the agricultural and industrial revolutions) and have dramatically increased the availability of omega-6 rich vegetable oils.[100] Further, the domestication of livestock and poultry, with its associated decrease in omega-3-rich grass feeding and increase in omega-6 rich grain-supplemented feeding, resulted in a shift in the polyunsaturated compartment of animal products to higher levels of omega-6 fatty acids and lower levels of omega-3 fatty acids.[101] During the 1960s the epidemic in coronary heart disease was attributed to the increased consumption of saturated fatty acids from animal products. High cholesterol was identified as a risk factor and every attempt was made to reduce cholesterol.[102] There was a public health campaign that declared a 'war on fat'. All Australians were urged to reduce fat consumption or at least to replace saturated fats with **omega-6 rich polyunsaturated fatty acids**, such as that from readily available vegetable oils.

Margarine was produced from vegetable oil by the partial hydrogenation of the omega-6 rich linoleic acid, which conveniently increased shelf life. The fact that commercial hydrogenation produced *trans*-isomers in the fatty acid molecule that are rarely found in nature was not considered relevant by manufacturers or health regulators at the time. *Trans*-fatty acids were cheap, easily added to pre-packaged foods and were not yet associated with heart disease, so they were ideal replacements for butter and lard.

The focus on reducing cholesterol by reducing dietary fat intake led to a new market range of 'low-fat' products. Natural products such as yoghurt were stripped of their fat content, which was replaced by a whole new range of synthetic additives, usually carbohydrate based. But this new Western diet, the combination of low fat and high carbohydrate intakes, over time has fed an epidemic of obesity and diabetes and the incidence of autoimmune diseases, especially type 1 diabetes, is rapidly rising.[103]

Carbohydrate intake in the Western diet is much higher than that of most traditional diets and there is a compelling argument that the modern high-carbohydrate diet is associated with negative health outcomes, including increased risk of various autoimmune diseases.[15] Grains may contain antinutrients, such as lectins, which not only reduce the absorption of micronutrients from the small intestine but have been shown to induce intestinal secretion of IFN-γ and up-regulate MHC class II expression in enterocytes, thereby exacerbating inflammation in coeliac disease.[104] The wheat protein gliadin was shown to inappropriately up-regulate MHC class II presentation in the presence of IFN-γ in inflammatory bowel disease.[105] Several gliadins are suspected of

DIETARY CONSIDERATIONS TO REDUCE PRO-INFLAMMATORY CYTOKINES

- Limit red meat to maximum of three meals per week.
- Reduce 'junk food', pre-packaged food, take-away meals and all foods containing vegetable oil, such as corn chips, mayonnaise and biscuits.
- Eat at least three fish meals per week, preferably oily fish.
- Reduce or eliminate the consumption of grains.
- Limit dairy intake to natural yoghurt only, with no added sugar.
- Limit simple sugars to those found naturally in fresh and dried fruits.
- Reduce salt intake, check the salt content of cans of tomatoes and tomato paste and choose 'no added salt' products.
- Snack on dried fruits and nuts.
- Have fresh vegetable juices daily.
- Cut out coffee while anxious. Replace with dandelion coffee and herbal teas.
- Virgin olive oil should replace the 'light' olive oil, which is 'light' only in the beneficial antioxidants.

molecular mimicry. Certain self-proteins, such as alpha-gliadin and the autoantigen BM 180, which has been isolated from the basement membrane of affected exocrine glands in Sjögren's syndrome, share an almost identical amino acid sequence.[15]

Low levels of **omega-3** intake, together with a high level of omega-6 intakes, creates an imbalance between n-6 and n-3 fatty acids that has been related to many modern-day diseases, from mental health problems to chronic inflammation and autoimmune disease. For instance, in habitually violent and impulsive male offenders with antisocial personality, plasma phospholipid DHA levels were significantly lower than controls, while the arachidonic acid metabolites PGE_2 and TXB_2 levels were elevated.[106] The raised level of arachidonic acid metabolites are evidence that the inflammatory pathways related to NF-κB and COX-2 have been activated, the former stimulating the up-regulation of the expression and activity of genes that code for the pro-inflammatory cytokines. According to one study,[107] the Palaeolithic diet consisted of an equal ratio of omega-6 and omega-3 fatty acids. This ratio is currently estimated at 10–15:1 in Australia, and 20–30:1 in the USA. The correction of the imbalance between the essential fatty acids has major clinical implications. For instance, the author of this study states that inflammation was reduced in patients with rheumatoid arthritis by reducing the ratio of n-6 to n-3 fatty acids to 2–3:1.

In broader evolutionary terms, the last century or two is an incredibly short period of time. While human protein-coding genes have not significantly changed, there has been a significant and dramatic change in our diet, corresponding with the rise of 'lifestyle' diseases such as chronic stress, heart disease, cancer, obesity, diabetes, depression and autoimmune diseases. Chronic inflammatory processes form an underlying component of all these diseases. Evidence is mounting that the modern Western diet, characterised by high caloric intake and high intake of carbohydrates, saturated, *trans*- and omega-6 fatty acids, and low intakes of antioxidants and omega-3 fatty acids in addition to an imbalanced omega-6:omega-3 fatty acid ratio, is a pro-inflammatory diet.

Early work in nutritional immunology showed that protein- and calorie-restricted diets were associated with dramatic and significant alterations in immune function, readily demonstrated in several animal models of autoimmune diseases.[108] In animal studies low-protein diets have delayed the onset of autoimmunity and blunted the clinical progression of autoimmune disease, and caloric restriction has more than doubled life span.[109] Protection from autoimmune disease by calorie restriction is thought to be associated with a reduction in T-cell proliferation and B-cell antigen formation when compared to a normal diet.[110] Based on these findings, a 25–40% caloric reduction has been recommended as a safe and effective preventive strategy and treatment for autoimmune diseases in humans. This is, however, a huge undertaking for most people and requires an extraordinary commitment over a very long period of time.

Caloric restriction in combination with omega-3 fatty acids has been shown to both delay the onset and improve the progression of autoimmune diseases. A proposed mechanism for omega-3 fatty acids is through up-regulation of protective antioxidant pathways, resulting in lower oxidative stress and reduced pro-inflammatory cytokine expression and activity.

Omega-3 fatty acids and the inflammatory cascade

Omega-3 fatty acids influence the production of inflammatory metabolites from the omega-6 polyunsaturated fatty acid, arachidonic acid. For instance, leukotriene B_4 (LTB_4) is derived from arachidonic acid and is a potent stimulator of pro-inflammatory cytokine production.[111] One mechanism that EPA uses to suppress pro-inflammatory cytokine production is via the suppression of the production of LTB_4.[112] Recently, the long-chain fatty acids have been shown to directly activate gene-transcription factors responsible for the regulation of gene expression and activity for cytokines, such as NF-κB and peroxisome proliferator activated receptors, respectively.

As a general rule omega-6 fatty acids promote while omega-3 fatty acids inhibit the expression, production and secretion, and target cell responsiveness, of pro-inflammatory cytokines, as illustrated in Figure 28.3.[113] When high levels of omega-6 fatty acids are present, however, the enzyme shifts its preference to favour omega-6 fatty acid metabolism.[114] This means that diets rich in omega-6 fatty acids reduce omega-3 metabolism while promoting the production of arachidonic acid derived eicosanoids.[115] Conversely, fish oil has also been shown to decrease the enzyme activity, suggesting the possibility of antagonistic inhibition of omega-6 metabolism by high levels of omega-3 fatty acids.[116] This has particular implications for vegetarians that rely on land-based omega-3 fatty acids.

Vegetarians and vegans rely heavily on the activity of these liver enzymes for the production of the long chain omega-3 fatty acids, as they do not consume them in their diet. Figure 28.4 illustrates some of the known influences on delta-6-desaturase. **Essential cofactors** include zinc, magnesium, niacin (vitamin B3), pyridoxine (vitamin B6) and vitamin C. The stress hormones, adrenaline, noradrenaline and cortisol, inhibit the enzyme as do high blood sugar levels and high levels of linoleic acid, as in the modern Western diet. DHA, as in those taking fish-oil supplements, also inhibits these enzymes, inhibiting the production of arachidonic-derived inflammatory mediators, such as prostaglandins and leukotrienes. The enzyme delta-6-desaturase is the rate-limiting step in eicosanoid synthesis (see Figure 28.4). The stress hormones cortisol and the catecholamines (adrenaline and noradrenaline) inhibit the enzyme. Dietary cofactors, such as zinc, magnesium, vitamins B3 and B6 and vitamin C are also required for optimal enzyme functioning.

Recently, the National Health and Medical Research Council (NHMRC) set targets for the daily intake of the long chain omega-3 fatty acids based on strong evidence of a protective effect from chronic disease at 610 mg for men and 430 mg for women

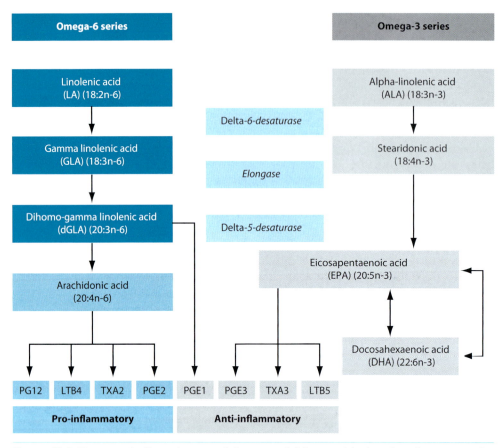

Figure 28.3 The metabolic pathways of the essential fatty acids showing the enzymatic competition for the desaturases and elongases and common food sources. Sunflower oil and most vegetable oils are rich in alpha-linolenic acid, while evening primrose oil capsules are rich in GLA, which is quickly metabolised into dGLA, a precursor for the anti-inflammatory PGE$_1$ eicosanoids.

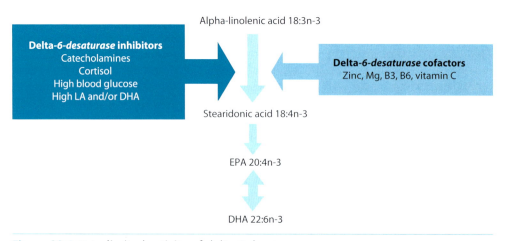

Figure 28.4 Rate-limited activity of delta-6-desaturase

(see the box below). In 2006, the Australian average intakes of omega-3 fatty acids were estimated from data collected during the 1995 National Nutrition Survey, taking into account the contribution of omega-3 fatty acids contained in red meat.[117] The average estimate for Australians was 246 mg per day, but the median daily intake was only 121 mg per day.[118] These data are alarming as they indicate that most Australians consume only about one-quarter of the daily requirements of these essential nutrients recommended for the prevention of chronic diseases.

In clinical trials, fish-oil supplements have shown beneficial outcomes in a range of autoimmune diseases. For instance, in a randomised, placebo-controlled, double-blind study of fish oil in systemic lupus erythematosus (SLE), 59 subjects were allocated into one of four groups. Subjects were given 3 × 1 g MaxEPA (180 mg EPA + 120 mg DHA) per day or 3 mg of copper (as copper di-glycinate amine acid complex) per day or both copper and fish oil or placebo (olive oil). The primary outcome measure was scores on the Systemic Lupus Activity Measure (SLAM-R), a routinely used, reliable and validated measure of disease activity. After 24 weeks of supplementation, participants in the fish-oil groups had significantly reduced scores on the SLAM-R ($p < 0.05$).[119] This study demonstrated that symptoms of SLE improved significantly compared with placebo after 6 months of high doses of fish oil.

Inhibition of nuclear factor-kappa B (NF-κB)

Nuclear transcription factor kappa B (NF-κB) is a protein that resides in the cytoplasm of B and T lymphocytes. In its latent form it is bound to an inhibitory protein (iκB). After activation by an inducer, iκB is degraded and NF-κB is released. Immediately, it moves quickly into the cell nucleus. Within minutes it up-regulates the expression of the genes for many pro-inflammatory mediators, such as the cytokines IL-2, IL-6, and IL-8. Inducers of NF-κB include, but are not limited to, the reactive oxygen species, pro-inflammatory cytokines, TNF-α and IL-1, bacteria, viruses, UV radiation, hypoxia and growth factors.[120]

Some nutritional factors may predispose an organism towards a pro-inflammatory state by up-regulation of NF-κB. **Zinc** deficiency is associated with increased NF-κB activation and subsequent increased incidences of diseases in the elderly.[121] These findings have been supported by animal studies that demonstrated that zinc was required for normal anti-inflammatory function of the cell.[122] However, some conflicting data have also been published, where zinc deficiency was shown to delay the onset and progression of autoimmune disease in early stage SLE in mice.[123] Until more research is conducted into the effects of zinc on the immune system in autoimmune disorders, it is probably best to ensure that zinc levels are within the normal range. In addition to zinc levels, normal range is also best advised for **iron** levels. Extremely low and high intakes of iron are associated with increased morbidity in mice models of SLE. While low iron levels are associated with immune dysfunction, high levels contribute to oxidative stress.[124] Both zinc and iron levels should therefore be maintained within normal range.

NHMRC OMEGA-3 GUIDELINES

- Women 430 mg/day
- Men 610 mg/day.
- Estimated intake: 121 mg/day

NF-κB is extremely sensitive to oxidative stress. Increased levels of reactive oxygen species activate NF-κB through the degradation of *i*κB, a mechanism which can be inhibited by antioxidants. Activation of NF-κB is involved in the pathogenesis of auto-immune diseases such as rheumatoid arthritis. Thus, agents which can block NF-κB activation, such as the glucocorticoids, are effective interventions in autoimmune diseases.[120] Docosahexaenoic acid (DHA) is an **omega-3 fatty acid** that was shown to block NF-κB activation.[125] Mice macrophage cells that were stimulated with the bacteria, lipopolysaccharides and IFN-γ increased NO production. Pre-treatment with various polyunsaturated fatty acids demonstrated that DHA had a marked dose-dependent inhibitory effect on NO production. The mechanism of effect for DHA was up-regulation of glutathione to a level high enough to effectively balance the oxidative stress and prevent the activation of NF-κB. It is interesting to note that the long-chain omega-3 fatty acids up-regulate antioxidant expression inside cells and assist the antioxidant protective mechanisms.

Antioxidants may mediate anti-inflammatory effects by preventing the activation of NF-κB in T-cells or via other mechanisms. The main polyphenol in **green tea**, epigallo-catechin-3-gallate (EGCG), has been shown to down regulate TNF-α gene expression and activity by preventing proteolysis of *i*κB, thus effectively blocking the activation of NF-κB. This coincided with reduced activation of autoantigen-specific T-cells in humans with multiple sclerosis.[126,127]

High levels of the **amino acids** arginine and glutamine were shown to inhibit NF-κB. In 10 patients with Crohn's disease, colonic biopsies were cultured with low or high (that is, physiological or pharmacological) amounts of arginine and glutamine, respectively. The formula with the pharmacological levels of both amino acids significantly reduced the production of the pro-inflammatory gene transcription factor NF-κB and the cytokines TNF-α, IL-1β, IL-6 and IL-8 in the culture medium.[128] The **citrus bioflavonoids** luteolin,[129] quercetin[130] and 3'-hydroxy-flavone have been shown to block activation of NF-κB.[131]

These studies indicate that there may be many nutritional factors that influence this important early stage of inflammation. This is an interesting area for the expansion of research. The most promising research thus far focuses on the inhibition of NF-κB activity by omega-3 fatty acids and various dietary antioxidants.

Antioxidants and pro-inflammatory cytokines

The build up of free radicals (reactive oxygen species) activates NF-κB to up-regulate the expression of pro-inflammatory cytokines such as TNF-α, IL-1β and IL-6. Antioxidants inhibit the production of such pro-inflammatory cytokines by blocking reactive oxygen intermediate-induced activation of NF-κB.[132] This prevents many major downstream inflammatory events, including the activation of COX-2, the subsequent production of the eicosanoids, especially LTB4, and the increased secretion of pro-inflammatory cytokines.[133]

Recent research suggests that a major underlying mechanism for the production of the pro-inflammatory cytokines as the third signal to induce a fully activated immune

ROLE OF OMEGA-3 FATTY ACIDS

Omega-3 fatty acids up-regulate antioxidants inside cells and thus prevent the activation of NF-κB.

response is via the generation of reactive oxygen species; and that disruption of the reactive oxygen species–cytokine pathway to the activation of the third signal has been shown to be an effective prevention of autoimmune disease.[134]

In a mouse model of type 1 diabetes, 10 mg/kg of antioxidants or placebo were injected several hours prior to immunisation with antigen and every day for 7 days post-immunisation. On day 8 the animals were sacrificed and spleen cells were incubated with antigen and TNF-α. The TNF-α was reduced by half in the presence of antioxidants compared with placebo. Antigen-specific T-cell proliferation and IFN-γ were also dramatically reduced compared with placebo. Spleen cells incubated in vitro with antigen demonstrated that both antigen-presenting cells and T-cells generate reactive oxygen species after exposure to an antigen, an effect that was substantially and significantly reduced by pre-treatment with antioxidants. The reduction of reactive oxygen species by antioxidants corresponded to reduced levels of TNF-α secretion from both T-cells and antigen-presenting cells. In vitro stimulation of spleen cells with antigen in the presence of TNF-α significantly reduced production of IFN-γ.[134]

Antioxidants therefore were able to substantially and significantly down-regulate the cytokine signals required for the activation of the autoimmune disease. Autoimmune-prone mice treated with antioxidants demonstrated reduced activation of naive T-cells in vivo, demonstrated by reduced levels of antigen-specific CD4+ T-cell proliferation and a 10-fold reduction of IFN-γ level in mice, compared with autoimmune prone mice that did not receive the antioxidants.[134] In autoimmune-prone mice, dietary antioxidants induced hyporesponsiveness of autoantigen-specific CD4+ T-cells, even in the presence of pro-inflammatory cytokines! Antioxidants therefore were able to prevent the full activation of an autoimmune response even in the presence of cytokine signalling.

Alpha-lipoic acid is a potent antioxidant that appears to work in a multitude of ways. It is a free radical scavenger, it regenerates other antioxidants such as vitamin C and E, and it raises intracellular glutathione. Alpha-lipoic acid is a cofactor in several enzyme systems during aerobic metabolism. As a type of fatty acid, it readily crosses cell membranes and the blood–brain barrier, and has been shown to be neuroprotective in cerebral ischaemia and other brain injury caused by free radicals.[135] Alpha-lipoic acid also has important anti-inflammatory properties.

In autoimmunity, alpha-lipoic acid has been shown to prevent the onset of disease in the mouse model of multiple sclerosis.[136] Mice were treated with alpha-lipoic acid in the drinking water from the same day the mice were inoculated with a peptide that activates myelin-specific autoreactive T-cells. When compared with controls that had only drinking water, alpha-lipoic acid mice had delayed onset of the disease and reduced severity of its progression.[137] This protective effect in clinical scores corresponded with a reduction in the infiltration of T-cells into the central nervous system and reduced demyelination of the central nervous system. In addition, a second group of mice were given alpha-lipoic acid or placebo from the onset of the first clinical signs; antigen-specific T-cells in the spleen and lymph nodes were significantly and substantially reduced by alpha-lipoic acid treatment. This demonstrates that alpha-lipoic acid is effective as both a prevention and an intervention in the animal model of multiple sclerosis.

ROLE OF ANTIOXIDANTS

Antioxidants prevented the full activation of an autoimmune response even in the presence of cytokine signalling.

While animal studies are indicative of possible therapeutic interventions, it is difficult to extrapolate these results to human studies, especially in terms of effective dosages and potential side effects. A pilot clinical trial of alpha-lipoic acid randomised subjects with multiple sclerosis into one of four treatment groups: a placebo group, and various doses of alpha-lipoic acid with 1200 mg/day as the highest dose. Subjects took the study medication before meals for 2 weeks.[138] Alpha-lipoic acid was quite well tolerated, with some reports of mild self-limiting adverse effects, such as nausea, on the gastrointestinal system. Two markers of leukocyte trafficking were used as outcome measures: matrix metalloproteinase-9 (MMP-9), which is produced by activated T-cells to facilitate leukocyte migration into the central nervous system, and intercellular adhesion molecule-1 (ICAM-1), which binds leukocytes and facilitates their migration into the brain. Stimulation of the production of MMP-9 and ICAM-1 is mediated by pro-inflammatory cytokines, and increased levels are associated with multiple sclerosis.

Alpha-lipoic acid was shown to suppress both molecules in a dose-dependent manner, with subjects on the highest dose showing the lowest levels of ICAM-1. There was also a negative correlation between peak alpha-lipoic acid serum levels and MMP-9. Therefore, this pilot study indicated that high doses of alpha-lipoic acid were able to reduce leukocyte trafficking into the brain of people with multiple sclerosis and may thus constitute a valid dietary intervention in multiple sclerosis.[136] While a pilot study does not have the statistical power to demonstrate conclusively that alpha-lipoic acid will be effective in people with multiple sclerosis, it provides good preliminary evidence of its safety and efficacy.

Genistein is an isoflavone with anti-inflammatory, antioxidant and apoptotic properties. Genistein binds to human oestrogen receptors on immune cells.[139] In a study using the mouse model for multiple sclerosis, mice were fed genistein (200 mg/kg body weight per day) for 7 days. In autopsied brain tissue, IL-12, IFN-γ and TNF-α were significantly lower and IL-10 was higher in genistein-fed mice compared with non-treated mice.[139] Thus genistein decreased inflammatory mediators and increased anti-inflammatory mediators during autoimmune pathology. This beneficial shift in cytokine biology corresponded to significant improvements in clinical signs of disease progression for the genistein-treated group, evident in less weight loss and lower total clinical score, reduced leukocyte trafficking and less endothelial adherence into the brain. Such animal studies suggest that genistein may offer effective protection at the blood-brain barrier by regulating cytokine profiles.

Quercetin is a phytoestrogenic flavanol with anti-inflammatory properties.[140] Quercetin reduced the severity and duration of paralysis as well as reductions of central nervous system demyelination and inflammation in animal models of multiple sclerosis.[73]

Resveratrol is a polyphenol compound with oestrogen-modulating, antioxidant and anti-inflammatory properties.[141] Its mechanisms of action includes inhibition of the production of pro-inflammatory cytokines and COX-2 via inhibition of NF-κB and the activator protein-1 (AP-1).[142] Resveratrol significantly delayed the onset of autoimmune pathology and halved the clinical symptoms in a dose-dependent manner in animal models. The reduction in the clinical scores corresponded with less inflammatory-related damage in the central nervous system. Pro-inflammatory cytokines in serum, including TNF-α, IFN-γ and IL-2, were reduced, but not significantly.[141] Serum IL-17 was significantly reduced in the resveratrol group, compared with placebos. Resveratrol also increased IL-6, compared with controls. Resveratrol was also found to induce cell death in activated autoreactive T-cells.[141]

In summary, promising research into the mechanisms for nutritional anti-inflammatory agents in autoimmune disease continues. Clinical trials are required to determine the optimal amount of these compounds required for effective interventions. However, it is likely that a diet rich in these and other anti-inflammatory compounds may have a cumulative effect, all helping to keep oxidative stress levels low, preventing the unnecessary activation of NF-κB and thereby keeping pro-inflammatory cytokine expression and activity at low levels. Other natural compounds, such as herbal medicines, have also been shown to have anti-inflammatory actions, many through the inhibition of NF-κB, as discussed below under 'Herbal medicine and inflammatory cytokines'. Before turning to Western herbal medicine, the anti-inflammatory effect of exercise, and the pro-inflammatory effect of psychological stress is discussed below.

Physical exercise and the immune system

There appears to be many mechanisms by which exercise mediates beneficial effects on the immune system.[143] Perhaps the most interesting is that skeletal muscle acts as a storehouse of the branched-chain amino acids, which supply nitrogen for the synthesis of glutamine by skeletal muscle. Skeletal glutamine supplies the rest of the body with glutamine as a precursor for the antioxidant, glutathione.

Cells that rapidly proliferate, such as immune cells especially during inflammation, are highly dependent on skeletal glutamine release via muscle contractions during physical exercise. This has particular implications for autoimmune diabetes, as pancreatic beta cells have reduced expression and activity of glutathione, and rely heavily on a systemic supply. Skeletal muscles release glutamine into the bloodstream after physical exercise at a very high rate.[144] Muscle contractions during physical exercise thus may offset pancreatic β-cell glutamine depletion, and subsequent increase in glutathione levels and antioxidant protective mechanisms.

Depletion of glutamine may cause the immunosuppression often observed after significant stressors such as major surgery or excessive exercise. Patients undergoing major surgery (coronary, vascular and colon) that received glutamine supplementation had significantly lower postoperative infection rates.[145] Studies using the stress of elite athletics found that glutamine supplementation immediately after a race and again 2 hours after the race protected against the immunosuppression that often follows a race.[146] In those athletes that drank the glutamine beverage, 81% reported no upper respiratory tract infection episodes in the 7 days after the race, compared with those that had the placebo drink, which contained maltodextrin, where only 49% reported no upper respiratory tract infections.

Metabolic acidosis may precipitate glutamate depletion as it increases the utilisation of glutamine in the kidney. Stress, strenuous physical exercise, starvation and major surgery are associated with depletion of plasma glutamine.[147] The stress hormones cortisol and adrenaline are both associated with increased glutamine utilisation and depletion.

Physical exercise elicits a cytokine response in the body. The type of physical exercise is a determinant of the particular cytokine response. The take-home message is that moderate physical exercise has been shown to induce anti-inflammatory cytokines (IL-1 receptor antagonist and IL-10), and offers protection against inflammation and autoimmune diseases.[148]

Psychological stress

Psychological and emotional stress increases the secretion of pro-inflammatory cytokines.[91,149–151] The clinical implications are that it is essential to address stress in order to effectively regulate cytokine biology. This may mean referral for counselling, meditation or relaxation training. Adaptogenic herbs and nutritional supplements are those that have been shown to be effective interventions in helping the organism cope with or adapt to stress. **Botanical adaptogens** and **tonics** that have received the most research attention include *Panax ginseng, Eleutherococcus senticosus,*[152–159] *Withania somnifera,*[160,161] *Bacopa monnieri*[162] and *Glycyrrhyza glabra*[163] (see the endocrine and nervous system sections for more detail). A multivitamin and mineral supplement also improved several parameters of stress in a randomised, placebo-controlled, double-blinded clinical trial.[164] **Lecithin** has demonstrated adaptogenic qualities in rats.[165] **Omega-3 fatty acids** have also been shown to inhibit cytokine production.[111,166,167]

Herbal medicine and inflammatory cytokines

Boswellia serrata has been used traditionally for treating a range of conditions, including inflammation. The anti-inflammatory agents in *Boswellia serrata* resin are the boswellic acids which have been shown to act as non-steroidal anti-inflammatory agents, inhibiting 5-lipoxygenase activity and thereby suppressing leukotriene production, such as the potent LTB4.[168–170] A systematic review of all randomised controlled trials (RCTs) of *Boswellia serrata* in inflammatory disease states has been published recently.[171] This review found seven RCTs using *Boswellia serrata* in inflammatory conditions. Of these, three were for osteoarthritis of the knee and one was for rheumatoid arthritis. The review concluded that there was 'encouraging but not compelling' evidence for the use of *Boswellia serrata* for inflammatory conditions. Adverse effects reported in the clinical trials were mild and self-limiting, and included nausea, heartburn and gastrointestinal disturbances. Although the study of rheumatoid arthritis patients did not find any significant differences between groups, the *Boswellia serrata* group reduced their NSAID use more than did the placebo group.[172] For more discussion on herbs in osteoarthritis of the knee, see Chapter 22 on osteoarthritis.

Indian trials in rheumatoid arthritis and CD demonstrated significant abatement of symptoms with administration of *Boswellia serrata* and, although the trials are difficult to obtain, they have been included in an Indian review of the literature.[173] The Indian review reported that in a series of clinical trials of moderate to severely affected patients with rheumatoid arthritis or aortic stenosis most (either bed-ridden or could not perform normal daily tasks) showed improvement in symptoms between 2 and 4 weeks of administration of *Boswellia serrata* extract.[174] When 17 patients were changed to the placebo, they all suffered re-onset of symptoms within 10 days.[173] Although it is not possible to fully evaluate the literature from a review, taken together these studies provide encouraging preliminary evidence for the use of *Boswellia serrata* as a potential intervention in autoimmune rheumatic conditions.

A note of caution: *Boswellia serrata* has been shown to inhibit in vitro all the major human drug detoxification enzymes, cytochrome P450 1A2/2C8/2C9/2C19/2D6 and 3A4 enzymes.[177] This has implications for herb–drug interactions, as these enzymes are involved in the metabolism of 95% of pharmaceutical drugs.[178] By inhibiting the metabolism of pharmaceuticals, *Boswellia serrata* may potentiate an overdose of other drugs. Until further research can clarify the clinical relevance of these interactions for therapeutic doses of *Boswellia serrata*, it may be best to avoid this herb in patients taking other medications.

Harpagophytum procumbens has been used traditionally for centuries to treat arthritic conditions, pain and a range of other conditions.[179] The extract from the roots is now a licensed medicine in Germany.[180] A thorough systematic review found there is good scientific evidence for the use of *Harpagophytum procumbens* in degenerative

HERBAL CYTOKINE MODULATION

A review article[175] showed that a number of herbs modulate one or more cytokines. While some herbs stimulated pro-inflammatory cytokine secretion, other herbs had suppressive actions on these cytokines, and some herbs were shown to do both, depending on dosage, cell type and type of stimulus.

Cytokine studies commonly use in vitro and in vivo models, so caution should be applied in extrapolating results to humans.

There are many factors that influence cytokine production, and by taking cells out of context, in vitro and ex vivo studies risk overlooking factors that regulate cytokine production in the plasma.

It is also difficult to extrapolate the human equivalent concentrations from herb concentrations that have been effective in vitro. Some herbs have been found to be suppressive at low concentrations and stimulatory at high concentrations in vitro.

Traditional herbal immune suppressants include *Hemidesmus indicus*, *Tylophora indica* and *Stephania tetrandra*.[176]

Herbal cytokine modulators are summarised in Chapter 6 on respiratory infections and immune insufficiency and in Appendix 10.

joint diseases and other chronic inflammatory diseases.[179] The key actives are the iridoid glycosides, especially harpagoside; however, the level of pharmacological activity reportedly differs significantly depending on geographical location, extraction methods and the presence of other constituents that may be synergistic or antagonistic. For instance, harpagoside was shown to inhibit COX-2 expression comparable with ibuprofen but harpagide, another pharmacologically active compound found in the extract, was shown to significantly stimulate COX-2 activity by twofold.[180] Therefore, the anti-inflammatory activity of an extract may depend on the ratios of the pharmacologically active constituents. These variables have been postulated as an explanation for inconsistency across studies aiming to demonstrate anti-inflammatory activity of extracts.[180]

The mechanism of action is not clear, but it has been shown to inhibit the secretion of the pro-inflammatory cytokines IL-1β and TNF-α, the pro-inflammatory enzymes COX-2 and iNOS, and other inflammatory mediators such as leukotriene C4, prostaglandin E2 and thromboxane B2.[181] An open study in people with rheumatic conditions in the UK aimed to assess the safety and efficacy of 960 mg (480 mg twice daily) of *Harpagophytum procumbens* in 259 patients over 8 weeks.[182] Significant improvements in global pain, stiffness and function were reported, and 66% of patients had reduced or stopped their pain medication by week 8.[182] The treatment was considered safe and well tolerated, with no serious adverse events. While this study provides evidence for its safety, the methodology used does not allow conclusions to be drawn about the efficacy of the herb, as the placebo effect was not estimated by inclusion of a control group.

A word about the safety of use: it has been reported that *Harpagophytum procumbens* is contraindicated in people with gastric and duodenal ulcer and gallstones due to its bitter taste, which increases gastric acid secretion. This would make it contraindicated in Crohn's disease and ulcerative colitis. As no data are available for pregnancy and lactation, it is best avoided during these times.[183] There is also some evidence that *Harpagophytum procumbens* may interact with anti-arrhythmic medications. In osteoarthritis studies, adverse effects were very mild gastrointestinal disturbances even at high doses (8100 mg) of extract. Most clinical trial dosages in osteoarthritis studies range from 960 mg to 2610 mg extract/day.[183]

Uncaria tomentosa has been used for centuries in Peru to support immune function.[184] It is widely used as an anti-inflammatory herb and has been shown to significantly inhibit the activation of NF-κB,[185] and inhibit the stimulated production of TNF-α by 65–85%.[186] There are two species, *U. tomentosa* and *U. guianensis*, which are used interchangeably in South America, but most Western preparations contain *U. tomentosa* due to its ease of standardisation.[187] In a study comparing the antioxidant and anti-inflammatory activity of the two species it was found that there were 35 times more alkaloids in *U. tomentosa* than in *U. guianensis*.[188] Interestingly, *U. guianensis* was the better antioxidant and stronger anti-inflammatory, challenging the widespread belief that oxindole alkaloids are responsible for its therapeutic actions. Others have identified the presence of quinic acids as having anti-inflammatory properties.[189] In a randomised, placebo-controlled, double-blinded study of freeze-dried *U. tomentosa* (1 capsule of 100 mg daily) in osteoarthritis of the knee, those taking the *U. tomentosa* had non-significant reductions in medically assessed osteoarthritis after 1 week of treatment that continued to become highly significant at the 2-week mark.[190] A review of the toxicology associated with oral administration of *U. tomentosa* noted that it had a low potential for acute toxicity.[191]

Curcuma longa and curcumin, the active constituent of *C. longa*, have demonstrated therapeutic effects in a wide range of autoimmune diseases.[192] In a randomised, placebo-controlled double-blinded clinical trial of curcumin compared with placebo in 89 patients with quiescent ulcerative colitis, 2 g/day curcumin was significantly better than placebo at preventing remissions, and improving the clinical activity index and endoscopic index.[89] Curcumin has been described as a non-steroidal anti-inflammatory agent, and found to be twice as potent as the NSAID phenylbutazone during acute inflammation, but only half as powerful during chronic inflammation.[193] Curcumin was shown to inhibit the ex vivo stimulated production of pro-inflammatory cytokines TNF-α by 58% and IL-8 by 30%.[194]

A study of 54 traditional Mexican Indian herbs found that only three were able to inhibit NF-κB, All belong to the *Asteraceae* family and are rich in sesquiterpene lactones.[195] *Tanacetum parthenium* contains high levels of the sesquiterpene lactone parthenolide, which has been shown to be anti-inflammatory by inhibiting the activation of NF-κB.[196,197] *Urtica dioica* has also been shown to be a potent inhibitor of NF-κB. A standardised extract used in Germany as a commercial drug preparation (IDS23, Rheuma-Hek) was shown to be effective as the inhibition of ex vivo TNF-α-induced NF-κB activation in human cells inhibits *i*κB degradation.[198] After oral administration of IDS23 for 7 and 21 days in 20 healthy volunteers, there was an inhibition in the ex vivo LPS stimulated TNF-α release of 14.6% and 24.0%, respectively, while IL-1β was inhibited by 19.2% and 39.3%, respectively.[199]

The leaves of *Tylophora indica* have been used in Ayurvedic medicine for the treatment of respiratory disorders such as asthma. In a series of studies comparing the effects of *Tylphora* spp. and placebo in mice after contact sensitivity with a noxious agent, *Tylphora* spp. significantly and reproducibly prevented the onset of the delayed hypersensitivity response. Although cytokines were not measured, these studies demonstrated that the mechanism of action involved suppression of cellular (T-cell) immunity.[200] For a review of studies into its effects in respiratory conditions see Chapter 6 on respiratory infections.

Hemidesmus indicus was shown to inhibit the ex vivo production of the pro-inflammatory cytokines TNF-α and IL-8 by 50%.[194] Anethole, a constituent of *Foeniculum vulgare*, has been shown to block TNF-α stimulated NF-κB activation.[201] In 14 renal patients with increased blood levels of TNF-α and reduced levels of IL-10, glomerular dysfunction and proteinuria, 900–1125 mg/day *Ganoderma lucidum* was shown to reduce TNF-α and increase IL-10 and correct renal dysfunction, including suppressing proteinuria.[202]

For a summary of a systematic review of herbal medicine on cytokines, see Appendix 2 at the end of the book.

Case Study

A 27-year-old woman has recently been **diagnosed with systemic lupus erythematosus** (SLE). She had been diagnosed after she had presented to a doctor's surgery with **fatigue, sleeping difficulties** and **increased swelling and stiffness in many joints of her hands,** with **reddish rash** over the bridge of her nose and the knuckles of her hands. Her doctor told her that her blood tests were normal except for a **high ESR** (a measure of inflammatory activity). She has been put on standard dosage of NSAIDs for her arthralgia and referred to a rheumatologist who had diagnosed SLE after finding positive serum antinuclear antibodies. She is also currently **trying to conceive,** and has some concerns about this.

SUGGESTIVE SYMPTOMS

- Female of childbearing age (↑ risk)
- Swollen and stiffness in small joints of hands in symmetrical pattern
- Butterfly-shaped rash across cheeks and nose
- Scaly disc-shaped rash on face, neck, ears, scalp, chest
- Sunlight sensitivity
- Fatigue
- Raynaud's phenomenon (digital ischaemia)
- Mouth sores, tongue sores, inside nose sores
- Chest pain (indicates serositis)

Aetiology of SLE

Systemic lupus erythematosus (SLE) is a chronic inflammatory connective tissue disease that predominately affects women of childbearing age, although men and children may also be affected. Immunologically, there is impairment in T-cell function with abnormal cytokine production—specifically the over-expression of the pro-inflammatory cytokines IL-17, IFN-γ[203] and TNF-α. Overproduction of IFN-γ has been linked with B-cell activation.[204] Autoantibody production by activated B cells results in positive serum antinuclear antibodies, often anti-DNA antibodies.

Example treatment

The patient was advised to find out more about living with lupus from appropriate support groups. She was advised to become familiar with her own early symptoms and trigger factors in order to minimise future flares. For instance, sunlight exposure may induce flares, and she reports her skin feeling strange after exposure to sun. She was encouraged to find an indoor pool and continue her swimming. Physical activity is not only good for helping deal with stress and tension, but also helps to boost the immune system. She was also advised that her condition would not necessarily affect her ability to have a baby, although she was advised to stabilise her condition before trying to conceive.

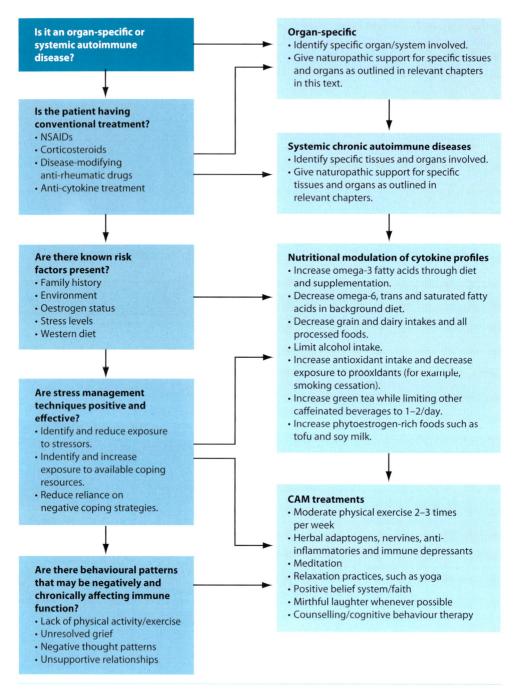

Is it an organ-specific or systemic autoimmune disease?

Organ-specific
- Identify specific organ/system involved.
- Give naturopathic support for specific tissues and organs as outlined in relevant chapters in this text.

Is the patient having conventional treatment?
- NSAIDs
- Corticosteroids
- Disease-modifying anti-rheumatic drugs
- Anti-cytokine treatment

Systemic chronic autoimmune diseases
- Identify specific tissues and organs involved.
- Give naturopathic support for specific tissues and organs as outlined in relevant chapters.

Are there known risk factors present?
- Family history
- Environment
- Oestrogen status
- Stress levels
- Western diet

Nutritional modulation of cytokine profiles
- Increase omega-3 fatty acids through diet and supplementation.
- Decrease omega-6, trans and saturated fatty acids in background diet.
- Decrease grain and dairy intakes and all processed foods.
- Limit alcohol intake.
- Increase antioxidant intake and decrease exposure to prooxidants (for example, smoking cessation).
- Increase green tea while limiting other caffeinated beverages to 1–2/day.
- Increase phytoestrogen-rich foods such as tofu and soy milk.

Are stress management techniques positive and effective?
- Identify and reduce exposure to stressors.
- Indentify and increase exposure to available coping resources.
- Reduce reliance on negative coping strategies.

CAM treatments
- Moderate physical exercise 2–3 times per week
- Herbal adaptogens, nervines, anti-inflammatories and immune depressants
- Meditation
- Relaxation practices, such as yoga
- Positive belief system/faith
- Mirthful laughter whenever possible
- Counselling/cognitive behaviour therapy

Are there behavioural patterns that may be negatively and chronically affecting immune function?
- Lack of physical activity/exercise
- Unresolved grief
- Negative thought patterns
- Unsupportive relationships

Figure 28.5 Naturopathic treatment decision tree—autoimmune disease

Stress is a trigger factor for many people with lupus, so she was advised to consider stress management techniques and/or counselling. Stress management techniques will depend on the type of stress that she is experiencing, which needs to be thoroughly teased out, and a referral for a course of counselling may be advised (see the referral section). Yoga and meditation practices would be a great way to re-learn how to relax in the body, as yoga may help to strengthen muscles and meditation would help to calm the mind.

Dietary modifications were the primary intervention for the first consultation. The fatty acid profile in the background diet was manipulated in order to reduce production of arachidonic acid inflammatory metabolites and the pro-inflammatory cytokines. Herbal medicines were also prescribed to support her through the period of increased stress (*Glycyrrhiza glabra*) and also to help reduce the chronic inflammation (*Boswellia serrata*, *Harpagophytum procumbens*, *Hemidesmus indicus* and *Uncaria tomentosa*). The combination of herbs, diet and exercise would be assessed at another consultation, scheduled for 1 month's time.

Herbal prescription

Uncaria tomentosa 1:2	30 mL
Harpagophytum procumbens 1:2	30 mL
Hemidesmus indicus 1:2	25 mL
Glycyrrhiza glabra 1:1	15 mL
5 mL t.d.s. before meals	100 mL

Boswellia complex tablets containing *Boswellia serrata*, turmeric, ginger, celery seed. Take 4 per day for 1 month, then review.

Teas

Green tea 3–4 cups per day
Dandelion coffee 1–2 cups per day

Nutritional prescription

Fish oil high strength (+ vitamin E) 4 g EPA + DHA per day
Multivitamin + mineral 1 per day
Alpha-lipoic acid 1000 mg 1 per day
All supplements to be taken with meals (preferably breakfast) to facilitate absorption. To be reviewed in 1 month.

INTEGRATIVE MEDICAL CONSIDERATIONS

Counselling

The patient was referred for counselling for support in dealing with stress relating to her diagnosis and family planning issues. Strong emotions usually accompany such a diagnosis but must be managed as chronic stress and depression can lead to deterioration of the condition in terms of increasing inflammation and the risk of flares.[205] Education about how to manage the disease, the medications and the role of emotions can help to cope with the diagnosis.[206]

Daily stress events have been shown to worsen symptoms of lupus more so than significant life events.[207] The patient was counselled on new ways of dealing with daily stress and distress through these sessions.

A brief pain and stress management program incorporating biofeedback and cognitive behaviour therapy was significantly more effective than symptom monitoring (placebo) or usual care (no intervention controls) at reducing pain and physical symptoms in 92 SLE patients in an American randomised, placebo-controlled trial.[208] Psychological functioning was improved in the active intervention group compared with placebo, while the usual care group (controls) actually deteriorated over time.

Physical exercise

The patient was recommended to think about getting fit on her own or getting a personal trainer to help her to develop an aerobic training program. In chronic inflammatory diseases, the conventional acute management strategy is to rest and medicate. However, in chronic diseases that wax and wane, it is important during times of remission to build muscle strength and increase range of motion.[209] Exercise should start as low-impact and gradually increase. The specific type of exercise is not important; instead a range of types incorporating aerobic and anabolic should be encouraged. It should start with stretching and gradually be built up.

Most women with SLE suffer from poor quality of sleep, contributed to by corticosteroid use, lack of exercise and depressed mood.[210] A clinical trial of a supervised exercise program showed significant improvement in quality of life, depression and aerobic fitness in 60 women with SLE that participated in either the training group (60 minutes' supervised training, three mornings per week for 12 weeks) or controls (did not participate in the training program).[211] The training session consisted of 10 minutes warm-up and stretching, 40 minutes walking and 10 minutes of cooling down. There is good preliminary evidence that physical exercise can help in a range of symptoms associated with SLE.[212] Exercise also improves mood outcomes.[213]

> **NATUROPATHIC TREATMENT AIMS**
> - Reduce inflammation:
>   - Reduce proinflammatory cytokine production.
>   - Reduce oxidative stress.
>   - Reduce psychological stress.
> - Prevent flare-ups:
>   - Identify and avoid known triggers.
> - Increase wellbeing:
>   - Increase physical exercise.
>   - Increase relaxation or meditation practice.

Homoeopathy

In a *Lancet* published meta-analysis of homoeopathy in clinical trials there was an overall trend towards an effect for homoeopathy.[214] Many people with autoimmune diseases believe that homoeopathy may be helpful. In a survey of 413 people with inflammatory bowel disease, 52% had tried CAM, and homoeopathy was the most frequently used (55% of CAM users).[215] A survey of people with multiple sclerosis showed a similar trend.[216] Part of the reasons for the common use of homoeopathy seems to be dissatisfaction with conventional treatment and its side effects, and the fact that homoeopathy can be used alongside conventional medicine.[217]

In a randomised, placebo-controlled trial of 112 patients using homoeopathy in rheumatoid arthritis, there were significant improvements in pain (18%) and articular index (24%) for both the placebo and active group. There was a huge drop-out rate in the 6-month study, causing some methodological issues. Most of the homoeopathic prescriptions were for Sulphur 30C and Rhus Tox 6C and 30C.[218] In an earlier, randomised, controlled trial using homoeopathy or placebo in rheumatoid arthritis in patients that were also using their own medication, those in the homoeopathy group had significant improvement in pain, articular index, stiffness and grip compared with the placebo group.[219]

This body of research is promising and provides some preliminary evidence for an effect for homoeopathy. There is obviously a need for much more research into the efficacy of homoeopathy in autoimmune conditions. These conditions are complex and require multifaceted approaches. Perhaps there is a role for homoeopathy, which may one day be validated with much stronger evidence than we have today.

Expected outcomes and follow-up protocols

The diagnosis of a chronic autoimmune disease, such as SLE, can be a stressful and disempowering experience. Empowerment through education and self-help strategies has been shown to improve outcomes for people with SLE on a range of parameters including feelings of uncertainty, self-worth and depression.[220] The major strategies that need to be monitored and continued are the stress management, the dietary modifications, the anti-inflammatory herbal intervention, the gradual build-up of aerobic fitness and the regular relaxation or meditation practice. Other activities that reduce stress and have beneficial outcomes on immune parameters should also be encouraged, such as laughter, meditation and activities such as choir singing and listening.

Most of the medications used to treat SLE involve a multitude of serious side effects that have to be monitored and minimised if possible. For instance NSAIDs are COX inhibitors, but cyclooygenase (COX) has two isoforms. The inhibition of COX-1 is associated with the serious side effects, particularly to the gut mucosa, causing nausea, and may lead to ulceration, which may be asymptomatic or may cause bleeding.[87] Some of these side effects are noted in the box above.[221] These effects may be minimised using slippery elm powder and probiotic supplementation. The traditional way is to take a teaspoon of slippery elm in yoghurt before breakfast.

During infection and inflammation, however, it is COX-2 that is substantially raised. COX-2 plays a key role in the mediation of inflammation in autoimmune diseases. Pro-inflammatory mediators are known to induce COX-2 and raise prostaglandin synthesis. It is COX-2 that the anti-inflammatory steroid hormones (the glucocorticoids) suppress. NSAIDs that selectively inhibit COX-2 inhibitors are just as effective as the traditional non-selective COX inhibitors, but without the serious side effects.[87] Further, small bowel permeability ('leaky gut') has been shown to be increased by the COX-1 inhibitors, but remains unaffected by COX-2 inhibitors.[87] Where possible, therefore, COX-2 inhibitors are the NSAID of choice.

A note of caution about COX-2 inhibitors is that the long-term use of certain COX-2 inhibitors is associated with increased risk of primary heart attacks and stroke (in people with no previous history of heart disease) and hence certain COX-2 drugs were withdrawn from the market in 2004–5.[222] Fortunately, it has been demonstrated that these complications can be reduced by combining fish-oil supplementation with COX-2 inhibitors.[223]

Lupus flares

Close management of flares should also be followed up. Has the patient experienced a flare since the last visit? What were the symptoms and what events preceded it? If it is possible (and it is not always) to identify the triggers of a flare, the triggers can be avoided in the future.

Many people with lupus experience periods when the symptoms return, or the disease 'flares' up. Indeed, 11% of all hospital admissions in the USA are due to SLE or lupus flares.[224] What causes them is not clear. One study set out to see whether T-cell activation could predict them. In a 4-year follow-up study, 60 patients (57 females) with SLE were tested at baseline for a urinary marker of a T-cell proliferation (T-bet).[225] By the 4-year mark 46.6% had experienced a flare; 28% were severe (organ involvement). Those with high urinary T-bet were eight times more likely to have a flare.

This study demonstrated that T-cell activation preceded a lupus flare. The T-cells were being activated long before the clinical manifestations appeared. This suggests that managing immune cell parameters to reduce the incidence of inflammation is of paramount

SIDE EFFECTS OF NSAIDs

- Nausea
- Vomiting
- Diarrhoea
- Cramping
- Abdominal pain
- Constipation
- Rash
- Dizziness
- Headache
- Drowsiness
- Tinnitus

importance in attempting to prevent flares. The protocol outline above aims to reduce inflammation. During periods of increased inflammation, these protocol should be strictly adhered to.

It is an important aspect of each individual's journey with lupus to identify the triggers that may combine to cause a flare. It may be useful to keep a journal for a while until some trigger factors become known. Most often they are lifestyle factors such as stress, infection, sunlight and some medications.[226]

The patient was advised to develop a strategy to deal with fatigue in order to minimise the risk of a flare. It is important to not get over-tired, to pay attention to the body signals and to rest often.[226] It was advised that the patient start a yoga or meditation practice and instigate a discipline of practice for 1 hour every morning and 1 hour every evening. This may mean a major restructuring of the patient's day and life to fit this in, but its importance must not be underestimated. The patient was also encouraged to build aerobic fitness by starting an exercise training program and building up to at least 30 minutes three times per week.

There is a known seasonal variation to lupus flares, with exposure to extremes of temperature best avoided to minimise the risk of flare.[227] Sunlight exposure is another known trigger of flare and can be minimised by wearing protective clothing and sunscreen. The patient was advised to cover up when walking or jogging outside in summer and to go early in the morning or later in the afternoon to avoid the midday sun. Similarly, sunscreen should be used while swimming outside.

Reducing infections

Infections may be viral, bacterial, fungal or parasitic, and acute or chronic.[228] Patients on immune-suppressive drugs and some patients with SLE are genetically more susceptible to opportunistic infections.[229] Chronic infections such as hepatitis C should be closely monitored.

Periodontal disease and gum infections should be considered and carefully managed. Mouth ulcers should be dealt with immediately. They are generally taken as a sign that the immune system is struggling but if they do not respond within days to zinc and vitamin C treatment, teaspoons of medical honey and herbal antibacterial mouthwashes, they may be a sign of an underlying infection. In SLE, high temperature or fever is a warning sign of infection, which increases the risk of flare.

It has to be stressed that all infections should be treated immediately. See Chapter 6 on respiratory infections for advice on treating respiratory tract infections, and Chapter 27 for advice on urinary tract infections and the fungal infection, candida. Probiotics may need to be supplemented from time to time to ensure healthy bowel flora and help to prevent infections. If the patient does not respond quickly to herbal medicine treatment (within a few days), then medical treatment for antibiotics may be required to reduce the risk of endocarditis (inflammation of the heart valves).[230] Sulfur antibiotics should be avoided as they are known to cause allergic reactions in 30% of SLE patients, and increase photosensitivity and skin rash.[230]

WARNING SIGNS AND SYMPTOMS OF A LUPUS FLARE-UP

- Increased fatigue
- Increased pain in joints
- Skin rash
- Sensitivity to the sun
- High temperature
- Mouth ulcers
- Headache
- Dizziness
- Abdominal discomfort

Infection in the SLE patient requires a much more rigorous approach than people without the disease. It may be prudent to refer early to a GP for antibiotics if a bacterial infection is suspected, as the consequences of an untreated infection can be devastating. The side effects of antibiotic therapy on the gut flora should be minimised by simultaneous supplementation with probiotics (see Section 1 on the gastrointestinal system). Every attempt should be made to avoid infection (see the box below for some ideas of prevention strategies).[230]

Pregnancy is known to trigger lupus flare in around 60% of women.[231,232] The patient was advised that, in women with stable SLE, pregnancy is safe for mother and child, although it does increase the risk of a flare.[233] Pregnancy requires a management strategy commencing with an assessment of pre-gestational risk factors before conception. In most cases of a lupus flare during pregnancy, the disease can be successfully managed under medical supervision with a multidisciplinary approach.[234] Hospitalisation may be required during the pregnancy. The miscarriage rate is about one in five in SLE, as opposed to one in 10 for normal pregnancies.[235] The contraceptive pill, on the other hand, has been shown in a double-blind, randomised, placebo-controlled clinical trial of 183 women using the lupus flare as the end point to *not* trigger a flare.[236]

Stress and infections may exacerbate a flare-up of disease activity. It is important for prevention of a flare that people living with SLE take every precaution to minimise these and other environmental triggers that may lead to an increased risk of a flare. If the patient follows the above detailed prescription, her condition is expected to gradually improve over the course of weeks and months. Autoimmune conditions often wax and wane in presentation, so it is important to counsel the patient that, while progress may be being made, there is a likely chance of an exacerbation at some point. Although complete remission is the ultimate goal, a more modest outcome is the lessening of the severity of symptoms, a reduction in the frequency of flares and an overall enhancement of the person's health and wellbeing.

REDUCING RISK OF INFECTION

- Wash hands before touching food and after touching people or animals.
- Avoid touching used dishcloths and other items that may contain bacteria.
- Avoid people with an infection, and avoid crowds.
- Avoid buildings with airconditioning.
- Take temperature daily to establish a normal baseline

Table 28.3 Review of the major evidence

INTERVENTION	KEY LITERATURE	SUMMARY OF RESULTS	COMMENT
Omega-3 fatty acids	Fortin et al. 1995:[237] American meta-analysis on fish oil in RA in 368 patients	3 months' supplementation significantly reduced morning stiffness (rate difference RD [95% CI] = −25.9 [−44.3 to −7.5] [$p < 0.01$]) and tender joint count [RD][95% CI] = −2.9 [−3.8 to −2.1][$p = 0.001$]) and as compared with heterogeneous dietary control oils.	This is the highest level of evidence and demonstrates conclusively that 3 months' supplementation with fish-oil supplements can cause a modest reduction in joint tenderness and a substantial reduction in morning stiffness.

(Continued)

Table 28.3 Review of the major evidence (*Continued*)

INTERVENTION	KEY LITERATURE	SUMMARY OF RESULTS	COMMENT
Omega-3 fatty acids	James and Cleland 1997:[90] Australian review of 12 randomised controlled clinical trials of fish oil in RA.	Found good evidence for modest beneficial effects of fish oils in RA. A possible confound that may underestimate the size of the effect is that most studies do not control for omega-6 levels in background diet.	In clinical practice, background dietary omega-6 levels should be considered when recommending fish-oil supplements or a high omega-3 diet.
Omega-3 fatty acids	Duffy et al. 2004:[119] Canadian double-blind, double-placebo-controlled trial on 3 × 1 g MaxEPA (180 mg EPA + 120 mg DHA) in 52 patients with SLE for 6 months	Significant improvement in disease activity compared with controls (Systemic Lupus Activity Measure (SLAM-R) score of 6.12 to 4.69 ($p < 0.05$)). There were no changes in immunological markers between the groups.	Researchers concluded that fish oil was beneficial for symptomatic relief.
Curcumin	Hanai et al. 2006:[89] Japanese randomised, multicentre, double-blind, placebo-controlled trial in 89 patients with quiescent UC, 2 g/day curcumin or placebo alongside usual medications (sulfasalazine or mesalamin) for 6 months	Prevents remissions and improves the clinical activity index and endoscopic index compared with placebo ($p < 0.05$).	This was a good study demonstrating that curcumin is a safe and effective complementary therapy in the prevention of relapse in people with UC.
Alpha lipoic acid	Yadav et al. 2005:[138] American pilot randomised-control trial in 37 patients with multiple sclerosis taking various amounts of alpha-lipoic acid ranging from 600 mg/day to 2400 mg/day for 2 weeks	1200 mg/day reduced two immunologic markers of multiple sclerosis activity (serum MMP-9 ($p = 0.04$) and sICAM-1 ($p = 0.03$)) which are indirectly associated with T-cell migration into the central nervous system.	Although a pilot study, these results provide good preliminary evidence for the safety and efficacy of lipoic acid as an intervention in people with multiple sclerosis.
Boswellia serrata	Sander et al. 1998:[172] Double-blind pilot study in outpatients with RA	Reduced use of NSAIDs in *Boswellia serrata* group compared to controls 5.8% (*Boswellia serrata*) and 3.1% (placebo).	Pilot study does not have the statistical power to find a significant effect. Abstract only available in English so cannot study methodology to work out the sample size, the primary outcome measures and other issues that may have confounded the results.

(*Continued*)

Table 28.3 Review of the major evidence (*Continued*)

INTERVENTION	KEY LITERATURE	SUMMARY OF RESULTS	COMMENT
Harpagophy-tum procumbens	Warnock et al. 2007:[182] UK open study of 960 mg (480 mg twice daily) in 259 patients with rheumatic disease over 8 weeks	Improvements in global pain, stiffness and function ($p < 0.0001$) and 66% of patients had reduced or stopped their pain medication by week 8.	The treatment was considered safe and well tolerated, with no serious adverse events. While this study provides evidence for its safety, the methodology used does not allow conclusions to be drawn about the efficacy of the herb, as the placebo effect was not estimated by inclusion of a control group.

KEY POINTS

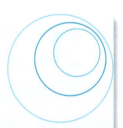

- Increase levels of omega-3s, preferably from marine sources.
- Decrease levels of omega-6s in the diet by reducing intake of products containing vegetable oils.
- Decrease oxidative stress by ensuring plenty of antioxidants in the diet.
- Decrease low-grade metabolic acidosis by moving towards the Palaeolithic diet—basically minimise intake of salt, grains and dairy.
- Increase physical exercise to release endorphins, antioxidant precursors and antiinflammatory cytokines, at least 30 minutes three times per week.
- Practise relaxation or meditation every day, at least 30 minutes per day.

Further reading

Brown AC. Lupus erythematosus and nutrition: a review of the literature. J Ren Nutr [Review] 2000;10(4):170–183.

Lupus Association, NSW. http://www.lupusnsw.org.au/

Lupus Foundation of America, Inc. http://www.lupus.org

Petri M. Treatment of systemic lupus erythematosus: an update. Am Fam Physician 1998;57(11):2753–2760.

Vliet Vlieland TPM. Non-drug care for RA—is the era of evidence-based practice approaching? Rheumatology (Oxford) [Review] 2007;46(9):1397–1404.

Wallace DJ. The lupus book. 3rd edn. New York: Oxford University Press, 2005.

References

1. Brickman CM, Shoenfeld Y. The mosaic of autoimmunity. Scand J Clin Lab Invest 2001;61(7):3–15.
2. Shoenfeld Y, et al. The mosaic of autoimmunity: hormonal and environmental factors involved in autoimmune diseases—2008. Isr Med Assoc J 2008;10(1):8–12.
3. Kuek A, et al. Immune-mediated inflammatory diseases (IMIDs) and biologic therapy: a medical revolution. Postgrad Med J 2007;83(978):251–260.
4. Kumar P, Clark M, eds. Clinical medicine. 5th edn. London: W.B. Saunders, 2002.
5. Porth CM. Pathophysiology: concepts of altered health states. 4 edn Philadelphia: J.B. Lippincott Company, 1994.
6. GPnotebook. Major histocompatibility antigen class II. Online. Available: http://www.gpnotebook.co.uk/simplepage.cfm?ID = -328531924&linkID = 21624&cook = yes. Accessed 4 February 2009.
7. Davidson A, Diamond B. Autoimmune diseases. N Engl J Med 2001;345(5):340–350.
8. GPnotebook. Hashimoto's thyroiditis. Online. Available: http://www.gpnotebook.co.uk/simplepage.cfm?ID = 342556680. Accessed 4 February 2009.

9. Ramagopalan SV, et al. Expression of the multiple sclerosis-associated MHC class II Allele HLA-DRB1*1501 is regulated by vitamin D. PLoS Genet 2009;5(2):e1000369.

10. Mackay IR. Science, medicine, and the future: tolerance and autoimmunity. BMJ 2000;321(7253):93–96.

11. Hill N, Sarvetnick N. Cytokines: promoters and dampeners of autoimmunity. Curr Opin Immunol 2002;14(6):791–797.

12. Sospedra M, Martin R. Immunology of multiple sclerosis. Annu Rev Immunol 2005;23(1):683–747.

13. Blass S, et al. The immunologic homunculus in rheumatoid arthritis. Arthritis Rheum 1999;42(12):2499–2506.

14. Head KA, Jurenka JS. Inflammatory bowel disease part 1: ulcerative colitis—pathophysiology and conventional and alternative treatment options. Altern Med Rev 2003;8(3):247–283.

15. Cordain L. Cereal grains: humanity's double-edged sword. World Rev Nutr Diet 1999;84:19–73.

16. Heyman M, Desjeux JF. Cytokine-induced alteration of the epithelial barrier to food antigens in disease. Ann N Y Acad Sci 2000;915:304–311.

17. Dimitrov JD, et al. Insight into the mechanism of the acquired antibody auto-reactivity. Autoimmun Rev 2008;7:410–414.

18. Frassetto L, et al. Diet, evolution and aging—the pathophysiologic effects of the post-agricultural inversion of the potassium-to-sodium and base-to-chloride ratios in the human diet. Eur J Nutr 2001;40(5):200–213.

19. Falcone M, Sarvetnick N. Cytokines that regulate autoimmune responses. Curr Opin Immunol 1999;11(6):670–676.

20. Grimble RF. Nutritional modulation of cytokine biology. Nutrition 1998;14(7–8):634–640.

21. Pert C. Molecules of emotion. USA: Simon & Schuster, 1997.

22. Leonard B. Stress and the immune system: immunological aspects of depressive illness. In: Schmoll HJ, Tewes U, eds. Psychoneuroimmunology—interactions between brain, nervous system, behaviour, endocrine and immune system. New York: Hogrefe & Huber Publishers, 1999:114–136.

23. Germain RN. T-cell development and the CD4-CD8 lineage decision. Nat Rev Immunol 2002;2(5):309–322.

24. Weaver CT, et al. IL-17 family cytokines and the expanding diversity of effector T cell lineages. Annu Rev Immunol 2007;25(1):821–852.

25. Swain SL. T cell subsets and the recognition of MHC class. Immunol Rev 1983;74(1):129–142.

26. Zola H, et al. CD molecules 2005: human cell differentiation molecules. Blood 2005;106(9):3123–3126.

27. Merck. Components of the immune system. Online. Available: http://www.merck.com/mmpe/sec13/ch163/ch163b.html#. Accessed 13 February 2009.

28. Elenkov IJ, et al. Cytokine dysregulation, inflammation and well-being. Neuroimmunomodulation 2005;12:255–269.

29. McEwen BS, et al. The role of adrenocorticoids as modulators of immune function in health and disease: neural, endocrine and immune interactions. Brain Res Brain Res Rev 1997;23(1–2):79–133.

30. Chang JT, et al. Regulation of interleukin (IL)-12 receptor beta 2 subunit expression by endogenous IL-12: a critical step in the differentiation of pathogenic autoreactive T cells. J Exp Med 1999;189(6):969–978.

31. O'Shea JJ, et al. Cytokines and autoimmunity. Nat Rev Immunol 2002;2(1):37–45.

32. Mills KHG. Induction, function and regulation of IL-17-producing T cells. Eur J Immunol 2008;38(10):2636–2649.

33. Annunziato F, et al. Phenotypic and functional features of human Th17 cells. J Exp Med 2007;204(8):1849–1861.

34. Daniels MD, et al. Recombinant cardiac myosin fragment induces experimental autoimmune myocarditis via activation of Th1 and Th17 immunity. Autoimmunity 2008;41(6):490–499.

35. Gaffen SL. An overview of IL-17 function and signaling. Cytokine 2008;43(3):402–407.

36. Ogura H, et al. Interleukin-17 promotes autoimmunity by triggering a positive-feedback loop via interleukin-6 induction. Immunity 2008;29(4):628–636.

37. Curtsinger JM, et al. Inflammatory cytokines provide a third signal for activation of naive CD4+ and CD8+ T cells. J Immunol 1999;162(6):3256–3262.

38. Vella AT, et al. CD28 engagement and proinflammatory cytokines contribute to T cell activation and long-term survival in vivo. J Immunol 1997;158(10):4714–4720.

39. Pape KA, et al. Inflammatory cytokines enhance the in vivo clonal expansion and differentiation of antigen-activated CD4+ T cells. J Immunol 1997;159(2):591–598.

40. Danke NA, et al. Autoreactive T cells in healthy individuals. J Immunol 2004;172(10):5967–5972.

41. Piccirillo CA, et al. CD4+Foxp3+ regulatory T cells in the control of autoimmunity: in vivo veritas. Curr Opin Immunol 2008;20(6):655–662.

42. Maloy KJ, Powrie F. Regulatory T cells in the control of immune pathology. Nat Immunol 2001;2(9):816–822.

43. Cope AP. Regulation of autoimmunity by proinflammatory cytokines. Curr Opin Immunol 1998;10(6):669–676.

44. Strom TB, Koulmanda M. Cytokine related therapies for autoimmune disease. Curr Opin Immunol 2008;20(6):676–681.

45. Cooper GS, et al. The role of genetic factors in autoimmune disease: implications for environmental research. Environ Health Perspect 1999;107(Suppl. 5):693–700.

46. Nancy AL, et al. Prediction and prevention of autoimmune skin disorders. Arch Dermatol Res 2009;301(1):57–64.

47. Svendsen AJ, et al. Relative importance of genetic effects in rheumatoid arthritis: historical cohort study of Danish nationwide twin population. BMJ 2002;324(7332):264.

48. Prelog M. Aging of the immune system: a risk factor for autoimmunity? Autoimmun Rev 2006;5(2):136–139.

49. Thewissen M, et al. Premature immunosenescence in rheumatoid arthritis and multiple sclerosis patients. Ann N Y Acad Sci 2005;1051:255–262.

50. University of Maryland Medical Center. Multiple sclerosis—risk factors. Online. Available: http:www.umm.edu/patiented/articles/who_gets_multiple_sclerosis_000017_5.htm

51. Münz C, et al. Antiviral immune responses: triggers of or triggered by autoimmunity? Nat Rev Immunol 2009;9(4):246–258.

52. Niller HH, et al. Regulation and dysregulation of Epstein-Barr virus latency: implications for the development of autoimmune diseases. Autoimmunity 2008;41(4):298–328.

53. Cutolo M, Straub RH. Stress as a risk factor in the pathogenesis of rheumatoid arthritis. Neuroimmunomodulation 2006;13(5–6):277–282.

54. Atkinson JP. Complement deficiency. Predisposing factor to autoimmune syndromes. Am J Med 1988;85(6A):45–47.

55. Tsutsumi A, et al. Mannose binding lectin: genetics and autoimmune disease. Autoimmun Rev 2005;4(6):364–372.

56. Grulich AE, et al. Altered immunity as a risk factor for non-Hodgkin lymphoma. Cancer Epidemiol Biomarkers Prev 2007;16(3):405–408.

57. Cerhan JR, et al. Association of aspirin and other non-steroidal anti-inflammatory drug use with incidence of non-Hodgkin lymphoma. Int J Cancer 2003;106(5):784–788.

58. Yavari N, et al. What role do occupational exposures play in RA? Studies have found significant associations and increased risk. J Musculoskeletal Med 2008;25(3):130.

59. Bártová J, et al. Dental amalgam as one of the risk factors in autoimmune diseases. Neuro Endocrinol Lett 2003;24(1–2):65–67.

60. Noonan CW, et al. Nested case-control study of autoimmune disease in an asbestos-exposed population. Environ Health Perspect 2006;114(8):1243–1247.

61. Parks CG, et al. Occupational exposure to crystalline silica and autoimmune disease. Environ Health Perspect 1999;107(Suppl. 5):793–802.

62. Chen RT, et al. Epidemiology of autoimmune reactions induced by vaccination. J Autoimmun 2001;16(3):309–318.

63. Mayes MD. Epidemiologic studies of environmental agents and systemic autoimmune diseases. Environ Health Perspect 1999;107(Suppl. 5):743–748.

64. Dow CT. Paratuberculosis and type I diabetes: is this the trigger? Med Hypotheses 2006;67(4):782–785.

65. Kamen DL, Aranow C. The link between vitamin D deficiency and systemic lupus erythematosus. Curr Rheumatol Rep 2008;10(4):273–280.

66. Coo H, Aronson KJ. A systematic review of several potential non-genetic risk factors for multiple sclerosis. Neuroepidemiology 2004;23(1–2):1–12.

67. Palma BD, et al. Effects of sleep deprivation on the development of autoimmune disease in an experimental model of systemic lupus erythematosus. Am J Physiol Regul Integr Comp Physiol 2006;291(5):R1527–R1532.

68. Beers MH, Berkow R, eds. The Merck manual of diagnosis and therapy. 17th edn New Jersey: Merck Research Laboratories, Division of Merck & Co., Inc., 1999.

69. Goemaere S, et al. Onset of symptoms of rheumatoid arthritis in relation to age, sex and menopausal transition. J Rheumatol 1990;17(12):1620–1622.

70. Hall GM, et al. A randomised controlled trial of the effect of hormone replacement therapy on disease activity in postmenopausal rheumatoid arthritis. Ann Rheum Dis 1994;53(2):112–116.

71. Carlsten H, Carlsten H. Immune responses and bone loss: the estrogen connection. Immunol Rev 2005;208:194–206.

72. Jansson L, Holmdahl R. Enhancement of collagen-induced arthritis in female mice by estrogen receptor blockage. Arthritis Rheum 2001;44(9):2168–2175.

73. Muthian G, Bright JJ. Quercetin, a flavonoid phytoestrogen, ameliorates experimental allergic encephalomyelitis by blocking IL-12 signaling through JAK-STAT pathway in T lymphocyte. J Clin Immunol 2004;24(5):542–552.

74. Klecha AJ. Immune-endocrine interactions in autoimmune thyroid diseases. Neuroimmunomodulation 2008;15(1):68–75.

75. Matos-Santos A, et al. Relationship between the number and impact of stressful life events and the onset of Graves disease and toxic nodular goitre [see comment]. Clin Endocrinol (Oxf) 2001;55(1):15–19.

76. Gold SM, et al. Stress and disease progression in multiple sclerosis and its animal models. Neuroimmunomodulation 2006;13(5–6):318–326.

77. Chida Y, et al. Social isolation stress exacerbates autoimmune disease in MRL/LPR mice. J Neuroimmunol 2005;158(1–2):138–144.

78. Sternberg EM. Neuroendocrine regulation of autoimmune/inflammatory disease. J Endocrinol 2001;169(3):429–435.

79. Jara LJ, et al. Immune-neuroendocrine interactions and autoimmune diseases. Clin Dev Immunol 2006;13(2–4):109–123.

80. Homo-Delarche F. Neuroendocrine immuno-ontogeny of the pathogenesis of autoimmune disease in the nonobese diabetic (NOD) mouse. ILAR J 2004;45(3):237–258.

81. Kumar R, et al. Immunoregulatory role of stress mediators in rheumatoid arthritis. Z Rheumatoly 1981;40:122–125.

82. Sternberg EM, et al. Inflammatory mediator-induced hypothalamic-pituitary-adrenal axis activation is defective in streptococcal cell wall arthritis-susceptible Lewis rats. Proc Natl Acad Sci U S A 1989;86:2374–2378.

83. Vally M, Pillarisetti S. Disease modification in rheumatoid arthritis and osteoarthritis current and emerging targets and therapeutics. Cur Med Chem Immunol Endocr Metab Agents 2005;5:259–268.

84. Choy EH, Panayi GS. Cytokine pathways and joint inflammation in rheumatoid arthritis. N Engl J Med 2001;344(12):907–916.

85. Brooks P. Rheumatoid arthritis. Herston: CMPMedica Australia Pty Ltd, 2006.

86. Kievit W, et al. The efficacy of anti-TNF in rheumatoid arthritis, a comparison between randomised controlled trials and clinical practice. Ann Rheum Dis 2007;66(11):1473–1478.

87. Brooks PM, Day RO. COX-2 inhibitors. Med J Aust 2000;173(8):433–436.

88. Fox RI. Mechanism of action of hydroxychloroquine as an antirheumatic drug. Semin Arthritis Rheum 1993;23(2 Suppl. 1):82–91.

89. Hanai H, et al. Curcumin maintenance therapy for ulcerative colitis: randomized, multicenter, double-blind, placebo-controlled trial. Clin Gastroenterol Hepatol 2006;4(12):1502–1506.

90. James MJ, Cleland LG. Dietary n-3 fatty acids and therapy for rheumatoid arthritis. Semin Arthritis Rheum 1997;27(2):85–97.

91. Maes M, et al. The effects of psychological stress on humans: increased production of pro-inflammatory cytokines and a Th1-like response in stress-induced anxiety. Cytokine 1998;10(4):313–318.

92. Kiecolt-Glaser JK, et al. Emotions, morbidity, and mortality: new perspectives from psychoneuroimmunology. Annu Rev Psychol 2002;53:83–107.

93. Salovey P, et al. Emotional states and physical health. Am Psychol 2000;55(1):110–121.

94. Yoshino S, et al. Effects of mirthful laughter on neuroendocrine and immune systems in patients with rheumatoid arthritis. J Rheumatol 1996;23(4):793–794.

95. Davidson RJ, et al. Alterations in brain and immune function produced by mindfulness meditation [see comment]. Psychosom Med 2003;65(4):564–570.

96. Solberg EE, et al. Meditation: a modulator of the immune response to physical stress? A brief report. Br J Sports Med 1995;29(4):255–257.

97. Seeman TE, et al. Religiosity/spirituality and health. A critical review of the evidence for biological pathways. Am Psychol 2003;58(1):53–63.

98. Prather AA, et al. Positive affective style covaries with stimulated IL-6 and IL-10 production in a middle-aged community sample. Brain Behav Immun 2007;21(8):1033–1037.

99. Kreutz G, et al. Effects of choir singing or listening on secretory immunoglobulin A, cortisol, and emotional state. J Behav Med 2004;27(6):623–635.

100. Miller JB, et al. The GI factor: the glucose revolution. 2nd edn. Sydney: Hodder Headline, 1996.

101. Simopoulos A. Essential fatty acids in health and chronic disease. Am J Clin Nutr 1999;70(3):560S–569S.

102. Muldoon MF, et al. Lowering cholesterol concentration and mortality: a quantitative review of primary prevention trials. BMJ 1990;301:309–314.

103. ABS. Diabetes mellitus. 41020—Australian Social Trends, 2007. Online. Available: http://www.abs.gov.au/ausstats/abs@.nsf/latestproducts/62051E65E97FF67BCA25732C002076F3?opendocument. Accessed 4 May 2009.

104. Lowes JR, et al. Characterisation and quantification of mucosal cytokine that induces epithelial histocompatibility locus antigen-DR expression in inflammatory bowel disease. Gut 1992;33(3):315–319.

105. Mothes T, et al. Effect of gliadin and other food peptides on expression of MHC class II molecules by HT-29 cells. Gut 1995;36(4):548–552.

106. Virkkunen MF, et al. Plasma phospholipid essential fatty acids and prostaglandins in alcoholic, habitually violent and impulsive offenders. Biol Psychiatry 1987;22:1087–1096.

107. Simopoulos AP. Omega-3 fatty acids in inflammation and autoimmune diseases. J Am Coll Nutr 2002;21(6):495–505.

108. Fernandes G. Progress in nutritional immunology. Immunol Res 2008;40(3):244–261.

109. Good RA, et al. Nutritional deficiency, immunologic function, and disease. Am J Pathol 1976;84(3):599–614.

110. Friend PS, et al. Dietary restrictions early and late: effects on the nephropathy of the NZB X NZW mouse. Lab Invest 1978;38(6):629–632.

111. Calder P. n-3 polyunsaturated fatty acids and cytokine production in health and disease. Ann Nutr Metab 1997;41:203–234.

112. Calder PC. Polyunsaturated fatty acids and inflammation. Prostaglandins Leukot Essent Fatty Acids 2006;75(3):197–202.

113. Endres S, von Schacky C. n-3 polyunsaturated fatty acids and human cytokine synthesis. Curr Opin Lipidol 1996;7(1):48–52.

114. Huang YS, Nassar BA. Modulation of tissue fatty acid composition, prostaglandin production and cholesterol levels by dietary manipulation of n-3 and n-6 essential fatty acid metabolites. In: Horrobin D, ed. Omega 6 essential fatty acids: pathophysiology and roles in clinical medicine. USA: Wiley-Liss, 1990:127–144.

115. Brenner R. Nutritional and hormonal factors influencing desaturation of essential fatty acids. Prog Lipid Res 1981;20:41–47.

116. Brenner RR, Peluffo RO. Inhibitory effect of docosa-4,7,10,13,16,19-hexaenoic acid upon the oxidative desaturation of linoleic into gamma-linolenic and of alpha-linoleic into octadeca-6,9,12,15-tetraenoic acid. Biochim Biophys Acta 1967;137:184–186.

117. Howe P, et al. Dietary intake of long-chain [omega]-3 polyunsaturated fatty acids: contribution of meat sources. Nutrition 2006;22(1):47–53.

118. Meyer BJ, et al. Dietary intakes and food sources of omega-6 and omega-3 polyunsaturated fatty acids. Lipids 2003;38(4):391–398.

119. Duffy EM, et al. The clinical effect of dietary supplementation with omega-3 fish oils and/or copper in systemic lupus erythematosus. J Rheumatol 2004;31(8):1551–1556.

120. Baldwin AS. The NF-kappa B and l kappa B proteins: new discoveries and insights. Annu Rev Immunol 1996;14(1):649–681.

121. Vasto S, et al. Inflammation, genes and zinc in ageing and age-related diseases. Biogerontology 2006;7(5–6):315–327.

122. Shen H, et al. Zinc deficiency induces vascular pro-inflammatory parameters associated with NF-kappaB and PPAR signaling. J Am Coll Nutr 2008;27(5):577–587.

123. Beach RS, et al. Nutritional factors and autoimmunity. III. Zinc deprivation versus restricted food intake in MRL/1 mice—the distinction between interacting dietary influences. J Immunol 1982;129(6):2686–2692.

124. Leiter LM, et al. Iron status alters murine systemic lupus erythematosus. J Nutr 1995;125(3):474–484.

125. Komatsu W, et al. Docosahexaenoic acid suppresses nitric oxide production and inducible nitric oxide synthase expression in interferon-[gamma] plus lipopolysaccharide-stimulated murine macrophages by inhibiting the oxidative stress. Free Radic Biol Med 2003;34(8):1006–1016.

126. Aktas O, et al. Green tea epigallocatechin-3-gallate mediates T cellular NF-kappa B inhibition and exerts neuroprotection in autoimmune encephalomyelitis. J Immunol 2004;173(9):5794–5800.

127. Wheeler DS, et al. Epigallocatechin-3-gallate, a green tea-derived polyphenol, inhibits IL-1beta-dependent proinflammatory signal transduction in cultured respiratory epithelial cells. J Nutr 2004;134(5):1039–1044.

128. Schreiber S, et al. Activation of nuclear factor kappa B in inflammatory bowel disease. Gut 1998;42(4):477–484.

129. Kim SH, et al. Luteolin inhibits the nuclear factor-kappa B transcriptional activity in Rat-1 fibroblasts. Biochem Pharmacol 2003;66(6):955–963.

130. Ruiz PA, et al. Quercetin inhibits TNF-induced NF-kappaB transcription factor recruitment to proinflammatory gene promoters in murine intestinal epithelial cells. J Nutr 2007;137(5):1208–1215.

131. Ruiz PA, Haller D. Functional diversity of flavonoids in the inhibition of the proinflammatory NF-kappaB, IRF, and AKT signaling pathways in murine intestinal epithelial cells. J Nutr 2006;136(3):664–671.

132. Ziegler-Heitbrock HW, et al. Pyrrolidine dithiocarbamate inhibits NF-kappa B mobilization and TNF production in human monocytes. J Immunol 1993;151(12):6986–6993.

133. Merrill JE, Murphy SP. Inflammatory events at the blood brain barrier: regulation of adhesion molecules, cytokines, and chemokines by reactive nitrogen and oxygen species. Brain Behav Immun 1997;11(4):245–263.

134. Tse HM, et al. Disruption of innate-mediated proinflammatory cytokine and reactive oxygen species third signal leads to antigen-specific hyporesponsiveness. J Immunol 2007;178(2):908–917.

135. Packer L, et al. Neuroprotection by the metabolic antioxidant alpha-lipoic acid. Free Radic Biol Med 1997;22(1–2):359–378.

136. Marracci GH, et al. Alpha lipoic acid inhibits T cell migration into the spinal cord and suppresses and treats experimental autoimmune encephalomyelitis. J Neuroimmunol 2002;131(1–2):104–114.

137. Morini M, et al. Alpha-lipoic acid is effective in prevention and treatment of experimental autoimmune encephalomyelitis. J Neuroimmunol 2004;148(1–2):146–153.

138. Yadav V, et al. Lipoic acid in multiple sclerosis: a pilot study. Mult Scler 2005;11(2):159–165.

139. De Paula ML, et al. Genistein down-modulates proinflammatory cytokines and reverses clinical signs of experimental autoimmune encephalomyelitis. Int Immunopharmacol 2008;8(9):1291–1297.

140. Miodini P, et al. The two phyto-oestrogens genistein and quercetin exert different effects on oestrogen receptor function. Br J Cancer 1999;80(8):1150–1155.

141. Singh NP, et al. Resveratrol (trans-3,5,4'-Trihydroxystilbene) ameliorates experimental allergic encephalomyelitis, primarily via induction of apoptosis in T cells involving activation of aryl hydrocarbon receptor and estrogen receptor. Mol Pharmacol 2007;72(6):1508–1521.

142. de la Lastra CA, Villegas I. Resveratrol as an anti-inflammatory and anti-aging agent: mechanisms and clinical implications. Mol Nutr Food Res 2005;49(5):405–430.

143. Pedersen BK, Toft AD. Effects of exercise on lymphocytes and cytokines. Br J Sports Med 2000;34(4):246–251.

144. Costa Rosa LFBP. Exercise as a time-conditioning effector in chronic disease: a complementary treatment strategy. Evid Based Complement Alternat Med 2004;1(1):63–70.

145. Estivariz CF, et al. Efficacy of parenteral nutrition supplemented with glutamine dipeptide to decrease hospital infections in critically ill surgical patients. J Parenter Enteral Nutr 2008;32(4):389–402.

146. Castell LM, et al. Does glutamine have a role in reducing infections in athletes? Eur J Appl Physiol 1996;73(5):488–490.

147. Castell LM. Glutamine supplementation in vitro and in vivo, in exercise and in immunodepression. Sports Med 2003;33(5):323–345.

148. da Silva Krause M. de Bittencourt PIH. Type 1 diabetes: can exercise impair the autoimmune event? The L-arginine/glutamine coupling hypothesis. Cell Biochem Funct 2008;26(4):406–433.

149. Anisman H, et al. Cytokines as a stressor: implications for depressive illness. Int J Neuropsychopharmacol 2002;5(4):357–373.

150. Arimura A, et al. Interactions between cytokines and the hypothalamic-pituitary-adrenal axis during stress. Ann N Y Acad Sci 1994;739:270–281.

151. De Kloet ER, et al. Cytokines and the brain corticosteroid receptor balance: relevance to pathophysiology of neuroendocrine-immune communication. Psychoneuroendocrinology 1994;19(2):121–134.

152. Banerjee U, Izquierdo JA. Antistress and antifatigue properties of *Panax ginseng*: comparison with piracetam. Acta Physiol Lat Am 1982;32(4):277–285.

153. Caso MA, et al. Double-blind study of a multivitamin complex supplemented with ginseng extract. Drugs Exp Clin Res 1996;22(6):323–329.

154. Dua PR, et al. Adaptogenic activity of Indian *Panax pseudoginseng*. Indian J Exp Biol 1989;27(7):631–634.

155. Grandhi A, et al. A comparative pharmacological investigation of ashwagandha and ginseng. J Ethnopharmacol 1994;44:131–135.

156. Kumar R, et al. Enhanced thermogenesis in rats by *Panax ginseng*, multivitamins and minerals. Int J Biometeorol 1996;39(4):187–191.

157. Leung KW, et al. Angiomodulatory and neurological effects of ginsenosides. Curr Med Chem 2007;14(12):1371–1380.

158. Nocerino E, et al. The aphrodisiac and adaptogenic properties of ginseng. Fitoterapia 2000;71(Suppl. 1):S1–S5.

159. Saito H, et al. Effect of *Panax ginseng* root on exhaustive exercise in mice. Jpn J Pharmacol 1974;24:119–127.

160. Bhattacharya SK, Muruganandam AV. Adaptogenic activity of *Withania somnifera*: an experimental study using a rat model of chronic stress. Pharmacol Biochem Behav 2003;75(3):547–555.

161. Dhuley JN. Adaptogenic and cardioprotective action of ashwagandha in rats and frogs. J Ethnopharmacol 2000;70(1):57–63.

162. Rai D, et al. Adaptogenic effect of *Bacopa monniera* (brahmi). Pharmacol Biochem Behav 2003;75(4):823–830.

163. Armanini D, et al. Affinity of licorice derivatives for mineralocorticoid and glucocorticoid receptors. Clin Endocrinol 1983;19:609–612.

164. Schlebusch L, et al. A double-blind, placebo-controlled, double-centre study of the effects of an oral multivitamin-mineral combination on stress. S Afr Med J 2000;90(12):1216–1223.

165. Kumar R, et al. Antistress and adaptogenic activity of lecithin supplementation. J Altern Complement Med 2002;8(4):487–492.

166. De Caterina R, et al. The omega-3 fatty acid docosahexaenoate reduces cytokine-induced expression of proatherogenic and proinflammatory proteins in human endothelial cells. Arterioscler Thromb 1994;14(11):1829–1836.

167. Maes M, et al. In humans, serum polyunsaturated fatty acid levels predict the response of proinflammatory cytokines to psychologic stress. Biol Psychiatry 2000;47(10):910–920.

168. Safayhi H, et al. Mechanism of 5-lipoxygenase inhibition by acetyl-11-keto-beta-boswellic acid. Mol Pharmacol 1995;47(6):1212–1216.

169. Ammon HP, et al. Inhibition of leukotriene B4 formation in rat peritoneal neutrophils by an ethanolic extract of the gum resin exudate of *Boswellia serrata*. Planta Med 1991;57(3):203–207.

170. Singh GB, Atal CK. Pharmacology of an extract of salai guggal ex- *Boswellia serrata*, a new non-steroidal anti-inflammatory agent. Inflamm Res 1986;18(3):407–412.

171. Ernst E. Frankincense: systematic review. BMJ 2008; 337:a2813.

172. Sander O, et al. [Is H15 (resin extract of *Boswellia serrata*, 'incense') a useful supplement to established drug therapy of chronic polyarthritis? Results of a double-blind pilot study]. Z Rheumatol 1998;57(1):11–16.

173. Shah BA, et al. Boswellic acids: a group of medicinally important compounds. Nat Prod Rep 2009;26(1):72–89.

174. Pachnanda VK, et al. Clinical evaluation of salai guggul in patients of arthritis. Indian J Pharmacol 1981;13:63.

175. Spelman K, et al. Modulation of cytokine expression by traditional medicines: a review of herbal immunomodulators. Altern Med Rev 2006;11(2):128–150.

176. Bone K. Clinical applications of Ayurvedic and Chinese herbs. Warwick: Phytotherapy Press, 1996.

177. Frank A, Unger M. Analysis of frankincense from various *Boswellia* species with inhibitory activity on human drug metabolising cytochrome P450 enzymes using liquid chromatography mass spectrometry after automated on-line extraction. J Chromatogr A 2006;1112(1–2):255–262.

178. Guengerich FP. Cytochromes P450, drugs, and diseases. Mol Interv 2003;3(4):194–204.

179. Brendler T, et al. Devil's claw (*Harpagophytum procumbens* DC): an evidence-based systematic review by the Natural Standard Research Collaboration. J Herb Pharmacother 2006;6(1):89–126.

180. Abdelouahab N, Heard C. Effect of the major glycosides of *Harpagophytum procumbens* (devil's claw) on epidermal cyclooxygenase-2 (COX-2) in vitro. J Nat Prod 2008;71(5):746–749.

181. Grant L, et al. A review of the biological and potential therapeutic actions of *Harpagophytum procumbens*. Phytother Res 2007;21(3):199–209.

182. Warnock M, et al. Effectiveness and safety of devil's claw tablets in patients with general rheumatic disorders. Phytother Res 2007;21(12):1228–1233.

183. Brien S, et al. Devil's claw (*Harpagophytum procumbens*) as a treatment for osteoarthritis: a review of efficacy and safety. J Altern Complement Med 2006;12(10):981–993.

184. Cat's Claw. Online. Available: http://nccam.nih.gov/health/catclaw/. Accessed 15 April 2009.

185. Sandoval-Chacon M, et al. Antiinflammatory actions of cat's claw: the role of NF-kappaB. Aliment Pharmacol Ther 1998;12(12):1279–1289.

186. Sandoval M, et al. Cat's claw inhibits TNF alpha production and scavenges free radicals: role in cytoprotection. Free Radic Biol Med 2000;29(1):71–78.

187. Hardin SR, Hardin SR. Cat's claw: an Amazonian vine decreases inflammation in osteoarthritis. Complement Ther Clin Pract 2007;13(1):25–28.

188. Sandoval M, et al. Anti-inflammatory and antioxidant activities of cat's claw (*Uncaria tomentosa* and *Uncaria guianensis*) are independent of their alkaloid content. Phytomedicine 2002;9(4):325–337.

189. Sheng Y, et al. An active ingredient of Cat's Claw water extracts identification and efficacy of quinic acid. J Ethnopharmacol 2005;96(3):577–584.

190. Piscoya J, et al. Efficacy and safety of freeze-dried cat's claw in osteoarthritis of the knee: mechanisms of action of the species *Uncaria guianensis*. Inflamm Res 2001;50(9):442–448.

191. Valerio Jnr LG, et al. Toxicological aspects of the South American herbs cat's claw (*Uncaria tomentosa*) and maca (*Lepidium meyenii*): a critical synopsis. Toxicol Rev 2005;24(1):11–35.

192. Jagetia GC, Aggarwal BB. Spicing up the immune system by curcumin. J Clin Immunol 2007;27(1):19–35.

193. Srimal RC, Dhawan BN. Pharmacology of diferuloyl methane (curcumin), a non-steroidal anti-inflammatory agent. J Pharm Pharmacol 1973;25(6):447–452.

194. Jain A, Basal E. Inhibition of *Propionibacterium acnes*-induced mediators of inflammation by Indian herbs. Phytomedicine 2003;10(1):34–38.

195. Bork PM, et al. Sesquiterpene lactone containing Mexican Indian medicinal plants and pure sesquiterpene lactones as potent inhibitors of transcription factor NF-kappaB. FEBS Lett 1997;402(1):85–90.

196. Hehner SP, et al. The antiinflammatory sesquiterpene lactone parthenolide inhibits NF-kappaB by targeting the I kappaB kinase complex. J Immunol 1999;163(10):5617–5623.

197. Kwok BH, et al. The anti-inflammatory natural product parthenolide from the medicinal herb feverfew directly binds to and inhibits I kappaB kinase. Chem Biol 2001;8(8):759–766.

198. Riehemann K, et al. Plant extracts from stinging nettle (*Urtica dioica*), an antirheumatic remedy, inhibit the proinflammatory transcription factor NF-kappaB. FEBS Lett 1999;442(1):89–94.

199. Teucher T, et al. Cytokine secretion in whole blood of healthy volunteers after oral ingestion of an *Urtica dioica* L. leaf extract. Zytokin-Sekretion im Vollblut gesunder Probanden nach oraler Einnahme eines *Urtica dioica* L-Blattextraktes 1996;46(9):906–910.

200. Ganguly T, Sainis KB. Inhibition of cellular immune responses by *Tylophora indica* in experimental models. Phytomedicine 2001;8(5):348–355.

201. Chainy GB, et al. Anethole blocks both early and late cellular responses transduced by tumor necrosis factor: effect on NF-kappaB, AP-1, JNK, MAPKK and apoptosis. Oncogene 2000;19(25):2943–2950.

202. Futrakul N, et al. *Ganoderma lucidum* suppresses endothelial cell cytotoxicity and proteinuria in persistent proteinuric focal segmental glomerulosclerosis (FSGS) nephrosis. Clin Hemorheol Microcirc 2004;31(4):267–272.

203. Crispin JC, et al. Expanded double negative T cells in patients with systemic lupus erythematosus produce IL-17 and infiltrate the kidneys. J Immunol 2008;181(12):8761–8766.

204. Harigai M, et al. Excessive production of IFN-gamma in patients with systemic lupus erythematosus and its contribution to induction of B lymphocyte stimulator/B cell-activating factor/TNF ligand superfamily-13B. J Immunol 2008;181(3):2211–2219.

205. Frieri M. Neuroimmunology and inflammation: implications for therapy of allergic and autoimmune diseases. Ann Allergy Asthma Immunol 2003;90(6 Suppl. 3):34–40.

206. Halverson PB, Holmes SB. Systemic lupus erythematosus: medical and nursing treatments. Orthop Nurs 1992;11(6):17–24.

207. Peralta-Ramirez MI, et al. The effects of daily stress and stressful life events on the clinical symptomatology of patients with lupus erythematosus. Psychosom Med 2004;66(5):788–794.

208. Greco CM, et al. Effects of a stress-reduction program on psychological function, pain and physical function of systemic lupus erythematosus patients: a randomized controlled trial. Arthritis Rheum 2004;51(4):625–634.

209. Minor MA, Lane NE. Recreational exercise in arthritis. Rheum Dis Clin North Am 1996;22(3):563–577.

210. Costa DD, et al. Determinants of sleep quality in women with systemic lupus erythematosus. Arthritis Rheum 2005;53(2):272–278.

211. Carvalho MR, et al. Effects of supervised cardiovascular training program on exercise tolerance, aerobic capacity and quality of life in patients with systemic lupus erythematosus. Arthritis Rheum 2005;53(6):838–844.

212. Ayan C, Martin V. Systemic lupus erythematosus and exercise. Lupus 2007;16(1):5–9.

213. Dua J, Hargreaves L. Effect of aerobic exercise on negative affect, positive affect, stress, and depression. Percept-Mot Skills 1992;75(2):355–361.

214. Linde K, et al. Are the clinical effects of homoeopathy placebo effects? A meta-analysis of placebo-controlled trials. Lancet 1997;350(9081):834–843.

215. Joos S, et al. Use of complementary and alternative medicine in Germany—a survey of patients with inflammatory bowel disease. BMC Complement Altern Med 2006;6:19.

216. Schwarz S, et al. Complementary and alternative medicine for multiple sclerosis. Mult Scler 2008;14(8):1113–1119.

217. Quattropani C, et al. Complementary alternative medicine in patients with inflammatory bowel disease: use and attitudes. Scand J Gastroenterol 2003;38(3):277–282.

218. Fisher P, Scott DL. A randomized controlled trial of homeopathy in rheumatoid arthritis. Rheumatology (Oxford) 2001;40(9):1052–1055.

219. Gibson RG, et al. Homeopathic therapy in rheumatoid arthritis: evaluation by double blind clinical therapeutic trial. Br J Clin Pharmacol 1980;9(5):453–459.

220. Braden CJ. Patterns of change over time in learned response to chronic illness among participants in a systemic lupus erythematosus self-help course. Arthritis Care Res 1991;4(4):158–167.

221. NonSteroidal Antiinflammatory Drugs (NSAIDs). MedicineNetcom. Online. Available: http://www.medicinenet.com/nonsteroidal_antiinflammatory_drugs/article.htm.

222. Foster M, et al. COX-2 inhibitor safety in the workers' compensation market. Lippincott's Case Manag 2005;10(4):217–220.

223. Das UN. Can COX-2 inhibitor-induced increase in cardiovascular disease risk be modified by essential fatty acids? J Assoc Physicians India 2005;53:623–627.

224. Krishnan E. Hospitalization and mortality of patients with systemic lupus erythematosus. J Rheumatol 2006;33(9):1770–1774.

225. Chan RW, et al. Expression of T-bet, a type 1 T-helper cell transcription factor, in the urinary sediment of lupus patients predicts disease flare. Rheumatology (Oxford) 2007;46(1):44–48.

226. Living With lupus. Online. Available: http://www.lupusnsw.org.au/lwlupus.html. Accessed 8 July 2009.

227. Szeto CC, et al. Climatic influence on the prevalence of noncutaneous disease flare in systemic lupus erythematosus in Hong Kong. J Rheumatol 2008;35(6):1031–1037.

228. Ramos-Casals M, et al. Acute viral infections in patients with systemic lupus erythematosus: description of 23 cases and review of the literature. Medicine (Baltimore) 2008;87(6):311–318.

229. Zandman-Goddard G, et al. Infections and SLE. Autoimmunity 2005;38(7):473–485.

230. Lupus and Infections. Better Health channel: healthier living. Online. Available: http://www.betterhealth.vic.gov.au/bhcv2/bhcarticles.nsf/pages/Lupus_and_infections. Accessed 11 July 2009.

231. Tincani A, et al. Pregnancy and autoimmunity: maternal treatment and maternal disease influence on pregnancy outcome. Autoimmun Rev 2005;4(7):423–428.

232. Petri M, et al. Frequency of lupus flare in pregnancy. The Hopkins Lupus Pregnancy Center experience [see comment]. Arthritis Rheum 1991;34(12):1538–1545.

233. Molad Y. Systemic lupus erythematosus and pregnancy. Curr Opin Obstet Gynecol 2006;18(6):613–617.

234. Khamashta MA. Systemic lupus erythematosus and pregnancy. Best Pract Res Clin Rheumatol 2006;20(4):685–694.

235. Lupus and pregnancy. Better health channel: healthier living. Online. Available: http://www.betterhealth.vic.gov.au/bhcv2/bhcarticles.nsf/pages/Lupus_and_pregnancy. Accessed 11 July 2009.

236. Petri M, et al. Combined oral contraceptives in women with systemic lupus erythematosus [see comment]. N Engl J Med 2005;353(24):2550–2558.

237. Fortin PR, et al. Validation of a meta-analysis: the effects of fish oil in rheumatoid arthritis. J Clin Epidemiol 1995;48(11):1379–1390.

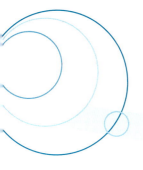

29
Cancer

Janet Schloss
ND, MNutrMed

AETIOLOGY

Cancer is a multifactorial disease that is still not completely understood. Many theories exist as to what may cause cancer and only a few cancers have definitive risk factors (for example, cigarette smoking and lung cancer,[1] or human papilloma (HPV) and cervical cancer).[2] However, even with these connections, not everyone who smokes gets lung cancer and not everyone with HPV gets cervical cancer. Table 29.1 shows some possible general theories incorporating medical and naturopathic causes of cancer.

Certain cancers have been linked with certain dietary and lifestyle choices (see Table 29.2).

CANCER PREVENTION

Cancer prevention is a very broad topic where a lot of information could be collated on different types of cancer. To simplify this, several areas of a person's life can be taken into consideration to aid trying to prevent this disease. It should be noted that a person may have all of these areas covered perfectly and could still end up with cancer. With such a multifactorial disease, people can only do the best they can to prevent its initiation and growth in their body.

A basic list of areas to consider in the prevention of cancer includes:
- diet—eat a balanced diet with lots of fresh fruit and vegetables (refer to the section on diet) and ensure adequate nutrition[32]
- exercise[32]
- maintenance of an optimal body weight[32,33]
- decrease of negative stress[34]
- adequate sleep[35]
- having fun and enjoyment in life[36]
- reducing alcohol intake, reducing or stopping smoking and illicit drug use[37]
- having safe sex[38]
- spirituality or religion or some form of belief[36]
- moderation in everything.

Table 29.1 Theorised causative factors in cancer

POSSIBLE CAUSE	EXPLANATION
Genetics	Certain cancers, such as breast, prostate and colon cancer, have been found to have hereditary links. There are certain genetic markers that the medical fraternity can test for to check if someone has the genetic markers for that cancer, e.g. the BRCA gene for breast cancer.[3]
Viruses and infection	Viruses such as the HPV have been linked with the development of certain cancers. Examples of these include human papillomavirus (cervical cancer);[2] Epstein-Barr virus (non-Hodgkin's lymphoma);[4] HIV (Kaposi's sarcoma, primary central nervous system lymphoma, invasive cervical cancer and non-Hodgkin's lymphoma);[5] hepatitis B virus (hepatocellular carcinomas);[6] retroviruses (adult T-cell leukaemia);[7] *Helicobacter pylori* (gastric cancer in people with certain polymorphisms);[8] simian virus 40 (non-Hodgkin's lymphoma)[9]
Mitochondrial dysfunction	Cancer progression has been linked with mitochondrial dysfunction. This can be a result of mitochondrial DNA (mtDNA) mutations and/or depletion. These mutations or mitochondrial depletions have also been linked with an increase of drug resistance within cells. This mitochondrial dysfunction has been found in certain cancers such as prostate cancer.[10]
Environmental influences	Over the years, an increase in cancer in the Western world has been found.[11] Epidemiological studies have found an association with this increase and the exposure to environmental toxins such as organochlorides and synthetic pesticides.[12] Further research is being conducted but it seems at this stage that fetuses, infants, children and young adults are most at risk.[12] There are specific cancers, such as mesothelioma, which have been directly linked with exposure to asbestos.[13]
Immune system	It has been postulated that a lowered immune system may increase the chance of cancer developing. The natural killer cells are the main surveillance system of the body, protecting against cancer formation and infection. These natural killer cells are a main part of the innate immune system and, if they are not functioning correctly, can allow tumours to develop through abnormal cell development.[14]
Cell cycle mitosis malfunction	In cell replication certain checkpoints and cellular activity maintain the health of the cell. If these checkpoints, such as p53, have mutations[15] or there are abnormal centrosomes in a cell, cancer cells may develop.[16] The elderly in particular are prone to malignant tumours that are related to the accumulation of damaged DNA from malfunctioning cell mitosis.[17]
Oxidative damage	There are several schools of thoughts that oxidative damage, especially to DNA and cellular components, can be attributed to the development of cancer. Reactive species such as ROS (reactive oxygen species) and RNS (reactive nitrogen species) are a natural by-product of normal biochemical and physiological reactions in the body. These reactive species can cause damage to the DNA, cellular membrane and cellular organelles, and can interfere with cellular regulators if there is not enough antioxidants to counteract reactive species damaging effect.[18]
Mind–body connection	A different way of looking at cancer is the psychological aspect. There are theories on a connection between the mind and the development of certain cancers, but this has not been confirmed. However, there is good evidence that mind–body medicine should be taken into consideration when addressing cancer.[19]

Table 29.1 Theorised causative factors in cancer *(Continued)*

POSSIBLE CAUSE	EXPLANATION
Polymorphisms	There are numerous studies on polymorphisms and genetic mutations increasing the risk of nearly all cancers. As this is a relatively new area of research, more studies will emerge on new polymorphisms that can be linked with certain cancers, and testing procedures will become more accessible and less expensive.[20–22]
Epigenetics	The increase of scientific knowledge on how chromatin organisation modulates gene transcriptions has highlighted how epigenetic mechanisms are involved in the initiation and progression of human cancer. These epigenetic changes have been found to affect nearly every step in tumour progression, especially the aberrant promoter hypermethylation that is associated with gene silencing.[23]

Table 29.2 Links between cancer and lifestyle

FOOD OR BEVERAGE	IMPLICATED CANCER
Smoking	• Lung cancer[1] • Cervical cancer in people with HPV[24] • Vulvar squamous cell carcinoma (SCC)[24]
Alcohol	• Total cancer risk[25] • Liver cancer[26] • Breast cancer—especially oestrogen-dependent cancers[27] • Colon cancer[28]
Low fruit and vegetable, fibre intake, high intake of processed meats, nitrosamines, highly salted foods	• Gastric cancer[29]
Obesity	• Gastric cancer[30] • Breast cancer—link with leptin regulation[31]

CONVENTIONAL TREATMENT

Traditional treatment of cancer is based on four forms of treatment: surgery, chemotherapy, radiation and hormone therapy. Any one or combination of these treatments may be used, depending on the type of tumour, the location, the aggressiveness, the age of the patient, and what has been found to be most effective.

The Cochrane database is an important source of information; there are many different Cochrane reviews of chemotherapy and radiation for a variety of different types of cancer and adjunct medications with cancer treatment. The information is quite extensive and beyond the scope of this chapter to list in detail. Entering 'chemotherapy' and 'radiation' separately into the Cochrane search engine will provide a broad overview of current effective treatments.

CAM TREATMENT OF COMMON SIDE EFFECTS OF CHEMOTHERAPY AND RADIATION

Table 29.3 provides specific evidence pertaining to integrative cancer treatment only; see the relevant chapters for generalised information.

Table 29.3 CAM treatment of common side effects of chemotherapy and radiation

SIDE EFFECT	CAM THERAPY
Mouth ulcers	Calcium phosphate, honey, zinc sulfate[39]
Diarrhoea	Glutamine[40]
Constipation	Senna[41]
Intestinal permeability	Glutamine[42]
Radiation enteritis or enteropathy	Hyperbaric oxygen chambers,[43] probiotics during radiation,[44] glutamine during radiation[45]
Neutrophilia	Vitamin E[46]
Anaemia	Iron[47]
Fibrosis	Lipoic acid[48]
Fatigue	L-carnitine,[49] coenzyme Q10[50]
Memory loss	Egg phosphocholine and low-dose vitamin B12[51]
Weight loss	Omega-3 fatty acids[52]
Weight gain	Dietary suggestions to keep BMI in range[53]
Stress/anxiety	l-theanine[54]
Peripheral neuropathy	Vitamin B1, B6, B12[55]
Cardiomyopathy	Coenzyme Q10[56]

POTENTIAL INTERACTIONS

Potential interactions between orthodox and complementary therapies need to be taken into consideration when treating a patient with cancer. As there are many different drugs used for cancer, it is important for the naturopath to address each drug and check for any possible interactions both beneficial and contradictory (see Figure 29.1). Unfortunately, most potential interactions of cancer drugs and complementary medicine still require clinical research as there is little human data (most studies are animal or in vitro based).[57] A chart of potential interactions between naturopathic medicines and chemotherapeutics is in the appendices at the back of the book.

There are, however, ways in which the potential risk for interaction with chemotherapy can be moderated. As many naturopathic medicines can protect and support not only the body from deleterious effects of chemotherapy but the cancerous tissue as well, it may be prudent to apply a cautionary approach to CAM prescription.[58] In principle it takes five half-lives to reach a steady state and five half-lives to eliminate virtually all of a drug in the body. Knowing both the half-lives of naturopathic medicine and chemotherapy can allow for a dosing regimen that can reduce risk of possible interactions (see Table 29.4).

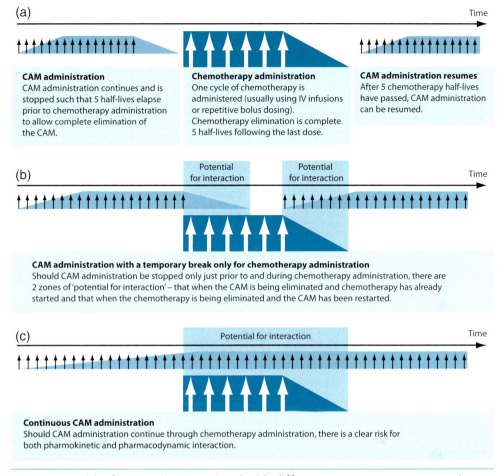

Figure 29.1 Risk of interactions associated with different CAM treatment protocols
Source: Seely D, et al[58].

Table 29.4 Selected antioxidant naturopathic medicines and their half-life[58]

NATUROPATHIC INTERVENTION	HALF-LIFE
Green tea	3.4 h ± 0.3 h
Curcumin	< 1 h
Selenium	102–252 days
Vitamin C	30 min

RISK FACTORS

The risk factors vary depending on the type of cancer. These may include diet and life-style factors, viruses, genetics, environmental exposure and lowered immune system. Other risk factors include lack of physical exercise,[59] high BMI/obesity,[59] exposure or lack of exposure to sun (due to low vitamin D),[60,61] nutrient deficiencies,[62] medication (in some cases medication can increase the risk of other cancers, such as Tamoxifen

COMMON TUMOUR MARKERS

PSA: prostate specific antigen. Range 0–4 ng/L
CEA: carcinoembryonic antigen for colon cancer, but can also indicate pancreatic, gastric, lung or breast cancer. Range < 2.5 ng/L in non-smoker, < 5 ng/L in a smoker
CA 19-9: mainly for pancreatic cancer, but can also be present in colon and gastric cancer
CA 125: ovarian cancer
AFP: alpha-fetoprotein for heptocellular carcinoma. Range < 10 μg/L
HCG: human chorionic gonadotropin, normally elevated in pregnancy, can also be found in gestational trophoblastic disease and germ cell tumours as well breast, lung and GIT tumours

causing endometrial carcinoma),[63] country/nationality,[64] stress,[65] gender (for example, prostate cancer in males and ovarian cancer in females), age[17] and occupation.[66–68]

TUMOUR MARKERS

Certain types of cancers have been found to release certain molecules in the blood or tissues; these markers can be measured or identified. They can be used to aid diagnosis or in the clinical management of a patient. Blood tests are used to ascertain these markers. Ideally, a positive result should only be found in a patient with the malignancy, and it should correlate with the stage of the cancer or the patient's response to treatment. Unfortunately, tumour markers can be used only as a guide as no tests meet all requirements.

Tumour markers have four purposes:
1. screening of a healthy population or a high risk population for the presence of cancer
2. aid making a diagnosis of cancer or of a specific type of cancer
3. determining the prognosis in a patient
4. monitoring a patient in remission or while receiving surgery, radiation or chemotherapy.

NATUROPATHIC APPROACHES TO CANCER PATHOPHYSIOLOGY

Cell mitosis

The regulation of cell division is the most important part of cell mitosis. Without the cell regulators, abnormal cell development can occur. There are three main areas to consider in cell mitosis: oncogenes and tumour-suppressor genes, p53 and p21 checkpoints and centrosomes. All three interact to allow abnormal cell development.

Oncogenes and tumour-suppressor genes

Oncogenic processes have long been associated with cancer development and progression. These genes stimulate the process of cell mitosis and DNA replication and studies have shown that these genes are altered in cancer. The two main genes that are focused on are the proto-oncogenes and tumour-suppressor genes.[69]

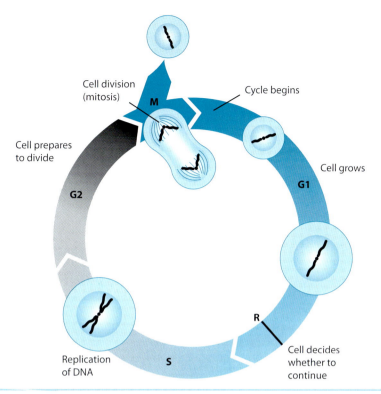

Figure 29.2 The cell cycle for normal cell division

Recent studies have identified a specific small class of RNA molecules called micro-RNAs (miRNAs). These miRNAs negatively regulate gene expression post-transcriptionally and aid the development of cell identity. These are important as they can affect cellular transformation, carcinogenesis and metastasis because they can act as an oncogene or tumour-suppressor gene.[70]

According to naturopathic treatment, keeping cellular oncogenes working efficiently without the development of cancer requires both dietary regulation and the maintenance of levels of particular nutrients in the body. Epidemiological and experimental data have found that Western diets that are high in fat and low in calcium and vitamin D can accelerate tumour growth by causing genetic manipulation.[71] Maintaining a diet low in detrimental fats and increasing calcium and vitamin D levels may therefore prevent gene alteration.

p53, p21

Abnormalities in the regulatory marker p53 have been found in most cancer cells. Cancer cells may have either mutations of the p53 gene or an accumulation of p53 proteins in the cells.[72,73] p21-activated kinases (Paks) aid controlling G(2)/M transition and mitosis and are tumour-suppressor genes regulated by p53. Therefore they are necessary for cell proliferation, mitotic progression and other regulators.[74,75]

A number of different nutrients can affect the p53 and p21 genes and be of benefit for cancer. Low levels of **folate** and **vitamin B6** can affect p53, increasing the risk of colorectal cancer.[76] The mechanism of this deficiency involves the mutation of the p53 gene, therefore changing its expression. It is recommended that people should consume over 400 μg of folate a day to prevent this occurring.

Resveratrol has also been found to modulate p53 to induce apoptosis (programmed cell death that is an integral part of normal biological processes to kill abnormal cell development) as well as knocking out excessive p53, having a beneficial effect in preventing cancer. Resveratrol has also been found to induce apoptosis via modulating other cellular molecules such as cyclin D1, p21, BCL2, BAX, Bcl XL, caspase 9 and p27.[77,78]

Green tea is another nutrient that has been found to affect p53 and p21. One study has found that green tea enhanced *Zizyphus jujuba*'s selective cytotoxic activity by causing cell death via up-regulation of p53 and p21 while decreasing cyclin E levels in HepG2 cells.[79] Green tea has also been found to inhibit tumour growth and angiogenesis as well as induce apoptosis.[80] **Genistein** has been found to influence p21 transcription by markedly inhibiting proliferative activity and inducing the expression of p21 plus ERbeta.[81]

Vitamin D also influences p53 and p21. Both p21 and p53 have vitamin D binding sites (VDR).[75] If a patient is deficient in vitamin D, both p53 and p21 may be affected, possibly influencing cancer development or progression. Flavonoids—such as **quercetin**—have also been found to influence p53 in relation to cancer. One study found that quercetin helped to stabilise p53 at both the mRNA and the protein level to reactive p53-dependent cell cycle arrest and apoptosis.[82] This was achieved by quercetin inducing p53 phosphorylation and total p53 protein, but not up-regulating p53 mRNA at transcription. It also stimulates p21 expression and suppresses cyclin D1 to activate cell cycle arrest. Quercetin was also found to inhibit p53 mRNA degradation post transcriptionally.

Centrosomes

These microtubules aid cell mitosis by creating the polar rejection force that pushes the chromosomes away from the spindle poles by wobbling at high frequencies. A rise in intracellular calcium aid the regulation of the polar force at the onset of chromosomal splitting. If this is defective, chromosomal instability (characteristic of most cancers) can occur.[83] It has also been found that cells that have dysfunctional p53s have more centrosomes.[84]

Vitamin A plays a key role in centrosomes and chromosome replication through the retinoblastoma protein, which is a regulating protein of cyclins D and E, cdk 4 and 6, cdk inhibitors p16, p15 and p53.[85] A **vitamin B12** deficiency has been associated with enlarged, disrupted centrioles in monocytes and neutrophils.[86]

Proteasomes play an important role in a variety of cellular processes such as cell cycle progression, signal transduction and the immune response, and are important in maintaining rapid turnover of short-lived proteins. They also prevent accumulation of misfolded or damaged proteins. **Zinc** increases proteasome substrates such as p5 and p21, as well as decreasing the enzyme that degrades these substrates in centrosomes.[87]

Folate also plays a critical role in the prevention of chromosome breakage and hypomethylation of DNA. A folate deficiency can cause centromere defects that can induce abnormal distribution of replicated chromosomes during mitosis. It has also been found to be a risk factor for chromosomes 17 and 21 aneuploidy, which has been observed in breast cancer and leukaemia.[88]

Glycolysis and p53

A common theory sometimes postulated in the naturopathic treatment of cancer is that tumours feed on sugar. In part this is true, as cancer cells work differently to other cells biochemically. Research has found that most cancer cells have higher rates of glycolysis than normal cells.[73] Research has found that, after a loss of functional p53, there were mitochondrial changes, up-regulation of rate-limiting enzymes and proteins in glycolysis and intracellular pH regulation, hypoxia-induced switching to anaerobic metabolism leading to higher lactic acid levels, and metabolic reprogramming.

Extrapolation of these results has led to various diets being developed to 'starve' the cancer. This theory has not yet been proven to work; however, it is still recommended that people with cancer decrease their sugar intake as it has been found that insulin-like growth factor 1 is involved in a number of cancers.[89,90] One animal study has shown delayed growth of gastric cancer cells with administration of a ketogenic diet high in omega-3 fats.[91]

The high usage of glycolysis by tumours is also why it is often recommended in traditional naturopathic theory to alkalise the body of a patient with cancer. It is hoped that the spread of cancer can be decreased by increasing buffers and trying to decrease the acidic environment. This theory has yet to be validated, though alkalising diets (higher fruit and vegetable intake, and lower meat intake) generally have positive effects in cancer.

Another theory (the Warburg effect) suggests 'oxygenating' the body, as cancer cells use more anaerobic glycolysis than normal cells do and normal cells use the aerobic system of the mitochondria.[92] Increasing oxygen availability (for example, through breathing exercises and circulatory stimulants) to cells more generally may aid the normal cells rather than the cancer cells and also aid the removal of toxins and carcinogens.

Inflammation

Inflammation has been linked with a variety of different cancers as inflammatory markers aid tumour progression, promotion and growth. It has been found that a cellular inflammatory microenvironment and an increased level of nitric oxide can stimulate or accelerate tumour development.[93] Cyclooxygenase enzymes such as prostaglandins and thromboxanes play an important role in cancer, particularly in gastrointestinal, oesophageal, gastric, liver, pancreatic and colorectal cancers.[94]

A key approach to cancer is to modulate the inflammatory cascade; this can have a positive effect on cancer initiation, promotion, progression and metastasis. **Anti-inflammatory nutrients** such as curcumin,[95] bromelain,[96] quercetin[96] and EPA/DHA[96] can decrease the progressive effect of the inflammation in cancer. **Herbal medicines** such as *Zingiber officinale*, *Curcuma longa*,[95] *Withania somnifera*[97] and *Boswellia serrata* may also be useful.[96]

Immunological factors

A functioning immune system appropriately monitors and attacks any foreign cells or pathogenic invaders. A dysregulated immune system can allow cancer cells to develop and spread.[98] States that can cause a dysregulated immune system affecting cancer include stress,[99,100] diabetes,[101] HIV (and other viruses)[102] and nutritional deficiencies.[103,104]

Nutrients and herbs that support immune function can be very important in assisting people with cancer. Those clinical **nutritional interventions** with particular benefit in cancer include vitamin D,[105] antioxidants,[106] vitamin C,[106] zinc[106] and medicinal mushrooms such as shiitake or reishi.[107,108] Herbal medicines which may be of benefit include *Astragalus membranaceus*,[109] *Uncaria tomentosa*,[110] *Eleutherococcus senticosus*,[111] *Rhodiola rosacea*,[111] *Schisandra chinensis*,[111] *Panax ginseng*[112] and *Echinacea* spp.[113]

Hormonal factors

Some specific cancers, including breast,[114] ovarian, endometrial,[115] cervical, prostate and testicular cancers, are well known to have hormonal influences.[116] Other cancers, including both gastric and lung cancer, may also have hormonal influences.[117,118]

Breast cancer can be stimulated by oestrogen and/or progesterone,[114] whereas ovarian, endometrial and cervical cancers may be oestrogen-stimulated via receptor sites on the cancer cells.[115] Testosterone is the key hormone related to prostate- or male genitalia-based cancers, whereas testicular cancer may be related to either oestrogen or androgens, and approximately 7–11% of males who get testicular cancer have also been found to have gynaecomastia.[116]

Oestrogen may have protective effects on gastric cancer, as the prevalence of gastric cancer is higher in men and lower in premenopausal women, women on hormone replacement and men undergoing oestrogen therapy.[117] The actual mechanism of protection is unclear, but it is thought that oestrogen may increase the expression of trefoil factor proteins, which have been found to protect mucous epithelia or inhibit the expression of c-erb-2 oncogene.

Lung cancer has also been found to have an oestrogen connection. Adenocarcinoma is the most common type of lung cancer in non-smokers, and it has been suggested that there is a distinct pattern concerning oestrogen beta receptors.[118]

A number of nutrients and herbs can have a positive effect in the integrative treatment of hormonal tumours. For oestrogen- and progesterone-stimulated tumours, cruciferous indoles—particularly **indole-3-carbonol**—aids in a number of different ways: it aids the induction of apoptosis in breast and cervical cancer cells by inducing DNA breakage in the nucleus of the cells,[119] and it alters the metabolism of active oestrogen hormones indicated in urinary excretion (16-oestrodiol to 2-oestrodiol).[120]

Other nutrients that have been found to be of assistance include **zinc** for testosterone via the enzyme 5 alpha-reductase;[121] **resveratrol** via inhibiting the cytochrome p450 19 enzymes—also called aromatase catalases—which are the rate limiting step of oestrogen synthesis;[122] and **genistein**, which, although controversial and having mixed results, has shown positive results by inhibiting cell proliferation and inducing apoptosis in breast cancer cell lines.[123] However, it has also been shown to stimulate growth in oestrogen-dependent human tumour cells, MCF-7, and may negate the inhibitory effect of Tamoxifen.[124]

Herbs that have shown to be of potential benefit include ***Serenoa repens*** for prostate cancer. Serenoa has been found to induce growth arrest of prostate cancer cells as well as increasing p21 and p53 in the prostate cells.[125] ***Cimicifuga racemosa*** has been found to improve symptoms associated with breast cancer by alleviating vasomotor symptoms associated with the decrease of oestrogen.[126]

Trifolium pratense has also been found to be of benefit for oestrogen-based cancers. The isoflavone constituent biochanin A has been found to inhibit cytochrome p19 (aromatase) activity and gene expression, therefore decreasing the effect of active oestrogen.[127]

Mitochondrial function

Mitochondrial dysfunction has been linked with the increased risk of cancer.[128] Most of the mitochondrial influence is via its link to apoptosis (p53) and anaerobic glycolysis; however, there may be another area in which mitochondrial function plays an important role. Cancer cells may have impaired mitochondria and mitochondrial activity, which may support Warburg's theory as to why cancer cells use the anaerobic glycolysis pathway rather than the aerobic system.[129] Concentrating on mitochondrial reprogramming and support may therefore assist in addressing cancer. **Nutrients** that have been found to assist mitochondrial function include coenzyme Q10,[130] lipoic acid,[131] carnitine[132] and B vitamins such as niacin (NAD).[133]

Angiogenesis

Angiogenesis (developing their own blood supply to aid their proliferation and growth) in tumours is well recognised.[128] Many chemotherapeutics currently target this angiogenic process. However, some naturopathic medicines have also been found to possess an anti-angiogenic action. These include intravenous vitamin C,[134] *Curcuma longa,*[135,136] *Artemisia annua, Viscum album, Scutellaria baicalensis,* resveratrol and proanthocyanidins, *Magnolia officinalis, Camellia sinensis, Ginkgo biloba,* quercetin, *Poria cocos, Zingiber officinales, Panax ginseng* and *Rabdosia rubescens hora.*[137] Using any number of these naturopathic medicines may aid the reduction of angiogenesis, by virtue of possibly having a positive effect on decreasing tumour initiation, promotion, progression and metastasis.

DIET AND CANCER

There have been a number of studies on diet and its effect on cancer. Certain dietary deficiencies have been associated with cancer development. Dietary factors account for approximately 30% of cancer cases in developed countries and 20% in developing nations, and are second only to tobacco as a preventable cause of cancer.[138] Other studies have been conducted on specific foods or beverages linked with cancer. There are also a multitude of diets that are promoted as 'anti-cancer diets', but most of these have not been studied specifically and are mostly based on broader empirical evidence.

The most common dietary link to cancer is the crude lack of fruit and vegetables.[139] An increased intake of fruit and vegetables has been found to be protective against lung,[140] oesophageal[141] and colon cancer.[142] Fruit and vegetable intake has also been suggested to be protective from breast and ovarian cancer although results at this stage state that the lack of fruit and vegetables is not a risk factor for either.[143,144]

In addition to an increased consumption of fruit and vegetables, a low intake of meat and potatoes has been found to be protective against colorectal and oesophageal cancer.[141,142] High meat consumption—particularly through adolescence—has also been found to be a risk factor for premenopausal breast cancer.[145] Both high meat consumption and high sugar intake have also been linked as risk factors for pancreatic cancer.[146] High poultry intake and high-fat dairy intake are associated with an increased risk of gastric cancer.[141] Adherence to a Western-style diet and high alcohol intake are also associated with an increased risk of gastric cancer.[147] A high intake of alcohol has been associated with not only gastric cancer but also breast[148] and liver cancer.[26]

Fat intake is another area of concern in relation to cancer. High-fat diets have been linked with numerous cancers, including breast, prostate and colon cancers.[149,150] Studies have also found that high fat intake increases the oxidation of DNA and encourages damaged cell proliferation.[149] However, specific fats, such as **omega-3 fatty acids** as found in fish oil, have demonstrated protective effects for breast, prostate and colon cancer.[149,150] The current Western diet has a disproportionate ratio of omega-6 fatty acids to omega-3 fatty acids compared to more traditional diets; this may result in increased risk of cancer development.[150]

Iodine has been studied for a number of cancers, including thyroid cancer and breast cancer. Both a deficiency and an excessive amount of iodine have been associated with an increased risk of thyroid cancer.[151,152] For breast cancer, recent studies have suggested that iodine may have a protective effect on breast tissue by inhibiting cancer development via the modulation of the oestrogen pathway.[152]

Green tea[153] has also been extensively studied for cancer with positive results, and **black tea**[154] and **coffee**[155] have also shown convincing beneficial effects. Green tea and black tea have demonstrated benefit across a broad range of cancers; however, coffee seems to be mainly beneficial in protection against liver cancer. The protective effect of coffee seems to be related to moderate intake with studies looking at only one coffee drink a day, or less than 250 mg of caffeine intake a day.[155]

Studies looking at vegetarian or plant-based diets have also achieved reasonable results, though nothing conclusive has been found at this stage. It seems that a vegetarian or plant-based diet or a macrobiotic diet may be of benefit, particularly for colorectal, prostate and breast cancer.[156,157] This may be related not merely to the vegetarian nature of the diet, but also to the increased proportions of fibre, fruit and vegetable intakes often associated with these diets.

Although most studies focus on specific components or diets, the general consensus is that broad improvements in diet are extremely beneficial in the prevention of and treatment of cancer. Increasing fruit and vegetable consumption has clear benefit. Patients should be encouraged to 'have a rainbow on their plate'—eating as many colours (often associated with specific phytochemical compounds) each day as they can. The less adventurous could be given the task of exploring a new fruit or vegetable each week. Increasing fibre and reducing the intake of simple carbohydrates also show great benefit, and these changes can be achieved by encouraging patients to experiment with lesser known grains such as buckwheat, quinoa, millet, brown rice and bulghur. Legumes can also be a beneficial addition in this respect. While these additions are clearly beneficial, they are in many cases large diversions from current eating habits, and patients may require practical support as well as suggestions if they are to implement these changes successfully.

INTEGRATIVE MEDICAL CONSIDERATIONS

Acupuncture

There are many studies proving the beneficial effects of acupuncture for cancer, for a variety of different reasons. Studies using acupuncture to treat cancer pain,[163] vasomotor and fatigue symptoms of both breast and prostate cancer[164,165] show that it boosts the immune system and decrease tumour growth[166] and is beneficial for the treatment of nausea and other side effects.[167] Acupuncture has had documented success in improving nausea symptoms associated with chemotherapy.[168–170] Electroacupuncture seems more effective than manual acupuncture for this purpose. Other studies on acupuncture and specific cancer conditions show benefit, suggesting it may be a beneficial adjuvant treatment.[128]

Psychosocial and mind–body interventions

Meditation can be of assistance to people with cancer by reducing stress, improving mood and quality of life and aiding sleep problems.[171] Counselling has been found to assist with the anxiety, depression and life decisions that these people experience.[172]

Yoga is another therapy that has growing support to assist with quality of life, sleep and mood. Other therapies that may be of assistance include creative therapies such as

ALTERATIVES/DEPURATIVES AND CANCER—ESSIAC

One of the best known CAM treatments used as a depurative for cancer is the Essiac® tea. It is a mixture of four herbs: *Arctium lappa*, *Rumex acetosella*, *Rheum officinale* and *Ulmus fulva*. It was originally a herbal formulation from the Ojibway Indians in Canada and was discovered in 1922 by Rene Caisse, who reports to have 'cured' hundreds of people with cancer with this formula.[158]

Rumex acetosella is said to destroy cancer cells while the other three herbs aid purifying the blood. A chiropractor, Gary Glum, stated that the burdock root also contains inulin, which is considered to be a powerful immune modulator.[158] Most of the information is anecdotal; however, there have been a few recent studies on the mechanism of action of Essiac, although there are also studies that found that there was no real benefit to Essiac.

The first real investigation of Essiac was in 2007 by the Department of Research and Clinical Epidemiology in the Canadian College of Naturopathic Medicine in Toronto.[159] This study comes about as a response to the negative recommendations from the Task Force on Alternative Therapies of the Canadian Breast Cancer Research Initiative, as very little research has been conducted on this formula.[159]

The activity of Essiac was measured using assays to establish the antioxidant, fibrinolytic, antimicrobial, anti-inflammatory, immune modulation, cell-specific cytotoxicity and effect on cytochrome P450 enzymes. It was found that Essiac exhibited significant antioxidant activity and had immunomodulating effects through stimulation of granulocyte phagocytosis, increasing CD8+ cell activation and moderately inhibiting inflammatory pathways. It also exhibited significant cell-specific cytotoxicity towards ovarian epithelial carcinoma cells. In regards to cytochrome P450 enzymes, it inhibited CYP1A2 and CYP2C19. Clot fibrinolytic activity was dose dependent.[159]

Two other in vitro studies found that Essiac had positive results, with one indicating inhibition of tumour growth in prostate cells.[160] However, one of the studies also showed that Essiac tea stimulated some pro-inflammatory molecules as well as nitric oxide.[161] This same study found that that it had no anti-proliferative affect on leukaemic cell lines but that it inhibited 50% of MCF7 breast cancer cell lines, as did Flor-Essence tea—a similar product containing *Arctium lappa*, *Rumex acetosella* and *Ulmus fulva*, but also containing *Nasturtium officinale*, *Rheum palmatum*, *Cnicus benedictus* and *Trifolium pratense*.[161]

Only one in vivo study has been conducted on animals (mice); the tea was administered orally, mimicking human intake. The result found that it did demonstrate a modest gastric protective effect by reducing ethanol-induced gastric ulceration. However, there was no demonstration of hepatoprotective, hypoglycaemic or immunomodulatory effects, not supporting the suggested actions of Essiac.[162]

There seems to be no toxicity associated with Essiac tea and in vitro studies seem to indicate potential positive anticancer properties. However, further studies on humans are required to scientifically support or discredit the use of Essiac tea in cancer treatment. However, there appears to be no or very little harm to patients with cancer if they consumed Essiac tea as an adjuvant.

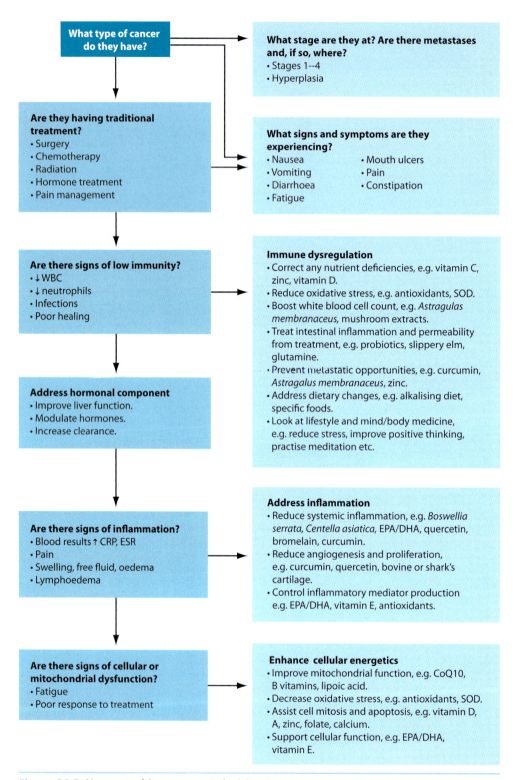

Figure 29.3 Naturopathic treatment decision tree—cancer

TREATMENT OF PEOPLE AT DIFFERENT STAGES OF CANCER AND LEVELS OF VITALITY

It is important for the naturopath to realise the condition and level of vitality of the patient when treating them. For example, someone with a stage 4 cancer who has been told they have little time left to live, or that they are in palliative care as there is nothing else that can be done, may react several ways. They may be ready to pass away and just want assistance in managing pain and quality of life; or they may not accept the diagnosis and want to fight. Either way, the naturopath needs to acknowledge this and support the patient in their decision.

Vitality at this stage is also important as some people who have been told they have a couple of months to live may actually have a lot of vitality and are able to take on a rigorous regimen to assist their health. Others may not have vitality and may be very sick, so taking on a rigorous regimen is not appropriate as their body is not able to withstand the regimen suggested. Nor in most cases do they have the energy or body function to allow it. An example of this is someone at end-stage cancer in extreme cachexia with or without the start of peripheral shutdown. This indicates that their body can take only very little stress and is very close to passing away. Normally they have no appetite, and have difficulty swallowing and performing normal bodily functions.

Another example is radiation enteropathy where the person has severe vomiting, diarrhoea and inflammation along their entire gastrointestinal tract. They normally go into severe cachexia very quickly and have problems keeping anything down. It is nearly impossible to prescribe anything orally to assist, so other options need to be considered.

Therefore, understanding the patient's level of vitality and emotional status is an essential aspect of treatment.

visual arts, painting, dance and music, which may help patients with cancer express their feelings and help them cope with what they are experiencing.[171] A review of 50 studies found that qi gong was mostly associated with positive outcomes in cancer patients.[173]

However, it should be noted that while such interventions, like support groups, can help cancer patients in numerous ways, evidence does not at this stage seem to suggest that this translates into prolonging their lives.[174] Religious or spiritual beliefs have been found to be of benefit for cancer patients. The supportive environment and thought of an afterlife can be very important for cancer patients;[175] however, this should not translate to the encouragement of false hope.

Homoeopathy

A Cochrane review on homoeopathy and cancer treatment involving eight controlled trials and a total of 664 participants found preliminary data to support the efficacy of topical homoeopathic Calendula treatment for prophylaxis of acute dermatitis during radiotherapy and the proprietary homoeopathic Traumeel S mouthwash in the treatment of chemotherapy-induced stomatitis.[176] They found no convincing evidence for the efficacy of homoeopathic medicines for other adverse effects of cancer treatment. Pilot studies from the UK hospitals have demonstrated positive patient outcomes when homoeopathy has been used in conjunction with conventional treatment.[177]

Massage

Massage has been found to give immediate beneficial effects for pain and improving mood for patients with cancer.[178] While positive outcomes have been found for stress and anxiety as well, adverse effects from massage therapy—including pathological fractures of metastatic bones and bruising in patients with coagulopathy—may be more likely in cancer patients.[179]

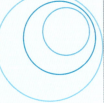

KEY POINTS

- Treat the person first, not the disease.
- Cancer is a complex condition with a myriad of different causes and interactions. It is important to address this multifactorial condition from many different aspects by addressing each stage rather than everything at once.
- Keep supplementation and diet simple, and don't overwhelm the patient with too many things to take, especially if they are also undergoing traditional treatment.
- Many nutritional and lifestyle factors can be involved with cancer and it is important to address the specific factors associated with the person as well as the type of cancer.
- Always address nutritional deficiencies and ensure a balanced body weight.
- Encourage a supportive environment and refer if required for psychological support.

Case Study 1: Colon Cancer

A female Buddhist yoga teacher, 55 years of age, presents with **colon cancer with secondaries**. She has **metastasis on the liver** (three spots), which was found first. The primary site has not been identified. The stool test was clear, with no rectal bleeding. She has a very healthy diet with no sugar, a good amount of fibre and vegetable juices daily and eats organic fruit, vegetables and organic, plus fish. She drinks over 3 litres of water a day as well as Japanese green tea, peppermint tea and fenugreek tea. Currently she has had a **porta cath** implanted in her chest and is having **chemotherapy** every 2 weeks (a slow drip through the porta cath for 24 hours). The chemotherapeutic is Oxyplatin and 5 FU.

MAIN SYMPTOMS

- Weight loss
- Side effects:
  - nerve ending neurotoxicity
  - haemorrhoids (may have lower gastrointestinal bleeding (red) or upper gastrointestinal bleeding (melena))
  - mouth ulcers
  - nose bleeds
  - very fatigued
- Metastasis lumps in the liver have decreased by about 20 mm each.
- CEA is 1.3 (range of 0–5).

Overview

The aetiology of cancer has been previously discussed; however, there are certain aspects that are more relevant to colon cancer. Diet and lifestyle are associated with the development of colon cancer, but the most clearly defined aetiological factors appear to be hereditary factors, inflammatory bowel disease, papillomavirus and acquired immunodeficiency syndrome (AIDS).[180]

Table 29.5 Review of the major evidence—colon cancer

INTERVENTION	METHODOLOGY	RESULT	COMMENT
Folate[181]	399 women with 22 years of follow up Laboratory immunohistochemically assayed p53 expression in paraffin-fixed colon cancer specimens	Compared with women with folate intake < 200 µg/day, the RR for p53-overexpressing (mutated) cancers were: • 0.54 (95% CI 0.36–0.81) for women who consumed 200–299 µg/day. • 0.42 (95% CI, 0.24–0.76) for women who consumed 300–399 µg/day. • 0.54 (95% CI, 0.35–0.83) for women who consumed ≥ 400 µg/day. Total folate intake had no influence on wild-type tumours. High vitamin B4 intake conferred a protective effect on p53-overexpressing cancers (top versus bottom quintile: RR, 0.57; 95% CI, 0.35–0.94; p(heterogeneity) = 0.01) but had no effect on p53 wild-type tumours.	This study was conducted after a RCT trial on folate supplementation showed that it didn't reduce the risk of adenoma recurrence. However, this study did show that low folate and vitamin B6 intake affected p53 expression in colon cancer. Therefore, maintaining folate intake of over 400 mg a day and a high vitamin B6 intake may decrease the risk of colon adenoma but not of wild type tumours.
Calcium and vitamin D[182]	In 2002 48,115 US women, free of colorectal cancer or polyps, completed a food frequency questionnaire in 1980, and then underwent endoscopy.	Colon cancers found included 2,747 cases of adenoma. Total calcium intake weakly associated with distal colorectal adenoma risk (RR − 0.88, 95% CI: 0.74, 1.04; p(trend) = 0.06), particularly for large adenoma (RR = 0.73, 95% CI: 0.56, 0.96; p(trend) = 0.02). Total vitamin D intake weakly associated with reduced risk of distal colorectal adenoma (RR = 0.79, 95% CI: 0.63, 0.99; p(trend) = 0.07), but more strongly with distal colon adenoma risk (RR = 0.67, 95% CI: 0.52, 0.87; p(trend) = 0.004).	Greater total calcium and vitamin D intakes were associated with reduced risk of colon cancer. The findings of reduced risk are most likely due to the vitamin D activity rather than the calcium, but this study did show that both are important in decreasing the risk of colon cancer.
Selenium[183]	Randomised 424 patients to 200 µg or 400 µg/day of selenium or to matched placebo since 1989	The 200 µg/day selenium treatment decreased total cancer incidence by a statistically significant 25%; however, 400 µg/day of selenium had no effect on total cancer incidence.	Higher intake of selenium was shown to increase selenium levels. As selenium can cause toxicity, a lower dose may be more beneficial (as shown in this study) than higher dosing.

(Continued)

Table 29.5 Review of the major evidence—colon cancer *(Continued)*

INTERVENTION	METHODOLOGY	RESULT	COMMENT
Fibre[184]	137-item food frequency question-naire using prostate, lung, colorectal and ovarian (PLCO) cancer screening trial 33,971 participants who were sigmoidoscopy-nega-tive for polyps 3591 cases with at least one histo-logically verified adenoma in the distal large bowel	High intakes of dietary fibre were associated with a lower risk of colorectal adenoma. Participants in the highest quintile of dietary fibre intake had a 27% (95% CI 14–38, p(trend) = 0.002) lower risk of adenoma than those in the lowest quintile. Risks were similar for advanced and non-advanced adenoma. Risk of rectal adenoma was not significantly associated with fibre intake.	The best dietary fibre that was found to be beneficial was from grains, cereals and fruits. It is not only the amount of fibre that is important, but also its type.
Echinacea[185]	15 people 1000 mg of standard-ized *E. purpurea* for 10 days. Faecal samples were collected at baseline, 10 days and 17–18 days. Tested for select aerobic and anaerobic bacteria.	Significant increases in total aerobic bacteria, *Bacteroides* group and *Bacteroides fragilis*. No alteration in the number of enteric bacteria, enterococci, lactobacilli, bifidobacteria or total anaerobic bacteria.	This study shows that echinacea supplemen-tation can alter the GI microbacteria. These changes may aid the reduction of the risk of colon cancer as well as other colon diseases.
Cabbage[186]	12 healthy volunteers 3 meals at 48 hour intervals containing raw cabbage, cooked cabbage or mustard. Watercress juice was also consumed to allow individual and temporal variation in postabsorptive iso-thiocyanate recovery to be measured. Volume of each urination for 24 h after each meal. Samples were analysed for N-acetyl cysteine conjugates of isothiocyanates.	Excretion of isothiocyanates was rapid and substantial after mustard. After raw cabbage, allyl isothiocyanate was rapidly excreted, although to a lesser extent. Cooked cabbage excretion of allyl isothiocyanate was considerably less and the excretion was delayed.	Cabbage contains glucosinolate sinigrin, which is hydrolysed by myrosinase to allyl isothiocyanates. These isothiocyanates are said to inhibit colon cancer cell develop-ment. From these results iso-thiocyanate production is more extensive after consumption of raw vegetables; they are still produced but to a lesser extent when the vegetables are cooked. This delayed excre-tion by the cooked cabbage may be due to the colon microflora catalysing glucosino-late hydrolysis of the cabbage.

Example treatment

Prescription

This patient has started with a very good diet and has adequate fibre intake, so minimal dietary changes are required. The dietary changes include adding cabbage to the juice she is consuming daily. Due to weight loss, it would be beneficial to drink a whey-based protein drink twice a day as well as increasing her intake of sardines and salmon for the omega-3 fatty acids. Using fats such as flax seed, chai seeds, nuts and seeds, olive oil and ghee in her diet will also be of benefit for both good fats and maintaining weight. She should drink at least 2–3 cups of sencha green tea, making sure to let it stand for 10 minutes before drinking to ensure catechin release.

For exercise she is advised to continue **yoga** on a daily basis. Her spiritual beliefs and supportive environment will be good for her wellbeing.

The herbal formula is aimed at increasing immunity and white blood cells during the chemotherapy as well as supporting the liver. It may also alleviate some of the fatigue she is experiencing. The nutrients are aimed at increasing the immunity, bowel health, cell mitosis and apoptosis of cancer cells, and the vitamin B6 is aimed at trying to decrease some of the neuropathy.

Herbal formula

Echinacea angustifolia 1:2	30 mL
Astragalus membranaceus 1:2	40 mL
Eleutherococcus senticosus 1:2	30 mL
5 mL t.d.s.	100 mL
Silybum marianum thistle 10 g 1 tablet b.d.	

Nutritional prescription

Folic acid tablet	500 mg/day
Selenium capsule	200 µg/day
Vitamin D3 capsule	1000 µg/day
Activated B6	50 mg/day

Note: No supplements should be taken the day before and 1–2 days after chemotherapy.

Other prescriptive options

When experiencing diarrhoea, slippery elm powder may be of benefit to assist slowing down the passage of faeces, adding bulk and healing the gut lining. Another nutrient that may be of assistance is beta glucan, which may increase the digestive immune system (GALT). For mouth ulcers, bicarbonate soda in water may be of benefit. Other options include manuka honey, zinc paste, glutamine mouth wash or a diluted calendula mouth wash.

Therapeutic considerations

One beneficial aspect for this patient is that sections of her bowel have not been removed so she does not experience bowel problems such as low transit time and poor absorption. However, as the metastasis is in the liver it can mean that certain foods or supplements may be reactive. The herbal mixture, with its alcohol base, could become an issue in this case. To counteract this, the naturopath could use glycertracts, non-alcohol-based herbal liquids, capsules or tablets.

Interactions with chemotherapy are another issue, especially as the patient's chemotherapy is a slow release over 2 days. First she may not feel very well those days and secondly, as there is no concrete evidence that the natural medicine will not interact with the chemotherapy, it is best to stop the day before and recommence a day or two after, depending on how the lady is feeling.

Lastly, taking a lot of supplements may become overwhelming for the patient, especially when they are going through treatment. It is best to keep this in mind and check if the patient is able to follow the prescription.

Expected outcomes and follow-up protocols

This patient has a very good state of mind and will to live, as well as a supportive environment that will benefit her greatly. However, as the primary site has not been found, her long-term results are quite difficult to predict. In all, the diet and supplements should decrease her side effects, increase her immune system, aid cellular function, decrease inflammation and support body functions. She has specific foods for bowel cancer and support for her liver.

Bowel cancer can be quite aggressive and liver metastasis is the most common secondary associated with this disease. Every patient is different when it comes to cancer and expected outcomes are difficult to predict.

KEY POINTS

- Colon cancer is a hereditary disease that can be influenced by diet and lifestyle.
- Nutritional deficiencies are associated with increased risk of colorectal cancer.
- Test patients for nutritional deficiencies such as vitamin D3, selenium and red cell folate.
- Many complex factors that interact can affect bowel cancer and all need to be taken into consideration depending on the patient.
- Focus on the pertinent cancer perspectives that affect that person.

Case Study 2: Breast Cancer

A female, 42 years of age, presents with breast cancer with secondaries. Her primary **breast cancer** was diagnosed 6 years ago and was a **ductal carcinoma in situ (DCIS) with a grade 3**. It was oestrogen positive and progesterone negative. She had a lumpectomy on the left breast with concurrent chemotherapy for 6 months, and 5 weeks of radiation. She then started on Tamoxifen. Two years later she was diagnosed with **metastasis in the liver, bone and lung**. She underwent further chemotherapy and started using natural therapies. She has been monitored since then and has been put on Xeloda continuously with a week's break every 2–3 weeks depending on status. She is following a **very strict diet** (suggested by a complementary doctor) that is alkaline with no grains, dairy, sugar, caffeine (except green tea) and stimulants and has limited fruit intake. She drinks 3 litres of water a day, green tea and vegetable juices and is taking a range of complementary supplements. She requires refinement of supplements and restructure of the diet.

MAIN SYMPTOMS

- Primary breast cancer 6 years ago
- Metastasis 2 years later in liver, lung and bone
- Oestrogen positive
- Surgery on liver metastasis 1 year ago

- Side effects of chemotherapy: burning and painful feet, mouth ulcers, general feeling of being unwell, digestive upsets, insomnia and anxiety

OVERVIEW

The aetiology of breast cancer is multifaceted. There are many suggested causes of this disease and there are a variety of different types of breast cancer from benign to hormone sensitive to inflammatory. Breast cancer can be oestrogen positive, progesterone positive or both. Research has found that longer exposure to oestrogen and higher levels of oestrogen exposure do increase the risk of developing breast cancer. Pregnancy, late menarche and early menopause are all considered to be protective factors.[187] High concentrations of oestrogen even as a fetus have been found to have an effect on breast cancer development.[188]

Another risk factor for breast cancer is an energy-rich diet during puberty and adolescence as it develops pre-cancerous lesions in the breast. Full-term pregnancy decreases these developments; however, continuation of an energy-rich diet late in life also contributes

Table 29.6 Review of the major evidence—breast cancer

INTERVENTION	METHODOLOGY	RESULT	COMMENT
Black cohosh Vitamin E Soy phytoestrogen[200]	10 RCT, double-blind clinical trials with 1581 women 3 placebo-controlled double-blind trials with 329 men 14 pilot trials with 350 people	Pilot trials found that further studies are warranted. Men studies found that hot flushes were markedly decreased by low doses of megestrol acetate, moderate by gabapentin but not by clonidine. Women studies found that hot flushes were markedly decreased by low dose progestational agents, moderate by venlafaxine, mildly by fluoxetine, vitamin E, soy phytoestrogen and black cohosh.	Although this study shows only limited affect for black cohosh, vitamin E and soy phytoestrogens, there are other studies, although not RCTs, that do indicate positive results in decreasing the vasomotor response in women. This study was indicated for both menopausal women and those with breast cancer. It was found that even those women on Tamoxifen had results with these. Further studies are required.
Vitamin D[192]	Meta-analysis of 1731 studies on Pubmed, Embase and Web of Science 6 studies had original data.	Overall, no association between amount of vitamin D and risk of breast cancer was found. Most studies found low intakes vitamin D (100–400 IU/day) ≥ 400 IU/day had less risk of breast cancer.	There are many studies linking low vitamin D to an increased risk of breast cancer, but there has been no RCT for this as it is very hard to do. The best studies would be those comparing vitamin D levels of women with breast cancer and those of women who don't. More studies are necessary.
Coenzyme Q10, vitamins B3 and B2[201,202]	CoQ10, niacin and riboflavin given with Tamoxifen for 90 days (no amounts given) Blood samples taken at baseline, days 45 and 90 78 untreated, sole TAM, and combination group with age 46 and sex matched controls Lipids, lipid peroxides, enzymes and antioxidants tested	Untreated group had increased oxidative stress and decreased AO. TAM group had slight increased oxidative stress and decreased antioxidants with severe hypertriglyceridaemia. Combination group had decreased oxidative stress and increased antioxidants.	Increased oxidative stress has been observed in breast cancer patients and can lead to promotion of cancer cells. Decreasing this oxidative stress and increasing antioxidant status is extremely beneficial in the prevention of further cancer development in these women. Combining CoQ10 and vitamins B1 and B2 with traditional treatment has great promise for breast cancer patients.

to an increase in obesity and growth of existing subclinical breast cancer lesions. The mechanism behind this dietary factor is through endocrine factors such as oestrogen.[189]

Other suggested risk factors include iodine deficiencies,[190,152] vitamin D deficiencies,[191,192] high intake of red meat,[145] environmental exposure to xenoestrogens[193] and organochlorides,[194,195] factors such as make-up, deodorants and creams,[196,197] low melatonin or sleep deprivation (including that from shiftworking)[198] and other diseases such as diabetes.[199]

Example treatment
Prescriptions
Diet: As this patient had a good diet; all she needed was more variety. Diet suggestions include increasing cold water oily fish, salmon or sardines four to five times a week, and including fruits such as berries, strawberries, paw paw, red apples, cherries, red grapes and pears. For grains, include quinoa, buckwheat or black rice porridge using coconut milk. She

can also include legumes such as chickpeas, akuzi beans and broad beans. She can use quinoa or brown rice for lunch and/or dinner for added grains. Organic red meat can be consumed 1–2 times a week if needed, low-mercury fish as much as she wants, and organic chicken 2–3 times a week. Almond or quinoa milk can be used where required. One drink of a red wine such as pinot noir a night for 3–4 nights or fewer a week if she wants (this is for resveratrol).

Lifestyle: Take up yoga or pilates at least once a week. Meditate every day for around 5–20 minutes, or more if possible. Look at getting massage when needed to aid relaxation. Look at stress management techniques.

Supplements: All supplements are explained above in the overview. Indole-3-carbinole (not discussed above) has been found to help the conversion of oestrogen to 16-hydroxyestrone (16-OHE1) instead of 2-hydroxyestrone (2-OHE1). Women with breast cancer have been found to have higher levels of 2-OHE1, which is considered to be detrimental as it is associated with the development of breast cancer.[203]

Note: No supplements are to be taken at least 3 hours before or after the chemotherapy tablet.

> **Herbal prescription**
>
> *Silybum marianum* thistle 10,000 mg/day in tablet form
>
> **Nutritional prescription**
>
> CoQ10 200–300 mg/day with food
> Lipoic acid 400 mg–600 mg/day with food
> Vitamin B complex 1 capsule a day after breakfast
> Quercetin 600 mg and vitamin C 3 g split throughout the day in between food
> 5-hydroxytryptophan 100 mg at night away from food, for anxiety
> Calcium 800 mg and vitamin D 5–100 µg at night before bed
> Indole-3-carbinole or diindolylmethane (DIM) 2–4 capsules a day

Other prescriptive options

Other herbs to consider if required would be *Cimicifuga racemosa* if hot flushes start. *Astragalus membranaceus*, *Panax ginseng*, *Eleutherococcus sentocosus*, *Zizyphus spinosa*, *Rhodiola rosea*, *Uncaria tomentosa* or *Withania somnifera* may all be used as adaptogens to assist general wellbeing, energy and immune system. *Passiflora incarnata*, *Scutellaria lateriflora*, *Withania somnifera*, *Bacopa monnieri* or *Centella asiatica* may all assist with the nervous system and anxiety. Many other herbs can be used; it depends on the patient which herbs are more suited. Lymphatic herbal medicines, including Essiac, have also been traditionally used.

Other nutrients that can be used are L-theanine for anxiety and sleep, resveratrol as a capsule instead of drinking red wine (as a capsule is a more concentrated form) and green tea as a capsule instead of drinking it (to get higher concentrations). Extra vitamin D3 may be required if the patient's blood levels are found to be on the low side.

Supplements that could be very beneficial and can be added later are calcium D-glucarate, which aids the excretion of environmental or pharmacological xenobiotics by increasing glucuronidation in phase II liver detoxification. Citrus pectin has been suggested to be of assistance, particularly in people with metastasis. Melatonin has many chemoprotective and antioxidant properties and has also been found to be beneficial for people with cancer. Mushroom extracts such as shiitake or reishi may be used to boost the immune system.

Depending on the digestive upsets, she should be taking a probiotic, possibly betaine hydrochloride as she shows signs of low stomach acid, and slippery elm, depending on chemotherapy.

Many other supplements, including liver nutrients, taurine, glutathione, mixed antioxidants and berry punches, can be used. It is important to ascertain which is most appropriate at each particular stage for the patient without overwhelming them.

Therapeutic considerations

This patient has everything to work towards and is very compliant. She has no real restrictions to compliance other than too many tablets, which could overwhelm her. Her husband is a doctor and is very supportive. It is best to work with the medical practitioners treating her.

There are many compliance issues that can restrict patients. One of the largest is knowing what to take and when; they can be overwhelmed with the treatment they are receiving medically and not know how to incorporate the complementary medicine with it. Ideally, the naturopath should understand what the patient is willing and able to do and work within that framework, rather than trying to give them everything at once. Another compliance issue is the oncologist with whom the patient is undergoing treatment, and the oncologist's feelings or opinions about using complementary therapies during treatment. These can cause a lot of people to choose not to take certain supplements during treatment, or follow dietary suggestions.

Expected outcomes and follow-up protocols

The expected outcome is realistically being able to extend this patient's life and quality of life. She has advanced breast cancer and it is possible that she could pass away from this disease. With hope and persistence, her life expectancy could be extended, but maintenance and constant treatment will be required. Her positive attitude and supportive environment will be of great assistance and her compliance will be very beneficial to her ability to beat this disease and live as long as possible.

KEY POINTS

- Breast cancer is extremely varied, from benign to hormone sensitive to inflammatory. Treatment will depending on what type and grade it is. Not all people with breast cancer are required to have their oestrogen levels decreased.
- Genetic involvement is very relevant for this type of cancer, so working on genetic factors to support cell mitosis and decrease DNA breakage is extremely important.
- Reduce as much as possible any negative environmental and dietary factors, for example radiation from microwaves and mobile phones (it should be noted that evidence in this area is currently inconclusive), as well as organochlorides and xenoestrogens.

Case Study 3: Prostate Cancer

A male, who is 56 years of age, married and owns his own company, presents with the **diagnosis of prostate cancer**. He has a **PSA of 7 with a Gleason score of 8**. At present, he has decided to try 3 months of natural therapies before deciding on any medical intervention such as surgery. His diet consists of meat every day, mostly red with some chicken, pork and seafood. He consumes limited vegetables, eats about two serves of fruit a day, has a mixture of white and wholemeal breads and grains, eats a lot of dairy products and has a lot of business lunches and dinners, which consist mainly of fried foods. He drinks around 1 litre of water, three or four brewed coffees a day (with 1 teaspoon of sugar and milk), has two or three beers most days and one to three glasses of wine every day.

KEY SYMPTOMS

- PSA of 7 (range < 2)
- Gleason score of 8 which means it is aggressive
- May develop difficult or painful urination or sexual dysfunction

Overview

Like the other cancers, the aetiology is not completely proven and is multifactorial. The one clear factor that has been linked with prostate cancer is testosterone and its active metabolite, dihydrotestosterone.[204] Genetic factors have also been found to be involved with prostate cancer. In this case, there is a complex interaction between genetic factors and the environment, which seem to be the predisposing factors for prostate cancer.[204]

Occupational factors that increase the risk of prostate cancer include jobs that have exposure to cadmium and other heavy metals in men with lower zinc levels. These include occupations such as farmers, miners, painters and printers.[204] The dietary factors associated with increased risk of prostate cancer include fats such as animal fats and alpha-linoleic vegetable fats. The fat on meats in particular has been found to be a high indicator.[204]

Sexual habits have also been linked with increased risk of prostate cancer. This includes the age of first intercourse, the number of sexual partners and a history of sexually transmitted diseases. All of these have been found to increase the risk; however, studies are still inconclusive.[204]

Conventional treatment is the same as all other cancers, except the new technology for radiation called 'brachytherapy' whereby radioactive tiny rods are inserted directly into the prostate. This directs radiation at the spot rather than going through other organs. There are two ways to implement brachytherapy: via permanent seed implantation or high-dose rate (HDR) temporary brachytherapy.

Permanent seed implantation is a technique where the doctors inject approximately 100 radioactive tiny rods into the prostate gland; these give off their radiation at a low dose for several weeks to months. The tiny rods stay in the prostate permanently. The HDR temporary brachytherapy involves placing very tiny plastic catheters into the prostate gland, and computer-controlled radiation is then given at a high dose through the catheters. The catheters are then pulled out and no radioactive rods are left in the gland.

Example treatment

Prescription

Diet: Alkalise the diet as much as possible, aiming for a low-fat, vegan-style diet with the exception of eating fish. It is important to include a lot of fruit and vegetables, especially cruciferous vegetables such as broccoli, cabbage, kale and brussels sprouts for the sulforazanes, as well as berries, especially raspberries. Cooked tomatoes is also important for lycopene, and carrots and high betacarotene foods are also beneficial. Garlic, onions, shallots as well as spices such as turmeric and cumin are also very good to include in the diet. Reduce as many animal products as possible, including fatty meats, cream and dairy. Increase fish as a protein, plus nuts, seeds and legumes. Recommend that he drink ginger punch, which has extra antioxidants in it, including turmeric, green tea and resveratrol. Suggest that he stops drinking alcohol for the 3 months,

Herbal formula

Uncaria tomentosa	1:2 50 mL
Andrographis paniculata	1:2 25 mL
Matricaria recutita	1:2 25 mL
5 mL t.d.s.	100 mL
Serenoa repens 3 g tablet b.d.	

Nutritional prescription

Selenium 200 µg/day
Zinc 30–50 mg/day
Antioxidant mix: vitamin C 3 g, vitamin E 500 IU, bioflavonoids 600 mg, vitamin D3 100 IU, vitamin A 5000IU, Coenzyme Q10 50 mg
Trace elements: including manganese 5 mg/day or a product that contains superoxide dismutase

Table 29.7 Review of the major evidence—prostate cancer

INTERVENTION	METHODOLOGY	RESULT	COMMENT
Selenium[183]	Randomised study on 1312 high-risk patients to 200 µg/day of selenium or matched placebo Another study began in 1989 with randomised 424 patients to 400 µg/day selenium or matched placebo Both studies had similar baseline selenium levels.	200 µg/day of selenium had a statistically significant effect on total cancer incidence with a decrease of 25%. 400 µg/day of selenium had no effect on total cancer incidence.	Selenium has been found to have an effect on many cancers, including prostate. Further specific studies need to be conducted; however, the positive results of selenium show that it is a beneficial supplement for prostate cancer. Continue to monitor selenium status through blood tests to avoid toxicity.
Manganese SOD and carotenoids such as lycopene[205]	Nested case control study with follow-up on 612 prostate cancer patients and 612 matched controls Invested MnSOD gene Ala16Val polymorphism and its joint association with plasma carotenoid concentrations in relation to total and aggressive prostate cancer (advanced stage or Gleason score ≥ 7)	No association was found between MnSOD genotype and risk of total and aggressive cancer. No statistically significant interactions were observed between MnSOD genotype and plasma carotenoids for risk of total and aggressive prostate cancer. An increased risk of aggressive prostate cancer was found in men with Ala/Ala genotype and low long-term lycopene status.	This study, although negative for association with genotypes, did confirm a significant finding that low antioxidant status, particularly with lycopene over a long period of time in men with a particular genotype, was associated with an increased risk of prostate cancer development. This shows that maintaining good antioxidant status and lycopene consumption should be imperative for men from about 30 years old onwards. Further studies are required, but this is a good baseline study.
Lycopene and soy products[206]	Small study on 41 men with recurrent, asymptomatic prostate cancer were randomised to 2 groups. Group A (n = 20) consumed tomato products (no soy) for weeks 0–4 (minimum 25 mg of lycopene). Group B (n = 21) consumed soy (no tomatoes) for weeks 0–4 (40 g of soy protein/day). For weeks 4–8 all men consumed a combined tomato-rich diet and soy supplement.	Serum PSA decreased between weeks 0 and 8 for 14/41 men (34%). Mean serum vascular endothelial growth factor for the entire group was reduced from 87 to 51 ng/mL over 8 weeks.	This study showed that a diet in tomato and soy products is easy for men to be compliant with. Combining both tomato and soy products was reasonably beneficial in decreasing PSA in mild prostate cases; however, further studies are required to determine the efficacy of lycopene and soy for prostate cancer prevention or management.

Table 29.7 Review of the major evidence—prostate cancer *(Continued)*

INTERVENTION	METHODOLOGY	RESULT	COMMENT
Very low-fat, vegan diet—protective effect of antioxidants, vitamins, carotenoids and fibre[207]	93 early stage prostate cancer patients in randomised controlled trial assigned to a very low-fat (10%) vegan diet supplemented with soy protein and lifestyle changes; the control was usual care. 3 day food records at baseline (*n* = 42 intervention, *n* = 43 control) and after 1 year (*n* = 37 in each group)	Intervention group compared to control showed increased dietary intake of macronutrients, vitamins, minerals, carotenoids and isoflavones. Fibre increased from mean 31 to 59 g/day. Lycopene increased from 8693 to 34,464 µg/day Saturated fatty acids decreased from 20 to 5 g/day. Cholesterol decreased from 200 to 10 mg/day.	This is a good study looking at dietary effects on cancer patients. These results indicate that a very low-fat vegan diet may be useful in increasing beneficial nutrients and decreasing detrimental nutrients. Further studies do need to be conducted to show the effect on the actual cancer and the diet's long-term effect.

decreases his coffee consumption to one 'real' coffee a day and changes to drinking a green tea such as sencha (remembering to let it sit for 10 minutes before drinking).

Lifestyle: Exercise at least three or four times a week, but incorporate relaxing exercise as well such as yoga or pilates. Incorporate stress management techniques, such as meditation and breathing exercises, as much as possible.

Supplements: The nutritional supplementation has been explained above. Although no RCT studies have been conducted on *Serenoa repens*, it has shown to be of benefit for prostate cancer patients.[125] *Andrographis paniculata* has been found to induce apoptosis of prostate cancer cells via the activation of caspase 3, up-regulation of bax, down-regulation of bcl-2 and inhibition of vascular endothelial growth factor.[208] *Matricaria recutita* has also been found to be antiproliferative and can induce apoptosis in cancer cells but not normal cells.[209] *Uncaria tomentosa* has also been found to have antiproliferative effects against cancer.[110] Monitoring the selenium and zinc as well as copper levels by blood tests on a regular basis, ideally every 2 months, is also advised.

Other prescriptive options

Other herbs that could be added later include immune herbs and adaptogens such as *Eleutherococcus senticosus*, *Astragulus membranaceus*, *Rhodiola rosea*, *Zizyphus spinosa* and *Schisandra chinensis*. Other herbs specific to the prostate also include *Epimedium grandiflorum*, *Urtica dioica* (root), *Smilax ornata*, *Arctostaphylos uva-ursi* and *Prunus africana*. Any mixture of these herbs can be added later or found in particular prostate herbal tablets. Herbal teas of any of these may be used.

As in the breast cancer case, supplements that could be very beneficial and can be added later include calcium D-glucarate, which aids the excretion of environmental or pharmacological xenobiotics by increasing glucuronidation in phase II liver detoxification. Citrus pectin has been suggested to be of assistance, particularly in people with metastasis. Melatonin has many chemoprotective and antioxidant properties that have been found to be beneficial for people with cancer. Mushroom extracts such as shitake or reishi may also be used to boost the immune system.

Many other supplements, including liver nutrients, taurine, glutathione and mixed antioxidants, can be used. It is important to ascertain which is most appropriate at each particular stage for the patient without overwhelming them.

Therapeutic considerations

As he is a businessman, the hardest part for him to alter may be his diet (decreasing coffee and stopping alcohol consumption, particularly with all his business lunches). It will be difficult to make sure he chooses foods correctly when he is out, and he may have to call ahead to ensure that food that he can eat is available.

Some men may rather take tablets or capsules rather than liquid herbals for convenience (and taste), so using combination tablets or capsules may assist compliance. The thought of cancer does scare a lot of people and compliance is normally very good because of this. Prostate cancer in older men is normally a very slow-growing cancer and they can thereby observe the impact of the treatment over time. However, younger men are often found to have a more aggressive cancer, so in these patients continual scrutiny of PSA and Gleason score is advised.

Men seem in general to be less compliant compared to women; however, as this client has a very supportive partner, she can assist him in making sure he has all the food and beverages necessary and remove all other foods and beverages he should not consume. This should help dramatically with compliance.

Expected outcomes and follow-up protocols

It is important to remember that every patient responds differently. This client has allowed 3 months to see what can happen and he could expect to see his PSA decrease but not to levels low enough for him not to consider other treatment. The decision remains the patient's; he may decide that as there has been enough of a decrease that he will continue with the CAM interventions rather than the orthodox for as long as possible. The older the patient, the more likely it seems that the PSA will decrease and that patients can continue with complementary therapies. However, younger men seem to not decrease their PSA as much and may be less inclined to continue complementary treatment alone.[128]

In either circumstance, it is important for the patient to continue with dietary advice and support even if they ultimately choose the surgical, hormone treatment or radiation options. Life expectancy in general is very good, especially if the cancer has not spread, and may not result in the ultimate reason for mortality.

KEY POINTS

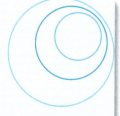

- Prostate cancer is normally more aggressive in younger men than in older men; this is identified by the Gleason score (the higher the score, the more aggressive the cancer).
- Prostate specific antigen (PSA) is one of the main tumour markers used to monitor prostate cancer. The higher the number, the higher the chance that the cancer has spread.
- A very low-fat, vegan or no-animal-product type diet should be implemented
- Always test mineral levels such as zinc and selenium before supplementation rather than making the assumption that they are low.

Further reading

Aggarwal BB, Harikumar KB. Potential therapeutic effects of curcumin, the anti-inflammatory agent, against neurodegenerative, cardiovascular, pulmonary, metabolic, autoimmune and neoplastic diseases. Int J Biochem Cell Biol 2009. In press.

Bartsch H, et al. Dietary polyunsaturated fatty acids and cancers of the breast and colorectum: emerging evidence for their role as risk modifiers. Carcinogenesis 1999;20(12):2209–2218.

Dewell A, et al. A very-low-fat vegan diet increases intake of protective dietary factors and decreases intake of pathogenic dietary factors. J Am Diet Assoc 2008;108(2):347–356.

Fleet JC. Molecular actions of vitamin D contributing to cancer prevention. Mol Aspects Med 2008;29(6):388–396.

Gissel T, et al. Intake of vitamin D and risk of breast cancer—a meta-analysis. J Steroid Biochem Mol Biol 2008;111(3–5):195–199.

Littrell J. The mind-body connection: not just a theory anymore. Soc Work Health Care 2008;46(4): 17–37.

Mumber, M, ed. Integrative oncology: principles and practice. London: Taylor & Francis, 2005.

Oh K, et al. Calcium and vitamin D intakes in relation to risk of distal colorectal adenoma in women. Am J Epidemiol 2007;165(10):1178–1186.

Reid ME, et al. The nutritional prevention of cancer: 400 mcg per day selenium treatment. Nutr Cancer 2008;60(2):155–163.

Schernhammer ES, et al. Folate and vitamin B6 intake and risk of colon cancer in relation to p53 expression. Gastroenterology 2008;135(3):770–780.

Mason M, Moffet L. Prostate cancer: the facts. New York: Oxford University Press, 2003.

Northrup C. Breast health CD set. ISBN: 1564553116.

Stoddard FR, et al. Iodine alters gene expression in the MCF7 breast cancer cell line: evidence for an anti-estrogen effect of iodine. Int J Med Sci 2008;5(4):189–196.

Urbaniak E. Healing your prostate: natural cures that work. Gig Harbor: Harbor Press, 1998.

Wallace JM. Nutritional and botanical modulation of the inflammatory cascade—eicosanoids, cyclooxygenases, and lipoxygenases—as an adjunct in cancer therapy. Integr Cancer Ther 2002;1(1):7–37.

References

1. Cancer Council NSW. Lung cancer: causes and symptoms. myDR Australian Government, 2002.
2. Krambeck WM, et al. HPV detection and genotyping as an earlier approach in cervical cancer screening of the female genital tract. Clin Exp Obstet Gynecol 2008;35(3):175–178.
3. Bourret P. BRCA patients and clinical collectives: new configurations of action in cancer genetics practices. Soc Stud Sci 2005;35(1):41–68.
4. Queiroga EM, et al. Viral studies in Burkitt lymphoma: association with Epstein-Barr virus but not HHV-8. Am J Clin Pathol 2008;130(2):186–192.
5. Nutankalva L, et al. Malignancies in HIV: pre- and post-highly active antiretroviral therapy. J Natl Med Assoc 2008;100(7):817–820.
6. Tao X, et al. The role of hepatitis B virus x gene in development of primary hepatocellular carcinoma. Sci China C Life Sci 2000;43(3):293–301.
7. Yoshida M. Identification of adult T-cell leukemia virus and its gene structure. Gan To Kagaku Ryoho 1983;10(2):680–689.
8. Zhou SZ, et al. [Association of single nucleotide polymorphism at interleukin-10 gene 1082 nt with the risk of gastric cancer in Chinese population]. Nan Fang Yi Ke Da Xue Xue Bao 2008;28(8):1335–1338.
9. Amara K, et al. Presence of simian virus 40 DNA sequences in diffuse large B-cell lymphomas in Tunisia correlates with aberrant promoter hypermethylation of multiple tumor suppressor genes. Int J Cancer 2007;121(12):2693–2702.
10. Moro L, et al. Mitochondrial DNA depletion reduces PARP-1 levels and promotes progression of the neoplastic phenotype in prostate carcinoma. Cell Oncol 2008;30(4):307–322.
11. Kamangar F, et al. Patterns of cancer incidence, mortality, and prevalence across five continents: defining priorities to reduce cancer disparities in different geographic regions of the world. J Clin Oncol 2006;24(14):2137–2150.
12. Newby JA, Howard CV. Environmental influences in cancer aetiology. J Nutr Environ Med 2006:1–59.
13. Frost G, et al. Occupational exposure to asbestos and mortality among asbestos removal workers: a Poisson regression analysis. Br J Cancer 2008;99(5):822–829.
14. Schmitt C, et al. NK cells and surveillance in humans. Reprod Biomed Online 2008;16(2):192–201.
15. Bell HS, Ryan KM. Targeting the p53 family for cancer therapy: 'big brother' joins the fight. Cell Cycle 2007;6(16):1995–2000.
16. Pelletier L. Centrosomes: keeping tumors in check. Curr Biol 2008;18(16):R702–R704.
17. Arai T, et al. Role of DNA repair systems in malignant tumor development in the elderly. Geriatr Gerontol Int 2008;8(2):65–72.
18. Hoye AT, et al. Targeting mitochondria. Acc Chem Res 2008;41(1):87–97.
19. Gordon JS. Mind-body medicine and cancer. Hematol Oncol Clin North Am 2008;22(4):683–708.
20. Ma Z, et al. Polymorphisms of fibroblast growth factor receptor 4 have association with the development of prostate cancer and benign prostatic hyperplasia and the progression of prostate cancer in a Japanese population. Int J Cancer 2008;123:2574–2579.

21. Mosor M, et al. Polymorphisms and haplotypes of the NBS1 gene in childhood acute leukaemia. Eur J Cancer 2008;44:627–630.

22. Zhang Z, et al. Genetic variants in RUNX3 and risk of bladder cancer: a haplotype-based analysis. Carcinogenesis 2008;29(10):1973–1978.

23. Jones PA, Baylin SB. The fundamental role of epigenetic events in cancer. Nat Rev Genet 2002;3:415–428.

24. Hussain SK, et al. Cervical and vulvar cancer risk in relation to the joint effects of cigarette smoking and genetic variation in interleukin 2. Cancer Epidemiol Biomarkers Prev 2008;17(7):1790–1799.

25. Inoue M, et al. Alcohol drinking and total cancer risk: an evaluation based on a systematic review of epidemiologic evidence among the Japanese population. Jpn J Clin Oncol 2007;37(9):692–700.

26. Gomaa AI, et al. Hepatocellular carcinoma: epidemiology, risk factors and pathogenesis. World J Gastroenterol 2008;14(27):4300–4308.

27. Deandrea S, et al. Alcohol and breast cancer risk defined by estrogen and progesterone receptor status: a case-control study. Cancer Epidemiol Biomarkers Prev 2008;17(8):2025–2028.

28. Mizoue T, et al. Alcohol drinking and colorectal cancer risk: an evaluation based on a systematic review of epidemiologic evidence among the Japanese population. Jpn J Clin Oncol 2006;36(9):582–597.

29. Liu C, Russell RM. Nutrition and gastric cancer risk: an update. Nutr Rev 2008;66(5):237–249.

30. Gravaghi C, et al. Obesity enhances gastrointestinal tumorigenesis in Apc-mutant mice. Int J Obes (Lond) 2008;32:1716–1719.

31. Perera CN, et al. Leptin regulated gene expression in MCF-7 breast cancer cells: mechanistic insights into leptin regulated mammary tumor growth and progression. J Endocrinol 2008;199(2):221–233.

32. Amin AR, et al. Perspectives for cancer prevention with natural compounds. J Clin Oncol 2009;27(16):12–25.

33. Thomas CC, et al. Endometrial cancer risk among younger, overweight women. Obstet Gynecol 2009;114(1):22–27.

34. Andrykowski MA, et al. Psychological health in cancer survivors. Semin Oncol Nurs 2008;24(3):193–201.

35. Blask DE. Melatonin, sleep disturbance and cancer risk. Sleep Med Rev 2009;13(4):257–264.

36. Mystakidou K, et al. Exploring the relationships between depression, hopelessness, cognitive status, pain, and spirituality in patients with advanced cancer. Arch Psychiatr Nurs 2007;21(3):150–161.

37. Frieden TR, et al. A public health approach to winning the war against cancer. Oncologist 2008;13(12):1306–1313.

38. Stanley M. Prevention strategies against the human papillomavirus: the effectiveness of vaccination. Gynecol Oncol 2007;107(2 Suppl 1):S19–S23.

39. Worthington HV, et al. Interventions for preventing oral mucositis for patients with cancer receiving treatment. Cochrane Database Syst Rev 2007;17(4):CD000978.

40. Daniele B, et al. Oral glutamine in the prevention of fluorouracil induced intestinal toxicity: a double blind, placebo controlled, randomized trial. Gut 2001;48(1):28–33.

41. Thorpe DM. Management of opioid-induced constipation. Curr Pain Headache Rep 2001;5(3):237–240.

42. Li Y, et al. Oral glutamine ameliorates chemotherapy-induced changes of intestinal permeability and does not interfere with the antitumor effect of chemotherapy in patients with breast cancer: a prospective randomized trial. Tumori 2006;92(5):396–401.

43. Marshall GT, et al. Treatment of gastrointestinal radiation injury with hyperbaric oxygen. Undersea Hyperb Med 2007;34(1):35–42.

44. Demirer S, et al. Effects of probiotics on radiation-induced intestinal injury in rats. Nutrition 2006;22(2):179–186.

45. Erbil Y, et al. The effect of glutamine on radiation-induced organ damage. Life Sci 2005;78(4):376–382.

46. Branda RF, et al. Vitamin E but not St John's wort mitigates leukopenia caused by cancer chemotherapy in rats. Transl Res 2006;148(6):315–324.

47. Wojtukiewicz MZ, et al. The Polish Cancer Anemia Survey (POLCAS): a retrospective multicenter study of 999 cases. Int J Hematol 2009;89(3):276–284.

48. Liu R, et al. Therapeutic effects of alpha-lipoic acid on bleomycin-induced pulmonary fibrosis in rats. Int J Mol Med 2007;10(6):865–873.

49. Cruciani RA, et al. Safety, tolerability and symptom outcomes associated with L-carnitine supplementation in patients with cancer, fatigue, and carnitine deficiency: a phase I/II study. J Pain Symptom Manage 2006;32(6):551–559.

50. Nicolson GL, Conklin KA. Reversing mitochondrial dysfunction, fatigue and the adverse effects of chemotherapy of metastatic disease by molecular replacement therapy. Clin Exp Metastasis 2008;25(2):161–169.

51. Masuda Y, et al. EGG phosphatidylcholine combined with vitamin B12 improved memory impairment following lesioning of nucleus basalis in rats. Life Sci 1998;62(9):813–822.

52. MacDonald N. Cancer cachexia and targeting chronic inflammation: a unified approach to cancer treatment and palliative/supportive care. J Support Oncol 2007;5(4):157–162.

53. Campbell KL, et al. Resting energy expenditure and body mass changes in women during adjuvant chemotherapy for breast cancer. Cancer Nurs 2007;30(2):95–100.

54. Yamada T, et al. Effects of theanine, r-glutamylethylamide, on neurotransmitter release and its relationship with glutamic acid neurotransmission. Nutr Neurosci 2005;8(4):219–226.

55. Caram-Salas NL, et al. Thiamine and cyanocobalamin relieve neuropathic pain in rats: synergy with dexamethasone. Pharmacology 2006;77(2):53–62.

56. Conklin KA. Coenzyme q10 for prevention of anthracycline-induced cardiotoxicity. Integr Cancer Ther 2005;4(2):110–130.

57. Engdal S, et al. Identification and exploration of herb-drug combinations used by cancer patients. Integr Cancer Ther 2009;8(1):29–36.

58. Seely D, et al. A strategy for controlling potential interactions between natural health products and chemotherapy: a review in pediatric oncology. J Pediatr Hematol Oncol 2007;29(1):32–47.

59. Moayyedi P. The epidemiology of obesity and gastrointestinal and other diseases: an overview. Dig Dis Sci 2008;53(9):2293–2299.

60. Dobbinson S, et al. Prevalence and determinants of Australian adolescents' and adults' weekend sun protection and sunburn, summer 2003–2004. J Am Acad Dermatol 2008;59:602–614.

61. Bouillon R, et al. Vitamin D and human health: lessons from vitamin D receptor null mice. Endocr Rev 2008;16:200–257.

62. Ames BN. Low micronutrient intake may accelerate the degenerative diseases of aging through allocation of scarce micronutrients by triage. Proc Natl Acad Sci U S A 2006;103(47):17589–17594.

63. Bläuer M, et al. Effects of tamoxifen and raloxifene on normal human endometrial cells in an organotypic in vitro model. Eur J Pharmacol 2008;592(1–3):13–18.

64. Moore M, et al. Cancer registration literature update (2006–2008). Asian Pac J Cancer Prev 2008;9(2):165–185.

65. Chan C, et al. Stress-associated hormone, norepinephrine, increases proliferation and IL-6 levels of human pancreatic duct epithelial cells and can be inhibited by the dietary agent, sulforaphane. Int J Oncol 2008;33(2):415–419.

66. Lahti TA, et al. Night-time work predisposes to non-Hodgkin lymphoma. Int J Cancer 2008;123(9):2148–2151.

67. Karunanayake CP, et al. Occupational exposures and non-Hodgkin's lymphoma: Canadian case-control study. Environ Health 2008;7(1):44.

68. Swiatkowska B, et al. [Occupational risk factors for lung cancer—a case-control study, Łódź industrial center]. Med Pr 2008;59(1):25–34.

69. Furney SJ, et al. Prioritization of candidate cancer genes—an aid to oncogenomic studies. Nucleic Acids Res 2008;36(18):e115.

70. Medina PP, Slack FJ. MicroRNAs and cancer: an overview. Cell Cycle 2008;7(16):2485–2492.

71. Yang K, et al. Dietary components modify gene expression: implications for carcinogenesis. J Nutr 2005;135(11):2710–2714.

72. Azarhoush R, et al. Relationship between p53 expression and gastric cancers in cardia and antrum. Arch Iran Med 2008;11(5):502–506.

73. Yeung SJ, et al. Roles of p53, MYC and HIF-1 in regulating glycolysis—the seventh hallmark of cancer. Cell Mol Life Sci 2008;65:3981–3999.

74. Maroto B, et al. P21-activated kinase is required for mitotic progression and regulates P1k1. Oncogene 2008;27(36):4900–4908.

75. Saramäki A, et al. Regulation of the human p21(waf1/cip1) gene promoter via multiple binding sites for p53 and the vitamin D3 receptor. Nucleic Acids Res 2006;34(2):543–554.

76. Schernhammer ES, et al. Folate and vitamin B6 intake and risk of colon cancer in relation to p53 expression. Gastroenterology 2008;135:770–780.

77. Cecconi D, et al. Induction of apoptosis in Jeko-1 mantle cell lymphoma cell line by resveratrol: a proteomic analysis. J Proteome Res 2008;7(7):2670–2680.

78. Chan JY, et al. Resveratrol displays converse dose-related effects on 5-fluorouracil-evoked colon cancer cell apoptosis: the roles of caspase-6 and p53. Cancer Biol Ther 2008;7(8).[Epub ahead of print]

79. Huang X, et al. Green tea extract enhances the selective cytotoxic activity of Zizyphus jujuba extracts in HepG2 Cells. Am J Chin Med 2008;36(4):729–744.

80. Lee SC, et al. Effect of a prodrug of the green tea polyphenol (-)-epigallocatechin-3-gallate on the growth of androgen-independent prostate cancer in vivo. Nutr Cancer 2008;60(4):483–491.

81. Matsumura K, et al. Involvement of the estrogen receptor beta in genistein-induced expression of p21(waf1/cip1) in PC-3 prostate cancer cells. Anticancer Res 2008;28(2A):709–714.

82. Tanigawa S, et al. Stabilization of p53 is involved in quercetin-induced cell cycle arrest and apoptosis in HepG2 cells. Biosci Biotechnol Biochem 2008;72(3):797–804.

83. Wells J. Do centrioles generate a polar ejection force? Riv Biol 2005;98(1):71–95.

84. Dutertre S, et al. The absence of p53 aggravates polyploidy and centrosome number abnormality induced by Aurora-C overexpression. Cell Cycle 2005;4(12):1783–1787.

85. Krämer A, et al. Centrosome replication, genomic instability and cancer. Leukemia 2002;16(5):767–775.

86. Crist WM, et al. Dysgranulopoietic neutropenia and abnormal monocytes in childhood vitamin B12 deficiency. Am J Hematol 1980;9(1):89–107.

87. Kim I, et al. Pyrrolidine dithiocarbamate and zinc inhibit proteasome-dependent proteolysis. Exp Cell Res 2004;298(1):229–238.

88. Wang X, et al. Folate deficiency induces aneuploidy in human lymphocytes in vitro-evidence using cytokinesis-blocked cells and probes specific for chromosomes 17 and 21. Mutat Res 2004;551(1–2):167–180.

89. Kuramoto H, et al. Immunohistochemical evaluation of insulin-like growth factor I receptor status in cervical cancer specimens. Acta Med Okayama 2008;62(4):251–259.

90. Haluska P, et al. HER receptor signaling confers resistance to the insulin-like growth factor-I receptor inhibitor, BMS-536924. Mol Cancer Ther 2008;7(9):2589–2598.

91. Otto C, et al. Growth of human gastric cancer cells in nude mice is delayed by a ketogenic diet supplemented with omega-3 fatty acids and medium-chain triglycerides. BMC Cancer 2008;8:122.

92. Samudio I, et al. The warburg effect in leukemia-stroma cocultures is mediated by mitochondrial uncoupling associated with uncoupling protein 2 activation. Cancer Res 2008;68(13):5198–5205.

93. Hussain SP, et al. Nitric oxide is a key component in inflammation-accelerated tumorigenesis. Cancer Res 2008;68(17):7130–7136.

94. Wang D, DuBois RN. Pro-inflammatory prostaglandins and progression of colorectal cancer. Cancer Lett 2008;267(2):197–203.

95. Aggarwal BB, Harikumar KB. Potential therapeutic effects of curcumin, the anti-inflammatory agent, against neurodegenerative, cardiovascular, pulmonary, metabolic, autoimmune and neoplastic diseases. Int J Biochem Cell Biol 2008;41:40–59.

96. Wallace JM. Nutritional and botanical modulation of the inflammatory cascade—eicosanoids, cyclooxygenases, and lipoxygenases—as an adjunct in cancer therapy. Integr Cancer Ther 2002;1(1):7–37.

97. Kaileh M, et al. Screening of indigenous Palestinian medicinal plants for potential anti-inflammatory and cytotoxic activity. J Ethnopharmacol 2007;113(3):510–516.

98. de Visser KE, et al. Paradoxical roles of the immune system during cancer development. Nat Rev Cancer 2006;6:24–37.

99. Caserta MT, et al. The associations between psychosocial stress and the frequency of illness, and innate and adaptive immune function in children. Brain Behav Immun 2008;22(6):933–940.

100. Littrell J. The mind body connection: not just a theory anymore. Soc Work Health Care 2008;46(4):17–37.

101. Bartella V, et al. Insulin-dependent leptin expression in breast cancer cells. Cancer Res 2008;68(12):4919–4927.

102. Silberstein J, et al. HIV and prostate cancer: a systematic review of the literature. Prostate Cancer Prostatic Dis 2008;12(1):6–12.

103. Pérez-López FR. Sunlight, the vitamin D endocrine system, and their relationships with gynaecologic cancer. Maturitas 2008;59(2):101–113.

104. Friedlander AH, et al. The relationship between measures of nutritional status and masticatory function in untreated patients with head and neck cancer. J Oral Maxillofac Surg 2008;66(1):85–92.

105. Fleet JC. Molecular actions of vitamin D contributing to cancer prevention. Mol Aspects Med 2008;29(6):388–396.

106. Maggini S, et al. Selected vitamins and trace elements support immune function by strengthening epithelial barriers and cellular and humoral immune responses. Br J Nutr 2007;98(Suppl 1):S29–S35.

107. Shen J, et al. Potentiation of intestinal immunity by micellary mushroom extracts. Biomed Res 2007;28(2):71–77.

108. Nozaki H, et al. Mushroom acidic glycosphingolipid induction of cytokine secretion from murine T cells and proliferation of NK1.1 alpha/beta TCR-double positive cells in vitro. Biochem Biophys Res Commun 2008;373(3):435–439.

109. Dong JC, Dong XH. [Comparative study on effect of astragalus injection and interleukin-2 in enhancing antitumor metastasis action of dendrite cells]. Zhongguo Zhong Xi Yi Jie He Za Zhi 2005;25(3):236–239.

110. Pilarski R, et al. Antiproliferative activity of various Uncaria tomentosa preparations on HL-60 promyelocytic leukemia cells. Pharmacol Rep 2007;59(5):565–572.

111. Kormosh N, et al. Effect of a combination of extract from several plants on cell-mediated and humoral immunity of patients with advanced ovarian cancer. Phytother Res 2006;20(5):424–425.

112. Choi KT. Botanical characteristics, pharmacological effects and medicinal components of Korean Panax ginseng C A Meyer. Acta Pharmacol Sin 2008;29(9):1109–1118.

113. Zhai Z, et al. Enhancement of innate and adaptive immune functions by multiple Echinacea species. J Med Food 2007;10(3):423–434.

114. Ogba N, et al. HEXIM1 regulates 17beta-estradiol/estrogen receptor-alpha-mediated expression of cyclin D1 in mammary cells via modulation of P-TEFb. Cancer Res 2008;68(17):7015–7024.

115. Tan DS, et al. ESR1 amplification in endometrial carcinomas: hope or hyperbole? J Pathol 2008;216:271–274.

116. Hassan HC, et al. Gynaecomastia: an endocrine manifestation of testicular cancer. Andrologia 2008;40(3):152–157.

117. Chandanos E, Lagergren J. Oestrogen and the enigmatic male predominance of gastric cancer. Eur J Cancer 2008;44(16):2397–2403.

118. Alì G, et al. Different estrogen receptor beta expression in distinct histologic subtypes of lung adenocarcinoma. Hum Pathol 2008;39(10):1465–1473.

119. Chen DZ, et al. Indole-3-carbinol and diindolylmethane induce apoptosis of human cervical cancer cells and in murine HPV16-transgenic preneoplastic cervical epithelium. J Nutr 2001;131(12):3294–3302.

120. Higdon JV, et al. Cruciferous vegetables and human cancer risk: epidemiologic evidence and mechanistic basis. Pharmacol Res 2007;55(3):224–236.

121. Om AS, Chung KW. Dietary zinc deficiency alters 5 alpha-reduction and aromatization of testosterone and androgen and estrogen receptors in rat liver. J Nutr 1996;126(4):842–848.

122. Wang Y, et al. A positive feedback pathway of estrogen biosynthesis in breast cancer cells is contained by resveratrol. Toxicology 2008;248(2–3):130–135.

123. Li Z, et al. Genistein induces cell apoptosis in MDA-MB-231 breast cancer cells via the mitogen-activated protein kinase pathway. Toxicol In Vitro 2008;22:1749–1753.

124. Ju YH, et al. Dietary genistein negates the inhibitory effect of letrozole on the growth of aromatase-expressing estrogen-dependent human breast cancer cells (MCF-7Ca) in vivo. Carcinogenesis 2008;29(11):2162–2168.

125. Yang Y, et al. Saw palmetto induces growth arrest and apoptosis of androgen-dependent prostate cancer LNCaP cells via inactivation of STAT 3 and androgen receptor signaling. Int J Oncol 2007;31(3):593–600.

126. Kanadys WM, et al. [Efficacy and safety of black cohosh (Actaeal Cimicifuga racemosa) in the treatment of vasomotor symptoms–review of clinical trials]. Ginekol Pol 2008;79(4):287–296.

127. Wang Y, et al. The red clover (Trifolium pratense) isoflavone biochanin A inhibits aromatase activity and expression. Br J Nutr 2008;99(2):303–310.

128. Mumber M, ed. Integrative oncology: principles and practice. London: Taylor & Francis, 2005.

129. Ortega AD, et al. Glucose avidity of carcinomas. Cancer Lett 2008;276:125–135.

130. Littarru GP, Tiano L. Bioenergetic and antioxidant properties of coenzyme Q10: recent developments. Mol Biotechnol 2007;37(1):31–37.

131. McCarty MF, et al. The 'rejuvenatory' impact of lipoic acid on mitochondrial function in aging rats may reflect induction and activation of PPAR-gamma coactivator-1alpha. Med Hypotheses 2009;72(1):29–33.

132. Inazu M, Matsumiya T. [Physiological functions of carnitine and carnitine transporters in the central nervous system]. Nihon Shinkei Seishin Yakurigaku Zasshi 2008;28(3):113–120.

133. Ahn BH, et al. A role for the mitochondrial deacetylase Sirt3 in regulating energy homeostasis. Proc Natl Acad Sci U S A 2008;05(38):14447–14452.

134. Mikirova NA, et al. Anti—angiogenic effect of high doses of ascorbic acid. J Transl Med 2008;6(1):50.

135. Anand P, et al. Biological activities of curcumin and its analogues (Congeners) made by man and Mother Nature. Biochem Pharmacol 2008;76:1590–1611.

136. Binion DG, et al. Curcumin inhibits VEGF mediated angiogenesis in human intestinal microvascular endothelial cells through COX-2 and MAPK inhibition. Gut 2008;57:1509–1517.

137. Sagar SM, et al. Natural health products that inhibit angiogenesis: a potential source for investigational new agents to treat cancer—part 2. Curr Oncol 2006;13(3):99–107.

138. Lock K, et al. The global burden of disease attributable to low consumption of fruit and vegetables: implications for the global strategy on diet. Bull World Health Organ 2005;83(2):100–108.

139. Riboli E, Norat T. Epidemiologic evidence of the protective effect of fruit and vegetables on cancer risk. Am J Clin Nutr 2003;78(3 Supp):559S–569S.

140. Wright ME, et al. Intakes of fruit, vegetables, and specific botanical groups in relation to lung cancer risk in the NIH-AARP Diet and Health Study. Am J Epidemiol 2008;168:1024–1034.

141. Navarro Silvera SA, et al. Food group intake and risk of subtypes of esophageal and gastric cancer. Int J Cancer 2008;123(4):852–860.

142. Flood A, et al. Dietary patterns as identified by factor analysis and colorectal cancer among middle-aged Americans. Am J Clin Nutr 2008;88(1):176–184.

143. van Gils CH, et al. Consumption of vegetables and fruits and risk of breast cancer. JAMA 2005;293(2):183–193.

144. Koushik A, et al. Fruits and vegetables and ovarian cancer risk in a pooled analysis of 12 cohort studies. Cancer Epidemiol Biomarkers Prev 2005;14(9):2160–2167.

145. Linos E, et al. Red meat consumption during adolescence among premenopausal women and risk of breast cancer. Cancer Epidemiol Biomarkers Prev 2008;17(8):2146–2151.

146. Hart AR, et al. Pancreatic cancer: a review of the evidence on causation. Clin Gastroenterol Hepatol 2008;6(3):275–282.

147. Bahmanyar S, Ye W. Dietary patterns and risk of squamous-cell carcinoma and adenocarcinoma of the esophagus and adenocarcinoma of the gastric cardia: a population-based case-control study in Sweden. Nutr Cancer 2008;54(2):171–178.

148. Duffy CM, et al. Alcohol and folate intake and breast cancer risk in the WHI Observational Study. Breast Cancer Res Treat 2008;168(9):1024–1034.

149. Bartsch H, et al. Dietary polyunsaturated fatty acids and cancers of the breast and colorectum: emerging evidence for their role as risk modifiers. Carcinogenesis 1999;20(12):2209–2218.

150. Berquin IM, et al. Multi-targeted therapy of cancer by omega-3 fatty acids. Cancer Lett 2008;269(2):363–377.

151. Dal Maso L, et al. Risk factors for thyroid cancer: an epidemiological review focused on nutritional factors. Cancer Causes Control 2008;42(2–3):53–61.

152. Stoddard 2nd, FR, et al. Iodine alters gene expression in the MCF7 breast cancer cell line: evidence for an anti-estrogen effect of iodine. Int J Med Sci 2008;5(4):189–196.

153. Ishii T, et al. Covalent modification of proteins by green tea polyphenol (−)–epigallocatechin-3-gallate through autoxidation. Free Radic Biol Med 2008;45:384–1394.

154. Arts IC. A review of the epidemiological evidence on tea, flavonoids, and lung cancer. J Nutr 2008;138(8):1561S–1566S.

155. Tao KS, et al. The multifaceted mechanisms for coffee's anti-tumorigenic effect on liver. Med Hypotheses 2008;71:730–736.

156. Young GP, Le Leu RK. Preventing cancer: dietary lifestyle or clinical intervention? Asia Pac J Clin Nutr 2002;11(Suppl 3):S618–S631.

157. Kushi LH, et al. The macrobiotic diet in cancer. J Nutr 2001;131(11 Suppl):3056S–3064S.

158. Majchrowicz MA. Essiac. Notes Undergr 1995;(29):6–7.

159. Seely D, et al. In vitro analysis of the herbal compound Essiac. Anticancer Res 2007;27(6B):3875–3882.

160. Ottenweller J, et al. Inhibition of prostate cancer-cell proliferation by Essiac. J Altern Complement Med 2004;10(4):687–691.

161. Cheung S, et al. Antioxidant and anti-inflammatory properties of ESSIAC and Flor-Essence. Oncol Rep 2005;14(5):1345–1350.

162. Leonard BJ, et al. An in vivo analysis of the herbal compound essiac. Anticancer Res 2006;26(4B):3057–3063.

163. Robb K, et al. A Cochrane Systematic Review of transcutaneous electrical nerve stimulation for cancer pain. J Pain Symptom Manage 2009;37(4):746–753.

164. Harding C, et al. Auricular acupuncture: a novel treatment for vasomotor symptoms associated with luteinizing-hormone releasing hormone agonist treatment for prostate cancer. BJU Int 2008;103(2):186–190.

165. Johnston MF, et al. Acupuncture and fatigue: current basis for shared communication between breast cancer survivors and providers. J Cancer Surviv 2007;1(4):306–312.

166. Lai M, et al. [Effects of electroacupuncture on tumor growth and immune function in the Walker-256 model rat]. Zhongguo Zhen Jiu 2008;28(8):607–609.

167. Naeim A, et al. Evidence-based recommendations for cancer nausea and vomiting. J Clin Oncol 2008;26(23):3903–3910.

168. Streitberger K, et al. Acupuncture for nausea and vomiting: an update of clinical and experimental studies. Auton Neurosci 2006;129:107–117.

169. Choo SP, et al. Electroacupuncture for refractory acute emesis caused by chemotherapy. J Altern Complement Med 2006;12:963–969.

170. Ezzo JM, et al. Acupuncture-point stimulation for chemotherapy-induced nausea or vomiting. Cochrane Database Syst Rev 2006;(2):CD002285.

171. Carlson L, Bultz B. Mind-body interventions in oncology. Curr Treat Options Oncol 2008;9(2–3):127–134.

172. Montazeri A. Health-related quality of life in breast cancer patients: a bibliographic review of the literature from 1974 to 2007. J Exp Clin Cancer Res 2008;27(1):32.

173. Chen K, Yeung R. Exploratory studies of Qigong therapy for cancer in China. Integr Cancer Ther 2002;1(4):345–370.

174. Smedslund G, Ringdal G. Meta-analysis of the effects of psychosocial interventions on survival time in cancer patients. J Psychosom Res 2004;57(2):123–131.

175. Breitbart W. Spirituality and meaning in supportive care: spirituality- and meaning-centered group psychotherapy interventions in advanced cancer. Support Care Cancer 2002;10(4):272–280.

176. Kassab S, et al. Homoeopathic medicines for adverse effects of cancer treatments. Cochrane Database Syst Rev 2009;15(2):CD004845.

177. Thompson EA, et al. Towards standard setting for patient-reported outcomes in the NHS homoeopathic hospitals. Homoeopathy 2008;97(3):114–121.

178. Kutner JS, et al. Massage therapy versus simple touch to improve pain and mood in patients with advanced cancer: a randomized trial. Ann Intern Med 2008;149(6):369–379.

179. Corbin L. Safety and efficacy of massage therapy for patients with cancer. Cancer Control 2005;12(3):158–164.

180. Ponz de Leon M, et al. Aetiology of colorectal cancer and relevance of monogenic inheritance. Gut 2004;53:115–122.

181. Schernhammer ES, et al. Folate and vitamin B6 intake and risk of colon cancer in relation to p53 expression. Gastroenterology 2008;135(3):770–780.

182. Oh K, et al. Calcium and vitamin D intakes in relation to risk of distal colorectal adenoma in women. Am J Epidemiol 2007;165(10):1178–1186.

183. Reid ME, et al. The nutritional prevention of cancer: 400 mcg per day selenium treatment. Nutr Cancer 2008;60(2):155–163.

184. Peters U, et al. Dietary fibre and colorectal adenoma in a colorectal cancer early detection programme. Lancet 2003;361(9368):1491–1495.

185. Hill LL, et al. *Echinacea purpurea* supplementation stimulates select groups of human gastrointestinal tract microbiota. J Clin Pharm Ther 2006;31(6):599–604.

186. Rouzaud G, et al. Hydrolysis of glucosinolates to isothiocyanates after ingestion of raw or microwaved cabbage by human volunteers. Cancer Epidemiol Biomarkers Prev 2004;13(1):125–131.

187. Key TJ, Verkasalo PK. Endogenous hormones and the aetiology of breast cancer. Breast Cancer Res 1999;1(1):18–21.

188. Swerdlow AJ, et al. Risks of breast and testicular cancers in young adult twins in England and Wales: evidence on prenatal and genetic aetiology. Lancet 1997;350(9093):1723–1728.

189. de Waard F, Trichopoulos D. A unifying concept of the aetiology of breast cancer. Int J Cancer 1988;41(5):666–669.

190. Patrick L. Iodine: deficiency and therapeutic considerations. Altern Med Rev 2008;13(2):116–127.

191. Blackmore KM, et al. Vitamin D from dietary intake and sunlight exposure and the risk of hormone-receptor-defined breast cancer. Am J Epidemiol 2008;168:915.

192. Gissel T, et al. Intake of vitamin D and risk of breast cancer—a meta-analysis. J Steroid Biochem Mol Biol 2008;111(3–5):195–199.

193. Fénichel P. B-DF. Breast risk cancer and environmental endocrine disruptors. Gynecol Obstet Fertil 2008.

194. Krieger N, et al. Breast cancer and serum organochlorines: a prospective study among white, black, and Asian women. J Natl Cancer Inst 1994;86(8):589–599.

195. Wolff MS, et al. Environmental exposures and puberty in inner-city girls. Environ Res 2008;107(3):393–400.

196. Darbre PD. Aluminium, antiperspirants and breast cancer. J Inorg Biochem 2005;99(9):1912–1919.

197. Darbre PD, Harvey PW. Paraben esters: review of recent studies of endocrine toxicity, absorption, esterase and human exposure, and discussion of potential human health risks. J Appl Toxicol 2008;28(5):561–578.

198. Korkmaz A, et al. Role of melatonin in the epigenetic regulation of breast cancer. Breast Cancer Res Treat 2009;115(1):13.

199. Hjartåker A, et al. Obesity and diabetes epidemics: cancer repercussions. Adv Exp Med Biol 2008;630:72–93.

200. Loprinzi CL, et al. Mayo Clinic and North Central Cancer Treatment Group hot flash studies: a 20-year experience. Menopause 2008;15(4 Pt 1):655–660.

201. Yuvaraj S, et al. Augmented antioxidant status in Tamoxifen treated postmenopausal women with breast cancer on co-administration with Coenzyme Q10, Niacin and Riboflavin. Cancer Chemother Pharmacol 2008;61(6):933–941.

202. van Dalen EC, et al. Cardioprotective interventions for cancer patients receiving anthracyclines. Cochrane Database Syst Rev 2008;(2):CD003917.

203. Dalessandri KM, et al. Pilot study: effect of 3,3'-diindolylmethane supplements on urinary hormone metabolites in postmenopausal women with a history of early-stage breast cancer. Nutr Cancer 2004;50(2):161–167.

204. O'Rielly PH. Aetiology and pathology of prostate cancer. Pharm J 1999;6:65–67.

205. Mikhak B, et al. Manganese superoxide dismutase (MnSOD) gene polymorphism, interactions with carotenoid levels, and prostate cancer risk. Carcinogenesis 2008;29(1):2335–2340.

206. Grainger EM, et al. A combination of tomato and soy products for men with recurring prostate cancer and rising prostate specific antigen. Nutr Cancer 2008;60(2):145–154.

207. Dewell A, et al. A very-low-fat vegan diet increases intake of protective dietary factors and decreases intake of pathogenic dietary factors. J Am Diet Assoc 2008;108(2):347–356.

208. Zhao F, et al. Anti-tumor activities of andrographolide, a diterpene from *Andrographis paniculata*, by inducing apoptosis and inhibiting VEGF level. J Asian Nat Prod Res 2008;10(5–6):467–473.

209. Srivastava JK, Gupta S. Antiproliferative and apoptotic effects of chamomile extract in various human cancer cells. J Agric Food Chem 2007;55(23):9470–9478.

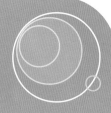

PART D
Clinical naturopathy across the life cycle

While clinicians focus on the treatment of people as individuals and their specific disease and health patterns, the broader context of practice takes into account the patient's stage of life. Although treatment protocols are not often altered due to a patient's age, the focus of treatment and prescription often is. This reflects the altered requirements that are necessary for growth, development and normal functioning at different stages of life. For example, common conditions observed in clinical practice vary considerably between paediatric and elderly populations, as does the dosage level or suitability of various biological interventions. Furthermore, prescriptive dietary and lifestyle advice is usually age-specific.

Clinical issues when treating children (aside from dosage variations) include special considerations regarding digestion, acute infections and developmental and emotional wellbeing. Compliance issues are of particular concern, as the prescription is effective only if applied or taken. Herbal medicines used in this population should have less potential for toxicity, and are usually more 'tolerable' to the palate. An overarching consideration when treating children is that they are a vulnerable group and therefore communication with the parents is a key factor in ethical treatment.

In adults of a fertile age wanting to conceive, the therapeutic focus is on pre- and antenatal care. While there is controversy and a dearth of definitive evidence regarding naturopathic interventions to improve fertility, the naturopath can help to ensure optimal health or correct underlying pathology—a healthy body is generally a fertile one. However, this special stage of life has specific needs, as does any other.

In treating elderly persons, the clinical focuses tend to be on improving and sustaining quality of life, managing chronic diseases and providing palliative care when required. Medication use, and therefore potential drug–CAM interactions, is more prevalent in this population, requiring increased diligence with respect to these matters.

This part focuses on the three major phases of the life cycle: childhood and adolescence; the fertile period; and old age.

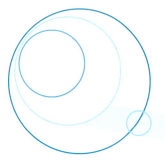

30
Paediatrics

Vicki Mortimer
ND, RN, RM

OVERVIEW OF PAEDIATRIC CONSIDERATIONS

Working with children can be extremely rewarding, but it is very different from treating adults. Children often face very different medical conditions to adults and require specialised care. Practitioners need to be aware of children's special needs, the sensitivity of the child, and the child's parents and their siblings. While many childhood conditions can be treated in the family home, it is wise to seek the help of medical intervention when a condition is worsening, and to do so as soon as possible because children (especially babies) can become gravely ill quite quickly. Conversely, they can recover quickly once appropriate intervention is commenced. Children's immune systems and nervous systems develop rapidly, and this also needs to be considered at all times when embarking on any health intervention.

The terminology for the classification of the paediatric patient is used in this chapter according to the definitions given at the International Conference on Harmonisation (ICH).[1] The ICH recommended age should be classified in completed days, months or years following the stage categories of:
1. preterm newborn infants
2. term newborn infants (0–27 days)
3. infants and toddlers (28 days to 23 months)
4. children (2–11 years)
5. adolescents (12 to 16 or 18 years depending on the region).

The United Nations' *Convention on the Rights of the Child* defines a 'minor' as anyone under the age of 18 years.[2]

The use of complementary and alternative medicine (CAM) in paediatric treatment is prevalent.[3–5] Studies have shown that the use of one or more CAM therapies for treatment of children range between 20% and 70% of cases. The rates for general paediatric patients are 20–30%, for adolescents 30–70% and for paediatric patients with chronic or recurrent conditions, including those considered to be incurable, 30–70%.[3,4] CAM practices used most commonly for children include infant massage, general massage and vitamin and herbal therapies. Demographic data for paediatric treatment reflect that seen in generalised populations, showing that the parents of children being given CAM therapies are often more educated and affluent. They choose to use CAM because they believe it is natural, lower cost, more effective, has been recommended by family or friends, are worried about possible side effects of conventional therapies, or conventional therapies have failed them in the past.[3,4,6]

Ethical and legal considerations

Cohen and Kemper raised some questions about the clinically appropriate use of CAM in paediatrics.[5] They suggested that the non-judicious use of various CAM therapies may cause direct harm (or indirect harm) by creating an unwarranted financial and emotional burden. They recommended a series of questions that practitioners treating paediatric patients could ask when deciding how to advise patients on the use of CAM. These questions are:

1. Do parents elect to abandon effective care when the child's condition is serious or life-threatening?
2. Will use of the CAM therapy otherwise divert the child from imminently necessary conventional treatment?
3. Are the CAM therapies selected known to be safe and/or effective?
4. Have the proper parties consented to the use of the CAM therapies?
5. Is the risk:benefit ratio of the proposed CAM therapy acceptable to a reasonable, similarly situated clinician, and does the therapy have at least minority acceptance or support in the medical literature?[5]

As the body of evidence concerning CAM increases, there will be more proof (or otherwise) as to the efficacy and safety of certain CAM therapies and these ethical considerations will become less clouded.

Cohen and Kemper also concluded that paediatric use of CAM therapies may raise legal as well as clinical concerns.[5] A cautious yet balanced approach ideally can help guide the specialised paediatric naturopath towards clinical advice (including referral) that is clinically responsible, ethically appropriate and legally defensible. Employing such an approach—one that embraces both clinical and legal concerns—can help to protect the child's welfare as new parameters for integrative health care unfold.

Most research on CAM therapies is being conducted on adults and may therefore not be directly applicable to paediatric populations. There are some specific considerations that need to be made when looking at the particular aspects of conducting clinical trials on the paediatric population. These include the ongoing changes to children's bodies (their metabolism and developmental stage), their changing social relationships and their vulnerability and dependence upon others.

Until there are much more reliable research data on CAM in paediatric populations, practitioners will need to continue to extrapolate data and adjust the adult information to the child, being mindful of the child's unique circumstances.

PAEDIATRIC MEDICATION CONSIDERATIONS

The consensus is that children do not equate to small adults.[7] There are marked differences in pathology, physiology, pharmacokinetics and pharmacodynamics between children and adults.[8–10] The efficacy of a medication depends on the practitioner selecting an appropriate preparation, calculating the correct dosage and motivating the family to ensure regular administration.[11]

There are some important considerations when deciding the dose of medications at different life stages. Drugs are metabolised very differently in neonates and children compared to adults. Absorption is affected by differences in gastric acid secretion, bile salt formation, gastric emptying, intestinal motility and microflora.[7] These are mostly reduced in a neonate and may also be reduced—though sometimes raised—in an ill child. The distribution of the volume of drugs in children can change with age because of the differences in the body's composition of minerals, lipids, proteins and water (see Figure 30.1 below); plasma protein binding capacity also changes with age. Drug elimination can be longer in babies than adults. So, when medicating babies and children less than 12 years old, body weight and age should be considered.[8] (See Table 30.1 with formulas below.)

Individual practitioners will have a preference for one formula over another when selecting a dose for children. Table 30.1 can be used to guide those in doubt when considering a herbal formula. Ausberger's rule and Clarke's rule for calculations of paediatric doses of medications are based on weight as opposed to age and may be more suitable to allow for the faster metabolism of children at certain ages.[12] Fried's rule and Young's rule are based on age alone.

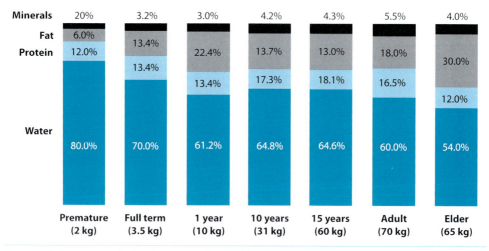

Figure 30.1 Changes in body proportions of body composition with growth and ageing
Source: Adapted from Puig M, Body composition and growth. In Walker WA. Watkins JB, eds. Nutrition in pediatrics. 2nd edn. Hamilton, Ontario, BC: Decker, 1996.

Table 30.1 Calculating medication dosages[12,13]

AGE	RULE	FORMULA
Birth to 12 months	Ausberger's rule	1.5 × weight in kg + 10 = % of adult dose
1–2 years	Fried's rule (or Ausberger's rule)	$\dfrac{\text{Age in months}}{150} \times \text{adults dose} = \text{child's dose}$
2–12 years	Young's rule or	$\dfrac{\text{Age in years}}{(\text{age}+12)} \times \text{adults dose} = \text{child's dose}$
	Ausberger's rule or	1.5 × weight in kg + 10 = % of adult dose
	Clarke's rule	$\dfrac{\text{Weight in kg}}{67} \times \text{adult dose} = \text{child's dose}$
12–16 years	Ausberger's rule	1.5 × weight in kg + 10 = % of adult dose
16+ years	Unless the teenager is of small stature, adult doses may be considered.	

Hepatic metabolism

Medications are metabolised by enzymatic and metabolic reactions. Phase I activity for drug metabolism is reduced in neonates, increases progressively during the first 6 months of life, slows during adolescence, and usually attains adult rates by late puberty.[8,9] Neonates metabolise medications much more slowly than adults do. By 6 months of age the immature reactions involving acetylation, glucuronidation and conjugation with amino acids have matured to adult levels.[9] The metabolic pathways for phase II reactions reach adult levels by 3–4 years of age.[9,14–16]

Digestive flora

Colonisation of the gastrointestinal tract begins at birth and is usually established by week 1. The type of microorganism will depend on hygiene and diet. *Bifidobacterium* is the most prolific organism in a breastfed baby.[13] It is estimated that the number of aerobic and anaerobic bacteria in newborns is up to a total of 10^{10}/g wet weight.[17] Implications of this altered flora are discussed in the chapters on irritable bowel syndrome, atopic skin disorders and asthma.

Nutrition in children

The physiological differences in children when compared to adults also result in differing nutritional requirements for children. This reflects the population's unique needs for growth and development, as well as their differing maintenance requirements due to higher metabolisms. The estimated average requirements for the main nutrients are listed in Tables 30.2 and 30.3.[18–20]

Herbal medicine in children

The conditions encountered in paediatric practice may be different from those encountered in general practice (for example, otitis media and colic). Therefore the herbal medicines most commonly used will also differ. Table 30.4 outlines common paediatric conditions and herbal medicines used to treat these conditions.

HERBAL MEDICINE CONSIDERATIONS IN PAEDIATRIC PRACTICE

- Keeping herbal medicines in a locked cupboard is essential.
- Consideration of metabolic rate, constitution and temperament is important.
- Start the dosage in the lower part of the therapeutic range for the herb or nutrient and increase if needed.
- The vitality of the child needs to be taken into consideration.
- Be particularly careful of sweetened medications with young children, and do not use honey as a sweetener in babies under 12 months of age.

COMMON PAEDIATRIC CONDITIONS

Generally, these conditions can be treated in a similar manner to the adult populations as suggested in appropriate chapters (while also paying attention to recommendations in this chapter). The more common conditions treated in infants and toddlers, children and adolescents are:[13,25]

- acne
- asthma

- allergies and food intolerances
- conjunctivitis
- constipation
- colic
- cough
- dermatitis
- diarrhoea
- ear infections
- enuresis
- fever and infectious diseases
- fussy eaters
- obesity
- otitis media
- recurrent colds
- stomach upset, food regurgitation and vomiting
- stress and adjustment issues
- tantrums and bad behaviour
- vaccination decisions and reactions.

OTITIS MEDIA

A study has shown that olive oil infused with extracts of *Allium sativum*, *Verbascum thapsus*, *Calendula officinalis* and *Hypericum perforatum* is effective in reducing pain in children with otitis media.[26]

Table 30.2 Vitamins

AGE GROUP AND GENDER	VITAMIN C (MG/DAY)	THIAMINE (MG/DAY)	RIBOFLA-VIN (MG/DAY)	NIACIN (MG/DAY) NIACIN EQUIVALENTS	VITAMIN B6 (MG/DAY)	VITAMIN B12 (µG/DAY)	FOLATE(µG/DAY) AS DIETARY FOLATE EQUIVALENTS
Infants 0–6 months	25	0.2	0.3	2	0.1	0.4	65
7–12 months	30	0.3	0.4	4	0.3	0.5	80
Children 1–3 years	25	0.4	0.4	5	0.4	0.7	120
4–8 years	25	0.5	0.5	6	0.5	1.0	160
Boys 9–13 years	28	0.7	0.8	9	0.8	1.5	250
14–18 years	28	1.0	1.1	12	1.1	2.0	330
Girls 9–13 years	28	0.7	0.8	9	0.8	1.5	250
14–18 years	28	0.9	0.9	11	1.0	2.0	330

(Continued)

Table 30.2 Vitamins *(Continued)*

AGE GROUP AND GENDER	PANTOTHENIC ACID (MG/DAY)	BIOTIN (MG/DAY)	CHOLINE (µG/DAY)	VITAMIN A (RETINOL EQUIVALENTS) (MG/DAY)	VITAMIN D (µG/DAY)	VITAMIN E α-TOCOPHEROL EQUIVALENTS (MG/DAY)	VITAMIN K (µMG/DAY)
Infants 0–6 months	1.7	5	125	250	5	4	2.0
7–12 months	2.2	6	150	430	5	5	2.5
Children 1–3 years	3.5	8	200	210	5	5	25.0
4–8 years	4.0	12	250	275	5	6	35.0
Boys 9–13 years	5.0	20	375	445	5	9	45.0
14–18 years	6.0	30	550	630	5	10	55.0
Girls 9–13 years	4.0	20	375	420	5	8	45.0
14–18 years	4.0	25	400	485	5	8	55.0

Table 30.3 Main minerals

AGE GROUP AND GENDER	CALCIUM (MG/DAY)	MAGNE-SIUM (MG/DAY)	IRON (MG/DAY)	POTASSIUM (MG/DAY)	SELENIUM (µG/DAY)	SODIUM (MG/DAY)	ZINC (MG/DAY)
Infants 0–6 months	210	30	0.2	400	12	120	2.0
7–12 months	270	75	7.0	700	15	170	2.5
Children 1–3 years	360	65	4.0	2000	20	200–400	2.5
4–8 years	520	110	4.0	2300	30	300–600	3.0
Boys 9–13 years	800–1050	200	6.0	3000	40	400–800	5.0
14–18 years	1050	340	8.0	3600	60	460–920	11.0
Girls 9–13 years	800–1050	200	6.0	2500	40	400–800	5.0
14–18 years	1050	300	8.0	2600	50	460–920	6.0

Table 30.4 Commonly used herbs in paediatrics according to herbal tradition[13,18,21–25]

MAIN CONDITIONS	MAIN TREATMENT ACTIONS	COMMON HERBS
Infants and toddlers		
Colic	Carminative	*Mentha piperita, Foeniculum vulgare, Matricaria recutita, Melissa officinalis* Essential oils: *Matricaria recutita* 2 drops plus 2 drops of *Foeniculum vulgare* or *Anaethum graveolens*
Common cold	Immune system-enhancing Circulatory stimulant Antiseptic	*Echinacea* spp., *Andrographis paniculata, Astragalus membranaceus* (not in the acute phase) *Zingiber officinale Verbascum thapsis* and *Thymus vulgaris Glycyrrhiza glabra*
Constipation	Laxatives Demulcent Spasmolytic Hydrative	*Iris versicolor, Angelica polymorpha, Rumex crispus, Taraxacum officinale* (radix), *Glycyrrhiza glabra Ulmus fulva Matricaria recutita, Melissa officinalis, Mentha piperita*
Children		
Respiratory tract infections	Anticatarrhals Respiratory demulcents Expectorants Mucolytics Antitussives Antiseptic Mucous membrane trophorestorative	*Solidago virgaurea, Hydrastis canadensis Althea officinalis, Chondus crispus Pelargonium sidoides, Grindelia camporum, Inula helenium Allium sativum, Amoracia rusticana Prunus serotina, Glycyrrhiza glabra Thymus vulgaris, Allium sativum, Inula helenium, Pelargonium sidoides Hydrastis canadensis*
Fever	Diaphoretics Cooling bitters	*Mentha piperita, Achillea millefolium, Sambucus nigra Taraxacum officinale, Gentiana lutea*
Allergy	Antiallergy	*Albizzia lebbeck, Scutellaria baicalensis*
Asthma	Bronchodilator Expectorant Bronchodilator Trophorestorative Anticatarrhal	*Adhatoda vasica Coleus forskohlii Hydrastis canadensis*
Adolescents		
Acne	Depurative Hypoglycaemic Immune modulating Anti-inflammatory	*Rumex crispus, Berberis aquifolium, Arctium lappa Galega officinalis, Gymnema sylvestre Echinacea* spp., *Andrographis paniculata Glycyrrhiza glabra, Buplurum falcatum, Rehmannia glutinosa*
Warts	Antiviral Immunomodulating	*Thuja occidentalis Echinacea* spp.

(Continued)

Table 30.4 Commonly used herbs in paediatrics according to herbal tradition (*Continued*)

MAIN CONDITIONS	MAIN TREATMENT ACTIONS	COMMON HERBS
Stress	Adrenal tonic Adaptogen Nervine	*Glycyrrhiza glabra* *Eleutherococcus senticosus, Withania somnifera* *Hypericum perforatum, Scutellaria lateriflora, Passiflora incarnata*

COMPLIANCE ISSUES

Babies

Babies clearly communicate differently to other populations until they grow and develop speech. Parents can quickly learn the different types of crying their baby has for hunger, pain or discomfort (including being wet or soiled), fear and frustration or being too hot or cold. If a baby requires medication it may be preferable to give the medicine in an adult dose to a breastfeeding mother, or in an appropriate baby's dose in a teat with just a little formula feed.

If a baby has thrush, the appropriate probiotic can be put on the nipple before feeding for a breastfed baby, or on the teat for a formula-fed infant.

Children

Children of all ages need to be given positive feedback on their progress and positive attitudes. Realistic goals should be set to increase the likelihood of compliance—for example, in the case of planned weight loss, planning to lose 1 of 10 kg by the next follow-up consultation if on a weight-loss plan, or having three different-coloured vegetables at least four times a week if diversifying their foods has been recommended.[8]

If changes to lifestyle such as dietary changes or physical activities and exercise have been recommended, the instructions given to the family should be simplified, and introduced incrementally where possible (an important exception to this would be the need to immediately remove a highly allergic food such as peanuts in children who have experienced an anaphylactic reaction to the peanuts or other dangerous or life-threatening situations).

Young children may find it difficult to swallow pills and may dislike the taste of tablets and liquids. A child disliking the taste of medication is a common problem and may result in most of the liquid herbal formula not being ingested by the time they return for the next consultation. By explaining ways of taking the medications or having a printed handout with suggestions the naturopath may minimise the non-compliance. Supplements and medications can be crushed where possible and added to other palatable foods, or mixed with a little apple or pear concentrate. Alternatively, as with liquid medications, they can be frozen into little ice blocks with a pleasant-tasting juice or fruit concentrate, and then they can be chipped into smaller pieces and easily swallowed.

Adolescents

Older children and teenagers may rebel to assert their independence. They may feel that they need to be in control of their treatment and their illness, and they need to be involved and take responsibility for the progress of the illness and treatment.[8] Open communications are to be encouraged; some rebellious behaviour is to be expected as adolescents learn to control their feelings and find their rightful place in their family and community.

Stomach upset
- Co-occurring anxiety
- Hunger, excitement
- Loss of appetite
- Functional abdominal pain
- Nausea, vomiting
- Constipation or diarrhoea

→

- Lifestyle advice, e.g., reduce stimulants and external stressors, moderate exercise and tailored relaxation techniques or massage. Referral for psychological treatment may also be helpful if the stress is prolonged or the child's behaviour changes remarkably
- Dietary increase of magnesium, B vitamins, folate, zinc containing foods, e.g. whole grains, leafy vegetables and lean protein. Avoid refined, highly processed and sugary foods. Determine if they are tolerating a high fibre diet. Try small, frequent, nutritious meals rather than 3 large meals.
- Use of anxiolytic and nervine herbal medicines, e.g. *Piper methysticum* (not for children under 12 years), *Passiflora incarnata, Scutellaria lateriflora, Withania somnifera* and *matricaria recutita*. Judicious use of carminatives, antinausea/vomiting herbs, sedatives, spasmolytics, possibly use of appetite stimulants and demulcents, e.g. *Mentha X piperita, Matricaria recutita, Melissa officinalis, Filipendula ulmaria, Foeniculum vulgare* and *Althea officinalis*
- Exclude organic causes – refer to a medical doctor especially if there is weight loss, frequent vomiting, loss of energy, fever, growth retardation, constant abdominal pain, abdominal mass or severe diarrhoea
- Recolonise the GIT with good bacteria, e.g. *Bifidobacterium* and *Lactobacillus*, if they have had a sugary diet, an illness or are on a course of antibiotics.

Stress and adjustment issues
- Loss of appetite
- Abdominal aches and pains
- Constipation or diarrhoea
- Mood reactivity/easily upset or angry or withdrawing
- Nail biting
- Nervousness and restlessness
- Secondary enuresis
- Headaches, worry, depression
- Tiredness, insomnia
- Anxiety, nightmares
- Poor concentration
- Worsening of any existing condition, e.g. eczema, asthma

→

- Use of anxiolytic and nervine herbal medicines, e.g. *Piper methysticum* (not for children under 12 years), *Passiflora incarnata, Scutellaria lateriflora, Withaonia somnifera, Matricaria recutita*.
- Supplement with calcium, magnesium, B vitamin complex, vitamin C and zinc.
- Lifestyle advice, e.g. encourage the child to talk about their feelings, reduce stimulants and external stressors, do moderate exercise but avoid excitement and physical activities before bed, and use tailored relaxation techniques or massage. Bathe with lavender, marjoram, ylang ylang, chamomile and clary sage aromatherapy oils. Use a hops and lavender herbal pillow. Referral for psychological treatment may also be helpful.
- Dietary increase of magnesium, B vitamins, folate, zinc, calcium and vitamin C–containing foods, e.g. whole grains, leafy vegetables and lean protein. Include foods that are therapeutic for the nervous system, e.g. oats, millet, brown rice, asparagus, onion, garlic, potatoes, turnips, carrots, lentils, kidney beans and the culinary herbs rosemary, nutmeg, marjoram and oregano.
- Exclude food allergies, fluctuating blood glucose levels and intestinal parasites.
- Inquire about bullying at school.

Atopic dermatitis/eczema
- Itchy skin condition occurring in the last 12 months plus at least three of the following:
  - onset before 2 years of age
  - history of flexural involvement
  - history of xerosis
  - history of other atopic conditions
  - visual flexural rash
- Predisposition to develop asthma and/or allergic rhinitis
- Indications of EFA deficiency
- Indications of micronutrient and antioxidant deficiency
- Indications of immune deficiency

→

- Pay careful attention to hygiene to minimise *Staphylococus aureus*.
- Check for candidiasis and recolonise the GIT with good bacteria, e.g. *Bifidobacterium lactis, Lactobacillus GG, Lactobacillus rhamnosus* and *Lactobacillus reuteri*.
- Detect and eliminate allergens, dietary and environmental – in particular investigate dairy products, eggs, peanuts, tomatoes, wheat, sugar, chocolate, yeast extracts, pork, beef, nightshades, nuts and food additives.
- Supplement with GLA and antioxidants (vitamins A, C , E and zinc in particular).
- Look for and correct hypochlorhydria.
- Behaviour modification/counselling for stress and scratching.
- Herbal medicines: consider using immunomodulating herbs, depuratives, digestives, adaptogens, anti-allergy and antioxidant classes of herbs, e.g. *Echinacea* spp., *Albizzia lebbeck, Hemidesmus indicus, Rumex crispus, Curcuma longa*.
- Topically: *Avena sativa* baths or poultices for the itch can give immediate relief and *Glycyrrhiza glabra* and *Matricaria recutita* mixed into a gentle cream base such as vitamin E cream b.d t.d.s. can give great relief. Experience shows that if the lesions are particularly advanced, applying wet packs over the cream and lesion and wrapping them in protective plastic can aid absorption.

Figure 30.2 **Examples of treatment options for common paediatric conditions**[13,21,23–28]

Children and adolescents of all ages may resist treatment regimens that take them away from activities or classes or make them appear different to their friends. Engaging the adolescent appropriately in the treatment process may reduce these compliance issues.

Parents

It is important to consider that, while the child is certainly the patient, treatment must often extend to the parent as well. Health issues in children are clearly a stressful and emotional time for parents, and they need to be supported throughout the treatment in a rational and appropriate manner. Parents need to be included in the treatment process and educated appropriately.

Parents may not fully understand the instructions and rationale of the prescription, for example the medications, dietary advice or physical therapy. Giving written instructions in a language they can understand is useful.

An early follow-up telephone call can be made to see if the family has any residual questions and can assist with adherence to a new regimen.[8] People under financial stress (a common occurrence when raising children) may have priorities other than paying for medicine. Ask the family to bring the medication bottles with them to each consultation and record the pill or liquid count or an estimation. Discrepancies could explain why expected results have not been achieved—many parents may simply not understand that under-dosing can reduce effectiveness. These considerations need to be taken into account when formulating a treatment plan.

Some parents may have beliefs or attitudes that deter or prevent them from giving children medications or other treatments.[8] These considerations also need to be taken into account, and potential problems can be resolved by actively engaging the parents in the treatment process. Concise but informative and easily understandable oral and written instructions should be given to the parents for each suggested medication or other treatment. The instruction should explain what the medication or treatment is for, how it will work and any possible side effects that might occur.[15]

There may be potential challenges working with the parents. For example, a parent may become defensive about a child's diet or activity level, and if the need for this is not explained in a gentle but educational manner there may be a loss of confidence in parenting skills, or a reduction in patient compliance.

Case Study: Nocturnal Enuresis

A **7-year-old male** who has recently moved house with his parents to a new area and a new school **presents with bedwetting**. He has been typically quite well, is current with all childhood vaccinations (to which he had no serious reactions), and is a little **inclined to anxiety** at times of change or stress in the family. He **presents with feeling upset in his stomach** and **not wanting to eat, constipation, and a history of bedwetting** since the family moved house (he had stopped wetting the bed a year ago at the age of 6), an **increase in crying episodes** and not wanting to meet new friends at school or play with other children after school.

SIGNS AND SYMPTOMS

- Intermittent urinary incontinence during sleep in the absence of physical disease in a child of a development age of 5 years or older
- Primary NE—a child has never been dry at night for more than 6 months
- Secondary NE—a child who has been dry previously for at least 6 months.

Classification, epidemiology and aetiology

Primary nocturnal enuresis (PNE) as defined by the International Continence Society[30] is the involuntary discharge of urine at night in children aged 5 years or older who do not have congenital or acquired defects of the central nervous system or urinary tract and have not experienced a dry period of more than 6 months. Secondary nocturnal enuresis (SNE) is defined as for PNE except that these children have had a period of dryness of more than 6 months and enuresis has started again.[30,31]

PNE is a common childhood problem. Epidemiological studies in Western countries show a prevalence of 13–20% of 5-year-olds, 7% of 7-year-olds, 5% of 10-year-olds, 2–3% of 12–14-year-olds and 1–2% aged 15 years and older wet the bed on average twice a week at night.[32,33] The prevalence of nocturnal enuresis (NE) decreases with age.[34,35] Without treatment, about 15% of enuretic children will become dry each year.[33,36]

The aetiology can be multifactorial and can include genetic factors,[33,37–39] physiological and psychological factors, a delay in the mechanism for bladder control maturation (antidiuretic hormone not increasing at night),[40] a delay in maturation of the nervous system and impaired cortical arousal.[38,39] Children with NE usually have normal bladder function and capacity but they can have a smaller nocturnal capacity.[37,41] There can be other contributing factors such as a diet with large volumes of fluids before bed, caffeinated or diuretic drinks, constipation, sleep apnoea and upper airway obstructions and emotional stress.[10,33,39] Constipation may result in bladder dysfunction. Urinary incontinence (46%) and NE (34%) has been reported in constipated children.[42]

Approximately 30% of all children with enuresis show clinically relevant behavioural disorders.[42] PNE overall has a low comorbidity and externalising disorders predominate, whereas nocturnal SNE has a high comorbidity when both emotional (internalising) and externalising disorders occur.[42]

Risk factors

The key risk factor for a child with enuresis (both nocturnal and daytime) is the possibility of damage to the child's self-esteem. These children can have low self-esteem, leading to a loss of confidence, poor school achievement and difficulty making friends.[43] Bedwetters can be sad, embarrassed and ashamed and are fearful that their peers may find out their secret. These factors may prevent adherence to a treatment plan.[42] Parents can feel anxious and guilty, and may lose confidence in their parenting skills and in the parent–child relationship.[44] Bedwetting has been reported as the second-commonest reason for child abuse (second to persistent crying).[45]

The two commonly prescribed pharmaceutical medications need to be treated with caution. The antidiuretic drug Desmopressin, sometimes used for enuresis, has been associated with seizures and two deaths possibly due to hyponatraemia. Symptoms of hyponatraemia include nausea, vomiting, fatigue, muscle cramps and weakness.[29] Imipramine, also used at times for enuresis, can have cardiotoxic side effects and death with overdose.[42]

Risk factors that might increase the risk of bedwetting can include anxiety, stress, shock, moving house and school (and away from established friendships), familial stress such as divorce or death in the family (including family pets) and a genetic component.

Conventional treatment

Current medical treatments concentrate on alarm therapy (a behavioural modification therapy where the child is woken by an alarm immediately on bedwetting),[31,37] pharmacological interventions (Desmopressin, oxybutynin, tolterodine and tricyclic antidepressants) and psychological interventions (such as counselling and psychotherapy—though there are no controlled trials),[37,43] as well as other behavioural interventions such as reward systems and scheduled awakening.[46]

There are a wide variety of responses including cure, poor response, potential side effects and relapses after discontinuing the treatment.[46–49] There is little high quality evidence for what is currently recommended for enuresis, but the majority of recommendations used by many health professionals are mentioned below.[50]

Enuresis alarm

This is the oldest specific therapy for enuresis. There are different types of alarm systems, but they all rely on the alarm alerting the child to void when the bladder is full.[51]

Desmopressin

Studies show that patients with NE placed on Desmopressin were 4.6 times more likely to achieve 14 consecutive dry nights than placebo and that response to Desmopressin (defined as a more than 50% reduction in the number of wet nights) was seen in 60–70% of patients.[51]

Anticholinergics

Oxybutynin or tolterodine can be used as a smooth muscle relaxant by blocking M2M3 muscarinic receptors in the detrusor muscle, leading to diminished detrusor overactivity and improvement of bladder storage function.[51]

Key treatment protocols

Secondary nocturnal enuresis (SNE) is associated with anxiety and social withdrawal. The constipation in this case could be a complicating and/or causative factor, and the recent stressful move to a new area and school could be contributing to his anxiety, poor appetite and stomach upset. Education and explanation are paramount. An understandable, child-friendly explanation of the causes and treatment options of enuresis is important.

> **NATUROPATHIC TREATMENT AIMS**
> - Discover and treat the cause/s to provide relief to the child and family.
> - Calm the nervous system and support psychologically.
> - Support a healthy appetite and normal bowel motions.
> - Provide a plan to reduce the recurrence of NE after cessation of treatment.

The main aim is to find and treat the underlying cause of the SNE; this can be difficult with a child who is withdrawing socially. It is important that the child feels confident to speak with their parents (and their practitioner) and know that their secret is safe. It is important that it is discussed with the practitioner, who will also keep the secret to be able to help the condition (not the 'problem'). The aim is for a happy and confident child who enjoys dry nights, restful sleep and the company of his peers. It may be wise to refer to a medical doctor or specialist clinic early to exclude any organic causative factors.

Concomitant conditions—in this case, the constipation, which may be partially or fully causing or exacerbating the condition, possibly contributing to the stomach upset and poor appetite—also need to be treated. Anxiety, which also may be causative or exacerbating the condition and contributing to the stomach upset, the lack of appetite and the social withdrawal, also requires treatment.

The practitioner needs to convey a sense of compassion and understanding to the child and family.[37] The parents and siblings need to be counselled that it is not appropriate to punish the child. Parental attitudes and experience should be taken into account in treatment plans as they can profoundly influence the outcomes.[42]

Treatment options

PNE and SNE are treated initially in the same way, and do not always require intensive treatment.[37] The family needs to see a practitioner if the parent or child are frustrated by the bedwetting; the child is at least 6 years old; the parent or sibling punish or are worried that they may punish the child; or the child wets or has bowel motions in their pants during the daytime.[35]

Nutritional supplements

Nutritional supplements can be of use when deficiency states are present. There can be compliance issues when giving children nutritional supplements. Supplementation for children should be on the advice of a health-care practitioner trained in the area.[52]

Selenium may be of use in this case. Low dietary intakes of selenium have been linked with greater incidence of anxiety, depression and tiredness, whereas higher intakes and short-term selenium supplementation have been shown to elevate mood and anxiety in particular, under double-blind, crossover test conditions.[18] In this case selenium 30 µg/day for 5 weeks for a 7-year-old (see Table 30.3) can be tried.

Herbal medicines

Most cases of nocturnal enuresis do not require medications, and this extends to herbal medicines.[35] However, treatment with short-term herbal medication may help comorbid conditions such as the constipation and anxiety associated with this case. If they are causative factors, then herbal medicine could potentially be very important in resolving the condition.

There is a scarcity of evidence-based information about the commonly used herbal medicines for NE but traditionally the **most commonly used herbs** for monosymptomatic NE are *Rhus aromatica*,[13] *Piper methysticum*,[13] *Plantago lanceolata*,[13] *Hypericum perforatum*,[13] *Viburnum opulus*,[13] *Thuja occidentalis*[21] and *Zea mays*.[13,21] *Piper methysticum* is not recommended by the Australian Therapeutic Goods Administration for use by children under 12 years of age, and may be restricted in certain jurisdictions.[13]

In accordance with naturopathic principles any underlying causes need to be treated as quickly as possible. Constipation and anxiety are both potential causes for NE and may be treated with appropriate herbal medicines. **Nervine tonic herbs** that help lift the mood and are calming for anxiety and stress in children include *Hypericum perforatum*, *Verbena officinalis*, *Melissa officinalis*, *Scutellaria lateriflora*, *Avena sativa*, *Turnera diffusa*, *Lavandula* spp., *Scutellaria baicalensis*, *Passiflora incarnata*, *Withania somnifera*[12] and *Matricaria recutita*. Appropriate **herbs for constipation** may include *Iris versicolor*, *Turnera diffusa*, *Angelica polymorpha*, *Rumex crispus*[12] and *Taraxacum officinale*.[21]

Lifestyle

Children require routines and need to know that they are loved, respected and are important enough to be involved in the treatment plan for their condition. They also need the appropriate amount of sleep for their age, appropriate diet, exercise, fluid intake and fun and play. These need to be incorporated into the treatment plan of NE.

The use of alarms to alert the child and parents that enuresis is starting is the most successful form of treatment[53] and effects a cure by itself in 80% of cases. A moisture-detecting mat placed on the bed is connected to a battery-powered alarm. Alarms can be used in combination with other forms of treatment. The child should be involved in the treatment and learn to turn the alarm on when they go to bed. When the child wets, the alarm sounds and the child should get up and go to the toilet to complete the micturition. It can take a couple of weeks to start having some dry nights. If the child is a deep sleeper, the parents may have to wake the child for the first few nights and take them to the toilet. The battery power is of low voltage and poses no danger to the child.[35] Personal alarms that attach to the child's clothing are also available.

In spite of NE the child should be encouraged to drink plenty of fluids during the day and extra when they are playing energetically or exercising. Diuretic and caffeine-containing fluids (such as tea, hot chocolate and colas) should be restricted in the evenings.[35]

Psychotherapy or counselling

If the parents are able to have the child discuss their concerns with them, it may not be necessary to seek professional counselling. However often the whole family is affected, and in this case parents, the affected child and any siblings may need counselling. If the child is sharing a room or a bed with siblings or parents this can exacerbate the stress on the family because of the disruptions in the middle of the night to change the bed linen and clean the child or others affected.[54]

It can be difficult to explain what stress is to a child, and the effect it can have on their body as well as their emotions and actions. Some of the subclinical psychological symptoms in children with NE are being unhappy, very unhappy, fitful, fearful, impatient, anxious and with feelings of inferiority.[37] There are other responses such as the social consequence of not being able to stay at a friend's house overnight, or have a friend stay; of affect being changed to feelings of sadness, shame or annoyance; of feeling isolated because they have a secret; and of the sensations of urine being unpleasant, cold, wet, itchy or nasty. A very small percentage of children reported the experience as an advantage such as liking the wet feeling or getting more attention from their mother.

When the child is ready to go to a friend's for a sleepover, discuss the situation with the other child's parent, and hide a pull-up nappy in the bag for the child to discreetly put on so that the child need not be embarrassed.[45]

Meditation may also be an effective tool for managing stress, and children benefit as much as adults.[55] There are many effective meditations for children and practising the meditations with the family can be a way of having family interactions that give health benefits and family cohesion.

Dietary considerations

In this case the child has a poor appetite and constipation since moving home. This is a common occurrence. Diet is very important to help in the treatment of constipation and, as this may be a causative or exacerbating factor in SNE, it may be prudent to work with their diet to encourage plentiful fluids (but not diuretic fluids in the evenings) and sufficient fibre.

In the case of a poor appetite, encourage small meals frequently rather than three larger meals a day, and encourage nutrient-dense foods. Foods rich in magnesium, calcium, zinc and essential fatty acids are of benefit to growing children and magnesium-rich foods are indicated for anxiety states where magnesium may be deficient.[18]

Food sensitivities should also be considered. One study of 21 children with migraine and/or hyperkinetic behaviour and NE that were placed on a restricted 'oligoantigenic' diet found significant remission of NE.[56] Twelve of the 21 had remission of their NE when on the diet. Nine of the responders were then challenged with reactive foods and later with non-reactive foods. Six children given reactive foods did have a return of their NE but none of the nine responded with NE when given non-reactive foods. Although the study provides tentative support for this dietary modification, it is worth consideration if food intolerances or allergies are suspected. Given the large numbers of children with NE, there is a need for more research in this area.

Integrative medical considerations
Hypnotherapy
Children generally are receptive to hypnosis, make good subjects for guided imagery and can have good results for a lot of conditions, including NE. Culbert et al.[38] reported four classic studies where hypnosis had better outcomes for bladder control than other treatments including pharmaceuticals, especially in the long term after cessation of treatments. Teaching children self-hypnosis is empowering for the child as they can take control of their own conditions.

Homoeopathy
There does not appear to be any published studies on the effects of homoeopathy and NE.[38] Homoeopathic texts list several remedies which when matched appropriately to the symptom picture may effect a cure: Cina 30, Causticum 200, Sepia Officinalis 200, Equisetum Hyemale 30, Verbascum Thapsus 30, Kreosotum 30 and Calcarea Carbonica 200.[57]

Acupuncture
Laser acupuncture may be a more gentle approach than needling when treating children. The literature published on acupuncture's effectiveness for treating NE is conflicting. Bower et al.[58] published a systematic review of acupuncture for paediatric NE. They evaluated 206 abstracts. Eleven were deemed eligible for data abstraction. The authors reported tentative evidence for the efficacy of the treatments, although they comment that the studies were of poor methodological quality.

Example treatment
Nutritional prescription
Foods rich in magnesium, calcium and zinc provide the building blocks for healthy growth and maturation for cells and metabolic pathways, for example almonds, cashews, cocoa, molasses, parsnips, soya beans and wholegrain cereals, meat, shellfish, yoghurt, salmon, tofu, sardines, spinach, baked beans, bok choi, snapper, tuna, barley.

> ### Herbal formula
>
> | | |
> |---|---|
> | *Turnera diffusa* 1:2 | 30 mL |
> | *Hypericum perforatum* 1:2 | 40 mL |
> | *Glycyrrhiza glabra* 1:1 | 30 mL |
> | | 100 mL |
>
> Dose (Young's rule) 2 mL t.d.s. a.c.
> Chamomile tea b.d. p.c.
>
> ### Nutritional treatment
>
> Selenium 30 µg/day for 5 weeks

Turnera diffusa acts as a nervine tonic, tonic and mild laxative. Its potential indications include nervous dyspepsia, constipation, nervousness, anxiety and depression.[12] There is no specific safety information available for its use in paediatrics, but it is used as a slimming tea in Mexico served to children.[13] *Hypericum perforatum* is prescribed for its nervine properties. Several human studies confirm the mood-modulating effect of St John's wort extract (see Section 4 on the nervous system) and it is well tolerated by children (there were no adverse effects in one trial with 101 children[13]). *Matricaria recutita* is sedative, calming on the stomach and improves

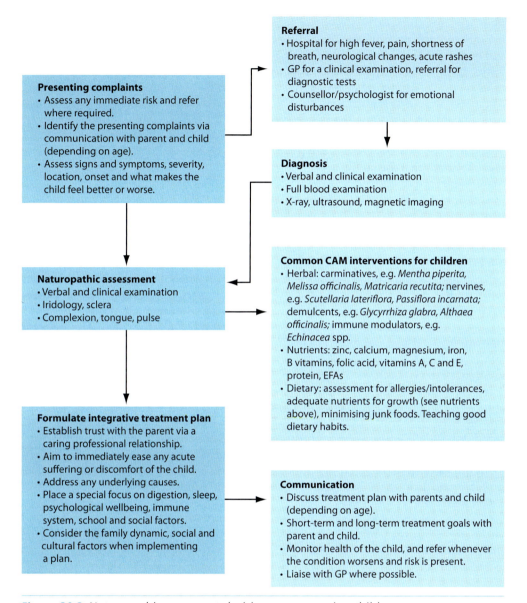

Presenting complaints
- Assess any immediate risk and refer where required.
- Identify the presenting complaints via communication with parent and child (depending on age).
- Assess signs and symptoms, severity, location, onset and what makes the child feel better or worse.

Referral
- Hospital for high fever, pain, shortness of breath, neurological changes, acute rashes
- GP for a clinical examination, referral for diagnostic tests
- Counsellor/psychologist for emotional disturbances

Diagnosis
- Verbal and clinical examination
- Full blood examination
- X-ray, ultrasound, magnetic imaging

Naturopathic assessment
- Verbal and clinical examination
- Iridology, sclera
- Complexion, tongue, pulse

Common CAM interventions for children
- Herbal: carminatives, e.g. *Mentha piperita, Melissa officinalis, Matricaria recutita;* nervines, e.g. *Scutellaria lateriflora, Passiflora incarnata;* demulcents, e.g. *Glycyrrhiza glabra, Althaea officinalis;* immune modulators, e.g. *Echinacea* spp.
- Nutrients: zinc, calcium, magnesium, iron, B vitamins, folic acid, vitamins A, C and E, protein, EFAs
- Dietary: assessment for allergies/intolerances, adequate nutrients for growth (see nutrients above), minimising junk foods. Teaching good dietary habits.

Formulate integrative treatment plan
- Establish trust with the parent via a caring professional relationship.
- Aim to immediately ease any acute suffering or discomfort of the child.
- Address any underlying causes.
- Place a special focus on digestion, sleep, psychological wellbeing, immune system, school and social factors.
- Consider the family dynamic, social and cultural factors when implementing a plan.

Communication
- Discuss treatment plan with parents and child (depending on age).
- Short-term and long-term treatment goals with parent and child.
- Monitor health of the child, and refer whenever the condition worsens and risk is present.
- Liaise with GP where possible.

Figure 30.3 Naturopathic treatment decision tree—treating children

mood.[18] It is considered safe when taken by children.[13] *Glycyrrhiza glabra* has a mild laxative effect, acts as an adrenal tonic and has a sweet flavour. Care should be taken that the child is not consuming the confectionery liquorice concomitantly so that excessive exposure is avoided.[13]

Additional prescriptive options

The diet may be improved more generally by encouraging a wide variety of colours and textures in foods with daily selections of vegetables, fruits, nuts and seeds to educate the children to good lifelong eating patterns. If this is coupled with appropriate physical activity, fun, laughter, love and respect, it may help the child recover. Rich selenium sources such as brewer's yeast, wheat germ, meats, fish, seafood, brazil nuts and garlic may also be useful as low dietary intakes of selenium have been linked with depression and anxiety.[18] Abdominal massage with a relaxing oil such as lavender after drinking a warm drink has been traditionally used to help relieve constipation. The gentle strokes must go up the ascending colon, across the transverse colon and down the descending colon. Chickweed is a nutritious food and traditional herbal medicine uses it to help with constipation. It should be avoided at night as it can have a mild diuretic effect.[18]

Therapeutic considerations

It is important that the family never punish the child for the condition as this may make the situation worse.

If the child is staying overnight at a friend or relative's house, discreetly add a pull-up nappy so the child can put it on privately. NE can lead to frictions in a family with tired, frustrated, worried parents. Children with the condition need lots of bedclothes, and an increase in washing added to an already busy routine can cause extra strain on the family and parents. Staying in nappies is unlikely to help the problem. It can cut down on washing, but the child has no incentive to wake up when the bladder is full. Neither will nappies work with alarms.[35] Ensure the parents understand and agree with the diagnosis, see it as serious, and believe that the treatment will eventually work. For some, this may involve directing them to research findings and connecting them with relevant institutions such as the Bedwetting Institute (http://www.bedwettinginstitute.com.au).

Expected outcomes and follow-up protocols

The best outcomes come from the child, parents and practitioner working together.[34] If there is compliance with herbs, diet and alarm, resolution may be expected within a few months.

NE is a significant problem from the perspective of both the child and their parents. Understanding their perceptions will help in formulating a successful treatment plan.[54] Giving positive reinforcement without being negative on the 'wet' days will assist the recovery and help the child raise their self-esteem. Aiming for achievable goals will lessen frustrations.[59]

Teaching relaxation or meditation to children may help with their self-identity and encourage calmness. Children often enjoy meditation and it may help to maintain the dry state after treatments have ceased.

Frequent follow-ups are important—with emotional support for both the parents and the child.[60]

The child needs to be very involved in their treatment if it is to work. It is important to recognise that there will be good and bad days. Have the child make a diary or chart to record the dry nights and encourage them to decide how it should be completed.[35]

Surprises are a good idea when they are making progress but it is not advisable to promise big rewards (like a new puppy or bicycle) because it may add to the stress, particularly if they do not succeed in staying dry.[35] The parents too sometimes need rewards during this process so suggest they plan to have a few nights alone.

It may be reasonably expected that this case of SNE will resolve quickly in a supportive familial environment. If the stress is managed and controlled, the child could be 'dry' every night in 2–3 months. Once this has occurred there is no need to continue the herbal and supplement treatment, but the dietary suggestions should continue. Other 'non-clinical' factors such as making new friends at the new school should help with the child's distress and treatment success.

Table 30.5 Review of the major evidence

INTERVENTION	KEY LITERATURE	RESULT	COMMENT
Acupuncture (Cochrane review)[33]	3 trials included a group receiving acupuncture. One small trial compared acupuncture with Desmopressin.	Numbers too small to demonstrate if acupuncture was effective.	More studies with larger samples are required.
Diet or restricted foods (Cochrane review)[33]	Two trials tested the effect of dietary manipulation on enuresis. In the first (Egger 1992) a subsample of children whose enuresis appeared to respond to a restricted diet of 'few foods' were tested in a double-blind randomised fashion by re-introducing test foods that were thought to affect enuresis.	Relapse occurred in 6/9 children given test foods compared with 0/9 given placebo (non-reactive) foods.	The numbers were too few for reliable comparison.
Hypnosis (Cochrane review)[33]	Two small trials addressed this comparison: versus imipramine in two and with or without suggestions or versus an untreated group in the other.	The number of children cured or improved was similar at the end of treatment in one trial; the high relapse (19/25 children) resulted in a lower combined failure or relapse rate than after hypnosis.	Data combining and small numbers do not prove to be statistically relevant.
Herbal medicine[38]	Culbert and Banez[38] 2008 and the author of this chapter have searched literature reviews and found no published studies in mainstream medical journals on the use of Western herbal medicine for NE	Herbal medicine lacks present evidentiary support from clinical trials.	Studies are urgently required using herbal medicines in NE.

KEY POINTS

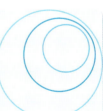

- Children are not 'little adults', but have their own specific requirements.
- Children's symptoms can exacerbate quickly, so that they often need urgent and appropriate attention.
- Parents and siblings may also require some form of treatment or support.
- Education, explanation and motivation should form the basis of treatment.
- Children of all ages require positive feedback on their progress.
- Encourage healthy attitudes to digestion and elimination in the early years as this may assist in providing lifelong health.
- Enuresis alarms are the treatment of choice for nocturnal enuresis.
- Give positive reinforcement for dry nights; do not be negative on the wet ones.
- Identify achievable goals.
- Use diet/activity/dry-night diaries with small treats, but do not promise large rewards. Encourage the child to make a chart and choose how to complete it.
- Reward the parents with a few nights on their own.

Further reading

Garth M. Starbright meditations for children. North Blackburn: Collins Dove 1992.

Garth M. Moonbeam meditations for children. North Blackburn: Collins Dove 1993.

Glazener C, Evans J, Cheuk D. Complementary and miscellaneous interventions for nocturnal enuresis in children. Cochrane Database Syst Rev 2005;(2):CD005230.

Robson W. Clinical practice. Evaluation and management of enuresis. N Engl J Med 2009;36014:1429–1436.

Santich R, Bone K. Phytotherapy essentials: healthy children: optimising children's health with herbs. Warwick: Phytotherapy Press, 2008.

United Nations. Conventions on the rights of the child. General Assembly resolution 44/25 of 20 November 1989. Geneva, Switzerland. Online. Available: http://www.unicef.org/crc. 1989

Useful resources

The Bedwetting Institute
http://www.bedwettinginstitute.com.au
PO Box 737 Glebe 2037 NSW Australia
Tel: 1300 135 796
International + 61 2 9518 8769
Fax: 02 82 105 125
International Fax: + 61 2 82 105 125
The Continence Foundation of Australia
http://www.continence.org.au
Helpline 1800 330 066
The National Continence Management Strategy
http://www.bladderbowel.gov.au/ncms/
The International Children's Continence Society
http://www.i-c-c-s.org/
Children's Hospital at Westmead
http://www.chw.edu.au/parents/factsheets/bedwetting.htm

References

1. International Conference on Harmonisation. Clinical investigation of medicinal products in the paediatric population E11. Online. Available: http://emea.europa. eu/htms/human/ich/ichefficacy.htm.
2. United Nations. Conventions on the rights of the child. General Assembly resolution 44/25 of 20 November 1989. Geneva, Switzerland. Online. Available: http://www. unicef.org/crc.
3. Kemper K. Complementary and alternative medicine for children: does it work? Archives of Disease in Children 2001;84:6–9.
4. Loman D. The use of complementary and alternative health care practices among children. J of Paediatric Health Care 2003;17:58–63.
5. Cohen M, Kemper K. Complementary therapies in paediatrics: a legal perspective. Paediatrics 2005;115(3):774–780.
6. Tillisch K. Complementary and alternative medicine for functional gastrointestinal disorders. GUT 2006;55:593–596.
7. Ethics Advisory Committee. Royal College of Paediatrics and Child Health. Guidelines for the ethical conduct of medical research involving children. Arch Dis Ch 2002;82(2):177–182.
8. Beers MH, et al, eds. Merck manual of diagnosis and therapy. Whitehouse Station: Merck Research Laboratories, 2006.
9. Suggs D. Pharmacokinetics in children: history, considerations, and applications. J of the American Academy of Nursing 2000;12(6):236–239.
10. Kurtz R, Gill D. Practical and ethical issues in pediatric clinical trials. Applied Clinical Trials 2003:September, article 79923. Online. Available: http://appliedclinicaltrialsonlinefindpharma.com/appliedclinicaltrials/author/authorDetail jsp?id+5124
11. Hull D, Johnston DI, eds. Essential paediatrics. 3rd edn. Edinburgh: Churchill Livingstone, 1993.
12. Bone K. A clinical guide to blending liquid herbs. Herbal formulations for the individual patient. Edinburgh: Churchill Livingstone, 2003.
13. Santich R, Bone K. Phytotherapy essentials: healthy children:optimising children's health with herbs. Warwick: Phytotherapy Press, 2008.
14. Zenk K. Challenges in providing pharmaceutical care for pediatric patients. American Journal of Hospital Pharmacy 1994;51:683–694.
15. Reed M. Principles of drug therapy. In: Nelson WE, Behrman RE, et al., eds. Textbook of pediatrics. 15th edn: W.B. Saunders Co., 1996.
16. Niederhauser V. Prescribing for children: Issues in pediatric pharmacology. American Journal of Primary Health Care 1997;22(3):16–30.
17. Millard R, et al. Clinical efficacy and safety of tolterodine compared to placebo in detrusor overactivity. Journal of Urology 1999;161:1551–1555.
18. Braun L, Cohen M. Herbs and natural supplements. An evidence-based guide. Sydney: Elsevier Australia, 2007.
19. NHMRC. Nutrient reference values for Australia and New Zealand including recommended dietary intakes. Australian Federal Government, 2006.

20. Shils M, et al, eds. Modern nutrition in health and disease. 10th edn. Philadelphia: Lippincott Williams & Wilkins, 2006.
21. Thomsen M. Phytotherapy desk reference. 2nd edn. Denmark: Michael Thomsen Publishing, 2005.
22. Mills S, Bone K. Principles and practice of phytotherapy. London: Churchill Livingstone, 2000.
23. Brewin L. Natural health for children. An A–Z of childhood ailments and how to treat them naturally. Australian Broadcasting Corporation, 2002.
24. Pizzorno J, et al. The textbook of natural medicine. Churchill Livingstone, 2008.
25. Scott J, Barlow T. Herbs in the treatment of children. Missouri: Churchill Livingstone, 2003.
26. Sarrell E, et al. Naturopathic treatment for ear pain in children. Pediatrics 2003;111(5):574–579.
27. Hyman P, Danda C. Understanding and treating childhood bellyaches. Pediatr Annals 2004;33(2):97–104.
28. Williams H. Epidemiology of atopic dermatitis. Clinical Exp Dermatol 2000;25(7):522–529.
29. Online. Available: http://www.medicinnet.com/script/main/art.asp?articlekey=85646
30. Norgarrd JP, et al. A standardization and definitions in lower urinary tract dysfunction in children. Br J Urol 1998;81(1) (Supplement 3):1–16.
31. Robson W. Clinical practice. Evaluation and management of enuresis. N Engl J Med 2009;360(14):1429–1436.
32. Nijman RJM, et al. Committee 10A. Conservative management of urinary incontinence in childhood. In: Abrams P, Cardozo L, Khoury S, Wein A, eds. Incontinence, in Proceedings of the Second International Consultation on Incontinence. Health Productions Ltd, 2002:513–551.
33. Glazener CMA, et al. Complementary and miscellaneous interventions for nocturnal enuresis in children. Cochrane Database of Systematic Reviews 2002;(2):CD005230.
34. Gumus B, et al. Prevalence of nocturnal enuresis and accompanying factors in children aged 7–11 years in Turkey. Acta Paediatr 1999;88:1369–1372.
35. Rural children's Hospital (melbarne). Bedwetting. Online. Available: http://www.rch.org.au/kidsinfo/factsheets.cfm?doc_id=3716
36. Freehan M, McGee R, Stanton W, Silva PA. A 6-year follow-up of childhood enuresis: prevalence in adolescence and consequences for mental health. J Paediatric Child Health 1990;26:75–79.
37. Hjalmas K, et al. Nocturnal enuresis: an international evidence based management strategy. Journal of Urology 2004;171(6 II):2545–2561.
38. Culbert T, Banez GA. Wetting the bed: integrative approaches to nocturnal enuresis. Journal of Science and Healing 2008;4(3):215–220.
39. Caldwell PHY, Ng C. Management of childhood enuresis. [online]. Med Today 2008;8:16–20:22–24.
40. Sobenin IA, et al. [Reduction of cardiovascular risk in primary prophylaxy of coronary heart disease]. Klin Med (Mosk) 2005;83(4):52–55.
41. Sheldon S. Sleep-related enuresis. In: Sheldon S, et al, eds. Principles and practice of pediatric sleep medicine. Philadelphia: Elsevier Saunders, 2005.
42. Hjalmas K, et al. Nocturnal enuresis: an international evidence based management strategy. Journal of Urology 2004;171(6, Part 2 of 2)2004:2545–2561.
43. Blackwell C. A guide to the treatment of enuresis for professionals. Bristol: Enuresis Resource and Information Centre, 1989.
44. Hagglof B, et al. Self esteem before and after treatment in children with nocturnal enuresis and urinary incontinence. Scand J Urol Nephrol Suppl 1997(183):79–82.
45. Dobson P. Enuresis. Bedwetting—the last taboo. Nurs Stand 1990;4:25–27.
46. Glazner CMA, Evans JHC. Desmopressin for nocturnal enuresis in children. Cochrane Database System Review 2002;(3): CD002238.
47. Glazner CMA, Evans JHC. Tricyclic and related drugs for nocturnal enuresis in children. Cochrane Database System Review 2003;(3):CD002117.
48. Glazner CMA, Evans JHC. Drugs for nocturnal enuresis in children (other than desmopressin and tricyclics). Cochrane Database System Review 2003;(4):CD002238.
49. Glazner CMA, et al. Complex behaviour and educational interventions for nocturnal enuresis in children. Cochrane Database System Review 2004;(1):CD004668.
50. Wicks GR. Bedwetting and toileting problems in children/ In reply. Medical Journal of Australia 2005;182(11):596.
51. Wright A. Evidence-based assessment and management of childhood enuresis. Paediatrics and Child Health 2008;18(12):561–567.
52. Mansberg G. Paediatric complementary medicine. J Complementary Medicine 2004;March/April:37–40.
53. Glazner CMA, et al. Alarm interventions for nocturnal enuresis in children. Cochrane Database System Review 2005;(2):CD002911.
54. Ng CFN, Wong SN. Primary nocturnal enuresis: patient attitudes and parental perceptions. HK J Paediatrics 2004;9(1):54–58.
55. Ott M. Mindfulness meditation in pediatric clinical practice. Pediatr Nurs 2002;28(5):487–490.
56. Egger J, et al. Effect of diet treatment on enuresis in children with migraine or hyperkinetic behaviour. Clin Pediatrics 1992;31:302–307.
57. Allen H. Keynotes: rearranged and classified with leading remedies of the materia medica and bowel nosodes. Delhi: B. Jain Publishers, 1999.
58. Bower WF, et al. Acupuncture for nocturnal enuresis in children. A systematic review and exploration of rationale. Neurourol Urodyn 2005;24:267–272.
59. Berry A. Helping children with nocturnal enuresis. AJN 2006;106(8):58–65.
60. Longstaffe MM, Whelan JC. Behavioural and self concept changes after six months of enuresis treatment: a randomised, controlled trial. Paediatrics 2000;105(4 pt 2), 935–940.

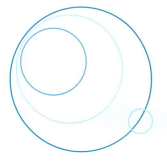

31

Fertility, preconception care and pregnancy

Jon Wardle
ND, MPH
Amie Steel
ND, MPH

PRECONCEPTION CARE

There is solid scientific evidence that infant health is inextricably linked to the health of the women who bear them, especially regarding preconception care.[1] Preconception care takes place prior to conception and focuses on the reduction of conception-related risk factors and increasing healthy behaviours. It can be said that preconception care epitomises the naturopathic principle to address the cause, not just the symptom, of illness. By ensuring health issues are addressed in both partners prior to conception, the aim is to improve the health of the infant at birth in a way that even early prenatal care can not.[2] Ideally, preconception care involves both partners as some risk factors affect both males and females. Furthermore, involving both partners may help promote equal involvement in the preparation for a major life transition. As with all naturopathic treatments, preconception care incorporates a holistic approach and, as such, supports the physical and psychological health of both partners.

The nature of a preconception care plan will differ between couples. For ease of understanding, preconception care can be categorised into two broad categories: health promotion and disease attenuation. Health promotion preconception care describes couples who have not yet attempted conception and have no diagnosed illnesses, but would like to ensure optimum health before their baby is conceived. Disease attenuation preconception care, in contrast, applies to couples with current diagnosed health conditions, or who have already had unsuccessful attempts to conceive. There may be some crossover between these two categories and, once disease attenuation has been addressed, it is quite common to incorporate health promotion into the plan prior to

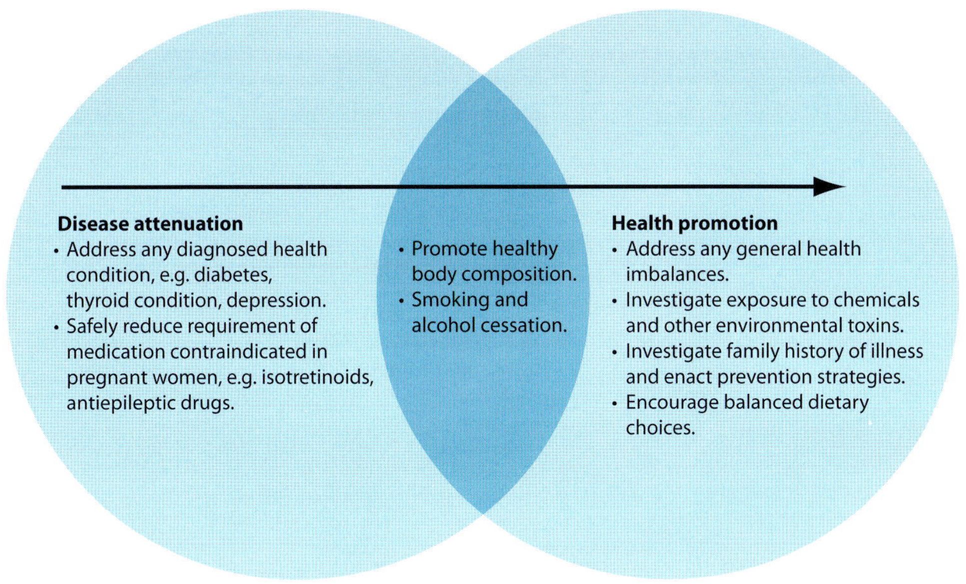

Disease attenuation
- Address any diagnosed health condition, e.g. diabetes, thyroid condition, depression.
- Safely reduce requirement of medication contraindicated in pregnant women, e.g. isotretinoids, antiepileptic drugs.

- Promote healthy body composition.
- Smoking and alcohol cessation.

Health promotion
- Address any general health imbalances.
- Investigate exposure to chemicals and other environmental toxins.
- Investigate family history of illness and enact prevention strategies.
- Encourage balanced dietary choices.

Figure 31.1 Approaches to preconception care

conception (see Figure 31.1). However, these are general guides only and the approach to the treatment plan should always be patient-centred, with the time and level of intervention required for each category determined based on couples' needs. As such, it is important to remind couples that, although many achieve conception soon after they commence attempting, for others patience is required

Infertility and subfertility

Impaired fertility affects approximately one in six couples.[3] In young, healthy couples, the probability of conception in one reproductive cycle is typically 20 to 25%, and in 1 year it is approximately 90%; however, this success rate can decline rapidly due to various age-related or health factors.[3]

Reproductive specialists use strict definitions of infertility.[4] Clinical infertility in a couple is defined as the inability to become pregnant after 12 months of unprotected intercourse. However, consensus is building that the diagnosis of clinical infertility should also be considered after six cycles of unprotected sex in women over 35 years of age.[5] Clinical infertility may also be considered when the female is incapable of carrying a pregnancy to full term. At this time further investigation becomes warranted to establish whether there are physical conditions hindering conception and, if so, what intervention may be appropriate. Infertility is not necessarily analogous to subfertility, which is often caused by other underlying conditions such as endometriosis or polycystic ovarian syndrome.

Causes of infertility and subfertility

Infertility can be considered to be primary or secondary. Couples with primary infertility have never been able to conceive, while secondary infertility is defined as difficulty conceiving after already having conceived (and either carried the pregnancy to term or had a miscarriage).[4] Secondary infertility is not considered as a diagnosis if there has been a change of partners.[4]

Table 31.1 Common causes of infertility in males and females

MALE	FEMALE
Low sperm count	Non-specific immune factors
Low percentage of progressively motile sperm	Irregular ovulation (e.g. polycystic ovarian syndrome)
Disorders of sperm morphology	Steroid hormone imbalance (may be influenced by insulin, thyroid function, stress, adiposity or exposure to hormone disrupting compounds)
High degree of abnormality on sperm	Hostile endometrial environment (may be influenced by hormonal imbalance, structural abnormalities, fibroids, infection or immunological factors)
Chromosome fragmentation	Genetic variations (such as MTHFR polymorphism)

Source: Adapted from Speroff and Fritz 2005[4]

Infertility may also be more broadly grouped into categories of sterility or relative infertility. Sterility can arise from various predominantly non-treatable underlying disorders involving lack of eggs (menopause, radiation damage or some autoimmune diseases); lack of sperm (infectious causes or immature sperm); fallopian tube obstruction (endometriosis, surgical or due to infection such as chlamydia) or hysterectomy. In contrast, infertility may be caused by other factors (see Table 31.1). Male causes of infertility include defective sperm production and/or insemination difficulties.[6] Female causes include ovulation factors (anovulation or infrequent ovulation), tubal damage, uterine factors such as adhesions, and cervical mucus 'hostility' (commonly due to an immunological defect).[6]

CONVENTIONAL TREATMENT

The conventional approach to preconception care does not differ greatly from the naturopathic approach. The focus is on increasing the general level of health and ceasing unhealthy behaviours. The factors identified as areas of concern for preconception care include chronic diseases, infectious diseases, reproductive issues, genetic/inherited conditions, medications and medical treatment, and personal behaviours or exposures.[2] Of these issues, a number have proposed clinical practice guidelines. Folic acid supplementation, for example, is considered essential to reduce the incidence of neural tube defects in the fetus, and thus supplementation ideally begins 3 months prior to conception.[2] Prevention of congenital defects due to rubella infection is also recommended through rubella vaccination, and a similar approach is taken to hepatitis B due to the potential for vertical transmission to infants and resulting organ damage.[2] Management of chronic diseases such as diabetes and hypothyroidism is also considered important in pregnancy to reduce the effects on the developing fetus. Likewise, conditions managed with medication such as isotretinoids and anti-epileptic medication need to be approached with lower dosages or alternative medication as these drugs are teratogens and as such can cause birth defects.[2]

If a couple have been attempting to conceive for at least 12 months, then initial assessment of hormone levels, ovulation, weight/body composition and semen analysis is undertaken. In the longer term, gynaecological examination to check for physical factors interfering with conception (e.g. scarring from previous STI or endometriosis) is conducted.

Once the diagnosis of infertility has been made, the conventional treatment approach varies depending on the diagnosed reason for the infertility. If the diagnosis is male infertility, then the treatment will depend on the seminal analysis. If azoospermia (absence of sperm) is diagnosed, then conception relies upon donor insemination.[6] However, if there is severe oligospermia (fewer than 5 million sperm), then a single spermatozoon is recovered from the epididymis and microinjected in the ovum. This has a 30% success rate.[6] There have been some attempts to increase the sperm count of men with oligospermia using hormonal therapy (testosterone analogues and antioestrogens) with limited documented benefit.[6] Another alternative in this situation is in vitro fertilisation.[6]

Alternatively, infertility may be due to female reproductive pathophysiology. Anovulation is managed by encouraging the woman to aim for an appropriate body composition, and use of an antioestrogen drug (clomifene), which has resulted in a 70% conception rate in amenorrhoeic women.[6] If tubal damage has been diagnosed, there are really only two options available: microsurgery to attempt to repair the fallopian tubes, or in vitro fertilisation. With a diagnosis of cervical hostility, the traditional conventional approach is to encourage the couple to use condoms for 6 months in the hope that the antibodies attacking the sperm will be eliminated. Other, more invasive approaches include ingestion of oral corticoids by the male in the first 10 days of the woman's cycle, the use of washed sperm, or in vitro fertilisation or gamete intrafallopian transfer techniques.[6]

RISK FACTORS

Like many conditions, factors that increase the risk of infertility can be both inherited and due to lifestyle. Lifestyle factors that contribute to infertility include common concerns such as cigarette smoking and alcohol misuse, but also extend to the use of certain prescription medications.

Cigarette smoking adversely affects fertility in both males and females.[7–10] Smoking affects sperm production, motility, morphology and incidence of DNA damage in males;[11] this may be explained by increased reactive oxygen species, which has been linked with lowered sperm concentration, motility and morphology.[12] Cigarette smoking in females may affect the follicular microenvironment, and may cause alteration of hormone levels in the follicular phase.[11] Both active and passive smoking have been demonstrated to increase zona pellucida thickness; this may make it more difficult for sperm to penetrate.[13] In active smokers, the effect of delayed conception is increased with the number of cigarettes smoked.[9] Despite these statistics, more than 10% of pregnant women continue to smoke cigarettes.[14]

Caffeine intake may also adversely affect fertility outcomes.[15] Some research has found that coffee and/or tea intake greater than six cups a day is associated with reduced fertility.[10] However, other researchers assert that coffee and tea consumption associated with reduced fertility rates in males and females is not dose related, and that constituents other than caffeine may also have an effect.[8] Other drug use, such as recreational drugs and alcohol, may also contribute to certain subtypes of infertility.[15]

Another lifestyle factor that may affect fertility is diet and its associated nutritional status. A range of dietary constituents have been linked with various aspects of infertility including *trans*-fatty acids,[16] iron,[17,18] antioxidants,[19,20] selenium[21] and zinc.[22] Increasing intake of vegetable protein and replacing animal protein may also reduce the ovulatory infertility risk.[23] Similarly, a high glycaemic load diet and overall high dietary carbohydrates have also been associated with increased ovulatory infertility.[24]

Psychological stress is an added risk factor for reduced fertility in females[25] and males.[26] Depression in males has been correlated with decrease in sperm concentration and poor coping mechanisms have been associated with increased occurrence of early miscarriage.[26]

Both maternal and paternal age have a bearing on the fertility level of a couple. Older women experience more difficulty achieving and maintaining pregnancy, and are less likely to deliver a healthy infant than younger women.[27] In females spontaneous cumulative pregnancy rates begin to decline as early as 31–35 years of age.[27] One-third of women aged 35–39 years of age will experience difficulty achieving pregnancy, and half of women aged 40–44 years will have an impaired ability to reproduce.[27] Increasing maternal age results in a decreased number of oocytes, decreased oocyte quality, uterine age-related changes affecting endometrial receptivity and neuroendocrine system ageing.[27]

Another general risk factor to consider when approaching preconception care is the presence of underlying disease. Women with a chronic disease such as diabetes have an increased risk of congenital abnormalities in their offspring, but are known to have improved birth outcomes when they plan their pregnancies and use preconception care.[28] Coeliac disease is another condition which is known to incur higher miscarriage rates, increased fetal growth restriction and lower birth weights.[29] Although not a disease, obesity may also affect fertility for both males[30] and females.[31] Sexually transmitted infections, particularly chlamydia and gonorrhoea, may lead to infertility.[15] Infection of any nature may be associated with reduced sperm motility.[32] Other conditions may affect fertility but, rather than the disease being detrimental, it is the medication used to manage the condition which is problematic. Several different types of medications, including hormones, antibiotics, antidepressants, pain-relieving agents, and aspirin and ibuprofen when taken in the middle of the cycle, have been reported to affect female fertility.[4] With this in mind, it is important to address any underlying health issues, resolving them where possible, to reduce reliance on medication. Alternatively, where the condition cannot be resolved, exploration of substitute medication may be necessary.

KEY TREATMENT PROTOCOLS

A key naturopathic principle to be considered when supporting couples with fertility issues is to treat the whole person. It is vital that the approach to the development of a treatment plan for such couples is patient-centred, and does not make assumptions about their individual needs without diligent exploration of their health history and current health complaints. Such exploration must go beyond reproductive health, as a number of conditions not directly linked to the reproductive system have been associated with infertility. Examples of such conditions are inflammatory bowel disease,[33] thyroid disease[34] and type 1 diabetes.[35] Other conditions more

NATUROPATHIC TREATMENT AIMS

- Address lifestyle related risk factors:
  - smoking
  - caffeine intake
  - body mass index (BMI)
  - stress
  - diet.
- Ensure sufficiency of key nutrients.
- Address confounding and high risk conditions:
  - PCOS
  - endometriosis
  - hormone imbalances
  - thyroid imbalances
  - semen parameters.

directly associated with the reproductive system which may need to be addressed include endometriosis[36] and polycystic ovarian syndrome.[37]

Underlying conditions aside, preconception care will still benefit many couples by promoting health. Many lifestyle factors dramatically affect fertility, birth success and infant health.[11] Preconception care must address these factors in order to promote fertility, conception and healthy pregnancy outcome. A study found that 81% of couples previously classified as infertile were able to conceive within 2 years of commencing an individualised preconception program.[38]

In general, due to the individual nature of preconception care, the treatment interventions used will vary significantly between couples; however, there are some remedies which are more commonly used. Common herbal medicines that may be useful when supporting couples during preconception care include **Vitex agnus-castus** and **Tribulus terrestris**. *Vitex agnus-castus*, or chaste berry, is used traditionally in fertility disorders, particularly for women with progesterone deficiency or luteal phase defects. No large studies have explored this role; however, a randomised, placebo-controlled trial (RCT) with 96 women with various fertility disorders (secondary amenorrhoea, luteal insufficiency and idiopathic insufficiency) taking *Vitex agnus-castus* for 3 months resulted in women with secondary amenorrhoea and luteal insufficiency achieving pregnancy twice as often as those in the placebo group.[39] Previous smaller trials show similar results.[40,41] *Tribulus terrestris* has also been associated with improving conception outcomes in women with endocrine sterility.[42]

Window of fertility

The first priority when approaching preconception care and couples with fertility issues is to establish the window of fertility. The window of fertility is probably best defined as the period in the 6 days leading up to ovulation, when in theory the oocytes and sperm should have maximum viability and survivability.[43,44] However, in an individual clinical setting this can be more accurately garnered through analysis of intermenstrual intervals, cervical mucus and basal body temperature charts (see Chapter 20 on polycystic ovarian syndrome). Intercourse is most likely to result in pregnancy when it occurs within the 3 days prior to ovulation.

Although certainly not a prerequisite for pregnancy to occur, the probability of conception is highest when cervical mucus (vaginal secretions) is slippery and clear (see Figure 31.2).[45–47] When combined with basal body temperature charts these simple and cheap analyses are able to predict peak fertility far better than menstrual charts alone. Cervical mucus analysis alone has been demonstrated to better predict peak fertility than either basal body temperature charts or biochemical ovulation detection kits based on LH.[48]

Monitoring cervical mucus may have other practical benefits as water-based vaginal lubricants can inhibit sperm motility by 60–100% in vitro.[50] Mineral oil, canola oil or hydroxyethylcellulose-based lubricants do not seem to have this effect.

Diet

Dietary change is an important intervention in any preconception plan and, although the focus is on a general healthy diet for couples, some specific dietary choices have been found to have direct benefits for fertility. Replacing animal protein with vegetable protein, for example, has been found to be beneficial in women seeking to get pregnant.[51] Similarly, low-fat dairy products have been connected with higher rates of anovulatory infertility, and higher dietary intake of *trans*-unsaturated fats have been linked with increased risk

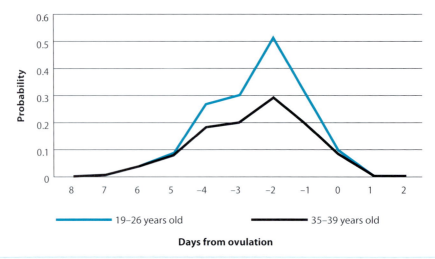

Figure 31.2 Probability of pregnancy by cycle day, involving recurrent intercourse, by age[49]

LET'S TALK ABOUT SEX

Trying to conceive is a stressful time for any couple and this stress can creep into the bedroom. Some couples may have forgotten to have intercourse as often as required or have turned it into a chore. Others may have been trying for so long that they even forget to have intercourse at all—except for once a month according to the calendar. This places further stress on the couple and may be ultimately counterproductive. Couples should maintain intimacy and engage in sexual activity as they desire, not purely based on ovulatory cycles. A well-timed weekend away or regular date night may improve both the relationship and the chances of a couple falling pregnant.

of ovulatory infertility.[52] **Organic food** may also be of benefit by reducing the potential exposure to environmental chemicals. Ultimately, the consensus seems to be that encouraging healthier eating habits more broadly improves fertility outcomes. As such, a healthy eating plan that includes foods with high levels of nutrients should be encouraged. High levels of **brightly coloured fruit and vegetables** to provide antioxidants plus **good protein sources** (meat if eaten, cheese, eggs, tofu if vegetarian; vegans need to be particularly careful with protein levels) and **good-quality carbohydrates** (wholemeal and wholegrain) should be routinely recommended (see Appendix 3, 'Food sources of nutrients').

Body composition

Overweight and obese women are less likely to conceive than those of normal weight.[15] These women also experience increased risk of pregnancy complications and adverse pregnancy outcomes in comparison to women who weigh less. Conversely, women who are very underweight may also experience problems conceiving.[15] Reproductive function can be affected by both obesity and low body weight, due to hormone imbalances and ovulatory dysfunction.[11] Overall, the relative risk of ovulatory infertility is increased for body mass index (BMI) below 20.0 kg/m^2 or above 24.0 kg/m^2.[53] There appears to be a 7% increase in the rate of fetal anomaly for each unit of BMI above 25.[54] Obesity affects fertility in ways that are complex and not well understood; however, the association with functional hyperandrogenism and hyperinsulinaemia is thought to play an important role.[55] Abdominal obesity in women with polycystic ovarian syndrome (PCOS) is considered to be co-responsible for the development of hyperandrogenism and chronic anovulation through mechanisms involving decreased concentrations of sex-hormone-binding globulin in the blood and insulin-mediated overstimulation of ovarian steroidogenesis.[55] Obesity may also contribute to reduced outcomes of IVF/ICSI procedures by promoting resistance to clomiphene and gonadotrophin-induced ovulation.[55] It has been demonstrated that weight loss in obese women can improve fertility through the recovery of spontaneous ovulation, and that others will have improved responses to ovarian stimulation in infertility treatment.[56,57]

Attenuating the hormonal imbalances resulting from high body fat can be achieved through both diet and exercise (as discussed in Chapter 20 on polycystic ovarian syndrome). Even after 12 weeks of dietary and exercise intervention, favourable menstrual and metabolic outcomes conducive to conception could be gained in infertile, overweight women.[58] In fact, lifestyle modification proved more effective than fertility drugs in inducing ovulation in women with anovulatory disorders.[59] However, it is important to note that weight loss needs to be approached responsibly, as rapid weight loss is understood to lower progesterone levels, slow follicular growth and inhibit the luteinising hormone surge, disallowing ovulation.[60]

Lifestyle activity

Maintaining an active lifestyle is beneficial in promoting both male and female fertility; however, moderation is very important. While moderate exercise may improve the chances of conceiving spontaneously or through fertility treatment,[11] excessive physical exercise is associated with a spectrum of reproductive dysfunctions in both males and females. Female fertility issues associated with excessive exercise range from luteal-phase defects to anovulation to infertility and finally to amenorrhoea.[53] Increase in vigorous activity (but not moderate activity) is associated with reduced relative risk of ovulatory infertility,[53] and has been linked to poor IVF outcomes.[61] This concern has also been found to affect male fertility, through subclinical changes in their reproductive hormone profile and semen parameters.[62] For example, male endurance runners have been found to have a reduction in total and free testosterone, alterations in luteinising hormone release, and in pituitary responses to gonadotrophin-releasing hormone.[62] Furthermore, there has been evidence of a change in the semen parameters of some endurance athletes, such as low normal sperm count, decreased motility and various morphological changes.[62]

This apparent contradiction between the benefits and risks of exercise can be best explained by the role of exercise in preventing and managing conditions that detrimentally effect fertility, such as polycystic ovarian syndrome and obesity.[63] In contrast, any level of activity which induces metabolic stress will interfere with the hypothalamus–pituitary–gonadal axis, and therefore affect fertility.[64] Overall, the focus when supporting couples prior to conception should be on moderate exercise that does not place undue stress on their systems.

Reduce risk factors

Factors such as smoking, caffeine intake and alcohol consumption may adversely affect fertility outcomes and should be reduced. Even if fertility is not yet a concern for a couple, these risk factors will still need to be addressed as they all have negative effects on the developing fetus and infant health. Maternal smoking during pregnancy, for example, has been linked to increased risk of wheezing in infants up to 2 years old[65] and reduced fetal brain development,[66] and may increase the infant's risk of adult development of diabetes, hypertension and metabolic syndrome.[67] Similarly, high alcohol consumption during pregnancy puts the developing fetus at risk of fetal alcohol syndrome.[68] Even lower-level intake can affect the neuroendocrine and behavioural functions of the offspring.[69]

Stress

The emotional journey of a subfertile couple is complex. Seemingly innocuous events such as friends falling pregnant, family events and birthdays may trigger underlying anxiety issues (see Figure 31.3).

The process of undergoing infertility treatment itself can also be stressful and exacerbate anxiety, depression and stress, often enough to negatively affect pregnancy outcomes.[72,73] This may be due to increased cortisol secretion, resulting from a normal stress response, down-regulating the hypothalamus–pituitary–gonadal (HPG) axis. It has been postulated that this may occur by inhibiting gonadotrophin-releasing hormone's (GnRH) release of follicle-stimulating hormone (FSH) and luteinising hormone (LH) from the pituitary.[74]

As such, **counselling** or **psychological support**, particularly interventions which focus on stress management and coping-skills training, should be strongly recommended throughout this process.[75] It is equally as important for the infertile couple to build a support network. Both attending support sessions and using cognitive behavioural interventions were equally effective in reducing the emotional aspects of infertility and improving the chances of pregnancy.[76] **Music therapy** has also been associated with positive pregnancy outcomes.[77] Overall, couples should be encouraged to take part in stress reduction activities at all stages of preconception and pregnancy. Anecdotal stories of previously infertile couples conceiving after ceasing trying or while on holiday are not to be ignored.[78]

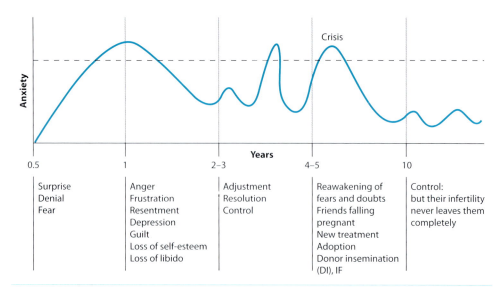

Figure 31.3 Emotional responses to infertility[70,71]

RELATIONSHIP ISSUES

Preconception can be an exciting time for a couple, but it can also be challenging. Sometimes in the lead-up to starting a family relationship issues that may not have been apparent previously can surface. The process of becoming pregnant can consume time and substantial resources—emotional, physical and financial. If fertility problems become apparent and assisted fertility in the way of procedures such as IVF is required, this can further add to feelings such as loss of control, distance between the couple and feelings of guilt or blame. All of these issues can be a significant source of stress in the relationship. It is important that a couple remember that the reason they want to bring a baby into the world is that they are two people in love. Nurturing the relationship by continuing to do things as a couple is very important. Small suggestions like a candlelit dinner occasionally or a walk along the beach together should be as much a part of the preconception prescription as any naturopathic medications. It is also important that a couple maintain intimacy by continuing the physical side of their relationship when they feel like doing that, and not only adhere to ovulation cycles and fertility plans.

Environmental concerns

Exposure to herbicides, fungicides, pesticides and other chlorinated hydrocarbons has been associated with decreased fertility and a higher risk of spontaneous miscarriage.[79,80] Further to this, it should be noted that, although over 140,000 chemicals are in common use in today's society, evaluation of the effects on reproduction of common physical and chemical agents has occurred in only 5% of substances.[81] With this in mind, it is important to investigate potential exposure to environmental chemicals such as pesticides, herbicides, household chemicals, paint and paint thinners, and plastics. Paradoxically many couples will subject themselves to high levels of environmental toxins during 'nesting' activities while trying to conceive or during pregnancy. While preparation for the child is certainly important, activities that include exposure to dust, paint or other chemicals and substances that release toxins, such as home renovations, may adversely affect pregnancy outcomes and should be considered carefully.

If exposure is identified, and particularly if it is occupational (for example, factory workers, tradesmen, farmers and horticulturalists), then protective measures must be taken. Such measures include appropriate occupation health and safety interventions like wearing protective clothing and masks.[82] Beyond this, the preconception treatment plan needs to incorporate suitable detoxification protocols (see the box on liver detoxification in Chapter 19 on endometriosis).

Immune dysfunction

Immune system imbalances may adversely affect fertility outcomes through a number of ways, including high generalised inflammation and antibodies targeted to key tissues. High levels of inflammatory prostaglandins, for example, may reduce uterine receptivity to fertilised embryos,[83] possibly by affecting the regulation of genes necessary for human endometrial receptivity.[84] Chronic inflammation may also contribute to the development of anatomic abnormalities such as pelvic adhesions and occluded fallopian tubes, as well as premature ovarian failure.[85] Causes of inflammation in reproductive tissues vary and may include sexually transmitted infections such as *Chlamydia trachomatis*,

INFLAMMATION AND HEALTHY REPRODUCTION

Inflammation is often approached as an undesirable adversary in the human body. In fact, inflammation is a mechanism necessary for the normal and healthy reproductive process. As the luteinising hormone (LH) surge occurs prior to ovulation, LH stimulates granulosa cells to secrete inflammatory mediators (prostaglandins and cytokines) and progesterone. These compounds all trigger the secretion of matrix metalloproteinases, which break down the extracellular matrix, thereby allowing for follicular rupture and ovulation.[85] As such, indiscriminate use of anti-inflammatory interventions in preconception care should be avoided.

endometriosis and autoimmune conditions.[85] Autoimmune conditions which can contribute to infertility may be non-specific, such as type 1 diabetes mellitus and Hashimoto's thyroiditis, or specific, such as antibodies that target FSH and LH and their receptors.[86,87] Another such example is antibodies that target ovaries and sperm.[84] It is worth noting, however, that the inflammatory response is also an important mechanism within healthy, normal reproductive function (see the box on inflammation and healthy reproduction). With this in mind, various measures to reduce inflammation systemically and specifically can be found in other relevant chapters.

Nutritional medicines

The primary conventional focus of nutrient supplementation in preconception care is on the role of **folic acid** in preventing neural tube defect.[88] The benefits attributed to folic acid in the prevention of this condition require maternal sufficiency in the first 28 days of gestation, before many women know they are pregnant.[88] It is this knowledge that has led to public health interventions such as folate fortification of bread flour and further supplementation of 400 µg/day for women of reproductive age.[88]

Folic acid is not the only nutrient required in preconception and the early stages of gestation. A recent longitudinal study[89] observed the effect of pregnancy on the micronutrient status of the mothers. It was noted that, while folate levels decreased slightly during pregnancy and remained decreased up to 6 weeks after delivery, **vitamin B12** progressively declined throughout gestation and reached marginal or deficient levels.[89] This is of particular concern, as vitamin B12 has been overlooked as an important nutrient for preconception supplementation. Low maternal vitamin B12 status has been associated with a threefold risk of neural tube defect.[90] This deviates from the previous approach to neural tube defect prevention, which has been firmly focused on folic acid supplementation and fortification of food. In fact, the focus on folic acid fortification of food, such as bread flour, may be contributing to a masking of vitamin B12 deficiency and an increased risk of neural tube defect[91] (see the box on vitamin B12 and folate).

Various multivitamin and antioxidant nutritional supplements have improved pregnancy rates in those undergoing assisted reproduction[92] or lowered time to conception in couples seeking preconception care.[92,93] Preconception multivitamin use has also been associated with a higher incidence of multiple births for unknown reasons.[94] Folate needs to be taken at least 3 months prior to conception for optimal benefit in reducing neural tube defects or leukaemia development in the fetus. However, it is also associated with decreased incidence of ovulatory infertility more generally.[95] Vitamin C

VITAMIN B12 OR FOLIC ACID?

Folic acid has been used for a number of years to prevent neural tube defect;[88] however, recent research has identified that vitamin B12 is also important in preventing this condition.[90] With this in mind, the most predictable course of action may be to incorporate vitamin B12 supplementation into standard preconception care approaches alongside folic acid. Unfortunately, just as some concerns regarding the risks of folic acid supplementation masking vitamin B12 deficiency have been raised,[91] excess vitamin B12 intake, resulting in potential cobalt toxicity,[97] may also be a concern. To avoid this, and to stay true to the naturopathic patient-centred approach, assessing the most appropriate nutrients required for supplementation and the relevant dosages are vital. Folic acid is found predominantly in legumes and green leafy vegetables, while vitamin B12 is found in its most bioavailable form in animal products.[98] As such, an assessment of a patient's diet will provide an initial indication as to whether supplementation of folic acid and/or vitamin B12 is required. In general, though, it is important to remember that the absorption of vitamin B12 is an incredibly complex process that relies on healthy gastric, pancreatic and intestinal function, and that dysfunction in any one of these organs can compromise B12 status.[98] A more thorough assessment of sufficiency of these nutrients can be gleaned through testing. The most accurate test to determine folic acid status is red blood cell folate, not the commonly used serum folate, which does not correlate with tissue stores.[99] Vitamin B12 status can be assessed using serum cobalamin, which is more specific and stable compared with serum folate; however, both pregnancy and folate deficiency can result in false low readings. A more accurate assessment, which is independent of both of these conditions, is that of methylmalonic acid. Unfortunately, this test is much more expensive and technically demanding.[100]

supplementation has also had improved fertility outcomes in women with luteal phase defects.[96]

The male partner

It is important to realise that in 20% of infertile couples males are the sole cause of infertility and are an important contributing factor in a further 20–40% of infertile couples.[101] Although many infertile men may have physical or structural conditions that require surgical intervention, many may have reversible issues that can be corrected with non-invasive measures. Men also experience declining fertility as they age—most profoundly after the age of 55 years but even men over the relatively young age of 35 years have half the chance of successfully inseminating as men under the age of 25 years.[102]

A decline in male fertility has been reported over the past few decades in a number of countries, though this has been controversial.[103] It has been suggested that environmental and lifestyle factors such as increased occupational chemical and pesticide exposure are at least partly responsible for this decline.[104–106] Oestrogen-like products are thought to be partly responsible. The fact that organic farmers have higher sperm counts than regular farmers or other exposed occupational groups lends further credence to this theory.[107] Other environmental and lifestyle factors that may be affecting fertility include wearing tight-fitting clothing, using hot baths and spas and having occupations that require long periods of sitting down, as these behaviours all increase scrotal temperature.[108] Dietary intake must also be considered, as it may affect semen quality. Men consuming diets high in meat and dairy products[109] and soy protein[110] have compromised semen parameters, whereas diets high in fruits and vegetables show benefit.[109] The advantage in a fruit- and vegetable-rich diet may be attributed to an increased antioxidant intake.[111]

Beyond diet and lifestyle, some specific nutrients have been identified to improve fertility in men. For example, there is evidence that **coenzyme Q10** supplementation can improve semen parameters in men,[112,113] while **vitamin C**, **vitamin E**, **beta caro-tene**, **folate** and **zinc** are important for semen quality.[4] A similar trial that identified increased pregnancy rates in couples with severe male infertility when taking an anti-oxidant supplement containing ascorbic acid, zinc, vitamin E, folate, lycopene, garlic oil and selenium has been conducted.[114] In contrast, selenium has been demonstrated to improve sperm quality and motility in subfertile men, but not those diagnosed with infertility,[115–117] or conversely with normal testicular selenium levels.[118,119] Similarly, L-carnitine has been associated with increased semen quality and sperm concentration, particularly in groups with lower baseline levels,[120–123] though one trial suggested that this may be true only in those with normal mitochondrial function.[124]

Assisted fertility procedures

Assisted reproductive technologies encompass a spectrum of methods and are valid options for infertile couples (see Table 31.2). However, the usefulness of these therapies needs to be considered by any prospective couple in the context of the costs and risks. For example, a systematic review of studies measuring the prevalence of birth defects in infants conceived using assisted reproductive technologies found a 30–40% increased risk.[125] Furthermore, the average cost of IVF for Australian women is $32,903,[126] while the success rate is 10% for a single IVF procedure, and increases to 40% if the procedure is repeated five times.[6] Finally, the process of IVF requires constant emotional adjust-ment through each phase of the process,[127] and can be debilitating for the woman in

Table 31.2 Types of assisted reproductive technologies

TYPE	PROCEDURE	PREGNANCY RATE*
Assisted insemination with husband's sperm (AIH)	Sperm are transferred by catheter into uterus or fallopian tube.	Up to 15% per cycle
In vitro fertilisation (IVF)	Fertilised eggs are transferred in to the uterus or fallopian tube.	10–25% per cycle; depends on maternal age
Gamete intrafallopian transfer (GIFT)	Unfertilised eggs and sperm are transferred into one or both fallopian tubes using laparoscopy or transvaginal ultrasound.	Up to 30–40% per cycle
Intracytoplasmic sperm injection (ICSI)	Sperm is injected into the egg.	More than 50% per cycle
Zygote intrafallopian transfer (ZIFT), tubal embryo stage transfer (TEST)	Zygote or early embryo is transferred into the fallopian tube using laparoscopy or transvaginal ultrasound the day after egg pick-up.	Up to 30–40% per cycle

*Adapted from Oats and Abraham 2005[6] Note that pregnancy rate is not the same as live birth rate. Naturopathic treatment of couples undergoing assisted reproductive techniques should not cease once these interventions have resulted in a successful pregnancy.

particular. To support this, a questionnaire study[128] found that financial burden (23%), psychological stress (36%) and lack of success (23%) were the most predominant reasons couples discontinued IVF programs. In particular, a combination of lack of success and psychological stress was noted in 18% of participants.

Often this course of action is used as a symptomatic approach to infertility and does not have the added benefit of preparing the body for a healthy pregnancy or allowing for improved success of subsequent births. In one study 65% of couples who had previously undergone multiple IVF cycles were able to conceive within 2 years of a preconception program.[38] However, there will be instances where referral to this procedure will be appropriate.

Most patients attending assisted reproduction will be using some form of complementary therapy and are likely to be consulting a complementary therapist; they are perhaps using several options concurrently.[129] Therefore it may be prudent to identify the broad scope of treatment the patient is undertaking so as to reduce the risk of negative interactions. Acupuncture on the day of embryo transfer is demonstrated to have a beneficial effect on live births.[130] L-arginine supplementation can improve the response rates of poor responder women undergoing assisted reproduction.[131]

Pregnancy

Pregnancy is one area that lends itself to naturopathic treatment for a number of reasons. Although it is not a disease state (though it has certainly been managed and thought of as one in the past) it is a significant life transition that encompasses the mind, body and spirituality of the mother. It is also a time when the power of nature and the abilities of the body are apparent and there is a greater recognition of the immediate need and benefit of optimal health. Pregnancy care is also a time in which the accepted aim of treatments is to be as minimally invasive as possible. Therefore the aim of the naturopath is to avoid unnecessary treatment of any kind and instead support optimal health for the mother and child.

The management of the pregnant woman should be in conjunction with a qualified specialist practitioner—a midwife and/or obstetrician. Midwifery and naturopathy have traditionally had a supportive relationship due to their shared belief that pregnancy and birth are normal physiological processes that can be supported through adequate nutrition, psychological and physical support when required and avoidance of harmful substances.

Decision making when supporting the pregnant woman requires careful thought. The potential for any therapy to do harm needs to be considered. This includes not only instances of possible direct harm to the fetus or mother (for example, the use of potentially teratogenic herbs—see 'Safety in pregnancy' below), but also the possibility of indirect harm. Indirect harm includes such things as potentially delaying a useful therapy (for example, in the progression of preeclampsia to toxaemia) or financially exploiting the patient through the use of unnecessary or ineffective therapies. It can be easy to overcomplicate treatment in the pregnant woman, and a simple approach is often best.

DIETARY REQUIREMENTS

Dietary requirements in pregnancy encompass nutrients that must be included and foods that should be avoided. Additional energy is needed in pregnancy and lactation to cover the needs of the growing fetus, the placenta and expanding maternal tissues, and additional maternal effort at rest and in physical activity, as well as the production of breast milk during lactation. Nothing additional over pre-pregnancy requirements is needed in the first trimester, though in the second trimester an extra 1.4 MJ/day and in the third trimester an extra 1.9 MJ/day over pre-pregnancy levels should be consumed.[132] **Protein** requirements also increase to 1.1 g/kg of body weight, as does the recommended daily intake of a number of nutrients including **folic acid**, **vitamin C**, **iron**, **zinc** and **calcium** (see Table 31.3).

Table 31.3 Key nutrients in pregnancy

NUTRIENT	EFFECT	COMMENT
DHA	Accumulates in the developing brain, and is important for prenatal and post-natal neurological development.	Can be easily converted via desaturases from α-linolenic acid.
Vitamin A	Important for the regulation of gene expression and for cell differentiation and proliferation.	Direct studies of vitamin A status are lacking, but excess retinol is a known teratogen. The threshold risk is still unclear, but the upper intake level is 3000 μg/day.
Folate	Required for normal cell division, and methylation during nucleotide synthesis. Associated with prevention of neural tube defect.	Supplementation still needs to be approached judiciously as the upper limit is only 1000 μg/day and some women already have folate-rich diets.
Vitamin B12	Supports methylation of nucleotides in conjunction with folate. Also essential for neurological function. Absorption decreases during pregnancy.	Although vitamin B12 can be stored in adults long term, only newly absorbed vitamin B12 is readily transported across the placenta. Vegan women will need to supplement.
Biotin	Animal studies imply that deficiency is teratogenic.	More evidence relating specifically to pregnant women is required to make confident clinical decisions.
Calcium	Required for bones, teeth, vascular contraction, vasodilation, muscle contraction, nerve transmission and glandular secretion.	Most fetal accretion occurs in the third trimester, and this is lower when maternal intake is low.
Chromium	Potentates the action of insulin.	Chromium is depleted throughout pregnancy and fetal tissue levels decline after birth, suggesting the need for deposition during pregnancy.
Iodine	Required for thyroid hormones, and therefore associated with myelination of the central nervous system and general metabolism. Most active in perinatal periods.	Deficiency is damaging to the developing brain and includes mental retardation, hypothyroidism and goitre.
Iron	Required for haem proteins and other iron-dependent enzymes.	Deficiency in pregnancy is associated with increased perinatal maternal and infant mortality, premature delivery and low birth weight
Zinc	A cofactor to nearly 100 enzymes, with catalytic, structural and regulatory functions.	Maternal zinc deficiency may lead to prolonged labour, intrauterine growth retardation, teratogenesis and embryonic or fetal death. Lower dietary intakes can lead to a higher incidence of premature deliveries.

Source: Adapted from Turner 2006[135]

A number of dietary practices should be avoided or limited.[133] Alcohol consumption during pregnancy is linked to a spectrum of disorders in the infant ranging from fetal alcohol syndrome through to alcohol-related birth defects or alcohol-related neuro-developmental disorders.[133] There is no safe level of alcohol intake during pregnancy, and as such pregnant women should be discouraged from any consumption (see the box on ethanol-based herbal extracts and pregnancy). Fish consumption must also be approached with care in pregnancy due to the risks associated with fetal exposure to methylmercury. In general, this compound accumulates from industrial pollution (although it also occurs naturally) in some of the larger, longer-lived fish, and those that consume other fish.[133] Examples include shark, swordfish, king mackerel and tuna.[133] In contrast, sardines and white fish have lower mercury levels and as much as 360 g can be safely consumed per week.[133] Another risk is food contamination with *Listeria monocytogenes,* which can cause spontaneous abortion, stillbirth and fetal infection (listeriosis).[133] To prevent this illness, pregnant women should avoid unpasteurised milk, undercooked or raw animal products, refrigerated smoked food, pâtés or meat spreads, soft cheeses, and unwashed fruit and vegetables.[133] Caffeine consumption must also be approached with caution during pregnancy, as it has been connected with fetal growth restriction and low birth weight infants.[134] One of the concerns surrounding caffeine is that the enzyme responsible for caffeine clearance, CYP1A2, is not present in fetal tissue, although caffeine can easily pass through the fetoplacental barrier.[134] For this reason, it is important that if the pregnant woman is going to consume caffeine their own phase 1 detoxification pathway is functioning at its optimum. This should be addressed in preconception treatment, however, not during pregnancy. It has been recommended that women should not consume more than 200 mg/day of caffeine throughout gestation.[134]

Appropriate weight gain

There should be relatively little maternal weight gain until the second and third trimesters, with the bulk of the weight gain in the third trimester (see Figure 31.4). Increased weight gain may lead to an increased risk of gestational diabetes, which has significant health implications for both mother and child.[4] High blood-sugar levels are used as an energy source by the growing baby and will therefore lead to increased birth weight. Although there are several negative health consequences for the baby associated with

ETHANOL-BASED HERBAL EXTRACTS AND PREGNANCY

It is recommended that all pregnant women minimise their alcohol consumption and abstain if possible.[133] But where does that leave the prescription of ethanol-based herbal extracts? If possible, other forms of herbal products should be prescribed to pregnant women to keep alcohol consumption to a minimum. This can include preformulated tablets, infusions, decoctions or glycetracts. However, the value in an individualised and extemporaneously dispensed formula of ethanol-based herbal extracts is well known to most practising naturopaths. If it is deemed that the best treatment for the individual is in the form of an ethanol-based herbal extract, then a useful approach is the addition of hot water to the tincture prior to each dose. This encourages evaporation of the alcohol and, although it may not eliminate the alcohol completely, it will reduce the amount remaining in the tincture.

high birth weight and gestational diabetes, one of the main concerns is the potential labour complications associated with giving birth to a larger baby. Patients should be made aware of these potentially alarming practical complications in addition to the negative health aspects.

Another potential cause of inappropriate weight gain is oedema, which may be linked to preeclampsia. Preeclampsia is a form of hypertension that occurs only in pregnancy, and is accompanied by proteinuria and excessive oedema.[133] Although obesity does increase the risk of developing preeclampsia,[133] it should not be assumed that weight gain is simply fat gain. Thorough dietary and physical assessment are needed to determine if fluid retention is an issue, or whether a high glycaemic, hypercaloric diet is the concern.

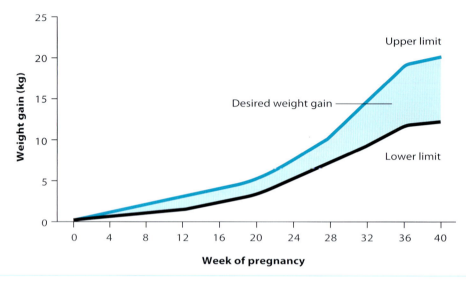

Figure 31.4 Appropriate weight gain in pregnancy

Anaemia

Maternal iron requirements increase in pregnancy because of the demands of the developing fetus, the formation of the placenta and the increasing maternal red cell mass.[136] Fetal iron requirements seem to come at the expense of maternal stores if there is insufficient intake. Even moderate iron deficiency is associated with a twofold risk of maternal death.[136] However, routine iron supplementation in women with normal haemoglobin is not associated with improved pregnancy outcomes. Furthermore, supplementation with high levels of iron increases the risk of oxidative stress, and should be approached with caution. With this in mind, one study[137] found that taking an iron supplement (60 mg **iron**, 200 µg **folic acid** and 1 µg **B12**) daily was no more beneficial than taking two tablets once per week. This may be an approach to reduce the risk of oxidative damage and still ensure iron sufficiency.

Safety in pregnancy

As the aim of pregnancy care is generally to move towards optimal health rather than treatment of particular disease states, herbal medicines and large doses of specific nutrients should generally be avoided during pregnancy (see Table 31.4). Even seemingly innocuous herbal medicines with hormonal activity or uterine activity are best avoided during pregnancy. Although uterine tonics may have a role to play in preparation for labour, even they need to be avoided at early stages of pregnancy.

There is still a high use of many different herbal and nutritional medicines by pregnant women, and nearly three-quarters of these women do not discuss this use with their conventional physician.[138,139] This may be due to the fact that specialist obstetricians generally have less favourable attitudes towards complementary medicines than women's non-obstetric physicians.[140]

To assist naturopaths to determine the safety of herbal medicines, a classification system[141] based on Therapeutic Goods Administration (Australia) and Food and Drug Administration (USA) categories for prescription medicines in pregnancy has been developed. Contraindicated herbs fit into categories D and X in this system (see Table 31.5). However, it is recommended that most herbal medicines be avoided during pregnancy unless absolutely necessary.

Partus preparator

Rubus idaeus has long been traditionally used as a 'partus preparator'—preparing the uterus for delivery and to facilitate labour.[145] Animal studies have suggested that *Rubus idaeus* may increase the regularity and decrease the frequency of uterine contractions.[146] Although no clinical studies have been conducted in humans, retrospective studies have

Table 31.4 Herbs contraindicated during pregnancy (bold indicates common herbs more likely to be encountered regularly in clinical practice)[141–144]

Abrus precatorius	*Daphne mezereum*	*Podophyllum resin*
Achillea millefolium	*Datura* spp.	*Pteridium aquilinum*
Aconitum spp.	*Digitalis* spp.	***Pulsatilla vulgaris***
Acorus calamus	*Dryopteris filix-mas*	*Rauwolfia* spp.
Adhatoda vasica	*Duboisia* spp.	*Rhamnus frangula*
Adonis vernalis	*Echium vulgare*	*Ricinus communis*
Aloe vera	*Ephedra* spp.	*Robinia pseudoacacia*
Ammi visnaga	*Erysimum* spp.	***Salvia officinalis***
Angelica archangelica	*Euonymus europaeus*	*Sarpthamnus scoparius*
Angelica sinensis	*Galega officinales*	*Schoenocaulon officinale*
Apocynum spp.	*Galanthus* spp.	***Schisandra sinensis***
Aristolochia spp.	*Gelsemium* spp.	*Scopolia carniolica*
Arnica spp.	*Heliotropium* spp.	*Semecarpus anacardium*
Artemisia spp.	*Helleborus* spp.	*Senecio* spp.
Arum maculatum	*Juglans canadensis*	*Solanum* spp.
Belladonna spp.	*Juniperus* spp.	*Sophora secundiflora*
Brugmansia spp.	*Hyoscyamus* spp.	*Spigelia marilandica*
Brunfelsia uniflora	*Lantana camara*	*Staphisagria* spp.
Calendula officinalis	*Larrea* spp.	*Strophanthus* spp.
Calotropis spp.	*Lathyrus sativus*	*Strychnos* spp.
Carbenia benedicta	*Lithospermum* spp.	*Strychnos gaulthieriana*
Caulophyllum thalictroides	*Lobelia* spp.	*Strychnos ignatii*
Catha edulis	*Mandragora* spp.	*Symphytum* spp.
Chenopodium ambrosioides	*Menispermum canadense*	*Tamus communis* fruit and root
Cicuta virosa	*Mentha pulegium*	***Tanacetum spp.***
Cimicifuga racemosa	*Oleander* spp.	*Teucrium* spp.
Cinchona spp.	*Opunita cylindrica*	*Thevetia* spp.
Colchicum spp.	***Panax quinqefolium***	***Thuja occidentalis***
Convallaria spp.	***Panax notoginseng***	*Toxicodendron radicans*
Coronilla spp.	*Papaver somniferum*	***Tribulus terrestris***
Corydalis ambigua	*Peganum harmala*	***Turnera diffusa***
Crotalaria spp.	*Petasites* spp.	*Tussilago farfara*
Croton spp.	*Peumus boldus*	***Viscum album***
Cynoglossum officinale	***Phytolacca spp.***	*Virola sebifera*
		Yohimbin spp.

Table 31.5 Examples of herbs classified for use in pregnancy[141]

CATEGORY	CATEGORY DEFINITION	RELEVANT HERBS
Category A	Drugs which have been taken by a large number of pregnant women and women of childbearing age without any proven increase in the frequency of malformations or other direct or indirect harmful effects on the fetus having been observed.	*Rubus idaeus* *Zingiber officinale* *Echinacea* spp. *Matricaria recutita* *Panax ginseng* *Vaccinium myrtillus* *Curcuma longa*
Category B1	Drugs which have been taken by only a limited number of pregnant women and women of childbearing age, without an increase in the frequency of malformation or other direct or indirect harmful effects on the human fetus having been observed. Studies in animals have not shown evidence of an increased occurrence of fetal damage.	*Astragalus membranaceus* *Valeriana officinalis* *Ginkgo biloba* *Hypericum perforatum* *Bupleurum falcatum*
Category B2	Drugs which have been taken by only a limited number of pregnant women and women of childbearing age, without an increase in the frequency of malformation or other direct or indirect harmful effects on the human fetus having been observed. Studies in animals are inadequate or may be lacking, but available data show no evidence of an increased occurrence of fetal damage.	*Barosma betulina*
Category B3	Drugs which have been taken by only a limited number of pregnant women and women of childbearing age, without an increase in the frequency of malformation or other direct or indirect harmful effects on the human fetus having been observed. Studies in animals have shown evidence of an increased occurrence of fetal damage, the significance of which is considered uncertain in humans.	*Andrographis paniculata*
Category C	Drugs which, owing to their pharmacological effects, have caused or may be suspected of causing harmful effects on the human fetus or neonate without causing malformations. These effects may be reversible. Accompanying texts should be consulted for further details.	*Arctostaphylos uva-ursi* *Hydrastis canadensis* *Glycyrrhiza glabra* *Aesculus hippocastanum* *Salvia mitorrhiza*
Category D	Drugs which have caused, are suspected to have caused or may be expected to cause an increased incidence of human fetal malformations or irreversible damage. These drugs may also have adverse pharmacological effects. Accompanying texts should be consulted for further details.	*Ruta graveolens* *Adhatoda* spp. *Tabebuia avellanedae* *Phytolacca* spp.
Category X	Drugs which have such a high risk of causing permanent damage to the fetus that they should not be used in pregnancy or when there is a possibility of pregnancy.	*Aristolochia* spp. *Senecia* spp. *Peumus boldus*

demonstrated that *R. idaeus* use is associated with a decreased rate of medical interventions required in childbirth.[147,148] One study found that *R. idaeus* shortened labour times and reduced the incidence of pre- and postterm labour,[149] while another suggested it reduced only the duration of second stage of labour. A recent literature review concluded that the evidence for the use of *R. idaeus* was scarce, and more research is needed.[150]

Chronic miscarriage

Conservative estimates suggest that 10% of first trimester pregnancies end in spontaneous abortion or miscarriage.[4] *Viburnum prunifolium* was traditionally used by the eclectic physicians of North America to prevent miscarriage,[151] and was embraced by obstetricians in the late 1800s for the same purpose.[152–155] *Dioscorea villosa* and *Chamaelirium luteum* have also been traditionally used in threatened miscarriage.[142] Unfortunately, more recent research into the efficacy of these herbs has not been conducted; furthermore, concerns over the accurate identification of the herb used in earlier interventions have been raised.[156]

Other underlying factors may need to be considered and treated in cases of recurrent or threatened miscarriage. For example, an increased risk of miscarriage in both naturally conceived pregnancies and following fertility treatment has been associated with extremes of BMI,[157] and interventions that have addressed elevated BMI have been found to reduce the incidence of miscarriage in high-risk women.[158]

Nausea and vomiting

Up to 80% of all pregnant women experience some nausea and vomiting,[159] commonly referred to as 'morning sickness'. It has been noted, however, that one of the possible causes of nausea and vomiting in early pregnancy is elevated prostaglandin E_2, stimulated by human chorionic gonadotrophin.[160] Due to the important functions PgE_2 performs in early stages of pregnancy, treatment of morning sickness in the first trimester needs to be tempered with respect for the natural process of gestation.

The most common naturopathic treatment for nausea and vomiting in pregnancy is *Zingiber officinale*. *Z. officinale* has been demonstrated to be an effective treatment for nausea and vomiting in early pregnancy according to a Cochrane review.[161] Since this review, other studies have also demonstrated positive effects,[162–164] but some authorities have expressed concern at the high levels of *Z. officinale* in commercial herbal supplements.[165] Ginger tea and candied ginger are also suitable therapeutic sources in the pregnant patient. *Z. officinale* is also effective for postoperative nausea associated with childbirth.[166]

Several large trials have demonstrated **vitamin B6** to be an effective treatment for the nausea and vomiting of pregnancy.[167–169] The optimum dose for this is thought to be between 30 and 75 mg daily.[161]

Preeclampsia

Obesity and stress are both associated with increased risk of preeclampsia.[170,171] Exercise can help reduce the incidence of preeclampsia.[172] Insufficient protein, magnesium, calcium, iron, pyridoxine (B6), vitamin C, vitamin E, essential fatty acids and folic acid have all been directly indicated in the pathogenesis of preeclampsia.[173] Rather than focusing on one particular nutrient, consensus is moving towards nutritional education more generally as a preventive measure.

Urinary tract infections

Women experience urinary tract infections more frequently during pregnancy. *Vaccinium macrocarpon* is an effective naturopathic treatment with a documented safety profile in pregnancy and therefore offers a valid therapeutic choice.[174,175]

Another potentially beneficial treatment option is the use of probiotics. The most direct route to increase the *Lactobacillus* spp. colony in vaginal mucosal tissue is through insertion of encapsulated probiotics, and should result in improved populations within 3 days.[176] If oral administration is preferred then 10×10^9 colony forming units are recommended, and will require 28–60 days to normalise vaginal colonies.[176] (See Chapter 27 on recurrent urinary tract infections.)

Childbirth

Childbirth is a culmination of between 37 and 42 weeks' gestation, and providing support to women at this important moment in time can prevent unnecessary interventions at later stages. Education and empowerment of women to trust their body and the birth process are paramount before labour begins.[177] This can be achieved successfully through group psychoeducation and support work to release fear surrounding the birth process.[178] It is also important that the woman feels supported by sensitive and nurturing birth companions at the time of birth.[177] Birth companions such as midwives[179–182] and doulas[183–186] have been associated with improved birth outcomes for women seeking low-intervention births.

Reducing interventions associated with birth not only benefits the birth experience of the woman if she desires a low-intervention birth, but may also benefit the health of the infant. For example, an induced labour frequently results in a cascade of interventions such as the use of intravenous lines, enforced bed rest, continuous electronic fetal heart monitoring, amniotomy, increased pain and discomfort, epidural analgesia, operative (caesarean) delivery and prolonged hospital stay.[187] Postbirth health risks associated with induction and the potentially resulting caesarean delivery included maternal depression and neonatal respiratory illness,[188] as well as longer term risks to the infant of atopic diseases such as allergic rhinitis,[189] eczema and asthma[190] (see Chapter 25 on inflammatory skin disorders). Interventions such as induction and operative delivery may still be indicated in high risk circumstances, but the importance lies not so much in avoiding the intervention as ensuring women are educated and empowered to feel in control of their birth process.[191]

Outside of the medical model, there are some low-intervention therapies which may benefit child birth. For example, **acupressure** has been used effectively to reduce pain or delivery time in labour.[192] A case report has also been published promoting the use of homoeopathic **Caulophyllum** in conjunction with nipple stimulation to induce and augment labour,[193] and a small randomised controlled-trial found that a combination of homoeopathic **Arnica** and **Bellis Perennis** resulted in an apparent reduction in postpartum blood loss.[194] Even less invasive models such as **muscle relaxation techniques** and **lower back massage** have been associated with reduced labour pain.[195]

Postnatal support
Lactation

The mammary glands develop during pregnancy, but the levels of progesterone and oestrogen secreted by the placenta prevent lactation occurring until 30–40 hours after birth.[196] Healthy and adequate lactation provides extensive health benefits to infants both at birth and later in life, and promoting efficient suckling and successful breastfeeding begins with timely skin-to-skin contact between mother and infant.[197] Furthermore, promotion of good health practices through preconception and pregnancy education reduces the risk of breastfeeding complications.[198] In contrast, delayed contact between mother and infant, washing the mother or infant prior to contact or the use of a pacifier before 6 weeks of age have all been shown to interfere with effective and successful breastfeeding.[197]

A number of **herbs** have been used traditionally to encourage lactation: *Trigonella foenum-graecum*, *Galega officinalis*, *Foeniculum vulgare*, *Pimpinella anisum*, *Cnicus benedictus*, *Silybum marianum*, *Asparagus racemosus* and *Urtica dioica*.[199,200]

Unfortunately, recent research into the efficacy and physiological activity of these herbs is scarce. Based on experimental data, increased milk production can generally be expected 24–72 hours after consumption of *F. vulgare*,[201] and *A. racemosus*'s traditional Ayurvedic use as a galactagogue has also been confirmed in a clinical trial.[202]

Formula feeding

There is an undeniable weight of evidence that 'breast is best', although in some instances breastfeeding may not be an option. Formula supplementation may also be required in the nutritionally compromised mother.

Soy proteins have been used as an alternative protein source for infants with allergies or food intolerances, although there is little evidence to support their use. A Cochrane review of five studies found only one study comparing soy to cow's milk formula noted a reduction in childhood allergy, asthma and allergic rhinitis.[203] The other four studies that fit the inclusion criteria reported no significant benefit for any allergy or food intolerance. Many infants allergic to cow's milk may also be allergic to soy milk,[204] suggesting a deeper underlying immunological issue. Furthermore, intestinal permeability is higher in infants fed formula than those fed breast milk;[205] this may contribute to the risk of the development of atopic disease (see Chapter 25 on inflammatory skin disorders). In these circumstances, **colostrum** supplementation in the initial feeding of formula-fed infants may offer some protection.[206]

No formula will ever be able to replicate the comprehensive and complex nutritional profile of human breast milk. In addition, any nutritional deficiencies will be compounded by exclusive use of one formula. Therefore several specific formulas should be rotated regularly to ensure that the effects of possible deficiencies are minimised.

Postnatal depression

Some women develop a severe depression after childbirth. Sleep deprivation and general tiredness may worsen these symptoms.[207,208] Recent research has also acknowledged that in 50% of couples, if women are depressed, their partners are depressed also.[209] Unfortunately, current family health systems do not effectively balance the postnatal support to both members of the parenting team.[209] If either partner is experiencing fatigue, promoting adequate sleep is important and may simply require sleeping when the baby sleeps. If there is difficulty sleeping during these odd hours, sleeping aids may be considered (see Chapter 14 on insomnia). **Omega-3 essential fatty acids** are also indicated in general postnatal depression (see Chapter 12 on depression). Other underlying issues, particularly those associated with the development of menstrual disorders, should be investigated, as women with a history of postnatal depression are more likely to develop menstrual difficulties and perimenstrual symptoms when menstruation recommences.[210]

INTEGRATIVE MEDICAL CONSIDERATIONS

Traditional Chinese medicine

Acupuncture on the day of embryo transfer is demonstrated to have a beneficial effect on live births.[130] Acupuncture has been demonstrated to be a safe and effective treatment tool for pelvic and back pain associated with pregnancy.[213] Similarly, acupressure, a less invasive therapy similar to acupuncture, has been associated with

Table 31.6 Review of the major evidence

INTERVENTION	METHODOLOGY	RESULT	COMMENT
Multivitamins	Prospective cohort study (Nurses Health Study II) [95]	Inverse association between multivitamin use and ovulatory infertility	116,671 female registered nurses enrolled in study and followed every 2 years with questionnaire.
Antioxidants	Self-reported retrospective food-frequency questionnaire[111]	High intake of antioxidants was associated with better semen quality (sperm concentration, motility and progressive motility) than low or moderate intake.	97 healthy male volunteers with at least 15 men from each age decade from 20 to 60 years of age. Volunteers completed Modified Block Food Frequency Question-naire and semen sample for analysis.
Diet	Prospective cohort study[52]	Increased intake of trans-unsaturated fats associated with increased risk of ovulatory infertility after adjustment for known and suspected risk factors for this condition.	18,555 married, premeno-pausal women without history of infertility who attempted a pregnancy or became pregnant over an 8-year period. Diet assessed twice during follow-up using food-frequency questionnaire.
Arginine	RCT ($n = 34$) of women under-going assisted reproduction were treated with stan-dard treatment plus placebo ($n = 17$) or standard treatment with oral L-arginine supplementation ($n = 17$)[131]	Arginine supplementation in poor responder patients improved ovarian response, endometrial receptivity and pregnancy rate (3/17 vs 0/17) (all $p \leq 0.05$).	No dose of L-arginine supplied. Success rates in pregnancy still low and all successful pregnancies still resulted in early pregnancy loss.
Smoking	Retrospective cohort study via questionnaire[8]	Cigarette smoking adversely affected fertility in both males and females.	Ontario Farm Family Health Study; 1898 couples with 2607 planned pregnancies conducted over 30 years.
	Population study via questionnaire[9]	Both active and passive smoking in women associated with delayed conception OR of 1.54 (95% CI 1.19–2.01) delayed conception > 12 months women who smoked compared to non-smokers; OR 1.14 (95% CI 0.92–1.42) for passive smokers). Heavy smoking in men independently associated with delayed conception. In active smokers, effect increased with number of cigarettes smoked.	All couples (14,893 preg-nant women) expected to deliver in Avon Health Authority area, UK, between April 1991 and Dec 1992. Main outcome measure: time taken to conceive.

(Continued)

Table 31.6 Review of the major evidence *(Continued)*

INTERVENTION	METHODOLOGY	RESULT	COMMENT
Body weight	Prospective cohort study (Nurses Health Study II)[53]	U-shaped association between body mass index (BMI) and relative risk of ovulatory infertility. Increased risk for BMI below 20.0 and above 24.0 kg/m².	Prospective data collected for 116,671 female registered nurses aged 25–42 years at cohort's inception; 830 cases of incident anovulatory infertility and 26,125 pregnancies.
Exercise	Prospective cohort study (Nurses Health Study II)[53]	Increase in vigorous physical activity associated with 7% (95% CI = 4–10%) lower relative risk of ovulatory infertility and a 5% (95% CI = 2–8%) reduction in relative risk per hour of weekly activity after adjustment for BMI.	Prospective data collected for 116,671 female registered nurses aged 25–42 years at cohort's inception; 830 cases of incident anovulatory infertility and 26,125 pregnancies.
Zinc	RCT (n = 45) men with asthenozoospermia were randomised to zinc only (n = 11), zinc + vitamin E (n = 2), zinc + vitamins E + C (n = 14), placebo (n = 8) for 3 months.[211]	All intervention groups had improved sperm parameters compared with placebo. There was also a measured reduction in oxidative stress, apoptosis and sperm DNA fragmentation in intervention groups.	The sample size of this study is quite small.
Selenium and n-acetyl cysteine	RCT (n = 468) men with idiopathic asthenoteratospermia were randomised to selenium 200 μg (n = 116), 600 μg NAC (n = 118), combination (n = 116), or placebo (n = 118) for 26 weeks followed by 30 week washout.[212]	Following treatment, FSH decreased and testosterone increased. Semen parameters significantly increased. The strongest correlation was noted between the combination therapy and mean sperm concentration, sperm motility and percentage normal morphology.	This is a well-constructed study, although baseline measurement of selenium and/or oxidative stress would have allowed for a more meaningful interpretation of results. However, the dosage used was within a therapeutic range and reflective of dosages used in clinical practice.

reduced pain and shorter delivery time in labour.[192] Moxibustion is a method used in traditional Chinese medicine as a method for cephalic version of breech babies;[214] however, due to methodological issues randomised controlled trials have not been completed.[215]

Antenatal classes

Antenatal classes can provide appropriate supervision and advice on antenatal exercises, back care, labour pain relief, relaxation skills and posture. An observational study involving 9004 women found that women who attended antenatal classes had a much lower risk of caesarean section and were half as likely to bottle feed in hospital, as well as being more satisfied with the experience of childbirth.[216] Furthermore, group psychoeducation classes, which focus on releasing the fear surrounding the birth process, can improve a woman's pain tolerance and coping mechanisms in childbirth.[178] Similarly, fathers attending antenatal classes felt they were more prepared for the birth and for their role as a support person.[217]

Homoeopathy

Individualised homoeopathic treatment in 45 subfertile men was found to improve semen parameters (sperm count and motility in addition to general health parameters) equal to conventional treatment.[218] Caulophyllum is a commonly used homoeopathic remedy for third trimester cervical ripening and induction of labour. A Cochrane review[219] evaluating this remedy identified two trials involving 133 women, but the results of the review were inconclusive due to a lack of information about the methodology used in the studies. Although a lower level of evidence, a case report has also been published promoting the use of this remedy.[193]

Aromatherapy

A pilot randomised-controlled feasibility study which took an individualised approach to the prescription of aromatherapy oils in childbirth found that the intervention group rated a lower pain perception, and a higher proportion of the control group had their infants transferred to the neonatal intensive care unit.[220]

Case Study

A 35-year-old female presents to the clinic, **wanting to fall pregnant**. She was diagnosed with **polycystic ovarian disease** 5 months ago, and unintentionally became pregnant 1 week later. She **miscarried** this pregnancy at 5 weeks. She and her partner have since been actively trying to conceive for 2–3 months. Her **BMI is 28.4**, and her **umbilical:hip ratio is 0.8**. Her **menstrual cycle is irregular**, and can vary between 26 and 47 day cycles. She also experiences **breast tenderness** and **depression premenstrually**. Her **libido has been diminished** and she has not menstruated since the miscarriage. She is feeling quite anxious about concieving and is waking 4–5 times per night.

SUGGESTIVE SYMPTOMS

- PCOD
- Elevated BMI
- Elevated umbilical:hip ratio
- Premenstrual symptoms

- Irregular menstrual cycle
- History of miscarriage
- Anxiety about fertility

Example treatment

The initial treatment for this case focused on supporting her nervous system and reproductive hormones, while further exploring her glucose tolerance. Due to the effects of physiological responses to stress on the reproductive hormones, anxiolytic, sedative and antidepressant herbs, such as *Matricaria recutita*, ***Hypericum perforatum***, *Melissa officinalis* and *Verbena officinalis* were included in the formula.[200] *Asparagus racemosus* was also included as a general nervine tonic, and for its capacity to support libido and conception.[221] The nervous system was also supported by the use of an individualised flower essence formula. (*Note:* Although popular in pregnancy and preconception, energetic medicines often require further evidentiary support.) The effect of her polycystic ovarian disease on potential fertility and capacity to carry to term was also acknowledged. She had already begun to modify her diet following the diagnosis 5 months ago, and reduced her dietary carbohydrate intake, with a focus on low glycaemic load carbohydrates, prior to her first appointment. It was recommended that, to support these changes, she resume regular exercise and aim for 20–30 minutes, three or four times per week. She had also begun weekly acupuncture treatment following the miscarriage, and was encouraged to continue. Prior to more aggressive treatment of her insulin sensitivity, a glucose-insulin tolerance test (GITT) was ordered. It was also recommended for her partner to join her for the next consultation.

Expected outcomes and follow-up treatments

Following this treatment, the next intended step would focus on more specific treatment of glucose metabolism, depending on the outcomes of the GITT. Depending upon the regularity of her menstrual cycle, *Vitex agnus-castus* would also be incorporated into her treatment plan. In this case, upon her return consultation, she was already 4.5 weeks pregnant. With this in mind, her liquid herbal formula was replaced with infusions of *Matricaria recutita* three times daily, and she was counselled to focus on maintaining a positive mindset.

Herbal formula	
Matricaria recutita 1:2	20 mL
Hypericum perforatum 1:2	15 mL
Melissa officinalis 1:2	15 mL
Verbena officinalis 1:2	20 mL
Asparagus racemosus 1:2	30 mL
Dosage: 10 mL twice daily	100 mL

Nutritional prescription

Pregnancy multivitamin
Dosage: 1 tablet daily

Flower essences

Dog rose of the wild forces, fringed violet, peach-flower tea tree, red Suva frangipani, she oak, Sturt desert pea, sunshine wattle

Lifestyle prescription

Exercise for 20–30 minutes 3–4 times per week
Glucose tolerance test via glucose-insulin tolerance test

The journey to conception for couples having difficulty can be quite tumultuous and unpredictable. It is important to have a plan in mind and encourage couples to allow sufficient time for good foundations to be laid before conceiving. However, this also needs to be tempered with the often-present impatience expressed by couples who have 'tried everything' prior to their first naturopathic consultation. Furthermore, naturopaths also need to be flexible with their treatment plan and be prepared to cancel intended treatment protocols and compromise certain stages in preconception care if this does not fit in with the timeline of the couple, or alternatively if the couple unexpectedly fall pregnant outside of the intended plan. Either way, it is important that the naturopath value and appreciate the powerful role counselling and dietary and lifestyle changes can have on conception and pregnancy outcomes, rather than placing all of their focus on supplements and other such interventions.

KEY POINTS

- Mothers should be reassured that pregnancy is a normal part of life and normal activities should be continued.
- Infertility or subfertility is rarely just a female issue. A coordinated approach involving both partners is necessary.
- There is no 'one-size-fits all' approach to preconception or pregnancy care, and an individualised approach is required.
- The treatment goal is the restoration of good health as often as it is treating infertility—in most cases a healthy body is a fertile body.
- Pregnancy is not a disease condition to be treated, but rather a natural process that needs to be supported.

Further reading

Atrash H, et al. Preconception care: a 2008 update. Curr Opin Obstet Gynecol 2008;20(6):581–589.

Derbyshire E. Dietary factors and fertility in women of childbearing age. Nutr Food Sci 2007;37(2): 100–104.

Gleicher N, Barad D. Unexplained infertility: does it really exist? Hum Reprod 2006;21(8):1951–1955.

Oats J, Abraham S. Fundamentals of obstetrics and gynaecology. Philadelphia: Elsevier Mosby, 2005.

Pairman S, et al., eds. Midwifery: preparation for practice. Sydney: Elsevier Churchill Livingstone, 2006.

References

1. Johnson K, et al. Recommendations to improve preconception health and health care—United States. A report of the CDC/ATSDR Preconception Care Work Group and the Select Panel on Preconception Care. MMWR Recomm Rep 2006;55:1–23.
2. Atrash HK, et al. Preconception care for improving perinatal outcomes: the time to act. Matern Child Health J 2006;10 Suppl 1:S3–S11.
3. Gnoth C, et al. Time to pregnancy: results of the German prospective study and impact on the management of infertility. Hum Reprod 2003;18:1959–1966.
4. Speroff L, Fritz M. Clinical gynecologic endocrinology and infertility. 7th edn. Philadelphia: Lippincott Williams & Wilkins, 2005.
5. Gnoth C, et al. Definition and prevalence of subfertility and infertility. Hum Reprod 2005;20:1144–1147.
6. Oats J, Abraham S. Fundamentals of obstetrics and gynaecology. Philadelphia: Elsevier Mosby, 2005.
7. Practice Committee of American Society for Reproductive Medicine. Smoking and infertility. Fertil Steril 2008;90 (5 Suppl):S254–S259.
8. Curtis K, et al. Effects of cigarette smoking, caffeine consumption and alcohol intake on fecundability. Am J Epidemiol 1997;146(1):32–41.
9. Hull M, et al. Delayed conception and active and passive smoking. Fertil Steril 2000;74(4):725–733.
10. Hassan M, Killick S. Negative lifestyle is associated with a significant reduction in fecundity. Fertil Steril 2004;81(2):384–392.
11. Homan G, et al. The impact of lifestyle factors on reproductive performance in the general population and those undergoing infertility treatment: a review. Hum Reprod Update 2007;13(3):209–233.
12. Agarwal A, et al. Reactive oxygen species as an independent marker of male factor infertility. Fertil Steril 2006;86(4):878–885.
13. Shiloh H, et al. The impact of cigarette smoking on zona pellucida thickness of oocytes and embryos prior to transfer into the uterine cavity. Hum Reprod 2004;19(1):157–159.
14. Martin J, et al. Births: final data for 2002. Natl Vital Stat Rep 2003;52:1–113.
15. Silva P, et al. Impact of lifestyle choices on female infertility. J Reprod Med 1999;44(3):288–296.
16. Chavarro JE, et al. Dietary fatty acid intakes and the risk of ovulatory infertility. Am J Clin Nutr 2007;85(1):231–237.
17. Chavarro JE, et al. Iron intake and risk of ovulatory infertility. Obstet Gynecol 2006;108:1145–1152.
18. Physicians F. Iron supplements may reduce risk for ovulatory infertility CME/CE. Obstet Gynecol 2006;108:1145–1152.
19. Ruder EH, et al. Oxidative stress and antioxidants: exposure and impact on female fertility. Hum Reprod Update 2008;14(4):345–357.
20. Verit FF, et al. Association of increased total antioxidant capacity and anovulation in nonobese infertile patients with clomiphene citrate–resistant polycystic ovary syndrome. Fertil Steril 2007;88(2):418–424.
21. Boitani C, Puglisi R. Selenium, a key element in spermatogenesis and male fertility. Molecular Mechanisms in Spermatogenesis 2008:65.
22. Yuyan L, et al. Are serum zinc and copper levels related to semen quality? Fertil Steril 2008;89(4):1008–1011.
23. Chavarro JE, et al. Protein intake and ovulatory infertility. Am J Obstet Gynecol 2008;198(2):210.
24. Chavarro JE, et al. A prospective study of dietary carbohydrate quantity and quality in relation to risk of ovulatory infertility. Human Reproduction 2007;22(5):1340–1347.
25. Hjolland N, et al. Distress and reduced fertility: a follow up study of first-pregnancy planners. Fertil Steril 1999;72(2):47–53.
26. Zorn B, et al. Psychological factors in male partners of infertile couples: relationship with semen quality and early miscarriage. J Andrology 2007;31(6):557–564.
27. Fitzgerald C, et al. Aging and reproductive potential in women. Yale J Biol Med 1998;71:367–381.
28. Ray J, et al. Preconception care and the risk of congenital anomalies in the offspring of women with diabetes mellitus: a meta-analysis. QJM 2001;94:435–444.
29. Eliakim R, Sherer DM. Celiac disease: fertility and pregnancy. Gynecol Obstet Invest 2001;51:3–7.
30. Sallmen M, et al. Reduced fertility among overweight and obese men. Epidemiology 2006;17(5):520–523.
31. Zain MM, Norman RJ. Impact of obesity on female fertility and fertility treatment. Women's Health 2008;4(2):183–194.
32. Diemer T, et al. Urogenital infection and sperm motility. Andrologia 2003;35(5):283–287.
33. Mahadevan U. Fertility and pregnancy in the patient with inflammatory bowel disease. Br Med J 2006;55(8):1198.
34. Poppe K, et al. Thyroid disease and female reproduction. Clin Endocrinol 2007;66(3):309–321.
35. Jonasson JM, et al. Fertility in women with type 1 diabetes. Diabetes Care 2007;30(9):2271–2276.
36. Kim HO, et al. Are IVF/ICSI outcomes of women with minimal to mild endometriosis associated infertility comparable to those with unexplained infertility? Fertil Steril 2007;88:215.
37. Franks S. Polycystic ovary syndrome. N Engl J Med 1995;333(13):853–861.
38. Ward N. Preconceptual care questionnaire research project. J Nutr Environ Med 1995;5:205–208.
39. Gerhard I, et al. Mastodynon(R) bei weiblicher Sterilität. Forsch Komplementarmed 1998;5(6):272–278.
40. Bubenzer R. Therapy with agnus castus extract (Strotan®). Therapiewoche 1993;43:32–33.
41. Bergmann J, et al. The efficacy of the complex medication Phyto-Hypophyson L in female, hormone-related sterility: a randomized, placebo-controlled clinical double-blind study. Forsch Komplementarmed Klass Naturheilkd 2000;7:190–199.
42. Tabakova P, et al. Clinical study of Tribestan® in females with endocrine sterility. Sofia: Bulgarian Pharmaclogy Group, 2000.
43. Wilcox A, et al. Timing of sexual intercourse in relation to ovulation-effects on the probability of conception, survival of the pregnancy, and sex of the baby. N Engl J Med 1995;333:1517–1521.

44. Brosens I, et al. Managing infertility with fertility-awareness methods. Sex Reprod Menopause 2006;4(1):13–16.

45. Scarpa B, et al. Cervical mucus secretions on the day of intercourse: an accurate marker of highly fertile days. Eur J Obstet Gynaecol Reprod Biol 2006;125:72–78.

46. Stanford J, et al. Timing intercourse to achieve pregnancy: current evidence. Obstet Gynecol 2002;100:1333–1341.

47. Stanford J, et al. Vulvar mucus observations and the probability of pregnancy. Obstet Gynecol 2003;101:1285–1293.

48. Bigelow J, et al. Mucus observations in the fertile window: a better predictor of conception than timing of intercourse. Hum Reprod 2004;19:889–892.

49. Stanford J, Dunson D. Effects of sexual intercourse patterns in time to pregnancy studies. Am J Epidemiol 2007;165:1088–1095.

50. Kutteh W, et al. Vaginal lubricants for the infertile couple: effect on sperm activity. Int J Fertil Menopausal Stud 1996;41:400–404.

51. Chavarro J, et al. Protein intake and ovulatory infertility. Am J Obstet Gynecol 2008;198(2):210.

52. Chavarro J, et al. Dietary fatty acid intakes and the risk of ovulatory infertility. Am J Clin Nutr 2007;85:231–237.

53. Rich-Edwards J, et al. Physical activity, body mass index, and ovulatory disorder infertility. Epidemiology 2002;13(2):184–190.

54. Nelson S, Fleming R. The preconceptual contraception paradigm: obesity and infertility. Hum Reprod 2007;22(4):912–915.

55. Pasquali R, et al. Obesity and reproductive disorders in women. Hum Reprod 2003;9(4):359–372.

56. Norman R, et al. Improving reproductive performance in overweight/obese women with effective weight management. Hum Reprod Update 2004;10(3):267–280.

57. Zain M, Norman R. Impact of obesity on female fertility and fertility treatment. Womens Health 2008;4(2):183–194.

58. Miller P, et al. Effect of short-term diet and exercise on hormone levels and menses in obese, infertile women. J Reprod Med 2008;53(5):315–319.

59. Karimzadeh M, Javedani M. An assessment of lifestyle modification versus medical treatment with clomiphene citrate, metformin, and clomiphene citrate-metformin in patients with polycystic ovary syndrome. Fertil Steril 2009:In press.

60. Wynn M, Wynn A. Slimming and fertility. Mod Midwife 1994;4:17–20.

61. Morris SN, et al. Effects of lifetime exercise on the outcome of in vitro fertilization. Obstet Gynecol 2006;108(4):938–946.

62. Arce JC, De Souza MJ. Exercise and male factor infertility. Sports med 1993;15(3):146–169.

63. Nelson SM, Fleming RF. The preconceptual contraception paradigm: obesity and infertility. Hum Reprod 2007;22(4):912–915.

64. Hill JW, et al. Hypothalamic pathways linking energy balance and reproduction. Am J Physiol Endocrinol Metab 2008;294(5):E827–E832.

65. Lannerö E, et al. Maternal smoking during pregnancy increases the risk of recurrent wheezing during the first years of life (BAMSE). Respir Res 2006;7(1):3.

66. Roza SJ, et al. Effects of maternal smoking in pregnancy on prenatal brain development. The Generation R Study. Eur J Neurosci 2007;25(3):611–617.

67. Hunt KJ, et al. Impact of parental smoking on diabetes, hypertension and the metabolic syndrome in adult men and women in the San Antonio Heart Study. Diabetologia 2006;49(10):2291–2298.

68. Guerri C, et al. Foetal alcohol spectrum disorders and alterations in brain and behaviour. Alcohol Alcohol 2009;44(2):108–114.

69. Weinberg J, et al. Prenatal alcohol exposure: foetal programming, the hypothalamic-pituitary-adrenal axis and sex differences in outcome. J Neuroendocrinol 2008;20(4):470–488.

70. Murtagh J. General practice. Sydney: McGraw-Hill, 2007.

71. Craig S. A medical model for infertility counselling. Aust Fam Physician 1990;19:491–500.

72. Burns L. Psychiatric aspects of infertility and infertility treatments. Psychiatr Clin North Am 2007;30(4):689–716.

73. Champagne D. Should fertilization treatment start with reducing stress? Hum Reprod 2006;21(7):1651–1658.

74. Damti OB, et al. Stress and distress in infertility among women. Harefuah 2008;147(3):256–260.

75. Cousineau TM, Domar AD. Psychological impact of infertility. Baillière's best practice and research. Clin obstet gynaecol 2007;21(2):293–308.

76. Domar A, et al. Impact of group psychological interventions on pregnancy rates in infertile women. Fertil Steril 2000;73(4):805–811.

77. Chang M, et al. Effects of music therapy on psychological health of women during pregnancy. J Clin Nurs 2008;17(19):2580–2587.

78. Kotz D. Success at last. Couples fighting infertility might have more control than they think. US News World Rep 2007;142(16):62–64.

79. Greenlee A, et al. Risk factors for female infertility in an agricultural region. Epidemiology 2003;14(4):429–436.

80. Hruska K, et al. Environmental factors in infertility. Clin Obstet Gynecol 2000;43(4):821–829.

81. Gold E, et al. Reproductive hazards. Occup Med 1994;9(3):363–372.

82. Claman P. Men at risk: occupation and male infertility. Sexuality, Reproduction and Menopause 2004;2(1):19–26.

83. Simon C, et al. Cytokines and embryo implantation. Reprod Immunol 1998;39:117–131.

84. Weiss G, et al. Inflammation in reproductive disorders. Reprod Sci 2009;16(2):216–219.

85. Weiss G, et al. Inflammation in reproductive disorders. Reprod Sci 2009;16(2):216.

86. Tuohy V, Altuntas C. Autoimmunity and premature ovarian failure. Curr Opin Obstet Gynecol 2007;19(4):366–369.

87. Altuntas C, et al. Autoimmune targeted disruption of the pituitary-ovarian axis causes premature ovarian failure. J Immunol 2006;177(3):1988–1996.

88. Johnston Jnr, RB. Folic acid: preventive nutrition for preconception, the fetus, and the newborn. Neo Rev 2009;10(1):e10.

89. Cikot R, et al. Longitudinal vitamin and homocysteine levels in normal pregnancy. Br J Nutr 2007;85(01):49–58.

90. Ray JG, et al. Vitamin B12 and the risk of neural tube defects in a folic-acid-fortified population. Epidemiology 2007;18(3):362–366.

91. Ray JG, et al. High rate of maternal vitamin B12 deficiency nearly a decade after Canadian folic acid flour fortification. QJM 2008;101(6):475–477.

92. Westphal LM, et al. A nutritional supplement for improving fertility in women: a pilot study. J Reprod Med 2004;49(4):289–293.

93. Czeizel A, et al. The effect of preconceptional multivitamin supplementation on fertility. Int J Vitam Nutr Res 1996;66(1):55–58.

94. Czeizel A, et al. The higher rate of multiple births after periconceptional multivitamin supplementation: an analysis of causes. Acta Genet Med Gemellol 1994;43(3–4):175–184.

95. Chavarro J, et al. Use of multivitamins, intake of B vitamins and risk of ovulatory infertility. Fertil Steril 2008;89(3):668–676.

96. Henmi H, et al. Effects of ascorbic acid supplementation on serum progesterone levels in patients with luteal phase defect. Fertil Steril 2003;80:459–461.

97. Karovic O, et al. Toxic effects of cobalt in primary cultures of mouse astrocytes: similarities with hypoxia and role of HIF-1alpha. Biochem Pharmacol 2007;73(5):694–708.
98. Kohlmeier M. Nutrient metabolism. San Diego: Academic Press, 2003.
99. Carmel R. Folic acid. In: Shils ME, et al., eds. Modern nutrition in health and disease. Philadelphia: Lippincott Williams & Wilkins, 2006:470–481.
100. Carmel R. Cobalamin (vitamin B12). In: Shils ME, et al., eds. Modern nutrition in health and disease. Philadelphia: Lippincott Williams & Wilkins, 2006:482–497.
101. Thonneau P, et al. Incidence and main causes of infertility in a resident population (1,850,000) of three French regions (1988–1989). Hum Reprod 1991;6(6):811–816.
102. Ford W, et al. Increasing paternal age is associated with delayed conception in a large population of fertile couples: evidence for declining fecundity in older men. The ALSPAC study team (Avon Longitudinal Study of Pregnancy and Childhood). Hum Reprod 2000;15:1703–1708.
103. Jorgensen N, et al. Regional differences in semen quality in Europe. Hum Reprod 2001;16:1012–1019.
104. Oliva A, et al. Contribution of environmental factors to the risk of male infertility. Hum Reprod 2001;16(8):1768–1776.
105. Kumar S. Occupational exposure associated with reproductive dysfunction. J Occupational Health 2004;46(1):1–19.
106. Swan S, et al. Semen quality in relation to biomarkers of pesticide exposure. Environ Health Perspect 2003;111(12):1478–1484.
107. Abell A, et al. High sperm density among members of organic farmers' association. Lancet 1994;343:1498.
108. Wang C, et al. Effect of increased scrotal temperature on sperm production in normal men. Fertil Steril 1997;68(2):334–339.
109. Mendiola J, et al. Food intake and its relationship with semen quality: a case-control study. Fertil Steril 2009;91(3):812–818.
110. Chavarro J, et al. Soy food and isoflavone intake in relation to semen quality parameters among men from an infertility clinic. Hum Reprod 2008;23(11):2584–2590.
111. Eskanzi B, et al. Antioxidant intake is associated with semen quality in healthy men. Hum Reprod 2005;20(4):1006–1012.
112. Lewin A, Lavon H. The effect of coenzyme Q10 on sperm motility and function. Mol Aspects Med 1997;18(Suppl):S213–S219.
113. Balercia G, et al. Coenzyme Q(10) supplementation in infertile men with idiopathic asthenozoospermia: an open, uncontrolled pilot study. Fertil Steril 2004;81(1):93–98.
114. Tremellen K, et al. A randomised control trial examining the effect of an antioxidant (Menevit) on pregnancy outcome during IVF-ICSI treatment [see comment]. Aust N Z J Obstet Gynaecol 2007;47(3):216–221.
115. Safarinejad M, Safarinejad S. Efficacy of selenium and/or N-acetyl-cysteine for improving semen parameters in infertile men: a double-blind, placebo controlled, randomized study. J Urol 2009;181(2):741–751.
116. Scott R, et al. The effect of oral selenium supplementation on human sperm motility. Br J Urol 1998;82(1):76–80.
117. Vézina D, et al. Selenium-vitamin E supplementation in infertile men. Effects on semen parameters and micronutrient levels and distribution. Biol Trace Elem Res 1996;53(1–3):65–83.
118. Hawkes W, et al. Selenium supplementation does not affect testicular selenium status or semen quality in North American men. J Androl 2009;30(5):525–533.
119. Iwanier K, Zachara B. Selenium supplementation enhances the element concentration in blood and seminal fluid but does not change the spermatozoal quality characteristics in subfertile men. J Androl 1995;16(5):441–447.
120. Lenzi A, et al. Use of carnitine therapy in selected cases of male factor infertility: a double-blind crossover trial. Fertil Steril 2003;79(2):292–300.
121. Costa M, et al. L-carnitine in idiopathic asthenozoospermia: a multicenter study. Italian Study Group on Carnitine and Male Infertility. Andrologia 1994;26(3):155–159.
122. Vitali G, et al. Carnitine supplementation in human idiopathic asthenospermia: clinical results. Drugs Exp Clin Res 1995;21(4):157–159.
123. Cavallini G, et al. Cinnoxicam and L-carnitine/acetyl-L-carnitine treatment for idiopathic and varicocele-associated oligoasthenospermia. J Androl 2004;25(5):761–770.
124. Garolla A, et al. Oral carnitine supplementation increases sperm motility in asthenozoospermic men with normal sperm phospholipid hydroperoxide glutathione peroxidase levels. Fertil Steril 2005;83(2):355–361.
125. Hansen M, et al. Assisted reproductive technologies and the risk of birth defects—a systematic review. Hum Reprod 2005;20(2):328–338.
126. Chambers GM, et al. Assisted reproductive technology treatment costs of a live birth: an age-stratified cost-outcome study of treatment in Australia. Med J Aust 2006;184(4):155–158.
127. Verhaak CM, et al. Women's emotional adjustment to IVF: a systematic review of 25 years of research. Hum Reprod update 2007;13(1):27–36.
128. Rajkhowa M, et al. Reasons for discontinuation of IVF treatment: a questionnaire study. Hum Reprod 2006;21(2):358–363.
129. Stankiewicz M, et al. The use of complementary medicine and therapies by patients attending a reproductive medicine unit in South Australia: a prospective survey. Aust N Z J Obstet Gynaecol 2007;47(2):145–149.
130. Cheong Y, et al. Acupuncture and assisted conception. Cochrane Database Syst Rev 2008;8(4):CD006920.
131. Battaglia C, et al. Adjuvant L-arginine treatment for in-vitro fertilization in poor responder patients. Hum Reprod 1999;14(7):1690–1697.
132. Food and Nutrition Board. Institute of Medicine. Dietary reference intakes for energy, carbohydrate, fiber, fat, fatty acids, cholesterol, protein and amino acids (macronutrients). Washington, DC: National Academy Press, 2002.
133. Moore MC. Nutritional assessment and care. Missouri: Elsevier Mosby, 2005.
134. Miles L, Foxen R. New guidelines on caffeine in pregnancy. Nutrition Bulletin 2009;34(2):203.
135. Turner RE. Nutrition during pregnancy. In: Shils ME, et al., eds. Modern nutrition in health and disease. Philadelphia: Lippincott Williams & Wilkins, 2006:771–783.
136. Food and Nutrition Board. Institute of medicine. Dietary reference intakes for vitamin A, vitamin K, arsenic, boron, chromium, copper, iodine, iron, manganese, molybdenum, nickel, silicon, vanadium, and zinc. Washington, DC: National Academy Press, 2001.
137. Casanueva E, et al. Weekly iron as a safe alternative to daily supplementation for nonanemic pregnant women. Arch Med Res 2006;37(5):674–682.
138. Holst L, et al. The use and the user of herbal remedies during pregnancy. J Altern Complement Med 2009;15(7):1–6.
139. Adams J, et al. Women's use of complementary and alternative medicine during pregnancy: a critical review of the literature. Birth 2009;36(3):237–245.
140. Adams J, et al. Complementary and alternative medicine and pregnancy: the attitudes and referral practices of obstetricians and other maternity care providers. Int J Gynecol Obstet 2009:In press.
141. Bone K. Safety considerations during pregnancy and lactation. In: Mills S, Bone K, eds. The essential guide to herbal safety. St Louis: Churchill Livingstone, 2005.
142. Scientific Committee of the British Herbal Medical Association. British herbal pharmacopoeia. 1st edn Bournemouth: British Herbal Medicine Association, 1983.

143. Blumenthal M, et al. In: Herbal medicine, ed. expanded commission E monographs (English translation). Austin: Integrative Medicine Communications, 2000.
144. European Scientific Cooperative on Phytotherapy. ESCOP Monographs. Stuttgart: Thieme, 2003.
145. McFarlin B, et al. A national survey of herbal preparation use by nurse-midwives for labor stimulation: review of the literature and recommendations for practice. J Nurse-Midwifery 1999;44(3):205–216.
146. Bamford D, et al. Raspberry leaf tea: a new aspect to an old problem. Br J Pharmacol 1970;40(1):161–162.
147. Simpson M, et al. Raspberry leaf in pregnancy: its safety and efficacy in labor. J Midwifery Womens Health 2001;46(2):51–59.
148. Parsons M, et al. Raspberry leaf and its effect on labour: safety and efficacy. J Aust Coll Midwives 1999;12(3):20–25.
149. Parsons M, et al. Raspberry leaf and its effect on labour: safety and efficacy. Aust Coll Midwives Inc J 1999;12(3):20–25.
150. Holst L, et al. Raspberry leaf—should it be recommended to pregnant women? Complement Ther Clin Prac 2009:In press.
151. Felter HW, Lloyd JU. King's American Dispensary. 18th edn Portland: Eclectic Medical Publications, 1905, reprinted 1983.
152. Chadwick CM. Embolus of the basilar artery. Br Med J 1886;1(1313):391.
153. Wilson JH. *Viburnum prunifolium*, or black haw, in abortion and miscarriage. Br Med J 1886;1(1318):640.
154. Napier ADL. *Viburnum prunifolium* in abortion. Br Med J 1886;1(1315):489.
155. Campbell WMF. Note on *Viburnum prunifolium* in abortion. Br Med J 1886;1(1313):391.
156. Bone K. A clinical guide to blending liquid herbs. Missouri: Churchill Livingstone, 2003.
157. Veleva Z, et al. High and low BMI increase the risk of miscarriage after IVF/ICSI and FET. Hum Reprod 2008;23(4):878–884.
158. Barclay L. Bariatric surgery before pregnancy may improve pregnancy outcomes in obese women CME. JAMA 2008;300:2286–2296.
159. Gadsby R, et al. A prospective study of nausea and vomiting during pregnancy. Br J Gen Pract 1993;43:245.
160. Gadsby P. Some functions of prostaglandin e2 in early pregnancy. Some reasons why prostaglandin e2 can be associated with nausea and vomiting in pregnancy 2000;50:4.
161. Jewell D, Young G. Interventions for nausea and vomiting in early pregnancy. Cochrane Database Syst Rev 2003;(4):CD000145.
162. Borrelli F, et al. Effectiveness and safety of ginger in the treatment of pregnancy-induced nausea and vomiting. Obstet Gynecol 2005;105:849–856.
163. Ozgoli G, et al. Effects of ginger capsules on pregnancy, nausea, and vomiting. J Altern Complement Med 2009;15(3):243–246.
164. Pongrojpaw D, et al. A randomized comparison of ginger and dimenhydrinate in the treatment of nausea and vomiting in pregnancy. J Med Assoc Thai 2007;90(9):1703–1709.
165. Danish Veterinary and Food Administration. [The Danish veterinary and food administration warn against food supplements containing ginger for pregnant women] [in Danish], 2008.
166. Chaiyakunapruk N, et al. The efficacy of ginger for the prevention of postoperative nausea and vomiting: a meta-analysis. Am J Obstet Gynecol 2006;194:95–99.
167. Sahakian V, et al. Vitamin B6 is effective therapy for nausea and vomiting of pregnancy: a randomized, double-blind placebo-controlled study. Obstet Gynecol 1991;78(1):33–36.
168. Schuster K, et al. Morning sickness and vitamin B6 status of pregnant women. Hum Nutr Clin Nutr 1985;39(1):75–79.
169. Vutyavanich T, et al. Pyridoxine for nausea and vomiting of pregnancy: a randomized, double-blind, placebo-controlled trial. Am J Obstet Gyneco 1995;173(3):881–884.
170. Wolf M, et al. Obesity and preeclampsia: the potential role of inflammation. Obstet Gynecol 2001;98:757–762.
171. Wergeland E, Strand K. Work place control and pregnancy health in a population-based sample of employed women in Norway. Scand J Work Environ Health 1998;24:206–212.
172. Weissgerber T, et al. The role of regular physical activity in preeclampsia prevention. Med Sci Sports Exerc 2003;36(12):2024–2031.
173. Roberts J, et al. Nutrient involvement in pre-eclampsia. J Nutr 2003;133 Supp:S1684–S1692.
174. Dugoua J, et al. Safety and efficacy of cranberry (vaccinium macrocarpon) during pregnancy and lactation. Can J Clin Pharmacol 2008;15(1):80–86.
175. Jepson R, et al. Cranberries for preventing urinary tract infections. Cochrane Database Syst Rev 2004(1):CD001321.
176. Barrons R, Tassone D. Use of *Lactobacillus* probiotics for bacterial genitourinary infections in women: a review. Clin Ther 2008;30(3):453–468.
177. Thorpe J, Anderson J. Supporting women in labour and birth. In: Pairman S, et al., eds. Midwifery: preparation for practice. Sydney: Elsevier Churchill Livingstone, 2006:393–415.
178. Saisto T, et al. Therapeutic group psychoeducation and relaxation in treating fear of childbirth. Acta Obstet Gynecol Scand 2006;85(11):1315–1319.
179. Janssen PA, et al. Outcomes of planned hospital birth attended by midwives compared with physicians in British Columbia. Obstet Gynecol Surv 2007;62(11):701.
180. Tan WM, et al. How do physicians and midwives manage the third stage of labor? Birth 2008;35(3):220–229.
181. Morano S, et al. Outcomes of the first midwife-led birth centre in Italy: 5 years' experience. Arch Gynecol Obstet 2007;276(4):333–337.
182. Johnson KC, Daviss BA. Outcomes of planned home births with certified professional midwives: large prospective study in North America. BMJ 2005;330(7505):1416.
183. Mottl-Santiago J, et al. A hospital-based doula program and childbirth outcomes in an urban, multicultural setting. Matern Child Health J 2008;12(3):372–377.
184. Campbell DA, et al. A randomized control trial of continuous support in labor by a lay doula. J Obstet Gynecol Neonatal Nurs 2006;35(4):456–464.
185. Nommsen-Rivers LA, et al. Doula care improves birth and breastfeeding outcomes for low-income, primiparous mothers. J Obstet Gynecol Neonatal Nurs 2009;38(2):157–173.
186. Moses MC, Potter RH. Use of doulas for inmates in labor: continuous supportive care with positive outcomes. Corrections Today 2008;70(3):4.
187. Thorogood C, Donaldson C. Disturbances in the rhythm of labour. In: Pairman S, et al., eds. Midwifery: preparation for practice. Sydney: Elsevier Churchill Livingstone, 2006:679–716.
188. Liston FA, et al. Neonatal outcomes with caesarean delivery at term. Arch Dis Child Fetal Neonatal Ed 2008;93(3):F176.
189. Pistiner M, et al. Birth by cesarean section, allergic rhinitis, and allergic sensitization among children with a parental history of atopy. J Allergy Clin Immunol 2008;122(2):274–279.
190. Thavagnanam S, et al. A meta-analysis of the association between caesarean section and childhood asthma. Clin Exp Allergy 2008;38(4):629–633.
191. Beebe KR, et al. The effects of childbirth self-efficacy and anxiety during pregnancy on prehospitalization labor. J Obstet Gynecol Neonatal Nurs 2007;36(5):410–418.

192. Lee MK, et al. Effects of SP6 acupressure on labor pain and length of delivery time in women during labor. J Altern Complement Med 2004;10(6):959–965.

193. Kistin SJ, Newman AD. Induction of labor with homeopathy: a case report. J Midwifery Women's Health 2007;52(3):303–307.

194. Oberbaum M, et al. The effect of the homeopathic remedies Arnica montana and Bellis perennis on mild postpartum bleeding—a randomized, double-blind, placebo-controlled study—preliminary results. Complement Ther Med 2005;13(2):87–90.

195. Davim RMB, et al. Effectiveness of non-pharmacological strategies in relieving labor pain. Rev Esc Enferm USP 2009;43:438–445.

196. Baddock S, Dixon L. Physiological changes in labour and the postnatal period. In: Pairman S, et al., eds. Midwifery: preparation for practice. Sydney: Elsevier Churchill Livingstone, 2006:375–392.

197. Henderson A, Scobbie M. Supporting the breastfeeding mother. In: Pairman S, et al., eds. Midwifery: preparation for practice. Sydney: Elsevier Churchill Livingstone, 2006:507–523.

198. Gartner L, et al. Breastfeeding and the use of human milk. Pediatrics 2005;115(2):496–506.

199. Abascal K, Yarnell E. Botanical galactagogues. Altern Complement Ther 2008;14(6):288–294.

200. Blumenthal M. British herbal pharmacopoeia. London: BHMA Publishing, 1996.

201. Gabay M. Galactogogues: medications that induce lactation. J Hum Lact 2002;18:274–279.

202. Sharma S, et al. Randomized controlled trial of Asparagus racemosus (shatavari) as a lactogue in lactational inadequacy. Indian Pediatr 1996;33(8):675–677.

203. Osborn D, Sinn J. Soy formula for prevention of allergy and food intolerance in infants. Cochrane Database Syst Rev 2004;(3):CD003741.

204. Allen L. Formulas and milks for infants and young children: making sense of it all. Mod Med 1999;42(6):24–30.

205. Taylor S, et al. Intestinal permeability in preterm infants by feeding type: mother's milk versus formula. Breastfeeding Med 2009;4(1):11–15.

206. Uruakpa FO, et al. Colostrum and its benefits: a review. Nutr Res 2002;22(6):755–767.

207. Hunter L, et al. A selective review of maternal sleep characteristics in the postpartum period. J Obstet Gynecol Neonatal Nurs 2009;38(1):60–68.

208. Ross L, et al. Sleep and perinatal mood disorders: a critical review. J Psychiatry Neurosci 2005;30(4):247–256.

209. Fletcher RJ, et al. Addressing depression and anxiety among new fathers. Med J Aust 2006;185(8):461–463.

210. Steiner M. Female-specific mood disorders. Clin Obstet Gynecol 1992;35(3):599–611.

211. Omu AE, et al. Indications of the mechanisms involved in improved sperm parameters by zinc therapy. Med Princ Pract 2008;17(2):108–116.

212. Safarinejad MR, Safarinejad S. Efficacy of selenium and/or N-acetyl-cysteine for improving semen parameters in infertile men: a double-blind, placebo controlled, randomized study. J Urol 2009;181(2):741–751.

213. Ee C, et al. Acupuncture for pelvic and back pain in pregnancy: a systematic review. Am J Obstet Gynecol 2008;198(3):254–259.

214. Ewies A, Olah K. Moxibustion in breech version—a descriptive review. Acupunct Med 2002;20(1):26–29.

215. Cardini F, et al. A randomised controlled trial of moxibustion for breech presentation. BJOG 2005;112(6):743–747.

216. Spinelli A, et al. Do antenatal classes benefit the mother and her baby? J Matern-Fetal Neonatal Med 2003;13(2):94–101.

217. Fletcher R, et al. New fathers' postbirth views of antenatal classes: Satisfaction, benefits, and knowledge of family services. J Perinat Educ 2004;13(3):18–26.

218. Gerhar I, Wallis E. Individualized homeopathic therapy for male infertility. Homeopathy 2002;91:133–134.

219. Smith CA. Homoeopathy for induction of labour. Cochrane Database Syst Rev 2003;(4):CD003399.

220. Burns E, et al. Aromatherapy in childbirth: a pilot randomised controlled trial. BJOG 2007;114(7):838–844.

221. Thakur RS, et al. Major medicinal plants of India. Lucknow: Central Institute of Medicinal and Aromatic Plants 1989;361.

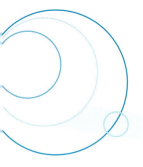

Ageing and cognition

Christina Kure
ND, BAppSci

OVERVIEW AND AETIOLOGY

Ageing is a multidimensional process comprising physical, psychological and social factors that vary and interact over the life span.[1,2] Normal ageing is characterised by organ and system changes that vary among individuals depending on the physical, emotional, psychological and social changes experienced during life.[3] These changes are influenced by such factors as genetics, physical and social environments, diet, health, stress and lifestyle choices. In the absence of disease the normal ageing process involves changes and impairment in systems of the body leading to structural and functional changes, some of which can be noticeable upon inspection of the older patient (refer to Figure 32.1). The focus of this chapter regards ageing in the latter stages of life, specifically in elderly people (65+ years). In the recent decades, individuals of this group in developed countries have experienced a dramatic increase in life expectancy, and a declining death rate, which has given rise to a vastly older population.

Over the past 20 years in Australia, life expectancy has improved by 6 years for males and 4.1 years for females; males and females born between 2005 and 2007 in Australia are expected to live 79 and 83.7 years, respectively.[4] In the year 2000, 10% of the global population was aged 60 years or older and this percentage is projected to reach 21% by 2050.[5] In 2007 13% of Australians were reported to be over the age of 65 years.[4] An increasingly older population leads to an increase in the number of individuals suffering from debilitating age-related diseases, including dementia, cardiovascular disease and cancer. In 2005, the global population suffering dementia was estimated at 24.3 million people, and there are around 4.6 million new cases diagnosed every year.[7] Furthermore, it is predicted that this population will double every 20 years with an alarming number of 81.1 million dementia patients in 2040.

A chief consequence of an ageing population is an increased burden on public health systems, as the elderly have higher rates of hospitalisation, surgery and visits to their physician than any other age group;[3] this has led to spiralling health-care costs. For example, health-care costs in the United States of America totalled around $3.6 billion in 1992,

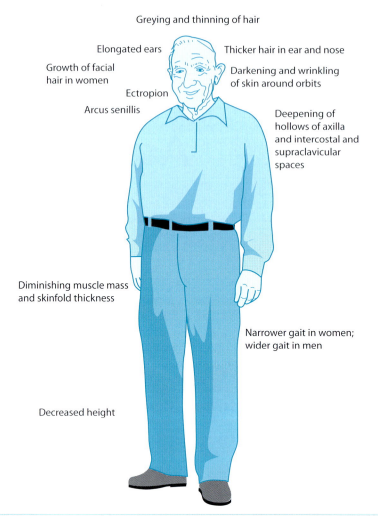

Greying and thinning of hair

Elongated ears

Thicker hair in ear and nose

Growth of facial
hair in women

Darkening and wrinkling
of skin around orbits

Ectropion

Arcus senillis

Deepening of
hollows of axilla
and intercostal and
supraclavicular
spaces

Diminishing muscle mass
and skinfold thickness

Narrower gait in women;
wider gait in men

Decreased height

Figure 32.1
Source: Eliopoulos 2005[3]

$12.7 billion in 1995, $1.4 trillion in 2001 and $1.9 trillion in 2004.[8] It is anticipated that these figures will increase to $2.8 trillion by 2011.[9] The holistic and preventive approach that is inherent in naturopathic practices suggest a clear role for these disciplines in the promotion of healthy ageing, and assisting in meeting the population and individual health challenges of the future. A comprehensive naturopathic system review will provide a detailed account of systems that are most affected during the ageing process for each individual. Furthermore, given that the pattern of ageing is unique to each individual,[3] naturopathic treatment needs to be tailored according to individual health and wellbeing needs.

Figure 32.2 indicates common diseases and illnesses seen in the elderly patient, such as cardiovascular disease, arthritis, diabetes, infections, cancer and gastrointestinal disturbances. (Refer to the respective chapters in this book for details on how to address these conditions holistically.)

Due to a number of changes in body composition, gastrointestinal function and sensory function, older people are prone to dysfunction in the digestive system and as a result are at risk of malnutrition.[10] In particular a poor production of digestive enzymes

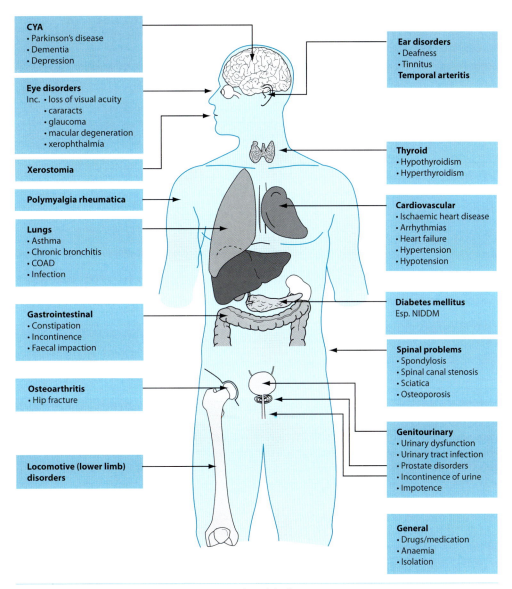

Figure 32.2 Common conditions seen in the elderly
Source: Murtagh J. General practice. 4th edn. Sydney: McGraw-Hill Australia, 2006.

may lead to inadequate digestion and assimilation of micronutrients to vital tissues and organs of the body, resulting in adverse consequences such as poor health, poor immunity and disability.[10] It is therefore vital to improve digestive functions and address resulting nutritional deficiencies (refer to the section on the digestive system). Other conditions commonly seen in the older population include osteoporosis, incontinence, visual and hearing difficulties, sleep disorders and depression (refer to Table 32.1).

Less salient ailments in the elderly population

While some conditions, such as those of the cardiovascular and neural systems, are commonly linked to the elderly other less salient conditions often mitigated by life changes can also affect their quality of life. Examples are leaving the workforce and entering the

Table 32.1 Common conditions seen in the elderly and naturopathic treatment approach, except cardio/cerebrovascular disease and cancer (see Section 3 on the cardiovascular system and Chapter 29 on cancer).

CONDITIONS COMMONLY SEEN IN THE ELDERLY	NATUROPATHIC TREATMENT APPROACH
Osteoporosis	Calcium and vitamin D are important for improving bone mass and preventing bone fractures and falls. RDAs For people aged 65+ years are:[11] • calcium 700–800 mg • vitamin D 400–800 IU. Increase dairy products (milk, yoghurts and cheese) and fish (sardines with bones).
Poor digestion[12]	This is the result of a decline in bifidobacteria and lactic-acid producing (LAB) bacteria in the gut, leading to microbial infections. Supplement with probiotics (bifidobacteria or lactobacilli) and address nutritional deficiencies. Use herbal medicines with bitter or aromatic properties.[13]
Urinary incontinence[14]	Seen in approximately 11.6% of 65+ year-olds living in the community. • Encourage adequate hydration. • Avoid caffeine and alcohol. • Address nutritional deficiencies, especially Mg, Zn and B12.
Sleep disorders	Effective treatments:[15] • melatonin (not available over the counter in Australia) for circadian disorders affecting sleep • valerian, tai chi, acupuncture, acupressure, yoga and meditation.

retirement years, widowhood and grandparenting, but other more gradual changes, such as becoming more dependent on family and social services in addition to requiring more acute care, have a substantial influence on the lives of the elderly. A recent review showed that loneliness is widespread amongst the elderly, and is linked to depression, high blood pressure, poor sleep, immune stress response and a decline in cognition.[16] Although sleep disturbances are not part of the normal ageing process, sleep becomes lighter with age and insomnia is prevalent in the older population with more than 49% of those aged 65 years and over experiencing sleep disturbances.[17] Inadequate sleep results in increased risk of falls, difficulties with concentration, impairments in memory and decrease in quality of life.[18] A large study ($n = 1506$) revealed that depression, heart disease, body pain and memory problems were associated with symptoms of insomnia in older adults, suggesting that sleep complaints are secondary to comorbidities in this population rather than due to ageing as such.[19] As a practitioner, it is therefore important to identify and understand the causes of sleep difficulties in the older patient (refer to Chapter 14 on insomnia).

Therapeutic considerations in the elderly

Age-related chronic diseases are often not successfully treated by conventional methods since these therapies often fail to provide long-term relief and have adverse side effects. Although the popularity of complementary and alternative medicine (CAM) use by the older population is unclear, the elderly (65 years or older) appear more likely than younger adults to discuss their CAM treatments with their doctors; clinical nutrition, chiropractic, massage therapy, meditation and herbal medicine were the most common forms of CAM used by the elderly.[6] Diagnosis of cognitive impairment in most countries must be made by a medical physician and be subsequently carefully monitored, and doctors need to be more active in initiating conversation about CAM use with their patients.

A medical history will help determine the timing of the disease onset, and assessment using the Minimental scales and measures of depression such as the geriatric depression scale[20] are valuable. Additionally, full blood cell count tests for thyroid, kidney and liver function, and serum level of vitamin B12 are recommended. A naturopathic treatment approach needs to consider the stage at which the elderly individual is, mentally and physically, in their ageing process. Each individual has been exposed to different factors in their lifetime that may either protect or increase the risk of developing cognitive decline and associated diseases. A detailed account of the presenting case and patient history will help determine an appropriate naturopathic treatment approach. The patient history will need to determine the likely risk factors that may have contributed to presenting cognitive complaints, and determine whether or not the presenting symptoms are due to normal or pathological ageing.

Wear and tear on the body over the years affects not only the brain and vascular system, but also other body parts. This may lead to knee replacements due to lack of cartilage, painful arthritic joints, loss of bone mass in the hips and lack of balance, leading to falls—and leading to reduced capacities overall.[21] Although not all elderly individuals are frail some operate slowly, walk slowly, experience difficulties hearing and may need time to stop and rest. It is therefore essential to consider these expected changes in the elderly person during the naturopathic consultations, and treat other chronic illnesses such as arthritis, diabetes or heart disease. It is also essential to support changes to systems of the body naturally seen in the elderly, such as improving gastrointestinal function (with bitters, protease/amylases/lipase and gut bacteria), supporting the cardiovascular system (with circulatory stimulants and cardiac tonics), regulating cholesterol levels, treating infections (with immune system stimulants), encouraging exercise to improve bone mass and muscle tone, supporting the genitourinary system (with urinary tonics) and seeking regular hearing and vision tests.

When the elderly suffer from various diseases and infections they are prone to using polypharmacy, so possible interactions with vitamins and herbs need to be well thought out prior to prescribing a naturopathic treatment regimen. Possible interactions with commonly used herbs, drugs and nutrients are outlined in drug–CAM interaction table in Appendix 1.

Keeping in mind that it is imperative to use a holistic approach to treating seniors whereby diseases and illness in each system of the body need to be addressed, this chapter focuses on age-associated cognitive decline with particular reference to the dementias of the vascular and Alzheimer's types.

Normal brain ageing

Cognition encompasses a broad range of brain processes, which are often taken for granted until they are lost, or at least decline in functional capacity, as is well documented in the ageing process. There is no universal definition to explain successful cognitive health in elderly individuals; however, the Critical Evaluation Study Committee defines cognitive health as 'the development and preservation of the multidimensional cognitive

HEAL THE HEALER

Due to the psychological (and in some cases physical) burden on the carer, practitioners should also consider treating the carer, especially in chronic situation of mental distress.

structure that allows the older adult to maintain social connectedness, an ongoing sense of purpose, and the abilities to function independently, to permit functional recovery from illness or injury, and to cope with residual functional deficits'.[22]

Cognitive functions such as learning, memory and attention can be affected by ageing, with some aspects of cognition being preserved while others decline.[23] Cognitive abilities can be classified as 'fluid' when they rely on short-term memory storage to process information, or 'crystallised' where knowledge and expertise accumulates and relies on long-term memory.[24] Fluid intelligence involves solving new problems, spatial manipulation, mental speed and identifying complex relations among stimulus patterns. Such fluid abilities are believed to peak in the mid 20s and then gradually decline until the age of 60 years, when the decline becomes more rapid.[24] In contrast, crystallised abilities increase during the life span through education, occupational and cultural experiences. Intellectual pursuits are thought to slow in late adulthood and may gradually decline from the age of 90 years (refer to Figure 32.3); they are affected by ageing and disease and often remain intact even in the early stages of dementia or after brain injury.[24]

Ageing significantly affects long-term memory for specific events (episodic memory), whereas some other aspects of long-term memory, such as procedural memory, are well maintained.[23] It is important for the naturopathic practitioner to detect signs of early cognitive decline in older patients and, using a combination of herbal, nutritional and lifestyle interventions together with appropriate referrals to other medical practitioners, prepare older patients for making decisions about their future care before they have lost the ability to do so.[25]

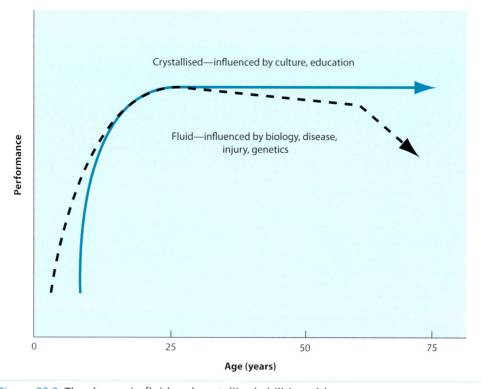

Figure 32.3 The change in fluid and crystallised abilities with age
Source: Anstey 2004[24]

Pathological cognitive decline

Individuals who experience cognitive decline are at a greater risk of developing dementia, and researchers suggest that early detection and intervention may be effective strategies to slow the progress of dementia.[22] Alzheimer's dementia (AD) is the most common of the subtypes of the dementias[26] characterised by the presence of amyloid-beta-protein (AβP) and intraneural deposition of neurofibrillary tangles in the brain; although this pathology is also seen in non-demented individuals, it is the distribution of these plaques in the brain that differentiates normal and abnormal brain changes.[27] Mild cognitive impairment (MCI) is a condition presenting with memory deficits that are below the defined norms and in the absence of other cognitive dysfunctions, and although it is thought to be a preclinical state of dementia[28] approximately half of MCI individuals go on to develop AD.[29] This again furnishes a role for naturopaths to work in conjunction with other medical professionals qualified to diagnose and monitor the progression of cognitive decline and provide a complementary treatment approach to prescribing holistic remedies proven to slow the progression of cognitive decline in these individuals.

Cerebrovascular conditions

Cerebrovascular disease (CVD) is defined as brain lesions caused by vascular disorders including cerebral infarction or acute cessation of blood flow to a localised area of the brain; brain haemorrhage caused by rupture in a vascular wall; and vascular dementia, caused by multiple small infarcts and subcortical Binswanger-like white-matter.[27] Vascular dementia (VaD) is recognised as the second most prevalent type of dementia. There is a large body of evidence linking cerebrovascular benefits with treatment of broader cardiovascular risk factors.[30] Older patients presenting with the problems of cognitive decline and depression should therefore have vascular risk assessed and treated more broadly.

Screening tools

When appropriate, naturopaths treating older patients are encouraged to arrange referrals to health professionals qualified to detect normal from abnormal brain ageing. Although there is no universally accepted measure to detect preclinical signs of AD, psychologists, psychiatrists and neuropsychologists are qualified to administer screening tools, which, by measuring patients' subjective or objective cognitive decline, can help distinguish normal from abnormal brain ageing, and the progression or stabilisation of cognitive decline.[25] Such screening tools include the Mini-Mental State Examination (MMSE), the Alzheimer's Disease Assessment Scale (ADAS-cog) and the *Diagnostic and Statistical Manual of Mental Disorders* (DSM-IV) (refer to Table 32.2).

Table 32.2 Cognitive screening tools[31-34]

SCREENING TOOL	DESCRIPTION
MMSE	A 30-point test that is commonly used to screen for dementia. The MMSE evaluates six areas of cognitive function: orientation, attention, immediate recall, short-term recall, language, and the ability to follow simple verbal and written commands. Scores: 20–26 = some cognitive impairment 10–19 = moderate to severe impairment < 10 = very severe impairment.
ADAS-cog	A screening test comprised of 11 tasks widely used to assess memory, language, praxis, attention and other cognitive abilities.
DSM-IV R	Criteria for dementia

RISK FACTORS

Several risk factors have been associated with the development of cognitive decline (for example, VaD and AD) including:[26,35-38]

- hypertension
- central obesity
- diabetes
- alcohol intake
- elevated homocysteine levels
- cigarette smoking
- inflammation
- a history of anxiety and depression.

Elevated blood pressure, for example, has been found to influence cognitive ability: hypertension increases the risk of vascular and endothelial damage and disrupts the blood–brain barrier,[26] and it has been proposed that a reduction in high blood pressure may be a preventive measure against stroke and cognitive decline in elderly patients.[39] Furthermore, increased central adipose tissue has been linked to vascular and metabolic factors that give rise to cognitive decline and dementia and there is emerging evidence suggesting that metabolic syndrome is associated with an increased risk of dementia. A greater waist to hip ratio (WHR) and age are significantly negatively correlated to hippocampal volumes, suggesting that a larger WHR may be related to neurodegenerative, vascular or metabolic processes that affect brain structures underlying cognitive decline and dementia.[36] Studies assessing the link between hypercholesterolaemia, atrial fibrillation, smoking and dementia have given more conflicting results.[40] Clinicians need to consider lifestyle interventions towards an early and effective cardiovascular risk-factor management to reduce the risk of cardiometabolic and the cognitive decline.[41]

A history of nervous disorders such as anxiety and depression has also been linked to poor cognitive health later on in life.[22] In particular, anxiety is a common feature of dementia, occurring in higher levels in VaD compared to AD, while people in severe stages of dementia tend to experience decreased levels of anxiety.[42] Furthermore, anxiety in dementia patients has been associated with poor quality of life and behavioural disturbances, even after controlling for depression.

CONVENTIONAL TREATMENT

Currently pharmacological treatments are available for the short-term symptoms of dementia through the use of cholinesterase inhibitors, rather than modifying the disease as such.[43] The central cholinergic system has a pertinent role in regulating cognitive functioning and a consistent deficit in the neurotransmitter acetylcholine (ACh) in the hippocampal area of the brain is a key feature of AD.[44] Inhibition of acetylcholinesterase (AChE), the main enzyme involved in the breakdown of ACh, is the key strategy for the short-term relief of symptoms commonly seen in AD. These therapies include the medications Donepezil, Tacrine and galantamine, in addition to drugs such as rivastigmine and, although these treatments delay the symptomatic progression associated with AD by 6 to 12 months,[43] they can cause adverse effects including gastrointestinal disturbances, diarrhoea, muscle cramps, fatigue, nausea, rhinitis, vomiting, anorexia and insomnia.[45] Additionally, ACh inhibitors such as galantamine, huperzine A, physostigmine and its derivatives have been used to increase the levels of ACh to improve neural functioning.[46]

Since there is no cure for AD, preventive measures are very important and are commonly prescribed by medical practitioners. To this end, some conventional medications, including non-steroidal anti-inflammatory, antidiabetic and hypertension medications are thought to be effective in preventing the onset of dementia. The therapeutic action of these medications targets the brain systems that scientists think are impaired in dementia and other age-related diseases including CVD.[47]

KEY TREATMENT PROTOCOLS

The causes of age-related cognitive decline and pathologies such as AD are not known. The underlying mechanisms associated with normal ageing need to be understood in order to understand abnormal ageing present in cognitive decline, and it is thought that cognitive decline may be a multifactorial process involving dietary, environmental, genetic and physiological mechanisms.[48]

Oxidative stress

Oxidative stress is strongly implicated in the ageing process in addition to various disease states, including cardiovascular conditions such as stroke, CVD and neurodegenerative diseases such as AD and dementia.[49,50] This process is most commonly explained by the 'free radical theory' of ageing, which was first proposed by Harman in the 1950s and holds that highly reactive chemicals in the body (free radicals) damage cells via chemical processes that accumulate over time and result in severe cell damage and cell death.[50] During normal metabolic processes highly reactive (free radical) species of oxygen (reactive oxygen species, ROS), nitrogen (reactive nitrogen species, RNS) and chorine (reactive chlorine species, RCS) are produced. Normally these reactive species (or oxidants) play important roles in the immune system, helping kill microorganisms and fight off diseases, but in excessive amounts free radicals initiate chemical reactions that damage proteins, carbohydrates, membrane lipids and DNA.[49,50] An inbuilt oxidative defence mechanism ordinarily protects the body against these oxidative reactions by counteracting the effects of these reactive molecules and preventing cellular destruction. However, when the body is unable to counteract the effects of these reactive substances they are left to destroy cellular processes disturbing physiological functions. **Antioxidant micronutrients** such as vitamin C, vitamin E and carotenoids are important in combating the effects of oxidative stress; inadequate dietary intake of these is thought to increase the risk of degenerative diseases including AD and MCI.[50] Rectifying deficiencies in these nutrients may be one aim of combating oxidative stress in the ageing individual.

Epidemiological evidence indicates that antioxidants such as **folate** also represent potentially beneficial nutritional

NATUROPATHIC TREATMENT AIMS

- Treat the presenting complaints using a holistic treatment approach.
- Prevent the onset of cognitive decline.
- If cognitive decline is evident then stem the progression of the decline.
- Monitor the patient's cognitive state and other health conditions throughout the ageing process.
- Address comorbid conditions (especially mood, anxiety and sleep disorders).
- Liaise regularly with patient's other health practitioners and carer.
- Address risk factors that are attributing to the presenting symptoms.
- Improve vascular stiffness and elasticity.
- Prevent the build-up of beta amyloid.
- Increase antioxidant status.
- Address non-cognitive symptoms, such as depression and anxiety.
- Address nutritional deficiencies.

components for AD. Vegetables, particularly those high in **vitamins C** and **E**, which have antioxidant properties, have also been linked to lowering the risk of AD.[51] High-dose vitamin E and vitamin C supplementation may lower the risk of AD. One study[52] examined the association between the use of vitamin E and vitamin C and the incidence of AD. A large sample of 633 participants aged 65 years and older were followed up an average of 4.3 years, and it was found that 91 of the participants with vitamin information met accepted criteria for the clinical diagnosis of Alzheimer's disease. None of the 27 vitamin E supplement users and none of the 23 vitamin C supplement users had AD. The authors concluded that the use of a high-dose vitamin E and vitamin C supplement may lower the risk of AD. Those with higher intakes of vitamin E from food sources may also reduce their risk of developing AD. Furthermore, a longitudinal population-based study (n = 2889; 65–102 years) found a 36% reduction in the rate of cognitive decline among high vitamin E consumers (from supplements and foods; median dose = 387.4 IU/day) compared with low vitamin E consumers (median dose = 6.8 IU/day intake from foods) (as measured by a food frequency questionnaire).

Elevated levels of F2-isoprostanes (metabolites indicative of free-radical oxidative damage) have been found to be present in patients with AD[53] and the finding that **pine bark extract** has significant beneficial effects on cognitive functioning and F2-isoprostanes following 90 days' administration (60–85 years; PYC 150 mg/day[54]) suggests the potential benefit of this treatment in improving cognition in the elderly.

Polyphenols are antioxidants found in fruits and vegetables and have been shown to have cognitive effects. The polyphenol **curcumin** has been shown to improve cognitive functioning in AD patients, and researchers suggest that this action is possibly due to curcumin's antioxidant, anti-inflammatory and lipophilic actions; and since curcumin is lipophilic nature it may possibly cross the blood–brain barrier and bind to amyloid plaques.[55] Additionally, preliminary human and animal studies show promising effects of polyphenols found naturally in **cocoa** as a treatment to delay age-related cognitive decline.[56–59] These studies suggest that flavonol-containing foods may be an effective part of treatment for delaying age-related cognitive deficits in normal ageing and for cerebrovascular ischaemia syndromes including dementias and stroke by improving vascular health.

Free radical mitochondrial theory

Mitochondrial dysfunction may play a key role underlying pathological changes associated with ageing, including brain ageing, and may be associated with the onset and development of neurodegenerative diseases.[48,60] Mitochondrial dysfunction can be caused by the oxidation of lipids, proteins and nucleic acid. The free radical mitochondrial theory of ageing asserts that cumulative oxidative injuries to the mitochondria cause the mitochondria to progressively become less efficient. **Coenzyme Q10** (CoQ10) is involved in mitochondrial functions including the manufacturing of adenosine triphosphate (ATP) and has been linked with improving cognitive functions. CoQ10 has been shown to have a neuroprotective effect in cognitive impairment and oxidative damage in the hippocampus and cerebral cortex in animals.[61] Investigation of an integrative treatment approach on cognitive performance using antidepressants, cholinesterase inhibitors, and vitamins and supplements (multivitamins, vitamin E, alpha-lipoic acid, omega-3 and CoQ10) was found to delay cognitive decline for 24 months and also improve cognition, especially frontal lobe activity and memory in patients with mild dementia and depression.[62]

Additionally, the important antioxidant **CoQ10** is readily used by the body and has been shown to delay the progression of neurodegenerative and heart conditions, though at present there is only a limited amount of research supporting this idea.

Alpha-lipoic acid (ALA) is a coenzyme involved in mitochondrial metabolism and is found in various food sources including meat and, at lower levels, in spinach, brewer's yeast and wheat germ. ALA and its derivatives improve the age-associated decline of memory, improve mitochondrial structure and function, inhibit the age-associated increase of oxidative damage, elevate the levels of antioxidants, and restore the activity of key enzymes.[48,60] Dihydrolipoic acid (DHLA)—a reduced form of ALA—is a strong antioxidant and has a key role in recycling other antioxidants including vitamins C and E, CoQ10 and glutathione. Additionally, DHLA chelates iron and copper.[60] Animal studies have found ALA to be beneficial for delaying the onset of neurodegenerative diseases such as AD; it improves age-associated cognitive dysfunction and neurodegenerative disease,[60] though human trials remain in their infancy.[63] Co-administration of ALA with other mitochondrial nutrients, such as acetyl-L-carnitine and coenzyme Q10, appears more effective in improving cognitive dysfunction and reducing oxidative mitochondrial dysfunction.[48,60]

Acetyl-L-carnitine (ALC) is derived from carnitine and has been reported to be an effective therapy for patients with Alzheimer's disease.[64] ALC acts on cholinergic neurons, enhances mitochondrial function and is involved with membrane stabilisation. Supplementation with ALC (2 g/day) in older individuals (> 65 years) with mild mental impairment has been associated with improved measures on behavioural scales, memory tests, attention barrage test and verbal fluency tests.[64] Additionally, a randomised, double-blind, placebo-controlled, parallel-group clinical trial[65] was carried out to compare 6 months of treatment with 1 g ALC twice daily and placebo in patients (*n* = 36) with dementia of the Alzheimer's type. Although no significant findings were observed, trends were apparent in the ALC group, who showed improvements in short-term memory. Findings suggest the importance of ALC in the treatment of elderly patients with mental impairment and clinical features of AD, particularly those related to short-term memory; however, these conclusions are based on small samples and larger studies are required to confirm these findings. Despite positive findings of these earlier studies, authors of a Cochrane review suggest that at present there is no evidence to recommend the routine use of ALC in clinical practice.[66]

Inflammatory markers

A number of molecules associated with inflammation are believed to be involved in the pathogenesis of AD. These include increases in inflammatory markers alpha 1-antichymotrypsin (ACT), interleukin-6 (IL-6), monocyte chemoattractant protein-1 (MCP-1) and oxidised low-density lipoprotein (oxLDL) in the plasma and cerebrospinal fluid in patients with AD.[67] It has also been established that centenarians have a higher frequency of genetic markers associated with better control of inflammation; such control appears to exert a protective effect against the development of age-related pathologies that have a strong inflammatory pathogenetic component.[67]

Bacopa monnieri is an Ayurvedic herb used traditionally for memory decline. *B. monnieri* contains bacosides A and B (steroidal saponins) believed to be essential for the clinical efficacy of the product. Although the exact mechanism of action of *B. monnieri* on cognitive processes has not yet been established, evidence suggests that it may modulate the cholinergic system and/or have antioxidant effects possibly via metal chelation,[68] remove β-amyloid deposits,[69] act as an anti-inflammatory,[70] anxiolytic[71] and antidepressant[72] and have adaptogenic properties.[73] Chronic administration of *B. monnieri* has been shown to increase the levels of endogenous antioxidants in the prefrontal cortex, striatum and hippocampus via a mechanism that resembles that of the antioxidant vitamin E.[68] *B. monnieri* supplementation has reduced specific amyloid peptides by as much as 60% while also improving a number of behavioural measures in an animal setting.[69]

Studies examining the effects of *B. monnieri* in healthy young adults have found significant improvements in the retention of new information, speed of visual information processing, speed of decision-making time, learning rate and memory consolidation, and improved performance on spatial working memory accuracy.[74,75,68] Measures of speed are one of the most prominent deficits to be shown in studies examining cognitive deterioration in the elderly. In conclusion, these findings suggest that *Bacopa monnieri* improves higher order cognitive processes such as learning and memory in healthy young individuals. Additionally, studies examining the effects of *B. monnieri* in older adults revealed that *B. monnieri* improves retention of new information and decreases the rate of forgetting of newly acquired information (40–65 years; 150 mg × 2/daily).[74] In addition, *B. monnieri* has been shown to improve depression and trait anxiety, and decrease heart rate in healthy elderly participants (65+ years) without clinical signs of dementia (300 g/day for 12 weeks).[76]

Vascular system and cognitive ageing

There is increasing evidence linking the role of vascular function to cognitive decline and dementia, so interventions that address these vascular factors may be effective in preventing cognitive impairments as seen in these individuals.[77] A review of the literature outlined the following vascular factors as possible causes involved in brain ageing and cognitive decline: a reduced cerebral blood flow, reduced cerebral blood volume, poor capillary elasticity and poor vasodilatory capacity.[48] Furthermore, cerebral blood flow (CBF) and volume (circulation) can be compromised by a number of factors, including age-reduced capillary elasticity and vasodilatory capacity, cholinergic deficits, vascular lesions and plaques, oxidative stress and glucose supply to the brain, which may affect the uptake and use of glucose and oxygen in the brain.[48] Furthermore, a relationship exists between arterial stiffness and cognitive impairment, suggesting that functional changes of the arterial system could be involved in the onset of dementia (VaD or AD types).[78] It is therefore reasonable to suggest that a strategy to prevent cognitive decline in the ageing individual may be to address the multiple mechanisms associated with brain ageing with appropriate supportive interventions, before normal age-related cognitive decline accelerates, potentially leading to impairments and eventual dementia.[48]

Elevated levels of the amino acid homocysteine are also associated with cognitive dysfunction in the elderly. **Folate** deficiency is associated with high blood levels of homocysteine, linked to the risk of arterial disease, dementia and Alzheimer's disease.[79] There is no current evidence showing benefits following folic acid supplementation with vitamin B12 on cognitive function and mood in healthy elderly people.[79] However, in another trial supplementation 800 μg/day folic acid over 3 years was associated with significant improvements in global functioning, memory storage and information-processing speed in healthy elderly individuals with high homocysteine levels. Folic acid supplementation has also been shown to significantly improve over-all response to cholinesterase inhibitors and scores on the Instrumental Activities of Daily Living and the Social Behaviour subscale of the Nurse's Observation Scale for Geriatric Patients in patients with AD.[79] However, supplementation with vitamin B12 did not show benefit in measures of cognitive function in participants with cognitive impairment.

Older subjects with greater intakes of **fruits** and **vegetables**, and the corresponding nutrients vitamin C and folate, have been shown to perform better on cognitive tests.[80].

Heavy metals

Levels of zinc, copper and iron are significantly altered in AD brain tissue, particularly in subcortical regions such as the hippocampus, amygdala and neocortex.[81] Recent findings suggest that metal complexing agents may have therapeutic benefits in AD.[82] **Curcumin**'s anti-inflammatory actions are believed to be due in part to its metal-chelating effects; it also has the ability to bind to heavy metals—particularly copper and iron—and as a result prevent neurotoxicity caused by such metals.[83] As already mentioned **B. monnieri** is believed to not only modulate the cholinergic system and/or have antioxidant effects, and remove β-amyloid deposits, but it also acts as a metal chelator.

Genetics

It has been suggested that genetic susceptibility is implicated in the cognitive impairment seen in ageing. For example, apolipoprotein E (Apo E) and ACE genes have been associated with cognitive impairments seen in ageing and dementia. Individuals carrying the Apo E epsilon4 allele exhibit lower memory performance on tests related to declarative (storing facts) and procedural (long-term) memory.[84] Furthermore, AD is an autosomal dominant disease involving four specific genes located on chromosomes 1, 14, 19 and 21; these genes have been associated with the progression of AD. Further research, however, is required to understand the relationship between Apo E and cognition.

Herbal cognitive enhancers

Chronic administration of **Panax ginseng** extracts has shown improvements in cognitive functioning and performance in healthy young and older individuals. Compared to a placebo group, 8–9 weeks' administration of a standardised *P. ginseng* extract (400 mg/day) in healthy older participants (> 40 years) resulted in significant improvements in performance on cognitive tasks, specifically related to executive processing.[85] Furthermore, 12 weeks of *P. ginseng* administration (G115) has been found to improve wellbeing.[86] Cognitive function has also been studied in acute administration of various ginseng doses. A study[87] examined the effects of 200, 400 and 600 mg *P. ginseng* (G115) following 1, 2.5, 4 and 6 hours post dose. These researchers found improvements in secondary memory factor for each dose, with more pronounced improvements seen with the 400 mg dose. Slowed performance was seen with the 200 and 600 mg doses, and the 200 and 400 mg doses were associated with declines in subjective alertness that reached significance by 6 hours post dose (the last testing session of the day). Additionally, various doses of *P. ginseng* (G115) and *G. biloba* extract (GK 501) combinations (320 mg, 640 mg and 960 mg) resulted in significant improvements in memory performance for the optimum dose of the combination (960 mg of the combined treatment) with this effect isolated to secondary memory, whereas lower doses (320 mg and 640 mg) resulted in deficiencies in speed on the attention tasks.[88]

G. biloba is one of the most widely researched herbs for the treatment and prevention of cognitive decline. The mechanisms by which *G. biloba* improves cognition are thought to be via platelet activating factor (PAF) antagonist activity,[89] free radical scavenger activity,[90,91,92] enhancing active choline uptake and improving cerebral blood flow. Although only a few trials have examined the effects of *G. biloba* in healthy cognitively intact older individuals, *G. biloba* has been shown to be effective in improving memory and cognitive function in healthy adults.[93,94,95] However, some trials have not replicated positive results.[94,96]

G. biloba has also been widely examined in elderly patients with and without dementia. A study[97] found that 6 weeks' daily administration of EGb 761 (180 mg) was effective in enhancing certain neuropsychological and memory processes in cognitively intact older individuals (*n* = 262; > 60 years). Furthermore, two large, randomised, placebo-controlled, multicentre trials[96,99] examined the effects of *G. biloba* EGb 761 on patients with mild to severe dementia of the Alzheimer's and vascular types. They found that treatment with 120 mg EGb 761 daily showed a statistically significant worsening in all domains of assessment and *G. biloba* was equivalent to stemming the course of the illness for 6 months.[96,99] A study[100] compared the effects of of *G. biloba* (EGb 761; 120 mg and 240 mg) administration to that of four cholinesterase inhibitors (donepezil, tacrine, rivastigmine and Metrifonate) in AD, and found that in all groups symptoms of dementia were delayed for similar periods of time and similar response rates were obtained. These findings suggest that both cholinesterase inhibitors and *G. biloba* (EGb 761) should be considered as equally effective in the treatment of mild to moderate AD.

Despite these positive findings, the results of the largest double-blind, placebo-controlled, randomised trial conducted on the cognitive effects of *G. biloba* present conflicting outcomes. Another study[101] investigated the effects of *G. biloba* (120 g b.d.; *n* = 1545) versus placebo (*n* = 1545) on reducing the incidence of dementia and AD in elderly individuals with normal cognition (*n* = 2587) and those with MCI (*n* = 482). In this multicentre trial, participants were assessed every 6 months for incident dementia for a mean number of 6.1 years. *G. biloba* was found to have no effect on the rate of progression to dementia in participants with normal cognition or those with MCI. Moreover, a *G. biloba* and *B. monnieri* administration over 4 weeks failed to find effects on cognitive function in healthy adults (18–68 years); however, it is possible that the dose was not sufficient or treatment duration was not long enough to produce a pharmacological effect.[102] Furthermore, the authors of a recent review of the literature regarding the therapeutic effects of *G. biloba* in patients diagnosed with cognitive impairment and dementia concluded that the pattern of results from clinical trials is inconsistent.[103] Although, compared to placebo, *G. biloba* appears to be safe and without adverse effects, the evidence indicating that *G. biloba* has a significant effect on patients with dementia or cognitive impairment is not convincing and further conventionally designed trials are unlikely to be useful.[103] Hence, further trials are necessary before any firm conclusions can be drawn on the utility of *G. biloba* in these groups.

Salvia officinalis contains antioxidant, oestrogenic and anti-inflammatory properties, inhibits butyryl and acetyl-cholinesterase and has been found to improve mnemonic performance in healthy young and elderly participants.[104] Furthermore, a 16-week administration of *S. officinalis* significantly improved scores on the ADAS-cog in patients with mild to moderate dementia.[105] **Melissa officinalis** has been shown to have cholinergic binding properties in vitro and may ameliorate cognitive decline associated with AD. A randomised, placebo-controlled, double blind, balanced crossover study[106] assessed the acute (1, 2.5, 4 and 6 h post dosing) cognitive and mood effects of three single doses of *M. officinalis* (LB 300 g, 600 g and 900 g) or matching placebo. Improvements were observed in accuracy of attention following 600 g LB and reductions in both secondary memory and working memory factors and self-rated 'calmness', as assessed by Bond-Lader mood scales, was elevated at the earliest time points by the lowest dose (LB 300 mg). Interestingly, alertness was significantly reduced at all time points following the highest dose. Although the research is still in its infancy, *S. officinalis* and *M. officinalis* are promising treatments for dementia.[104]

INTEGRATIVE MEDICAL CONSIDERATIONS

Cognitively stimulating activities and psychosocial factors

Numerous epidemiological studies of activity in older adults have observed that frequent participation in cognitively stimulating activities such as reading, playing mental games and doing crossword puzzles were associated with reduced dementia risk.[107,108] Psychosocial factors including emotional support, social engagements and social networks also prevent cognitive decline.[22] Anxiety, depression and poor quality of life are common symptoms in the elderly population suffering from AD. Therefore, counselling and support from social networks needs to be considered as part of a holistic treatment approach.

Dietary and lifestyle advice

Human epidemiological studies provide convincing evidence that dietary patterns practised during adulthood are important contributors to age-related cognitive decline and dementia risk.[109] Diets high in fat, especially *trans-* and saturated fats, adversely affect cognition, while those high in fruits, vegetables, cereals and fish are associated with better cognitive function and lower risk of dementia. A study[110] reviewed functional food approaches to preventing chronic diseases and healthy ageing, and linked dysfunctions of the mitochondria (including membrane leakage, oxidation and release of metals) and free radical discharge to pathological events involved in cardiovascular disease, neurodegenerative disease and carcinogenic processes. The **Mediterranean diet** is purported to be particularly useful for preventing the cognitive decline associated with ageing, as well as cognitive decline of the vascular and Alzheimer's types.[111] Fibre-rich foods and wheat germ oil are rich sources of tocopherols, which act as antioxidants and have anti-inflammatory actions, preventing the risk of Alzheimer's disease.[12] Additionally, polyphenols found in grapes and wine possess antioxidant activity and may potentially modify certain risk factors associated with atherogenesis and cardiovascular disease. Grape-skin extracts also contain **natural antioxidants** such as resveratrol, catechins, myricetin, caffeic acid and rutin. There is increasing evidence to suggest that cognitive impairment and dementia in older subjects might be positively influenced by a diet including seafood. A large trial (*n* = 2031; 70–74 years) found that daily fish intake was associated with a lower prevalence of poor cognitive performance, and the association between total fish intake and cognition was dose-dependent with the greatest effect seen in those consuming 75 g fish per day. The effects were more pronounced for non-processed lean fish and fatty fish.[112]

The Mediterranean herbs such as *Salvia officinalis* and *Rosmarinus officinalis* that have been well proven for memory protection may be added to the diet. *Allium*

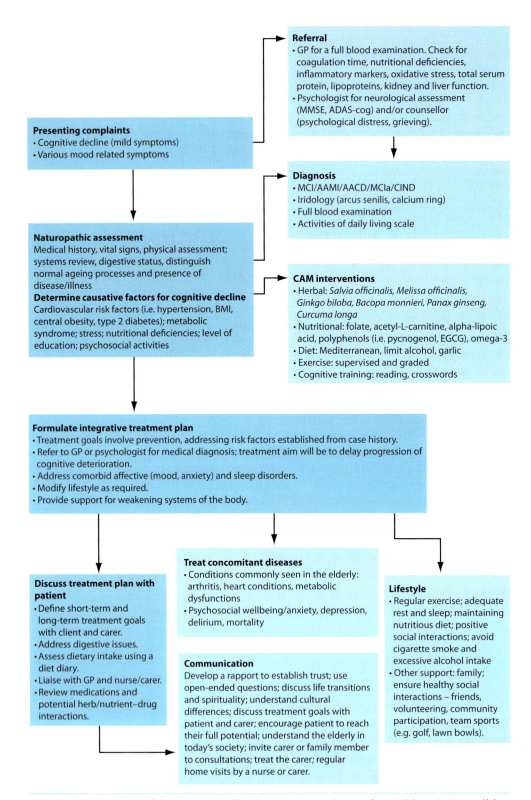

Presenting complaints
- Cognitive decline (mild symptoms)
- Various mood related symptoms

Referral
- GP for a full blood examination. Check for coagulation time, nutritional deficiencies, inflammatory markers, oxidative stress, total serum protein, lipoproteins, kidney and liver function.
- Psychologist for neurological assessment (MMSE, ADAS-cog) and/or counsellor (psychological distress, grieving).

Diagnosis
- MCI/AAMI/AACD/MCIa/CIND
- Iridology (arcus senilis, calcium ring)
- Full blood examination
- Activities of daily living scale

Naturopathic assessment
Medical history, vital signs, physical assessment; systems review, digestive status, distinguish normal ageing processes and presence of disease/illness
Determine causative factors for cognitive decline
Cardiovascular risk factors (i.e. hypertension, BMI, central obesity, type 2 diabetes); metabolic syndrome; stress; nutritional deficiencies; level of education; psychosocial activities

CAM interventions
- Herbal: *Salvia officinalis, Melissa officinalis, Ginkgo biloba, Bacopa monnieri, Panax ginseng, Curcuma longa*
- Nutritional: folate, acetyl-L-carnitine, alpha-lipoic acid, polyphenols (i.e. pycnogenol, EGCG), omega-3
- Diet: Mediterranean, limit alcohol, garlic
- Exercise: supervised and graded
- Cognitive training: reading, crosswords

Formulate integrative treatment plan
- Treatment goals involve prevention, addressing risk factors established from case history.
- Refer to GP or psychologist for medical diagnosis; treatment aim will be to delay progression of cognitive deterioration.
- Address comorbid affective (mood, anxiety) and sleep disorders.
- Modify lifestyle as required.
- Provide support for weakening systems of the body.

Discuss treatment plan with patient
- Define short-term and long-term treatment goals with client and carer.
- Address digestive issues.
- Assess dietary intake using a diet diary.
- Liaise with GP and nurse/carer.
- Review medications and potential herb/nutrient–drug interactions.

Treat concomitant diseases
- Conditions commonly seen in the elderly: arthritis, heart conditions, metabolic dysfunctions
- Psychosocial wellbeing/anxiety, depression, delirium, mortality

Communication
Develop a rapport to establish trust; use open-ended questions; discuss life transitions and spirituality; understand cultural differences; discuss treatment goals with patient and carer; encourage patient to reach their full potential; understand the elderly in today's society; invite carer or family member to consultations; treat the carer; regular home visits by a nurse or carer.

Lifestyle
- Regular exercise; adequate rest and sleep; maintaining nutritious diet; positive social interactions; avoid cigarette smoke and excessive alcohol intake
- Other support: family; ensure healthy social interactions – friends, volunteering, community participation, team sports (e.g. golf, lawn bowls).

Figure 32.4 Naturopathic treatment decision tree—ageing and cognition. MCI = mild cognitive impairment, AACI = age-associated cognitive impairment, AACD = age-associated cognitive decline, CIND = cognitive impairment, no dementia

sativum decreases low-density lipoprotein (LDL), is an anti-thrombotic and suppresses platelet aggregation. *Allium sativum* also exhibits an antioxidant action by increasing the levels of cellular antioxidant enzymes, such as superoxide dismutase, catalase and glutathione peroxidase, and scavenging reactive oxygen species.[113] Finally, monounsaturated fatty acid (MUFA) consumption from olive oil (> 100 g per day) appears to be associated with a high protection against cognitive decline, though it remains unknown whether the protective effect of olive oil is due to the high MUFA intake or to the presence of antioxidant compounds in the diet or both.

Case Study

A 68-year-old widow presents with **concerns about forgetting daily** tasks, and has reduced tolerance of other people. She also **reports feeling agitated, anxious** and **despondent**. She **wakes at night** with **worrying thoughts** and cannot get back to sleep, and **gets tired easily**.

SUGGESTIVE SYMPTOMS

- Forgetfulness
- Depression
- Anxiety
- Insomnia
- Decreased attention
- Fatigue

Physical activity

Regular exercise can be a protective factor for cognitive decline and dementia. A study[114] found that, compared with no exercise, regular physical activity was associated with lower risks of cognitive impairment and dementia, particularly AD, suggesting that regular physical activity may be an important protective factor for cognitive decline and dementia in the elderly.

Example treatment

Herbal and nutritional prescription

Given the patient's age it is possible that changes to her physiology are due to years of oxidative stress, build-up of inflammatory markers, build-up of heavy metals and/or impairments in cerebrovascular flow, which may be contributing to her mild memory impairment. It is possible that she is suffering from age-associated cognitive decline; however, a referral to her GP for a full blood examination and to a psychologist for cognitive assessments will provide an accurate medical diagnosis. Until an accurate diagnosis is determined the primary treatment objective is to address the early signs of memory impairment as this may also be affecting her anxiety and low mood. *G. biloba* and *B. monnieri* should improve cognitive functioning, with *B. monnieri*

Herbal formula

Bacopa monniera 1:2	35 mL
Ginkgo biloba 2:1	25 mL
Melissa officinalis 1:2	20 mL
Salvia officinalis 1:2	20 mL
5 mL t.d.s.	100 mL

Green tea 1 cup per day.

Panax ginseng tablets 1 g b.d.

Sleep mix: *Passiflora incarnata* and *Scutellaria lateriflora*

2.5 mL 1 hour before bedtime

Nutritional prescription

Alpha-lipoic acid

Antioxidant complex (with vitamins C and E)

Folic acid

providing added anxiolytic effects. *S. officinalis* and *M. officinalis* will provide additional anti-cholinesterase effects, with *S. officinalis* also functioning as an anti-oxidant. Traditionally used as a nervine tonic, *M. officinalis* may be beneficial for decreasing the patient's agitation and anxiety. For nutritional deficiencies, supplementation with antioxidant compounds such as alpha-lipoic acid and vitamins C, E and B, including folic acid, will provide additional therapeutic support. Furthermore, a sleep mix including *Passiflora incarnata* and *Scutellaria lateriflora* may improve quality of sleep and in turn combat feelings of tiredness.

Dietary and lifestyle advice

A diet that follows the principles of a Mediterranean diet (rich in olive oil, vegetables, legumes, cereals and fruit, and low in animal fats and products, moderate to high consumption of fish, low consumption of dairy and moderate amounts of wine) is recommended. To increase compliance to any dietary modifications it is important to incorporate a patient's favourite foods into their diet and, if they have dentures, increase the amount of soft foods in their diet. Furthermore, green tea and foods rich in vitamins C and E and the B vitamins including folate need to be increased. Lifestyle changes should include regular social interaction through leisure activities with friends and family to elevate moods and decrease anxiety, and participation in cognitively stimulating activities such as reading the newspaper and crosswords. Regular exercise such as bowling, walking or swimming should be encouraged to improve mood, assist with sleep, strengthen the vascular system and improve blood flow to the brain.

To get an account of the patient's understanding of the treatment regimen and compliance, ask the older patient to repeat the treatment regimen, address any possible challenges they might experience with incorporating the treatment regimen into their current lifestyle (such as cultural differences or lack of mobility) and ask the patient to return any surplus prescriptions at the next consultation. Ensure the patient's carer (family or nurse) understands the naturopathic treatment regimen and, if deemed appropriate, offer home and/or telephone consultations.

Expected outcomes and follow-up protocols

An improvement in memory should be seen 4–6 weeks after commencing the treatment, and sleep patterns would be expected to improve after 1 week. The treatment should be continued for 6–12 months and changes in cognitive function and mood, sleep and fatigue carefully monitored over time, with regular visits to a psychologist who will be able to administer neuropsychological tests and monitor changes in cognitive function. The treatment formula needs to be modified according to improvements or exacerbations in mood (thymoleptics, B vitamins), sleep (hypnotics), anxiety (nervines, anxiolytics, magnesium) and fatigue (adrenal tonics, B vitamins). By treating the insomnia, symptoms of anxiety, attention and forgetfulness are expected to improve. The treatment protocol needs to be reassessed if deterioration is observed in any aspect of cognitive function or mood. Once presenting symptoms have improved, the long-term treatment goals will be to treat (and prevent) any comorbid diseases and/or illnesses (such as arthritis, cardiovascular disease, infections and gastrointestinal function); encourage engagement in social activities and exercise; discuss changes in their ability to undertake daily tasks, future planning (such as nominating a carer if and when required) and transitional phases with the older patient.

ADDITIONAL THERAPEUTIC OPTIONS

Nutraceuticals
- It has been suggested that ageing is in part associated with decreased levels of DHA and that a high intake of **omega-3 polyunsaturated fatty acids** may be protective against age-related cognitive decline and decreased risk of AD.[115]
- Randomised clinical trials have found conflicting evidence.
- Data from a cross-sectional population-based study (n = 1613; 45–70 years) indicated that marine omega-3 PUFA (EPA and DHA) and fatty fish consumption are inversely related to the risk of impaired overall cognitive function and speed.[116]
- Compared to a control group, 26 weeks of EPA-DHA treatment showed no significant effects on cognitive performance in cognitively healthy (Mini-Mental State Examination score > 21) individuals aged 65 years or older.[117]
- A study[118] examined the association between lean and fatty fish (as measured by a food frequency questionnaire) on dementia, AD and VD, and found that lean fish consumption had no protective effect against dementia. However, eating two serves or more of fatty fish per week was associated with a 28% decreased risk of dementia.
- A 6-month omega-3 fatty acid (1.7 g DHA and 0.6 g EPA) administration did not delay the rate of cognitive decline as measured by the MMSE or the cognitive portion of the ADAS-cog in patients with mild to moderate AD who were also receiving acetyl cholinesterase inhibitor treatment.[119] Positive effects, however, were observed in a small group of patients with very mild AD (MMSE > 27 points).

Herbal medicine
- Green tea (*C. sinensis*) polyphenols and catechins (epigallocatechin gallate) have metal-chelating, antioxidant, anti-inflammatory and neuroprotectant properties.[120–121]
- Preliminary studies in animal models have indicated that **grape seed** extract may have a role in enhancing cognition in older rats. However, research on grape seed extracts is limited.
- A large study conducted on a Japanese population revealed that a higher consumption of **green tea** is associated with a lower prevalence of cognitive impairment in humans.[123]
- *Centella asiatica* has been used in traditional Ayurvedic medicine for centuries for enhancing memory and is listed as a treatment for dementia in the ancient Indian Ayurvedic medical text, *Caraka Susmita*.[124]
- Despite limited placebo controlled trials, a recent study revealed that 2 months' daily administration of a high dose (750 mg) of *Centella asiatica* enhances working memory and improves self-related mood (alertness and calmness) in healthy elderly participants (mean age = 65.05 ± 3.56 years; n = 28).[125]

Homoeopathy
- Authors of a Cochrane review to evaluate the safety and efficacy profile of homoeopathic treatments in dementia failed to find any randomised trials with a sample size of more than 20 to be considered in the review and therefore concluded that there is insufficient evidence to comment on the use of homoeopathy in treating dementia.[126]
- Homoeopathy may still be considered for treating comorbid conditions.

Table 32.3 Review of the major evidence

INTERVENTION	METHODOLOGY	SUMMARY OF RESULTS	COMMENT
Ginkgo biloba RCTs *Acute dosing*: Kennedy et al. 2000[95] (*n* = 20)	GK501, Pharmaton, SA 200 mg, 240 mg and 360 mg 1, 2.5, 4 and 6 hours post dose	Improvements in speed of attention factor following both 240 mg and 360 mg GB extract following 2.5 hours and this effect was still present after 6 hours.	Acute administration of GB is capable of producing a sustained improvement in atten- tion in healthy young volunteers
Chronic dosing: Stough et al. 2001[75] (*n* = 61; 18–40 years)	30 day GB (Ginkgo- forte™; 180 mg) vs pla- cebo in cognitively intact individuals.	Significant improvements found in the speed of information processing, working memory and executive processing attributed to GB.	Chronic GB treatment improves memory processes.
DeKosky et al. 2008[101] (*n* = 3,690; 75+ years); nor- mal cognition (*n* = 2587) or MCI (*n* = 482)	Participants were assessed every 6 months for incidence of demen- tia (median follow-up of 6.1 years); GB extract (120 mg twice daily) or placebo (*n* = 1524); inci- dence of dementia and AD was determined by expert panel consensus.	523 participants developed dementia (246 Plb and 277 GB) with 92% of the dementia cases classified as possible or probable AD, or AD with evidence of vascular disease of the brain; GB had no effect on the rate of progression to dementia in participants with MCI (RR, 1.13; 95% CI, 0.85–1.50; p = 0.39).	120 mg of GB twice a day was not effective in reducing either the overall incidence rate of dementia or AD incidence in elderly individuals with nor- mal cognition or those with MCI.
Bacopa monnieri RCTs Roodenrys et al. 2002[74] (*n* = 76; 40–65 years)	Keenmind® 300 mg for people < 90 kg and 450 mg for people > 90 kg vs placebo; 12 weeks Keenmind® 300 mg/day vs placebo; 12 weeks	BM decreases the rate of forgetting of newly acquired information.	BM improves higher order cognitive pro- cesses in healthy young individuals.
Stough et al. 2001[93] (*n* = 46; 18–65 years)		Significant improvement in speed of visual informa- tion processing, decision- making time, learning rate and memory consolidation (p < 0.05) and state anxiety (p < 0.001) with maximum effects after 12 weeks; improvements in spatial working memory accuracy.	Further studies are required to ascertain the effective dos- age range, the time required to attain ther- apeutic levels and the effects over a longer term of administration.
Polyphenols Review article Mishra & Pala- nivelu[55] 2008	Review of the various mechanisms of actions of curcumin in AD and pathology.	Due to its antioxidant, anti-inflammatory and lipophilic action curcumin improves the cognitive functions in patients with AD.	Overall, curcumin improves memory in patients with AD.
Francis et al. 2006[59]	fMRI was used to mea- sure blood oxygenation level-dependent (BOLD) responses to a cognitive task following 5 days of cocoa flavanols (150 mg) administration.	An increase in the BOLD signal intensity in response to a cognitive task follow- ing ingestion of flavanol- rich cocoa.	Cocoa flavanols may potentially be used for the treatment of vascular impairment, including dementia and strokes, and for maintaining cardiovas- cular health.

(Continued)

Table 32.3 Review of the major evidence (Continued)

INTERVENTION	METHODOLOGY	SUMMARY OF RESULTS	COMMENT
Sorond et al. 2008[58] (n = 34; 59–83 years)	Transcranial Doppler (TCD) ultrasound was used to measure mean blood flow velocity (MFV) in the middle cerebral artery (MCA) of healthy elderly volunteers in response to the regular intake of flavonol-rich cocoa (FRC) or flavonol-poor cocoa (FPC).	In response to 2 weeks of FRC intake, MFV increased by 8% ± 4% at 1 week ($p = 0.01$) and 10% ± 4% ($p = 0.04$) at 2 weeks. In response to 1 week of cocoa, significantly more subjects in the FRC as compared with the FPC group had an increase in their MFV ($p < 0.05$).	Regular cocoa flavanol consumption may have a promising role in the treatment of cerebrovascular ischaemic syndromes, including dementias and stroke.
B vitamins/folic acid Cochrane review Malouf & Evans 2008[79]	Folic acid supplements with or without vitamin B12 were compared with placebo in healthy elderly people or people with dementia or cognitive impairment.	3-year folic acid supplementation (800 μg/day) showed that healthy elderly people with high homocysteine levels experienced significant benefits in global functioning, memory storage and information-processing speed.	Folic acid was well tolerated and no adverse effects were reported. More studies are required.
Alpha-lipoic acid Hager et al. 2001[63] (n = 9; AD patients and related dementias)	Open-label, non-randomised trial; 600 mg ALA as an adjunct with standard AChE inhibitor medication.	Following a treatment period of 337 ± 80 days on average, cognitive function in patients who received ALA had stabilised.	Although the study sample was small and not randomised these results are the first indication that treatment with ALA might be a successful neuroprotective therapy option for AD and related dementias.
Vitamins E and C Morris et al. 1998[52] (n = 633; 65 years and over)	A random sample was selected from a disease-free population. At base line, all vitamin supplements taken in the previous 2 weeks were identified by direct inspection.	After an average follow-up period of 4.3 years 91 of the sample participants had the clinical diagnosis of Alzheimer's disease. None of the 27 vitamin E supplement users and none of the 23 vitamin C supplement users had Alzheimer's disease.	High-dose vitamin E and vitamin C supplement may lower the risk of Alzheimer's disease.

Note: RCT = randomised controlled trial; GB = Ginkgo biloba; BM = Bacopa monnieri; MCI = mild cognitive impairment; ALA = alpha-lipoic acid

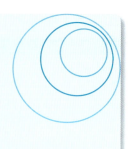

KEY POINTS

- Brain ageing is a multifactorial process.
- There is no universally accepted method to diagnose age-related cognitive decline.
- Early detection and intervention may be the key to delaying the onset of age-related cognitive impairment.
- The elderly are unique members of our society who need to be encouraged to reach their full potential.

Further reading

Anderson MA. Caring for older adults holistically. 4th edn Utah: F. A. Davis Company, 2007.

Anstey KJ, Low LF. Normal cognitive changes in ageing. Aust Fam Physician 2004;33(10):783–787.

Ames D, et al. Cerebrovascular disease, cognitive impairment and dementia. 2nd edn London: Informa Healthcare, 2003.

Eliopoulos C. Gerontological nursing. 6th edn. Philadelphia: Lippincott Williams & Wilkins, 2005.

MacKenzie ER, Rakel B. Complementary and alternative medicine for older adults. New York: Springer Publishing Company, 2006.

References

1. Baltes MM, Carstensen LL. The process of successful ageing: selection, optimization, and compensation. In: Staudinger UM, Lindenberger UER, eds. Understanding human development: dialogues with lifespan psychology. Boston, London: Kluwer Academic Publishers, 2003.
2. Kumar P, Clark M, eds. Clinical medicine. 5th edn. London: WB Saunders, 2002.
3. Eliopoulos C. Gerontological nursing. 6th edn. Philadelphia: Lippincott Williams & Wilkins, 2005.
4. Australian Bureau of Statistics. Deaths, Australia 2007. Online. Available: http://www.abs.gov.au/ausstats/abs@.nsf/mf/3302.0. Accessed 17 December 2008.
5. World Health Organization. Gender, health and ageing. 2003. Online. Available: http://www.who.int/gender/documents/en/Gender_Ageing.pdf. Accessed 5 November 2008
6. Xue CCL, et al. Complementary and alternative medicine use in Australia: a national population-based survey. Journal of Alternative and Complementary Medicine 2007;13(6):643–650.
7. Ferri CP, et al. Global prevalence of dementia: a Delphi consensus study. Lancet 2005;366(9503):2112–2117.
8. Smith C, et al. National health spending in 2004: recent slowdown led by prescription drug spending. Health Affairs 2006;25(1):186–196.
9. Heffler S, et al. Health spending projections for 2001–2011: the latest outlook. Health Affairs 2002;21(2):207–218.
10. Brownie S. Why are elderly individuals at risk of nutritional deficiency? International Journal of Nursing Practice 2006;12(2):110–118.
11. Gennari C. Calcium and vitamin D nutrition and bone disease of the elderly. Public Health Nutrition 2001;4(2 B):547–559.
12. Remacle C. Functional foods, ageing and degenerative disease. Cambridge: Woodhead Publishing Limited, 2004.
13. Mills S, Bone K. Principles and practice of phyto therapy. London: Churchill Livingstone, 2000.
14. Campbell AJ, et al. Incontinence in the elderly: prevalence and prognosis. Age Ageing 1985;14(2):65–70.
15. Gooneratne NS. Complementary and alternative medicine for sleep disturbances in older adults. Clinics in Geriatric Medicine 2008;24(1):121–138.
16. Luanaigh CÃ, Lawlor BA. Loneliness and the health of older people. International Journal of Geriatric Psychiatry 2008;23(12):1213–1221.
17. Foley DJ, et al. Sleep complaints among elderly persons: an epidemiologic study of three communities. Sleep 1995;18(6):32–425.
18. Ancoli-Israel S, et al. Sleep in the elderly: Normal variations and common sleep disorders. Harvard Review of Psychiatry 2008;16(5):279–286.
19. Foley D, et al. Sleep disturbances and chronic disease in older adults: results of the 2003 National Sleep Foundation Sleep in America Survey. Journal of Psychosomatic Research 2004;56(5):497–502.
20. Montorio I, Izal M. The geriatric depression scale: a review of its development and utility. International Psychogeriatrics 1996;8(1):103–112.
21. Anderson MA. Caring for older adults holistically. 3rd edn. Utah: F. A. Davis Company, 2003.
22. Hendrie HC, et al. The NIH Cognitive and Emotional Health Project. Alzheimer's and Dementia 2006;2(1):12–32.
23. Riddle DR, Schindler MK. Brain aging research. Reviews in Clinical Gerontology 2007;17(4):225–239.
24. Anstey KJ, Low LF. Normal cognitive changes in aging. Aust Fam Physician 2004;33(10):783–787.
25. Qualls SH, Smyer MA. Changes in decision-making capacity in older adults: assessment and intervention. New York: John Wiley & Sons, Inc., 2008.
26. Kalaria RN, et al. Alzheimer's disease and vascular dementia in developing countries: prevalence, management, and risk factors. Lancet Neurology 2008;7(9):812–826.
27. Thal DR, Del Tredici K, Braak H. Neurodegeneration in normal brain aging and disease. Science of aging knowledge environment. Sci Aging Knowl Environ 2004;23:26.

28. Akhtar S, et al. Are people with mild cognitive impairment aware of the benefits of errorless learning? Neuropsychol Rehabil 2006;16(3):329–346.

29. Palmer K, et al. Early symptoms and signs of cognitive deficits might not always be detectable in persons who develop Alzheimer's disease. Int Psychogeriatr 2008;20(2):252–258.

30. Flicker L. Vascular factors in geriatric psychiatry: time to take a serious look. Current Opinion in Psychiatry 2008;21(6):551–554.

31. Folstein MF, et al. 'Mini-mental state'. A practical method for grading the cognitive state of patients for the clinician. J Psychiatr Res 1975;12(3):189–198.

32. Rosen WG, et al. A new rating scale for Alzheimer's disease. American Journal of Psychiatry 1984;141(11):1356–1364.

33. Fioravanti M, et al. The Italian version of the Alzheimer's Disease Assessment Scale (ADAS): psychometric and normative characteristics from a normal aged population. Archives of Gerontology and Geriatrics 1994;19(1):21–30.

34. Erkinjuntti T, et al. The effect of different diagnostic criteria on the prevalence of dementia. New England Journal of Medicine 1997;337(23):1667–1674.

35. Whitmer RA, et al. Central obesity and increased risk of dementia more than three decades later. Neurology 2008;71(14):1057–1064.

36. Jagust W, et al. Central obesity and the aging brain. Archives of Neurology 2005;62(10):1545–1548.

37. Pavlovic DM, Pavlovic AM. Dementia and diabetes mellitus. Srpski arhiv za celokupno lekarstvo 2008;136 (3–4):170–175.

38. Xu G, et al. Alcohol consumption and transition of mild cognitive impairment to dementia. Psychiatry and Clinical Neurosciences 2008;63(1):43–49.

39. Pedelty L, Gorelick PB. Management of hypertension and cerebrovascular disease in the elderly. American Journal of Medicine 2008;121(8 Suppl 1):S23–S31.

40. Duron E, Hanon O. Vascular risk factors, cognitive decline, and dementia. Vascular Health and Risk Management 2008;4(2):363–381.

41. Milionis HJ, et al. Metabolic syndrome and Alzheimer's disease: a link to a vascular hypothesis? CNS Spectrums 2008;13(7):606–613.

42. Seignourel PJ, et al. Anxiety in dementia: a critical review. Clinical Psychology Review 2008;28(7):1071–1082.

43. Grutzendler J, Morris JC. Cholinesterase inhibitors for Alzheimer's disease. Drugs 2001;61(1):41–52.

44. Mukherjee PK, et al. Acetylcholinesterase inhibitors from plants. Phytomedicine 2007;14:289–300.

45. Pratt RD, et al. Donepezil: tolerability and safety in Alzheimer's disease. Int J Clin Pract 2002;56(9):710–717.

46. Houghton PJ, Howes MJ. Natural products and derivatives affecting neurotransmission relevant to Alzheimer's and Parkinson's disease. NeuroSignals 2005;14(1–2):6–22.

47. Desai AK, Grossberg GT. Diagnosis and treatment of Alzheimer's disease. Neurology 2005;64(12 Suppl 3):S34–S39.

48. Reynolds J, et al. Retarding cognitive decline with science-based nutraceuticals. JAMA 2008;11(1):23–31.

49. Mariani E, et al. Oxidative stress in brain aging, neurodegenerative and vascular diseases: an overview. J Chromatogr B Analyt Technol Biomed Life Sci 2005;827(1):65–75.

50. Polidori MC. Antioxidant micronutrients in the prevention of age-related diseases. Journal of Postgraduate Medicine 2003;49:229–235.

51. Engelhart M, et al. Dietary intake of antioxidants and risk of Alzheimer disease. JAMA 2002;287(24):3223–3229.

52. Morris MC, et al. Vitamin E and vitamin C supplement use and risk of incident Alzheimer disease. Alzheimer Dis Assoc Disord 1998;12(3):121–126.

53. Tuppo EE, et al. Sign of lipid peroxidation as measured in the urine of patients with probable Alzheimer's disease. Brain Res Bull 2001;54(5):565–568.

54. Ryan J, et al. An examination of the effects of the antioxidant Pycnogenol® on cognitive performance, serum lipid profile, endocrinological and oxidative stress biomarkers in an elderly population. Journal of Psychopharmacology 2008;22(5):553–562.

55. Mishra S, Palanivelu K. The effect of curcumin (turmeric) on Alzheimer's disease: an overview. Annals of Indian Academy of Neurology 2008;11(1):13–19.

56. Bisson JF, et al. Effects of long-term administration of a cocoa polyphenolic extract (Acticoa powder) on cognitive performances in aged rats. British Journal of Nutrition 2008;100(1):94–101.

57. Faridi Z, et al. Acute dark chocolate and cocoa ingestion and endothelial function: a randomized controlled crossover trial. American Journal of Clinical Nutrition 2008;88(1):58–63.

58. Sorond FA, et al. Cerebral blood flow response to flavanol-rich cocoa in healthy elderly humans. Neuropsychiatric Disease and Treatment 2008;4(2):433–440.

59. Francis ST, et al. The effect of flavanol-rich cocoa on the fMRI response to a cognitive task in healthy young people. Journal of Cardiovascular Pharmacology 2006;47(Suppl 2):S215–S220.

60. Liu J, The effects and mechanisms of mitochondrial nutrient alpha-lipoic acid on improving age-associated mitochondrial and cognitive dysfunction: an overview. Neurochemical Research 2008;33(1):194–203.

61. Ishrat T, et al. Coenzyme Q10 modulates cognitive impairment against intracerebroventricular injection of streptozotocin in rats. Behavioural Brain Research 2006;171(1):9–16.

62. Bragin V, et al. Integrated treatment approach improves cognitive function in demented and clinically depressed patients. American Journal of Alzheimer's Disease and Other Dementias 2005;20(1):21–26.

63. Hager K, et al. Alpha-lipoic acid as a new treatment option for Alzheimer type dementia. Archives of Gerontology and Geriatrics 2001;32(3):275–282.

64. Passeri M, et al. Acetyl-L-carnitine in the treatment of mildly demented elderly patients. Int J Clin Pharmacol Res 1990;10(1–2):75–79.

65. Rai G, et al. Double-blind, placebo-controlled study of acetyl-l-carnitine in patients with Alzheimer's disease. Current Medical Research and Opinion 1990;11(10):638–647.

66. Hudson S, Tabet N. Acetyl-L-carnitine for dementia. Cochrane Database of Systematic Reviews 2003;(2):CD003158.

67. Sun YX, et al. Inflammatory markers in matched plasma and cerebrospinal fluid from patients with Alzheimer's disease. Dement Geriatr Cogn Disord 2003;16(3):136–144.

68. Stough C, et al. Examining the nootropic effects of a special extract of Bacopa monniera on human cognitive functioning: 90 day double-blind placebo-controlled randomized trial. Phytotherapy Research 2008;22(12):1629–1634.

69. Holcomb LA, et al. Bacopa monniera extract reduces amyloid levels in PSAPP mice. J Alzheimers Dis 2006;9(3):243–251.

70. Channa S, et al. Anti-inflammatory activity of Bacopa monniera in rodents. J Ethnopharmacol 2006;104(1–2):286–289.

71. Bhattacharya SK, Ghosal S. Anxiolytic activity of a standardized extract of Bacopa monniera: an experimental study. Phytomedicine 1998;5(2):77–82.

72. Sairam K, et al. Antidepressant activity of standardized extract of Bacopa monniera in experimental models of depression in rats. Phytomedicine 2002;9(3):207–211.

73. Rai D, et al. Adaptogenic effect of *Bacopa monniera* (brahmi). Pharmacol Biochem Behav 2003;75(4):823–830.

74. Roodenrys S, et al. Chronic effects of brahmi (*Bacopa monnieri*) on human memory. Neuropsychopharmacology 2002;27:279–281.

75. Stough C, et al. The chronic effects of an extract of *Bacopa monnieri* (brahmi) on cognitive function in healthy human subjects. Psychopharmacology (Berl) 2001;156(4):481–484.

76. Calabrese C, et al. Effects of standardized *Bacopa monnieri* extract on cognitive performance, anxiety, and depression in the elderly: a randomized, double-blind, placebo-controlled trial. Journal of Alternative and Complementary Medicine 2008;14(6):707–713.

77. Alagiakrishnan K, et al. Treating vascular risk factors and maintaining vascular health: is this the way towards successful cognitive ageing and preventing cognitive decline? Postgraduate Medical Journal 2006;82(964):101–105.

78. Hanon O, et al. Relationship between arterial stiffness and cognitive function in elderly subjects with complaints of memory loss. Stroke 2005;36(10):2193–2197.

79. Malouf R, Grimley Evans J. Folic acid with or without vitamin B12 for the prevention and treatment of healthy elderly and demented people. Cochrane Database of Systematic Reviews 2008;(4):CD004514.

80. Morris MC, et al. Associations of vegetable and fruit consumption with age-related cognitive change. Neurology 2006;24;67(8):1370–1376.

81. Atwood CS, et al. Role of free radicals and metal ions in the pathogenesis of Alzheimer's disease. Met Ions Biol Syst 1999;36:309–364.

82. Cuajungco MP, et al. Metal chelation as a potential therapy for Alzheimer's disease. Ann N Y Acad Sci 2000;920:292–304.

83. Hatcher H, et al. Curcumin: from ancient medicine to current clinical trials. Cellular and Molecular Life Sciences 2008;65(11):1631–1652.

84. Bartres-Faz D, et al. Apo E influences declarative and procedural learning in age-associated memory impairment. Neuroreport 1999;10(14):2923–2927.

85. Sørensen H, Sonne J. A double-masked study of the effects of ginseng on cognitive functions. Current Therapeutic Research—Clinical and Experimental 1996;57(12):959–968.

86. Wiklund I, et al. A double-blind comparison of the effect on quality of life of a combination of vital substances including standardized ginseng G115 and placebo. Current Therapeutic Research—Clinical and Experimental 1994;55(1):32–42.

87. Kennedy DO, et al. Dose dependent changes in cognitive performance and mood following acute administration of ginseng to healthy young volunteers. Nutritional Neuroscience 2001;4(4):295–310.

88. Kennedy DO, et al. Differential, dose dependent changes in cognitive performance following acute administration of a *Ginkgo biloba/Panax ginseng* combination to healthy young volunteers. Nutr Neurosci 2001;4(5):399–412.

89. Smith PF, et al. The neuroprotective properties of the *Ginkgo biloba* leaf: a review of the possible relationship to platelet-activating factor (PAF). J Ethnopharmacol 1996;50(3):131–139.

90. Maitra I, et al. Peroxyl radical scavenging activity of *Ginkgo biloba* extract EGb 761. Biochem Pharmacol 1995;49(11):1649–1655.

91. Kristofikova Z, Klaschka J. In vitro effect of *Ginkgo biloba* extract (EGb 761) on the activity of presynaptic cholinergic nerve terminals in rat hippocampus. Dement Geriatr Cogn Disord 1997;8(1):43–48.

92. Gold PE, et al. *Ginkgo biloba*. A cognitive enhancer? Psychological Science in the Public Interest 2002;3(1):2–11.

93. Stough C, et al. Neuropsychological changes after 30-day *Ginkgo biloba* administration in healthy participants. Int J Neuropsychopharmacol 2001;4(2):131–134.

94. Elsabagh S, et al. Differential cognitive effects of *Ginkgo biloba* after acute and chronic treatment in healthy young volunteers. Psychopharmacology (Berl) 2005;179(2):437–446.

95. Kennedy DO, et al. The dose-dependent cognitive effects of acute administration of *Ginkgo biloba* to healthy young volunteers. Psychopharmacology (Berl) 2000;151(4):416–423.

96. Nathan PJ, et al. The acute nootropic effects of *Ginkgo biloba* in healthy older human subjects: a preliminary investigation. Human Psychopharmacology 2002;17(1):45–49.

97. Mix JA, Crews WD Jr. A double-blind, placebo-controlled, randomized trial of *Ginkgo biloba* extract EGb 761 in a sample of cognitively intact older adults: neuropsychological findings. Hum Psychopharmacol 2002;17(6):267–277.

98. Le Bars PL, et al. A placebo-controlled, double-blind, randomized trial of an extract of *Ginkgo biloba* for dementia. North American EGb Study Group. JAMA 1997;278(16):1327–1332.

99. Le Bars PL, et al. A 26-week analysis of a double-blind, placebo-controlled trial of the *Ginkgo biloba* extract EGb 761 in dementia. Dement Geriatr Cogn Disord 2000;11(4):230–237.

100. Wettstein A. Cholinesterase inhibitors and gingko extracts—are they comparable in the treatment of dementia? Comparison of published placebo-controlled efficacy studies of at least six months' duration. Phytomedicine 2000;6(6):393–401.

101. DeKosky ST, et al. *Ginkgo biloba* for prevention of dementia: a randomized controlled trial. JAMA 2008;300(19):2253–2262.

102. Nathan PJ, et al. Effects of a combined extract of *Ginkgo biloba* and *Bacopa monniera* on cognitive function in healthy humans. Human Psychopharmacology 2004;19:91–96.

103. Birks J, Grimley Evans J. *Ginkgo biloba* for cognitive impairment and dementia (review). Cochrane Database of Systematic Reviews 2008;(1):CD003120.

104. Kennedy DO, Scholey AB. The psychopharmacology of European herbs with cognition-enhancing properties. Curr Pharm Des 2006;12(35):4613–4623.

105. Akhondzadeh S, et al. *Salvia officinalis* extract in the treatment of patients with mild to moderate Alzheimer's disease: A double blind, randomized and placebo-controlled trial. Journal of Clinical Pharmacy and Therapeutics 2003;28(1):53–59.

106. Kennedy DO, et al. Modulation of mood and cognitive performance following acute administration of *Melissa officinalis* (lemon balm). Pharmacology Biochemistry and Behavior 2002;72(4):953–964.

107. Wilson RS, et al. Participation in cognitively stimulating activites and risk of incident Alzheimer Disease. JAMA 2002;287(6):742–748.

108. Wilson RS, et al. Relation of cognitive activity to risk of developing Alzheimer disease. Neurology 2007; 69(20):1911–1920.

109. Parrott MD, Greenwood CE. Dietary influences on cognitive function with aging: from high-fat diets to healthful eating. Ann N Y Acad Sci 2007;1114:389–397.

110. Ferrari CKB. Functional foods, herbs and nutraceuticals: towards biochemical mechanisms of healthy aging. Biogerontology 2004;5(5):275–289.

111. Panza F, et al. Mediterranean diet and cognitive decline. Public Health Nutrition 2004;7(7):959–963.

112. Nurk E, et al. Cognitive performance among the elderly and dietary fish intake: the Hordaland Health Study. American Journal of Clinical Nutrition 2007;86(5):1470–1478.

113. Qi R, Wang Z. Pharmacological effects of garlic extract. Trends in Pharmacological Sciences 2003;24(2):62–63.

114. Laurin D, et al. Physical activity and risk of cognitive impairment and dementia in elderly persons. Archives of Neurology 2001;58(3):498–504.
115. Uauy R, Dangour AD. Nutrition in brain development and aging: Role of essential fatty acids. Nutrition Reviews 2006;64(5 Pt 2):S24–S33.
116. Kalmijn S, et al. Dietary intake of fatty acids and fish in relation to cognitive performance at middle age. Neurology 2004;62(2):275–280.
117. van de Rest O, et al. Effect of fish oil on cognitive performance in older subjects: a randomized, controlled trial. Neurology 2008;71(6):430–438.
118. Huang TL, et al. Benefits of fatty fish on dementia risk are stronger for those without APOE epsilon4. Neurology 2005;65(9):1409–1414.
119. Freund-Levi Y, et al. Omega-3 fatty acid treatment in 174 patients with mild to moderate Alzheimer disease: OmegAD study—a randomized double-blind trial. Archives of Neurology 2006;63(10):1402–1408.
120. Choi Y, et al. The green tea polyphenol (–)-epigallocatechin gallate attenuates beta-amyloid-induced neurotoxicity in cultured hippocampal neurons. Life Sciences 2001;70(5):603–614.
121. Weinreb O, et al. A novel approach of proteomics and transcriptomics to study the mechanism of action of the antioxidant–iron chelator green tea polyphenol (–)-epigallocatechin-3-gallate. Free Radical Biology and Medicine 2007;43(4):546–556.
122. Mandel S, et al. Green tea catechins as brain-permeable, natural iron chelators—antioxidants for the treatment of neurodegenerative disorders. Mol Nutr Food Res 2006;50(2):229–234.
123. Kuriyama S, et al. Green tea consumption and cognitive function: a cross-sectional study from the Tsurugaya Project. Am J Clin Nutr 2006;83(2):355–361.
124. Dhanasekaran M, et al. *Centella asiatica* extract selectively decreases amyloid beta levels in hippocampus of Alzheimer's disease animal model. Phytotherapy Research 2008;23(1):14–19.
125. Wattanathorn J, et al. Positive modulation of cognition and mood in the healthy elderly volunteer following the administration of *Centella asiatica*. Journal of Ethnopharmacology 2008;116(2):325–332.
126. McCarney R, et al. Homeopathy for dementia. Cochrane Database of Systematic Reviews 2003;(1):CD003803.

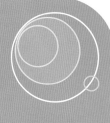

PART E
Integrative naturopathic practice

The worlds of naturopathy and conventional orthodox medicine are increasing merging as both sides develop appreciation for the other's respective strengths and awareness of their weaknesses. Naturopathic medicine provides time-tested temperate healing methods and interventions that are usually safe, while conventional medicine provides a stronger interventionist approach that is often required for serious medical conditions. The CAM approach to healing has the ability to effectively address chronic conditions (that are often lifestyle-based), while orthodox medicine is suited to addressing acute medical emergencies. In some conditions, medical diagnosis and intervention (such as pharmacotherapy or surgery) may be most effective, while the use of CAM interventions (herbal medicine, dietary and lifestyle modification or acupuncture) may enhance the healing process, prevent recurrence and improve the person's wellbeing.

The term 'integrative medicine' applies to different aspects of clinical practice. In many countries naturopaths have, or are gaining, new rights to study and practise medical-based techniques (or at the very least to refer for medical diagnosis). Legal factors (depending on the country) may, however, preclude some naturopaths from using many methods of conventional diagnosis and practice. Medical practitioners may desire to practise more 'integratively' or to use CAM products, while integrative practice may occur in a clinical setting, with various practitioners with diverse and complementing training practising together.

The potency of combining both approaches to the treatment of a patient is that the patient potentially benefits from the strengths of both paradigms. Regardless, a fundamental difference exists between these paradigms. A conventional medical practitioner that uses CAM products without an understanding of the core CAM principles is not practising integratively. True integrative medicine applies the principles of holistic medicine, not just the use of the product; it will incorporate an understanding to treat the underlying causes and the 'whole person'; will aim to use the least harmful interventions; and will seek to educate the patient by promoting prevention and the concept of wellbeing and vitality. This needs to occur via a therapeutic relationship that has adequate time to flourish.

The chapters contained within this part explore some key conditions that are ethically required to be treated with a conventional medical approach. This does not, however, preclude the use of naturopathic medicine in such cases, as the adjuvant use of CAM interventions often provides an effective supportive role. The diseases discussed—HIV, bipolar disorder, ADHD and chronic fatigue—are conditions that have a profoundly detrimental effect on society (and on the diagnosed individuals), and are all suited to an integrative approach. The final chapter is based on two vital areas that are often neglected in naturopathic education: how to practically address potential drug–CAM interactions; and pain management. Readers will note that the formatting of these chapters is slightly different to that of the preceding chapters in order to accommodate an integrative clinical approach.

33

Bipolar disorder with psychotic symptoms

James H. Lake
MD

EPIDEMIOLOGY, AETIOLOGY AND CLASSIFICATION

Bipolar disorder (BD) is a heritable mental illness. Approximately 1% of US adults experience persisting mood swings and fulfill criteria for a DSM-IV diagnosis of BD.[1] First-degree relatives of bipolar individuals are significantly more likely to develop the disorder than the population at large. Bipolar illness in one identical twin corresponds to a 70% risk that the other twin will also have the disorder and the concordance risk is estimated at 15% in non-identical twins.[2] Recent findings from genetic studies suggest that decreased expression of RNA coding for mitochondrial proteins results in dysregulations of energy metabolism in the brain, and especially in the hippocampus.[3] Dysregulations in hypothalamic circuits involved in maintaining normal circadian rhythms probably cause the affective and behavioural symptoms described in Western psychiatric nosology as bipolar disorder I and bipolar disorder II. It has been suggested that both phases of BD may be manifestations of chronic folate deficiency;[4] however, the aetiology of BD is varied and complex. Acutely manic patients frequently have abnormal EEG activity which may predict responsiveness to conventional pharmacological treatments.[5]

According to conventional Western psychiatric nosology, mania is a complex symptom pattern that may encompass disparate affective, behavioural and cognitive symptoms, including pressured speech, racing thoughts, euphoric or irritable mood, agitation, inflated self-esteem, distractibility, excessive or inappropriate involvement in pleasurable activities, increased goal-directed activity, diminished need for sleep and, in severe cases, psychosis.[6] According to the *DSM-IV-TR*,[6] a manic episode is diagnosed when elevated or irritable mood persists for at least 1 week, is accompanied by at least three of the above symptoms, is associated with severe social or occupational impairment, and cannot be adequately explained by a pre-existing medical or psychiatric disorder or the effects of substance abuse. In contrast to frank mania, the diagnosis of a hypomanic episode requires sustained irritable or euphoric mood lasting at least 4 days but does not cause severe impairment in social or occupational functioning; three or more of the above symptoms; and exclusion of medical or psychiatric disorders that may manifest as these symptoms. According to the *DSM-IV*, bipolar I is diagnosed when an individual has experienced one or more manic episodes, while one or more hypomanic episodes are required for a diagnosis of bipolar II disorder. Bipolar I disorder can be diagnosed after only one manic episode; however, the typical bipolar I patient has had several manic episodes, and at least 80% of patients who experience mania will have recurring manic episodes.[7] According to the *DSM-IV*, a history of depressive episodes is not required for a formal diagnosis of bipolar I disorder. In contrast, bipolar II disorder can be diagnosed only in cases when at least one hypomanic episode and at least one depressive episode have been documented. In both disorders moderate or severe depressive episodes typically alternate with manic symptoms; however, in 'mixed mania' symptoms of mania and depressed mood overlap. Another variant called rapid cycling is diagnosed when at least four complete cycles of depressed mood and mania occur during any 12-month period. A mild variant of bipolar disorder is called cyclothymic disorder. Cyclothymic disorder is diagnosed when several hypomanic and depressive episodes take place over a 2-year period in the absence of severe manic, mixed or depressive episodes. It is estimated that individuals diagnosed with bipolar I disorder are symptomatic approximately 50% of the time. Bipolar patients experience depressive symptoms three times more often than mania, and five times more often than rapid cycling or mixed episodes.[8]

Distinguishing between transient episodes of mania and acute agitation caused by a medical or psychiatric disorder can pose diagnostic challenges. A careful history is needed to establish a persisting pattern of mood changes fluctuating between depression and mania or hypomania. Conventional laboratory tests and functional brain imaging studies are used to rule out the presence of medical disorders that can mimic symptoms of depressed mood or mania including, for example, thyroid disease, strokes (especially in the right frontal area of the brain), multiple sclerosis, (rarely) seizure disorders, and other neurological disorders. Irritability or euphoria alternating with periods of depressed mood is also associated with chronic abuse of stimulants, marijuana or other drugs. It is often difficult to establish a primary diagnosis of bipolar disorder after ruling out pre-existing psychiatric or medical disorders because of the variety of symptoms that can take place during a manic episode. For example, symptoms of irritability, agitation and emotional lability are frequent concomitants of chronic drug or alcohol abuse, psychotic disorders and personality disorders. Ongoing debate over the construct validity of BD will probably result in new diagnostic criteria in the next edition of the *DSM*, which is scheduled for completion in 2012.[9] For example, it has been suggested that the 'rapid cycling' variant of bipolar disorder may more accurately correspond to a severe personality disorder than BD or other mood disorders.

RISK FACTORS

Several risk factors contribute to the rate of relapse and response to treatment in patients diagnosed with BD. A diagnosis of BD is one of the largest risk factors for suicide.[10] Fewer than half of patients who take conventional maintenance treatments following an initial manic episode report sustained control of their symptoms.[11] Furthermore, as many as 40% of bipolar patients who adhere to pharmacological treatment experience recurring manic or depressive mood swings while taking medications at recommended doses.[11] As many as one-quarter of bipolar I patients attempt suicide, and many eventually succeed. Treatment of bipolar disorder should be maintained on a consistent, long-term basis to reduce the rate of re-hospitalisation and increase chances of full remission.[12] Failure to initiate effective treatment that is well tolerated in the early stages of illness significantly increases the risk of relapse with associated increased risk of suicide.[13] In patients with diagnosed BD, stressors, seasonal change, reduced sleep and stimulants or recreational drug use may provoke an episode of hypomania or mania (although sometimes the trigger may not appear to have a cause).[14] Regular exercise, good nutrition, a strong social support network and a predictable, low-stress environment help reduce relapse risk.[15,16]

CONVENTIONAL TREATMENT

Medication management

The American Psychiatric Association endorses the use of different conventional pharmacological agents, including mood stabilisers (e.g. lithium carbonate and valproate), antidepressants, antipsychotics and sedative-hypnotics, to treat BD.[17] Antipsychotics are used to treat agitation and psychosis, which occur frequently in acute mania. Sedative hypnotics are prescribed for the severe insomnia that accompanies mania as well as for daytime management of agitation and anxiety.[18] A significant percentage of bipolar patients must rely on conventional antidepressants to control depressive mood swings. Repetitive transcranial magnetic stimulation (rTMS) is an emerging treatment of both the acute manic phase and the depressive phase of bipolar disorder and does not risk mania induction; however, findings of controlled trials to date are highly inconsistent.[19] Mania associated with psychosis is approached differently to a mixed episode that includes both manic and depressive symptoms. Conventional antipsychotics are appropriate first-line treatments of the auditory hallucinations that occur during an acute manic episode, while mixed episodes are often managed using a combination of two mood stabilisers or a mood stabiliser and antipsychotic.[14]

Psychotherapy and psychosocial interventions

Psychotherapy and psychosocial interventions in stable bipolar patients may potentially reduce relapse risk by providing psychological support, enhancing medication adherence, and helping patients address warning signs of recurring depressive or manic episodes before more serious symptoms emerge.[20] A review of randomised studies on adjunctive psychotherapy and psychosocial interventions in bipolar patients concluded that adjunctive psychotherapy reduces symptom severity and improves functioning.[20] Family therapy and interpersonal therapy were most effective in preventing relapse when started following an acute manic or depressive episode. Cognitive behavioural therapy and group psychoeducation were effective strategies for relapse prevention when initiated during stable periods. Psychotherapies and psychosocial interventions emphasising medication adherence and early recognition of mood symptoms were more effective in preventing recurrences of mania, and cognitive and interpersonal approaches had greater success in preventing depressive relapses. A specialised psychological intervention called 'enhanced relapse prevention' is aimed at recognising and managing the early warning signs of depressive or manic episodes by improving patients' understanding of BD, enhancing therapist–patient relationships, and optimising ongoing treatment. A study using qualitative interviews found that both therapists and their bipolar patients believe that enhanced relapse prevention increases awareness of early warning signs of recurring illness, leading to effective changes in medication management and fewer relapses.[21]

CLINICAL CONSIDERATIONS

- When patients present with depression, be aware that this may be a depressive phase of bipolar disorder.
- Always screen for the previous or current presence of hypomanic or manic signs.
- If involved in the management of a patient with bipolar hypomania or mania, be aware that a depressive phase may occur after the 'high' has resolved.

INTEGRATIVE MEDICAL DIAGNOSIS AND TREATMENT OPTIONS

A significant percentage of individuals diagnosed with bipolar disorder use non-pharmacological modalities together with prescription medications; however, there is relatively little evidence for the safety and efficacy of most non-conventional treatments.[22,23] The most appropriate and effective integrative treatment approach is determined by the type and severity of symptoms, the presence of comorbid medical or psychiatric disorders, response to previous treatments, patient preferences and constraints on cost and availability of treatments. When prominent symptoms of anxiety, psychosis or agitation are present, effective integrative strategies should prioritise treatment of those symptoms. For example, reasonable integrative approaches when managing an acutely manic patient who is agitated and extremely anxious include an initial loading dose of valproic acid or another conventional mood stabiliser, high potency benzodiazepines, an antipsychotic that is sedating (at bedtime), and possibly also amino acids known to have calming or sedating effects, such as L-tryptophan, 5-HTP or L-theanine.

INTEGRATIVE MEDICAL TREATMENT AIMS

- Confirm diagnosis of bipolar disorder and rule out comorbid psychiatric or medical disorders.
- Document conventional, CAM and integrative therapies that have already been tried.
- Identify core symptoms that will be the focus of clinical attention for treatment.
- Stabilise the patient as rapidly as possible, starting with conventional or integrative treatment protocols.
- Start with most validated conventional or integrative treatment protocols (see discussion below).
- When more substantiated modalities are not effective, consider less validated modalities with the patient's informed consent.
- After hypomania or mania has resolved, be aware of any relapse into a depressive phase and treat accordingly.

While CAM interventions appear to have limited activity in treating the hypomanic or manic phase of BD, they may have benefit in treating BD depression as monotherapies or as adjuvant treatments with synthetic antidepressants.[24]

Nutritional medicines

Adding **L-tryptophan** 2–3 g/day or 5-HTP 25 to 100 mg up to three times a day may have beneficial effects on anxiety associated with mania.[25,26] L-tryptophan 2 g can be safely added to mood stabilisers at bedtime and may improve sleep quality in agitated manic patients. Doses as high as 15 g may be required when insomnia is severe (although this should be closely monitored, and this dosage may be restricted in some countries).[27] When added to sedating antidepressants (such as trazodone) taken at bedtime L-tryptophan 2 g may accelerate antidepressant response and improve sleep quality.[28] Serious adverse effects have not been reported using this protocol. **L-theanine** reduces state anxiety by increasing alpha activity and increasing synthesis of GABA.[29,30] Noticeable anxiety reduction is generally achieved within 30 to 40 minutes and effective doses range between 200 mg and 800 mg/day.

Countries where there is high fish consumption have relatively lower prevalence rates of BD.[31] A systematic review of controlled trials on **omega-3 fatty acids** in BD that used rigorous inclusion criteria identified only one study in which omega-3s used adjunctively with a mood stabiliser showed a differential beneficial effect on depressive but not manic symptoms.[32] The reviewers cautioned that any conclusions about the efficacy of omega-3 fatty acids in bipolar disorder must await larger controlled studies of improved methodological quality. Large doses of omega-3 fatty acids may be more effective in the depressive phase of the illness.[33] Rare cases of increased bleeding times, but not increased risk of bleeding, have been reported in patients taking aspirin or anti-coagulants together with omega-3s. Some studies suggest that the omega-3 essential fatty acid EPA at doses between 1 and 4 g/day may have beneficial adjuvant effects when added to certain atypical antipsychotics;[34,35] however, one placebo-controlled trial did not confirm an adjuvant effect.[36] In contrast, the appropriate management of a severely depressed bipolar patient might include an integrative regimen that combines a mood stabiliser with an antidepressant and omega-3 fatty acids. Gradually titrating stable bipolar patients on a proprietary nutrient formula (see Table 33.1 for review of the evidence) while continuing them on their conventional mood stabiliser may result in improved outcomes, reductions in therapeutic doses in some cases, lower adverse effects rates and improved treatment adherence.

Magnesium may be an effective adjunctive therapy for treatment of acute mania or rapidly cycling bipolar disorder. In a small open trial, oral magnesium supplementation had comparable efficacy to lithium in rapid cycling bipolar patients.[37] In a small case series intravenous magnesium sulfate used adjunctively with lithium, haloperidol and a benzodiazepine in bipolar patients with severe treatment-resistant mania resulted in significant improvement in global functioning and reduction in the severity of mania.[38] Many patients treated with IV magnesium sulfate remained stable on lower doses of conventional medications.

A **proprietary 36-ingredient formula of vitamins and minerals** may significantly reduce symptoms of mania, depressed mood and psychosis in bipolar patients when taken alone or used adjunctively with conventional mood stabilisers.[39,40,41] Researchers believe the formula works by correcting inborn metabolic errors that result in bipolar-like symptoms in genetically predisposed individuals when certain micronutrients are deficient in the diet.[40] In one series, 11 bipolar patients who completed a 6-month protocol were able to reduce their conventional mood stabilisers by half while improving clinically. In another case series, 13 out of 19 bipolar patients who continued on the nutrient formula remained stable after discontinuing conventional mood stabilisers.[42] Some patients stopped taking the formula because of nausea and diarrhoea and three patients resumed conventional mood stabilisers because of recurring manic symptoms. Two randomised placebo-controlled double-blind studies are ongoing at the time of writing with the goal of determining whether the nutrient formula is an effective standalone treatment and identifying the most efficacious combination of nutrients and optimum dosing strategies for different phases of bipolar illness. Recent concerns have been raised over safety problems reported when the nutrient formula is taken together with a conventional mood stabiliser.[39]

Bipolar patients may be genetically susceptible to mood swings when certain amino acids are unavailable in the diet. Findings of two small randomised controlled trials (RCTs) suggest that certain **branch-chain amino acids** may rapidly improve acute mania by interfering with synthesis of norepinephrine and dopamine.[43,44] In one study 25 bipolar patients randomised to a special tyrosine-free amino acid drink (60 g/day) versus placebo experienced significant reductions in the severity of mania within 6 hours.[44] Improvements in mania were sustained with repeated administration of the amino acid drink. Restricting or excluding L-tryptophan from the diet may increase the susceptibility of bipolar patients to depressive mood swings; however, research findings to date are highly inconsistent.[45]

Choline is necessary for the biosynthesis of acetylcholine (Ach) and abnormal low brain levels of acetylcholine may cause some cases of mania.[46] Findings of a small RCT suggest that phosphatidylcholine (15 g to 30 g/day) may reduce the severity of mania and depressed mood in bipolar patients.[47] Findings of a RCT suggest that supplementation with **folic acid** 200 μg/day may enhance the beneficial effects of lithium carbonate in acutely manic patients.[4] Many case reports and case series suggest that choline (a B complex vitamin) reduces the severity of mania. It has been postulated that abnormal low brain levels of Ach are a primary cause of mania.[46] In a small case study of treatment-refractory, rapid-cycling bipolar patients who were taking lithium, four out of six people responded to the addition of 2000–7200 mg/day of free choline. It should be noted that two non-responders were also taking hypermetabolic doses of thyroid medication. Clinical improvement correlated with increased intensity of the basal ganglia choline signal as measured on proton magnetic resonance imaging (MRI). The effect of choline on depressive symptoms was variable.[47] Case reports, open trials and one small double-blind study suggest that supplementation with phosphatidylcholine 15 g to 30 g/day reduces the severity of both mania and depressed mood in bipolar patients, and that symptoms recur when phosphatidylcholine is discontinued.[46,47] Findings of a double-blind study suggest that folic acid 200 μg/day may enhance the beneficial effects of lithium carbonate in acutely manic patients.[4,48]

Findings of a small open study suggest that patients diagnosed with bipolar disorder who exhibit mania or depressed mood respond to low doses (50 μg with each meal) of a natural lithium preparation.[49] Posttreatment serum lithium levels were undetectable in patients who responded to **trace lithium supplementation**. Findings of a small pilot study suggest that magnesium supplementation 40 mEq/day may be as effective as lithium in the treatment of rapidly cycling bipolar patients.[37]

Findings from animal research and a small open study suggest that bipolar patients who take **potassium** 20 mEq twice daily with their conventional lithium therapy experience fewer side effects, including tremor, compared to patients who take lithium alone.[50] No changes in serum lithium levels were reported in patients taking potassium. Pending confirmation of these findings by a larger double-blind trial, potassium supplementation may provide a safe, cost-effective integrative approach for the management of bipolar patients who are unable to tolerate therapeutic doses of lithium due to tremor and other adverse effects. Patients who have cardiac arrhythmias or are taking antiarrhythmic medications should consult with their physicians before considering taking a potassium supplementation.

Herbal medicines

A meta-analysis of placebo-controlled trials comparing ***Hypericum perforatum*** to placebo or conventional antidepressants suggests that hypericum and standard antidepressants have similar beneficial effects.[51] This herb may be beneficial in the depressive phase of BD; however, no studies on this have currently been conducted. Several case reports of mania induction with *H. perforatum*[52,53] and potential serious interactions with many drugs[54] have resulted in limited use of this herbal for the treatment of BD. Findings of a large 12-week placebo-controlled trial suggest that a **proprietary Chinese compound herbal formula** consisting of at least 11 herbals may be a beneficial adjuvant of conventional mood stabilisers for treatment of the depressive phase of bipolar disorder.[55] Bipolar depressed (but not manic) patients randomised to the herbal formula plus a conventional mood stabiliser experienced significantly greater reductions in the severity of depressed mood compared to matched patients receiving a mood stabiliser only. These findings were replicated in a subsequent study, which confirmed that bipolar depressed patients treated with the herbal formula only improved more than patients treated with a placebo.[56] Early studies suggested that the Ayurvedic herbal ***Rauwolfia serpentina*** was an effective treatment of bipolar disorder that augmented the antimanic efficacy of lithium without risk of toxic interactions.[57,58] However, use of this herbal in Western countries is now very restricted because of safety concerns.

Therapeutic considerations

Conventional pharmacological treatments of the depressive and manic phases of BD have a mixed record of success. This is due to both high rates of treatment discontinuation and limited efficacy when treatment is adhered to. Furthermore, less severe symptoms of mania are often unreported or mis-diagnosed as anxiety disorders or sleep disorders, resulting in erroneous diagnoses of agitated depressed mood or other psychiatric disorder and, subsequently, inappropriate and ineffective treatment.[59] Fewer

Case Study

A 29-year-old single unemployed woman presents with diagnosed **bipolar type I disorder**. About 1 month ago, shortly following a suicide attempt, she was psychiatrically hospitalised, and found to be acutely **manic and psychotic**. In the emergency room she was found to be **paranoid**, and was internally preoccupied and was hearing voices. Her mood was **euphoric** and she had been unable to sleep for 1 week. Her **speech was pressured, her thoughts were racing** and her **thought process was derailed**. After being diagnosed with bipolar disorder I, she started on a conventional mood stabiliser and an atypical antipsychotic. After 3 days she was discharged without acute manic or psychotic symptoms. Three months later she presents with **moderate depression** and wishes to find a 'natural way' to reduce her medication and improve her wellbeing and mental health.

SUGGESTIVE SYMPTOMS

- Diminished need for sleep
- Euphoric or agitated mood
- Racing thoughts
- Flight of ideas (grandiosity)
- Talks excessively
- Inappropriate sexual behaviour
- Spends excessively beyond means
- May experience auditory hallucinations or frank delusions depending on severity
- May experience depressive mood symptoms concurrently (so-called 'mixed' state)

than half of patients who take conventional maintenance treatments following an initial manic episode report sustained control of their symptoms.[60] Furthermore, as many as 40% of bipolar patients who adhere to pharmacological treatment experience recurring manic or depressive mood swings while taking medications at recommended doses.[61] Only about half of all conventional medications used to treat BD are supported by strong evidence.[62] As many as half of all bipolar patients who take mood stabilisers do not experience good control of their symptoms or refuse to take medications, and approximately 50% discontinue their medications because of serious adverse effects including tremor, weight gain, elevated liver enzymes and others.[63] Due to this CAM therapies may have a potential role in improving quality of life, reducing side effects and improving compliance.

A significant percentage of bipolar patients relapse while taking conventional mood stabilisers for long-term maintenance. A systematic review of RCTs comparing valproic acid with lithium carbonate and other mood stabilisers found that valproic acid has equivocal efficacy as a long-term maintenance therapy of BD.[64] A systematic review of placebo-controlled trials of adjunctive pharmacological treatments of bipolar disorder concluded that combining a mood stabiliser with a conventional antidepressant does not improve outcomes compared to outcomes obtained with a single mood stabiliser.[65] An emerging conventional treatment of BD, repetitive transcranial magnetic stimulation (rTMS), may be an effective treatment of the depressive phase of BD; however, the findings of sham-controlled trials are inconsistent.[66,67]

Example treatment

Due to the patient being diagnosed with bipolar I, an integrative treatment plan that includes pharmaceutical medication is required. Lithium carbonate and a sedating atypical antipsychotic (at bedtime) are example synthetic treatments for BP I, while omega-3 essential fatty acids, a B-vitamin complex (high in folic acid) may provide adjuvant support. Preliminary evidence suggests that listening to soothing music or binaural sounds can also signifi-

> **Pre-prescribed pharmaceuticals**
>
> Lithium carbonate 1200 mg
> Risperidone 4 mg
>
> **Adjuvant prescription**
>
> Omega-3 fatty acids 3 g BD
> (EPA 1 g/DHA 0.8 g per day)
> High-potency B-complex including 500 µg of folic acid

cantly reduce symptoms of anxiety.[68,69] Consideration of antidepressant medications (natural or synthetic) may be advised to treat her depression; however, she would be needed to be closely monitored for potential 'switching' to a manic phase. If her sleep pattern is poor, various herbal or nutritional interventions in addition to sleep hygiene advice may be of benefit (see the case in Chapter 14 on insomnia).

Expected outcomes and follow-up protocols

When approaching an acutely manic patient the principal treatment goals are patient safety and rapid stabilisation, frequently requiring psychiatric hospitalisation. Atypical antipsychotics are probably the most effective and efficient conventional treatments of severe mania and accompanying psychosis, and generally result in stabilisation within hours or days. 'Loading' a manic patient with a conventional mood stabiliser (such as lithium or valproic acid) to rapidly achieve a therapeutic serum level is an effective strategy for the management of acute mania. Omega-3 fatty acids can be used adjunctively during the initial stages of treatment and may permit lower effective doses of

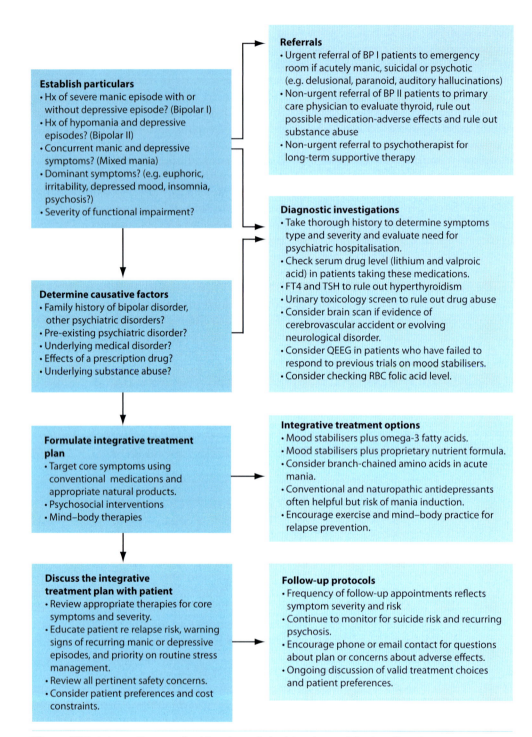

Establish particulars
- Hx of severe manic episode with or without depressive episode? (Bipolar I)
- Hx of hypomania and depressive episodes? (Bipolar II)
- Concurrent manic and depressive symptoms? (Mixed mania)
- Dominant symptoms? (e.g. euphoric, irritability, depressed mood, insomnia, psychosis?)
- Severity of functional impairment?

Referrals
- Urgent referral of BP I patients to emergency room if acutely manic, suicidal or psychotic (e.g. delusional, paranoid, auditory hallucinations)
- Non-urgent referral of BP II patients to primary care physician to evaluate thyroid, rule out possible medication-adverse effects and rule out substance abuse
- Non-urgent referral to psychotherapist for long-term supportive therapy

Diagnostic investigations
- Take thorough history to determine symptoms type and severity and evaluate need for psychiatric hospitalisation.
- Check serum drug level (lithium and valproic acid) in patients taking these medications.
- FT4 and TSH to rule out hyperthyroidism
- Urinary toxicology screen to rule out drug abuse
- Consider brain scan if evidence of cerebrovascular accident or evolving neurological disorder.
- Consider QEEG in patients who have failed to respond to previous trials on mood stabilisers.
- Consider checking RBC folic acid level.

Determine causative factors
- Family history of bipolar disorder, other psychiatric disorders?
- Pre-existing psychiatric disorder?
- Underlying medical disorder?
- Effects of a prescription drug?
- Underlying substance abuse?

Formulate integrative treatment plan
- Target core symptoms using conventional medications and appropriate natural products.
- Psychosocial interventions
- Mind–body therapies

Integrative treatment options
- Mood stabilisers plus omega-3 fatty acids.
- Mood stabilisers plus proprietary nutrient formula.
- Consider branch-chained amino acids in acute mania.
- Conventional and naturopathic antidepressants often helpful but risk of mania induction.
- Encourage exercise and mind–body practice for relapse prevention.

Discuss the integrative treatment plan with patient
- Review appropriate therapies for core symptoms and severity.
- Educate patient re relapse risk, warning signs of recurring manic or depressive episodes, and priority on routine stress management.
- Review all pertinent safety concerns.
- Consider patient preferences and cost constraints.

Follow-up protocols
- Frequency of follow-up appointments reflects symptom severity and risk
- Continue to monitor for suicide risk and recurring psychosis.
- Encourage phone or email contact for questions about plan or concerns about adverse effects.
- Ongoing discussion of valid treatment choices and patient preferences.

Figure 33.1 Integrative medical treatment decision tree—bipolar disorder

Table 33.1 Review of the major evidence

INTERVENTION	METHODOLOGY	RESULT	COMMENT
Omega-3 fatty acids	Systematic review of five RCTs on omega-3s in bipolar disorder[32]	Only one adjunctive study found differential beneficial effect over placebo for depressive but not manic symptoms.	Possibly beneficial for BP depression. No efficacy in BP mania. Uneven quality of studies. Need larger controlled studies with improved quality.
Magnesium	RCT oral magnesium as adjunctive to verapamil (n = 20, adults with mania)[70]	Greater improvement with magnesium than placebo; verapamil + magnesium group improved more than verapamil + placebo	Large prospective trials needed
	Open trial magnesium vs lithium (n = 9, adults with rapid cycling)[37]	Beneficial effects in 7 patients	Oral magnesium and lithium had equivalent effects in over half of patients
	Small case series IV magnesium sulfate with lithium, haloperidol and a benzodiazepine in bipolar patients with severe treatment-resistant mania.[38]	Resulted in significant improvement in global functioning and reduction in the severity of mania.[38]	Many patients treated with IV magnesium sulfate remained stable on lower doses of conventional medications.
Proprietary 36-ingredient nutrient formula	Case series (n = 11, adults)[40] Case series (n = 22, children and adults)[39]	Improvement in both depressive and manic symptoms; some patients stable on reduced doses of mood stabilisers	Large prospective trials needed Some subjects discontinue treatment due to recurring mania
	Case series (n = 19, adults)[41]	Improvement in 19; 11 of 15 previously on medications remained stable without them Improvement in 16; 13 remained stable off conventional mood stabilisers	Adverse effects causing drop out include nausea and diarrhoea Safety problems reported when nutrient formula is taken with conventional mood stabiliser
Branch chain amino acids	RCT (n = 25) special tyrosine-free amino acid drink (60 g/day) vs placebo[44]	Significant reductions in mania within 6 hours; sustained with continued use	Large prospective trials needed
Choline and phosphatidyl-choline	Small RCT phosphatidylcholine (15 g to 30 g/day)[47]	May reduce the severity of mania and depressed mood in bipolar patients	Large prospective trials needed
Folic acid	RCT folic acid 200 μg/day + lithium vs lithium alone[4]	Differential improvement over lithium alone in acute mania	Large prospective trials needed

mood stabilisers, reduced incidence of treatment-emergent adverse effects and improved medication compliance over the long term. Residual symptoms of insomnia can be managed using melatonin, improved sleep hygiene and guided imagery. Regular exercise and a mind–body practice provide a healthy preventative framework for bipolar patients. After stabilisation has been achieved with conventional medications it may be possible to gradually reduce doses of conventional medications in bipolar patients who are responding to adjunctive therapies, including a proprietary multinutrient formula and omega-3 essential fatty acids. In such cases, clinical management decisions should always be made in the context of close monitoring for treatment-emergent adverse effects or interactions, and warning signs of recurring manic or depressive episodes. Ongoing psychoeducation or psychosocial interventions enhance treatment adherence and help bipolar patients recognise and respond to early warning signs of relapse.

KEY POINTS

- Diverse genetic and metabolic factors probably contribute to the pathogenesis of bipolar disorder.
- Conventional pharmacological treatments of bipolar disorder have limited efficacy and significant safety issues, resulting in high rates of non-response, partial response and medication non-compliance.
- Emerging evidence suggests that omega-3 fatty acids play an important adjunctive role and may be an effective stand alone therapy in some cases of bipolar illness.
- Preliminary findings suggest that a proprietary nutrient formula may be an effective adjunctive therapy for bipolar disorder in combination with mood stabilisers; however, large RCTs are required to confirm efficacy claims and potentially serious safety issues need to be addressed before integrative regimens that include the formula can be generally recommended in bipolar disorder.
- Certain branch chained amino acids (IV or oral), magnesium, choline and *Hypericum perforatum* may be beneficial in some cases of bipolar disorder. More studies are needed.
- Regular exercise, relaxation training, yoga or other mind–body practices may help reduce relapse risk in some cases of bipolar disorder.

Further reading

American Psychiatric Association. Practice guidelines for treatment of patients with bipolar disorder. Am J Psychiatry 1994;151(12, Supplement): iv, 1–36.

Andreescu C, et al. Complementary and alternative medicine in the treatment of bipolar disorder—a review of the evidence. Journal of Affective Disorders 2008;110(1):16–26.

Lake J. Textbook of integrative mental health care. New York: Thieme Medical Publishers, 2006.

Sarris J, et al. Adjuvant use of nutritional and herbal medicines with antidepressants, mood stabilisers and benzodiazepines. Journal of Psychiatric Research 2009; 44(1):32–41.

References

1. Robins L, Regier D, eds. Psychiatric disorders in America: the epidemiologic catchment area study. New York: Free Press, 1991.
2. Gurling H. Linkage findings in bipolar disorder Nat Genet 1995;8–9:10.
3. Konradi C, et al. Molecular evidence for mitochondrial dysfunction in bipolar disorder. Arch Gen Psychiatry 2004;61: 300–308.
4. Hasanah CI, et al. Reduced red-cell folate in mania. Journal of Affective Disorders 1997;46:95–99.
5. Small JG, et al. Topographic EEG studies of mania. Clinical Electroencephalography 1998;29(2):59–66.
6. American Psychiatric Association. Diagnostic and statistical manual of mental disorders. 4th edn. Arlington: American Psychiatric Association, 2000.
7. Winokur G, et al. Manic depressive illness. St Louis: C.V. Mosby, 1969.
8. Judd L, et al. The long-term natural history of the weekly symptomatic status of bipolar I disorder. Arch Gen Psychiatry 2002;59(6):530–537.
9. Vieta E, Phillips ML. Deconstructing bipolar disorder: a critical review of its diagnostic validity and a proposal for DSM-V and ICD-11. Schizophr Bull 2007;33(4):886–892.
10. Ilgen MA, et al. A collaborative therapeutic relationship and risk of suicidal ideation in patients with bipolar disorder. J Affect Disord 2008;115(1):246–251.
11. Culver JL, et al. Bipolar disorder: improving diagnosis and optimizing integrated care. J Clin Psychol 2007;63(1):73–92.
12. Perlick DA, et al. Symptoms predicting inpatient service use among patients with bipolar affective disorder. Psychiatr Serv 1999;50(6):806–812.
13. Altamura AC, Goikolea JM. Differential diagnoses and management strategies in patients with schizophrenia and bipolar disorder. Neuropsychiatr Dis Treat 2008;4(1):311–317.

14. Miklowitz DJ, Johnson SL. The psychopathology and treatment of bipolar disorder. Annu Rev Clin Psycholz 2006;2:199–235.
15. Benjamin AB. A unique consideration regarding medication compliance for bipolar affective disorder: exercise performance. Bipolar Disord 2007;9(8):928–929.
16. Lakhan SE, Vieira KF. Nutritional therapies for mental disorders. Nutr J 2008;21(7):2.
17. American Psychiatric Association. Practice guidelines. Treatment of patients with bipolar disorder. 7th edn. Available: http://www.psychiatryonline.com/pracGuide/pracGuideTopic_8.aspx
18. Cousins DA, Young AH. The armamentarium of treatments for bipolar disorder: a review of the literature. Int J Neuropsychopharmacol 2007;10(3):411–413.
19. Rodriguez-Martin JL, et al. Transcranial magnetic stimulation for treating depression. Cochrane Depression Anxiety and Eurosis Group. Cochrane Database Syst Rev 2001;(4):CD003493.
20. Miklowitz DJ. Adjunctive psychotherapy for bipolar disorder: state of the evidence. Am J Psychiatry 2008;165(11):1408–1419.
21. Pontin E, et al. Enhanced relapse prevention for bipolar disorder: a qualitative investigation of value perceived for service users and care coordinators. Implement Sci 2009;9(4):4.
22. Ernst E. Complementary medicine: where is the evidence? J Fam Pract 2003;52:630–634.
23. Dennehy E, et al. Self-reported participation in non-pharmacologic treatments for bipolar disorder. Journal of Clinical Psychiatry 2004;65(2):278.
24. Sarris J, et al. Adjuvant use of nutritional and herbal medicines with antidepressants, mood stabilizers and benzodiazepines. Journal of Psychiatric Research 2009:In press.
25. Soderpalm B, Engel JA. erotonergic involvement in conflict behavior. Eur Neuropsychopharmacol 1990;1(1):7–13.
26. Kahn RS, et al. Effect of a serotonin precursor and uptake inhibitor in anxiety disorders; a double-blind comparison of 5 hydroxytryptophan, clomipramine, and placebo. Int Clin Psychopharmacol 1987,2(1):33–45.
27. Schneider-Helmert D, Spinweber CL. Evaluation of L-tryptophan for treatment of insomnia: a review. Psychopharmacology (Berl) 1986;89(1):1–7.
28. Levitan RD, et al. Preliminary randomized double-blind placebo-controlled trial of tryptophan combined with fluoxetine to treat major depressive disorder: antidepressant and hypnotic effects. Journal of Psychiatry and Neuroscience 2000;4:337–346.
29. Kakuda T, et al. Inhibiting effects of theanine on caffeine stimulation evaluated by EEG in the rat. Biosci Biotechno Biochem 2000;64:287–293.
30. Mason R. 200 mg of Zen; L-theanine boosts alpha waves, promotes alert relaxation. Alternative and Complementary Therapies 2001;7:91–95.
31. Hibbeln JR. Seafood consumption, the DHA content of mothers' milk and prevalence rates of postpartum depression: a cross-national, ecological analysis. J Affect Disord 2002;69:15–29.
32. Montgomery P, Richardson AJ. Omega-3 fatty acids for bipolar disorder. Cochrane Depression, Anxiety and Neurosis Group. Cochrane Database Syst Rev 2008;(2):CD005169.
33. Chiu CC, et al. Omega-3 fatty acids are more beneficial in the depressive phase than in the manic phase in patients with bipolar I disorder. J Clin Psychiatry 2005;66:1613–1614.
34. Emsley R, et al. Randomized, placebo-controlled study of ethyl-eicosapentaenoic acid as supplemental treatment in schizophrenia. Am J Psychiatry 2002;1859:1596–1598.
35. Peet M, Horrobin DF. (E-E Multicentre Study Group). A dose-ranging exploratory study of the effects of ethyl-eicosapentaenoate in patients with persistent schizophrenic symptoms. J Psychiatr Res 2002;36(1):7–18.
36. Fenton WS, et al. A placebo-controlled trial of omega-3 fatty acid (ethyl eicosapentaenoic acid) supplementation for residual symptoms and cognitive impairment in schizophrenia. Am J Psychiatry 2001;158(12):2071–2073.
37. Chouinard G, et al. A pilot study of magnesium aspartate hydrochloride (Magnesiocard) as a mood stabilizer for rapid cycling bipolar affective disorder patients. Progress in Neuropsychopharmacology Biology and Psychiatry 1990;4:171–180.
38. Heiden A, et al. Treatment of severe mania with intravenous magnesium sulphate as a supplementary therapy. Psychiatry Res 1999;89(3):239–246.
39. Popper C. Do vitamins or minerals (apart from lithium) have mood-stabilizing effects? J Clin Psychiatry 2001;62(12):933–935.
40. Kaplan BJ, et al. Effective mood stabilization with a chelated mineral supplement: an open-label trial in bipolar disorder. J Clin Psychiatry 2001;62:936–944.
41. Simmons M. Nutritional approach to bipolar disorder [Letter to the editor]. Jour Clin Psychiatry 2002;64:338.
42. Simmons M. Nutritional approach to bipolar disorder. Journal of Clinical Psychiatry 2003;64(3):338.
43. Barrett S, Leyton M. Acute phenylalanine/tyrosine depletion: a new method to study the role of catecholamines in psychiatric disorders. Primary Psychiatry 2004;11(6):37–41.
44. Scarna A, et al. Effects of a branched-chain amino acid drink in mania. British Journal of Psychiatry 2003;182:210–213.
45. Hughes J, et al. Effects of acute tryptophan depletion on cognitive function in euthymic bipolar patients. Eur Neuropsychopharmacology 2002;12(2):123–128.
46. Leiva D. The neurochemistry of mania: a hypothesis of etiology and rationale for treatment. Prog Neuropsychopharmacol Biol Psychiatry 1990;14(3):423–429.
47. Stoll AL, et al. Choline in the treatment of rapid-cycling bipolar disorder: clinical and neurochemical findings in lithium-treated patients. Biol Psychiatry 1996;40:382–388.
48. Coppen A, et al. Folic acid enhances lithium prophylaxis. Journal of Affective Disorders 1986;10(1):9–13.
49. Fierro A. Natural low dose lithium supplementation in manic-depressive disease. Nutr Perspectives 1988:10–11.
50. Tripuraneni B. Clin Psychiatry News 1990;18(10):3: presented to the 143rd Annual Meeting of the American Psychiatric Association, 12–17 May 1990, abstracts NR 100 and NR 210.
51. Linde K, et al. St John's wort for major depression. Cochrane Database Syst Rev 2008;(4):CD000448.
52. Moses EL, Mallinger AG. St. John's Wort: three cases of possible mania induction. J Clin Psychopharmacol 2000;20(1):115–117.
53. Fahmi M, et al. A case of mania induced by hypericum. World J Biol Psychiatry 2002;3(1):58–59.
54. Izzo AA. Drug interactions with St. John's Wort (Hypericum perforatum): a review of the clinical evidence. Int J Clin Pharmacol Ther 2004;42(3):139–148.
55. Zhang ZJ, et al. Adjunctive herbal medicine with carbamazepine for bipolar disorders: a double-blind, randomized, placebo-controlled study. J Psychiatr Res 2007;41(3–4):360–369.
56. Zhang ZJ, et al. The beneficial effects of the herbal medicine Free and Easy Wanderer Plus (FEWP) for mood disorders: double-blind, placebo-controlled studies. J Psychiatr Res 2007;41:828–836.
57. Bacher NM, Lewis HA. Lithium plus reserpine in refractory manic patients. Am J Psychiatry 1979;136(6):811–814.
58. Berlant JL. Neuroleptics and reserpine in refractory psychoses. J Clin Psychopharmacol 1986;6(3):180–184.
59. Benazzi F. Prevalence of bipolar II disorder in outpatient depression: a 203-case study in private practice. J Affect Disord 1997;43(2):163–166.

60. Tohen M, et al. Outcome in mania: a 4-year prospective follow-up on 75 patients utilizing survival analysis. Arch Gen Psychiatry 1990;47:1106–1111.

61. Strober M, et al. Relapse following discontinuation of lithium maintenance therapy in adolescents with bipolar I illness: a naturalistic study. Am J of Psychiatry 1990;147:457–461.

62. Boschert S. Evidence-based treatment largely ignored in bipolar disorder. Clinical Psychiatry News June 2004;1.

63. Fleck DE, et al. Factors associated with medication adherence in African American and white patients with bipolar disorder. J Clin Psychiatry 2005;66:646–652.

64. Macritchie KA, et al. Valproic acid, valproate and divalproex in the maintenance treatment of bipolar disorder. Cochrane Depression, Anxiety and Neurosis Group Cochrane Database Syst Rev 2008;(3):CD003196.

65. Ghaemi SN, et al. Effectiveness and safety of long-term antidepressant treatment in bipolar disorder. Journal of Clinical Psychiatry 2001;62(7):565–569.

66. Nahas Z, et al. Left prefrontal transcranial magnetic stimulation (TMS) treatment of depression in bipolar affective disorder: a pilot study of acute safety and efficacy. Bipolar Disorders 2003;5(1):40–47.

67. Kaptsan A, et al. Right prefrontal TMS versus sham treatment of mania: a controlled study. Bipolar Disorders 2003;5(1):36–39.

68. Kerr T, et al. Emotional change processes in music-assisted reframing. Journal of Music Therapy 2001;38(3):193–211.

69. Atwater, F. The Hemi-Sync process. Research Division, The Monroe Institute, 1999. Online. Available: http://store.hemisyncforyou.com/v/hemisync-cd-process.html

70. Giannini AJ, et al. Magnesium oxide augmentation of verapamil maintenance therapy in mania. Psychiatry Research 2000;93:83–87.

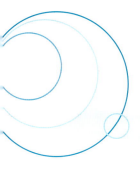

34
Attention deficit and hyperactivity disorder (ADHD)

James H. Lake
MD

EPIDEMIOLOGY, AETIOLOGY AND CLASSIFICATION

The worldwide prevalence rate of attention deficit and hyperactivity disorder (ADHD) has been estimated at between 2 and 29%.[1] The rate at which ADHD is diagnosed and treated in both children and adults has dramatically increased since the syndrome was first recognised as a specific disorder in the *Diagnostic and Statistical Manual of Mental Disorders* (DSM) in the 1970s. In the United States of America as many as 10% of males and 4% of females have been diagnosed with ADHD.[2] An objective epidemiological or scientific basis for the rapidly increasing prevalence of ADHD in general and the higher incidence of the syndrome in boys compared to girls is highly controversial and may reflect social issues and changes in diagnostic criteria more than actual changes in prevalence rates.[3]

The causes of ADHD are multifactorial. Data from twin studies show that ADHD is a highly heritable disorder[4] and the risk of developing this disorder is probably influenced by genes that affect CNS transport of dopamine and serotonin.[5] Other causes of ADHD include problems associated with premature birth, birth trauma, childhood illness and environmental toxins.[6] Increased risk of ADHD is associated with in-utero exposure to alcohol, tobacco smoke and lead. Up to 20% of ADHD cases are probably caused by brain injury around the time of birth. Certain food preservatives exacerbate the symptoms of ADHD, but probably do not actually cause the disorder.[7] Some cases of ADHD may be associated with delayed development of certain areas of the frontal and temporal lobes and relatively rapid maturation of motor areas of the brain.[8] Children diagnosed with ADHD frequently experience disturbed sleep including restlessness, sleep walking, night terrors and restless leg syndrome; however, a causal relationship between sleep disorders and

ADHD has not been clearly established.[9] Early childhood neglect or abuse probably also increase the risk of developing ADHD. Most cases of ADHD probably result from multiple genetic, developmental, physiological, environmental and psychosocial factors.[10]

With respect to diagnosis, according to the DSM a diagnosis of ADHD requires the presence of at least six symptoms of hyperactivity or inattention that begin before the age of 7 years, persist for at least 6 months, are maladaptive, inconsistent with the child's development level, and are not better explained by a pre-existing medical or psychiatric disorder. Specific symptoms of inattention may include careless mistakes in schoolwork, difficulty sustaining attention in school-related tasks or play, failure to follow through with instructions, difficulty organising tasks and activities, reluctance to engage in tasks requiring sustained attention, and being distracted easily by extraneous stimuli. Specific symptoms of hyperactivity or impulsivity may include fidgeting with hands or feet or squirming while sitting, frequently getting up in a classroom or other situation in which remaining seated is expected, running or moving in inappropriate or disruptive ways, or (in adults) subjective 'feelings of restlessness', difficulty engaging in quiet leisure activities and talking excessively.

Three subtypes of ADHD are recognised in the DSM, depending on the type and severity of symptoms:
1. predominantly inattentive type
2. predominantly hyperactive type
3. combined type (inattentive and hyperactive).

Symptoms of inattention, impulsivity or hyperactivity must cause clinically significant impairment in at least two spheres including social, academic or occupational functioning. Neuropsychological testing is frequently employed to assess inattention, processing speed and neurocognitive deficits. A diagnosis of ADHD should be made in childhood only after other childhood disorders, including pervasive developmental disorders, learning disorders and anxiety disorders, have been ruled out.[11] Many children diagnosed with ADHD also meet criteria for conduct disorder. When evaluating adults a thorough medical history is important to rule out medical or psychiatric disorders that mimic symptoms or functional impairments that resemble ADHD. These include, for example, bipolar disorder, absence seizures, hypothyroidism, obsessive-compulsive disorder and chronic sleep deprivation.[12]

RISK FACTORS

The hyperactivity of ADHD often resolves by late adolescence or adulthood; however, symptoms of distractibility may not lessen with age. It has been estimated that fewer than one-fifth of adults with ADHD have been correctly diagnosed and appropriately treated, resulting in significant social and occupational risk. ADHD is highly comorbid with oppositional-defiant disorder and learning disorders in children, and with major depressive disorder, anxiety disorders and substance abuse in adults.[13] It has been estimated that almost half of individuals diagnosed with ADHD never graduate from high school and fewer than 5% complete a 4-year university degree program.[14] The high prevalence rate of ADHD significantly affects employment statistics. A large population survey of US adults found that a diagnosis of ADHD was associated with 35 days of lost work on average. Extrapolating these findings to the population suggests that US$19 billion in lost productivity and 120 million lost work days annually are attributable to ADHD.[15]

CONVENTIONAL TREATMENT

Stimulant medications are the standard Western treatment of ADHD; however, SSRIs and other antidepressants are also used with varying degrees of success. Extended-release forms of stimulants are better tolerated and less often lead to abuse. Approximately one-third of children and adolescents who take stimulants experience significant adverse effects, including abdominal pain, decreased appetite and insomnia, and 10% experience serious adverse effects.[16] Because stimulants are classified as scheduled or restricted medications (depending on the country), prescriptions are usually limited to a short supply; this can result in treatment interruptions and transient symptomatic worsening when refills are not obtained on time. One-third of all individuals who take stimulants for ADHD report significant adverse effects, including insomnia, decreased appetite and abdominal pain.[16] Sporadic cases of stimulant-induced psychosis have been reported.[17] Neurotoxic effects associated with long-term stimulant use have not been fully elucidated; however, chronic amphetamine use in childhood is associated with slowing in growth. Stimulants and other conventional treatments of adulthood ADHD may be only half as effective as they are in children.[13]

Short-acting stimulants are the most prescribed conventional treatments of adult ADHD. Controlled-release stimulants, buproprion and the SSRI antidepressants are being increasingly used in the adult ADHD population; however, research findings suggest these medications may not be as efficacious as fast-released stimulants.[18] The non-stimulant medication atomoxetine has less potential for abuse, but may not be as efficacious as stimulants.[19] Although atomoxetine is the only non-amphetamine medication approved by the US Food and Drug Administration for the treatment of childhood ADHD, there are growing concerns about its adverse effects, including hypertension, tachycardia, nausea and vomiting, liver toxicity and possibly increased suicide risk.[20,21] In Australia atomoxetine is registered for use by the Therapeutic Goods Administration.

Growing concerns about inappropriate or over-prescribing by physicians of stimulant medications and incomplete understanding of risks associated with their long-term use have led to increasing acceptance of emerging non-conventional therapies.[22,23] In addition to conventional prescription medications, behavioural modification is a widely used conventional treatment of ADHD in children. Psychotherapy and psychosocial support help reduce the anxiety and feelings of loss of control that frequently accompany ADHD.

INTEGRATIVE MEDICAL DIAGNOSIS AND TREATMENT OPTIONS

Many individuals diagnosed with ADHD use alternative therapies alone or adjunctively with conventional pharmacological treatments.[24] Over half of parents of children diagnosed with ADHD treat their children's symptoms using one or more CAM therapies, including vitamins, dietary changes and expressive therapies, but few disclose this to their child's paediatrician.[25] Most CAM therapies for ADHD are supported by limited evidence; however, when any herbal or other naturopathic therapy is used to treat ADHD it is regarded as the primary treatment over 80% of the time.[25] Appropriate CAM and integrative treatment strategies for ADHD will depend on the subtype of ADHD that is being addressed, symptom severity, previous treatment outcomes using conventional or CAM modalities, adverse effect issues, psychiatric or medical comorbidities, patient preferences, the availability of qualified CAM practitioners and access to reputable brands of specific supplements. Dietary modifications, including reduced sugar and caffeine intake and specialised restrictive diets, are reasonable first-line strategies in ADHD-diagnosed children who are predominantly hyperactive. There are no contraindications to taking stimulant medications while following a restrictive diet; however, parents of ADHD children should first consult their child's paediatrician before initiating a strict dietary regimen, and ideally with a nutritionist who can provide them with expert guidance. Preliminary findings suggest that omega-3 essential fatty acids in doses up to 16 g/day are effective adjuvants when combined with stimulants for both hyperactivity and inattention; however, more studies are needed to confirm this. Preliminary findings suggest that a standardised extract of the bark of the French maritime pine tree may be beneficial in some cases of ADHD; however, it is not clear whether this product has adjunctive benefits when combined with stimulants. Zinc supplementation may enhance the efficacy of prescription stimulants permit-

> ### INTEGRATIVE MEDICAL TREATMENT AIMS
>
> Confirm the diagnosis of ADHD, including symptoms starting in childhood, and rule out underlying primary psychiatric or medical causes:
>
> - Take a complete history to determine the possible relationship between diet, food allergies and so on (including food colourings or additives) and ADHD symptoms.
> - Document conventional and CAM treatments (including doses, durations and brands of natural products) that have been tried, including patient's response and adverse effects.
> - Develop an integrative treatment plan with the patient (or parent if the patient is younger than 18 years), including dietary changes if appropriate, behavioural therapy and psychosocial interventions, the use of select nutrients (such as essential fatty acids), trace elements, homoeopathic remedies and EEG biofeedback.
> - Monitor symptoms using standardised symptom-rating scales and modify the treatment plan using conventional or CAM modalities until consistent improvement is achieved.

ting reductions in stimulant doses in some cases, and preliminary findings suggest that acetyl-L-carnitine at doses up to 1500 mg/day may significantly ameliorate symptoms of inattention, but not hyperactivity. Other reasonable integrative treatment strategies for ADHD combine specific EEG biofeedback protocols with restrictive diets, the above supplements and stimulants. When EEG biofeedback training is pursued on a regular basis, effective doses of conventional stimulants can sometimes be reduced, resulting in fewer adverse effects, improved treatment adherence and better outcomes.

Dietary modification

Early studies on a **restrictive diet** that eliminates all processed foods reported promising findings in children with ADHD;[26] however, a review of controlled studies failed to support these findings.[27] The **oligoantigenic diet** (**OAD**) is a highly restrictive multiple elimination diet that excludes food colourings and additives, in addition to dairy products, sugar, wheat, corn, citrus, eggs, soy, yeast, nuts and chocolate. Most OAD research protocols consist of two lean meats, two fruits, two sources of complex carbohydrates, some vegetables, water and salt. Studies involve several phases requiring many weeks to complete. During phase I, which typically lasts 4 weeks, specific food items are withheld from the diet and the patient is monitored using standardised symptom rating scales. In cases where symptoms improve during the initial treatment phase, specific foods are gradually re-introduced in phase II. A third phase follows a placebo-controlled crossover design in which the patient is randomised to a food item that initially caused symptoms or an acceptable placebo for 1 week, followed by a washout period, and subsequently exposed to either placebo or a specific food item or additive for an additional week.

THE PUTATIVE ROLE OF SUGAR IN ADHD

Sugar is often regarded as a causative or exacerbating factor in ADHD; however, research findings are inconsistent. In a 9-week RCT, non-ADHD children randomised to high-sucrose diets vs aspartame or saccharin showed no differences in behaviour.[32]

This study failed to adequately control for fruits, juices or other high-glycaemic foods. Future studies are needed to investigate a possible link between high glycaemic index foods and hyperactivity.[33]

Parental expectations may bias perceptions of children's behaviour following consumption of large quantities of sugar. Mothers who believed their children had eaten sugar were more likely to label their child's behaviour as hyperactive.[34]

Large prospective studies on the therapeutic efficacy of dietary restrictions in ADHD are challenging because of difficulties controlling eating behaviour.[3]

Several studies on the OAD regimen reported significant reductions in hyperactivity in children diagnosed with ADHD when specific food items were eliminated from the diet using the above protocol.[28,29,30] In all of these studies behavioural symptoms improved during the elimination and placebo phases and recurred when children were subsequently challenged with the eliminated food item following a blinded protocol. Although these results are promising they cannot be used to develop general ADHD treatment protocols because of study design flaws, including heterogeneity of patient populations, absence of standardised outcome measures, high drop-out rates and, in some studies, non-blinded researchers.[31]

EEG biofeedback

Many individuals diagnosed with ADHD have abnormal patterns of brain electrical activity, including 'under-arousal' in frontal and midline cortical regions and frontal 'hyper-arousal' that is more frequent in stimulant non-responders.[36] Electroencephalographic (**EEG**) **biofeedback** is aimed at normalising EEG activity in order to correct the brain's state of relative under-arousal and improve cognitive and behavioural functioning.[37] Two EEG biofeedback protocols have been extensively evaluated as treatments of ADHD. Sensorimotor rhythm (SMR) training reinforces EEG activity in the faster 'beta' frequency range (16–20 Hz) in the midline cortical regions with the goal of reducing symptoms of impulsivity and hyperactivity. 'Theta suppression' reduces EEG activity in the slower 'theta' frequency range (4–8 Hz) and is primarily used to treat symptoms of inattention. Controlled studies comparing EEG biofeedback to a stimulant medication versus a waitlist report positive clinical effects and EEG normalisation with select protocols have been conducted; however, it has not yet been established whether improved alertness is associated with increased or decreased alpha activity (12–18 Hz).[38,39] The significance of research findings is limited by small study sizes, heterogeneous populations, absence of a control group, inconsistent outcome measures and limited or absent follow-up. Large studies in which patients are randomly allocated to true versus sham biofeedback are needed to rule out positive group expectation effects. The use of sophisticated QEEG analysis with reference to a normative database may help future clinicians select the most efficacious treatment protocols for a particular ADHD symptom pattern.

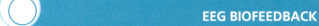

EEG BIOFEEDBACK

An EEG biofeedback protocol directed at suppressing theta activity (4–8 Hz) over the midline regions is probably the most effective strategy when treating primarily symptoms of distractibility and inattention.

Nutritional medicines

Children diagnosed with ADHD have lower plasma concentrations of certain **essential fatty acids** compared to the average population.[40] Findings to date on controlled trials of essential fatty acids in ADHD are inconsistent. One study of EFAs as an adjunctive therapy to stimulants found no differential benefit of essential fatty acids compared to stimulants plus a placebo.[41] Another adjunctive study found only modest improvements over placebo in disruptive behaviour and attention.[42] In a placebo-controlled trial on EFAs as a stand-alone treatment of ADHD, parents of children in the treatment group reported more improvement than parents of children receiving a palm oil placebo.[43] This study has been criticised because a high drop-out rate biases findings in a positive direction.[33] The use of olive oil as a placebo may mask the beneficial clinical effects of essential fatty acids because an active constituent of olive oil is converted into oleamide, which is known to affect brain function.[44] The short durations and low doses of essential fatty acids used in most studies may not be adequate to result in the long-term changes in neuronal membrane structure required for clinical improvement.[41] The issue of dosing has been addressed by a small open-label study ($n = 9$) in which ADHD children were supplemented with high dose EPA/DHA concentrates (16.2 g/day) while continuing on stimulant medications. Most children were rated by a blinded psychiatrist as having significant improvements in both inattention and hyperactivity that correlated with reductions in the AA:EPA ratio at the end of an 8-week treatment period.[45] Large prospective trials are needed to replicate these findings.

Some children diagnosed with ADHD may have abnormally low plasma **zinc** levels, which may interfere with optimal information processing and result in difficulties maintaining attention.[46,47] Findings of studies on zinc in ADHD are inconsistent. In a large 12-week prospective controlled randomised trial (PCRT) ($n = 400$), children and adolescents randomised to zinc (150 mg/day) experienced significant improvements in hyperactivity and impulsivity, but not inattention, over placebo.[48] A high drop-out rate limits the significance of findings. In another study adding zinc to a stimulant resulted in greater improvement than stimulant alone.[49] Large prospective studies are needed to replicate these preliminary findings and confirm the optimum dosing of zinc sulfate.[50]

Abnormally low serum ferritin levels may be associated with hyperactivity in non-anaemic ADHD children, but not with deficits in cognitive performance.[51] In an open trial non-iron-deficient children given oral **iron** for 1 month were perceived as less hyperactive and distractible by teachers but not by parents.[52] In a small 12-week randomised PCRT non-anaemic ADHD children with abnormally low serum ferritin levels randomised to oral iron (ferrous sulfate 80 mg/day) showed progressive improvements in ADHD symptoms over placebo that were comparable to improvements obtained with stimulants.[53]

Acetyl-L-carnitine (ALC) is required for energy metabolism and synthesis of fatty acids. Findings of one small study suggested that L-carnitine significantly reduces the severity of ADHD symptoms; however, design flaws limit the significance of these findings.[54] In a multi-site 16-week pilot study 112 ADHD children were randomised to placebo versus ALC (500 to 1500 mg b.i.d). Children in the ALC group with predominantly inattentive type ADHD experienced greater improvement over placebo, but there was no differential benefit in children with combined type ADHD. Significant adverse effects were not reported. Large prospective trials are needed to replicate this finding before ALC can be recommended for ADHD.

Herbal medicines

In a 4-week open study involving 36 children diagnosed with ADHD, a herbal preparation containing **Ginkgo biloba** and **Panax quinquefolium** was added to their existing ADHD medication.[55] Beneficial effects were observed in children taking the herbal combination after 4 weeks. It should be noted, however, that the absence of a placebo group (or a stimulant-only group) and the small size of the study limit the significance of findings. Findings of open studies suggest that a standardised extract of **Pinus pinaster** bark is beneficial in ADHD; however, only one PCRT has been published to date. Sixty-one children and adolescents randomised to a standardised bark extract (Pycnogenol™) 1 mg/kg/day for 1 month experienced significant improvements in hyperactivity, inattention and visual–motor coordination over placebo; these returned to pretreatment baseline levels after a 1-month washout.[56] Only one case of mild gastric discomfort was reported. These findings should be regarded as preliminary pending replication by large prospective studies. **Bacopa monnieri** is an Ayurvedic herbal used as a tonic and memory enhancer. In one randomised controlled trial (RCT) ($n = 85$) healthy men and women randomised to a extract containing *G. biloba* and *B. monnieri* did not perform better than a placebo group in tests of short-term memory, working memory, executive processing, planning, problem solving and information processing speed.[57] These findings cannot be generalised to ADHD; however, they suggest that this herbal formula does not ameliorate the core symptoms of ADHD.

Homoeopathic remedies

A systematic review of PRCTs on homoeopathic remedies in ADHD found no evidence of beneficial effects of homoeopathy on symptom severity, core symptoms or the course of ADHD.[58] These findings have been criticised because conventional PCRT study designs may not permit the demonstration of measurable clinical effects of homoeopathic remedies for ADHD. Long-term studies that include an initial open-label phase are needed to determine the 'optimal' homoeopathic remedy for each unique patient over several months. In a subsequent placebo-controlled phase individuals could then be randomised to their 'optimum' remedy versus a randomly selected homoeopathic preparation.[59]

Yoga and massage

In a small pilot study ADHD children randomised to yoga experienced greater improvement over time compared to children who exercised. Children who continued on stimulants while practising yoga experienced the greatest improvements.[60] Two small controlled studies suggest that yoga and regular massage therapy may reduce the severity of ADHD symptoms.[61,62]

Therapeutic considerations

Stimulant abuse is an established risk factor in long-term prescription stimulant use among adults; however, a meta-analysis of six controlled trials found that when stimulants are used to treat childhood ADHD the risk of subsequent substance abuse actually *decreases*.[65] Although the American Academy of Paediatrics endorses the use of stimulants as safe and effective, considerable controversy surrounds their widespread use, especially

'GREEN' PLAY ENVIRONMENTS

ADHD may result from 'attention fatigue' caused by limited contact with 'green spaces' during early childhood.

Findings of a large observational study suggest that ADHD children who spend more time playing outdoors in natural environments may experience fewer and less severe symptoms.[63]

These findings have been criticised because of design flaws, such as a heterogeneous population that included children with comorbid oppositional-defiant disorder and the absence of independent raters.[64]

among children, and their long-term safety has not been clearly established.[66] Several cases of sudden cardiac death in children and adults taking mixed amphetamine salts resulted in the temporary withdrawal of this stimulant from the Canadian marketplace in 2005, and led to American Heart Association guidelines recommending a baseline electrocardiogram (ECG) and monitoring of blood pressure and pulse before starting stimulant therapy and during the course of therapy in children, adolescents and adults.[67]

ADHD remains a highly controversial diagnosis among mental health professionals and parents because of many unresolved issues, and some claim that the disorder does not even exist.[68,69] In spite of considerable research there is still no strong evidence of a genetic or physiological basis for the disorder.[70] Diagnostic criteria required to diagnose ADHD continue to evolve, suggesting that there is no consensus on the symptoms that constitute ADHD. Finally, although there is probably little abuse potential when stimulants are used to treat childhood ADHD, this remains a central concern among parents.[71]

Case Study

A 55-year-old divorced woman comments during the therapy session that she is currently getting treatment for ADHD. She says she used to get **distracted easily** and has **problems being on time** and **staying organised**. She says she does not have a learning disorder but recalls having **difficulty focusing that began in early childhood**. In primary school she was frequently scolded for **disruptive behaviour** in class and turning in homework assignments late. The patient has been taking a stimulant medication for several years; this has significantly increased her ability to focus, but she **sometimes experiences headaches, loss of appetite** and **insomnia**. She wants to know of any other treatment in addition to her medication that may be helpful.

SUGGESTIVE SYMPTOMS

Primarily inattentive type
- Short attention span
- Easily distractible
- Difficulty organising tasks
- Reluctant to engage in tasks requiring sustained mental effort
- May be irritable or explosive

Primarily hyperactive type
- May fidget with hands or feet
- Difficulty engaging in leisure activities
- Talks excessively
- Poor impulse control
- Often 'on the go' as if driven internally

Example treatment

In the above example case, the use of EEG biofeedback, dietary and lifestyle modifications, and nutritional treatments may be effective in enhancing her focus and improving her mood. If her serum ferritin level is in the low range, iron supplementation may be

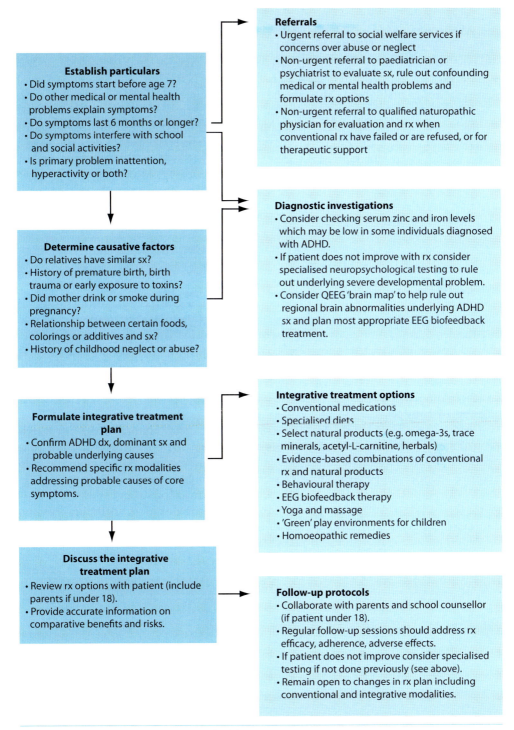

Referrals
- Urgent referral to social welfare services if concerns over abuse or neglect
- Non-urgent referral to paediatrician or psychiatrist to evaluate sx, rule out confounding medical or mental health problems and formulate rx options
- Non-urgent referral to qualified naturopathic physician for evaluation and rx when conventional rx have failed or are refused, or for therapeutic support

Establish particulars
- Did symptoms start before age 7?
- Do other medical or mental health problems explain symptoms?
- Do symptoms last 6 months or longer?
- Do symptoms interfere with school and social activities?
- Is primary problem inattention, hyperactivity or both?

Diagnostic investigations
- Consider checking serum zinc and iron levels which may be low in some individuals diagnosed with ADHD.
- If patient does not improve with rx consider specialised neuropsychological testing to rule out underlying severe developmental problem.
- Consider QEEG 'brain map' to help rule out regional brain abnormalities underlying ADHD sx and plan most appropriate EEG biofeedback treatment.

Determine causative factors
- Do relatives have similar sx?
- History of premature birth, birth trauma or early exposure to toxins?
- Did mother drink or smoke during pregnancy?
- Relationship between certain foods, colorings or additives and sx?
- History of childhood neglect or abuse?

Integrative treatment options
- Conventional medications
- Specialised diets
- Select natural products (e.g. omega-3s, trace minerals, acetyl-L-carnitine, herbals)
- Evidence-based combinations of conventional rx and natural products
- Behavioural therapy
- EEG biofeedback therapy
- Yoga and massage
- 'Green' play environments for children
- Homoeopathic remedies

Formulate integrative treatment plan
- Confirm ADHD dx, dominant sx and probable underlying causes
- Recommend specific rx modalities addressing probable causes of core symptoms.

Discuss the integrative treatment plan
- Review rx options with patient (include parents if under 18).
- Provide accurate information on comparative benefits and risks.

Follow-up protocols
- Collaborate with parents and school counsellor (if patient under 18).
- Regular follow-up sessions should address rx efficacy, adherence, adverse effects.
- If patient does not improve consider specialised testing if not done previously (see above).
- Remain open to changes in rx plan including conventional and integrative modalities.

Figure 34.1 Integrative treatment decision tree—ADHD. sx = symptoms, rx = treatment dx = diagnosis

beneficial. The supplementation of EFAs and ALC may provide an adjuvant effect on ameliorating her ADHD symptoms. EEG biofeedback training on a weekly basis using a protocol aimed at suppressing theta activity in frontal brain regions may also be beneficial. If these protocols are found to be effective, she may be able to cut back on her psychostimulant medication. This may reduce her headaches and improve her sleep.

Expected outcomes and follow-up protocols

In spite of their adverse effects and associated risk of substance abuse stimulants continue to be the most widely used conventional treatments of ADHD. When stimulants fail to result in significant reductions in symptom severity or when adverse effects, toxicities or comorbid substance abuse preclude their use, EEG biofeedback and select naturopathic treatments should be considered. Amelioration of ADHD symptoms usually requires several weeks of specialised EEG biofeedback training protocols, specifically SMR training or theta suppression (see above). Restrictive diets are reasonable interventions in cases where impulsivity and distractibility may be related to sugar intake or food allergies. When therapeutic doses of stimulants cannot be achieved with acceptable tolerance the adjunctive use of essential fatty acids, and select herbals including *G. biloba*, *Panax quinquefolium*, *P. pinaster* and *B. monnieri* may improve response. The adjunctive use of acetyl-L-carnitine, zinc and iron may be beneficial; however, these treatments are not substantiated by strong research findings. Regular yoga and massage therapy may also help improve attention and hyperactivity in some cases. In cases where an individual diagnosed with ADHD fails to respond to established pharmacological and alternative treatments it is prudent to rule out confounding psychiatric disorders, including learning disorders, depressed mood and anxiety disorders, which are frequently comorbid with the syndrome and may significantly affect treatment outcomes.

Pre-prescribed pharmaceuticals

Methylphenidate 20 mg per day

Diet

Restrictive diet (excludes sugar, chocolate, food additives and colourings)

Nutritional supplements

EFAs 6 g per day
(1.2 g EFA, 0.8 g DHA)
Iron (amino acid chelate)
24 mg elemental per day
Acetyl-L-carnitine 500 mg per day

Lifestyle

Regular massage therapy (twice weekly)

Table 34.1 Review of the major evidence

INTERVENTION	METHODOLOGY	RESULT	COMMENT
Dietary changes	Double-blind placebo-controlled challenge crossover trial (n = 300 ADHD children) Phase I elimination, phase II challenge[72] Double-blind placebo-controlled challenge crossover trial (n = 56 children ages 4–12 years with behavioural problems) phase I open elimination followed by challenge[73]	75% improved with restricted diet but symptoms recurred when food colourings, additives re-introduced Improved behaviour and attention scores	No description of recruitment or eligibility of non-reactors in phase 2 More restrictive than Feingold but less restrictive than OAD protocol

(Continued)

Table 34.1 **Review of the major evidence** *(Continued)*

INTERVENTION	METHODOLOGY	RESULT	COMMENT
EEG biofeedback	1-year clinical trial stimulants vs EEG biofeedback plus stimulants[37] (*n* = 100, ages 6–19 years)	Symptoms improved on stimulants but only biofeedback group sustained improvement without stimulants at 1-year follow-up.	Group assignments based on parental preference. Average of 43 sessions required for sustained improvement
	12-week clinical trial EEG biofeedback SMR and beta rhythms 3×/week vs stimulants (*n* = 34, boys aged 8–12 years)[74]	TOVA and Conners scores significantly improved in EEG biofeedback group	Group assignments based on parental preference
Herbal medicine	4-week open study (*n* = 34) ADHD children randomised Ginkgo + American ginseng added to ongoing stimulant medication[55]	Improvements in ADHD symptoms were found after 4 weeks of treatment.	No comparison group treated with stimulants only
	1-month RCT (*n* = 61) standardised extract of French maritime pine bark 1 mg/kg/day.[56]	Significant improvements in hyperactivity, inattention and visual–motor coordination	Large studies needed to replicate findings
	RCT (*n* = 85 healthy men and women) extract of *gingko biloba* and *Bacopa monnieri* vs placebo[57]	No improvements over placebo in short-term memory, working memory, executive processing, etc.	Study population consisted of normal individuals. Large prospective dose-finding trials on ADHD patients needed
Trace elements	12-week RCT (*n* = 400 children and adolescents) high dose zinc (150 mg/day) vs placebo.[48]	Significant improvement in hyperactivity and impulsivity but *not* inattention	High drop out rate limits significance
	12-week RCT non-anaemic ADHD children with low serum ferritin treated with oral iron (80 mg/day) vs placebo.[53]	Improvements with iron comparable to stimulants	Large prospective studies needed to confirm efficacy and determine optimal dosing
Other natural products (omega-3 fatty acids)	2-month double-blind placebo controlled randomised trial (*n* = 40, ages 6–12) diet consisted of DHA-enriched foods vs olive-oil enriched foods[75]	Short-term memory improved and commission errors decreased in control but not DHA group. No differences in parent or teacher ratings of behavioural or cognitive symptoms	Olive oil may not be inert (see text). Serum EFA levels were not measured. Some subjects had comorbid Asperger's syndrome, conduct disorder, learning disorders and mood disorders.
(acetyl-L-carnitine)	8-week open pilot study (*n* = 9) children given high dose EPA/DHA concentrates (16.2 g/day) then rated by blinded psychiatrist[45]	Significant improvements in behaviour and inattention, correlating with reduced AA:EPA ratio and global severity of illness scores. No serious adverse effects were reported.	No placebo group; some subjects had comorbid conduct disorder or oppositional-defiant disorder (which also improved during study). Dietary intake not recorded at baseline or during study. Supplement intake not closely monitored.
	16-week pilot study (*n* = 112 ADHD children) randomised to ALC (500 to 1500 mg b.i.d.) vs placebo.[54]	ALC superior to placebo in inattentive type children but not combined type ADHD.	Large prospective trials needed

(Continued)

Table 34.1 Review of the major evidence *(Continued)*

INTERVENTION	METHODOLOGY	RESULT	COMMENT
Yoga and massage	In 2 small controlled studies ADHD children stable on medications were randomised to yoga or regular massage therapy[61,62]	Regular yoga and massage may reduce severity of ADHD symptoms.	Possible group expectation effects. Large prospective studies needed

KEY POINTS

- Take into account the unique causes of the syndrome in each patient, including genetic factors, perinatal insults or toxic exposure, food sensitivities and social factors.
- Stimulants and non-stimulant medications are beneficial and well-tolerated conventional treatments of ADHD for a significant percentage of children, adolescents and adults.
- Restrict food colourings, additives, sugar or specific foods to significantly reduce symptoms of hyperactivity in some cases.
- Use validated EEG biofeedback protocols including SMR training for primarily hyperactive type ADHD and theta suppression for primarily inattentive type ADHD as first-line treatments when stimulants are not effective, cannot be tolerated or are refused.
- Zinc supplementation may be helpful when hyperactivity and impulsive behaviour do not respond to stimulants alone. Supplement with iron and ALC for the core symptoms of distractibility and inattention. More studies are needed.
- High doses of omega-3 essential fatty acids (up to 16 g/day) may have therapeutic effects on symptoms of both inattention and hyperactivity. More studies are needed.
- *Ginkgo biloba*, *Panax quinquefolium*, *Pinus pinaster* and *Bacopa monnieri* may be beneficial in ADHD; however, conclusive findings from large prospective controlled trials are needed before any of these can be recommended as adjunctive or first-line treatments.

Further reading

Biederman J, Faraone SV. Attention-deficit hyperactivity disorder. Lancet 2005;366(9481):237–248.

Lake J, Spiegel D, eds. Complementary and alternative treatments in mental health. Washington: American Psychiatric Press Inc. 2007.

Sears W, Thompson L. The A.D.D. Book. USA: Little, Brown and Company, 1998.

Shannon SM. Please don't label my child. USA: Rodale Inc. 2007.

References

1. Barkley RA. Attention-deficit hyperactivity disorder: a handbook for diagnosis and treatment. 2nd edn. New York: Guilford Press, 1998.
2. Centers for Disease Control. National Health Interview survey, 2002 Atlanta: Centers for Disease Control, 2004.
3. Biederman J, Faraone SV. The Massachusetts General Hospital studies of gender influences on attention-deficit/hyperactivity disorder in youth and relatives. Psychiatr Clin North Am 2004;27(2):225–232.
4. Biederman J, Faraone SV. Attention-deficit hyperactivity disorder. Lancet 2005;366(9481):237–248.
5. Wallis D, et al. Review: Genetics of attention deficit/hyperactivity disorder. J Pediatr Psychol 2008;33(10):1085–1099.
6. Swanson JM, et al. Etiologic subtypes of attention-deficit/hyperactivity disorder: brain imaging, molecular genetic and environmental factors and the dopamine hypothesis. Neuropsychol Rev 2007;17(1):39–59.
7. McCann D, et al. Food additives and hyperactive behaviour in 3-year-old and 8/9-year-old children in the community: a randomised, double-blinded, placebo-controlled trial. Lancet 2007;370(9598):1560–1567.
8. Brennan AR, Arnsten AF. Neuronal mechanisms underlying attention deficit hyperactivity disorder: the influence of arousal on prefrontal cortical function. Ann N Y Acad Sci 2008;1129:236–245.
9. Silvestri R, et al. Sleep disorders in children with attention-deficit/hyperactivity disorder (ADHD) recorded overnight by video-polysomnography. Sleep Med 2009 Jun 13. [Epub ahead of print].

10. Di Michele F, et al. The neurophysiology of attention-deficit hyperactivity disorder. Int J Psychophysiol 2005;58(1):81–93.

11. American Psychiatric Association. Diagnostic and statistical manual of mental disorders. 4th edn. Arlington: American Psychiatric Association, 2000.

12. Pearl P, el al. Medical mimics of ADHD. In: Wasserstein J, ed. ADHD in adults: brain mechanisms and behavior. Ann NY Acad Sci 2001:99–111.

13. Newcorn JH, et al. The complexity of ADHD: diagnosis and treatment of the adult patient with comorbidities. CNS Spectr 2007;12(8 Suppl 12):1–14.

14. Cimera R. Making ADHD a gift: teaching Superman how to fly. Lanham: Scarecrow Press, Inc., 2002:16.

15. Kessler RC, et al. The prevalence and effects of adult attention deficit/hyperactivity disorder on work performance in a nationally representative sample of workers. J Occup Environ Med 2005;47(6):565–572.

16. Schachter HM, et al. How efficacious and safe is short-acting methylphenidate for the treatment of attention-deficit disorder in children and adolescents? A meta-analysis. CMAJ 2001;165(11):1475.

17. Berman SM, et al. Potential adverse effects of amphetamine treatment on brain and behavior: a review. Mol Psychiatry 2009;14(2):123–142.

18. Slatkoff J, Greenfield B. Pharmacological treatment of attention-deficit/hyperactivity disorder in adults. Expert Opin Investig Drugs 2006;15(6):649–667.

19. Findling RL. Evolution of the treatment of attention-deficit/hyperactivity disorder in children: a review. Clin Ther 2008;30(5):942–957.

20. Miller MC. What is the significance of the new warnings about suicide risk with Strattera? Harv Ment Health Lett 2005;22(6):8.

21. Nissen SE. ADHD drugs and cardiovascular risk. N Engl J Med 2006;354(14):1445–1448.

22. Stubberfield T, Parry T. Utilization of alternative therapies in attention-deficit hyperactivity disorder. J Paediatr Child Health 1999;35(5):450–453.

23. Anderson SL, Navalta CP. Altering the course of neurodevelopment: a framework for understanding the enduring effects of psychotropic drugs. Int J Deve Neurosci 2004;22(5–6):40–423.

24. Bussing R, et al. Use of complementary and alternative medicine for symptoms of attention-deficit hyperactivity disorder. Psychiatr Serv 2002;53(9):1096–1102.

25. Chan E, et al. Complementary and alternative therapies in childhood attention and hyperactivity problems. J Dev Behav Pediatr 2003;24(1):4–8.

26. Feingold B. Why your child is hyperactive. New York: Random House, 1975.

27. Wender EH. The food additive-free diet in the treatment of behavior disorders: a review. J Dev Behav Pediatr 1986;7(1):35–42.

28. Egger J, et al. Controlled trial of hyposensitization in children with food-induced hyperkinetic syndrome. Lancet 1992;339:1150–1153.

29. Carter CM, et al. Effects of a new food diet in attention-deficit disorder. Arch Dis Child 1993;69:564–568.

30. Schmidt MH, et al. Does oligoantigenic diet influence hyperactive/conduct-disordered children: a controlled trial. Eur Child Adolesc Psychiatry 1997;6:88–95.

31. Rojas NL, Chan E. Old and new controversies in the alternative treatment of attention-deficit hyperactivity disorder. Ment Retard Dev Disabil Res Rev 2005;11(2):116–130.

32. Wolraich S, et al. Effects of diets high in sucrose or aspartame on the behavior and cognitive performance of children. N Engl J Med 1994;330(5):301–307.

33. Weber W, Newmark S. Complementary and alternative medical therapies for attention-deficit/hyperactivity disorder and autism. Pediatr Clin North Am 2007;54(6):983–1006, xii.

34. Hoover DW, Milich R. Effects of sugar ingestion expectancies on mother-child interactions. J Abnorm Child Psychol 1994;22(4):501–515.

35. Cormier E, Elder JH. Diet and child behavior problems: fact or fiction? Pediatr Nurs 2007;33(2):138–143.

36. Butnik SM. Neurofeedback in adolescents and adults with attention deficit hyperactivity disorder. J Clin Psychol 2005;61(5):621–625.

37. Monastra VJ, et al. The effects of stimulant therapy, EEG biofeedback, and parenting style on the primary symptoms of attention-deficit/hyperactivity disorder. Appl Psychophysiol Biofeedback 2002;27(4):231–249.

38. Monasstra VJ, et al. Electroencephalographic biofeedback in the treatment of attention-deficit/hyperactivity disorder. Applied Psychophysiology and Biofeedback 2005; 30(2):95–114.

39. Ramirez P, et al. EEG biofeedback treatment of ADD: a viable alternative to traditional medical intervention? Ann NY Acad Sci 2001;931:342–358.

40. Gedik Y, et al. Relationships between serum free fatty acids and zinc, and attention deficit hyperactivity disorder: a research note. J Child Psychol Psychiatry 1996;37: 225–227.

41. Voigt RG, et al. A randomized, double-blind, placebo-controlled trial of docosahexaenoic acid supplementation in children with attention-deficit/hyperactivity disorder. J Pediatr 2001;139(2):189–196.

42. Stevens LJ, et al. Essential fatty acid metabolism in boys with attention-deficit hyperactivity disorder. Am J Clin Nutr 1995;62(4):761–768.

43. Sinn N, Bryan J. Effect of supplementation with polyunsaturated fatty acids and micronutrients on learning and behavior problems associated with child ADHD. J Dev Behav Pediatr 2007;28(2):82–91.

44. Richardson AJ, Puri BK. A randomized double-blind, placebo-controlled study of the effects of supplementation with highly unsaturated fatty acids on ADHD-related symptoms in children with specific learning difficulties. Prog Neuropsychopharmacol Biol Psychiatry 2002;26:233–239.

45. Sorgi PJ, et al. Effects of an open-label pilot study with high-dose EPA/DHA concentrates on plasma phospholipids and behavior in children with attention deficit hyperactivity disorder. Nutrition Journal 2007;6:16.

46. Yorbik O, et al. Potential effects of zinc on information processing in boys with attention deficit hyperactivity disorder. Prog Neuropsychopharmacol Biol Psychiatry 2008;32(3): 662–667.

47. Arnold LE, et al. Serum zinc correlates with parent- and teacher-rated inattention in children with attention-deficit/hyperactivity disorder. Child Adolesc Psychopharmacol 2005;15(4):628–636.

48. Bilici M, et al. Double-blind, placebo-controlled study of zinc sulfate in the treatment of attention deficit hyperactivity disorder. Prog Neuropsychopharmacol Biol Psychiatry 2004;28(1):181–190.

49. Akhondzadeh S, et al. Zinc sulfate as an adjunct to methylphenidate for the treatment of attention deficit hyperactivity disorder in children: a double blind and randomized trial [ISRCTN64132371]. BMC Psychiatry 2004;4(1):9.

50. Arnold LE, DiSilvestro RA. Zinc in attention-deficit/hyperactivity disorder. Child Adolesc Psychopharmacol 2005;15(4):619–627.

51. Oner O, et al. Relation of ferritin levels with symptom ratings and cognitive performance in children with attention deficit-hyperactivity disorder. Pediatr Int 2008;50(1):40–44.

52. Sever Y, et al. Iron treatment in children with attention deficit hyperactivity disorder: a preliminary report. Neuropsychobiol 1997;35:178–180.

53. Konofal E, et al. Effects of iron supplementation on attention deficit hyperactivity disorder in children. Pediatr Neurol 2008;38(1):20–26.

54. Van Oudheusden LJ, Scholte HR. Efficacy of carnitine in the treatment of children with attention-deficit hyperactivity disorder. Prostaglandins Leukot Essent Fatty Acids 2002;67(1):33–38.

55. Lyon MR, et al. Effect of the herbal extract combination *Panax quinquefolium* and *Ginkgo biloba* on attention-deficit hyperactivity disorder: a pilot study. J Psychiatry Neurosci 2001;26(3):221–228.

56. Trebaticka J, et al. Treatment of ADHD with French maritime pine bark extract Pycnogenol[R]. Eur Child Adolesc Psychiatry Sept 2006;15(6):329–335.

57. Nathan PJ, et al. Effects of a combined extract of *Ginkgo biloba* and *Bacopa monnieri* on cognitive function in healthy humans. Hum Psychopharmacol 2004;19(2):91–96.

58. Coulter MK, Dean ME. Homeopathy for attention deficit/hyperactivity disorder or hyperkinetic disorder. Cochrane Database System Reviews 2007;(4):CD005648.

59. Frei H, et al. Randomised controlled trials of homeopathy in hyperactive children: treatment procedure leads to an unconventional study design. Experience with open-label homeopathic treatment preceding the Swiss ADHD placebo controlled, randomised, double-blind, cross-over trial. Homeopathy 2007;96(1):35–41.

60. Haffner J, et al. The effectiveness of body-oriented methods of therapy in the treatment of attention-deficit hyperactivity disorder (ADHD): results of a controlled pilot study]. Z Kinder Jugendpsychiatr Psychother 2006;34(1):37–47.

61. Jensen PS, Kenny DT. The effects of yoga on the attention and behavior of boys with attention-deficit/hyperactivity disorder (ADHD). J Atten Disord 2004;7(4):205–216.

62. Khilnani S, et al. Massage therapy improves mood and behavior of students with attention-deficit/hyperactivity disorder. Adolescence 2003;38(152):623–638.

63. Kuo FE, Taylor AF. A potential natural treatment for attention-deficit/hyperactivity disorder: evidence from a national study. Am J Public Health 2004;94(9):1580–1586.

64. Canu W, Gordon M. Mother nature as treatment for ADHD: overstating the benefits of green. Am J Clin Nutr 2005;95:371.

65. Faraone SV, Wilens T. Does stimulant treatment lead to substance use disorders? J Clin Psychiatry 2003;64(Suppl 11):9–13.

66. Lerner M, Wigal T. Long-term safety of stimulant medications used to treat children with ADHD. Pediatric Annals 2008;37(1):37–45.

67. Vetter VL, et al. Cardiovascular monitoring of children and adolescents with heart disease receiving stimulant drugs: a scientific statement from the American Heart Association Council on Cardiovascular Disease in the Young Congenital Cardiac Defects Committee and the Council on Cardiovascular Nursing. Circulation 2008;117(18):2407–2423.

68. Mayes R, et al. ADHD and the rise in stimulant use among children. Harv Rev Psychiatry 2008;16(3):151–166.

69. Foreman DM. Attention deficit hyperactivity disorder: legal and ethical aspects. Arch Dis Child 2006;91(2):192–194.

70. US Department of Health and Human Services. Treatment of attention-deficit/hyperactivity disorder. US Department of Health and Human Services, 1999.

71. Jadad AR, et al. The treatment of attention-deficit hyperactivity disorder: an annotated bibliography and critical appraisal of published systematic reviews and metaanalyses. Canadian Journal of Psychiatry. Revue Canadienne de Psychiatrie 1999;44(10):1025–1035.

72. Rowe KS, Rowe KJ. Synthetic food coloring and behavior: a dose response effect in a double-blind, placebo-controlled, repeated-measures study. J Pediatr 1994;125(5 Pt 1):691–698.

73. Dengate S, Ruben A. Controlled trial of cumulative behavioural effects of a common bread preservative. J Paediatr Child Health 2002;38(4):373–376.

74. Fuchs T, et al. Neurofeedback treatment for attention-deficit/hyperactivity disorder in children: a comparison with methylphenidate. Appl Psychophysiol Biofeedback 2003;28(1):1–12.

75. Hirayama S, et al. Effect of docosahexaenoic acid-containing food administration on symptoms of attention-deficit/hyperactivity disorder—a placebo-controlled double-blind study. Eur J Clin Nutr 2004;58(3):467–473.

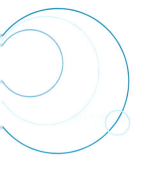

35

Chronic fatigue syndrome

Gary Deed
MBBS (Hons I)

OVERVIEW

Chronic fatigue syndrome (CFS) is a complex yet defined spectrum disorder. It is characterised by expert consensus to include persistent disabling fatigue lasting more than 6 months with other symptoms as listed in the box below. This definition is based upon the USA's Centers for Disease Control's description of this illness.[1] Importantly there are medical conditions by their nature that may mimic CFS and need to be excluded prior to making an accurate diagnosis. These include untreated thyroid disease, sleep disorders such as sleep apnoea, alcohol abuse, major depressive disorders and schizophrenia. The presence of past and treated malignancy or unresolved infectious hepatitis is also considered exclusive of CFS.[1-4] However, the persistence of symptoms despite adequate treatment of the above conditions, including thyroid conditions or infections such as Lyme disease, fibromyalgia and anxiety disorders, may possibly co-exist with a diagnosis of CFS.[2] CFS presents significant difficulties in diagnosis and assessment, as there is no single laboratory or clinically significant specific diagnostic test. Patients often appear

CDC CRITERIA FOR THE DIAGNOSIS OF CFS[1,2,3,4]

- Patients have severe chronic fatigue of 6 months or longer duration with other known medical conditions excluded by clinical diagnosis.
- Patients concurrently have four or more of the following symptoms: substantial impairment in short-term memory or concentration; sore throat; tender lymph nodes; muscle pain; multi-joint pain without swelling or redness; headaches of a new type, pattern or severity; unrefreshing sleep; and post-exertional malaise lasting more than 24 hours.
- The symptoms must have persisted or recurred during 6 or more consecutive months of illness and must not have predated the fatigue.
- The condition must also be defined by excluding other organic or psychiatric causes including that covered in Chapter 15 on adrenal exhaustion.

clinically well, though express profound deterioration of social and occupational functioning and have significant physical and psychological distress.

AETIOLOGY

Infectious agents

Clinically it is well known that many patients commence their illness after what appears to be an infectious episode. Certainly no single agent has been shown consistently to create all CFS cases; however, the CDC state 'the possibility remains that CFS may have multiple causes leading to a common endpoint, in which case some viruses or other infectious agents might have a contributory role for a subset of CFS cases, and infection with Epstein-Barr virus, Ross River virus and *Coxiella burnetti* will lead to a postinfective condition that meets the criteria for CFS in approximately 12% of cases'.[4]

Further research pointing to an infectious origin include:

- enterovirus in muscle biopsies of 20.8% of CFS patients, but not controls[5]
- *Mycoplasma* spp. (52%), *Chlamydia pneumoniae* (7.5%) and HHV 6 (30.5%)[6]
- mycoplasma infection[7]
- multiple active viral infections—HHV6; HHV 7; parvovirus B 19[8]
- tick-borne illnesses and borreliosis[9]
- gram-negative enterobacteria causing increased intestinal permeability.[10]

Immunologic abnormalities

CFS quite possibly may be the result of a complex interplay between an infectious insult and/or a disordered immune response in a susceptible individual. This complexity is revealed in research in the area of immunity and CFS; it clearly has not shown any one consistent abnormality (concerning interleukin abnormalities and altered cell-mediated immunity).[11-13] Combined with the consistently observed possibility of multiple infectious aetiological agents and the possibility of persistent or relapsing infections, the resulting immunologic disorders such as elevated pro-inflammatory cytokines 'may explain some of the manifestations such as fatigue and flu-like symptoms and influence NK activity'.[14]

Neuroendocrine abnormalities

Hypoactivity of the hypothalamic–pituitary–adrenal (HPA) axis combined with hyperactivity of the serotonergic system has been postulated as a cause of CFS.[15,16] Other research suggests that up-regulation of hypothalamic serotonergic receptors may be the cause some of the HPA disorders—distinctly different from depression[17] and 'adrenal exhaustion'. With respect to the HPA axis, lowered levels of dehydroepiandrosterone (DHEA, an adrenal steroidal hormone) have been assessed in CFS patients.[18] The interplay of dysfunctional immunity, cytokine imbalances leading to subtle neurotransmitter changes is demonstrated in Figure 35.1. Importantly, as mentioned above, depression and its manifestations are distinctly different from CFS both in psychological distress and in physiological dysfunctioning (see Section 4 on the nervous system for treatment details).[19]

Orthostatic intolerance

Patients with CFS have been shown to have abnormal autonomic responses to prolonged standing or even sitting for long periods.[20] This 'orthostatic intolerance' manifests as fatigue plus elevated pulse rates, often associated with faintness when the above

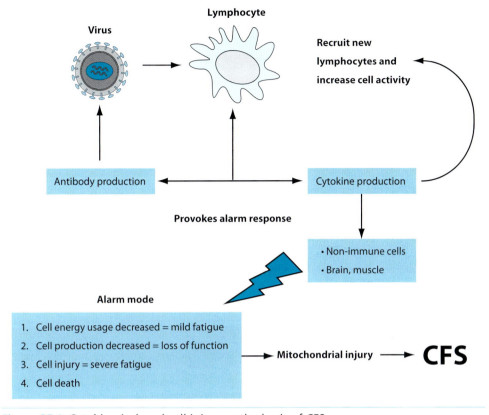

Figure 35.1 Cytokine-induced cell injury as the basis of CFS

activities occur. The condition is diagnosable with a severe hypotensive response to 'tilt table' testing, where a patient is subjected to a head tilt when lying flat.[21]

Nutritional causes

As the diagnosis is defined by the absence of other medical conditions, the fatigue that arises from iron deficiency, vitamin B and B12 deficiency is necessarily excluded as a cause. However, lowered levels of essential fatty acids, L-carnitine and magnesium have been assessed in patients with CFS.[17] Interestingly, these nutrients give direct support to mitochondrial function—an essential pathway for the production of cellular energy.[22] Empiric research has shown that vitamin B12 injections may improve energy and cognitive ability and mood often with normal serum B12 levels.[23,24] Serum folic acid levels have been assayed in patients with CFS and 50% of 60 patients have been shown to have lowered levels.[25] Oral nicotinamide (NADH) has been shown in a randomised placebo-controlled trial to give benefit to 31% of CFS patients treated.[26]

RISK FACTORS

No single risk factor has been strongly associated with CFS. With a spectrum disorder with multiple aetiological factors it seems prudent to individually assess the clinical case as it presents. However study has commenced on what makes a person vulnerable to CFS with the general consensus based upon observation that disordered immunity

Table 35.1 Predictive risks factors for developing CFS[27]

Older age	Female > male (4:1)
Low or middle rather than high educational level	The presence of an anxiety disorder
Mood disorder (pre-morbid or 2 months postinfection)	Personality trait—emotional instability
Musculoskeletal pain	Low fitness 2 months postinfection
Lower physical functioning at baseline assessment	The presence of fatigue at time of viral illness
Fatigue severity	Other family members with symptoms of CFS

and infectious agents intervene in a susceptible individual. A summary of the recent researched factors is shown in Table 35.1.

Very recent research has revealed that childhood trauma—abuse of sexual or emotional type—may predispose an individual to developing CFS in the presence of other initiating factors.[28] Neuroendocrine dysfunction, as discussed in Chapter 15 on adrenal exhaustion, explains how the combination of these factors develop as a definite risk for CFS.[29]

CONVENTIONAL TREATMENT

There remains much contention in some medical services about the existence of CFS, let alone its management. Fatigue is a common presentation to general practice; however, CFS is a unique and separate entity that requires understanding and knowledge of the condition itself and those things that may mimic it. Confusion arises because of the lack of a definitive laboratory test, plus uncertainty about management options available to patients.[17] Thus much conventional therapy is directed to symptomatic control of distress in the absence of single or definitive interventions. Key areas of conventional therapy that are summarised in one study[30] include:

- sedating antidepressants such as tricyclic antidepressants, and serotonergic reuptake inhibitors for sleep disorders[31,32]
- simple analgesia and non-steroidal anti-inflammatory agents for ongoing pain management
- serotonergic modulators such as fluoxetine or similar agents in this class for psychological support, especially reactive mood disorder with or without anxiety.

Note: It is important the patient has had a careful medical assessment to exclude those conditions that mimic CFS.

KEY TREATMENT PROTOCOLS

The primary clinical protocol is to be supportive and patient, and to address the individual needs of the person with CFS. Negotiate a personalised plan recognising the person knows the effect of their illness better than anyone else. The following discussion provides choices that may be individually assessed as appropriate to the person's needs.

Decrease suffering
Reduce pain and stiffness

Conventional therapies to reduce pain and suffering include regular doses of paracetamol and the use of a nocturnal dose of a tricyclic anti-depressant such as amitryptylline—10–50 mg at night.[31,32]

Integrative interventions most favoured by people with CFS include massage and chiropractic therapies.[33] Recent research suggests that, in the presence of accompanying myofascial pain, manual therapies such as manipulation and myofascial trigger point therapy may have some benefit.[34]

Nutritional interventions such as magnesium is a nutrient that is an essential cofactor in enzymes of energy metabolism; it acts on muscle tissue as a relaxant (through its calcium channel blocking actions), and

> **INTEGRATIVE MEDICAL TREATMENT AIMS**
> - Individualisation of therapies allows a patient centred approach.
> - Decrease suffering:
>   – reduce pain and stiffness
>   – improve sleep.
> - Increase physical condition:
>   – increase graded physical activity goals
>   – use nutritional and herbal therapies for fatigue and weakness.
> - Improve immune dysfunction:
>   – assess for infection, allergy and toxicity or deficiency
>   – use nutrition and phytotherapy.
> - Improve psychological symptoms:
>   – cognitive behavioural therapy
>   – nutrition and phytotherapy.

also is an essential cofactor in neurotransmitter regulation of pain.[35] In CFS it has been used by injection of either magnesium sulfate or oral chelates (such as citrate) at 500 mg two or three times a day to assist pain management.[36]

Herbal interventions may include combinations of *Curcuma longa*, *Boswellia serrata*, *Zingiber officinale* and *Apium graveolens*[41] with an emphasis on management of pain and stiffness.

Improve sleep

Conventional therapies aimed at managing sleep include hypnotic agents such as low-dose benzodiazepines or selective serotonin reuptake inhibitors, and **melatonin**, a naturally produced sleep hormone 5 mg 1–2 in evening.

Nutritional interventions include the use of **5-hydroxytryptophan**, which may increase serotonin production and melatonin production, at a dose of 50–100 mg at night, increasing to a maximum of 250 mg, being careful of nausea and also interactions with conventional antidepressants,

Herbal interventions include:
- **Withania somnifera**, an adaptogen that may also promote sleep normalisation, 600 mg of dry root extract up to four times a day[38]
- **Valeriana officinalis**, which may assist in management of insomnia, irritability and restlessness, 700 mg of the dry root and rhizome three times a day[39]
- **Zizyphus jujuba**, synergistic with *Valeriana officinalis* in helping nocturnal irritability and anxiety, 900 mg of the dry seed up to three times a day[39]
- **Passiflora incarnata**, synergistic with *Valeriana officinalis* to assist sleep and nervous agitation, 500 mg of the dry herb up to three times a day.[39]

Increase physical conditioning
Graded physical activity

Negotiate a balanced and achievable exercise plan with the patient (after a medical check-up). A graded exercise program supervised by a qualified health professional e.g. exercise physiologist or equivalent. Two reviews[40,42] of research show that, after 3 months of exercise intervention, physical function improved and less fatigue was experienced by those who participated. However improved responses were seen when education was combined with exercise therapy but not when anti-depressants were also used in combination.[40] Additionally the exercise intervention may be less palatable to some groups of patients than other interventions.[40]

Nutritional interventions
- **Acetyl carnitine** 500 mg three times a day has been shown to improve energy especially mental fatigue in an open labelled randomised trial.[43]
- In orthostatic intolerance and neurally mediated hypotension, increased intake of salt (**sodium chloride**) 600 mg twice to three times a day with increased water intake may assist the control of this syndrome.[21]
- **Magnesium citrate** 500 mg three times a day may assist energy metabolism.[36]
- **Nicotinamide** (NADH) 10 mg a day may assist energy metabolism.[26]
- **Essential fatty acids** have been trialled, with reported benefit in patients treated with high dose 1000 mg omega-3 marine oil four times a day.[44,45]
- Other interventions used with less evidence in CFS include **Co Q10**, with anecdotal evidence of improved exercise tolerance at 100 mg a day.[46]

Herbal interventions
- *Eleutherococcus senticosus* has been shown to assist physical labour and mental tasks, and reduces sick days in workers studied. It has been studied in a randomised controlled trial in CFS with improvements shown in treated, moderately fatigued CFS patients.[37]
- *Panax ginseng* is an adaptogenic (improves adaptation to stress) and tonic herb that increases stamina and helps normalise the hypothalamic–pituitary–adrenal axis.[47]
- *Withania somnifera* is adaptogenic but a non-stimulant and helps normalise sleep.[48]
- *Rhodiola rosea* is a tonic herb, improving cognitive performance, stamina and recall. The dose is 600 mg of the dry root up to four times a day or 3–4 mL of the alcoholic extract twice a day.[49]

Herbal treatments for orthostatic intolerance
- *Glycyrrhiza glabra* contains glycyrrhizin and glycyrrhetinic acid, which have adrenal steroidal anti-inflammatory effects, plus elevation of blood pressure due to the promotion of sodium retention from the kidney.[22] The dose is 1–2 mL of the 1:1 alcoholic extract up to three times a day.
- *Rehmannia glutinosa* supports the adrenal gland and acts in a similar way to liquorice without the potential for hypertensive effect. It is traditionally used for fatigue in traditional Chinese medicine.[50,51] The dose is 350 mg of the dry root up to four times a day.
- *Ruscus aculeatus* has been shown to assist the management of orthostatic hypotension.[52] Dose is 800 mg of the dry herb up to three times a day. It may be more effective when combined with *Aesculus hippocastanum*.

Improve immune dysfunction
Assess first for allergy and environmental toxicity (see Table 35.2).[45,46,54] Dysfunctional immunity has been demonstrated in CFS;[55,56] this may manifest as sensitivity to environmental agents such as foods, pollens, dust mites and other agents. Assessment may range from skin prick/patch testing for inhalant allergens, foods and mites to immunoglobulin G testing for food sensitivity.

Table 35.2 Tests for infection, allergy and environmental toxicity[45,46]

TESTS	FUNCTIONAL OUTCOME	MANAGEMENT RECOMMENDATION
Assess for infection	Detect any 'occult' or latent infections, e.g. *Mycoplasma*, *Chlamydia*, *Rickettsia*, virus or parasites	Requires specialised assessment and advice, but nutritional and herbal immune support can be used as a basis of management
Heavy metal assessment Tests to consider: • hair analysis • chelation challenge • porphyrin assessment	Elevated heavy metals	• Stabilise metal detoxification—improve digestion, antioxidants, replace displaced minerals—zinc, selenium etc. • Specific chelation agents
Liver detoxification profile	• Impaired phase 1 and/or phase 2 detoxification • Uncoupled phase 1 to phase 2	Enhance appropriate detoxification through nutritional support: • phase 1—vitamin B, phase 2—amino acid support • antioxidants
Food allergy assessment: • skin/patch test • IgG$_4$ blood test for food • digestive stool analysis or faecal bacterial DNA assessment	Identification of possible triggers for persistent immune dysfunction	• Elimination diet and challenge after exclusion • Digestive support through probiotic supplementation, digestive enzymes

Toxicity may involve allergy as mentioned above, but also the possibility of immunological or metabolic injury from heavy metals and chemicals. The effects may range from displacement of energy cofactors such as copper antagonising zinc bioavailability, or mercury displacing selenium. Other effects may be from enzyme induction or inhibition, leading to altered metabolic clearance or the production of physiological energy cofactors. An example of the latter is alteration of liver detoxification pathways.

Nutritional interventions
- **Omega-3 fatty acids** 1000 mg three times a day may rebalance eicosanoid pathways.[44,52]
- **Zinc** chelate 220 mg at night may have direct effects on immune cell proliferation and function. An observational study[54] found that serum zinc levels correlated with fatigue in 18 patients with CFS compared with 18 controls. The higher the zinc level, the less the fatigue.
- **Glutamine** 500 mg three times a day has been shown to modulate lymphocyte proliferation and assist immune outcomes.[57]
- **Digestive enzymes** may assist the reduction in ability to digest protein and complex carbohydrates (see Chapter 5 on food intolerances).
- **Probiotics** may be needed if there are significant abnormalities on digestive bacterial analysis (see Chapter 3 on irritable bowel syndrome).

Herbal interventions
- *Astragalus membranaceus* contains polysaccharides and saponins that may be indicated for chronic immune enhancement and recurrent viral illness. A recent study of 6 weeks found that its effects in CFS involved its ability to balance abnormal cytokine levels.[41] The dose is 4–5 mL t.d.s. of 1:2 alcoholic extract.
- *Hemidesmus indicus* contains essential oils and triterpenoid saponins, which are indicated for immune system suppression in cases of autoimmune conditions. The dose is 3–6 mL a day of 1:2 alcoholic extract or 500 mg up to four times a day of the dry root.

- *Echinacea* **spp.** is immunomodulatory for viral illness and immune disorders. The dose is 3–5 mL twice daily of the 1:2 alcoholic extract (mixed *augustifolia/purpurea*) or 600 mg of the tablets containing dried herbs of mixed species up to three times a day.[58]
- *Rehmannia glutinosa* supports the adrenal gland and acts in a similar way to liquorice without the potential for hypertensive effect. The dose is 350 mg of the dry root up to four times a day.[51]
- *Hypericum perforatum* assists mild mood disorders and depression. It may have activity against encapsulated viruses such as Epstein Barr. In a randomised controlled trial in 1994 39 patients treated with St John's wort showed significant improvement in symptoms after 4 weeks.[59] The dose is 1.8 g of the dry herb (standardised to 990 µg of hypericin) up to 3 times a day or 2.5 mL up to twice daily of the 1:2 alcoholic extract.[59]

Improve psychological symptoms
Conventional therapies
- Short-term studies have shown that **cognitive behavioural therapy** (CBT) is effective in reducing fatigue compared with other psychological therapies including relaxation, counselling and education/support.[60] This intervention has also shown benefit in randomised controlled studies in children and young adults. The long-term follow-up of CBT has shown benefits in fatigue, symptom reduction, physical functioning and school and work absences. It warrants further research.[27,30,31,60]
- **Antidepressants** may help regulate pain, sleep disorders (tricyclic antidepressants) or severe reactive depression. Possible side effects may limit their use and individual variations may occur in response. Research has failed, however, to show a consistent effect in most patients with CFS.[32,61]

Nutritional interventions
- **B12** replenishes CNS methylation imbalance. Improved cognitive function at doses of 1000 µg intramuscularly, titrated to patient response (weekly to monthly).[23,24]
- **S-adenosylmethionine** may relieve mood disorder plus joint pains, 200 mg three times a day.[22]

Herbal Interventions
Hypericum perforatum improves mild depressive symptoms. It has been postulated to have antiviral activity as well. It may be helpful for reactive depression. Care should be taken with possible interactions with prescription antidepressants.[53,59]

Case Study

A 25-year-old male presents with a 5-year history of developing **recurrent and relapsing severe fatigue, muscle aches with morning stiffness worsening after any physical exertion**. His fatigue escalates for about 48 hours after simple activity such as a brisk prolonged walk. He has **difficulty with concentration and memory** at tasks over 30 minutes. **His illness initially commenced after a viral episode of high fevers, glandular swelling, headache.** He feels he has **never fully recovered** from it with his energy levels being rated at 4–5/10 every day.

SUGGESTIVE SYMPTOMS
- Fatigue worsening after activity lasting more than 6 continual months
- Muscle ache and pains
- Headache
- Poor concentration and memory

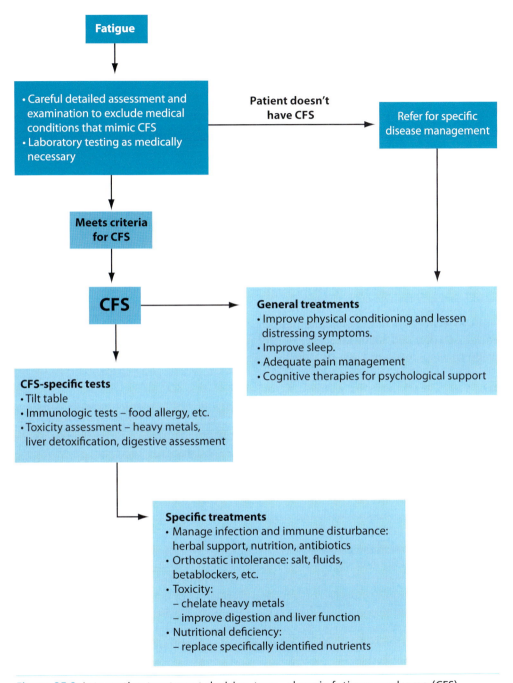

Figure 35.2 Integrative treatment decision tree—chronic fatigue syndrome (CFS)

Example treatment

Prescription

The patient with CFS was assisted to develop a plan for the next 3 months of management, to be reviewed every 4 weeks:

- psychological supportive sessions with cognitive behavioural therapy (CBT), supervised by a psychologist
- a graded exercise program to improve fitness and his physical stamina, supervised by an exercise physiologist or physiotherapist
- two herbal formulas—see the treatment box for immunological support and sleep stabilisation and stamina
- acetyl carnitine 500 mg three times a day for stamina and energy.

  Note: Create a plan. Negotiate this with the patient.

  Be flexible—people with CFS have fluctuating symptoms and needs.

Review the patient for not just physical symptoms but also psychological distress, social isolation and financial stress. Nutritional intervention may require follow-up to assess their response and adjustment.

> **Herbal prescription**
>
> | | |
> |---|---|
> | *Rhodiola rosea* 1:1 | 20 mL |
> | *Rehmannia glutinosa* 1:2 | 30 mL |
> | *Astragalus membranaceus* 1:2 | 35 mL |
> | *Glycyrrhiza glabra* 1:1 | 15 mL |
> | 5 mL t.d.s. | 100 mL |
> | *Withania somnifera* 600 mg | |
> | *Panax ginseng* 125 mg 2 tablets b.d. | |
>
> **Nutritional prescription**
>
> Acetylcarnitine—500 mg t.d.s. before meals
>
> CoQ10—100 mg per/day

Expected outcomes and follow-up protocols

CFS is a chronic condition that may take months to resolve, so patience is required. The patient with CFS has a spectrum of needs. Management of such a spectrum disorder may necessitate different team members at different times in the illness. Such team members may be a psychologist, exercise physiologist, dietician, physiotherapist and massage therapist, even a physician. Note that consideration of orthostatic intolerance may necessitate earlier assessment via tilt table testing. If a positive result is obtained, then additional assessment to exclude hypoadrenal function (fasting salivary cortisol) may be necessary with the addition of salt and fluid loading. Conventional therapy may include the use of a low dose beta-blocker. Interventions that may assist are liquorice, *Rehmannia glutinosa* and *Ruscus aculeatus* (see above). Fluctuations may occur with immunological symptoms (fluctuating fevers or glandular swelling, inflammatory symptoms such as joint pains and regional or diffuse muscle pain) require careful assessment. Exclusion of persistent infection through specific assessment for infectious agents and immunological disorders may be required. Exclusion of toxic exposure or persistent toxins such as heavy metals needs to be considered. In addition the possibility of detoxification disorders of the liver may be excluded through appropriate functional liver detoxification studies.

Table 35.3 Review of the major evidence

INTERVENTION	METHODOLOGY	RESULT	COMMENT
Cognitive behavioural therapy (CBT) 3 RCTs Deale et al 1997[62]	$n = 60$; 5-year follow-up after 26-week intervention[62]	All RCTs for CBT showed significantly different positive effects for the intervention compared to controls. The 5-year follow-up study showed improvements remained for global improvements, but not for physical functioning and fatigue scores.	More participants withdrew from this intervention than in other trial interventions (19% vs 13% average) across most studies, possibly indicating that this therapy does not meet the needs of some patients with CFS.
Prins et al 2001[63]	$n = 278$; 61-week follow-up after 35-week intervention[63]		
Sharpe et al 1996[31]	$n = 60$; 52-week follow-up[31]		
Graded exercise programs Fulcher & White 1997[64]	$n = 66$; follow-up 12 weeks[64]	All trials showed significantly better results in overall benefit from this intervention. No great side effects from these programs were reported.	A combined RCT with an antidepressant (fluoxetine) showed no significant additional benefit.
Powell et al. 2001[65]	$n = 148$; follow-up at 52 weeks after 26 weeks intervention[65]		
Wearden et al. 1998[66]	$n = 136$; follow-up at 26 weeks[66]		
Magnesium Cox et al. 1991[36]	$n = 32$; treated for 6 weeks; 15 patients with IMI magnesium sulfate and 17 with placebo[36]	12 of 15 treated patients experienced benefit versus 3 of the placebo arm. Improvements were energy level, less pain and better emotional state.	Study has been replicated without showing the same degree of benefit.
Omega-3 Behan et al. 1990[67]	$n = 63$; follow-up to 13 weeks[67]	8 by 500 mg marine based omega fatty acids were given to active patients versus placebo. At 1 month 74% of active treated versus 23% placebo had benefit with the 3-month effect at 85% active versus 17% placebo ($p = 0.0001$)[67]	Appears to have potential benefit in chronic fatigue syndrome. Larger studies are advised to validate these findings.

(Continued)

Table 35.3 Review of the major evidence *(Continued)*

INTERVENTION	METHODOLOGY	RESULT	COMMENT
Warren et al. 1999[53]	*n* = 50; follow-up to 13 weeks[53]	50 participants were randomised to EFAs = supplementation versus placebo showed some improvement of symptoms in treated group but did not reach significance.[53]	The study[53] using the Beck's depression score and a physical function questionnaire may have adequate 'quality of life' data to assess a true effect of the intervention.
Oral NADH Forsyth et al. 1999[68]	*n* = 26; follow-up to 12 weeks[68]	26 active versus 26 placebos. 4 weeks' intervention with 10 mg NADH and then 4 weeks' washout with a crossover treatment for 4 weeks 31% versus 8% placebo had benefit[68]	These are small studies that need replication.
Santaella et al. 2004[26]	*n* = 31; follow-up to 24 months[26]	12 actively treated patients had initial 3-month improvement versus placebo (*p* < 0.0001) on mean symptom scores of fatigue but this was not maintained at 24 months.[26]	
Homoeopathy Weatherley-Jones et al. 2004[69]	*n* = 103; follow-up to 26 weeks	47 patients versus 42 placebo participants completed this triple-blinded randomised controlled trial. There was a weak but significant difference in effect.	There appears to be some overall benefit from this intervention, but further trials may be needed to elucidate these outcomes.
Massage therapy Field et al. 1997[70]	*n* = 20; follow-up to 5 weeks	This small RCT showed beneficial effect to 5 weeks.	The study is considered flawed because comparisons were taken from within intervention groups rather than between them.

KEY POINTS

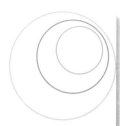

- Chronic fatigue syndrome is a complex disorder distinctive from depression and fatigue or other causes including 'adrenal exhaustion'.
- A spectrum of causes and symptom manifestations may require individualised management.
- Management should engage the patient through the use of a negotiated plan to address their physical and psychological needs while accepting that the patient is in charge of their health.
- Always observe and treat comorbid health conditions.
- An integrative approach using psychological, herbal, nutritional and lifestyle therapies should benefit the treatment of CFS, though pharmacotherapies may also be advised.

Further reading

Bruce M, Carruthers A, Kumar J, De Meirleir KL, et al. Myalgic encephalomyelitis/chronic fatigue syndrome: clinical working case definition, diagnostic and treatment protocols. J Chronic Fatigue 2003;11(1):7–116.

Shomon MJ. Living well with chronic fatigue syndrome and fibromyalgia. New York: HarperCollins, 2004.

References

1. Centers for Disease Control and Prevention diagnosis of chronic fatigue syndrome: http://www.cdc.gov/cfs/cfsdiagnosisHCP.htm
2. Centers for Disease Control and Prevention definition of chronic fatigue syndrome: http://www.cdc.gov/cfs/cfsdefinitionHCP.htm#conditions_exclude
3. Merck Manual definition of chronic fatigue syndrome: http://www.merck.com/mmpe/sec22/ch334/ch334b.html
4. Centers for Disease Control and Prevention causes of chronic fatigue syndrome: http://www.cdc.gov/CFS/cfscauses.htm
5. Lane RJ, et al. Enterovirus related metabolic myopathy: a postviral fatigue syndrome. J Neurol Neurosurg Psychiatry 2003;74(10):1382–1386.
6. Nicolson GL, et al. Multiple co-infections (*Mycoplasma, Chlamydia,* human herpes virus-6) in blood of chronic fatigue syndrome patients: association with signs and symptoms. Apmis 2003;111:557–566.
7. Endresen GK. *Mycoplasma* blood infection in chronic fatigue and fibromyalgia syndromes. Rheumatol Int 2003;23:211–215.
8. Koelle DM, et al. Markers of viral infection in monozygotic twins discordant for chronic fatigue syndrome. Clin Infect Dis 2002;35:518–525.
9. Gustaw K. Chronic fatigue syndrome following tick-borne diseases. Neurol Neurochir Pol 2003;37:1211–1221.
10. Maes M, et al. Increased serum IgA and IgM against LPS of enterobacteria in chronic fatigue syndrome (CFS): indication for the involvement of gram-negative enterobacteria in the etiology of CFS and for the presence of an increased gut–intestinal permeability. Journal of Affective Disorders 2006;99(1):237–240.
11. http://www.cdc.gov/CFS/cfscauses.htm
12. Lloyd AR, et al. Immunity and the pathophysiology of chronic fatigue syndrome. Ciba Found Symp 1993;173:176–187:discussion 187–192.
13. Lloyd A, et al. Cell-mediated immunity in patients with chronic fatigue syndrome, healthy control subjects and patients with major depression. Clin Exp Immunol 1992;87(1):76–79.
14. Lorusso L, et al. Immunological aspects of chronic fatigue syndrome. Autoimmun Rev 2009;8(4):287–291.
15. Smith AK, et al. Genetic evaluation of the serotonergic system in chronic fatigue syndrome. Psychoneuroendocrinology 2008;33(2):188–197.
16. Shephard RJ. Chronic fatigue syndrome: a brief review of functional disturbance and potential therapy. Journal of Sports Medicine and Physical Fitness 2005;45:381–392.
17. Griffith JP, Zarrouf AA. Systematic review of chronic fatigue syndrome: don't assume it's depression. Prim Care Companion J Clin Psychiatry 2008;10(2):120–128.
18. Kuratsune H, et al. Dehydroepiandrosterone sulfate deficiency in chronic fatigue syndrome. Int J Mol Med 1998;1(1):143–146.
19. Morriss RK, et al. The relation of sleep difficulties to fatigue, mood and disability in chronic fatigue syndrome. J Psychosom Res 1997;42(6):597–605.
20. Schondorf R, Freeman R. The importance of orthostatic intolerance in the chronic fatigue syndrome. Am J Med Sci 1999;317(2):117–123.
21. Rowe PC, Calkins H. Neurally mediated hypotension and chronic fatigue syndrome. Am J Med 1998;28:105(3a):15s–21s.
22. Braun L, Cohen M. Herbs and natural supplements: an evidence based guide. Sydney: Churchill Livingstone, 2007.
23. Lapp C. Using vitamin B12 for the management of CFS. CFIDS Chronicle 1999(Nov/Dec):14–16.
24. Pall ML. Cobalamin used in chronic fatigue syndrome therapy is a nitric oxide scavenger. J CFS 2001;8(2):39–44.
25. Jacobson W, et al. Serum folate and chronic fatigue syndrome. Neurology 1993;43(12):2645–2647.
26. Santaella ML, et al. Comparison of oral nicotinamide adenine dinucleotide (NADH) versus conventional therapy for chronic fatigue syndrome. P R Health Sci J 2004;23(2):89–93.
27. Hempel S, et al. Risk factors for chronic fatigue syndrome/myalgic encephalomyelitis: a systematic scoping review of multiple predictor studies. Psychological Medicine 2008;38:915–926.
28. Heim C, et al. Childhood trauma and risk for chronic fatigue syndrome: association with neuroendocrine dysfunction. Arch Gen Psychiatry 2009;66(1):72–80.
29. Nater UM, et al. Attenuated morning salivary cortisol concentrations in a population-based study of persons with chronic fatigue syndrome and well controls. Clin Endocrinol Metab 2008;93(3):703–709.
30. Rimes KA, Calder T. Treatments for chronic fatigue syndrome. Occupational Medicine 2005;55:32–39.
31. Sharpe M, et al. Cognitive behaviour therapy for the chronic fatigue syndrome: a randomised controlled trial. BMJ 1996;312:22–26.
32. Whiting P, et al. Interventions for the treatment and management of chronic fatigue syndrome. A systematic review. JAMA 2001;286(11):1360–1401.
33. Jones JF, et al. Complementary and alternative medical therapy utilization by people with chronic fatiguing illnesses in the United States. BMC Complement Altern Med 2007;7:12.
34. Vernon H, Schneider M. Chiropractic management of myofascial trigger points and myofascial pain syndrome: a systematic review of the literature. J Manipulative Physiol Ther 2009;32(1):14–24.
35. Murray ME. Brain and CSF magnesium concentrations during magnesium deficit in animals and humans. Magnesium Res 1992;5:303–313.
36. Cox IM, et al. Red blood cell magnesium and chronic fatigue syndrome. Lancet 1991;337:757–760.
37. Hart AJ, et al. Randomised controlled trial of Siberian ginseng for chronic fatigue. Psychological Medicine 2004;34:51–61.
38. Kulkarni SK, Dhira A. *Withania somnifera*: an Indian ginseng. Progress in Neuro-Psychopharmacology and Biological Psychiatry 2008;32(5):1093–1105.
39. Burgoyne B. Herbal treatment of insomnia. Modern Phytotherapist 2002;7(1):12–21.
40. Larun L, et al. Exercise therapy for chronic fatigue syndrome. Cochrane Database of Systematic Reviews 2004(3):CD003200.
41. Bone K. Chronic fatigue syndrome and its herbal treatment. Townsend Letter for Doctors and Patients, 1 November 2001.

42. Edmonds M, et al. Exercise therapy for chronic fatigue syndrome. Cochrane Database Syst Rev 2004;(3):CD003200.
43. Ruud C, et al. Exploratory open label, randomized study of acetyl- and propionylcarnitine in chronic fatigue syndrome. Psychosomatic Medicine 2004;66:276–282.
44. Behan PO, et al. Effect of high doses of essential fatty acids on the postviral fatigue syndrome. Acta Neurol Scand 1990;82:209–216.
45. Regland B, et al. Nickel allergy is found in a majority of women with chronic fatigue syndrome and muscle pain—and may be triggered by cigarette smoke and dietary nickel intake. Journal of Chronic Fatigue Syndrome 2001;8(1):57–65.
46. Racciatti D, et al. Chronic fatigue syndrome following a toxic exposure. Sci Total Environ 2001;270(1–3):27–31.
47. Morgan M, Bone K. Herbs to enhance energy and performance. A phytotherapist's perspective. Queensland: Mediherb, 2008:124.
48. Mishra LC, et al. Scientific basis for the therapeutic use of Withania somnifera (ashwagandha): a review. Altern Med Rev 2000;5(4):334–346.
49. Rhodiola rosea. Monograph. Altern Med Rev 2002;7(5):421–423.
50. Redman D. Rusculus aculeatus (butcher's broom) as a potential treatment for orthostatic hypotension with a case report. J Alt Compl Med 2000;6(6):539–549.
51. PDRhealth. Online. Available: http://www.pdrhealth.com
52. Chen R, et al. Traditional Chinese medicine for chronic fatigue syndrome. eCAM, doi:10.1093/ecam/nen017.
53. Warren G, et al. The role of essential fatty acids in chronic fatigue syndrome: a case controlled study of red-cell membrane essential fatty acids (EFA) and a placebo-controlled treatment study with high dose of EFA. Acta Neurol Scand 1999;99:112–116.
54. Graham, B. Associations between zinc/copper, metabolic rate and disability scales in chronic fatigue syndrome. Unpublished data, 2005. http://www.nutritional-healing.com
55. Tirelli U, et al. Immunological abnormalities in patients with chronic fatigue syndrome. Scand J Immunol 1994;40(6):601–608.
56. Racciatti D, et al. Study of immune alterations in patients with chronic fatigue syndrome with different etiologies. Int J Immunopathol Pharmacol 2004;17(2 Suppl):57–62.
57. Roth E. Immune and cell modulation by amino acids. Clin Nutr 2007;26(5):535–544.
58. Leigh E. Echinacea—Green paper 2001. Boulder: Herb Research Foundation, 2001; Leigh E. Ginseng—Green paper 1997-2001. Boulder: Herb Research Foundation, 2001.
59. Hübner WD, et al. Hypericum treatment of mild depressions with somatic symptoms. J Geriatr Psychiatry Neurol 1994;7(Suppl 1):S12–S14.
60. Price JR, et al. Cognitive behaviour therapy for chronic fatigue syndrome in adults. Cochrane Database Syst Rev 2008;(3):CD001027.
61. Chambers D, et al. Interventions for the treatment, management and rehabilitation of patients with chronic fatigue syndrome/myalgic encephalomyelitis: an updated systematic review. J R Soc Med 2006;99:506–520.
62. Deale A, et al. Cognitive behavior therapy for chronic fatigue syndrome: a randomized controlled trial. Am J Psychiatry 1997;154:408–414.
63. Prins J, et al. Cognitive behaviour therapy for chronic fatigue syndrome: a multicentre randomised controlled trial. Lancet 2001;357:841–847.
64. Fulcher KY, White PD. Randomised controlled trial of graded exercise with the chronic fatigue syndrome. BMJ 1997;314:1647–1652.
65. Powell P, et al. Randomised controlled trial of patient education to encourage graded exercise in chronic fatigue syndrome. BMJ 2001;322:387–392.
66. Wearden AJ, et al. Randomised, double-blind, placebo-controlled treatment trial of fluoxetine and graded exercise for chronic fatigue syndrome. Br J Psychiatry 1998;172:485–492.
67. Behan WM, Horrobin D. Effect of high doses of essential fatty acids on the postviral fatigue syndrome. Acta Neurol Scand 1990;82:209–216.
68. Forsyth LM, et al. Therapeutic effects of oral NADH on the symptoms of patients with chronic fatigue syndrome. Ann Allergy Asthma Immunol 1999;82:185–191.
69. Weatherley-Jones E, et al. A randomised, controlled, triple-blind trial of the efficacy of homeopathic treatment for chronic fatigue syndrome. Journal of Psychosomatic Research 2004;56(2):189–197.
70. Field TM, et al. Massage therapy effects on depression and somatic symptoms in chronic fatigue syndrome. J Chronic Fatigue Syndrome 1997;3:43–51.

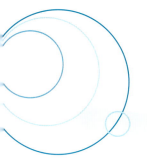

36
Human immunodeficiency virus

Jennifer Hillier
ND

AETIOLOGY

Human immunodeficiency virus (HIV; see Figure 36.1) is the infective agent behind the spectrum of symptoms involving the immune system and leading to the diagnosis of the acquired immunodeficiency syndrome (AIDS).[1] HIV attacks cells that have CD4 markers on their surface, most particularly T4 lymphocytes, also known as helper T cells. Helper T cells are the part of the immune system responsible for alerting the body to infection. Subverting these cells, the retrovirus avoids detection and uses the helper T cells to produce more HIV, leading to a greater viral load in the body. Initial infection produces a flu-like illness that is self-limiting and non-specific for HIV, so it often goes undiagnosed.[2] Symptoms may include night sweats, weight loss, fever and swollen lymph nodes. HIV infection then enters a latent stage that may last upwards of 10 to 20 years. As the lymphoid tissue and the T-cells get destroyed by HIV, AIDS may be diagnosed if the CD4 count is less than 200 copies/mm[3]. Symptoms at this point are usually due to the effects of opportunistic infections that take advantage of the inability of the body to combat invasion.[3]

RISK FACTORS

The greatest risk factor that currently predisposes an individual to contracting HIV is gender. Women and girls comprise the fastest-growing population of seropositive individuals in the world.[4] Anatomically this is due to the greater surface area of genital mucosa exposed to HIV-positive body fluids. Current World Health Organization estimates state that 50% of all HIV-positive individuals are female, a huge rise from the formerly male-dominated population of just a few years ago.[5] The highest occurrence of HIV worldwide is in sub-Saharan Africa, which currently reports 35% of new infections and 38% of AIDS deaths.[6] High-risk activities that may increase exposure to HIV

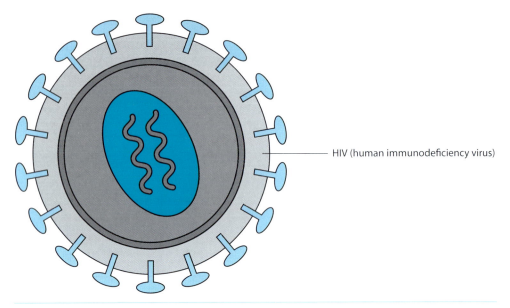

HIV (human immunodeficiency virus)

Figure 36.1 HIV virus

include any activity in which body fluids may be exchanged, including injection drug use, blood transfusions and unprotected sexual activity. It is also possible that pregnant women may pass HIV to their fetus during the pregnancy or birth and potentially while breastfeeding.[7]

CONVENTIONAL TREATMENT

Conventional medications are constantly evolving, and the prescribed drugs change often, depending upon the most recent research in this dynamic field. The aim of primary therapy is to increase CD4 count and to reduce the viral load down to an undetectable level. The most popularly prescribed agents for this task are grouped under the heading of highly active antiretroviral therapy (HAART) and include drugs from several classes.[8]

Each of these prescriptions works to target specific sites critical to the viral replication pathway. The most common classes of drugs include nucleoside/nucleotide reverse transcriptase inhibitors (NRTIs), which insert faulty messages into the reverse transcriptase process; non-nucleoside reverse transcriptase inhibitors (NNRTIs), which bind to reverse transcriptase and halt the production of viral DNA; protease inhibitors (PIs) which are responsible for targeting the construction of new HIV; and fusion inhibitors, which block binding of the virus to the cell. Often prescribed alongside these drugs are agents to combat the systemic effects of HIV, including lipid-lowering agents, antidepressants and sedatives.[9]

HAART AND CAM

HAART medication should never be withdrawn in favour of CAM interventions. CAM offers a beneficial role in supporting medical treatment by improving the patient's wellbeing and quality of life, and ameliorating the side effects of medications.

KEY TREATMENT PROTOCOLS

Optimise digestion and liver function

Common side effects of HIV and HIV medications can include a spectrum of gastrointestinal (GI) disorders, including diarrhoea, nutrient malabsorption, abdominal pain, GI bleeding and hepatomegaly.[10] Malnutrition and wasting are hallmarks of HIV infection,[11] making the need for optimal digestion critical for all individuals diagnosed with HIV. Opportunistic infections of the GI may also compound these symptoms and can seriously impact quality of life.[12] Supporting the gut in optimal functioning and promoting nutrient absorption can greatly improve an individual's ability to cope with the stresses of HIV.[13] Nutrients that support the gastric and intestinal mucosa include **L-glutamine**, **probiotics** and **dietary fibre**.[14]

> ### NATUROPATHIC TREATMENT AIMS
>
> - Treat underlying deficiencies that may lead to opportunistic infection.
> - Optimise nutrition that will negate mitochondrial damage and oxidation.
> - Regulate digestion and support liver function, especially if on medications.
> - Address the side effects of the HIV medications.
> - Improve vitality by strengthening the organ systems.
> - Focus on normalising blood lipids in order to decrease long-term cardiovascular damage.
> - Support the immune system in order to maintain high CD4 counts and low viral load.

Reducing mitochondrial toxicity

Although the drugs prescribed to combat HIV infection can greatly improve the quality of life of people living with HIV, mitochondrial toxicity is a problematic side effect regularly observed with NRTI therapy.[15] Lipodystrophy (LD) is a disorder of metabolism that cause fat deposition in atypical sites, causing fat loss in the limbs and face, and excess fat deposits on the trunk. The appearance of thin limbs and wasted face combined with abdominal obesity are often seen as identifying stigma for medicated individuals. In addition to the physical appearance, mitochondrial toxicity is also responsible for the intense fatigue present in some patients. Mitochondrial toxicity combined with the effects of increased cellular oxidation causes an accelerated rate of ageing and an increase in the risk of age-related comorbidities.[16] Additional effects of mitochondrial toxicity have been found to include lactic acidosis, pancreatitis and peripheral neuropathy.[17] Treatment of these side effects can slow the progression of adverse events and can greatly improve quality of life for individuals on NRTIs. Supplements that can reduce mitochondrial toxicity include **coenzyme Q10**, **riboflavin** and **thiamine**.[18] It has been noted that the levels of coenzyme Q10 are lower in individuals with advanced HIV, and that supplementation improves biochemical markers of health.[19] Supplements that can function as antioxidants, immune stimulants and can aid in the treatment of mitochondrial toxicity are highly efficacious and include N-acetyl cysteine, L-glutamine, L-carnitine and alpha-lipoic acid.[20] By acting as a sulphur donor, **N-acetyl cysteine** normalises lymphocyte glutathione production and thereby decreases the number of free radicals produced by the cell. This normalisation leads to improved CD4 levels and decreases progression to AIDS in clinical trials.[21–23]

    Glutamine deficiency is prevalent in HIV infection as it serves as the preferred fuel for lymphocytes, macrophages and enterocytes and, since it is primarily stored in muscle tissue, a deficiency exhibits as muscle wasting and overall weight loss.[24] It has been shown that supplementation at 40 g daily can reverse muscle wasting in HIV and increase weight gain in patients suffering from wasting syndrome.[25]

L-carnitine acts as an antioxidant and aids the production of energy by supporting the mitochondria and decreasing oxidation. Studies show that L-carnitine has an analgesic effect in the treatment of HIV peripheral neuropathy and can also improve peripheral nerve function by supporting several mechanisms, including nerve regeneration.[26] **Alpha-lipoic acid** is also used to support glutathione levels in the blood and therefore decrease free radical activity generated by HIV infection. One study demonstrated that 300 mg t.i.d. normalised blood glutathione and increased lymphocyte reactivity to T-cell mitogens.[27] In addition, alpha-lipoic acid had been used with success to treat the peripheral neuropathy of HIV by decreasing oxidative stress and inflammation of the involved nerves.[28]

Nutrient deficiencies

The elevated oxidation of cells in HIV infection, the side effects of therapeutic drugs and the increased stress on the body lead to the accelerated use of nutrients and subsequent deficiencies. Working to stay ahead of nutritional requirements is an integral part of treating individuals with HIV. Glutathione deficiency is a key source of immune dysfunction, muscle wasting and cellular oxidation as measured in multiple studies, but is not absorbable by the target tissues as a raw material.[22] Rather, the production of glutathione must be supported by precursors, which include glutamine and cysteine. Selenium, alpha-lipoic acid[27] and tryptophan are also important in increasing intracellular glutathione levels. Activities such as smoking,[29] excessive exercise and drinking excessive alcohol[30] can further deplete glutathione, so reducing exposure may, along with supplementation, lead to improved intracellular glutathione levels. Enhanced glutathione levels can lead to significant improvement in physical and quality of life markers, but research suggests that the benefits are present only while supplementation continues.[31] It has been observed that gastrointestinal issues common in HIV may exacerbate nutrient deficiencies via malabsorption. Vitamin B12, vitamin A, beta-carotene, zinc, selenium and folate may all be affected by decreased transit time, dysbiosis and gut inflammation due to HIV or HAART.[32] **Antioxidants** are also used at an increased rate in HIV, leading to the depletion of vitamin A, vitamin E and vitamin C.[33] Supplementing these nutrients, along with other antioxidant compounds, has been shown to improve lymphocyte proliferation and apoptosis.[34] Some research has been done with varying probiotic strains, but little clinical data exist to support their use in the general HIV population. Theoretically, introducing bacteria into an immunocompromised system may be harmful, and the benefits of supplementation should be carefully weighed against the inherent risk of infection.[35,36] Minerals are also depleted through various mechanisms involved in HIV pathogenesis. Supplementation with **minerals** such as zinc,[37] selenium,[38] magnesium and copper[39] have been shown to improve health outcomes and aid other nutrients in antioxidant functions.

Medication side effects

HAART is a life-saving intervention that can prolong an individual's life, improve CD4 count and decrease viral load.[40] Unfortunately these benefits often come at a physical price (see Table 36.1 and Figure 36.2). From liver toxicity and chronic diarrhoea, to insomnia and lipodystrophy, the symptoms are varied and can be so severe that people will stop taking the medications just to avoid the side effects. The primary target of naturopathic therapy is often the large number of adverse reactions to drugs. Making individuals more comfortable while they undergo therapy and stabilising their digestion, mood, sleep and cardiovascular health can have a profound influence upon quality of life and ultimately survival.

Table 36.1 Common side effects of HIV medications[41]

MEDICATION	COMMON SIDE EFFECTS
Nucleoside reverse transcriptase inhibitors and non-nucleoside reverse transcriptase inhibitors	Lactic acidosis, hepatitis, pancreatitis, anaemia, lipoatrophy
Protease inhibitors	Increased cholesterol and triglycerides, diabetes, lipodystrophy and lipoatrophy, osteoporosis and osteonecrosis
Fusion inhibitors	Pain at injection site, rashes, bad taste in mouth, increased occurrence of pneumonia

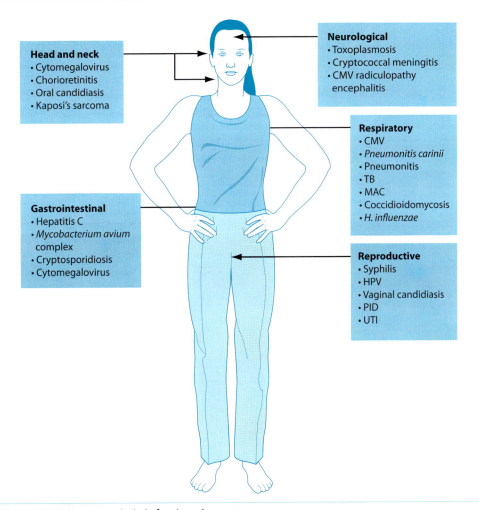

Head and neck
- Cytomegalovirus
- Chorioretinitis
- Oral candidiasis
- Kaposi's sarcoma

Neurological
- Toxoplasmosis
- Cryptococcal meningitis
- CMV radiculopathy encephalitis

Respiratory
- CMV
- *Pneumonitis carinii*
- Pneumonitis
- TB
- MAC
- Coccidioidomycosis
- *H. influenzae*

Gastrointestinal
- Hepatitis C
- *Mycobacterium avium* complex
- Cryptosporidiosis
- Cytomegalovirus

Reproductive
- Syphilis
- HPV
- Vaginal candidiasis
- PID
- UTI

Figure 36.2 Opportunistic infections by system

Cardiovascular risk

HIV not only affects the immune system, but it also has a considerable effect upon metabolism and in turn the cardiovascular system, and has been found to contribute to arteriosclerosis in infected individuals.[42] Protease inhibitors, NNRTIs or both are also contributing factors in developing cardiovascular pathologies. Dyslipidaemia, blood sugar abnormalities, inflammation and decreased fibrinolysis may all increase the occurrence of adverse cardiovascular events.[43] In addition to drug side effects, HIV pathogenesis has also been found to contribute to arteriosclerosis. Fortunately interventions that include **dietary and lifestyle changes** along with exercise can have a positive effect on lipid levels and cardiovascular markers.[44] It has also been found that the use of **omega-3 fish oils** in combination with exercise can lead to a reduction in triglyceride levels, and would therefore be an important addition to any treatment protocol.[45] In current research, another intervention that has been proven to change HIV-mediated cardiovascular markers is **vitamin E**.[46] Acting as an antioxidant, vitamin E reduces lipoprotein peroxidation, thus decreasing the potential for damage due to elevated blood lipids. Vitamin E also acts to decrease platelet aggregation, reducing the likelihood of vessel blockage and subsequent cardiovascular events.[47] In conclusion, suggesting a lower fat diet that includes high quality vegetable and protein sources, along with a moderate exercise schedule and metabolic support including fish oils and vitamin E, can help to decrease the risk of adverse cardiovascular events.

Opportunistic infections

Often the first indicator that may trigger the clinician to run an HIV test is the presence of an opportunistic infection. Though any microorganism may take advantage of a beleaguered immune system, there are certain opportunistic infections that occur more often in the presence of HIV (see Figure 36.3).

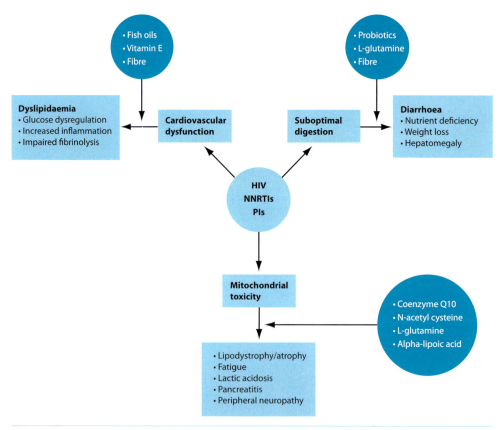

Figure 36.3 HIV/HAART side effects and nutritional interventions

Maintaining vitality (tonics and adaptogens)

One of the greatest challenges of treating HIV is that of keeping the vital force of the patient strong. Dealing with the mental and emotional stresses, along with the physical effects of the disease, can drain an individual and decrease their ability to cope with change. Patients can get extremely overwhelmed by the volume of new information that comes with a diagnosis of HIV, and with the continued therapies involved in their care. Health maintenance becomes the main goal, and keeping physical as well as mental health balanced can be the most effective approach of all. Adaptogenic therapies can be extremely useful as an adjunct to other more aggressive medicines. The focus of adaptogenic medicines needs to be not only on supporting the adrenal glands, but also targeting the immune system. Herbs such as *Withania somnifera*,[48] *Eleutherococcus senticosus*, *Panax ginseng*, *Ganoderma lucidum* and *Glycyrrhiza glabra* can all support the immune system while increasing tolerance to stress. **Withania somnifera**, in one study, was prescribed as an extract at 6 mL b.i.d. for 4 days with a result of stimulating an increase in the expression of CD4 and natural killer cells, demonstrating its stimulatory effect on the immune system.[49] **Eleutherococcus senticosus** extracts have been found to increase CD4 counts and lymphocyte populations when used in healthy subjects.[50] Studies have also shown that *Eleutherococcus senticosus* aids in adrenal function through decreasing adrenal hypertrophy and increasing adrenal vitamin C levels.[51] **Panax ginseng** is a popular botanical used in traditional Chinese medicine and has demonstrated a broad range of effects on the immune system by enhancing both B- and T-cell mediated responses while acting as an antimicrobial against *Heliobacter pylori* and *Staphylococcus aureus*,[52] which can lead to infection in HIV-positive individuals. In addition, one animal study found it to increase CD4 cell function against the challenge of an induced systemic candida infection,[53] which is one of the main opportunistic infections found in HIV/AIDS. **Ganoderma lucidum**, a fungus traditionally used in Chinese medicine, has been proven to reduce physical and mental fatigue, while improving the function of the immune system.[54] **Glycyrrhiza glabra**, as an extract, has been shown to decrease infective capability of *Candida albicans* strains.[55] It has also been studied as a compound that interferes with the infective abilities and replication of HIV, in addition to its anti-inflammatory and adrenal support functions.[56] Prescribing a botanical medicine based not only on its adaptogenic properties but also on its antimicrobial and immunosupportive qualities can help HIV-positive patients to maintain a high quality of life and improve their overall health.

Other lifestyle interventions, such as moderate exercise,[57] alternating hot and cold showers[58] and a daily meditation practice,[59,60] also round out a treatment protocol for enhancing energy and boosting perceived quality of life.

Mental health support

Supporting the body includes supporting the mind as well. A diagnosis of HIV can be a devastating occurrence and often triggers acute anxiety and depression. Long-term treatment fatigue can also take its toll as the constant reminder of illness counteracts attempts to live a meaningful and productive life.[61] Creating support networks of friends, healthcare providers and others living with HIV can validate and empower people to optimise their own health and that of the community.[62] Depression is of particular risk to adherence to medications and to risk behaviour in HIV-positive people. Individuals who perceive that they have nothing to lose are more likely to engage in high-risk activities and be less compliant with therapies.[63] It is important to recognise the symptoms of clinical depression and to treat or refer accordingly. Community support groups for people with HIV are particularly helpful in providing long-term coping strategies and creating a support network specific to HIV issues.

Drug–CAM interactions

It is important to recognise that there is a potential for interaction between the medications used for HAART and the botanical and nutraceutical supplements that naturopathic doctors use on a daily basis. Though there is limited research on interactions, proper individual research must go into any supplement that is being considered for a person on HAART. The literature recognises that botanicals that interact with CYP3A4 or P-glycoprotein can negatively affect the circulating levels of drugs in the system. Once such interaction occurs between *Hypericum perforatum* and PIs and NNRTIs, reducing their concentration in the body and promoting therapeutic failure.[64] There is promising research examining the potential for *Hypericum perforatum* to decrease HIV-1 transcription and replication,[65] but relatively few studies have pursued it due to interactions with traditional HIV drugs. A negative interaction also occurs between large amounts of garlic (*Allium sativum*) and ritonavir.[66] Criticism lies in the fact that most of the studies involve the supplements in combination with a single drug, a situation rarely seen in current HIV therapy, and therefore may not be an accurate reflection of the interactions occurring in patients using drugs and CAM.[67] Other natural compounds have been tested, but often with conflicting results between studies, thereby yielding no conclusive evidence.[68] More high-quality, effective research is needed to create a database of information for those treating HIV, but until this exists it is up to the practitioner to thoroughly assess and monitor any individual undergoing treatment, including the frequent assessment of CD4 and viral load levels.

INTEGRATIVE MEDICAL CONSIDERATIONS

Traditional Chinese medicine

Acupuncture is a very popular and effective method of treating the symptoms of HIV and the side effects of HAART. Due to the low probability of interaction between acupuncture and medical therapies and the cost-effective nature of this modality, it is a widely used tool in the treatment of HIV. One study recognised the value of acupuncture during structured treatment interruptions, where the group receiving the intervention during the interruption exhibited the suppression of viral load rebounds and the maintenance of immune function.[69] Many models exist to capture the effect that HIV has upon the energetic balance of the body. One model postulates that the infection is an invasion of Toxic Heat, which leads to a Stomach/Spleen disharmony and potentially then to Liver Qi stagnation or Blood Deficiency,[70] while another cites deficiencies in Blood and Yin as responsible for the spectrum of symptoms.[71] Regardless of the specifics of how the retrovirus presents in the greater population, treating a person for their symptoms while also addressing the root of the imbalance can lead to a greater quality of life and a decrease in physical discomfort.[72] Evidence exists to support the use of acupuncture for a variety of complaints associated with HIV/AIDS, including insomnia, diarrhoea, fatigue, malaise and neuropathic pain associated with HIV peripheral neuropathy.[73] As with all patients, it is important to follow universal precautions when dealing with body fluids and employ sterile technique during acupuncture sessions.

Homoeopathy

Cost-effective, widely available and demonstrating a reduced risk of interactions with medications, homoeopathy is another very popular option for people living with HIV. Working with the vital force while a person is fighting systemic infection and being treated with an arsenal of antiretroviral agents can be daunting, but using homoeopathy to help clear acute

Table 36.2 Progression of HIV to AIDS: treatment aims

CLINICAL OBSERVATIONS	NO SYMPTOMS OF HIV	SYMPTOMS OF HIV
Timeline	Latent period: average of 10 years CD4 > 200	Progression from HIV → AIDS: average of 4–20 years AIDS = CD4 < 200 + opportunistic infection
Primary actions of treatment aims	Screen for other sexually transmitted infections, including hepatitis C. Strengthen immune function, use antiretroviral botanicals. Optimise nutrition and digestive function. Develop spiritual and social support.	Treat opportunistic infections. Address medication side effects. Support cardiovascular health. Use adaptogenic therapies to reduce fatigue and improve immune function.

symptoms and support the constitution can engender profound change. Little research evidence exists, but one study that demonstrated improved health outcomes was found.[74]

With acute symptoms that can be found in multiple 'provings', researching conditions like explosive diarrhoea, nausea and anxiety can yield many remedies that are applicable to the set of symptoms a patient may present. The correct remedy given with frequent dosing and careful monitoring for aggravation can yield positive results. It is important to take a complete case, including what the person was like before the diagnosis and medications, to properly create a collection of information worthy of adding to the homoeopathic repertoire. As an individual progresses in the disease or is prescribed increasing amounts of medications, it becomes increasingly difficult to effect health using natural medicines like homoeopathy, which can be subtle and dependent upon the body's ability to adapt to change.

Therapeutic considerations in HIV

It is important to approach patients in an individualised way, taking into account their personal and spiritual beliefs, their preferences for treatment and their physical needs. Often women with young children and those of lower socioeconomic standing have difficulties with compliance to complex medication regimens and rigorous consultation schedules, and may lack access to costly supplement protocols. When working with an individual who is accessing additional faith- or cultural-based care, the botanical, nutritional or homoeopathic treatments applied must be understood in order to ascertain whether interactions might occur.

Case Study

A 34-year-old female patient presents to your clinic complaining of shortness of breath and **repeated chest infections** that have been **getting worse over the past three years.** She has been on multiple courses of antibiotics and has noticed an **increase in the occurrence of vaginal and oral yeast infections.** Over the past three years she has also noticed **increased fatigue and poor sleep,** punctuated by **hot flushes** which now occur nightly. She is has just been **diagnosed as HIV positive** and has **commenced HAART.**

SUGGESTIVE SYMPTOMS

- Repeated occurrence of infection
- Increasing fatigue
- Hot flushes and night sweats
- Infection by opportunistic pathogens, e.g. *Candida albicans, Pneumocystis carinii*

Initial presentation
- Build network of support (networks of friends, healthcare providers, others living with HIV/AIDS).
- Educate on risk activities and counsel on options available (such as still being able to be sexually active in a safe manner).
- Refer to other health services where appropriate—be particularly aware of mental health challenges (psychologist, support groups, conventional practitioner).

Does the patient exhibit symptoms of HIV infections?
CD4 count > 200

No →

Other issues
- Screen for other sexually transmitted infections (e.g. hepatitis C)
- Strengthen immune function (tonics, diet, lifestyle).
- Optimise nutrition and digestion (improve liver function; support gut function with glutamine, probiotics and fibre).

Yes

As per before symptoms were apparent, plus:
- Prevent and treat opportunistic infection (reduce exposure to pathogens in contaminated food or water, reduce public exposure during flu season, use immune tonics).
- Start adaptogenic therapies to reduce fatigue and improve immune function (*Withania somnifera, Eleutherococcus, Panax, Ganoderma*, glutathione, moderate exercise and other lifestyle factors).
- Address increased cardiovascular risk (omega-3 fatty acids, vitamin E, moderate exercise, lifestyle factors).
- Treat long-term considerations (fatigue, increased gastrointestinal symptoms, mental health considerations).

Is the patient on medication?

No

Counsel on conventional as well as complementary options and refer for appropriate treatment.

Yes

- Address medication side effects: diarrhoea, insomnia, lipodystrophy, traditional Chinese medicine—Toxic Heat leading to Liver Qi Stagnation or Blood Deficiency or Yin Deficiency common for broad reduction of symptoms; psychological as well as physical support for side effects such as lipodystrophy.
- Reduce mitochondrial toxicity associated with NRTI therapy (coenzyme Q10, B1, B2, carnitine, glutamine).
- Explore potential drug–CAM interactions (for example, *Hypericum perforatum* or *Allium sativum*; consider homoeopathy where appropriate to reduce risk of interaction).

Figure 36.4 Naturopathic treatment decision tree—HIV/AIDS

Example treatment

Prescription

The treatment focuses on ameliorating side effects associated with HAART and aims to improve overall health and vitality, potentially reducing comorbid conditions. *Withania somnifera*,[49] *Eleutherococcus senticosus*,[50] *Panax ginseng*,[53] *Ganoderma lucidum*[54] and *Glycyrrhiza glabra*[56] are prescribed as tonics that will support the body/mind and the immune system (see Chapter 15 on adrenal fatigue and Chapter 6 on immune insufficiency). *Gentiana lutea* is prescribed as a bitter digestive to aid the stimulation of digestion.[75]

Herbal formula	
Withania somnifera 1:1	25 mL
Eleutherococcus senticosus 1:2	25 mL
Panax ginseng 1:2	15 mL
Ganoderma lucidum 1:4	20 mL
Glycyrrhiza glabra 1:1	10 mL
Gentiana lutea 1:2	5 mL
5 mL t.d.s.	100 mL

Nutritional prescription
Antioxidant supplement including vitamin A, C, E and selenium b.d.
L-glutamine powder 15 g b.d.
Omega-3 fish oil 3 g b.d.

Antioxidant supplements including vitamins A, C and E and selenium are prescribed to reduce the toxicity associated with HIV medication and to improve resistance to viral load.[33,76] L-glutamine powder 15 g b.i.d. is prescribed to support optimal gut functioning and nutrient absorption.[25] Omega-3 fish oils are prescribed to reduce the risk of cardiovascular pathology from medication and infection.[77–79]

The patient is also provided dietary education, and the patient was advised to include 5–10 servings of brightly coloured fruits and vegetables, especially those that are red, yellow and orange, to increase the antioxidant and fibre content of diet. Daily exercise tailored to patient ability[57] and weekly acupuncture sessions to address imbalance[69] are also prescribed to improve immunity and quality of life. Though there is little research done on the effects of castor oil packs, this therapy may be beneficial in promoting a sense of wellbeing, decreasing insomnia and regulating digestion, and can be trialled in the patient.

Expected outcomes and follow-up protocols

In the Antiretroviral Therapy (ART) Cohort Collaboration study[80] it was determined that, taking all variables into account, patients had a 12% probability of progression to AIDS or death within 5 years of starting HIV treatment and 5% progressed to death within the same time period. The most positive outcomes were related CD4 levels above 350 copies/mm^3 and a viral load below 100,000 copies/mL at the beginning of treatment.[80] Patients who are newly diagnosed as HIV positive and are not yet in need of HAART, due to high CD4 counts and low viral loads, are best served by prescribing more aggressive herbs targeting the HIV replication process; however, the majority of patients who seek care are already receiving HAART. Herbs high in coumarins, alkaloids and flavonoids can affect several steps in the viral replication pathway[81] and can be useful in treatment-naive individuals. The longer a patient can be supported before they have a need for HAART, the longer the period of time that they will have to progress through the medication hierarchy, thus extending life expectancy.

The course of HIV is variable, and thus no exact prognosis can be offered to anxious patients and families. Those who optimise their overall health exhibit significant improvement in many determinants of quality of life. Once a patient is put on a well-researched protocol of antioxidants and adaptogens, with a good plan for proper nutrition and stress reduction, regular visits are often structured around acute complaints related to the disease or the medications. Many patients seen in a naturopathic clinical practice have already been prescribed HAART, and the real strength of naturopathic medicine lies in reducing side effects, improving vitality and empowering the patients to become part of the healing process. Though interventions can truly seem miraculous at times, with patients feeling greatly improved, it must be remembered that HIV effects a volatile and erratic course of symptoms. Patients who may appear strong and healthy in a naturopath's office today could be debilitated and in intensive care tomorrow. Fortunately, the opposite is also possible. It is important to remember that, even when physical systems may be shutting down, there is always room for healing, and therefore for hope in the face of this pandemic.

Table 36.3 Review of the major evidence

INTERVENTION	METHODOLOGY	RESULT	COMMENT
Probiotics, soluble fibre and L-glutamine[82]	12-week RCT ($n = 35$) of HIV-positive males taking nelfinavir or lopinavir/ritonavir, exhibiting diarrhoea. Probiotics (1.2 g/day), soluble fibre (11 g/day) and L-glutamine (30 g/day) if diarrhoea persisted at week 4 vs standard of care.	Diarrhoea resolved in 36% of treated subjects ($p < 0.01$). In 15 of 28 treated subjects with unresolved diarrhoea mean number of stools declined and loose BM decreased ($p < 0.05$). No change in weight, CD4 or HIV RNA.	Short-term treatment yields improvement in symptom profile. Longer-term monitoring of patients may show a significant effect upon the immune markers. Immune and digestive systems are also supported by the interventions. Further investigation is required.
Antioxidant therapy[76]	12-week-single centre, prospective, dose comparison study ($n = 48$). β-carotene, vitamin E, vitamin C, selenium, CoQ10 high dose vs same supplements at lower dose.	Antioxidant supplementation significantly improved markers of oxidative defence. No difference in effectiveness noted between high and low doses.	A significant difference in baseline antioxidant status was present between the two groups of participants. Future studies may account for this difference by grouping similar antioxidant baseline levels together for comparison of treatments.
Omega-3 fatty acid supplementation[77–79]	Three studies have been done examining the effect of omega-3 fatty acid supplementation in the form of fish oil on the mean triglyceride levels in HIV-positive individuals receiving HAART.	Significant reduction in the levels of triglycerides were found in each clinical trial, with 9 g of fish oil q.d., 2 g of fish oil t.i.d. and 3 g of fish oil b.i.d. prescribed as the studied intervention.	These studies included individuals receiving statin therapy and other lipid-lowering agents, providing a realistic representation of a HAART-prescribed population. Even factoring in the actions of these agents, omega-3 fatty acid supplementation in the form of fish oil still provided a statistically significant lipid-lowering effect.
Alpha CD4-pokeweed antiviral protein (PAP) immunoconjugate[83,84]	22 strains of HIV-1 were exposed to CD4-PAP in vitro and compared to the same strains exposed to zidovudine.	Zidovudine was ineffective in 5 of the 22 HIV-1 strains, whereas all strains were inhibited by treatment with CD4-PAP.	CD4-PAP was effective at eradicating all strains of HIV-1 in contrast to zidovudine, though it was found that more advanced stages of HIV infection required a higher concentration of CD4-PAP to exhibit inhibition. No damage to bone marrow was noted, even at high doses. Further studies are examining the potential for CD4-PAP to be used as an intra-vaginal antiviral microbicide.

KEY POINTS

- Educate patients with potential risk of HIV infection—IV drug users and those with promiscuous sexual activity.
- Support body/mind with herbal tonics, adaptogens and nervines, and prescribe nutrients in cases of deficiency.
- Reduce exposure to potential sources of pathogens via raw food, poor preparation or contaminated water, and excess public exposure in flu season.
- Support optimal digestion and nutrition (with a healthy diet and whole foods).
- Be sensitive to cultural beliefs and potential socioeconomic barriers.
- Stay alert to elevated cardiovascular risk, gastrointestinal symptoms and mental health challenges.
- Assist in establishing a network of care resources and make sure that psychological support is provided to the patient.

Acknowledgment

The author would like to acknowledge David Casteleijn for his assistance with herbal medicine approaches to HIV/AIDS.

Further reading

AIDSinfo website. Online. Available:http://www.aidsinfo.nih.gov/

Bodeker G, et al. HIV/AIDS: traditional systems of health care in the management of a global epidemic. In: Bodeker G, Burford G, eds. Traditional, complementary and alternative medicine: policy and public health perspectives. London: Imperial College Press, 2006.

Body Health Resources Corporation. TheBody.com. New York: Body Health Resources Corporation. Online. Available: http://thebody.com/

Canadian AIDS Treatment Information Exchange website. Online. Available: http://www.catie.ca/

Canadian Aboriginal AIDS Network website. Online. Available: http://www.caan.ca/english

References

1. World Health Organization HIV/AIDS. Online. Available: http://www.who.int/topics/hiv_aids/en/index.html 9 May 2009
2. Mandell GL, Bennett JE, Dolin R, eds. Natural history of human immunodeficiency virus infection. Principles and practice of infectious diseases. 6th edn. New York: Churchill Livingstone.
3. Hoffmann C, Bartlett J. Acute retroviral syndrome and general management of the human immunodeficiency virus. In: Piccini JP, Nilsson KR, eds. The Osler medical handbook. 2nd edn. Baltimore: Johns Hopkins University.
4. National Institute of Allergy and Infectious Diseases. HIV infection in women. Online. Available: http://www.niaid.nih.gov/factsheets/womenhiv.htm May 2006
5. World Health Organization. Gender, Women and Health. Online. Available: http://www.who.int/gender/hiv_aids/en 23 September 2008
6. World Bank. HIV/AIDS regional update—Africa. Online. Available: http://web.worldbank.org/WBSITE/EXTERNAL/COUNTRIES/AFRICAEXT/EXTAFRHEANUTPOP/EXTAFRREGTOPHIVAIDS 24 June 2009
7. World Health Organization. HIV/AIDS Online Q&A. Online. Available: http://www.who.int/features/qa/71/en/ 24 June 2009
8. What is antiretroviral therapy (ART)? Fact Sheet 403. AIDS Infonet. Online. Available: http://www.aidsinfonet.org/fact_sheets/view/403 24 April 2009
9. AIDSmeds and Poz. Currently approved drugs for HIV: a comparative chart. Online. Available: http://www.aidsmeds.com/articles/DrugChart_10632.shtml 11 February 2008
10. Wilcox CM. Gastrointestinal consequences of infection with human immunodeficiency virus. In: Feldman M, Friedman LS, Brandt LJ, eds. Sleisenger and Fordtran's gastrointestinal and liver disease. 8th edn. Philadelphia: WB Saunders.
11. Mandell GL, et al, eds. Special populations—human immunodeficiency virus/acquired immunodeficiency syndrome. Principles and practice of infectious diseases, 6th edn. Philadelphia: Churchill Livingstone. .
12. First consult: HIV/AIDS-associated opportunistic infections. MD Consult. Online. Available: http://www.mdconsult.com.ezproxy.ccnm.edu/das/pdxmd/body/146167088-4/0?type=med&eid=9-u1.0-_1_mt_5091503 26 June 2009
13. Fields-Gardner C. A review of mechanisms of wasting in HIV disease. Nutr Clin Pract 1995;10(5):167–176.
14. Fitch KV, et al. Effects of a lifestyle modification program in HIV-infected patients with the metabolic syndrome. AIDS 2006;11;20(14):1843–1850.
15. Mallewa JE, et al. HIV-associated lipodystrophy: a review of underlying mechanisms and therapeutic options. J Antimicrob Chemother 2008;62(4):648–660.
16. Caron M, et al. Contribution of mitochondrial dysfunction and oxidative stress to cellular premature senescence induced by antiretroviral thymidine analogues. Antivir Ther 2008;13(1):27–38.

17. Wester CW, et al. Higher-than-expected rates of lactic acidosis among highly active antiretroviral therapy-treated women in Botswana: preliminary results from a large randomized clinical trial. J Acquir Immune Defic Syndr 2007;46(3):318–322.

18. Bowers JM, Bert-Moreno A. Treatment of HAART-induced lactic acidosis with B vitamin supplements. Nutr Clin Pract 2004;19(4):375–378.

19. Folkers K, et al. Biochemical deficiencies of coenzyme Q10 in HIV-infection and exploratory treatment. Biochem Biophys Res Commun 1988;153(2):888–896.

20. Patrick, Lyn. Nutrients and HIV: N-acetylcysteine, alpha-lipoic acid, L-glutamine, and L-carnitine. Townsend Letter for Doctors and Patients April 2002;225:60.

21. De Rosa SC, et al. N-acetylcysteine replenishes glutathione in HIV infection. European Journal of Clinical Investigation 2000;30(10):915–929.

22. Droge W, Breitkreutz R. Glutathione and immune function. Proceedings of the Nutrition Society 2000;59:595–600.

23. Wu G, et al. Glutathione metabolism and its implications for health. J Nutr 2004;134(3):489–492.

24. Curi R, et al. Molecular mechanisms of glutamine action. Journal of Cellular Physiology 2005;204:392–401.

25. Shabert JK, et al. Glutamine-antioxidant supplementation increases body cell mass in AIDS patients with weight loss: a randomized, double-blind controlled trial. Nutrition 1999;15(11–12):860–864.

26. Chiechio S, et al. Acetyl-L-carnitine in neuropathic pain: experimental data. CNS Drugs 2007 (Suppl);21:31–38.

27. Jariwalla RJ, et al. Restoration of blood total glutathione status and lymphocyte function following alpha-lipoic acid supplementation in patients with HIV infection. J Altern Complement Med 2008;14(2):139–146.

28. Head K. Peripheral neuropathy: pathogenic mechanisms and alternative therapies. Alternative Medicine Review 2006;11(4):294–329.

29. Cole SB, et al. Oxidative stress and antioxidant capacity in smoking and nonsmoking men with HIV/acquired immunodeficiency syndrome. Nutr Clin Pract 2005;20(6):662–667.

30. Colell A, et al. Selective glutathione depletion of mitochondria by ethanol sensitizes hepatocytes to tumor necrosis factor. Gastroenterology 1998;115(6):1541–1551.

31. Namulema E, et al. When the nutritional supplements stop: evidence from a double-blinded, HIV clinical trial at Mengo Hospital, Kampala, Uganda. Journal of Orthomolecular Medicine 2008;23(3):130–132.

32. Singhal N. A clinical review of micronutrients in HIV infection. J Int Assoc Physicians AIDS Care 2002;1(2):63–75.

33. Fawzi W. Micronutrients and human immunodeficiency virus type 1 disease progression among adults and children. Clinical Infectious Diseases 2003;37(Suppl 2):S112–S116.

34. Winkler P, et al. Lymphocyte proliferation and apoptosis in HIV-seropositive and healthy subjects during long-term ingestion of fruit juices or a fruit-vegetable-concentrate rich in polyphenols and antioxidant vitamins. Eur J Clin Nutr 2004;58(2):317–325.

35. Cunningham-Rundles S, et al. Probiotics and immune response. Am J Gastroenterol 2000;95(1 Suppl):S22–S25.

36. Wolf BW, et al. Safety and tolerance of Lactobacillus reuteri supplementation to a population infected with the human immunodeficiency virus. Food Chem Toxicol 1998;36(12):1085–1094.

37. Bobat R, et al. Safety and efficacy of zinc supplementation for children with HIV-1 infection in South Africa: a randomised double-blind placebo-controlled trial. Lancet 2005;366(9500):1862–1867.

38. Ferencík M, Ebringer L. Modulatory effects of selenium and zinc on the immune system. Folia Microbiol (Praha) 2003;48(3):417–426.

39. Evans P, Halliwell B. Micronutrients: oxidant/antioxidant status. Br J Nutr 2001;85(Suppl 2):S67–S74.

40. Street E, Curtis H, Sabin CA, Monteiro EF, Johnson MA. British HIV Association (BHIVA) national cohort outcomes audit of patients commencing antiretrovirals from naïve. HIV Medicine 2009 Jul;10(6):337–342.

41. Oelklaus MW, et al. Managing long-term side of effects of HIV therapy. Test Positive Aware Network. Online. Available from: http://www.thebody.com/content/treat/art40471.html March2007

42. Schillaci G, et al. Aortic stiffness in untreated adult patients with human immunodeficiency virus infection. Hypertension 2008;52(2):308–313.

43. Grinspoon S, Carr A. Cardiovascular risk and body-fat abnormalities in HIV-infected adults. N Engl J Med 2005;6:352(1):48–62.

44. Triant VA, et al. Increased acute myocardial infarction rates and cardiovascular risk factors among patients with human immunodeficiency virus disease. J Clin Endocrinol Metab 2007;92(7):2506–2512.

45. Wohl DA, et al. Randomized study of the safety and efficacy of fish oil (omega-3 fatty acid) supplementation with dietary and exercise counseling for the treatment of antiretroviral therapy–associated hypertriglyceridemia. Clinical Infectious Diseases 2005;41(10):1498–1504.

46. Gavrila A, et al. Exercise and vitamin E intake are independently associated with metabolic abnormalities in human immunodeficiency virus-positive subjects: a cross-sectional study. Clin Infect Dis 2003;36(12):1593–1601.

47. Clarke MW, et al. Vitamin E in human health and disease. Crit Rev Clin Lab Sci 2008;45(5):417–450.

48. Rege NN, et al. Adaptogenic properties of six rasayanan herbs used in Ayurvedic medicine. Phytotherapy Research 1999;14(4):275–291.

49. Mikolai J, et al. In vivo effects of ashwagandha (Withania somnifera) extract on the activation of lymphocytes. Journal of Alternative and Complementary Medicine 2009;15(4):423–430.

50. Bohn B, et al. Flow-cytometric studies with eleutherococcus senticosus extract as an immunomodulatory agent. Arzneimittel-Forschung 1987;37(10):1193–1196.

51. Eleutherococcus senticosus monograph. Alternative Medicine Review 2006;11(2):151–155.

52. Tan BK, Vanitha J. Immunomodulatory and antimicrobial effects of some traditional Chinese medicinal herbs: a review. Curr Med Chem 2004;11(11):1423–1430.

53. Lee JH, Han Y. Ginsenoside Rg1 helps mice resist to disseminated candidiasis by Th1 type differentiation of CD4+ T cell. International Immunopharmacology 2006;6(9):1424–1430.

54. Bone K. Phytotherapy Review and Commentary. Townsend Letter; Aug/Sep2007:289/290:69–71.

55. Pellati D, et al. In vitro effects of glycyrrhetinic acid on the growth of clinical isolates of Candida albicans. Phytotherapy Research 2009;23(4):572–574.

56. Glycyrrhiza glabra monograph. Alternative Medicine Review 2005;10(3):230–237.

57. Hand GA, et al. Moderate intensity exercise training reverses functional aerobic impairment in HIV-infected individuals. AIDS Care 2008;20(9):1066–1074.

58. Goedsche K, et al. Repeated cold water stimulations (hydrotherapy according to Kneipp) in patients with COPD. Forsch Komplementmed 2007;14(3):158–166.

59. Creswell JD, et al. Mindfulness meditation training effects on CD4+ T lymphocytes in HIV-1 infected adults: a small randomized controlled trial. Brain Behav Immun 2009;23(2):184–188.

60. Fitzpatrick AL, et al. Survival in HIV-1 positive adults practicing psychological or spiritual activities for one year. Altern Ther Health Med 2007;13(5):18–20, 22–24.

61. Reisner SL, et al. A review of HIV antiretroviral adherence and intervention studies among HIV-infected youth. Top HIV Med 2009;17(1):14–25.

62. Mosack KE, et al. Influence of coping, social support, and depression on subjective health status among HIV-positive adults with different sexual identities. Behav Med 2009;34(4):133–144.

63. Seth P, et al. Psychological distress as a correlate of a biologically confirmed STI, risky sexual practices, self-efficacy and communication with male sex partners in African-American female adolescents. Psychology, Health and Medicine 2009;14(3):291–300.

64. Lee LS, et al. Interactions between natural health products and antiretroviral drugs: pharmacokinetic and pharmacodynamic effects. Clinical Infectious Diseases 2006;43(8):1052–1059.

65. Darbinian-Sarkissian N, et al. p27(SJ), a novel protein in St John's Wort, that suppresses expression of HIV-1 genome. Gene Ther 2006;13(4):288–295.

66. Patel J, et al. In vitro interaction of the HIV protease inhibitor ritonavir with herbal constituents: changes in P-gp and CYP3A4 activity. Am J Ther 2004;11(4):262–277.

67. Mills E, et al. Natural health product–HIV drug interactions: a systematic review. Int J STD AIDS 2005;16(3):181–186.

68. van den Bout-van den Beukel CJ, et al. Possible drug–metabolism interactions of medicinal herbs with antiretroviral agents. Drug Metab Rev 2006;38(3):477–514.

69. Zhao HX, et al. Effects of traditional Chinese medicine on CD4+ T cell counts and HIV viral loads during structured treatment interruption in highly active antiretroviral therapy. Zhongguo Yi Xue Ke Xue Yuan Xue Bao 2006;28(5):658–661.

70. Cohen M. Toxic heat and the human immunodeficiency virus: understanding HIV disease from the Chinese perspective. Online. Available: http://docmisha.com/applying/hiv/toxic-heat.htm 25 January 2009

71. Ryan MK. Development of a traditional Chinese medical model of HIV/AIDS. IEP Newsletter Spring 1995. Online. Available: http://www.iepclinic.com/model.html 25 January 2009

72. Acupuncture Research Resource Centre. Briefing Paper No 6: HIV infection and traditional Chinese medicine, the evidence for effectiveness. British Acupuncture Council. Online. Available: http://www.acupuncture.org.uk/content/Library/doc/hiv_bp6.pdf February 2000

73. Burke A. The essential role of acupuncture, herbs and related therapies in HIV care. American Acupuncturist 2007;41:26–28.

74. Rastogi DP, et al. A double blind placebo controlled study: homoeopathy in HIV infection. Natl J Homoeopathy 2001;3(5):318–325.

75. Aktay G, et al. Hepatoprotective effects of Turkish folk remedies on experimental liver injury. J Ethnopharmacol 2000;73(1–2):121–129.

76. Batterham M, et al. Preliminary open label dose comparison using an antioxidant regimen to determine the effect on viral load and oxidative stress in men with HIV/AIDS. Eur J Clin Nutr 2001;55(2):107–114.

77. Carter VM, et al. A randomised controlled trial of omega-3 fatty acid supplementation for the treatment of hypertriglyceridemia in HIV-infected males on highly active antiretroviral therapy. Sex Health 2006;3:287–290.

78. De Truchis P, et al. Reduction in triglyceride level with N-3 polyunsaturated fatty acids in HIV-infected patients taking potent antiretroviral therapy: a randomized prospective study. J Acquir Immune Defic Syndr 2007;44:278–285.

79. Gerber JG, et al. Fish oil and fenofibrate for the treatment of hypertriglyceridemia in HIV-infected subjects on antiretroviral therapy: results of ACTG A5186. J Acquir Immune Defic Syndr 2008;47(4):459–466.

80. The Antiretroviral Therapy (ART) Cohort Collaboration. Prognosis of HIV-1-infected patients up to 5 years after initiation of HAART: collaborative analysis of prospective studies. AIDS 2007;21:1185–1197.

81. Hoffman D. Medical herbalism, the science and practice of herbal medicine. Vermont: Healing Arts Press, 2003:165.

82. Heiser CR, et al. Probiotics, soluble fiber, and L-glutamine (GLN) reduce nelfinavir (NFV)-or lopinavir/ritonavir (LPV/r)-related diarrhea. J Int Assoc Physicians AIDS Care 2004;3(4):121–129.

83. Erice A, et al. Anti-human immunodeficiency virus type 1 activity of an anti-CD4 immunoconjugate containing pokeweed antiviral protein. Antimicrob Agents Chemother 1993;37(4):835–838.

84. D'Cruz OJ, et al. Mucosal toxicity studies of a gel forumulation of native pokeweed antiviral protein. Toxicol Pathol 2004;32(2):212–221.

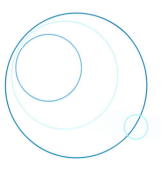

37

Polypharmacy and pain management

Justin Sinclair
ND, MHerbMed

OVERVIEW

Herbal medicines and other complementary therapies are currently experiencing a renewed interest and popularity in developed nations worldwide.[1–3] This increased trend in usage suggests that adverse drug–herb interactions may be of significant public health consequence,[4] and highlights the importance of sustained pharmacovigilance and evidence based appraisal with the concurrent use of herbs and drugs in a clinical setting.[5]

Statistics

The Adverse Drug Reactions Advisory Committee (ADRAC) of the Australian Therapeutic Goods Administration received their first report of an adverse drug reaction from a complementary medicine in 1979. Since this time, some 988 reports of suspected adverse drug reactions to herbal medicine have been collected in Australia. As of September 2008, there have been 205,787 reported adverse drug reactions to all forms of medicine.[6] While reported statistics on documented herbal adverse drug reactions can be viewed as being comparatively low in contrast to orthodox medications, this may be a reflection of both the relative safety of complementary medicines and the under-reporting of potential drug–herb interactions to regulatory agencies.[7,8] Complementary practitioners must remain assiduous in identifying and reporting suspected adverse drug reactions to the regulatory authorities.

Drug–herb interaction mechanisms

Given the multifarious array of substances currently used as medicines it is not surprising that this correlates with many complex factors that can modify drug responses. Current pharmacological opinion suggests that three heterogeneous interaction mechanisms exist: pharmacokinetic, pharmacodynamic and physicochemical models[7,9] (see Figure 37.1).

'Pharmacokinetics' is defined as the quantitative study of the absorption, distribution, metabolism and excretion of a medicine by the body (that is, the effects the body has on the medicine).[10] Pharmacokinetic interactions occur when there is a modification to any of the four aforementioned processes, resulting in a change in the concentration

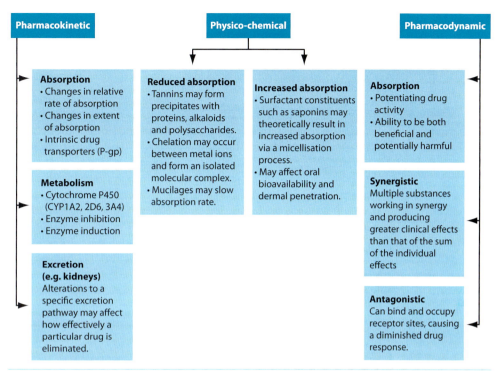

Figure 37.1 Interaction mechanisms
Source: Adapted from Braun L, Cohen M. Herbs and natural supplements. 2nd edn. Sydney: Churchill Livingstone, 2007.

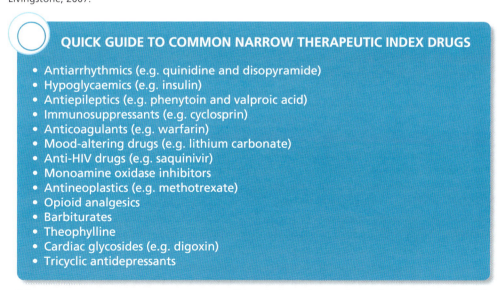

of drug at target tissues or receptor sites.[7] Herbal medicines have the ability to modify the pharmacokinetic profile of a drug by either increasing or reducing its availability within the body and therefore modifying biochemical and physiological responses. Representative examples of pharmacokinetic interactions include the inhibition/induction of certain isoenzymes of the hepatic cytochrome P450 system (particularly 1A2, 2D6 and 3A4), or the inhibition/induction of the drug transporter P-glycoprotein (P-gp).

As interactions of this model are largely unpredictable[11] they are of far greater clinical concern in patients taking pharmaceutical medicines, especially those with a narrow therapeutic index (see the box above). Other factors such as age-related changes to pharmacokinetics due to physiological deterioration, individual variability, patient constitution, reduced homeostatic mechanisms, gender, body composition, pregnancy and organ function can also affect drug response,[9,12–15] and should be carefully considered in the assessment of potential drug–herb interactions.[16]

'Pharmacodynamics' is concerned with the biochemical and physiological effect the drug has upon the body and includes the relationship between drug concentration and the magnitude of drug effect. Pharmacodynamic interactions transpire when one drug alters the sensitivity or responsiveness of tissues to another drug via receptor binding affinity and intrinsic activity, resulting in additive (agonistic), synergistic or antagonistic drug effects.[7] These drug effects have both positive and negative clinical repercussions, with synergistic and additive interactions frequently being used to improve patient outcomes.[17] Different to pharmacokinetic interactions, pharmacodynamic interactions may be theoretically predictable and can be identified by analysing the therapeutic profiles and mechanisms of action of both the drugs and the herbs used.

The physicochemical model represents the interaction of substances that have conflicting physical or chemical properties. Physicochemical interactions can have a positive or negative effect upon the absorption of one or both substances and their subsequent assimilation within the body. Examples of this type of interaction extend to herbal substances high in tannins, polyphenols, mucilages and saponins,[17] and also metal ions via the process of chelation. Decreases or increases in absorption based on these substances are of particular importance when narrow therapeutic index drugs and alkaloid-based herbs or medications are being used.

Challenges

The evidence available to guide naturopaths in the decision-making process for the assessment of drug–herb interactions is multifaceted and incorporates a variety of resources including human clinical trials, in vivo studies and adverse drug reaction database entries (see Table 37.1). Clinical adverse events that have been ascribed to drug–herb interactions are further complicated by such realities as botanical substitution (i.e. either intentional or accidental) of a different plant species and contamination of the herb with pharmaceutically derived medications or other non-herbal substances,[4] which should be taken into consideration before jumping to conclusions. This helps separate what one study[4] aptly termed true 'interaction from overreaction'.

With conclusive evidence to substantiate drug–herb interactions often lacking, it is usually the clinician that is left to speculate on a potential interaction between a herb and a drug.[4] Current academics in the field of herbal pharmacology suggest that much greater research and funding to assess the clinical significance of drug–herb interactions is required, and that until such a database exists it is wise to closely monitor patients who are elderly, taking multiple medications,[4] taking narrow therapeutic index drugs or suffering from serious diseases, conditions or disorders.

APPROACHING PATIENTS ON MEDICATIONS

Dealing with patients taking medications is one of the most challenging areas of complementary medicine practice, especially where polypharmacy is concerned.[9] A methodical and systematic approach (the INQUIRE method) to prescribing complementary

Table 37.1 Comparison of the evidence from studies of herb–drug interactions

STUDY DESIGN	ADVANTAGES	DISADVANTAGES
Controlled clinical trial in patients	• High internal validity and generalisability to patients of interest	• Controlled trial may not reflect clinical reality • Difficult to implement (logistics, cost, ethics) • Increased sample size may be required to account for expected variability
Controlled clinical trial in healthy subjects	• High internal validity • Allows a full and rigorous assesment of herb-drug interaction mechanisms	• As above • May not predict significance of interaction in patients with diseases, organ dysfunction, and/or other medications
Open label clinical trial	• Controlled patient group for comparison	• As above • Confounded by subjective endpoints
Case reports of series	• Informative and realistic information obtained in the patient group of interest • Generates hypotheses	• Uncontrolled observational study which may overestimate significance given the many possible confounders • May lead to over-reporting of cases with no insight into the clinical significance
Animal studies	• Allows a rigorous investigation of integrated pharmacological effects	• Some interspecies differences in drug response and metabolism may confound • Not possible to assess clinical significance
In vitro studies in animal or human tissues	• Provides mechanistic information and allows fundamental understanding of interaction cause	• Isolated tissues may not reflect in vivo response • Concentrations of constituents may not reflect concentration or metabolites in vivo
Adverse event database entries	• Provides immediate reporting of potentially dangerous interactions • Provides an international perspective on the incidence of serious but rare interactions • Hypothesis generating	• Often cannot be evaluated due to non-existent or inaccessible extraneous data for critical interpretation

Source: Coxeter PD, McLachlan AJ, Duke CC, Roufogalis BD. Herb–drug interactions: an evidence based approach. Current Medicinal Chemistry 2004;11:1513–1525.

medicines to patients taking pharmaceutical medications is proposed by this author as being best practice (see the box below). The method was designed specifically for students of herbal and naturopathic medicine to reduce the potential for oversight and to implement foundational skills that can be honed while under supervision. The INQUIRE method is discussed in more detail below.

Investigate: All medications must be suitably researched and investigated to provide a rational foundation to identify potential interactions using appropriate pharmacological resources (e.g. MIMS). This allows the naturopath to be cognisant of

PROTOCOL FOR THE ASSESSMENT OF PATIENTS ON MEDICATIONS

I: Investigate all aspects of the current medications the patient is taking (mechanisms of action, safety, adverse reactions, cautions, contraindications and interactions).

N: Note the posology of the medications taken by the patient (dosage, when taken and duration of administration)

Q: Qualify and rationalise the strengths and limitations of complementary medicines in being able to efficaciously assist in the management of the presenting conditions/disorders of the patient.

U: Understand. Armed with the information obtained from research of the medications and case history, the naturopath can develop a treatment protocol/regimen specific to the patient.

I: Identify any potential interactions with the intended treatment using reputable evidence-based texts and resources.

R: Remember to contact the GP or medical practitioner (with patient consent) to outline the treatment plan if required.

E: Educate the patient. Part of the strength of complementary medicine therapies lies in empowering and educating the patient to take an active role in their own health.

particularly problematic medications and therefore assists the selection of appropriate CAM therapies. Should the naturopath still be uncertain or need clarification, they should contact their local pharmacist for an expert opinion. Pertinent questions include:

- What types of medication are being taken? Are they prescription only (S4) or over-the-counter?
- Is there potential for interaction based on available pharmacodynamic/pharmacokinetic information for the drug?
- What are the cautions, side effects and contraindications of the drug?
- Is the drug known to be of narrow therapeutic index? If so, the naturopath should use caution in their treatment strategy.

Note: Understanding the medication is only one part of this process, as posology is equally important. Significant questions include:

- What is the dosage of the drug?
- What is the frequency of dosing? Is it b.i.d., t.i.d. or other (see the box below)?
- When is the drug taken? Is it taken before meals or after?
- How long has the patient been taking the medication?
- Is the patient taking any other supplements? Certain patients do not think of natural supplements as medicines. Many naturopaths ask their patients to bring all of their current medications and supplements with them to the consultation.

Qualify: There are many conditions and diseases which benefit from complementary medicine treatment. Conversely, there are also conditions which are considered too serious and beyond the scope of complementary medicine practice. Questions that can be asked are:

- Is there adequate evidence to support the use of complementary medicines in the patient's case?
- Should complementary medicines be applied as adjunct (supportive) rather than primary therapy?

QUICK GUIDE TO MEDICAL PRESCRIBING TERMS

q.d.: every day (*quaque die*, once daily)
b.i.d.: twice daily (*bis in die*)
t.d.s.: to be taken three times a day—used for oral medications
(*ter die sumendus*)
t.i.d.: thrice daily—used for external medications (*ter in die*)
q.i.d.: four times daily (*quater in die*)
p.r.n.: as required (*pro re nater*)
hs: at bedtime
ac: before meals (*ante cibum*)
cc: with meals (*circa cibum*)
pc: after meals (*post cibum*)

Understand: Armed with a thorough understanding of the case and the patient's medication, and taking into account the constitution, general health and age of the patient, a treatment outline can be developed. Potentially beneficial pharmacodynamic interactions (synergy or additive effects) can be explored further.

Identify: Once the treatment outline has been determined, it is now time to use complementary medicine-specific, evidence-based texts and other resources to identify any known drug–herb interactions (see the drug–CAM interaction chart in the appendices). In many cases, this can be done concurrently with the development of the treatment outline. At the conclusion of this, a prescription can be written.

Remember: If the patient is taking prescription-only drugs, or is being managed for a condition by a medical practitioner, it is wise for the naturopath to contact that practitioner before initiating treatment, out of professional courtesy. This is paramount if the patient desires to reduce their prescription medications. It also establishes an open channel of communication between the medical practitioner and the naturopath and reduces the likelihood of the naturopath being unaware of a medication or management plan alteration, thus increasing patient safety due to the decreased chance of a potential drug–herb interaction. The naturopath must obtain patient consent before initiating contact, due to confidentiality issues.

Educate: One of the key differences between complementary medicine and orthodox medicine is the role the naturopath has in educating the patient and getting them actively involved in their own health. Key points of importance here are factors such as:
• foods, supplements and herbs to avoid or include
• potential interactions that could occur
• the importance of compliance
• the time it will take before noticeable effects are experienced
• empowering the patient and using positive reinforcement.

PAIN MANAGEMENT

Pain is a disagreeable subjective physiological and psychosocial experience that often serves a biological purpose (warning of injury).[18–20] It incorporates both the perception of a painful stimulus and the response to the aforementioned perception.[21] Physiologically, it can be classified into either somatogenic (organic) or psychogenic (non-organic) origin.[22] Somatogenic pain occurs as a result of a direct physiological mechanism or insult (such as osteoarthritis) and can be further divided into nociceptive pain (for example, ongoing activation of visceral nociceptors) or neuropathic pain (neurological dysfunction such as nerve compression).[22] Pain can further be explained by duration of effect, being either acute (lasting less than 4 weeks) or chronic (pain lasting longer than 12 weeks).

Further compounding the deleterious physiological effects of pain are social, emotional and psychological[23] ramifications, which are especially prevalent in chronic pain, causing debilitating sequelae such as affective disorders and comorbid depression.[22] Factors such as age, gender, race and socioeconomic status are also important to consider in pain perception.[24] Pain sufferers are often impaired in their ability to initiate or maintain fundamental daily activities such as eating, shopping and cleaning,[25] further isolating the patient and increasing morbidity scales (decreasing quality of life).

The perception of pain is physiologically mediated mainly by myelinated A-delta (Aδ) fibre and unmyelinated C-fibre terminal nerve endings, in combination with the neurotransmitter glutamate.[18,24] In response to mechanical stimuli and subsequent chemical release at the site of injury, these nerve endings increase firing rates and cause pain by either direct stimulation or sensitising nerve endings.[18] Both A-delta and C-fibres transmit electrical impulses from the peripheral nervous supply through the dorsal root and into the dorsal horn of the spinal cord.[24] Myelination causes the A-delta fibres to transmit impulses extremely quickly, compared to the slower travelling unmyelinated C-fibres. Acute and sharp pain travels via the A-delta fibres in contrast to the more chronic, dull pain generally associated with C-fibre transmission.[18] Other fibres, such as silent nociceptors and A-beta fibres, occur in joints and the periosteum, and can also augment the pain response.[26]

Our physiological understanding of the source of pain, especially in osteoarthritis, is not well understood,[24] yet seems to encompass a wide range of contributing local and systemic factors. Examples of such mechanisms include the loss of hyaline articular cartilage and subsequent joint space narrowing, inflammatory mediators (such as bradykinin, histamine, prostaglandins, lactic acid, substance P, vasoactive intestinal peptide and calcitonin gene related peptide), nerve innervation, pain sensitisation and the cortical experience[27] of pain.

With such a mixture of factors potentially implicated in the pain response, both orthodox and complementary management plans use multiple treatment options. This provides a unique opportunity for collaboration and integration between both systems of medicine to provide the best patient outcomes. Figure 22.3 in Chapter 22 elaborates on the current medical management of osteoarthritis to include other complementary medicine modalities and outlines the potential for this integrated relationship. Benefits of such an approach include the potential to reduce current workloads on GPs (for mild to moderate patient presentations) and lessen the side effects experienced by many patients limited to drug therapy alone.

Certain key evidence-based and clinically relevant treatments specific to pain management associated with osteoarthritis of the knee are outlined below.

Acupuncture

With a history of use spanning millennia, acupuncture has proven a useful alternative treatment option for pain management in a variety of conditions. Clinical evidence suggests acupuncture, in combination with primary care when required, is associated with marked clinical improvement in patients with chronic osteoarthritis-associated pain of the knee or hip.[28] Improvement in WOMAC scores, increase in joint mobility and function,[29,30] and quality of life improvements have all been identified through clinical studies.[31] One review,[32] however, suggests that acupuncture requires more evidence of effectiveness in osteoarthritis and what evidence exists is dubious.

Exercise

Reduced mobility has been correlated with an increase in osteoarthritis progression and pain. Findings[33] identify high levels of evidence to support land-based therapeutic exercise as being beneficial in reducing knee pain and increasing physical function in osteoarthritis participants. The treatment effect was considered small, but was still comparable to previous reports specific to NSAID based trials.[33] Further research comparing both high and low intensity aerobic exercise in osteoarthritis symptoms found similar efficacy in improving pain, aerobic capacity, gait and patient functional status between the two groups.[34]

Aquatic exercise does not share similar long-term symptomatic benefits in contrast to land-based exercise regimens; however, it does appear to have some beneficial short-term effects for patients with osteoarthritis of the knee or hip.[35] Based on these findings, clinicians should consider encouraging patients to undergo aquatic exercise as the first stage of a longer exercise program for patients with arthritic conditions.[35]

Herbal medicines

Herbal medicines have a long established traditional usage in complaints such as osteoarthritis. **Plasters of chilli (*Capsicum* spp.)** have been applied topically for centuries, with modern research now identifying the proposed mechanism of action. Capsaicin, an alkaloidal constituent in the chilli plant, is able to reversibly deplete C-fibre afferent neurons of the neuropeptide substance P,[36] which leads to subsequent nerve desensitisation[37] in amounts of just 0.025% in topical creams. A clinical study including glyceryltrinitrate in combination with capsaicin in a topical preparation found a potentially synergistic additive effect in reducing pain,[38] with participants experiencing less discomfort than capsaicin alone.

Many herb-based medicines for internal ingestion share similar positive findings. Preparations of **Phytodolor** (an alcohol-based formulation containing *Populus tremula*, *Fraxinus excelsior* and *Solidago virgaurea*),[39,40] *Harpagophytum procumbens*,[41] *Zingiber officinale*,[41] *Rosa canina*[41] and avocado/soy bean unsaponifiables[40–42] have all shown benefit in the symptomatic management of osteoarthritis. Furthermore, apart from a long traditional history of use in managing pain and fever, ***Salix alba*** preparations have shown improvement in pain scores in osteoarthritis when standardised to salicin content.[43]

Traditional evidence should not be discounted. Herbs such as *Eschscholzia californica*, *Piscidia erythrina*, *Corydalis ambigua*, *Uncaria tomentosa*[44] and *Urtica dioica folia* have a long history of use for pain and joint disorders and are worthy of inclusion in treatment plans; however, from a scientific perspective they require more clinical studies to demonstrate efficacy.

Pharmaceutical medicines

Numerous medications are currently used by medical practitioners in the management of osteoarthritis and its associated pain. These drug classes typically include:

- non-steroidal anti-inflammatory drugs (NSAIDs) such as selective COX-2 inhibitors like celecoxib
- simple analgesics (for example, acetaminophen)

- narcotic analgesics (for example, tramadol)
- opiate analgesics (hydrocodone, oxycodone and so on)
- selective serotonin reuptake inhibitors (SSRIs)
- corticosteroids.

Clinical evidence obtained from Cochrane systematic reviews suggests improvements in pain associated with osteoarthritis of the knee and patient quality of life for drugs such as diacerein,[45] tramadol,[46] rofecoxib,[47] acetaminophen,[48] viscosupplementation (hyaluronan and hylan derivatives)[49] and corticosteroids.[50]

A statistically significant difference was noted between diacerein and placebo in relation to pain measured by the visual analogue scale, with further evidence suggestive of a slowing of disease progression (in hip osteoarthritis only).[45] Likewise, tramadol was shown to reduce pain intensity (a reduced WOMAC score), improve joint function and address symptomatic relief; however, the benefits were described as minimal by the research team.[45]

Twenty-six randomised controlled trials (RCTs) were included in the rofecoxib (Vioxx) review. Evidence indicated that rofecoxib was more effective than placebo but was associated with higher amounts of adverse events.[47] Rofecoxib and valdecoxib were withdrawn from the worldwide market in 2004 due to evidence that they increased the risk of heart attack and stroke.[47] As such they are no longer clinically relevant.

Fifteen RCTs met inclusion criteria for the systematic review of acetaminophen with a total of 5986 participants. Trials compared acetaminophen (paracetamol) to either placebo or NSAIDs such as diclofenac, naproxen sodium, ibuprofen and celecoxib.[48] Acetaminophen was found to be superior to placebo, but less effective than NSAIDs in moderate to severe disease presentations.[48]

As has been demonstrated, a key detrimental factor associated with medication usage is adverse events. Side effects such as diarrhoea (42% of participants), heartburn, soft stools, stomach pain and frequent bowel movements were reported in the diacerein[45] study, with nausea, vomiting, dizziness, constipation, tiredness and headache being reported with tramadol usage.[46] Adverse events of tramadol often caused participants to stop taking the medication, therefore limiting medication efficacy.[46] For this reason, it would be considered more beneficial to patient welfare to try complementary medicine therapy first for mild to moderate presentations of the disease before having to resort to drug therapy.

Nutraceuticals

Substances such as glucosamine, chondroitin, fish oils and methylsulfonylmethane have varied amounts of clinical evidence to support use in reducing inflammation and pain in conditions such as osteoarthritis.

Glucosamine is the best-studied substance out of the previously listed interventions. A randomised, placebo-controlled clinical trial with 1500 mg of glucosamine sulfate on osteoarthritis progression found that responders within the treatment group experienced significant improvement in pain via the WOMAC scale, as well as reductions in joint stiffness and limitations of physical function.[51] Evidence to support this has been provided by various other research teams[52–54] and a Cochrane review.[55] The Cochrane meta-analysis comprised 25 RCTs with a total of 4963 patients. Results favoured glucosamine with a 22% (change from baseline) improvement in pain (SMD –0.47; 95% CI –0.72 to –0.23) and a 11% (change from baseline) improvement in function using the Lequesne index.[56] Glucosamine was also considered as safe as placebo in terms of the number of adverse events experienced by participants. Some research is also supportive of glucosamine having the ability to modify joint space narrowing[57] via a supposed chondroprotective activity.

Chondroitin sulfate has been shown to exhibit an anti-inflammatory activity[58] and exhibit positive benefits in osteoarthritis management alone or in combination with glucosamine.[59] One study suggested that this anti-inflammatory effect potentially occurs via mechanisms such as diminishing the expression of phospholipase A2 and COX-2 and also reducing concentrations of prostaglandin E_2, which may reduce pain.[58] Clinical trials on chondroitin sulfate have demonstrated that, at doses between 800 mg and 1 g per day, reduction in pain and improved joint function[60–62] have been experienced, along with prevention of knee joint space narrowing.[60,62] While chondroitin sulfate has been classified as a slow-acting chondroprotective agent for osteoarthritis, some authors feel that more conclusive evidence is required.[63]

The lipids derived from **fish oils**, rich in both eicosapentaenoic acid (EPA) and docosahexaenoic acid (DHA), exhibit anti-inflammatory activity, providing support for their use in osteoarthritis pain management. Research suggests that fish oils inhibit the formation of the cyclooxygenase products thromboxane A_2 (TXA_2) and prostaglandin E_2 (PGE_2) derived from arachidonic acid.[64] Arthritic patients should be encouraged to supplement with fish oil, along with weight loss and exercise to retain muscle mass, to see if they experience any symptom amelioration.[65]

Methylsulfonylmethane has implied analgesic and anti-inflammatory activities,[66] and is a popular arthritic supplement in the United States of America. Pilot clinical trial results suggest that methylsulfonylmethane caused statistically significant reductions in WOMAC pain and physical function impairment without notable adverse events.[67] A systematic review supports the idea that methylsulfonylmethane is superior to placebo for osteoarthritis, yet also highlights the need for more rigorous clinical studies to be conducted.[68]

Surgical interventions

In patients with moderate to severe pain due to unicompartmental osteoarthritis of the knee, a Cochrane review based on 13 studies concluded that valgus high tibial osteotomy improved knee function and reduced pain.[69] In stark contrast, a controlled trial investigating arthroscopic lavage and debridement of the knee in osteoarthritis patients versus sham surgery revealed no difference in outcome measures being experienced between the two groups.[70] A systematic review of arthroscopic debridement found gold-level evidence that arthroscopic debridement provides no benefit in either mechanical or inflammatory osteoarthritis.[71]

Over 35,000 total knee replacement surgeries are performed in the United States of America every year.[72] This surgery has numerous short- and long-term benefits, with relief in pain and improvement in joint function being experienced in over 90% of patients.[73] The prosthetic replacements last for over 10 years in 90% of patients and the surgery has an incredibly low mortality rate (< 1%).[73] A study pointed out that total knee replacement surgeries should not always be viewed as a last resort, but rather should be investigated when the patient's quality of life is compromised sufficiently to make the risks of surgery worth the gain in function and reduction in pain.[73]

Non-surgical interventions

Numerous non-surgical interventions are currently used in the management of osteoarthritis, each with mixed outcomes. Results from a systematic review investigating the effectiveness of therapeutic ultrasound in osteoarthritis patients (n = 294) versus placebo or active therapy showed that there was no difference in range of motion, pain or gait velocity after 4 weeks of treatment.[74]

Viscosupplementation injections of either hyaluronan or hylan derivatives have been extensively studied in clinical trials for knee osteoarthritis. Over 76 studies on viscosupplementation met systematic review inclusion criteria, comparing against placebo (saline), intraarticular corticosteroids, NSAID usage and physical therapy.[75] Results indicated that viscosupplementation has benefit in reducing pain and improving joint function, with longer therapeutic benefit than corticosteroids and fewer systemic adverse events.[75]

Twenty-eight trials (n = 1973) comparing intraarticular corticosteroid use against placebo, intraarticular hyaluronan/hylan derivatives, joint lavage and against other intraarticular corticosteroids were included in a systematic review.[50] Outcome measures indicated that while the short-term benefits of corticosteroids such as pain reduction are well established, viscosupplementation appears more durable[50] in the long-term management of osteoarthritis.

Physiotherapy

Physiotherapy is a well-recognised allied health modality that has a strong history of success in managing mild to moderate symptomatic osteoarthritis pain. Objective improvements in knee strength (47%), reduced pain (76%) and range of motion (53%) have been observed in studies using manual physiotherapy for osteoarthritis.[76] Other adjunctive therapies such as balneotherapy,[77] pulsed electromagnetic fields[78] and transcutaneous electrical nerve stimulation (TENS)[79] may also provide short-term relief and improvement in function,[80] although more studies of better methodological quality are needed. Further studies investigating orthotics and braces have also shown minor benefit.[81]

Case Study

A 67-year-old female presents with severe persistent asthma, chronic pain from bilateral osteoarthritis of the knees and insomnia. Recent results from a bone scan are also suggestive of early stage osteoporosis. She is currently **heavily medicated on prednisolone, salbutamol, paracetamol with codeine, diazepam** and a **statin**. She asks for **advice on which complementary medicines may improve her health** and assist her in safely reducing medication, and **any that she should avoid**. Help with **pain management** is also sought.

Key treatment protocols

The above case study represents a clinical example of a patient trying to manage multiple health conditions and pain, in addition to a cocktail of pharmaceuticals. The presenting patient, currently on long-term prednisolone and salbutamol therapy, suggests she has severe and persistent asthma.[82] With a general paucity of evidence-based research in herbal medicines and severe asthma, and after consultation with the patient's GP, the following was decided:

- Routine blood tests would be ordered to assess any age-related changes to organ function, including liver function tests (ALT, AST, albumin, ALP, γ-glutamyltransferase, P4 bilirubin, globulins and total protein, LD and PT); BUN, electrolytes (HCO_3^-, Cl^-, K^+ and Na^+) and creatinine to assess kidney function; blood glucose; and FBE.[83] Lung function tests will also be conducted (PEF, spirometry).[84]

- The prednisolone usage is to be reduced slowly in a tapered manner. This must be done to reduce the likelihood of sudden severe withdrawal symptoms such as adrenal crisis. The dosage of prednisolone (30 mg) will be reduced over a period of 2–3 weeks by the patient's doctor, with the introduction of an inhaled corticosteroid (e.g. beclomethasone,[85,86] budesonide[87,88] or fluticasone)[89] and a concurrent long-acting β$_2$-agonist (LABA) such as salmeterol. Recent research has shown an increase risk of serious adverse events with LABA usage,[90] although this risk was reduced when co-administered with inhaled corticosteroid therapy, and requires close patient monitoring. The use of a short-acting β$_2$-adrenergic receptor agonist (SABA), such as salbutamol, as a reliever may be used as required (p.r.n.).
- During the period of prednisolone withdrawal, the patient will be making weekly visits to the GP for close monitoring. Compliance and patient education are reinforced as being crucial for positive outcomes.
- Long-term administration of prednisolone was considered a potential contributing factor to the early osteoporosis. Inhaled corticosteroid research shows minimal change to bone density or other markers of bone metabolism in long-term use.[91] Calcium supplementation is to be started immediately.

With long-term reliance upon paracetamol with codeine for analgesia, the potential for habit formation exists. Abruptly stopping this medication may cause a substantial increase in perceived pain. Based on this, the following treatment plan was initiated:

- Naproxen sodium (250 mg q.i.d.) or Ibuprofen (200 mg q.i.d.) is to be introduced to replace paracetamol. These drugs will achieve anti-inflammatory activity within 3 days, while the paracetamol with codeine dosage was halved and eventually stopped within 7 days.
- Glucosamine sulfate, 500 mg t.i.d., was started for its anti-inflammatory and chondroprotective activity.[51–54] Pain relief from responders to glucosamine sulfate usually occurs within 4–6 weeks. Naproxen sodium will address pain relief until the glucosamine sulfate and herbal medicines take effect, at which time it will be used for rescue medication only. The potential exists for a beneficial interaction between the naproxen sodium and glucosamine sulfate or herbs,[7] and drug dosage may require downward adjustment.
- *Harpagophytum procumbens*, *Zingiber officinale* and *Curcuma longa* were prescribed in liquid form. These herbs exhibit mild to moderate anti-inflammatory activity,[92,93] with ginger and turmeric also providing gastroprotective (anti-ulcer) activity to counter NSAID side effects.[94,95]
- Reduction of acid-forming foods in the diet is to be encouraged, with increases in alkaline foods such as fresh fruit and vegetables.[96]
- Zostrix (capsaicin 0.025%) topical analgesic cream (apply 3–4 times per day to affected area) is to be started immediately.

Herbal formula

Harpagophytum procumbens 1:2	50 mL
Zingiber officinale 1:2	15 mL
Curcuma longa 1:1	35 mL
5 mL t.i.d./a.c.	100 mL

Valeriana officinalis and *Humulus lupulus* combination 1 tablet (before bed)

Capsaicin 0.025% topical analgesic cream (apply 3–4 times per day to affected area)

Nutritional prescription

Glucosamine sulfate 750 mg b.i.d.
Calcium (Hydroxyapatite) 500 mg t.i.d.
Coenzyme Q10 (Ubiquinone) 50 mg b.i.d.

- Patient was also counselled to increase physical activity, as there is an increase in arthritis progression with immobility. Water aerobics (twice a week) is to be started until pain management is stable, then 15–20-minute walks are to be introduced into the daily regimen as it becomes possible.
- The patient is counselled to avoid self-medicating with nutritional and herbal medicines without prior approval from the consulting practitioner.

Much akin to systemic corticosteroids, diazepam should not be stopped abruptly due to the risk of side effects. The dosage of diazepam was halved from 5 mg to 2.5 mg for 2 weeks, then taken every other day with the inclusion of *Valeriana officinalis* equivalent dry root 1.25 g and *Humulus lupulus* equivalent dry fruit 360 mg 1 × tablet before bed for 2 weeks on alternate days due to the potential for an additive effect. After this time, diazepam can be removed from the management plan and dosage of the herbal combination may be increased as required.

As the patient is being withdrawn from prednisolone, diazepam and paracetamol with codeine within the first month of treatment, statin withdrawal will be withheld until the patient is stabilised on her new management regimen. The use of *Zingiber officinale* and *Curcuma longa* in this initial treatment plan carries secondary advantages as they are known hypocholesterolaemics,[94,95] which may require a reduction in statin dosage. To complement this hypocholesterolaemic activity, and to further offset the known coenzyme Q10 depletion caused by HMG-Co-reductase inhibitors,[97–99] a supplement of coenzyme Q10 will also be added to this patient's management plan. After 2 months of treatment, blood tests can be re-ordered to assess the impact of the CoQ10, and a decision made as to whether herbs such as *Cynara scolymus* and *Allium sativum* should be incorporated as the statin usage is lowered and eventually withdrawn.

Expected outcome and follow-up protocols

After 1 month since her initial consultation with a medical practitioner, the patient is expected to do well on her new asthma therapy. Blood test results and spirometry are aimed to be within acceptable limits. With good kidney function, the diuretic herb *Urtica dioica folia* could be included in her regimen as an infusion to increase the clearance of metabolic waste (in line with traditional naturopathic treatment principles for osteoarthritis). Good compliance is desired in all areas of diet, medication, supplementation and exercise. Both paracetamol with codeine and diazepam are aimed to be reduced or stopped (with medical consultation). Signposts of improvement are a reduction of knee pain to the point of it being manageable, and her sleep to be of better quality, with less grogginess in the mornings. A general increase in her appetite and energy levels is ideal, with increased ambulation (within the limitations of discomfort). Two months into treatment if the patient is progressing well, a reduction of rescue medication (naproxen) may be achieved. If her sleep patterns are stabilised, her valerian and hops prescriptions may be required only 3–4 nights per week. Blood tests to investigate total cholesterol, triglycerides and HDL:LDL ratio can be ordered to assess whether the herbal formulation and CoQ10 have had any effect on lipid profile. The new focus of treatment can now be concentrated around replacement of atorvastatin for her cholesterol management, building immune function and integrating supportive herbs such as *Albizzia lebbeck* into her asthma management.

KEY POINTS

- Managing patients on multiple medications is one of the greatest challenges to modern naturopaths and herbalists today, and requires excellent communication between the CAM practitioner, the primary physician and the patient to reduce the likelihood of a drug–herb interaction or adverse event.
- Many factors can have an influence on drug response: age, individual variability, patient constitution, reduced homeostatic mechanisms, gender, body composition, pregnancy and organ function.
- The use of complementary medicines and therapies (such as acupuncture) for the management of mild to moderate pain is well represented, and in many cases an integrated approach to pain management can be explored to obtain optimum results for patients.

Further reading

Blumenthal M, ed. Herbal medicine: expanded Commission E monographs. Massachusetts: Integrative Medicine Communications, 2000.

Braun L, Cohen M. Herbs and natural supplements: an evidence-based guide. 2nd edn. Sydney: Churchill Livingstone, 2007:91–105.

Coxeter PD, et al. Herb–drug interactions: an evidence based approach. Curr Med Chem 2004;11:1513–1525.

ESCOP Monographs. European Scientific Cooperative on Phytotherapy. 2nd edn. Stuttgart and New York: Exeter and G. Thieme Verlag, 2003.

Mills S, Bone K. The essential guide to herbal safety. St Louis: Churchill Livingstone:50–87.

Stargrove M, et al. Herb, nutrient, and drug interactions—clinical implications and therapeutic strategies. St Louis: CV Mosby.

WHO monographs on selected medicinal plants. Vol 1. Geneva: World Health Organization, 1999.

References

1. MacLennan AH, et al. The escalating cost and prevalence of alternative medicine. Prev Med 2002;35:166–173.
2. Thomas K, et al. Use and expenditure on complementary medicine in England: a population based survey. Complement Ther Med 2001;9:2–11.
3. Eisenberg D, et al. Trends in alternative medicine use in the United States, 1990-1997: results of a follow-up national survey. JAMA 1998;280(18):1569–1575.
4. Coxeter PD, et al. Herb–drug interactions: an evidence based approach. Curr Med Chem 2004;11:1513–1525.
5. Patel J, Gohil KJ. Herb–drug interactions: a review and study based on assessment of clinical case reports in literature. Indian J Pharmacol 2007;39(3):129–139.
6. Personal communication, 2008. Adverse Drug Reaction Advisory Committee: Canberra.
7. Braun L, Cohen M. Herbs and natural supplements: an evidence-based guide. 2nd edn. Sydney: Churchill Livingstone, 2007.
8. Farnsworth N. Relative safety of herbal medicines. Herbal-Gram 1993;29:36.
9. Bryant B, et al. Pharmacology for health professionals. Marrickville NSW Australia: Elsevier, 2003.
10. Mills S, Bone K. Principles and practice of phytotherapy. London UK: Churchill Livingstone, 2000.
11. Mills S, Bone K. The essential guide to herbal safety. St Louis: Churchill Livingstone, 2005:684.
12. Schmucker D. Liver function and phase I drug metabolism in the elderly: a paradox. Drugs Aging 2001;18(11):837–851.
13. Bressler R, Bahl JJ. Principles of drug therapy for the elderly patient. Mayo Clin Proc 2003;78(12):1564–1577.
14. Klotz U. Effect of age on pharmacokinetics and pharmacodynamics in man. Int J Clin Pharmacol Ther 1998;36(11):581–585.
15. Turnheim K. When drug therapy gets old: pharmacokinetics and pharmacodynamics in the elderly. Exp Gerontol 2003;38(8):843–853.
16. Mallet L, et al. A prescribing in elderly people 2: the challenge of managing drug interactions in elderly people. Lancet 2007;370(9582):185–191.
17. Braun L, Cohen M. Herbs and natural supplements: an evidence-based guide. Marrickville: Elsevier Australia, 2005.
18. Kumar P, Clark M, eds. Clinical medicine. 6th edn. Edinburgh: Elsevier Saunders, 2005.
19. Fauci AS, et al. eds. Harrison's principles of internal medicine. 17th edn. New York: McGraw Hill Medical, 2008.
20. Tortora GJ, Derrickson B, eds. Principles of anatomy and physiology. New York: John Wiley & Sons, Inc, 2009.
21. Thomas CL, ed. Pain. In: Thomas CL, Taber CW eds. Taber's cyclopedic medical dictionary. Philadelphia: F. A. Davis Company, 1993.
22. Beers MH, Berkow R, eds. The Merck manual of diagnosis and therapy. 17th edn. Whitehouse Station New York: Merck Research Laboratories, 1999.
23. Keefe FJ, et al. Recent advances and future directions in the biopsychosocial assessment and treatment of arthritis. J Consult Clin Psychol 2002;70(3):640–655.
24. Hunter DJ, et al. The symptoms of osteoarthritis and the genesis of pain. Med Clin North Am 2008;93(1):83–100.
25. Katz PP. The impact of rheumatoid arthritis on life activities. Arthritis Care Res 1995;8:272–278.
26. Schaible H, et al. Pathophysiology and treatment of pain in joint disease. Adv Drug Deliv Rev 2006;58(2):323–342.

27. Treede R-D, et al. The cortical representation of pain. Pain 1998;79:105–111.
28. Witt CM, et al. Acupuncture in patients with osteoarthritis of the knee or hip: a randomized, controlled trial with an additional nonrandomized arm. Revista Internacional de Acupuntura 2007;1(1):40–41.
29. Witt C, et al. Acupuncture in patients with osteoarthritis of the knee: a randomised trial. Lancet 366(9480): 136–143.
30. Berman BM, et al. The evidence for acupuncture as a treatment for rheumatologic conditions. Rheum Dis Clin North Am 2000;26(1):103–115.
31. Ezzo J, et al. Acupuncture for osteoarthritis of the knee: a systematic review. Arthritis Rheum 2001;44(4):819–825.
32. Ernst E. Acupuncture: what does the most reliable evidence tell us? J Pain Symptom Manage 2009;37(4):709–714.
33. Fransen M, McConnel S. Exercise for osteoarthritis of the knee. Cochrane Database Syst Rev 2008;(4):1–133.
34. Brosseau L, et al. Intensity of exercise for the treatment of osteoarthritis. Cochrane Database Syst Rev 2003;(2): 1–16.
35. Bartels E, et al. Aquatic exercise for the treatment of knee and hip osteoarthritis. Cochrane Database Syst Rev 2007;(4):1–47.
36. Rains C, Bryson HM. Topical capsaicin. A review of its pharmacological properties and therapeutic potential in post-herpetic neuralgia, diabetic neuropathy and osteoarthritis. Drugs Aging 1995;7(4):317–328.
37. Hayman M, Kam PC. Capsaicin: a review of its pharmacology and clinical applications. Curr Anaesth Crit Care 2008;19(5–6):338–343.
38. McCleane G. The analgesic efficacy of topical capsaicin is enhanced by glyceryl trinitrate in painful osteoarthritis: a randomised, double blind, placebo controlled study. Eur J Pain 2000;4:355–360.
39. Ernst E, Chrubasik S. Phyto-anti-inflammatories. A systematic review of randomized, placebo-controlled, double-blind trials. Rheum Dis Clin North Am 2000;26:13–27.
40. Hochberg M. Non-conventional treatment of osteoarthritis by herbal medicine. Osteoarthritis Cartilage 2008;16(Suppl 1):S2–S4.
41. Chrubasik J, et al. Evidence of effectiveness of herbal antiinflammatory drugs in the treatment of painful osteoarthritis and chronic low back pain. Phytother Res 2007;21:675–683.
42. Little C, et al. Herbal therapy for treating osteoarthritis. Cochrane Database Syst Rev 2000;1:CD002947.
43. Schmid B, et al. Efficacy and tolerability of a standardized willow bark extract in patients with osteoarthritis: randomized, placebo-controlled, double blind clinical trial [translated from German]. Z Rheumatol 2000;59: 314–320.
44. Hardin S. Cat's claw: an Amazonian vine decreases inflammation in osteoarthritis. Complement Ther Clin Pract 2007;13:25–28.
45. Fidelix T, et al. Diacerein for osteoarthritis. Cochrane Database Syst Rev 2006;1:CD005117.
46. Cepeda M, et al. Tramadol for osteoarthritis. Cochrane Database Syst Rev 2006;3:CD005522.
47. Garner S, et al. Rofecoxib for osteoarthritis. Cochrane Database Syst Rev 2005;1:CD005115.
48. Towheed T, et al. Acetaminophen for osteoarthritis. Cochrane Database Syst Rev 2006;(1):1–76.
49. Bellamy N, et al. Viscosupplementation for the treatment of osteoarthritis of the knee. Cochrane Database Syst Rev 2005;2:CD005321.
50. Bellamy N, et al. Intraarticular corticosteroid for treatment of osteoarthritis of the knee. Cochrane Database Syst Rev 2006;2:CD005321.
51. Reginster JY, et al. Long-term effects of glucosamine sulphate on osteoarthritis progression: a randomised, placebo-controlled clinical trial. Lancet 2001;357:251–256.
52. Pavelka K, et al. Glucosamine sulfate use and delay of progression of knee osteoarthritis: a 3-year, randomised, placebo-controlled, double-blind study. Arch Intern Med 2002;162:2113–2123.
53. Bruyere O, et al. Correlation between radiographic severity of knee osteoarthritis and future disease progression. Results from a 3-year prospective, placebo-controlled study evaluating the effect of glucosamine sulfate. Osteoarthritis Cartilage 2003;11:1–5.
54. Anon. Glucosamine sulfate. Altern Med Rev 1999;4(3): 193–195.
55. Towheed T, et al. Glucosamine therapy for treating osteoarthritis. Cochrane Database Syst Rev 2005;2:CD002946.
56. Towheed T, et al. Glucosamine therapy for treating osteoarthritis. Cochrane Database Syst Rev 2009;1:1–76.
57. Pavelka K, et al. Glucosamine sulfate use and delay of progression of knee osteoarthritis: a 3-year, randomised, placebo-controlled, double-blind study. Arch Intern Med 2002;162:2113–2123.
58. Iovu M, et al. Anti-inflammatory activity of chondroitin sulfate. Osteoarthritis Cartilage 2008;16(Suppl 3):S14–S18.
59. Clegg D, et al. Glucosamine, chondroitin sulfate, and the two in combination for painful knee osteoarthritis. N Engl J Med 2006;354(8):795–808.
60. Uebelhart D, et al. Intermittent treatment of knee osteoarthritis with oral chondroitin sulfate: a one-year, randomized, double-blind, multicenter study versus placebo. Osteoarthritis Cartilage 2004;12(4):269–276.
61. Mazieres B, et al. Chondroitin sulfate in osteoarthritis of the knee: a prospective, double blind, placebo controlled multicenter clinical study. J Rheumatol 2001;28(1): 173–181.
62. Uebelhart D, et al. Effects of oral chondroitin sulfate on the progression of knee osteoarthritis: a pilot study. Osteoarthritis Cartilage 1998;6(Suppl A):39–46.
63. Distler J, Anguelouch A. Evidence-based practice: review of clinical evidence on the efficacy of glucosamine and chondroitin in the treatment of osteoarthritis. J Am Acad Nurse Pract 2006;18:487–493.
64. Zurier RR, RG. Botanical and marine oils for treatment of arthritis. In: Watson, R, ed. Complementary and Alternative Therapies and the Aging Population. USA: Elsevier, 2009;Chapter 1:1–14.
65. Rayman M, Pattison DJ. Dietary manipulation in musculoskeletal conditions. Best Pract Res Clin Rheumatol 2008;22(3):535–561.
66. Debi R, et al. The role of MSM in knee osteoarthritis: a double blind, randomized prospective study. Osteoarthritis Cartilage 2007;15(Suppl 3):C231.
67. Kim L, et al. Efficacy of methylsulfonylmethane (MSM) in osteoarthritis pain of the knee: a pilot clinical trial. Osteoarthritis Cartilage 2006;14(3):286–294.
68. Brien S, et al. Systematic review of the nutritional supplements dimethyl sulfoxide (DMSO) and methylsulfonylmethane (MSM) in the treatment of osteoarthritis. Osteoarthritis Cartilage 2008;16(11):1277–1288.
69. Brouwer RW, et al. Osteotomy for treating knee osteoarthritis. Cochrane Database Syst Rev 2007;3:CD004019.
70. Moseley J, et al. A controlled trial of arthroscopic surgery for osteoarthritis of the knee. N Engl J Med 2002;347: 81–88.
71. Laupattarakasem W, et al. Arthroscopic debridement for knee osteoarthritis. Cochrane Database Syst Rev 2008;(1):1–48.
72. Healthcare Cost and Utilisation Project. Agency for healthcare research and quality. Rockville Maryland USA 2002.
73. Katz J. Total joint replacement in osteoarthritis. Best Pract Res Clin Rheumatol 2006;20(1):145–153.
74. Welch V, et al. Therapeutic ultrasound for osteoarthritis of the knee. Cochrane Database Syst Rev 2001;(3):1–17.

75. Bellamy N, et al. Viscosupplementation for the treatment of ostearthritis of the knee. Cochrane Database Syst Rev 2005;2:CD005321.

76. Marks R, Cantin D. Symptomatic osteoarthritis of the knee: the efficacy of physiotherapy. Physiotherapy 1997;83(6):306–312.

77. Verhagen A, et al. Balneotherapy for osteoarthritis. Cochrane Database Syst Rev 2003;4:CD000518.

78. Hulme J, et al. Electromagnetic fields for the treatment of osteoarthritis. Cochrane Database Syst Rev 2002;1:CD003523.

79. Osiri M, et al. Transcutaneous electrical nerve stimulation for knee osteoarthritis. Cochrane Database Syst Rev 2000;4:CD002823.

80. Fransen M. When is physiotherapy appropriate? Best Pract Res Clin Rheumatol 2004;18(4):477–489.

81. Brouwer R, et al. Braces and orthoses for treating osteoarthritis of the knee. Cochrane Database Syst Rev 2005;1:CD004020.

82. Beers MH, Berkow R, eds. The Merck manual of diagnosis and therapy. 17th edn. Whitehouse Station New Jersey: Merck Research Laboratories, 1999.

83. McPherson J, ed. Manual of use and interpretation of pathology tests. Sydney: The Royal College of Pathologists of Australasia, 1997.

84. Kumar P, Clark M, eds. Clinical medicine. 6th edn. Edinburgh: Elsevier, 2005.

85. Adams NP, et al. Beclomethasone versus placebo for chronic asthma. Cochrane Database Syst Rev 2004;4:CD002738.

86. Otulana BA, et al. High dose nebulized steroid in the treatment of chronic steroid-dependent asthma. Respir Med 1992;86(2):105–108.

87. Adams N, et al. Budesonide versus placebo for chronic asthma in children and adults. Cochrane Database Syst Rev 2001;1:CD000195.

88. Adelroth E, et al. High dose inhaled budesonide in the treatment of severe steroid-dependent asthmatics. A two-year study. Allergy 1985;40(1):58–64.

89. Abdullah AK, Khan S. Evidence-based selection of inhaled corticosteroid for treatment of chronic asthma. J Asthma 2007;44(1):1–12.

90. Cates CJ, Cates MJ. Regular treatment with salmeterol for chronic asthma: serious adverse events. Cochrane Database Syst Rev 2008;3:CD006363.

91. Boulet LP, et al. Effects of long-term use of high-dose inhaled steroids on bone density and calcium metabolism. J Allergy Clin Immunol 1994;94(5):796–803.

92. Blumenthal M, ed. Herbal medicine: expanded Commission E monographs. Newton: Integrative Medicine Communications, 2000.

93. WHO monographs on selected medicinal plants. Vol 1. Geneva: World Health Organization, 1999.

94. Barnes J, et al. Herbal medicines. 3rd edn. London: Pharmaceutical Press, 2007.

95. ESCOP Monographs. 2nd edn. Exeter: European Scientific Cooperative on Phytotherapy, 2003.

96. Mills S, Bone K. Principles and practice of phytotherapy. London: Churchill Livingstone, 2000:602.

97. Bargossi AM, et al. Exogenous CoQ10 supplementation prevents plasma ubiquinone reduction induced by HMG-CoA reductase inhibitors. Mol Aspects Med 1994;15:s187–s193.

98. Folkers K, et al. Lovastatin decreases coenzyme Q levels in humans. Proc Natl Acad Sci U S A 1990;87(22):8931–8934.

99. Mortensen SA, et al. Dose-related decrease of serum coenzyme Q10 during treatment with HMG-CoA reductase inhibitors. Mol Aspects Med 1997;18:s137–s144.

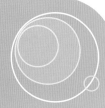

PART F
Appendices

Appendix 1

Drug–herb interaction chart

Justin Sinclair

ND, MHerbMed

This chart is a designed as a quick reference only. Further investigation may be required before making a clinical decision. This chart has been compiled using evidence-based texts, journal articles and monographs to give a current summary of known drug–herb interactions. Where applicable, supportive evidence has been referenced to allow for further investigation. The chart has been designed using a colour-coded system to highlight the different levels of supportive evidence and clinical significance. The table uses drug class as major headings for ease of information retrieval, and provides a summary of important or clinically relevant information at the end of each heading.

	Implies a serious interaction with known potential to cause harm or decreased drug effectiveness. Avoid concurrent use.
	Use caution. Interactions have some supportive evidence. Concurrent medical supervision or avoidance is advised.
	Observe. Interactions are largely theoretical and of unknown clinical significance and/or minimal supportive evidence.
	Implies a potential beneficial interaction. Interactions are largely theoretical and of unknown clinical significance and/or supportive evidence.

DRUG	HERB NAME	POTENTIAL ACTION	SUPPORTIVE EVIDENCE AND RECOMMENDATIONS
5-alpha-reductase inhibitors			
5-α-reductase inhibitors, e.g. Finasteride	Nettle (root) *Urtica dioica*	Additive effect	Nettle root has demonstrated in clinical studies to improve the micturition symptoms of BPH.[1,2] Potential beneficial interaction. Monitor patient symptoms.
	Pygeum *Pygeum africanum*	Additive effect	A standardised preparation of *Pygeum africanum* may be a useful treatment option for men with lower urinary symptoms consistent with benign prostatic hyperplasia.[3] Potential beneficial interaction. Monitor patient symptoms.
	Saw palmetto *Serenoa serrulata*	Additive effect	In vitro tests confirm saw palmetto inhibits 5-alpha reductase activity. A meta-analysis demonstrated saw palmetto as being beneficial in BPH.[1] Potential beneficial interaction. Monitor patient symptoms.
Summary	ESCOP states that nettle root and saw palmetto are used for the symptomatic management of micturition disorders (polyuria, nocturia, dysuria, urgency and hesitancy)[2,4] in BPH at stages I and II as defined by Alken, or stages II and III as defined by Vahlensieck.[2] Dosage of herb comparable to that used in clinical studies is advised to maximise therapeutic outcomes.		
Alcohol			
Alcohol (general)	Andrographis *Andrographis paniculata*	Decreased side effects	Based on the pharmacological activity of andrographis, the potential exists to reduce hepatic injury caused by alcohol.[1] Potential beneficial interaction.

DRUG	HERB NAME	POTENTIAL ACTION	SUPPORTIVE EVIDENCE AND RECOMMENDATIONS
	Kava kava *Piper methysticum*	Additive effect	Kava has demonstrated in vivo CNS sedative effects.[1] However, a clinical study reported no such effect on CNS depression in human subjects. Observe patients with moderate to high alcohol consumption and concurrent kava use.
	Ginseng, Korean *Panax ginseng*	Decreased side effects	Based on the pharmacological activity of Korean ginseng, the potential exists to reduce hepatic injury caused by alcohol.[1] Increased alcohol clearance has been observed. In mice, ginseng increases the activity of alcohol dehydrogenase and aldehyde dehydrogenase.[5] Potential beneficial interaction.
	Schisandra *Schisandra chinensis*	Decreased side effects	Based on the pharmacological activity of schisandra, the potential exists to reduce hepatic injury caused by alcohol.[1] Potential beneficial interaction.
	St Mary's thistle *Silybum marianum*	Decreased side effects	Based on the pharmacological activity of St Mary's thistle, the potential exists to reduce hepatic injury caused by alcohol.[1,6] Potential beneficial interaction.
Summary	The use of hepatotonics and hepatotrophorestoratives may benefit patients consuming moderate to high levels of alcohol. Observe patients taking kava concurrently. Consider that hydroethanolic extracts may alter blood alcohol levels (important for L- or P-plate drivers) and may not be appropriate for recovering alcoholics, so consider alternative dosage forms or tailor dosage regimen as required.		
Alkaloid-based medications			
Alkaloids (general)	Tannin-containing herbs	Decreased absorption of drug	Physicochemical interaction based on the known ability of tannins to precipitate alkaloids.[7] Take tannin-containing herbs a minimum of 2 hours away from drug.[7]
Summary	This interaction also applies to other alkaline drugs. This physicochemical interaction is of particular importance in the extemporaneous dispensing of liquid hydroethanolic extracts, yet also applies to other liquid dosage forms (infusions, decoctions, etc.).		
Anaesthetics			
General anaesthetics, e.g. halothane	St Mary's thistle *Silybum marianum*	Decreased side effects	In vivo animal studies suggest the herb may help to reduce liver toxicity of an aesthetics.[8] Uncertain clinical significance. Potential beneficial interaction.
Summary	The hepatoprotective/trophorestorative effects of milk thistle are well established. This area of research requires more investigation to substantiate usage in the field of anaesthesia.		

(Continued)

DRUG	HERB NAME	POTENTIAL ACTION	SUPPORTIVE EVIDENCE AND RECOMMENDATIONS
Analgesics (narcotics)			
Codeine	Adhatoda *Adhatoda vasica*	Additive effect	Based on the pharmacological activity of adhatoda, the potential exists to increase the antitussive activity of codeine.[1] Potential beneficial interaction.
	Ivy *Hedera helix*	Additive effect	Based on the antitussive, mucolytic and spasmolytic activity of ivy leaf preparations,[2] the potential exists to increase the antitussive activity of codeine. Potential beneficial interaction.
	Kava kava *Piper methysticum*	Additive effect	Kava may theoretically increase the CNS depressant activity of codeine.[1] Close patient monitoring and medical supervision are advised.
Morphine	Kava kava *Piper methysticum*	Additive effect	Kava may theoretically increase the CNS depressant activity of morphine.[1] Close patient monitoring and medical supervision are advised.
	Withania *Withania somnifera*	Reduced drug tolerance/dependence	Withania has demonstrated inhibited morphine tolerance and dependence in vivo with repeated administration (100 mg/kg),[1] so may be applicable to opium withdrawal. Uncertain clinical significance. Potential beneficial interaction.
Summary	Ivy-leaf preparations have a long history of use in Europe and should be standardised to hederacoside C if possible.[2] The use of withania in opium withdrawal requires further investigation to be of greater clinical significance.		

Analgesics (simple) and antipyretics

DRUG	HERB NAME	POTENTIAL ACTION	SUPPORTIVE EVIDENCE AND RECOMMENDATIONS
Simple analgesics and antipyretics (general)	Meadowsweet *Filipendula ulmaria*	Additive effect	Based on the pharmacological activity of meadowsweet, the potential exists to cause additive anti-inflammatory and analgesic effects.[1] Potential beneficial interaction.
	Willow *Salix alba*	Additive effect	Based on the pharmacological activity of willow, the potential exists to cause additive anti-inflammatory and analgesic effects.[1] Potential beneficial interaction.

DRUG	HERB NAME	POTENTIAL ACTION	SUPPORTIVE EVIDENCE AND RECOMMENDATIONS
Aspirin	Grape seed *Vitis vinifera*	Additive effect	Based on the pharmacological activity of grape seed, the potential exists to cause additive anti-inflammatory and antiplatelet effects.[1] Grape seed is rich in polyphenolics, and has the ability to inhibit platelet aggregation.[9] **Caution:** May increase risk of bleeding.
	Meadowsweet *Filipendula ulmaria*	Additive effect	Based on the pharmacological activity of meadowsweet, the potential exists to cause additive anti-inflammatory effects.[1] Potential beneficial interaction. **Caution:** May also enhance antiplatelet effects and increase risk of bleeding.
	Willow *Salix alba*	Additive effect	Based on the pharmacological activity of willow, the potential exists to cause additive anti-inflammatory and antiplatelet effects.[1] A clinical study demonstrated willow to have antiplatelet activity.[7] Higher doses than 240 mg/day of salicin may have a more significant effect.[1] Monitor patient closely in higher dosage. Potential beneficial interaction. **Caution:** May increase risk of bleeding.
Paracetamol	Andrographis *Andrographis paniculata*	Reduced drug side effects	Based on the pharmacological activity of andrographis, the potential exists to protect against paracetamol induced liver damage.[1] Potential beneficial interaction.
	Garlic *Allium sativum*	Reduced drug side effects	Based on the pharmacological activity of garlic, the potential exists to protect against paracetamol induced liver damage.[1] Potential beneficial interaction.
	Schisandra *Schisandra chinensis*	Reduced drug side effects	Based on the pharmacological activity of schisandra, the potential exists to protect against paracetamol induced liver damage.[1] Potential beneficial interaction.
	St Mary's thistle *Silybum marianum*	Reduced drug side effects	Based on the pharmacological activity of St Mary's thistle, the potential exists to protect against paracetamol induced liver damage.[1,6] Potential beneficial interaction.
Summary	Due to the potential additive anti-inflammatory and analgesic effect of the abovementioned herbs, drug modification may be required. Use caution with high doses of grape seed, meadowsweet or willow due to increased risk of bleeding. Observe patient for signs of increased bleeding (bruising, purpura, etc.).		

(Continued)

DRUG	HERB NAME	POTENTIAL ACTION	SUPPORTIVE EVIDENCE AND RECOMMENDATIONS
Antiarrhythmics			
Antiarrhythmics, e.g. quinidine	Dong quai *Angelica sinensis*	Additive effect	Dong quai has a quinidine-like action on the heart.[10] It can prolong the refractory period and correct experimental atrial fibrillation induced by atropine.[10] Interaction is theoretical and of uncertain clinical significance.
	Astragalus *Astragalus membranaceus*	Additive effect	In a clinical study, IV administration of astragalus significantly shortened ventricular late potentials in a study of 313 patients.[11] Astragalus has been shown to have a positive inotropic action in vivo.[10] Uncertain clinical significance for oral dosage forms of this herb.[1]
	Devil's claw *Harpagophytum procumbens*	Additive effect	In vitro tests show that harpagoside showed a significant, dose-dependent protective action against arrhythmias induced by reperfusion.[11] Interaction is theoretical and of uncertain clinical significance.[1]
	Hawthorn *Crataegus monogyna*	Addltive effect	Hawthorn has demonstrated in in vitro and in vivo tests that it has an effect similar to class III antiarrhythmic drugs (by blocking repolarising potassium currents in ventricular myocytes).[11] Interaction is theoretical and of uncertain clinical significance.[1]
	Lily-of-the-valley *Convallaria majalis*	Increased drug toxicity	Concurrent administration of quinidine and *Convallaria* may enhance both drug effects and side effects.[11] Lily-of-the-valley is currently a scheduled (S4) medicine. Avoid concurrent use.
Summary	Due to the seriousness of the underlying condition being managed, administration of any herb that can potentially alter the effects of antiarrhythmic medication should be considered only after consultation with the patient's medical practitioner.		
Antibiotics			
Antibiotics Quinolones	Dandelion *Taraxacum officinale*	Reduced drug effectiveness	Experimental studies have shown reduced drug absorption when administered simultaneously. Separate doses by a minimum of 2 hours.[1]
Triple therapy for *H. pylori* infection	Garlic *Allium sativum*	Additive effect	*Helicobacter pylori* growth was inhibited by garlic in in vitro and in vivo tests, with 2 clinical studies suggesting garlic has a synergistic effect with omeprazole.[1]

DRUG	HERB NAME	POTENTIAL ACTION	SUPPORTIVE EVIDENCE AND RECOMMENDATIONS
	Golden seal *Hydrastis canadensis*	Additive effect	Based on the mucous membrane trophorestorative activity of golden seal, the potential exists to have additive therapeutic effects. Potential beneficial interaction. Interaction is theoretical and of uncertain clinical significance.
Summary	Adjunct use of immune-stimulating herbs during infections may be of benefit.		

Anticoagulants and antiplatelets

DRUG	HERB NAME	POTENTIAL ACTION	SUPPORTIVE EVIDENCE AND RECOMMENDATIONS
Anticoagulants and antiplatelets	Andrographis *Andrographis paniculata*	Increased bleeding risk	Andrographis has shown ex-vivo antiplatelet activity.[7] Andrographolide has been shown to inhibit PAF induced platelet aggregation.[1] Monitor patient.
	Bilberry *Vaccinium myrtillus*	Increased bleeding risk	At doses lower than 100 mg/day of anthocyanins, bilberry usage with concurrent administration of anticoagulants should be observed. **Caution:** Avoid high doses of the herb (> 100 mg/day anthocyanins) with concurrent use.[7]
	Celery *Apium graveolens*	Increased bleeding risk	Celery contains furanocoumarins,[11,12] which may increase risk of bleeding with concurrent use. Interaction is theoretical and of uncertain clinical significance.
	Cranberry *Vaccinium macrocarpon*	Increased bleeding risk	Case reports have suggested potential to increase risk of bleeding with concurrent usage.[7] **Caution:** Avoid high doses of the herb with concurrent use.
	Dan shen *Salvia miltiorrhiza*	Increased bleeding risk	Case reports suggest dan shen can increase INR and prolong PTT.[7,13–15] In vitro studies have shown dan shen to possess anticoagulant and fibrinolytic activity.[10] Avoid concurrent use.
	Devil's claw *Harpagophytum procumbens*	Increased bleeding risk	A case of purpura was reported in a patient taking concurrent devil's claw and warfarin.[7] Due to lack of other medications, doses and duration of use in this case report, the clinical significance is questionable. Monitor patient.
	Dong quai *Angelica sinensis*	Increased bleeding risk	Concurrent use may increase risk of bleeding as dong quai may potentiate effects of warfarin.[7,11,16] IV administration of dong quai caused prothrombin time to be significantly longer.[11] Uncertain clinical significance for oral dosage forms of this herb. Monitor patient.

(Continued)

DRUG	HERB NAME	POTENTIAL ACTION	SUPPORTIVE EVIDENCE AND RECOMMENDATIONS
	Evening primrose (oil) *Oenothera biennis*	Increased bleeding risk	Evening primrose oil contains gamma-linoleic acid, which can affect prostaglandin synthesis and lead to inhibition of platelet aggregation.[1] Avoid high doses of the oil with concurrent use. Interaction is theoretical and of uncertain clinical significance.
	Fenugreek *Trigonella foenum-graecum*	Increased bleeding risk	Fenugreek contains trigomethyl coumarin. Clinical trial found no detrimental effect upon platelet aggregation or fibrinolytic activity.[1] Interaction is theoretical and of uncertain clinical significance.
	Feverfew *Tanacetum parthenium*	Increased bleeding risk	While in vitro and in vivo studies have shown feverfew to inhibit platelet aggregation, this was not seen in clinical trials.[1] High doses of feverfew may increase bleeding complications when combined with anticoagulants.[11]
	Garlic *Allium sativum*	Additive effect	Case reports have suggested that garlic may increase INR in patients on warfarin.[2,17–19] Poses a potential risk for postoperative bleeding.[20] Caution should be exercised with patients taking any anticoagulant medication.[21] Avoid high doses of the herb (> 4 g/day equiv. fresh) and monitor patient.
	Ginger *Zingiber officinale*	Increased bleeding risk	Ginger has been shown to inhibit platelet aggregation in high dose. Conflicting results in studies of platelet antagonism in human trials have been noted.[22] Daily doses of 2 g/day of ginger should not be exceeded in pregnancy.[12] Avoid high dose (> 10 g/day) unless under medical supervision;[1] a study suggested > 4 g/day dried ginger requires supervision.[7] Monitor patient closely or avoid concurrent use.
	Ginkgo *Ginkgo biloba*	Increased bleeding risk	Isolated studies and case reports have reported increased bleeding tendency for both warfarin and aspirin.[7,23–26] Recent clinical studies show ginkgo has no significant effect on warfarin.[1,27]
	Ginseng, Korean *Panax ginseng*	Increased bleeding risk	Inhibits platelet aggregation in in vitro and in vivo tests.[1] Case reports suggest it can lower INR in a previously stabilised patient.[11] Monitor closely or avoid concurrent use.

DRUG	HERB NAME	POTENTIAL ACTION	SUPPORTIVE EVIDENCE AND RECOMMENDATIONS
	Ginseng, Siberian *Eleutherococcus senticosus*	Increased bleeding risk	3,4-dihydroxybenzoic acid was isolated from Siberian ginseng and shown to be an antiplatelet aggregatory substance.[28] Interaction is theoretical and of uncertain clinical significance.
	Goji *Lycium barbarum*	Additive effect	Case report suggested increase in INR.[7] Avoid high doses of the herb. Monitor patient.
	Grape seed *Vitis vinifera*	Increased bleeding risk	Grape seed is rich in polyphenolics, and has the ability to inhibit platelet aggregation.[9] **Caution** with high doses of the herb. Interaction is theoretical and of uncertain clinical significance.
	Green tea *Camellia sinensis*	Reduced drug effectiveness	One case report of decreased INR. Epidemiological studies have not confirmed this finding.[7] **Caution** with high doses of the herb (c. 2–4 L green tea daily).[1]
	Guarana *Paullinia cupana*	Increased bleeding risk	In vitro and in vivo antiplatelet activity has been established.[1,11] Interaction is of uncertain clinical significance.
	Guggul *Commiphora mukul*	Increased bleeding risk	In vitro and clinical data suggest that guggul increased coagulation and prothrombin time, decreased platelet adhesiveness, increased fibrinolytic activity and inhibited platelet aggregation.[10,29] Unlike myrrh, use cautiously due to suggestive evidence.
	Horseradish *Amoracia rusticana*	Increased bleeding risk	Horseradish contains coumarins, which could theoretically interact with anticoagulant medication.[1] Interaction is theoretical and of uncertain clinical significance. Observe patient if taking high-dose supplements.
	Liquorice *Glycyrrhiza glabra*	Increased bleeding risk	In vitro and in vivo tests suggest glycyrrhizin inhibits prothrombin and isoliquiritigenin inhibits platelet aggregation.[1] **Caution** with high doses of this herb. Interaction is of uncertain clinical significance.
	Meadowsweet *Filipendula ulmaria*	Increased bleeding risk	In vivo studies suggest meadowsweet has anticoagulant activity.[1,7] Interaction is of uncertain clinical significance.

(Continued)

DRUG	HERB NAME	POTENTIAL ACTION	SUPPORTIVE EVIDENCE AND RECOMMENDATIONS
	Myrrh *Commiphora molmol*	Increased bleeding risk	While inhibition of platelet aggregation was observed, and other haematological parameters were affected by guggul, how this effects myrrh preparations is as yet unknown.[10] Interaction is of uncertain clinical significance.
	Pau d'arco *Tabebuia avellanedae*	Additive effect	Prolonged prothrombin time was observed in a clinical trial with a dose > 2 g/day of lapachol.[7] Interaction is of uncertain clinical significance.
	Saw palmetto *Serenoa* spp.	Additive effect	Case report suggestive that saw palmetto can increase INR.[7] Interaction is of uncertain clinical significance.
	St John's wort *Hypericum perforatum*	Reduced drug effectiveness	Reduced blood levels of warfarin have been noted in case reports from concurrent administration of *Hypericum* preparations.[1,2,4,7,30] St John's wort is a known inducer of CYT P450 enzymes, causing increased drug metabloism. Avoid concurrent use.
	St Mary's thistle *Silybum marianum*	Additive effect	Due to St Mary's thistle having inhibitive effects on the CYT P450 system, a potential increase in drug levels is possible.[1] Interaction is of uncertain clinical significance. Monitor patient closely.
	Sweet clover *Melilotus officinalis*	Increased bleeding risk	Sweet clover contains coumarins, which may theoretically increase bleeding risk.[7] Interaction is of uncertain clinical significance.
	Turmeric *Curcuma longa*	Increased bleeding risk	Curcumin, a key constituent of turmeric, has been shown to inhibit platelet aggregation in vitro.[31] Caution with doses > 15 g per day.[7]
	Willow *Salix alba*	Increased bleeding risk	Clinical study observed willow to have antiplatelet activity[7] Higher doses than 240 mg of salicin per day may have a more significant effect.[1] Monitor patient closely in higher dosage.
Summary	Administration of any herb that can potentially alter INR or increase bleeding risk should only be considered after consultation with the patient's medical practitioner. Avoid the concurrent use of herbs with known evidence of increased bleeding risk or reduced drug effectiveness.		

DRUG	HERB NAME	POTENTIAL ACTION	SUPPORTIVE EVIDENCE AND RECOMMENDATIONS
Anticonvulsants			
Anticonvulsants (general)	Ginkgo *Ginkgo biloba*	Reduced drug effectiveness	In vivo animal studies and 2 case reports suggest a potential interaction is possible with concurrent use of ginkgo, causing reduced drug effects.[7] Monitor patient.
	St John's wort *Hypericum perforatum*	Reduced drug effectiveness	St John's wort is known to induce the CYT P450 system, resulting in increased drug metabolism. This may lead to reduced drug effectiveness and poor clinical outcomes. Avoid concurrent use.
Carbamazepine	Ginkgo *Ginkgo biloba*	Reduced drug effectiveness	In vivo animal studies and 2 case reports suggest a potential interaction is possible with concurrent use of ginkgo causing reduced drug effects.[7] Monitor patient.
	St John's wort *Hypericum perforatum*	Reduced drug effectiveness	St John's wort is known to induce the CYT P450 system, resulting in the increased metabolism of multiple drugs. Carbamazepine is known to be metabolised by the isoenzyme 3A4, which St John's wort is known to induce.[1] This may lead to reduced drug effectiveness and poor clinical outcomes. Avoid concurrent use.
	St Mary's thistle *Silybum marianum*	Additive effect	St Mary's thistle has been shown to inhibit CYT P450 3A4, therefore reducing drug metabolism. This may lead to increased blood levels of carbamazepine (a NTI drug) and associated adverse effects.[1]
Phenobarbitone	Celery *Apium graveolens*	Increased drug duration of action	In vivo test on rats found that celery juice prolonged the action of phenobarbitone.[1] Interaction is of uncertain clinical significance.
	Kava kava *Piper methysticum*	Increased sedative effects	Isolated methysticin reversibly blocked epileptiform activity in various in vitro seizure models, showing anticonvulsant activity.[2] Interaction is of uncertain clinical significance.
Phenobarbitone and phenytoin	Kava kava *Piper methysticum*	Increased sedative effects	Isolated methysticin reversibly blocked epileptiform activity in various in vitro seizure models, showing anticonvulsant activity.[2] Interaction is of uncertain clinical significance.

(Continued)

DRUG	HERB NAME	POTENTIAL ACTION	SUPPORTIVE EVIDENCE AND RECOMMENDATIONS
	St John's wort *Hypericum perforatum*	Reduced drug effectiveness	St John's wort is known to induce the CYT P450 system, resulting in the increased metabolism of multiple drugs. This may lead to reduced drug effectiveness and poor clinical outcomes. No known adverse events have been reported with concurrent use of phenytoin or other anticonvulsants and St John's wort use.[12]
Summary	Administration of any herb that can potentially reduce drug effectiveness or alter serum levels, such as St John's wort, should be avoided or used only under medical supervision. Exercise caution in using any of the abovementioned herbs with patients on anticonvulsant medications.		
Antidepressants			
Antidepressants, e.g. SSRIs, SNRIs	Albizzia *Albizzia lebbeck*	Additive effect	Albizzia has been shown to increase serotonin levels in vivo.[1] The potential to cause serotonergic syndrome therefore exists. Interaction is of uncertain clinical significance.
	Ginkgo *Ginkgo biloba*	Reduced drug side effects	A clinical study reports reduced sexual function side effects.[1] A case report in a patient with Alzheimer's disease suggested a possible increase in the function of GABA receptors leading to sedation with concurrent use of trazodone.[7] Observe patient with concurrent use.
	St John's wort *Hypericum perforatum*	Additive effect	Potential for serotonergic syndrome with concurrent use.[1,2,7,32–36] Avoid if possible, or use only under close medical supervision.
Tricyclics	Yohimbe *Pausinystalia yohimbe*	Additive effect	Yohimbine alone can cause hypertension, but lower doses cause hypertension when combined with tricyclic antidepressants.[17,37,38] Effect is stronger in hypertensive than normotensive individuals.
	Andrographis *Andrographis paniculata*	Reduced drug side effects	Tricyclic drugs have the potential to cause liver damage. Theoretical beneficial interaction due to the hepatoprotective activity of andrographis.[1] Interaction is of uncertain clinical significance.
	St John's wort *Hypericum perforatum*	Additive effect	St John's wort may decrease tricyclic drug plasma levels, and also may increase available serotonin.[1] Avoid if possible, or use only under close medical supervision.

DRUG	HERB NAME	POTENTIAL ACTION	SUPPORTIVE EVIDENCE AND RECOMMENDATIONS
	St Mary's thistle *Silybum marianum*	Reduced drug side effects	Tricyclic drugs have the potential to cause liver damage. Theoretical beneficial interaction due to the hepatoprotective activity of St Mary's thistle.[1] Interaction is of uncertain clinical significance.
Summary	The use of herbal antidepressants is indicated only for the management of mild to moderate depression, not severe depressive states. Remember that it can take between 3 and 4 weeks for the full therapeutic effect of herbs such as St John's wort to take effect.[2] Administration of any abovementioned herb with a patient on antidepressant medication should be considered only after consultation with the patient's medical practitioner.		
Antihistamines			
Antihistamines (general)	Albizzia *Albizzia lebbeck*	Additive effect	Based on Albizzia's antiallergic activity via a stabilising effect on mast cells, a beneficial interaction may be possible.[1,10] Interaction is of uncertain clinical significance.
	Baical skullcap *Scutellria baicalensis*	Additive effect	Baical skullcap has known anti-inflammatory and antiallergic activity. Flavonoids present have been shown to inhibit prostaglandin production and histamine release by mast cells in vitro.[10] A beneficial interaction may be possible. Interaction is of uncertain clinical significance.
	Perilla *Perilla frutescans*	Additive effect	Perilla extract (seed) has known antiallergic activity and has been shown to inhibit histamine release from mast cells dose dependently.[1] A beneficial interaction may be possible. Interaction is of uncertain clinical significance.
Fexofenadine	St John's wort *Hypericum perforatum*	Reduced drug effectiveness	A clinical study demonstrated the potential for St John's wort to decrease drug levels.[7] Monitor patient.
Summary	The use of the abovementioned additive herbs concurrently with antihistamine medication may increase antiallergic activity, and is generally considered of low risk. Avoid St John's wort usage with Telfast (fexofenadine) if possible, based on clinical evidence.		
Antihypertensives			
Antihypertensives (general)	Coleus *Coleus forskohlii*	Additive effect	Forskolin has been shown in vitro to lower blood pressure.[7] Interaction may be beneficial, but is of uncertain clinical significance.
	Garlic *Allium sativum*	Additive effect	Clinical trials have demonstrated the ability for garlic to lower blood pressure. Potentially beneficial interaction,[1] but is of uncertain clinical significance. Monitor patient as drug requirements may need modification.

(Continued)

DRUG	HERB NAME	POTENTIAL ACTION	SUPPORTIVE EVIDENCE AND RECOMMENDATIONS
	Ginseng, Korean *Panax ginseng*	Reduced drug effectiveness	Due to CNS stimulatory activity the potential for reduced drug effectiveness exists. High doses may lead to Ginseng abuse syndrome, which is characterised by hypertension, nervousness, euphoria and skin eruptions.[12] Interaction is of uncertain clinical significance.
	Guarana *Paullinia cupana*	Reduced drug effectiveness	Due to CNS stimulatory activity from caffeine content, the potential for reduced drug effectiveness exists.[7] Interaction is of uncertain clinical significance.
	Hawthorn *Crataegus monogyna*	Additive effect	Hawthorn has demonstrated mild to moderate hypotensive activity. Higher OPC content extracts may have increased effect. Potentially beneficial interaction.[1] Monitor patient as drug requirements may need modification.
	Liquorice *Glycyrrhiza glabra*	Reduced drug effectiveness	High dose administration for longer than 4–6 weeks may result in pseudoaldosteronism and BP increase.[7] Avoid long-term use at doses > 100 mg/day of glycyrrhizin.[7] Monitor patient.
	Oats (as cereal) *Avena sativa*	Additive effect	A 73% decrease in blood pressure was observed in a clinical trial with patients ingesting oat-based cereals. Potentially beneficial interaction.[1] Monitor patient as drug requirements may need modification.
	Olive leaf *Olea europa*	Additive effect	Olive leaf extract has shown hypotensive activity.[49] Interaction is beneficial, but of unknown clinical significance. Drug dosage modification may be required.
	Yohimbe *Pausinystalia yohimbe*	Reduced drug effectiveness	Yohimbe has been shown to increase blood pressure in healthy male subjects.[11] Caution with concurrent use.
Felodipine	Peppermint (oil) *Mentha piperita*	Additive effect	Animal studies have shown the oil of peppermint to increase felodipine bioavailability.[1] Monitor patient as drug dosage requirement may need modification.
Diltiazem	Guggul *Commiphora mukul*	Reduced drug effectiveness	Guggulipid reduces bioavailability based on a clinical trial. Uncertain clinical significance for myrrh.[1] Monitor patient.

DRUG	HERB NAME	POTENTIAL ACTION	SUPPORTIVE EVIDENCE AND RECOMMENDATIONS
Propranolol	Guggul *Commiphora mukul*	Reduced drug effectiveness	Clinical trials reports that guggulipid reduced bioavailability of propranolol.[1] Uncertain clinical significance for myrrh.[1] Monitor patient.
Summary	The use of herbal medicines in pre-hypertension and stage I hypertension, along with dietary modification and exercise, generally has good clinical outcomes. Administration of any abovementioned herb with a patient currently taking hypotensive medication should be considered only after consultation with the patient's medical practitioner. Other herbs with hypotensive activity may decrease blood pressure further (e.g., *Viscum album, Astragalus membranaceus, Olea europea, Leonurus cardiaca* etc.). Monitor patient.		
Antipsychotics			
Haloperidol	Ginkgo *Ginkgo biloba*	Additive effect and reduced side effects	Clinical trial demonstrated that ginkgo administered at 250 mg/kg over 12 weeks had additive effect and also reduced drug side effects.[1] Interaction may be beneficial, but is of uncertain clinical significance and requires medical supervision. Use caution.
Phenothiazines	Evening primrose (oil) *Oenothera biennis*	Reduced drug effectiveness	Case reports suggest that the oil of evening primrose may reduce seizure threshold and reduce drug effectiveness in patients with schizophrenia being administered phenothiazines.[1] Avoid concurrent use until safety profile is established.[1]
Summary	Due to the seriousness of the condition being treated, avoid concurrent use or use only while patient is under close medical supervision. Avoid use of evening primrose oil based on current clinical evidence.		
Antivirals (including HIV protease inhibitors and non-nucleoside transcriptase inhibitors)			
Acyclovir	St John's wort *Hypericum perforatum*	Reduced drug effectiveness	Case report suggestive that the effective dose was lowered. Monitor patient and be prepared to shorten treatment or reduce dose.[7]
Non-nucleoside transcriptase inhibitors, e.g. nevirapine	St John's wort *Hypericum perforatum*	Reduced drug effectiveness	St John's wort is known to reduce drug levels via the CYT P450 and P-gp systems, resulting in reduced drug effectiveness and poor clinical outcomes.[1,7] Avoid concurrent use.
Protease inhibitors, e.g. indinavir or saquinivir	St Mary's thistle *Silybum marianum*	Reduced drug effectiveness	St Mary's thistle may reduce indinavir levels.[39] Use only under close medical supervision.
	St John's wort *Hypericum perforatum*	Reduced drug effectiveness	St John's wort is known to reduce drug levels via the CYT P450 and P-gp systems, resulting in reduced drug effectiveness and poor clinical outcomes.[1,7] Avoid concurrent use

(Continued)

DRUG	HERB NAME	POTENTIAL ACTION	SUPPORTIVE EVIDENCE AND RECOMMENDATIONS
	Garlic *Allium sativum*	Reduced drug effectiveness	Garlic has demonstrated in a clinical study to reduce serum levels of saquinivir and drug effectiveness, resulting in poor clinical outcomes.[1,40] Avoid concurrent use.
Summary	The use of any herb known to effect antiviral effectiveness, especially with non-nucleoside transcriptase or protease inhibitors should be avoided due to reduced drug effectiveness.		
Barbiturates (CNS depressants)			
Barbiturates (general)	Albizzia *Albizzia lebbeck*	Additive effect	In vivo studies demonstrated a potentiation of phenobarbitone-induced sleeping time.[1] Interaction may be beneficial, but is of uncertain clinical significance and requires medical supervision. Use caution.
	Andrographis *Andrographis paniculata*	Additive effect	In vivo studies demonstrated a potentiation of effects.[1] Interaction may be beneficial, but is of uncertain clinical significance and requires medical supervision. Use caution.
	Kava kava *Piper methysticum*	Additive effect	Potential to increase sedative effects.[1,41] Interaction may be beneficial, but is of uncertain clinical significance and requires medical supervision. Drug dosage modification may be required. Use caution.
	Lemon balm *Melissa officinalis*	Additive effect	Potential to increase sedative effects.[1] Interaction may be beneficial, but is of uncertain clinical significance and requires medical supervision.
	Passionflower *Passiflora incarnata*	Additive effect	Potential to increase sedative effects.[1] Interaction may be beneficial, but is of uncertain clinical significance and requires medical supervision. Use caution.
	St John's wort *Hypericum perforatum*	Reduced drug effectiveness	St John's wort is known to induce the CYT P450 system and P-gp,[1] resulting in reduced drug levels and poor clinical outcomes. Avoid concurrent use
	Valerian *Valeriana officinalis*	Additive effect	Potential to increase sedative effects.[1] Interaction may be beneficial, but is of uncertain clinical significance and requires medical supervision. Use caution.
	Withania *Withania somnifera*	Additive effect	Theoretically increases sedative effects.[1] Interaction may be beneficial, but is of uncertain clinical significance and requires medical supervision.
Summary	Administration of any abovementioned herb with a patient currently taking barbiturate medication should be considered only if under close medical supervision to modify drug dose if required. Avoid concurrent use of St John's wort based on clinical evidence.		

DRUG	HERB NAME	POTENTIAL ACTION	SUPPORTIVE EVIDENCE AND RECOMMENDATIONS
Benzodiazapines (CNS depressants)			
Benzodiazapines (general)	German chamomile *Matricaria recutita*	Additive effect	Theoretically increases sedative effects.[1] Interaction may be beneficial, but is of uncertain clinical significance. Monitor patient.
	Kava kava *Piper methysticum*	Additive effect	Kava can be used to ease symptoms of benzodiazepine withdrawal if done under medical supervision.[1] Potential beneficial interaction. Drug dosage modification may be required.
	Passionflower *Passiflora incarnata*	Additive effect	Potential to increase sedative effects.[1] Interaction may be beneficial, but is of uncertain clinical significance and requires medical supervision.
	St John's wort *Hypericum perforatum*	Reduced drug effectiveness	A clinical study demonstrated reduced drug levels with concurrent midazolam and St John's wort use.[7] Avoid concurrent use unless under medical supervision. Drug dosage modification may be required.
	Valerian *Valeriana officinalis*	Additive effect	Valerian may be used to ease symptoms of benzodiazepine withdrawal under medical supervision.[1] Potential beneficial interaction. Drug dosage modification may be required.
	Withania *Withania somnifera*	Additive effect	Potential to increase sedative effects.[1] Interaction may be beneficial, but is of uncertain clinical significance and requires medical supervision.
Summary	Administration of any abovementioned herb with a patient currently taking benzodiazapine medication should be considered only if under close medical supervision to modify drug dose if required. Avoid concurrent use of St John's wort based on clinical evidence.		
Bronchospasmolytics/bronchodilators			
Prednisone and salbutamol	Betel nut *Areca catechu*	Reduced drug effectiveness	Betel nut is known to contain a cholinergic alkaloid, arecoline. Arecoline challenge caused dose-related bronchoconstriction in six asthma patients.[17,42] Avoid concurrent use unless under medical supervision.
Theophylline	Chilli *Capsicum* spp.	Increased drug absorption	Chilli may increase the bio-availability and absorption of theophylline.[17,43] Due to the NTI status of this drug, caution is advised.

(Continued)

DRUG	HERB NAME	POTENTIAL ACTION	SUPPORTIVE EVIDENCE AND RECOMMENDATIONS
	St John's wort *Hypericum perforatum*	Reduced drug effectiveness	St John's wort is known to reduce drug levels via the CYT P450 system[44] and P-gp. Case reports show herb can decrease serum levels.[1,2,4,7,44,45] Avoid concurrent use.
Summary	Avoid concurrent use of St John's wort based on clinical evidence. Based on the ability for St John's wort to decrease drug levels, caution should also be exercised with other asthma/COPD medications such as inhaled corticosteroids (ICS) and systemic corticosteroids (e.g. prednisolone), especially in severe, persistent asthmatic patients. Monitor patient closely.		

Cardiac glycosides

DRUG	HERB NAME	POTENTIAL ACTION	SUPPORTIVE EVIDENCE AND RECOMMENDATIONS
Digoxin	Guar gum *Cyamopsis tetragonolobus*	Reduced drug absorption	Guar gum may slow the absorption of digoxin and paracetamol, Guar gum prolongs gastric retention.[17,46] Ensure doses separated by a minimum of 2 hours.
	Aloe *Aloe vera*	Increased drug toxicity	Oral use of aloe long-term may deplete potassium levels, lowering the threshold for digoxin toxicity[1,7] Avoid concurrent long-term use unless under medical supervision.
	Cascara *Cascara sagrada*	Increased drug toxicity	Avoid excessive use of laxative herbs as enhanced digoxin toxicity caused by lowered potassium levels is possible.[7] Avoid concurrent long-term use unless under medical supervision.
	Hawthorn *Crataegus monogyna*	Additive effect	In vitro and in vivo studies demonstrate hawthorn as having a positively inotropic and chronotropic activity.[1] Interaction may be beneficial, but is of uncertain clinical significance and requires medical supervision.
	Ginseng, Siberian *Eleutherococcus senticosus*	Assay interference	Siberian ginseng has the potential to interfere with digoxin assay,[7,47] and may produce false-positive test results.[1] Consult patient's medical practitioner.
	Guarana *Paullinia cupana*	Increased drug toxicity	Long-term use of high-dose guarana can deplete potassium levels, which lowers the threshold for digoxin toxicity.[1] Avoid concurrent long-term use unless under medical supervision.
	Liquorice *Glycyrrhiza glabra*	Increased drug toxicity	Long-term use of high dose liquorice can deplete potassium levels, lowering the threshold for digoxin toxicity.[1,7] Avoid concurrent use.
	Lily-of-the-valley *Convallaria majalis*	Increased drug toxicity	Concurrent administration of digoxin and *Convallaria* may enhance drug effects and side effects.[11] Use only under medical supervision.

DRUG	HERB NAME	POTENTIAL ACTION	SUPPORTIVE EVIDENCE AND RECOMMENDATIONS
	Senna *Cassia angustifolia*	Increased drug toxicity	Avoid excessive use of laxative herbs as enhanced digoxin toxicity caused by lowered potassium levels is possible.[7] Avoid concurrent long-term use unless under medical supervision.
	St John's wort *Hypericum perforatum*	Reduced drug effectiveness	St John's wort is known to reduce drug levels via the CYT P450[48] system and P-gp,[1] resulting in the increased metabolism of digoxin. A clinical study demonstrated that St John's wort significantly decreased serum levels of digoxin within 10 days of concurrent use.[1] Avoid concurrent use.[2,4,11]
Summary	Long-term use of laxative herbs that have the ability to deplete potassium levels requires prior consultation with the patient's medical practitioner. Due to the seriousness of the condition being treated, and the fact that digoxin is an NTI drug, avoid concurrent use or use only while patient is under close medical supervision.		
Chemotherapeutics (cancer medications)			
Chemotherapy (general)	Ginseng, Siberian *Eleutherococcus senticosus*	Improved treatment tolerance	Coadministration may increase drug tolerance and improve patient immune function.[1] Interaction may be beneficial, but is of uncertain clinical significance and requires medical supervision.
	Rosemary *Rosmarinus officinalis*	Increased drug effects of P-gp substrates	Rosemary inhibits P-glycoprotein so may affect the bioavailability of P-gp substrates.[49]
	St John's wort *Hypericum perforatum*	Reduced drug effectiveness	Clinical studies have shown St John's wort may decrease drug levels resulting in poor clinical outcomes.[7] Avoid concurrent use.
	Withania *Withania somnifera*	Reduced drug side effects	In vivo studies suggest that withania may be beneficial as adjunct treatment during chemotherapy to prevent drug-induced bone marrow suppression.[1]
Cisplatin	St Mary's thistle *Silybum marianum*	Increased drug effects	Research suggests that St Mary's thistle may reduce toxicity effects[1] but may reduce drug efficacy.[50] Interaction may be beneficial yet requires medical supervision.
Doxorubicin	Ginkgo *Ginkgo biloba*	Reduced drug side effects	In vivo studies suggest that ginkgo can prevent doxorubicin-induced cardiotoxicity.[1] Interaction may be beneficial, but is of uncertain clinical significance and requires medical supervision.

(Continued)

DRUG	HERB NAME	POTENTIAL ACTION	SUPPORTIVE EVIDENCE AND RECOMMENDATIONS
Irinotecan	St John's wort *Hypericum perforatum*	Reduced drug effectiveness	Clinical studies have shown St John's wort may decrease drug levels resulting in poor clinical outcomes.[7] Avoid concurrent use.
Paclitaxel	Liquorice *Glycyrrhiza glabra*	Additive effect	In vitro studies suggest an isolated constituent in liquorice has been found to significantly potentiate the effects of paclitaxel.[1] Interaction may be beneficial, but is of uncertain clinical significance and requires medical supervision.
Summary	Due to the seriousness of the conditions being managed, avoid concurrent use or use only while patient is under close medical supervision.		
CNS stimulants			
CNS stimulants, e.g. caffeine	Ginseng, Korean *Panax ginseng*	Additive effect	Based on the pharmacological activity of Korean ginseng, the potential to increase stimulating effects exists. Interaction is of uncertain clinical significance.
	Guarana *Paullinia cupana*	Additive effect	Based on the pharmacological activity of Korean ginseng, the potential to increase stimulating effects exists. Interaction is of uncertain clinical significance.
Summary	The use of CNS-stimulant herbs may theoretically have an additive effect. Avoid concurrent use if possible.		
Contraceptives (see 'Hormone-based medication')			
Corticosteroids			
Corticosteroids (general)	Liquorice *Glycyrrhiza glabra*	Additive effect	Concurrent use of liquorice preparations has been shown to increase the effects of both topical and oral corticosteroids (e.g. prednisolone).[1,51,52] Glycyrrhizin has been shown to inhibit prednisolone metabolism in clinical studies.[7] May be useful in minimising requirements of corticosteroids or aiding in their tapered withdrawal. Interaction may be beneficial, but is of uncertain clinical significance.
Topical corticosteroids, e.g. hydrocortisone	Aloe (gel) *Aloe vera*	Additive effect	Animal studies have demonstrated that aloe vera gel increases the absorption of hydrocortisone by hydrating the stratum corneum. It also inhibits hydrocortisone's antiwound healing activity and increases the wound's tensile strength.[1] *Aloe vera* gel also possesses anti-inflammatory and demulcent activity. Interaction may be beneficial, but is of uncertain clinical significance.

DRUG	HERB NAME	POTENTIAL ACTION	SUPPORTIVE EVIDENCE AND RECOMMENDATIONS
	Liquorice *Glycyrrhiza glabra*	Additive effect	Concurrent use of liquorice preparations has been shown to increase the effects of both topical and oral corticosteroids (e.g. prednisolone).[1] Glycyrrhizin has been shown to inhibit prednisolone metabolism in clinical studies.[7] May be useful in minimising requirements of corticosteroids or aiding in their tapered withdrawal. Interaction may be beneficial, but is of uncertain clinical significance.
Summary	Administration of any abovementioned herb with a patient currently taking corticosteroids requires prior consultation with the patient's medical practitioner. Drug modification may be required.		

Diuretics

Diuretics (general)	Aloe *Aloe vera*	Increased K^+ excretion	Oral use of aloe long-term may deplete potassium levels.[7] Monitor patient.
	Cascara *Cascara sagrada*	Increased K^+ excretion	Oral use of cascara long-term may deplete potassium levels.[7] Monitor patient.
	Dandelion (leaf) *Taraxacum officinale*	Additive effect	Due to its diuretic activity, dandelion leaf may theoretically increase diuresis.[1] Interaction is theoretical and of uncertain clinical significance.
	Guarana *Paullinia cupana*	Additive effect	Guarana may theoretically increase diuresis while also decreasing hypotensive activity.[1] Interaction is of uncertain clinical significance.
	Liquorice *Glycyrrhiza glabra*	Increased K^+ excretion	Long-term use of high dose liquorice can deplete potassium levels[1,7] Avoid doses > 100 mg glycyrrhizin/day for periods > 2 weeks.[1] Monitor patient.
	Senna *Cassia angustifolia*	Increased K^+ excretion	Oral use of senna long-term may deplete potassium levels.[7] Monitor patient.
	Stinging nettle (leaf) *Urtica dioica*	Additive drug effects	Due to its diuretic activity, nettle leaf may theoretically increase diuresis.[1] Interaction is theoretical and of uncertain clinical significance.
Summary	Caution should be used with the concurrent administration of any of the abovementioned herbs, especially with long-term use. May be necessary to place patients on a high potassium diet.[7]		

Dopaminergics

Levodopa	Kava kava *Piper methysticum*	Reduced drug effectiveness	Dopamine antagonistic effects have been reported.[1,53] Avoid concurrent use unless under medical supervision.
Summary	Due to the potential for dopamine antagonism, it is best to avoid using kava-based preparations. Use cautiously also in the elderly.[12]		

(Continued)

773

DRUG	HERB NAME	POTENTIAL ACTION	SUPPORTIVE EVIDENCE AND RECOMMENDATIONS
Drugs of dependence			
Methadone	Kava kava *Piper methysticum*	Additive effect	Based on the pharmacological activity of kava, concurrent use may theoretically increase sedation.[1] Interaction is theoretical and of uncertain clinical significance.
	St John's wort *Hypericum perforatum*	Reduced drug effectiveness	St John's wort may decrease serum levels of methadone.[1] Avoid concurrent use.
Summary	Administration of any abovementioned herb with a patient currently on methadone treatment requires medical supervision. Drug dosage modification may be required.		
Erectile dysfunction medication			
Sildenafil	Ginseng, Korean *Panax ginseng*	Additive effect	Korean ginseng has been shown to increase NO release from the corpus cavernosum.[7] Interaction is theoretical and of uncertain clinical significance.
Summary	Patient observation advised, especially if high doses of Korean ginseng are being used.		
Hormone-based medication			
Cortisol	See 'Corticosteroids'.		
Oestrogen	Hops *Humulus lupulus*	Additive effect	Based on the mild oestrogenic activity of hops, the potential to interact with preparations containing oestrogen exists.[1] Interaction is theoretical and of uncertain clinical significance.
	Red clover *Trifolium pratense*	Reduced drug effectiveness	Red clover contains phytoestrogens and if taken in large doses may compete with synthetic oestrogen for receptor binding.[1] Interaction is of uncertain clinical significance.
Oral contraceptives (OCP)	Chaste tree *Vitex agnus-castus*	Reduced herb effect	Speculation exists as to whether chaste tree is effective when OCPs are being taken. Clinical studies conducted in women taking OCPs have confirmed that chaste tree still reduces symptoms of PMS.[1]
	Liquorice *Glycyrrhiza glabra*	Increased side effects	OCPs may increase sensitivity to glycyrrhizin, increasing side effects such as hypertension, fluid retention and hypokalaemia.[17,54,55] Monitor patient and avoid doses > 100 mg glycyrrhizin/day for periods > 2 weeks.[1]

DRUG	HERB NAME	POTENTIAL ACTION	SUPPORTIVE EVIDENCE AND RECOMMENDATIONS
	St John's wort *Hypericum perforatum*	Reduced drug effectiveness	Breakthrough bleeding has been reported in 12 cases; this is suggestive of reduced drug effectiveness.[1,17] Reports from Britain and Sweden suggest unwanted pregnancies have occurred with concurrent use.[12] Avoid use with low-dose OCP (< 50 μg of oestrogen) if possible.[1,2]
Testosterone	Liquorice *Glycyrrhiza glabra*	Altered testosterone effect	Contradictory evidence suggests a possible effect on testosterone levels. Monitor testosterone levels.[1] Interaction is of uncertain clinical significance.
Thyroid hormones, e.g. levothyroxine	Bladderwrack *Fucus vesiculosis*	Additive effect	Based on the pharmacological activity of bladderwrack, the potential to interact with preparations containing thyroid hormones exists.[12]
	Bugleweed *Lycopus virginicus*	Reduced drug effectiveness	Based on the pharmacological activity of bugleweed, the potential to interact with preparations containing thyroid hormones exists.[12] Avoid concurrent use. Bugleweed may also interfere with thyroid diagnostic procedures that use radioactive isotopes.[12]
	Celery *Apium graveolens*	Reduced drug effectiveness	A case report suggested that celery extract may reduce drug effects.[1] Interaction is of uncertain clinical significance.
	Horseradish *Amoracia rusticana*	Increased drug requirement	Horseradish contains isothiocyanates, which may inhibit thyroxine formation and be goitrogenic.[1] Interaction is theoretical and of uncertain clinical significance.
	Motherwort *Leonurus cardiaca*	Reduced drug effectiveness	Based on the pharmacological activity of motherwort, the potential to interact with preparations containing thyroid hormones exists.[12] Avoid concurrent use.
	Withania *Withania somnifera*	Additive effect	In vivo tests suggested that daily administration of withania root extract enhanced serum T4 concentration.[1] Interaction is of uncertain clinical significance.
Summary	Administration of any abovementioned herb with a patient currently taking hormone-based medication requires prior consultation with the patient's medical practitioner. Drug dosage modification may be required.

(Continued)

DRUG	HERB NAME	POTENTIAL ACTION	SUPPORTIVE EVIDENCE AND RECOMMENDATIONS
Hypoglycaemics			
Hypoglycaemics (general)	Aloe *Aloe vera*	Additive effect	*Aloe vera* may have hypogly-caemic activity.[1] Interaction is theoretical and of uncertain clinical significance. Monitor patient's BSL.
	Andrographis *Andrographis paniculata*	Additive effect	Andrographis has shown hypo-glycaemic activity in vivo compa-rable to metformin.[1] Interaction is theoretical and of uncertain clinical significance. Monitor patient's BSL.
	Green tea *Camellia sinensis*	Additive effect	Oolong tea decreased concen-tration of plasma glucose and fructosamine in a clinical trial of patients with type II diabetes.[11] Monitor patient's BSL.
	Bilberry *Vaccinium myrtillus*	Additive effect	An in vivo animal study identi-fied the constituent myrtillin as exerting hypoglycaemic actions.[1] Interaction is theoretical and of uncertain clinical significance. Monitor patient's BSL.
	Damiana *Turnera diffusa*	Additive effect	Oral administration of damiana infusion resulted in hypoglycae-mic activity in an experimental model.[12] Interaction is theoreti-cal and of uncertain clinical sig-nificance. Monitor patient's BSL.
	Fenugreek *Trigonella foenum-graecum*	Additive effect	Fenugreek reduces BSL, but the exact mechanism of action is unclear.[11] Monitor patient's BSL. Drug dose modification may be required.
	Goats' rue *Galega officinalis*	Additive effect	Galegine, an alkaloid from goat's rue, has been shown to have hypoglycaemic proper-ties. Use cautiously and monitor patient's BSL regularly.[7] Drug dose modification may be required.
	Ginseng, Siberian *Eleutherococcus senticosus*	Additive effect	Siberian ginseng has shown hypoglycaemic activity in vitro. Interaction is theoretical and of uncertain clinical significance. Monitor patient's BSL.
	Gymnema *Gymnema sylvestre*	Additive effect	Gymnema has a well-documented hypoglycaemic activity causing the enhanced reduction of blood glucose. Use cautiously and monitor patient's BSL regularly.[7] Drug dose modification may be required.

DRUG	HERB NAME	POTENTIAL ACTION	SUPPORTIVE EVIDENCE AND RECOMMENDATIONS
	High-fibre herbs (Psyllium, linseed, etc.)	Reduced drug requirement	Clinical trials suggest that herbs such as psyllium may reduce the need for insulin, although the effect depends on the type of fibre ingested.[7] Monitor patient's BSL.
	Myrrh *Commiphora molmol*	Additive effect	Two furanosesquiterpenes isolated from myrrh exhibited hypoglycaemic activity in vivo in normal and diabetic models.[12] Interaction is theoretical and of uncertain clinical significance. Monitor patient's BSL.
Summary	If using herbal hypoglycaemics concurrently with hypoglycaemic medication, alert patients to the fact that they must check BSLs regularly and warn them of potential hypoglycaemia.[7] Contact patient's medical practitioner before administration as drug dosage modification may be required.		
Hypolipidaemics			
Hypolipidaemics (general)	Garlic *Allium sativum*	Additive effect	A meta-analysis of 13 clinical trials concluded that garlic can significantly reduce cholesterol levels.[1] ESCOP suggested garlic is useful for the prophylaxis of atherosclerosis and for treatment of elevated blood lipids non-responsive to dietary modifications.[2] Interaction may be beneficial. Drug dosage modification may be required.
	Globe artichoke *Cynara scolymus*	Additive effect	Based on the hypolipidaemic activity of globe artichoke, the potential to cause additive effects exists. Globe artichoke is used as an adjuvant to a low-fat diet in the treatment of mild to moderate hyperlipidaemia.[2] Interaction may be beneficial, but is of uncertain clinical significance. Drug dosage modification may be required.
	Guggul *Commiphora mukul*	Additive effect	Guggul prevented hypercholesterolaemia and atheroma in vivo. Clinical trials suggest that guggul can decrease total cholesterol, LDL cholesterol and triglycerides.[10] Interaction may be beneficial and require drug dosage modification. Uncertain clinical significance for myrrh.[1]
	Oats (as cereal) *Avena sativa*	Additive effect	Clinical trials suggest that oats-based cereals reduce total cholesterol levels.[1] Interaction may be beneficial and require drug dosage modification.

(Continued)

DRUG	HERB NAME	POTENTIAL ACTION	SUPPORTIVE EVIDENCE AND RECOMMENDATIONS
	Psyllium *Plantago ovata*	Additive effect	Psyllium is used as an adjuvant to a low-fat diet in the treatment of mild to moderate hypercholester-olaemia.[2] Due to its mucilaginous properties, doses of psyllium and pharmaceutical medications should be separated by at least 2 hours if possible. Psyllium may delay absorption. Interaction may be beneficial and require drug dosage modification.
HMG CoA-reductase inhibitors, e.g. simvastatin	Peppermint (oil) *Mentha piperita*	Additive effect	In vivo animal studies demon-strated that peppermint oil can increase the oral bioavailability of simvastatin.[1] Drug dosage modification may be required.
	St John's wort *Hypericum perforatum*	Reduced drug effectiveness	St John's wort increases the metabolism of simvastatin, and therefore drug dosage modifica-tion may be required.[1]
	St Mary's thistle *Silybum marianum*	Increased drug effect	St Mary's thistle may reduce simvastatin metabolism, result-ing in increased serum levels and associated adverse events.[1] Interaction is of uncertain clinical significance.
Summary	Administration of any abovementioned herb with a patient currently taking hypolipidaemic medication requires prior consultation with the patient's medi-cal practitioner as drug dosage modification may be required. Remember that mucilaginous herbs with hypolipidaemic activity should be separated from doses of other supplements or pharmaceutical prescription medications by a minimum of 2 hours.		
Immunosuppressants			
Immunosuppres-sants (general)	Andrographis *Andrographis paniculata*	Reduced drug effectiveness	Due to the known immunos-timulant activity of the herb, a potential for reduced drug effectiveness theoretically exists. Interaction is of uncertain clinical significance.
	Astragalus *Astragalus membranaceus*	Reduced drug effectiveness	Due to the known immuno-stimulant activity of the herb, a potential for reduced drug effectiveness theoretically exists. Interaction is of uncertain clinical significance.
	Cat's claw *Uncaria tomentosa*	Reduced drug effectiveness	Due to the known immuno-stimulant activity of the herb, a potential for reduced drug effec-tiveness theoretically exists. The manufacturers of products stan-dardised to pentacyclic oxindole alkaloids (POAs) warn against the use of cat's claw in patients receiving immunosuppressive medications.[7] Interaction is of uncertain clinical significance.

DRUG	HERB NAME	POTENTIAL ACTION	SUPPORTIVE EVIDENCE AND RECOMMENDATIONS
	Echinacea *Echinacea* spp.	Reduced drug effectiveness	Due to the known immuno-stimulant activity of the herb, a potential for reduced drug effectiveness theoretically exists.[7] Interaction is of uncertain clinical significance.
	Garlic *Allium sativum*	Reduced drug effectiveness	Due to the known immuno-stimulant activity of the herb,[1] a potential for reduced drug effectiveness theoretically exists. Interaction is of uncertain clinical significance.
	Ginseng, Korean *Panax ginseng*	Reduced drug effectiveness	Due to the known immuno-stimulant activity of the herb, a potential for reduced drug effectiveness theoretically exists. Interaction is of uncertain clinical significance.
	Ginseng, Siberian *Eleutherococcus senticosus*	Reduced drug effectiveness	Due to the known immuno-stimulant activity of the herb, a potential for reduced drug effectiveness theoretically exists. Interaction is of uncertain clinical significance.
	Pau d'arco *Tabebuia avellanedae*	Reduced drug effectiveness	Due to the known immuno-stimulant activity of the herb, a potential for reduced drug effectiveness theoretically exists. Interaction is of uncertain clinical significance.
	Pokeroot *Phytolacca decandra*	Reduced drug effectiveness	Due to the known immuno-stimulant activity of the herb, a potential for reduced drug effectiveness theoretically exists. Interaction is of uncertain clinical significance.
Cisplatin	St Mary's thistle *Silybum marianum*	Increased drug effects	Research suggests that St Mary's thistle and cisplatin may reduce toxicity effects.[1] Interaction may be beneficial, yet requires medical supervision.
Cyclosporine	Peppermint (oil) *Mentha piperita*	Additive effect	Peppermint oil has been shown in animal studies to increase the oral bioavailability of cyclosporine.[1] Interaction is of uncertain clinical significance.
	St John's wort *Hypericum perforatum*	Reduced drug effectiveness	St John's wort is known to induce the CYT P450 system and P-gp. Case reports suggest it may reduce drug effectiveness.[7,56–59] Avoid concurrent use.

(Continued)

DRUG	HERB NAME	POTENTIAL ACTION	SUPPORTIVE EVIDENCE AND RECOMMENDATIONS
	St Mary's thistle *Silybum marianum*	Reduced drug effectiveness and side effects	St Mary's thistle may decrease drug levels of cyclosporine; this is potentially dangerous for transplant recipients.[60] May also protect the pancreas from cyclosporine toxicity[61] and nephrotoxicity.[62] Use only under close medical supervision or avoid concurrent use.
Tacrolimus	St John's wort *Hypericum perforatum*	Reduced drug effectiveness	St John's wort is known to induce the CYT P450 system and P-gp. Herb decreases drug serum levels.[1] Avoid concurrent use
Summary	Due to the seriousness of the conditions being managed, specifically organ rejection, avoid concurrent use of any immunostimulant herbs or use only while patient is under close medical supervision and after previous consultation.		

Iron supplements

Iron supplements	Herbs high in tannins, polyphenolics or flavonoids	Decrease in Fe absorption	Clinical studies have shown the ability for tannins and other polyphenolics to reduce Iron absorption. Separate doses of iron by 2 hours. Caution in patients suffering from anaemia.
Summary	This physicochemical interaction applies to all dosage forms (infusions, decoctions, liquid extracts, etc.).		

Mood stabilisers

Lithium	Psyllium *Plantago ovata*	Reduced drug effectiveness	A case report suggested decreased lithium concentrations with concurrent administration of psyllium,[7,17,63] resulting in reduced drug effectiveness. Ensure dosage is separated by a minimum of 2 hours.
Summary	As with all demulcent/mucilage-containing herbs, separate dose of herb from any pharmaceutical medication by a minimum of 2 hours.		

Non-steroidal anti-inflammatory drugs (NSAIDs)

Aspirin Acetylsalicylic acid	Grape seed extract *Vitis vinifera*	Additive effect	May potentially enhance antiplatelet and anti-inflammatory effects of aspirin. May increase risk of bleeding.[1] Interaction may be beneficial, but is of uncertain clinical significance.
	Meadowsweet *Filipendula ulmaria*	Additive effect	May potentially enhance antiplatelet and anti-inflammatory effects of aspirin. May increase risk of bleeding.[1] Interaction may be beneficial, but is of uncertain clinical significance.

DRUG	HERB NAME	POTENTIAL ACTION	SUPPORTIVE EVIDENCE AND RECOMMENDATIONS
	Willow bark *Salix alba*	Additive effect	May potentially enhance anti-platelet and anti-inflammatory effects of aspirin. May increase risk of bleeding.[1] Interaction is of unknown clinical significance. Clinical study observed willow to have antiplatelet activity.[7] Higher doses than 240 mg of salicin per day may have a more significant effect.[1] Monitor patient closely in higher dosage. Interaction may be beneficial, but is of uncertain clinical significance.
Diclofenac sodium	Liquorice *Glycyrrhiza glabra*	Additive effect	The addition of glycyrrhizin enhanced the topical absorption of diclofenac sodium in vitro.[1] Interaction is of unknown clinical significance.
NSAIDs	Devil's claw *Harpagophytum procumbens*	Additive effect	A clinical study has reported anti-inflammatory activity.[1] In vitro studies suggested that devil's claw extract may inhibit the synthesis of prostaglandins by inhibiting cyclooxygenase 2 and inhibit release of TNF-α in human monocytes.[12] Drug dosage modification may be required. Interaction may be beneficial, but is of uncertain clinical significance.
	Ginger *Zingiber officinale*	Additive effect	In vitro and in vivo models have suggested that ginger exerts anti-inflammatory activity by inhibiting both cyclooxygenase and lipoxygenase pathways.[12] Ginger may enhance the anti-inflammatory activity effect of the drug, especially in high doses.[1] Drug dosage modification may be required. Interaction may be beneficial, but is of uncertain clinical significance.
	Nettle (leaf) *Urtica dioica*	Additive effect	In vitro tests suggested that nettle leaf and its constituents demonstrated anti-inflammatory activity by inhibiting cyclooxygenase and 5-lipoxygenase derived reactions.[12] Drug dosage modification may be required.[1] Interaction may be beneficial, but is of uncertain clinical significance.

(Continued)

DRUG	HERB NAME	POTENTIAL ACTION	SUPPORTIVE EVIDENCE AND RECOMMENDATIONS
	Turmeric *Curcuma longa*	Additive effect	Curcumin has been found to be a dual inhibitor of arachidonic acid metabolism, inhibiting both cyclo-oxygenase and 5-lipoxygenase enzymes.[12] Drug dosage modification may be required. Interaction may be beneficial, but is of uncertain clinical significance.
	Willow bark *Salix alba*	Additive effect	May potentially enhance anti-inflammatory effects.[12] Interaction may be beneficial, but is of uncertain clinical significance.
Summary	With concurrent administration with NSAIDs, drug dosage modification may be required. Caution is advised with high-dose preparations of herbs concurrently in patients using aspirin for anticoagulant effect. A further beneficial interaction may be observed with ginger and turmeric use, due to the gastroprotective qualities they exert; this is clinically relevant due to NSAID side effects.		
Pharmaceutical medications (all)			
Pharmaceuticals (all medications)	Herbs rich in mucilage	Reduced drug absorption	Mucilages may reduce the absorption of pharmaceutical medications. This is of particular importance in drugs that have a NTI. Separate doses by a minimum of 2 hours.
Summary	Avoid concurrent administration of herbs rich in mucilage and pharmaceutical medications where possible, especially NTI medications.		
Psoralen + UVA therapy			
Psoralen + UVA therapy	Celery *Apium graveolens*	Additive effect	Celery contains psoralens, but does not seem to be photosensitising even after large oral doses. May increase the risk of phototoxicity with concurrent PUVA therapy.[1] Interaction is of uncertain clinical significance.
	St John's wort *Hypericum perforatum*	Additive effect	Hypericin may increase sensitivity to UV radiation.[1] Use caution, especially in preparations containing high hypericin content. Interaction is of uncertain clinical significance.
Summary	Use caution in using the abovementioned herbs concurrently with patients receiving PUVA therapy.		
Vaccinations			
Vaccines Influenza virus vaccine	Ginseng, Siberian *Eleutherococcus senticosus*	Reduced drug side effects	Siberian ginseng may reduce the risk of postvaccine reactions. Interaction may be beneficial, but is of uncertain clinical significance.
Summary	Evidence is minimal to support the use of Siberian ginseng in reducing post-vaccine reactions. Observe patient.		

References

1. Braun L, Cohen M. Herbs and natural supplements: an evidence-based guide. Marrickville: Elsevier Australia, 2005.
2. ESCOP Monographs. 2nd edn Exeter: European Scientific Cooperative on Phytotherapy, 2003.
3. Wilt T, et al. *Pygeum africanum* for benign prostatic hyperplasia. Cochrane Database Syst Rev 2002;1:CD001044.
4. WHO monographs on selected medicinal plants Vol 2. Geneva: World Health Organization, 2003.
5. Lee F, et al. Effects of *Panax ginseng* on blood alcohol clearance in man. Clin Exp Pharmacol Physiol 1987;14:543–546.
6. Muriel P, et al. *Silymarin* protects against paracetamol-induced lipid peroxidation and liver damage. J Appl Toxicol 1992;12:439–442.
7. Mills S, Bone K. The essential guide to herbal safety. St Louis: Churchill Livingstone, 2005:684.
8. Siegers CP. Influence of dithiocarb, (+)-catechin and silybine on halothane hepatotoxicity in the hypoxic rat model. Acta Pharm Toxicol 1983;53:125–129.
9. Shanmuganayagam D, et al. Grape seed and grape skin extracts elicit a greater antiplatelet effect when used in combination than when used individually in dogs and humans. J Nutr 2002;132(12):3592–3598.
10. Bone K. Clinical applications of Ayurvedic and Chinese herbs: monographs for the Western herbal practitioner. Phytotherapy Professional Development. Warwick: Phytotherapy Press, 1996.
11. Gruenwald J, et al. Physicians desk reference for herbal medicines. 3rd edn. Montvale: Thomson PDR, 2004:988.
12. Bone K. A clinical guide to blending liquid herbs: herbal formulations for the individual patient. St Louis: Churchill Livingstone, 2003:531.
13. Chan K, et al. The effects of danshen (*Salvia miltiorrhiza*) on warfarin pharmacodynamics and pharmacokinetics of warfarin enatiomers in rats. J Pharm Pharmacol 1995;47:402–406.
14. Tam L, et al. Warfarin interactions with Chinese Traditional medicines: danshen and methyl salicylate medicated oil. Austr N Z J Med 1995;25:257.
15. Yu C, et al. Chinese Herbs and warfarin potentiation by danshen J Inter Med 1997;241:337–339.
16. Page R, Lawrence JD. Potentiation of warfarin by dong quai. Pharmacotherapy 1999;19:870–876.
17. Fugh-Berman A. Herb–drug interactions. Lancet 2000;355:134–137.
18. Rose K, et al. Spontaneous spinal epidural hematoma with associated platelet dysfunction from excessive garlic ingestion: a case report. Neurosurgery 1990;26(5):880–882.
19. German K, et al. Garlic and the risk of TRUP bleeding. Br J Urol 1995;76(4):518.
20. Burnham E. Garlic as a possible risk for postoperative bleeding. Plast Reconstr Surg 1995;95(1):213.
21. WHO monographs on selected medicinal plants Vol 1. Geneva: World Health Organization, 1999.
22. Valli G, Giardina E-G. Benefits, adverse effects and drug interactions of herbal therapies with cardiovascular effects. J Am Coll Cardiol 2002;39(7):1083–1095.
23. Lamant V, et al. Inhibition of the metabolism of platelet activating factor by three specific antagonists from *Ginkgo biloba*. Biochem Pharmacol 1987;36(27):49–52.
24. Rowin J, Lewis SL. Spontaneous bilateral subdural hematomas associated with chronic *Ginkgo biloba* ingestion. Neurology 1996;46:1775–1776.
25. Vale S. Subarachnoid haemorrhage associated with *Ginkgo biloba*. Lancet 1998;352:36.
26. Matthews M. Association of *Ginkgo biloba* with intracerebral hemorrhage. Neurology 1998;50:1933.
27. Coxeter PD, et al. Herb–drug interactions: an evidence based approach. Curr Med Chem 2004;11:1513–1525.
28. Yun-Choi, et al. Potential inhibitors of platelet aggregation from plant sources, III. J Nat Prod 1987;50(6):1059–1064.
29. Satyavati GV. Gum guggul (*Commiphora mukul*): the success story of an ancient insight leading to a modern discovery. Indian J Med Res 1988;87:327–335.
30. Blumenthal M, et al. The ABC clinical guide to herbs. 1st edn. Austin: American Botanical Council, 2003.
31. Mills S, Bone K. Principles and practice of phytotherapy. London: Churchill Livingstone, 2000:602.
32. Barbenel DM, et al. Mania in a patient receiving testosterone replacement postorchidectomy taking St John's wort and sertraline. J Psychopharmacol 2000;14(1):84–86.
33. Beckman SE, et al. Consumer use of St John's wort: a survey on effectiveness, safety, and tolerability. Pharmacotherapy 2000;20(5):568–574.
34. Dannawi M. Possible serotonin syndrome after combination of buspirone and St John's wort. J Psychopharmacol 2002;16(4):401.
35. Lantz MS. St John's wort and antidepressant drug interactions in the elderly. J Geriatr Psychiatry Neurol 1999;12(1):7–10.
36. Parker V, et al. Adverse reactions to St John's wort. Can J Psychiatry 2001;46(1):77–79.
37. De Smet P. Yohimbe alkaloids, in adverse effects of herbal drugs. In: De Smet PAGM. *Borago officinalis*. In De Smet PAGM, Keller K, Hansel R, Chandler RF, eds. Adverse effects of herbal drugs, vol II. Berlin: Springer-Verlag, 1997:181–206.
38. Lacombiez L, et al. Effect of yohimbine on blood pressure in patients with depression and orthostatic hypertension induced by clomipramine. Clin Pharmacol Ther 1989;45:241–251.
39. Piscitelli SC, et al. Effect of milk thistle on the pharmacokinetics of indinavir in healthy volunteers. Pharmacotherapy 2002;22(5):551–556.
40. Piscitelli SC, et al. The effect of garlic supplements on the pharmacokinetics of saquinavir. Clin Infect Dis 2002;34(2):234–238.
41. Anke J, Ramzan I. Pharmacokinetic and pharmacodynamic drug interactions with kava (*Piper methysticum* Forst.). J Ethnopharmacol 2004;93:153–160.
42. Taylor R, et al. Betel-nut chewing and asthma. Lancet 1992;339:1134–1136.
43. Bouraoui A, et al. Influence de l'alimentation épicée et piquante sur l'absorption de la théophylline. Therapie 1986;41:467–471.
44. Nebel A, et al. Potential metabolic interaction between St John's wort and theophylline. Ann Pharmacother 1999;33:502.
45. Sarkar MA, et al. Characterization of human liver cytochromes P-450 involved in theophylline metabolism. Drug Metab Dispos 1992;20(1):31–37.
46. De Smet P, D'Arcy PF. Drug interactions with herbal and other non-toxic remedies. Mechanism of drug interactions. Berlin: Springer-Verlag, 1996.
47. McRae S. Elevated serum digoxin levels in a patient taking digoxin and Siberian ginseng. CMAJ 1996;155:293–295.
48. Johne A, et al. Pharmacokinetic interaction of digoxin with an herbal extract from St John's wort *(Hypericum perforatum).* Clin Pharmacol Ther 1999;66:338–345.
49. Braun L, Cohen M. Herbs and natural supplements: an evidence-based guide. 2nd edn. Marrickville: Elsevier, 2007.
50. Gaedeke J, et al. Cisplatin nephrotoxicity and protection by silibinin. Nephrol Dial Transplant 1996;11(1):55–62.
51. Chen M-F, et al. Effect of oral administration of glycyrrhizin on the pharmacokinetics of prednisolone. Endocrinol Jpn 1991;38:167–175.
52. Chen M-F, et al. Effect of glycyrrhizin on the pharmacokinetics of prednisolone following low dosage of prednisolone hemisuccinate. Endocrinol Jpn 1990;37:331–341.

53. Schelosky L, et al. Kava and dopamine antagonism. J Neurol Neurosurg Psychiatry 1995;58:639–640.

54. Bernardi M, et al. Effects of prolonged graded doses of licorice by healthy volunteers. Life Sci 1994;55:864–872.

55. De Klerk G, et al. Hypokalaemia and hypertension associated with use of liqourice flavoured chewing gum. BMJ 1997;314:731–732.

56. Kronbach T, et al. Cyclosporine metabolism in human liver: identification of a cytochrome P-450III gene family as the major cyclosporine-metabolizing enzyme explains interactions of cyclosporine with other drugs. Clin Pharmacol Ther 1988;43(6):630–635.

57. Barone GW, et al. Herbal supplements: a potential for drug interactions in transplant recipients. Transplantation 2001;71:239–241.

58. Ruschitzka F, et al. Acute heart transplant rejection due to Saint John's wort. Lancet 2000;355(9203):548–549.

59. Bauer S, et al. Alterations in cyclosporin A pharmacokinetics and metabolism during treatment with St John's wort in renal transplant patients. Br J Clin Pharmacol 2003;55:203–211.

60. Pal D, Mitra AK. MDR-and CYP3A4-mediated drug-herbal interactions. Life Sci 2006;78:2131–2145.

61. von Schonfeld J, et al. Silibinin, a plant extract with antioxidant and membrane stabilizing properties, protects exocrine pancreas from cyclosporine A toxicity. Cell Mol Life Sci 1997;53:917–920.

62. Zima T, et al. The effect of silibinin on experimental cyclosporine nephrotoxicity. Ren Fail 1998;20(13):471–479.

63. Perlman B. Interaction between lithium salts and ipsaghula husk. Lancet 1990;335:416.

Appendix 2

Chemotherapy drugs and concurrent complementary therapy

Janet Schloss

ND, MNutrMed

CHEMOTHERAPY DRUG	PRIMARY INDICATIONS	SIDE EFFECTS AND MAJOR TOXICITIES	NUTRIENT/HERBS	ACTION INVOLVED
Alkalising agents—substitute alkyl chemical structure for a hydrogen atom in DNA resulting in cross-linking of each strand of DNA and preventing cell division				
Nitrogen mustards				
Chlorambucil (Leukeran)	Chronic lymphocytic leukaemia (CLL), Hodgkin's and non-Hodgkin's lymphomas	Bone-marrow suppression, toxicity to mucous membranes	Avoid glutathione during actual treatment, but have on non-chemo days.[1]	Increases cell resistance.[2]
			Immune herbs, e.g. Echinacea, Andrographis, Astragalus membranaceous	Reduces side effects, but could reduce drug effectiveness. Use with caution.[3]
Cyclophosphamide (Cytoxan)	Acute and chronic leukaemias, ovary and breast cancer, neuroblastomas, retinoblastomas, lymphomas, multiple myeloma, mycosis fungoides	Bone-marrow suppression, haemorrhagic cystitis, nausea, vomiting, anorexia, darkening of skin and nails, diarrhoea, facial flushing, headache, increased sweating, swollen lips, rash, hair loss, gonadal suppression, no menstruation, leukopenia, dizziness, weakness, hyperglycaemia, cardiotoxicity	Avoid glutathione during actual treatment, but have on non-chemo days.[1]	Increases cell resistance.[4]
			Vitamin C	Enhances effectiveness, reduces side effects.[5]
			Vitamin A	Improves effectiveness, reduces side effects.[6]
			Folic acid	Improves survival, improves efficacy.[7]
			Beta-carotene	Reduces toxicity, increases effectiveness.[8]
			Genistein	Aids killing tumour cells.[9,10]
			Withania somnifera	Reduces side effects, but may stimulate stem cell proliferation. Use with caution.[11]
Ifosfamide (Ifex)	Testicular tumours	Bone marrow suppression, nausea, vomiting, encephalopathy, mucous membrane toxicity	Avoid glutathione during actual treatment, but have on non-chemo days.[1]	Increases cell resistance.[4]
			Beta-carotene	Reduces toxicity, increases effectiveness[8]
			Taurine	Reduces renal toxicity[12]

(Continued)

CHEMOTHERAPY DRUG	PRIMARY INDICATIONS	SIDE EFFECTS AND MAJOR TOXICITIES	NUTRIENT/HERBS	ACTION INVOLVED
Mechlorethamine (Mustargen)	Lung cancers, Hodgkin's and non-Hodgkin's lymphomas, chronic leukaemia, malignant effusions, mycosis fungoides, polycythemia vera	Bone-marrow suppression, severe nausea and vomiting, diarrhoea, anorexia, metallic taste, neurotoxicity, weakness, hair loss, leukopenia, hyperuricaemia, gonadal suppression or missing menstrual period, peptic ulcers	Avoid glutathione during actual treatment, but have on non-chemo days.[13]	Increases cell resistance[4]
			Immune herbs, e.g. *Echinacea* spp., *Andrographis paniculata*, *Astragalus membranaceus*	Reduces side effects, but could reduce drug effectiveness. Use with caution.[3,13]
Melphalan (Alkeran)	Multiple myeloma, ovarian cancer	Bone marrow suppression, allergic reactions, mucous membrane toxicity	Avoid glutathione during actual treatment, but have on non-chemo days.[1]	Increases cell resistance.[4]
			Vitamin E	Enhances inhibition of oestrogen-dependent tumour growth.[14-16]
			Beta-carotene	Reduces toxicity, increases effectiveness.[8]
Uracil mustard (Uracil)	CLL, CML, non-Hodgkin's, mycosis fungoides	Leukopenia, thrombocytopenia, mucous membrane toxicity	Avoid glutathione during actual treatment, but have on non-chemo days.[1]	Increases cell resistance.[4]
Nitrosureas				
Carmustine (BiCNU)	Primary brain tumours, multiple myeloma	Bone marrow suppression, lung fibrosis, nephrotoxicity	Avoid glutathione during actual treatment, but have on non-chemo days.[1]	Increases cell resistance.[4]
			Vitamin C	Makes drug more effective through oxidative stress.[16,17]
			Maitake mushroom (beta-glucan)	Aids in inducing apoptosis making drug more effective.[18]
			Vitamin E	Aids in protecting non-cancer cells in low glutathione levels with vitamin C[17]

Drug	Used for	Side effects	Complementary therapy	Effects
Cisplatin (Platinol)	Bladder, ovarian and testicular carcinomas	Nephrotoxicity, severe nausea and vomiting, bone marrow suppression, neurotoxicity, blurred vision, dizziness, anorexia, depression, anaemia	Melatonin	Reverses adverse drug effects, esp. mylosuppression, cachexia and neurotoxicity.[34,35,47]
			Glutamine	Improves drug effectiveness, reduces mucosal injury in the gut and mouth 4 g/day.[48,49]
			Beta-carotene	Reduces toxicity, increases effectiveness[8,15]
			Magnesium	Reduces side effects of drug, and Mg deficiency associated with drug.[50,51]
			Potassium	Decreases deficiency associated with drug.[52,53]
			Green tea	Reduces drug resistance by inhibiting P-glycoprotein, improves drug effectiveness.[52]
			Carnitine	Reduces side effects, 4 g/day for 7 days reduced fatigue.[38]
			Selenium	Reduced side effects—nephrotoxicity, myeloid suppression and weight loss.[38]
			Calcium	Increases effectiveness and decreases gastrointestinal toxicity.[32]
			Vitamin D	Increases effectiveness and decreases gastrointestinal toxicity.[32]
			Silybum marianum	Increased drug effectiveness, reduced side effects.[53]
			Avoid Vitamin B6	Although it decreases neurotoxicity, it decreases duration effect of drug.[54]

CHEMOTHERAPY DRUG	PRIMARY INDICATIONS	SIDE EFFECTS AND MAJOR TOXICITIES	NUTRIENT/HERBS	ACTION INVOLVED
Lomustine (CeeNU)	Primary brain tumours and Hodgkin's lymphomas	Bone marrow suppression, anorexia, nausea, vomiting, neurotoxicity, nephrotoxicity, hepatotoxicity, fibrosis	Avoid glutathione during actual treatment, but have on non-chemo days[1]	Increases cell resistance[4]
			Vitamin C	Decreases side effects[19]
			Vitamin A	Decreases side effects[19]
			Vitamin E	Aids in protecting non-cancer cells in low glutathione levels with vitamin C.[17] Protects bacteria toxicity.[20]
Streptoztocin (Zanosar)	Pancreatic cancer	Nephrotoxicity, nausea, vomiting	Avoid glutathione during actual treatment, but have on non-chemo days.[1]	Increases cell resistance.[4]
			Vitamin C	Decreases excessive oxidation.[21]
			Vitamin E	Decreases excessive oxidation.[4]
			Quercetin	Decreases oxidative damage.[22]
			Lipoic acid	Increases reduced glutathione.[23]
			Fish oils HAD/EPA	Increases reduced glutathione.[23]
Pipobroman (Vercyte)	Chronic granulocytic leukaemia	Bone marrow suppression, nausea, vomiting, diarrhoea	Avoid glutathione during actual treatment, but have on non-chemo days[1]	Increases cell resistance.[4]

(Continued)

Drug	Cancer types	Side effects	Complementary therapy	Action
Thiotepa (Thioplex)	Breast, ovarian, bladder cancers, lymphomas, malignant effusions	Bone marrow suppression	Avoid glutathione during actual treatment, but have on non-chemo days[1]	Increases cell resistance.[4]
			Calcium	Improves efficacy of drug.[31]
			Vitamin D	Works synergistically with drug and improves efficacy.[27–30]
			Vitamin A	Increases efficacy of drug via DNA replication.[55]
			Vitamin E	Increases efficacy of drug via DNA replication, decreases side effects.[55]
			Vitamin C	Increases cytotoxicity of drug.[56]
Other				
Busulfan (Myleran)	CML	Bone marrow suppression, hyperpigmentation, gynaecomastia	Avoid glutathione during actual treatment, but have on non-chemo days.[1]	Increases cell resistance[4] Note: Cysteine levels were not depleted and aided glutathione levels after.[24]
			Quercetin	Aids antiproliferative action.[25]
			Vitamin E	Stops depletion and cell damage during bone transplantation.[24]
			Vitamin C	Stops depletion and cell damage during bone transplantation.[24]
			Zinc	Stops depletion and cell damage during bone transplantation.[24]
			Avoid iron	Overload levels can occur before and during bone transplantation.[26]

(Continued)

CHEMOTHERAPY DRUG	PRIMARY INDICATIONS	SIDE EFFECTS AND MAJOR TOXICITIES	NUTRIENT/HERBS	ACTION INVOLVED
Carboplatin (Paraplatin)	Ovarian carcinoma, prostate cancer, brain tumours, neuroblastomas	Bone marrow suppression, nausea, vomiting, neurotoxicity, neuropathies, ototoxicity	Avoid glutathione during actual treatment, but have on non-chemo days.[1]	Increases cell resistance.[4]
			Vitamin D	Works synergistically with drug and improves efficacy.[27-30]
			Calcium	Improves efficacy of drug,[31] decreases gastrointestinal toxicity.[32]
			Vitamin A	Decreases side effects[33]
			Melatonin	Reverses adverse drug effects, esp. myelosuppression, cachexia and neurotoxicity.[34-36]
Cisplatin (Platinol)	Bladder, ovarian and testicular carcinomas	Nephrotoxicity, severe nausea and vomiting, bone marrow suppression, neurotoxicity, blurred vision, dizziness, anorexia, depression, anaemia	Avoid glutathione during actual treatment, but have on non-chemo days[1]	Increases cell resistance.[4]
			Vitamin C	Enhances effectiveness, reduces side effects.[5,15,16,37]
			Vitamin E	Enhances drug, aids inhibition of oestrogen, 300 mg/day taken before treatment and continued for 3 months reduced the severity of neurotoxicity.[15,16,38,39]
			Vitamin A	Improves effectiveness, reduces side effects.[33,40,41]
			Lipoic acid	Inhibits NF-$\varkappa$B, reduces drug resistance and side effects,[2] aids in reducing peripheral neuropathy.[42]

			DHA/EPA	Reduces late radionecrosis, improves blood perfusion, increases cell-kill count[43]
			Quercetin	Potentiates drug activity, inhibits P-glycoprotein, reduces drug resistance.[44, 45]
			Zinc	Chemopotentiating agent as it aids in DNA repair.[46]
Antimetabolites—interfere with the synthesis of DNA and RNA, specifically S phase				
Cytarabine (Cytosar-U)	AML, ALL	Bone-marrow suppression, anorexia, oral and GI ulceration, mucositis, conjunctivitis	Calcium	Improves efficacy of drug.[57]
			Vitamin D	Improves drug efficacy.[57–59]
			Vitamin A	Improves drug efficacy.[58]
			Quercetin	Potentiates drug activity, inhibits P-glycoprotein, reduces drug resistance.[45]
			Glutamine	Improves drug effectiveness, reduces mucosal injury in the gut and mouth 4 g/day.[48,49]

CHEMOTHERAPY DRUG	PRIMARY INDICATIONS	SIDE EFFECTS AND MAJOR TOXICITIES	NUTRIENT/HERBS	ACTION INVOLVED
5-Fluorouracil (Adrucil, 5-FU)	Colon, rectum, breast, stomach and pancreatic cancers, head and neck cancers, ovarian	Diarrhoea, stomatitis, bone marrow suppression, oesoph-agopharyngitis, leukopenia, thrombocytopenia, GI ulceration, dermatitis, anorexia, alopecia, weakness, dry skin, diarrhoea, phlebitis, mucositis	Vitamin C	Enhances effectiveness, reduces side effects.[9]
			Vitamin E	Enhances drug.[16]
			Vitamin B6	Reduces pain in palms and feet,[60,61] may ↓ toxic side effect of palmar plantar erythro-dysesthesia (PPE).[62]
			Vitamin A	Reduces dose, improves anti-tumour effect,[63] reduces side effects.[16]
			Bromelain	Can reduce dose of drug to result in cancer regression.[64]
			Glutamine	Improves drug effectiveness, reduces mucosal injury in the gut and mouth 4 g/day.[48,49]
			Folic acid—use with caution. Do not use during days of chemotherapy.	Improves survival, improves efficacy.[4] Drug can deplete folate levels and certain polymorphisms may affect treatment. Only to be used in non-chemo weeks.[65,66]
			Quercetin	Aids apoptosis.[67,68]
Floxuridine (FUDR)	GI adenocarcinoma with liver metastasis	Bone-marrow suppression, stomatitis, anaphylaxis	Vitamin C	Aids drug efficacy.[69]
Fludarabine (Fludara)	CLL	Bone-marrow suppression, fever, chills, nausea, vomiting, infection	Similar to 5-FU	No studies located.

(Continued)

Drug	Cancer types	Side effects	Complementary therapy	Effect
Mercaptopurine (Purinethol)	ALL, AML	Bone-marrow suppression, anorexia, cholestasis	Similar to 5-FU	No studies located.
Methotrexate (Folex)	Breast, head and neck, lung, trophoblastic, renal, ovarian, bladder and testicular cancers, ALL, non-Hodgkin's lymphomas, meningeal leukaemia, mycosis fungoides, osteosarcoma	Bone-marrow suppression, diarrhoea, stomatitis, nausea, vomiting, anorexia, acne, boils, skin rash or itching, loss of hair, GI ulcers and bleeding, leukopenia, infections, thrombocytopenia, pharyngitis, liver toxicity, pneumonitis, pulmonary fibrosis, renal failure, hyperuricaemia, cutaneous vasculitis	Folic acid—use with extreme caution or avoid	Drug binds with dihydrofolate reductase to inhibit DNA and RNA synthesis.[4]
			Vitamin A	Improves effectiveness, reduces side effects.[16,70,71]
			Glutamine	Improves WBC count, improves drug effectiveness, reduces mucosal injury in the gut and mouth 4 g/day.[48,49]
			Adenosine	Chemoprotective action, improves WBC recovery. Can be taken with chemotherapy[72,73]
			Green tea (EGCG and ECG)	Inhibits DHFR, therefore increases efficacy of drug.[74]
			Enterococcus faecium (probiotic bacteria)	Improves anti-inflammatory effects of drug.[75]
			N-acetyl cysteine	Decreases gastrotoxicity.[75]
			Vitamin E	Decreases side effects.[70,76]
Thioguanine	Acute nonlymphocytic leukaemia (ANLL)	Bone-marrow suppression		

Antibiotics—interfere with DNA functioning by blocking the transcription of new DNA or RNA. They delay or inhibit mitosis.

Drug	Cancer types	Side effects	Complementary therapy	Effect
Bleomycin (Blenoxane)	Squamous cell carcinoma, lymphomas, testicular cancer	Chills, fever, pneumonitis, mucositis, lung fibrosis, hyperpigmentation, pulmonary toxicity, hypersensitivity reactions	Vitamin C	Enhances effectiveness, reduces side effects.[16]
			Vitamin E	Enhances drug.[16]
			Beta-carotene	Reduces toxicity, aids effectiveness.[8]

(Continued)

CHEMOTHERAPY DRUG	PRIMARY INDICATIONS	SIDE EFFECTS AND MAJOR TOXICITIES	NUTRIENT/HERBS	ACTION INVOLVED
Dactinomycin (Cosmegen)	Wilm's tumour, Ewing's sarcoma, choriocarcinoma, rhabdomyosarcoma	Bone-marrow suppression	Similar to doxorubicin	No studies located.
(DaunoXome)	HIV, Kaposi's sarcoma	Bone-marrow suppression, cardiomyopathy, severe mucositis	Vitamin D	Improved drug efficacy.[59]
Doxorubicin (Adriamycin)	Acute leukaemia, Wilm's tumour, soft tissue and bone sarcomas, Hodgkin's disease, lymphomas, breast and various other carcinomas	Bone-marrow suppression, cardiomyopathy, severe mucositis, darkening of soles, palms anc nails, diarrhoea, red urine, loss of hair (alopecia), leukopenia, thrombocytopenia, stomatitis, oesophagitis, cellulitis, nephropathy, hyperuricaemia	Vitamin C	Enhances effectiveness, reduces side effects.[16]
			Vitamin E	Enhances drug, decreases side effects, esp. alopecia.[77–80]
			Vitamin A	Improves effectiveness, reduces side effects.[16,80]
			Selenium	Reduces lipid peroxide induced cardiotoxicity.[80]
			Genistein	Aids killing tumour cells.[9,81,82]
			Coenzyme Q10	Maintains cellular energetics,[9] decreases cardiotoxic side effects.[83]
			Lipoic acid	Reduces side effects.[84]
			DHA/EPA	Reduces late radionecrosis, improves blood perfusion, increases cell-kill count.[42]
			Melatonin	Reverses adverse drug effects, esp. mylosuppression, cachexia and neurotoxicity.[34,35]

Drug	Use	Toxicity	Complementary agent	Interaction
			Quercetin	Potentiates drug activity, inhibits P-glycoprotein, reduces drug resistance.[45]
			Beta-carotene	Reduces toxicity, aids effectiveness.[8]
			Carnitine	Reduced side effects, esp. those cardiotoxic.[85,86]
			Ginkgo biloba	Prevents cardiotoxicity (only animal studies).[87]
			Vitamin B6	May ↓ toxic side effect of palmar plantar erythrodysesthesia (PPE).[62]
Idarubicin (Idamycin)	AML	Severe bone-marrow, suppression, infection, alopecia, nausea, vomiting, haemorrhage	No studies located.	
Mitomycin (Mutamycin)	Disseminated adenocarcinomas of pancreas or stomach	Bone-marrow suppression	Selenium	Decreased chromosomal mutations from chemotherapy.[88]
			Vitamin B2	Aids drug under radiation, having a radio-protective effect.[89]
			Vitamin C	Aids drug under radiation having a radio-protective effect.[89-91]
			Vitamin E	Potentiates drug under radiation.[90]
			Beta carotene	Potentiates drug under radiation.[90]
			Quercetin	Protects non-cancer cells DNA from damage.[92]
			Rutin	Protects non-cancer cells DNA from damage.[92]
			Green tea	Increases efficacy of drug.[93]

(Continued)

CHEMOTHERAPY DRUG	PRIMARY INDICATIONS	SIDE EFFECTS AND MAJOR TOXICITIES	NUTRIENT/HERBS	ACTION INVOLVED
Mitoxantrone (Novantrone)	Acute nonlymphocytic leukaemia (ANLL)	Cardiotoxicity, severe myelosuppression	Melatonin	Decreases side effects and immunosuppression.[34]
			Similar to doxorubicin	
Pentostatin (Nipent)	Hairy cell leukaemia	Bone-marrow suppression, renal toxicity, rash	Adenosine	Aids efficacy of the drug.[94]
Plicamycin (Mithracin)	Testicular tumours, hypercalcaemia	Epistaxis, haemorrhage, nausea, bone-marrow suppression, stomatitis, vomiting, diarrhoea	No studies located.	
Mitotic inhibitors—plant alkaloids that block cell division in metaphase				
Etoposide (VePesid)	Refractory testicular tumours, small cell lung cancer	Bone-marrow suppression, alopecia, hypotension with rapid infusion	Genistein	Aids killing, reduces multi-drug resistance.[8,81]
			Beta-carotene	Reduces toxicity, aids effectiveness.[8]
			Melatonin	Reverses adverse drug effects esp. mylosuppression, cachexia and neurotoxicity.[34,35]
			Vitamin A	Improves effectiveness, reduces side effects.[16,33]
			Vitamin D	Improved drug efficacy.[59]
Teniposide (Vumon)	ALL	Bone-marrow suppression, mucositis, alopecia		
Vinblastine (Velban)	Breast and testicular cancer, Hodgkin's and non-Hodgkin's lymphomas, Kaposi's sarcoma, mycosis fungoides	Leukopenia, alopecia, muscle pain, hyperuricaemia, neurotoxicity, nausea, vomiting, hair loss, cellulitis, stomatitis, rectal bleeding, haemorrhagic colitis	Vitamin C	Enhances effectiveness, reduces side effects.[16]
			Quercetin	Potentiates drug activity, inhibits P-glycoprotein, reduces drug resistance.[45]
			Glycyrrhiza glabra	Additive effects.[95]

Drug	Cancers	Side effects	Complementary agent	Effect
Vincristine (Oncovin)	ALL, rhabdomyosarcoma, neuroblastoma, Wilm's tumour and various other carcinomas	Mild to severe paresthesias, jaw pain, ataxia, muscle wasting, constipation, anorexia, nausea, vomiting, autonomic toxicity, neurotoxicity, painful urination, bed wetting, constipation, orthostatic hypotension, lack of sweating	Vitamin E	Enhances drug.[16]
			Vitamin A	Improves effectiveness, reduces side effects.[16]
			Lipoic acid	Inhibits NF-KB, reduces drug resistance and side effects.[2,96]
			DHA/EPA	Reduces dose, reduces late radionecrosis, improves blood perfusion, increases cell-kill count.[42]
			Bromelain	Can reduce dose of drug to result in cancer regression.[64]
			Glutamine	Improves drug effectiveness, reduces mucosal injury in the gut and mouth 4 g/day.[48,49]
Vinorelbine (Navelbine)	Non-small cell lung cancer	Bone-marrow suppression, nausea, vomiting, asthenia	Resveratrol	Increases apoptosis and cell necrosis, decreases dose of drug.[97]
			Propolis	Increases apoptosis and cell necrosis, decreases dose of drug.[97]
			GLA	Increases chemosensitivity.[98]

(Continued)

CHEMOTHERAPY DRUG	PRIMARY INDICATIONS	SIDE EFFECTS AND MAJOR TOXICITIES	NUTRIENT/HERBS	ACTION INVOLVED
Miscellaneous antineoplastic agents				
Hormones—used in neoplasms sensitive to hormonal growth controls in the body. Apparently they interfere with the growth-stimulating receptors on target tissues.				
Corticosteriods, e.g. prednisone, dexamethasone	Lymphocytic leukaemias and lymphomas—both Hodgkin's and non-Hodgkin's, breast and brain cancer. Also used in conjunction with radiotherapy to decrease oedema	Nausea, vomiting, anorexia, diarrhoea, gastric irritation, headaches, vertigo, insomnia, restlessness, ↑sweating, ↑bruising, purpura	Vitamin D	Works synergistically with drug and improves efficacy,[30] aids calcium absorption.[100]
			Calcium	Minimises bone demineralisation from the drug,[100] reduces side effects.[3]
			Vitamin C	Enhances drug efficacy and decreases dose of drug.[99] Increases wound healing.[99]
			Vitamin E	Enhances drug efficacy and decreases dose of drug.[99]
			Selenium	Enhances drug efficacy and decreases dose of drug.[99]
			Fibre (FOS)	Enhances drug efficacy and decreases dose of drug.[99]
			Fish oils (DHA/EPA)	Enhances drug efficacy and decreases dose of drug.[99]
			Chromium	Reduced side effects,[3] drug linked with increased urinary loss.[101]
			Glycyrrhyza glabra	Potentiates drug effects.[3]

Anti-androgens

Drug	Cancer	Side effects	Complementary therapy	Effect
Bicalutamide (Casodex)—inhibits androgens from receptors binding to target tissues	Prostate cancer	Hot flushes, pruritis, breast tenderness, gynaecomastica, hepatic disturbances, depression, alopecia, ↓ libido, haematuria	Vitamin E	Aids drug efficacy.[102]
			Zinc	May assist anti-androgen affect.[103]
			Arginine	Aids presentation of cells for drug action,[104] aids androgen-receptor inhibition.[105]
			Serine	Aids presentation of cells for drug action.[104]
			Lysine	Aids presentation of cells for drug action.[104]
			B12, B6, folate, SAMe or methionine	Aids in methylation of amino acids to assist drug's action.[104]
Flutamide (Eulexin)—orally, inhibits the uptake or binding of androgens to target tissues	Ovarian cancer, testicular steroidogenesis, prostate cancer	Diarrhoea, impotency, hepatotoxicity, anorexia, insomnia, leukopenia, anaemia, thrombocytopenia, macrocytic anaemia, oedema, photosensitivity	I3C-indole-3-carbonol	Potent chemotherapy agent that controls growth of prostate cell growth.[106]
			Vitamin E	Decreases toxic effects of PCBs on prostate cells, thus aiding drug's effect.[107]
			Vitamin C	Depleted by drug.[108]
			Vitamin D	Decreases bone demineralisation.[109]
			Calcium	Decreases bone demineralisation.[109]
Nilutamide (Nilandron)—blocks testosterone effects on androgen receptors	Metastatic prostatic cancer	Nausea, alcohol intolerance, dark/light adaptation problems, dizziness, impotence, ↓ libido, hot flushes, body hair loss, sweating, ↑ transaminases	L-cysteine (or glutathione)	Decreases toxicity of drug.[110]
			Vitamin E	Aids in glutathione levels and decreasing toxicity of drug.[110]
			Vitamin B3	No research but traditionally used to help with alcohol detoxification.[3]

(Continued)

CHEMOTHERAPY DRUG	PRIMARY INDICATIONS	SIDE EFFECTS AND MAJOR TOXICITIES	NUTRIENT/HERBS	ACTION INVOLVED
Goserelin (Zoladex)—inhibitor of pituitary gonadotropins	Prostate carcinoma	Hot flushes, sexual dysfunction, decreased erections, fertility impairment, impotence, sweating, blood pressure changes, oedema, breast pain, temporary bone pain, ↓ BMD, nausea	Vitamin E	May be low in prostate cancer patients, may aid drug efficacy.[111]
			Vitamin D	Decreases bone demineralisation.[109,112,113]
			Calcium	Decreases bone demineralisation.[109,112,113]
Oestrogens, e.g. diethylstilbestrol (DES), polyestradiol, ethinyl estradiol, estramustine	Androgen sensitive prostatic cancer, advanced breast cancer in post-menopausal women	Inducing thrombosis	Quercetin	Reduces DNA damage.[114,115]
			Resveratrol	Acts as an agonist for the drugs, acts on NF-KB.[116–118]
			Melatonin	Anti-proliferative affect.[119]
Anti-oestrogens				
Tamoxifen—synthetic anti-oestrogen that binds to receptors	Breast cancer	Nausea, vomiting, headaches, hot flushes, weight gain, impotency, endometrial cancer, thromboembolism, ocular toxicity, hepatotoxic	Avoid genistein	Interacts with drug's action.[4,120–123]
			Avoid red clover	Interacts with drug's action.[125]
			Diadazen	Aids drug in decreasing carcinogenesis.[124]
			Vitamin C (also works with other antioxidants)[15]	Enhances effectiveness, reduces side effects.[16]
			Melatonin	Reverses adverse drug effects, esp. cachexia and neurotoxicity.[34,35]
			Resveratrol	Anti-inflammatory aids drug effectiveness.[122,126]

Drug	Cancer type	Side effects	Complementary therapy	Action
			Quercetin	Anti-inflammatory effect aids drug effectiveness,[122,126] potentiates drug by anti cell proliferation and prevention of angiogenesis.[127]
			Green tea	Aids in cancer prevention, aids apoptosis.[128-130]
			Coenzyme Q10	Increases antioxidant activity, decreases carcinogenesis.[131,132]
			Niacin (B3)	Increases antioxidant activity.[132]
			Riboflavin (B2)	Increases antioxidant activity.[132]
			Folate, vitamin B12, methionine	Methylation helps to decrease homocysteine levels linked with ↑ CVD.[133, 134]
			Cimicifuga racemosa	May work synergistically to have a cytotoxic affect against cancerous cell growth.[135]
Raloxifene (Evista)	Breast cancer	Hot flushes, leg cramps, thromboembolism, headaches, nausea, diarrhoea, oedema, arthralgia, sinus, rhinitis, weight gain	Genistein	Decreases bone demineralisation.[136, 137]
			Vitamin D	Decreases bone demineralisation.[138]
			Calcium	Decreases bone demineralisation.[138]
			Resveratrol	Decreases vaginal stratification, preserves neuronal function while on drug.[139,140]
			Quercetin	Aids in inhibition of aromatase.[142]
			Folate, vitamin B12, methionine	Methylation helps to decrease homocysteine levels linked with ↑ CVD.[133, 134]

(Continued)

CHEMOTHERAPY DRUG	PRIMARY INDICATIONS	SIDE EFFECTS AND MAJOR TOXICITIES	NUTRIENT/HERBS	ACTION INVOLVED
Toremifene (Fareston)—similar to tamoxifen	Metastatic breast cancer in postmenopausal women	Hypocholesterolaemic, thromboembolism (possible), hypercalcaemia, hot flushes, sweating, dizziness, GI upset, leucorrhoea, vaginal bleeding, oedema, pain, endometrial hypotrophy	Same as tamoxifen	
Anastrozole (Arimidex)—inhibits steroid aromatase, reducing oestrone synthesis in the adrenal glands	Palliative therapy of advanced breast cancer in post menopausal women	Hot flushes, vaginal dryness, bleeding, hair thinning, joint pain, stiffness, back and breast pain, peripheral oedema, cough, pharyngitis, asthenia, somnolence, insomnia, headache, rash, GI upset, ↑ cholesterol, weight gain, depression	Calcium	Increases bone mineral density.[142]
			Vitamin D	Increases bone mineral density.[142]
Testolactone (Teslac)—aromatase inhibitor	Premenopausal women with non-terminated or terminated ovarian function	Hot flushes, decreased bone mineral density	Relatively new drug; no studies of interactions with vitamins or herbs have been conducted as of yet.	
Progestins, e.g. Medroxyprogesterone (Depo-Provera) and megestrol (Megace)	Advanced endometrial cancer, advanced carcinoma of the breast, advanced renal carcinoma	Menstrual irregularities, ↓ BMD, anaphylaxis, thromboembolism, ocular effects, adrenal disturbances, abscesses, urticaria, pruritus, rash, acne, hirsutism, alopecia, sweating, nausea, breast tenderness, cervical changes, weight gain, abdominal pain	Calcium	Decreases risk of oesteoporosis.[143]
			Vitamin D	Decreases risk of oesteoporosis.[144]
			Genistein—avoid high doses	High doses may have detrimental affects in stimulating tumour growth.[145]
			Vitamin E	Protective effect against endometrial cell wall damage.[146]
			Vitamin B12	Drug reduces levels so corrects deficiency.[147]
			Vitamin A	Protective effect.[148]

Other agents

Drug	Use	Side effects	Complementary therapy	Comments
Altretamine (Hexalen)	Palliative treatment of persistent or recurrent ovarian cancer	Nausea, vomiting, neurotoxicity, myelosuppression, CNS changes—ataxia, dizziness, mood alterations	Avoid vitamin B6	Although decreases neurotoxicity, it decreases duration effect of drug.[54]
			Zinc	Drug depletes zinc stores, so aids mineral deficiency.[54]
Topotecan (Hycamtin)—topoisomerase inhibitor	Multiple myeloma, relapsed or refractory metastatic carcinoma of the ovary after failure of other therapies	Neutropenia, leukopenia, thrombocytopenia, anaemia, headache, diarrhoea, stomach pain, nausea, vomiting, alopecia, tiredness, dyspnoea, neuromuscular pain	Quercetin	Sensitiser to chemo drug, aids effect.[149]

VEGF inhibitor (vascular endothelial growth factor—anti-angiogenesis)—interferes with the growth of cancer by blocking the formation and growth of new blood vessels in the tumour.

Drug	Use	Side effects	Complementary therapy
Avastin (Bevacizumab) – recombinant humanised monoclonal IgG₁ antibody	Colon, rectum, lung or breast cancer	Reaction to injection, bleeding, GIT perforations, haemorrhage, hypertension, fistula formation, proteinuria, epistaxis, headache, rhinitis, taste alteration, dry skin, rectal haemorrhage, lacrimation disorder, exfoliative dermatitis	No studies located.
Erbitux (Cetuximab)—recombinant humanised monoclonal IgG₁ antibody	Colon and rectum cancer, sometimes head and neck cancers	Reaction to injection, acne like skin rash, severe skin rash, slow heart rate, weak pulse, fainting, slow breathing, chest pain, heavy feeling, fever, chills, flu symptoms, easy bruising, bleeding, hot dry skin, white patches or sores in mouth, headaches, dryness	No studies located.

(Continued)

CHEMOTHERAPY DRUG	PRIMARY INDICATIONS	SIDE EFFECTS AND MAJOR TOXICITIES	NUTRIENT/HERBS	ACTION INVOLVED
Miscellaneous agents				
Asparaginase (Elspar, Kidrolase)—reduces asparagines to aspartic acid	ALL	Hyperammonaemia, headaches, anorexia, nausea, vomiting, abdominal cramps, decreases blood clotting factors, allergic reactions, liver toxicity, pancreatitis and anaphylaxis	Glutamine—use with caution	Deamination of glutamine assists drug's action.[150,151]
Caelyx (contains doxorubicin)	Ovarian cancer, Kaposi's sarcoma	See doxorubicin	See doxorubicin.	
Cladribine (Leustatin)	Hairy cell leukaemia	Severe anaemia, infection, skin rash, bleeding or bruising, anorexia, headache, nausea, vomiting, fatigue	Glucosamine hydrochloride	Increases B cell apoptosis.[152]
Dacarbazine (DTIC-Dome)	Malignant melanoma, Hodgkin's disease	Flu-like syndrome, anorexia, nausea, vomiting, diarrhoea, cardiotoxicity, alopecia	Green tea	Inhibits melanoma growth and metatasis.[153]
			Vitamin C	Aids growth inhibitory effect.[15]
			Vitamin E	Aids growth inhibitory effect in combination with other antioxidants.[15]
			Beta-carotene	Aids growth inhibitory effect in combination with other antioxidants.[15]
			Vitamin A	Aids growth inhibitory effect in combination with other antioxidants.[15]
			Quercetin—avoid	Inhibits liver enzyme P450 (CYP1A2), which helps make the drug active.[154]

Drug	Cancer type	Side effects	Complementary therapy	Effect
Docetaxel (Taxotere)	Advanced breast cancer	Bone-marrow suppression, nausea, diarrhoea, stomatitis, fever, skin reactions, myalgia, fluid retention neurotoxicity, alopecia	GLA	If given together for 24–48 hours before and during drug treatment, it works in synergy with drug.[155]
			Vitamin E	Prevents oxidisation of GLA to assist synergy with drug.[155]
			Vitamin B6	May ↓ toxic side effect of palmar plantar erythrodysesthesia (PPE).[62]
			Vitamin D	Aids anti-neoplastic effect.[156–158]
Gemcitabine (Gemzar)—pyrimidine nucleoside antimetabolite	Adenocarcinoma of the pancreas, kidney and bladder cancers, non-small cell lung cancer	Dyspnoea, peripheral oedema, a flu-like syndrome, nausea, vomiting, diarrhoea, rash, paresthesia, stomatitis, myelosuppression	DHA/EPA	Doesn't interfere and may potentiate drug.[159]
			Quercetin	Sensitiser for chemo drug.[149]
Hydroxyurea (Hydrea)	Head, neck, ovarian carcinoma, chronic myelocytic leukaemia, malignant melanoma	Bone-marrow suppression, diarrhoea, anorexia, nausea, vomiting, drowsiness	Vitamin D	Improved drug efficacy.[59]
			Calcium	Improves efficacy of drug.[57]
			Vitamin E	Aids in increasing low vitamin E levels in CML patients after treatment,[160] decreases toxicity damage.[161]
			Vitamin C	Decreases toxic side effects with vitamin E.[162]
			Zinc	Enhances drug's effect.[163,164]
			Quercetin	Aids drug in DNA synthesis inhibition.[165]
Irinotecan (Camptosar)—topoisomerase I inhibitor	Metastatic colorectal cancer, rectal cancer	Severe diarrhoea, myelosuppression, nausea, vomiting	Zinc	Chemopotentiating agent as it aids in DNA repair.[46,166]
			Selenium	Decreases side effects and toxicity.[167,168]
			Quercetin	Aids action of drug.[169]
			Glutamine	Decreases diarrhoea side effect.[48]

(Continued)

CHEMOTHERAPY DRUG	PRIMARY INDICATIONS	SIDE EFFECTS AND MAJOR TOXICITIES	NUTRIENT/HERBS	ACTION INVOLVED
Levamisole (Ergamisol)—anthelmintic	Colorectal cancer	Bone-marrow suppression, nausea, diarrhoea, metallic taste, arthralgia, flu-like syndrome	Selenium—11.3 mg	Prevents weight loss and increased glutathione levels.[170]
			Cobalt—7.2 mg	Prevents weight loss.[170]
Mitotane (Lysodren)	Inoperable adrenal cortex cancer	Adrenal gland insufficiency, dark skin, diarrhoea, anorexia, depression, nausea, vomiting, weakness, drowsiness, light headedness	No studies located.	
Paclitaxel (Taxol)	Metastatic ovarian cancer, metastatic breast cancer	Severe allergic reactions, bone-marrow suppression, peripheral neuropathy, muscle pain, alopecia, gastric distress	Vitamin C	Enhances effectiveness, reduces side effects.[16,171]
			Glycyrrhiza glabra	Potentiates the effects of paclitaxel.[95]
			Vitamin D	Works synergistically with drug and improves efficacy.[30,32]
			Calcium	Increases effectiveness and decreases gastrointestinal toxicity.[32]
			Glutamine	Decreases side effects.[48,49]
			Vitamin E	Enhances drug absorption and utilisation, decreases neurotoxicity.[171-174]
			Beta-carotene	Decreases side effects.[8,171]
			Quercetin	Aids drug absorption and plasma concentrations.[175]
			Andrographis paniculata, Astragalus membranaceus, Scutellaria baicalensis, Allium spp., Panax ginseng, Eleutherococcus senticosus, Echinacea spp.	Reduces side effects (use with caution).[3,176]
			Lipoic acid	Aids in reducing peripheral neuropathy.[42]

Drug	Indication	Side effects	Complementary therapy	Notes
Aldesleukin (Proleukin)	Renal cell carcinoma	Oedema, anaemia, thrombocytopenia, hypotension	No studies located.	
Epirubicin (Ellence)	Metastatic breast cancer, mesothelioma	Cardiotoxicity, dehydration, alopecia, transient ECG changes, nausea, vomiting, diarrhoea, mucositis, myelosuppression, mild anaemia	Melatonin	Decreases toxicity and increases efficacy of drug.[34,35,177]
			Avoid glutathione	Increases drug resistance.[178,179]
			Coenzyme Q10	Protective effect against cadiotoxicity.[180,181]
G-CSF (Neupogen)	Used to decrease the potential for infection in people receiving myelosuppressive agents	Nausea, vomiting, hair loss, diarrhoea, fevers, mucositis, anorexia, fatigue, bone pain	Vitamin C	Works in synergy to increase vitamin C uptake.[182,183]
			Vitamin A	Works in synergy with drug.[184,185]
			Vitamin E	Works with drug and vitamin A to normalise neutrophils, improve platelets and RBC.[186,187]
Granulocyte-macrophage colony-stimulating factor (pro-inflammatory cytokine)	Acute lymphoblastic anaemia, Hodgkin's disease, non-Hodgkin's lymphoma	Redness/pain at the site of injection, fever, rapid or irregular heartbeat, sores on skin, wheezing, chest pain	Vitamin C	Decreases ROS produced from the drug.[188,189]
			Vitamin A	Inhibited the differentiation and maturation of cord blood dendritic cells in bone marrow.[190,191]
			Adenosine	Increases GM-CSF in bone marrow[192]

(Continued)

CHEMOTHERAPY DRUG	PRIMARY INDICATIONS	SIDE EFFECTS AND MAJOR TOXICITIES	NUTRIENT/HERBS	ACTION INVOLVED
Imatinib (Gleevec)— phosphotyrosine kinase inhibitor	Gastrointestinal cancers, glioblastomas, adenoid cystic cancers, prostate cancers, leukaemia	Myelosuppression, hepatotoxicity, oedema, bleeding	Vitamin C	Restores sensitivity to drug.[182]
			Flavonoids, e.g. quercetin	Aids drug in inhibiting cyclin-dependent kinases, inhibits angiogenic mediators and induces apoptosis.[193]
			Vitamin D	Effects cytokines in leukaemic cells and aids in control of apoptotic-gene expression in synergy with drug and vitamin A.[194]
			Vitamin A	Effects cytokines in leukaemic cells and aids in control of apoptotic-gene expression in synergy with drug and vitamin E.[194]
Interferon	Hairy cell leukaemia, genital warts, AIDS, Kaposi's sarcoma, bladder cancer, chronic active hepatitis	Flu-like syndrome, fever, chills, muscle pain, loss of appetite, lethargy, myelosuppression, nausea, vomiting, neurotoxicity, cardiotoxicity	Carnitine	Reduces fatigue associated with treatment: 2 g/day[195]
			Scutellaria baicalensis	Use with caution: reports of acute pneumonitis due to allergic-immunological mechanism.[3]
			Vitamin C	Aids growth inhibitory effect.[15,16]
			Vitamin E	Aids growth inhibitory effect in combination with other antioxidants.[15,16]
			Beta-carotene	Aids growth inhibitory effect in combination with other antioxidants.[15,16]
			Vitamin A	Aids growth inhibitory effect in combination with other antioxidants.[15,16]

Drug	Cancer type	Side effects	Complementary agent	Effect
Oxaliplatin (Eloxatin)	Colorectal cancer	Neurologic toxicity, myelosuppression	Lipoic acid	Aids efficacy of drug.[196]
Pegaspargase (Oncasper)	ALL	Hypersensitivity reactions, hepatotoxicity, coagulopathies, cardiotoxicity	No studies located.	
Pemetrexed (Alimta)—inhibits several folate-dependent enzymes that play roles in purine and pyrimidine synthesis	Lung cancer, mesothelioma	Neutropenia, diarrhoea, nausea/vomiting, mucositis, and skin rash, spermatoxicity	Folic acid Vitamin B12	Decreases side effects.[197-200] Decreases side effects.[197-200]
Procarbazine (Matulane)—alkylating and weak MAOI	Hodgkin's disease	Bone-marrow suppression, pneumonitis, nausea, vomiting, weakness, drowsiness, myalgia, muscle twitching, insomnia, nightmares, increased nervousness	Vitamin C Vitamin C N-acetyl cysteine	Enhances effectiveness, reduces side effects.[16] Decrease spermatoxicity of drug.[201] Decrease spermatoxicity of drug.[201]
Rituximab (Rituxan)	B cell non-Hodgkin's lymphoma	Fever, chills, weakness, headache, angio-oedema, hypotension, myalgia, nausea, vomiting, leukopenia, pruritus, rash	No studies located.	
Temozolomide (Temodar)	Melanoma, intermediate-grade gliomas	Myelosuppression, GI upset, thrombocytopenia, infertility, fatigue, headache, nausea, vomiting, constipation, anorexia, rash, alopecia	Resveratrol Zinc	Aids in apoptosis in the S phase of cell mitosis.[202] Chemopotentiating agent as it aids in DNA repair.[46, 66]
Tretinoin (Vesanoid)—a retinoid	Acute promyelocytic leukaemia	Headaches, fever, increased weakness, malaise, shivering, infections, haemorrhage, peripheral oedema	No studies located.	
Combination therapy				
Folfox—combination name for treatment with folinic acid, fluorouracil and oxaliplatin.	Colon cancer	Increased risk of infection, headaches, aching muscles, cough, sore throat, tiredness, breathlessness, bruising more easily than normal, anaemia	Calcium and magnesium Lipoic acid Glutathione	Decreases neurotoxicity.[203] Decreases neurotoxicity[203] Aids in decreasing neurotoxicity.[203]

General supplementation for chemotherapy

DRUG	NUTRIENT/HERB	POTENTIAL OUTCOME	RECOMMENDATION	EVIDENCE/ COMMENTS
Chemotherapy in general	*Eleutherococcus senticosus*	Improved treatment tolerance	Use with caution; however, possible beneficial interaction.	Co-administration may increase drug tolerance and improve immune function.[3]
	Withania somnifera	Reduced side effects	Observe: beneficial interaction.	May prevent drug-induced bone-marrow suppression.[3]
	Adenosine	Increases WBC	Use in conjunction with treatment and up to 1 month after chemo.	Acts as a chemo-protective agent.[2]
	Ganoderma spp./ *Lentinula* spp.	Increases WBC	Use in conjunction with treatment and up to 1–3 months after chemo.	Increase or support immune response.[2]
	Selenium	Chemoprotective	Used mainly in breast, prostate, colon and lung cancer.	Has protective effects from various sources of chemo and has a variety of effects.[204]
	Digestive enzymes	Increased absorption of nutrients	Decreased GIT function and GIT toxicity is common during chemotherapy.	Aids absorption of nutrients.[2]
	Liver support	Decreased systemic damage from drugs	During chemotherapy use low dose as you don't want to increase clearance of drug too soon. Increase dose for liver protection and function.	Decreases liver toxicity and congestion plus increases liver function.[2]

References

1. Frischer H, Ahmad T. Severe generalized glutathione reductase deficiency after antitumour chemotherapy with BCNU*[1,3-bis(chloroethyl)-1-nitrosourea]. J Lab Clin Med 1977;89(5):1080–1091.
2. Osiecki H. Cancer: a nutritional/biochemical approach. 2nd edn. Brisbane: BioConcepts Publishing, 2003.
3. Braun L, Cohen M. Herbs and natural supplements, an evidence-based guide. Sydney: Elsevier, 2005.
4. Salerno E. Pharmacology for health professionals. St Louis: Mosby, 1999.
5. Kurbacher CM, et al. Ascorbic acid (vitamin C) improves the antineoplastic activity of doxorubicin, cisplatin, and paclitaxel in human breast carcinoma cells in vitro. Cancer Lett 1996;103(2):183–189.
6. Tsutani H, et al. Pharmacological studies of retinol palmitate and its clinical effect in patients with acute non-lymphocytic leukemia. Leuk Res 1991;15(6):463–471.
7. Branda RF, et al. Nutritional folate status influences the efficacy and toxicity of chemotherapy in rats. Blood 1998;92(7):2471–2476.
8. Teicher BA, et al. In vivo modulation of several anticancer agents by beta-carotene. Cancer Chemother Pharmacol 1994;34(3):235–241.
9. Conklin A. Dietary antioxidants during cancer chemotherapy: impact on chemotherapeutic effectiveness and development of side effects. Nutr Cancer 2000;37(1):1–18.
10. Wietrzyk J, et al. Antiangiogenic and antitumour effects in vivo of genistein applied alone or combined with cyclophosphamide. Anticancer Res 2001;21(6A):3893–3896.
11. Davis L, Kuttan G. Effect of *Withania somnifera* on cyclophosphamide-induced urotoxicity. Cancer Lett 2000;148(1):9–17.
12. Badary OA. Taurine attenuates Fanconi syndrome induced by ifosimide without compromising its antitumour activity. Oncol Res 1998;10(7):355–360.

13. Mills S, Bone K. The essential guide to herbal safety. St Louis: Churchill Livingstone, 2005.

14. Heisler T, et al. Peptide YY and vitamin E inhibit hormone-sensitive and -insensitive breast cancer cells. J Surg Res 2000;91(1):9–14.

15. Prasad KN, et al. Modification of the effect of tamoxifen, cis-platin, DTIC, and interferon-alpha 2b on human melanoma cells in culture by a mixture of vitamins. Nutr Cancer 1994;22(3):233–245.

16. Prasad KN, et al. High doses of multiple antioxidant vitamins: essential ingredients in improving the efficacy of standard cancer therapy. J Am Coll Nutr 1999;18(1):13–25.

17. Nakagawa Y, et al. Relationship between ascorbic acid and alpha-tocopherol during diquat-induced redox cycling in isolated rat hepatocytes. Biochem Pharmacol 1991;25:42(4):883–888.

18. Fullerton SA, et al. Induction of apoptosis in human prostatic cancer cells with beta-glucan (maitake mushroom rythrocytese). Mol Urol 2000;4(1):7–13.

19. Georgian L, et al. The protective effect of vitamin A and vitamin C on the chromosome-damaging activity of CCNU. Morphol Embryol (Bucur) 1986;32(4):241–245.

20. Gadjeva V, et al. Spin labeled antioxidants protect bacteria against the toxicity of alkylating antitumor drug CCNU. Toxicol Lett 2003;144(3):289–294.

21. Blasiak J, et al. Genotoxicity of streptozotocin in normal and cancer cells and its modulation by free radical scavengers. Cell Biol Toxicol 2004;20(2):83–96.

22. Mahesh T, Menon VP. Quercetin allievates oxidative stress in streptozotocin-induced diabetic rats. Phytother Res 2004;18(2):123–127.

23. Yilmaz O, et al. Effects of alpha lipoic acid, ascorbic acid-6-palmitate, and fish oil on the gluthione, malonaldehyde, and fatty acid levels in rythrocytes of streptozotocin induced diabetic male rats. J Cell Biochem 2002;86(3):530–539.

24. Jonas CR, et al. Plasma antioxidant status after high dose chemotherapy: a randomised trial of parenteral nutrition in bone marrow transplantation patients. Am J Clin Nutr 2000;72(1):181–189.

25. Hoffman R, et al. Enhanced anti-proliferative action of busulphan by quercetin on the human leukaemia cell line K562. Br J Cancer 1989;59(3):347–348.

26. Durken M, et al. Deteriorating free radical-trapping capacity and antioxidant status in plasma during bone marrow transplantation. Bone Marrow Transplant 1995;15(5):757–762.

27. Beer TM, et al. High-dose calcitriol and carboplatin in metastatic androgen-independent prostate cancer. Am J Clin Oncol 2004;27(5):535–541.

28. Wigington DP, et al. Combination study of 1,24(S)-dihydroxyvitamin D2 and chemotherapeutic agents on human breast and prostate cancer cell lines. Anticancer Res 2004;24(5A):2905–2912.

29. Trump DL, et al. Anti-tumor activity of calcitriol: pre-clinical and clinical studies. J Steroid Biochem Mol Biol 2004; 89–90(1–5):519–526.

30. Johnson CS, et al. Vitamin D-related therapies in prostate cancer. Cancer Metastasis Rev 2002;21(2):147–158.

31. Saunders DE, et al. Additive inhibition of RL95-2 endometrial carcinoma cell growth by carboplatin and 1,25 dihydroxyvitamin D3. Gynecol Oncol 1993;51(2): 155–159.

32. Meara DJ, et al. Role of calcium in modulation of toxicities due to cisplatin and its analogs: a histochemical approach. Anticancer Drugs 1997;8(10):988–999.

33. Lovat PE, et al. Synergistic induction of apoptosis of neuroblastoma by fenretinide or CD437 in combination with chemotherapeutic drugs. Int J Cancer 2000;88(6):977–985.

34. Lissoni P, et al. Treatment of cancer chemotherapy-induced toxicity with the pineal hormone melatonin. Support Care Cancer 1997;5(2):126–129.

35. Jung B, Ahmad N. Melatonin in cancer management: progress and promise. Cancer Res 2006;66(20):9789–9793.

36. Ghielmini M, et al. Double-blind randomized study on the myeloprotective effect of melatonin in combination with carboplatin and etoposide in advanced lung cancer. Br J Cancer 1999;80(7):1058–1061.

37. Antunes LM, et al. Protective effects of vitamin C against cisplatin-induced nephrotoxicity and lipid peroxidation in adult rats: a dose dependent study. Pharmacol Res 2000;41(4):405–411.

38. Ali BH, Al Moundhri MS. Agents ameliorating or augmenting the nephrotoxicity of cisplatin and other platinum compounds: some recent research. Food Chem Toxicol 2006;44(8):1173–1183.

39. Pace A, et al. Neuroprotective effect of vitamin E supplementation in patients treated with cisplatin chemotherapy. J Clin Oncol 2003;21(5):927–931.

40. Weisman RA, et al. Phase I trial of retinoic acid and cis-platinum for advanced squamous cell cancer of the head and neck based on experimental evidence of drug synergism. Otolaryngol Head Neck Surg 1998;118(5):597–602.

41. Kalemkerian GP, et al. A phase II study of all-trans-retinoic acid plus cisplatin and etoposide in patients with extensive stage small cell lung carcinoma: an Eastern Cooperative Oncology Group Study. Cancer 1998;83(6):1102–1108.

42. Melli G, et al. Alpha-lipoic acid prevents mitochondrial damage and neurotoxicity in experimental chemotherapy neuropathy. Exp Neurol 2008;214(2):276–284.

43. Bougnoux P. n-3 polyunsaturated fatty acids and cancer. Curr Opin Clin Nutr Metab Care 1999;2(2):121–126.

44. Jakubowicz-Gil J, et al. The effect of quercetin on pro-apoptotic activity of cisplatin in HeLa cells. Biochem Pharmacol 2005;69(9):1343–1350.

45. Francescato HD, et al. Protective effect of quercetin on the evolution of cisplatin-induced acute tubular necrosis. Kidney Blood Press Res 2004;27(3):148–158.

46. Sliwinski T, et al. Zinc salts differentially modulate DNA damage in normal and cancer cells. Cell Biol Int 2009;33(4): 542–547.

47. Lissoni P, et al. A randomized study of chemotherapy with cisplatin plus etoposide versus chemo-endocrine therapy with cisplatin, etoposide and the pineal hormone melatonin as a first-line treatment of advanced non-small cell lung cancer in patients in a poor clinical state. J Pineal Res 1999;23(1):15–19.

48. Savarese DM, et al. Prevention of chemotherapy and radiation toxicity with glutamine. Cancer Treat Rev 2003;29(6): 501–513.

49. Anderson PM, et al. Oral glutamine reduces the duration and severity of stomatitis after cancer chemotherapy. Cancer 1998;83:1433–1439.

50. Buckley JE, et al. Hypomagnesemia after cisplatin combination therapy. Arch Intern Med 1982;144:2347.

51. Van de Loosdrecht AA, et al. Seizures in a patient with disseminated testicular cancer due to cisplatin-induced hypomagnesaemia. Acta Oncol 2000;39:239–240.

52. Sadzuka Y, et al. Modulation of cancer chemotherapy by green tea. Clin Cancer Res 1998;4(1):153–156.

53. Sonnenbichler J, et al. Stimulatory effects of silibinin and silicristin from the milk thistle Silybum marianum on kidney cells. J Pharmacol Exp Ther 1999;290(3):1375–1383.

54. Slavik M, et al. Changes in serum copper and zinc during treatment with anticancer drugs interfering with pyridoxal phosphate. Adv Exp Med Biol 1989;258:235–242.

55. Radu I, et al. The combined action of thiotepa and lomustine cytostatics, of estradiol hormone and of vitamins E and A on Walker tumor chromatin structure. Rom J Endocrinol 1993;31(3–4):149–153.

56. Lialiaris T, et al. Enhancement and attenuation of cytogenetic damage by vitamin C in cultured human lymphocytes exposed to thiotepa or L-ethionine. Cytogenet Cell Genet 1987;44(4):209–214.

57. Studzinski GP, et al. Potentiation by 1-alpha, 25 dihydroxyvitamin D3 of cytotoxicity to HL-60 cells produced by cytarabine and hydroxyurea. J Natl Cancer Inst 1986;76(4):641–648.

58. Kim CH. Increased expression of N-acetylglucosaminyltransferase-V in human hepatoma cells by retinoic acid and 1alpha,25-dihydroxyvitamin D3. Int J Biochem Cell Biol 2004;36(11):2307–2319.

59. Makishima M, et al. Growth inhibition and differentiation induction in human monoblastic leukaemia cells by 1alpha-hydroxyvitamin D derivatives and their enhancement by combination with hydroxyurea. Br J Cancer 1998;77(1):33–39.

60. Vukelja SJ, et al. Pyridoxine for the palmar-plantar erythrodysesthesia syndrome. Ann Intern Med 1989; 111(8):688–689.

61. Fabian CJ, et al. Pyridoxine therapy for palmar-plantar erythrodysesthesia associated with continuous 5-fluorouracil infusion. Invest New Drugs 1990;8(1):57–63.

62. Nagore E, et al. Antineoplastic therapy-induced palmar plantar erythrodysesthesia ('hand-foot') syndrome. Incidence, recognition and management. Am J Clin Dermatol 2000;1(4):225–234.

63. Nakashima T, et al. Phase 1 study of concurrent radiotherapy with TS-1 and vitamin A (TAR therapy) for head and neck cancer. Gan To Kagaku Tyoho 2005;32(6):803–807.

64. Lotz-Winter H. On the pharmacology of bromelain: an update with special regard to animal studies on dose-dependent effects. Planta Med 1990;56(3):249–253.

65. Toffoli G, Cecchin E. Uridine diphosphoglucuronosyl transferase and methylenetetrahydrofolate reductase polymorphisms as genomic predictors of toxicity and response to irinotecan-, antifolate- and fluoropyrimidine-based chemotherapy. [Review] J Chemother 2004;16 Suppl 4:31–35.

66. Etienne MC, et al. Thymidylate synthase and methylenetetrahydrofolate reductase gene polymorphisms: relationships with 5-fluorouracil sensitivity. Br J Cancer 2004;90(2):526–534.

67. Zhong X, et al. [Effects of quercetin on the proliferation and apoptosis in transplantation tumor of breast cancer in nude mice]. Sichuan Da Xue Xue Bao Yi Xue Ban 2003;34(3):439–442.

68. Koide T, et al. Influence of flavonoids on cell cycle phase as analyzed by flow-cytometry. Cancer Biother Radiopharm 1997;12(2):111–115.

69. Yuan H, Zhang Z. Some factors affecting sister-chromatid differentiation (SCD) and sister-chromatid exchange (SCE) in Hordeum vulgare. Mutat Res 1992;272(2): 125–131.

70. Pyrhonen S, et al. Randomised comparison of fluorouracil, epidoxorubicin and methotrexate (FEMTX) plus supportive care with supportive care alone in patients with non-resectable gastric cancer. Br J Cancer 1995;71(3):587–591.

71. Nagai Y, et al. Vitamin A, a useful biochemical modulator capable of preventing methotrexate damage during methotrexate treatment. Pharmacol Toxicol 1993;73:69–74.

72. Fishman P, et al. Adenosine acts as a chemoprotective agent by stimulating G-CSF production: a role for A1 and A3 adenosine receptors. J Cell Physiol 2000;183(3): 393–398.

73. Ohana G, et al. Differential effect of adenosine on tumour and normal cell growth: focus on the A3 adenosine receptor. J Cell Physiol 2001;186(1):19–23.

74. Navarro-Peran E, et al. Kinetics of the inhibition of bovine liver dihydrofolate reductase by tea catechins: origin of slow-binding inhibition and pH studies. Biochemistry 2005;44(20):7512–7525.

75. Rovensky J, et al. The effects of Enterococcus faecium and selenium on methotrexate treatment in rat adjuvant-induced arthritis. Clin Dev Immunol 2004;11 (3–4):267–273.

76. Mivazono Y, et al. Oxidative stress contributes to methotrexate-induced small intestinal toxicity in rats. Scand J Gastroenterol 2004;39(11):1119–1127.

77. Perez JE, et al. High-dose alpha-tocopherol as a preventive of doxorubicin-induced alopecia. Cancer Treat Rep 1986;70(10):1213–1214.

78. Shinozawa S, et al. Effect of high dose alpha-tocopherol and alpha-tocopherol pretreatment on adriamycin (doxocurbicin) induced toxicity and tissue distribution. Physiol Chem Med NMR 1988;20(4):329–335.

79. Ripoll EA, et al. Vitamin E enhances the chemotherapeutic effects of adriamycin on human prostatic carcinoma cells in vitro. J Urol 1986;136(2):529–531.

80. Quiles JL, et al. Antioxidant nutrients and adriamycin toxicity. Toxicology 2002;180(1):79–95.

81. Versantvoort CH, et al. Genistein modulates the decreased drug accumulation in non-P-glycoprotein mediated multidrug resistant tumour cells. Br J Cancer 1993;68(5):939–946.

82. Monti E, Sinha BK. Antiproliferative effect of genistein and adriamycin against estrogen-dependent and -independent human breast cell carcinoma lines. Anticancer Res 1994;14(3):1221–1223.

83. Conklin KA. Coenzyme Q10 for prevention of anthracycline-induced cardiotoxicity. Integr Cancer Ther 2005; 4(2):110–130.

84. Dovinova I, et al. Combined effect of lipoic acid and doxorubicin in murine leukaemia. Neoplasma 1999;46(4):237–241.

85. Mijares A, Lopez JR. L-carnitine prevents increase in diastolic [Ca^{2+}] induced by doxocurbicin in cardiac cells. Eur J Pharmacol 2001;425(2):117–120.

86. Waldner R, et al. Effects of doxocuribicin-containing chemotherapy and a combination with L-carnitine on oxidative metabolism in patients with non-Hodgkin lymphoma. J Cancer Res Clin Oncol 2006;132(2):121–128.

87. Yeh YC, et al. A standardized extract of Ginkgo biloba suppresses doxorubicin-induced oxidative stress and p53-mediated mitochondrial apoptosis in rat testes. Br J Pharmacol 2009;156(1):48–61.

88. Hu Q, et al. Antimutagenicity of selenium-enriched rice on mice exposure to cyclophosphamide and mitomycin C. Cancer Lett 2005;220(1):29–35.

89. Fuga L, et al. Vitamin B2 (riboflavin) and a mixture of vitamin B2 and C affects MMC efficiency in aerated media under irradiation. Anticancer Res 2004;24(6):4031–4034.

90. Kammerer C, Getoff N. Synergistic effect of dehydroascorbic acid and mixtures with vitamin E and beta-carotene on mitomycin C efficiency under irradiation in vitro. In Vivo 2004;18(6):795–798.

91. Krishnaia AP, Sharma NK. Ascorbic acid potentiates mitomycin C-induced micronuclei and sister chromatid exchanges in human peripheral blood lymphocytes in vitro. Teratog Carcinog Mutagen 2003; Suppl 1:99–112.

92. Undeger U, et al. The modulating effects of quercetin and rutin on the mitomycin C induced DNA damage. Toxicol Lett 2004;151(1):143–149.

93. Kurita T, et al. A dosage design of mitomycin C tablets containing finely powdered green tea. Int J Pharm 2004;275 (1–2):279–283.

94. Niitsu N, Homma Y. Adenosine analogs as possible differentiation-inducing agents against acute myeloid leukemia. [Review] Leuk Lymphoma 1999;34(3–4):261–271.

95. Rafi MM, et al. Modulation of bcl-2 and cytotoxicity by licochalcone-A, a novel estrogenic flavonoid. Anticancer Res 2000;20(4):2653–2658.

96. Berger M, et al. Effect of thioctic acid (alpha-lipoic acid) on the chemotherapeutic efficacy of cyclophosphamide and vincristine sulphate. Arzneimittelforschung 1983;33(9):1286–1288.

97. Scifo C, et al. Resveratrol and propolis as necrosis or apoptosis inducers in human prostate carcinoma cells. Oncol Res 2004;14(9):415–426.

98. Menendez JA, et al. Synergistic interaction between vinorelbine and gamma-linolenic acid in breast cancer cells. Breast Cancer Res Treat 2002;72(3):203–219.

99. Seidner DL, et al. An oral supplement enriched with fish oil, soluble fiber, and antioxidants for corticosteroid sparing in ulcerative colitis: a randomized, controlled trial. Clin Gastroenterol Hepatol 2005;3(4):358–369.

100. Nesbitt LT. Minimizing complications from systemic glucocorticosteroid use. Dermatol Clin 1995;13(4):925–939.

101. Ravina A, et al. Reversal of corticosteroid-induced diabetes mellitus with supplemental chromium. Diabet Med 1999;16(2):164–167.

102. Thompson TA, Wilding G. Androgen antagonist activity by the antioxidant moiety of vitamin E, 2,2,5,7,8-pentamethyl-6-chromanol in human prostate carcinoma cells. Mol Cancer Ther 2003;2(8):797–803.

103. Jiang F, Wang Z. Identification and characterization of PLZF as a prostatic androgen-responsive gene. Prostate 2004;59(4):426–435.

104. Kang Z, et al. Coregulator recruitment and histone modifications in transcriptional regulation by the androgen receptor. Mol Endocrinol 2004;18(11):2633–2648.

105. Juniewicz PE, et al. Effects of androgen and antiandrogen treatment on canine prostatic arginine esterase. Prostate 1990;17(2):101–111.

106. Zhang J, et al. Indole-3-carbinol induces a G1 cell cycle arrest and inhibits prostate-specific antigen production in human LNCaP prostate carcinoma cells. Cancer 2003;98(11):2511–2520.

107. Mi Y, Zhang C. Toxic and hormonal effects of polychlorinated biphenyls on cultured testicular germ cells of embryonic chickens. Toxicol Lett 2005;155(2):297–305.

108. Mathur PP, Chattopadhyay S. Involvement of lysosomal enzymes in flutamide-induced stimulation of rat testis. Andrologia 1982;14(2):171–176.

109. Diamond T, et al. The effect of combined androgen blockade on bone turnover and bone mineral densities in men treated for prostate carcinoma: longitudinal evaluation and response to intermittent cyclic etidronate therapy. Cancer 1998;83(8):1561–1566.

110. Fau D, et al. Mechanism for the hepatotoxicity of the antiandrogen, nilutamide. Evidence suggesting that redox cycling of this nitroaromatic drug leads to oxidative stress in isolated hepatocytes. J Pharmacol Exp Ther 1992;263(1):69–77.

111. Iynem AH, et al. The effect of prostate cancer and antiandrogenic therapy on lipid peroxidation and antioxidant systems. Int Urol Nephrol 2004;36(1):57–62.

112. Diamond TH, et al. Osteoporosis and spinal fractures in men with prostate cancer: risk factors and effects of androgen deprivation therapy. J Urol 2004;172(2):529–532.

113. Hatano T, et al. Incidence of bone fracture in patients receiving luteinizing hormone-releasing hormone agonists for prostate cancer. BJU Int 2000;86(4):449–452.

114. Cemeli E, et al. Modulation by flavonoids of DNA damage induced by estrogen-like compounds. Environ Mol Mutagen 2004;44(5):420–426.

115. Kitson TM, et al. Interaction of sheep liver cytosolic aldehyde dehydrogenase with quercetin, resveratrol and diethylstilbestrol. Chem Biol Interact 2001;130–132(1–3):57–69.

116. Gehm BD, et al. Estrogenic effects of resveratrol in breast cancer cells expressing mutant and wild-type estrogen receptors: role of AF-1 and AF-2. J Steroid Biochem Mol Biol 2004;88(3):223–234.

117. Morris GZ, et al. Resveratrol induces apoptosis in LNCaP cells and requires hydroxyl groups to decrease viability in LNCaP and DU 145 cells. Prostate 2002;52(4):319–329.

118. Cho DI, et al. Effects of resveratrol-related hydroxystilbenes on the nitric oxide production in macrophage cells: structural requirements and mechanism of action. Life Sci 2002;71(17):2071–2082.

119. Karasek M, et al. Melatonin inhibits growth of diethylstilbestrol-induced prolactin-secreting pituitary tumor in vitro: possible involvement of nuclear RZR/ROR receptors. J Pineal Res 2003;34(4):294–296.

120. Jones JL, et al. Genistein inhibits tamoxifen effects on cell proliferation and cell cycle arrest in T47D breast cancer cells. Am Surg 2002;68(6):575–577;discussion 577–578.

121. Ju YH, et al. Dietary genistein negates the inhibitory effect of tamoxifen on growth of estrogen-dependent human breast cancer (MCF-7) cells implanted in athymic mice. Cancer Res 2002;62(9):2474–2477.

122. Ravindranath MH, et al. Anticancer therapeutic potential of soy isoflavone, genistein. [Review] Adv Exp Med Biol 2004;546:121–165.

123. Liu B, et al. Low-dose dietary phytoestrogen abrogates tamoxifen-associated mammary tumour prevention. Cancer Res 2005;65(3):879–886.

124. Constantinou AL, et al. The soy isoflavone daidzein improves the capacity of tamoxifen to prevent mammary tumours. Eur J Cancer 2005;41(4):647–654.

125. Herbal Medicine Research and Education Centre. Herbs used in menopause. Complementary Medicine 2005;4(4):51.

126. Donnelly LE, et al. Anti-inflammatory effects of resveratrol in lung epithelial cells: molecular mechanisms. Am J Physiol Lung Cell Mol Physiol 2004;287(4):L774–L783.

127. Ma ZS, et al. Reduction of CWR22 prostate tumor xenograft growth by combined tamoxifen-quercetin treatment is associated with inhibition of angiogenesis and cellular proliferation. Int J Oncol 2004;24(5):1297–1304.

128. Fujiki H, et al. Cancer prevention with green tea and monitoring by a new biomarker, hnRNP B1. [Review] Mutat Res 2001;480–481:299–304.

129. Suganuma M, et al. Mechanisms of cancer prevention by tea polyphenols based on inhibition of TNF-alpha expression. Biofactors 2000;13(1–4):67–72.

130. Suganuma M, et al. Combination cancer chemoprevention with green tea extract and sulindac shown in intestinal tumor formation in Min mice. J Cancer Res Clin Oncol 2001;127(1):69–72.

131. Perumal SS, et al. Combined efficacy of tamoxifen and coenzyme Q10 on the status of lipid peroxidation and antioxidants in DMBA induced breast cancer. Mol Cell Biochem 2005;273(1–2):151–160.

132. Perumal SS, et al. Augmented efficacy of tamoxifen in rat breast tumorigenesis when gavaged along with riboflavin, niacin, and CoQ10: effects on lipid peroxidation and antioxidants in mitochondria. Chem Biol Interact 2005;152(1):49–58.

133. De Leo V, et al. Menopause, the cardiovascular risk factor homocysteine, and the effects of treatment. [Review] Treat Endocrinol 2004;3(6):393–400.

134. Palomba S, et al. Lipid, glucose and homocysteine metabolism in women treated with a GnRH agonist with or without raloxifene. Hum Reprod 2004;19(2):415–421.

135. Al Akoum M, et al. Synergistic cytotoxic effect of tamoxifen and black cohosh on MCF-7 and MDA-MB-231 human breast cancer cells: an in vitro study. Can J Physiol Pharmacol 2007;85(11):1153–1159.

136. Rickard DJ, et al. Phytoestrogen genistein acts as an estrogen agonist on human osteoblastic cells through estrogen receptors alpha and beta. J Cell Biochem 2003;89(3):633–646.

137. Rliwinski L, et al. Differential effects of genistein, estradiol and raloxifene on rat osteoclasts in vitro. Pharmacol Rep 2005;57(3):352–359.

138. Antoniucci DM, et al. Vitamin D insufficiency does not affect bone mineral density response to raloxifene. J Clin Endocrinol Metab 2005;90(8):4566–4572.

139. Hascalik S, et al. Effects of resveratrol, raloxifene, tibolone and conjugated equine estrogen on vaginal squamous cell maturation of ovariectomized rats. Gynecol Obstet Invest 2005;60(4):186–191.

140. Celik O, et al. Magnetic resonance spectroscopic comparison of the effects of resveratrol (3,4′,5-trihydroxy stilbene) to conjugated equine estrogen, tibolone and raloxifene on ovariectomized rat brains. Eur J Obstet Gynecol Reprod Biol 2005;120(1):73–79.

141. Fiorelli G, et al. Estrogen synthesis in human colon cancer epithelial cells. J Steroid Biochem Mol Biol 1999;71(5–6):223–230.

142. Paterson AH. Evaluating bone mass and bone quality in patients with breast cancer. Clin Breast Cancer 2005;5 Suppl 2:S41–S45.

143. Lindsay R, et al. Bone response to treatment with lower doses of conjugated estrogens with and without medroxyprogesterone acetate in early postmenopausal women. Osteoporos Int 2005;16(4):372–379.

144. Brodowska A. [The influence of hormonal replacement therapy on bone density in postmenopausal women depending on polymorphism of vitamin D receptor (VDR) and estrogen receptor (ER) genes]. Ann Acad Med Stetin 2003;49:111–130.

145. Day JK, et al. Dietary genistein increased DMBA-induced mammary adenocarcinoma in wild-type, but not ER alpha KO, mice. Nutr Cancer 2001;39(2):226–232.

146. Subakir SB, et al. Oxidative stress, vitamin E and progestin breakthrough bleeding. Hum Reprod 2000;15 Suppl 3:18–23.

147. Barnes JF, et al. Effects of two continuous hormone therapy regimens on C-reactive protein and homocysteine. Menopause 2005;12(1):92–98.

148. Meram I, et al. Trace elements and vitamin levels in menopausal women receiving hormone replacement therapy. Clin Exp Obstet Gynecol 2003;30(1):32–34.

149. Sliutz G, et al. Drug resistance against gemcitabine and topotecan mediated by constitutive hsp70 overexpression in vitro: implication of quercetin as sensitiser in chemotherapy. Br J Cancer 1996;74(2):172–177.

150. Panosyan EH, et al. Deamination of glutamine is a prerequisite for optimal asparagines deamination by asparaginases in vivo (CCG-1961). Anticancer Res 2004;24(2C):1121–1125.

151. Rotoli BM, et al. Inhibition of glutamine synthetase triggers apoptosis in asparaginase-resistant cells. Cell Physiol Biochem 2005;15(6):281–292.

152. Myszka H, et al. Synthesis and induction of apoptosis in B cell chronic leukemia by diosgenyl 2-amino-2-deoxy-beta-D-glucopyranoside hydrochloride and its derivatives. Carbohydr Res 2003;338(2):133–141.

153. Liu JD, et al. Inhibition of melanoma growth and metastasis by combination with (-)-epigallocatechin-3-gallate and dacarbazine in mice. J Cell Biochem 2001;83(4):631–642.

154. Reid JM, et al. Metabolic activation of dacarbazine by human cytochromes P450: the role of CYP1A1, CYP1A2, and CYP2E1. Clin Cancer Res 1999;5(8):2192–2197.

155. Menendez JA, et al. Omega-6 polyunsaturated fatty acid gamma-linolenic acid (18:3n-6) enhances docetaxel (Taxotere) cytotoxicity in human breast carcinoma cells: relationship to lipid peroxidation and HER-2/neu expression. Oncol Rep 2004;11(6):1241–1252.

156. Beer TM, et al. Rationale for the development and current status of calcitriol in androgen-independent prostate cancer. [Review] World J Urol 2005;23(1):28–32.

157. Beer TM, Myrthue A. Calcitriol in cancer treatment: from the lab to the clinic. [Review] Mol Cancer Ther 2004;3(3):373–381.

158. Beer TM, et al. Quality of life and pain relief during treatment with calcitriol and docetaxel in symptomatic metastatic androgen-independent prostate carcinoma. Cancer 2004;100(4):758–763.

159. Wynter MP, et al. Effect of n-3 fatty acids on the antitumour effects of cytotoxic drugs. In Vivo 2004;18(5):543–547.

160. Ghalaut PS, et al. Serum vitamin E levels in patients of chronic myeloid leukaemia. J Assoc Physicians India 1999;47(7):703–704.

161. Przybyszewski WM, et al. Protection of L5178Y cells by vitamin E against acute hydroxyurea toxicity does not change the efficiency of ribonucleotide reductase-mediated hydroxyurea-induced cytotoxic events. Cancer Lett 1987;34(3):337–344.

162. Malec J, et al. Hydroxyurea-induced toxic side-effects in animals and an attempt at reducing them with vitamins E and C. Neoplasma 1989;36(4):427–435.

163. Makaroy AA, et al. Zinc(II)-mediated inhibition of ribonuclease Sa by an N-hydroxyurea nucleotide and its basis. Biochem Biophys Res Commun 2004;319(1):152–156.

164. Higgin JJ, et al. Zinc(II)-mediated inhibition of a ribonuclease by an N-hydroxyurea nucleotide. Bioorg Med Chem Lett 2003;13(3):409–412.

165. Wong WS, McLean AE. Effects of phenolic antioxidants and flavonoids on DNA synthesis in rat liver, spleen, and testis in vitro. Toxicology 1999;139(3):243–253.

166. Miknyoczki SJ, et al. Chemopotentiation of temozolomide, irinotecan, and cisplatin activity by CEP-6800, a poly(ADP-ribose) polymerase inhibitor. Mol Cancer Ther 2003;2(4):371–382.

167. Fakih M, et al. Selenium protects against toxicity induced by anticancer drugs and augments antitumor activity: a highly selective, new, and novel approach for the treatment of solid tumors. Clin Colorectal Cancer 2005;5(2):132–135.

168. Cao S, et al. Selective modulation of the therapeutic efficacy of anticancer drugs by selenium containing compounds against human tumor xenografts. Clin Cancer Res 2004;10(7):2561–2569.

169. Yoshikawa M, et al. Transport of SN-38 by the wild type of human ABC transporter ABCG2 and its inhibition by quercetin, a natural flavonoid. J Exp Ther Oncol 2004;4(1):25–35.

170. Bremner I, et al. Control of selenium and cobalt deficiency in lambs by supplementation of oral anthelmintics. Vet Rec 1988;123(9):217–218.

171. Pathak AK, et al. Chemotherapy alone vs chemotherapy plus high dose multiple antioxidants in patients with advanced non small cell lung cancer. J Am Coll Nutr 2005;24(1):16–21.

172. Varma MV, Panchagnula R. Enhanced oral paclitaxel absorption with vitamin E-TPGS: effect on solubility and permeability in vitro, in situ and in vivo. Eur J Pharm Sci 2005;25(4–5):445–453.

173. Siewinski M, et al. Determination of cysteine peptidases-like activity and their inhibitors in the serum of patients with ovarian cancer treated by conventional chemotherapy and vitamin E. J Exp Ther Oncol 2004;4(3):189–193.

174. Argyriiou AA, et al. Vitamin E for prophylaxis against chemotherapy-induced neuropathy: a randomized controlled trial. Neurology 2005;64(1):26–31.

175. Choi JS, et al. Enhanced paclitaxel bioavailability after oral administration of paclitaxel or prodrug to rats pretreated with quercetin. Eur J Pharm Biopharm 2004;57(2):313–318.

176. Taixiang W, et al. Chinese medical herbs for chemotherapy side effects in colorectal cancer patients. Cochrane Database Syst Rev 2005;1:CD004540.

177. Reiter RJ, et al. Melatonin: reducing the toxicity and increasing the efficacy of drugs. J Pharm Pharmacol 2002;54(10):1299–1321.

178. Kinnula K, et al. Endogenous antioxidant enzymes and glutathione S-transferase in protection of mesothelioma cells against hydrogen peroxide and epirubicin toxicity. Br J Cancer 1998;77(7):1097–1102.

179. Jarvinen K, et al. Antioxidant defense mechanisms of human mesothelioma and lung adenocarcinoma cells. Am J Physiol Lung Cell Mol Physiol 2000;278(4):L696–L702.

180. Shinozawa S, et al. Protective effects of various drugs on adriamycin (doxorubicin)-induced toxicity and microsomal lipid peroxidation in mice and rats. Biol Pharm Bull 1993;16(11):1114–1117.

181. Solaini G, et al. Inhibitory effects of several anthracyclines on mitochondrial respiration and coenzyme Q10 protection. Drugs Exp Clin Res 1985;11(8):533–537.

182. Tarumoto T, et al. Ascorbic acid restores sensitivity to imatinib via suppression of Nrf2-dependent gene expression in the imatinib-resistant cell line. Exp Hematol 2004;32(4):375–381.

183. Vera JC, et al. Colony-stimulating factors signal for increased transport of vitamin C in human host defense cells. Blood 1998;91(7):2536–2546.

184. Higucki T, et al. Induction of differentiation of retinoic acid-resistant acute promyelocytic leukemia cells by the combination of all-trans retinoic acid and granulocyte colony-stimulating factor. Leuk Res 2004;28(5):525–532.

185. Matsui W, et al. Requirement for myeloid growth factors in the differentiation of acute promyelocytic leukaemia. Br J Haematol 2005;128(6):853–862.

186. Ganser A, et al. Improved multilineage response of hematopoiesis in patients with myelodysplastic syndromes to a combination therapy with all-trans-retinoic acid, granulocyte colony-stimulating factor, erythropoietin and alpha-tocopherol. Ann Hematol 1996;72(4):237–244.

187. Maurer AB, et al. Changes in erythroid progenitor cell and accessory cell compartments in patients with myelodysplastic syndromes during treatment with all-trans retinoic acid and haemopoietic growth factors. Br J Haematol 1995;89(3):449–456.

188. Carcamo JM, et al. Vitamin C inhibits granulocyte macrophage-colony-stimulating factor-inducing signaling pathways. Blood 2002;99(9):3205–3212.

189. Vera JC, et al. Colony-stimulating factors signal for increased transport of vitamin C in human host defense cells. Blood 1998;91(7):2536–2546.

190. Tao YH, Yang Y. [Effects of vitamin A on the differentiation, maturation and functions of dendritic cells from cord blood]. Zhonghua Er Ke Za Zhi 2004;42(5):340–343.

191. Hengesbach LM, Hoag KA. Physiological concentrations of retinoic acid favor myeloid dendritic cell development over granulocyte development in cultures of bone marrow cells from mice. J Nutr 2004;134(10):2653–2659.

192. Fishman P, et al. The A3 adenosine receptor as a new target for cancer therapy and chemoprotection. Exp Cell Res 2001;269(2):230–236.

193. Faderl S, Estrov Z. Commentary: effect of flavonoids on normal and leukemic cells. Leuk Res 2003;27(6): 471–473.

194. Mogattash S, Lutton JD. Leukemia cells and the cytokine network: therapeutic prospects. Exp Biol Med 2004; 229(2):121–137.

195. Neri S, et al. L-carnitine decreases severity and type of fatigue induced by interferon-alpha in the treatment of patients with hepatitis C. Neuropsychobiology 2003;47(2):94–97.

196. Gedlicka C, et al. Effective treatment of oxaliplatin-induced cumulative polyneuropathy with alpha-lipoic acid. J Clin Oncol 2002;20(15):3359–3361.

197. Socinski MA, et al. The evolving role of pemetrexed (Alimta) in lung cancer. [Review] Semin Oncol 2005;32(2 Suppl 2):S16–S22.

198. Buddle LS, Hanna NH. Antimetabolites in the management of non-small cell lung cancer. [Review] Curr Treat Options Oncol 2005;6(1):83–93.

199. Adjei AA. Pharmacology and mechanism of action of pemetrexed. [Review] Clin Lung Cancer 2004;5 Suppl 2:S51–S55.

200. Fossella FV. Pemetrexed for treatment of advanced non-small cell lung cancer. [Review] Semin Oncol 2004;31(1 Suppl 1):100–105.

201. Horstman MG, et al. Separate mechanisms for procarbazine spermatotoxicity and anticancer activity. Cancer Res 1987;47(6):1547–1550.

202. Fuggetta MP, et al. In vitro antitumour activity of resveratrol in human melanoma cells sensitive or resistant to temozolomide. Melanoma Res 2004;14(3):189–196.

203. Grothey A. Clinical management of oxaliplatin-associated neurotoxicity. Clin Colorectal Cancer 2005;5 Suppl 1: S38–S48.

204. El-Bayoumy K, Sinha R. Molecular chemoprevention by selenium: a genomic approach. Mutat Res 2005;591(1–2): 224–236.

Appendix 3

Food sources of nutrients

Order is roughly indicative of ranking of content.

NUTRIENT	COMMON FOOD SOURCE
Vitamins	
A	Liver, sweet potato, carrots, spinach, butternut pumpkin, dandelion greens, butter, eggs
B1	Whole grains, pork, sunflower seeds, nuts, legumes
B2	Liver, other organ meats, mushrooms, ricotta cheese, milk, meats, eggs, cheese, whole grains, oysters
B3	Tuna, liver, chicken, beef, halibut, mushrooms, nuts, whole grains
B5	Egg yolk, liver, kidney, brewer's yeast—widespread in most foods
B6	Steak, legumes, potato, salmon, bananas, whole grains, other meats and fish
B12	Meat, fish, shellfish, eggs, cheese, milk, oysters, fermented foods
Folate	Brewer's yeast, leafy greens, asparagus, wholegrain cereals, legumes, nuts, liver
C	Pawpaw, oranges, rockmelon, broccoli, Brussels sprouts, tomatoes, grapefruit, cabbage, strawberries
D	Fatty and canned fish, butter, margarine, cream, cheese, eggs—also synthesised in skin upon exposure to sunlight
E	Vegetable oils, nuts, olive oil, wheat germ, avocado, egg, fatty fish and small amounts in wholegrain cereals and green vegetables
K	Green vegetables, cheese, soy, butter, pork, eggs—also synthesised by healthy intestinal microflora
Biotin	Brewer's yeast, liver, kidney, legumes, eggs, chard, bitter greens—also synthesised by healthy intestinal microflora
Minerals	
Boron	Legumes, nuts, whole grains, fruits and vegetables, beer, wine, cider
Calcium	Yoghurts and cheeses, sesame seeds (tahini), milk, bony fish (particularly sardines), clams, oysters, broccoli, nuts, dried fruit
Chromium	Brewer's yeast, mushrooms, prunes, asparagus, organ meats, whole grains, tea, cheese
Copper	Liver, shellfish, whole grains, legumes, eggs, meats, fish
Fluoride	Tea, bony fish—very small amounts in most food sources
Iodine	Seafood, sea vegetables, iodised table salt, sunflower seeds, liver, mushrooms—nutrient soil-dependent in other sources
Iron	Organ meats, other meats, oysters, nuts, legumes, leafy greens, whole grains, eggs
Magnesium	Nuts, legumes, whole grains, soy, parsnips, molasses, cocoa mass, corn, peas, leafy greens
Manganese	Whole grains, nuts, leafy greens, tea, blueberries, pineapple
Molybdenum	Soy, legumes, buckwheat, oats, whole grains, nuts, meat
Phosphorus	Meats, fish, poultry, eggs, milk, cheese, nuts, legumes, whole grains
Potassium	Avocadoes, bananas, dried fruits, oranges, peaches, potatoes, legumes, tomatoes, wheat bran, eggs, apricots, nuts
Selenium	Brazil nuts, kidney, tuna, crab, lobster—nutrient particularly soil-dependent

(Continued)

NUTRIENT	COMMON FOOD SOURCE
Sulfur	Most protein foods
Zinc	Oysters, wheat germ, meats, liver, whole grains, pumpkin seeds, nuts
Phytonutrients	
Anthocyanins	Red, blue and purple berries, red and purple grapes, red wine
Carotenoids	Carrots, pumpkin, butternut pumpkin, sweet potato, pawpaw, red and yellow capsicum, corn, kale, leafy greens, tomatoes, rockmelon, paprika, peas
Chlorophyll	Spinach, parsley, watercress, beans, rocket, leeks
Cruciferous indoles	Cruciferous vegetables (broccoli, Brussels sprouts, cabbage, kale, turnip, radish, swedes, horseradish, watercress)
Flavanols	Tea, cocoa, berries, grapes, apples
Hesperidin and rutin	Citrus fruits and juices (especially grapefruit and blood oranges)
Isoflavones	Soy, legumes
Isothiocyanates	Cruciferous vegetables, garlic
Lignans	Linseed, sesame seeds, kale, broccoli, apricots, cabbage
Lutein and zeaxanthin	Spinach, kale, leafy greens, peas, squash, butternut pumpkin, broccoli, Brussels sprouts, corn
Luteolin and other flavones	Parsley, thyme, celery, chillies
Lycopene	Tomato paste, tomato puree, watermelon, tomatoes, pink grapefruit
Quercetin and other flavonols	Onions, shallots, kale, broccoli, apples, berries, tea
Fats	
Omega-3	Oily fish, oysters, linseed, walnuts

Appendix 4

Laboratory reference values

The reference values and ranges for these blood tests are given in the system of international units (SI) and are based on guidelines from the Royal College of Pathologists of Australasia. They may vary from laboratory to laboratory. When paediatric reference ranges may differ from adult ranges they are indicated by an asterisk (*). Further information and resources can be found at the online manual of the Royal College of Pathologists of Australasia at http://www.rcpamanual.edu.au/.

INVESTIGATION/APPLICATION	REFERENCE VALUE	POTENTIAL INCREASED LEVEL	POTENTIAL DECREASED LEVEL
Electrolytes			
Potassium Monitoring status with diuretic usage, acid–base balance or mineralocorticoid status*	3.5–5.0 mmol/L	Acidosis, tissue damage, renal failure and mineralocorticoid deficiency Drugs such as ACE inhibitors, NSAIDs, diuretics	Alkalosis, vomiting or diarrhoea, mineralocorticoid excess Drugs such as insulin, diuretics, salbutamol
Sodium Monitoring fluid and electrolyte status	135–145 mmol/L	Dehydration, vomiting or diarrhoea, kidney disease, excess mineralocorticoids, excess salt intake or retention	Low salt intake, high blood glucose, mineralocorticoid or thyroid deficiency, excess water intake, kidney, heart or liver failure
Sodium:potassium ratio	28–34	> 34 + raised sodium → potassium deficiency	< 28 → sodium deficiency, also low magnesium and vitamin E
Chloride Assess cause of acid–base imbalance	95–107 mmol/L	High sodium and metabolic acidosis	Low sodium and metabolic alkalosis
Bicarbonate Acid–base imbalance and metabolic abnormalities	23–32 mmol/L	Metabolic alkalosis, compensated respiratory acidosis, potassium deficiency, excess laxatives or vomiting	Metabolic or diabetic acidosis, excess lactic acid, alcohol or aspirin, fasting
Kidney function			
Urea Renal function	3.0–8.0 mmol/L	Excess protein, renal failure, kidney stones, congestive heart failure, enlarged prostate, GI bleeding, diarrhoea or vomiting, dehydration or sweating	Low protein intake, water retention, urea cycle defects, poisoning or severe liver damage < 5.0 → dietary protein deprivation
Urate Gout, pregnancy induced hypertension*	M 0.17–0.45 mmol/L F 0.12–0.40 mmol/L	Gout, pregnancy induced hypertension, renal failure, fasting, excess lactate or ketones Drugs such as diuretics, low dose salicylates	Protein insufficiency and poor nucleotide synthesis

(Continued)

INVESTIGATION/APPLICATION	REFERENCE VALUE	POTENTIAL INCREASED LEVEL	POTENTIAL DECREASED LEVEL
Creatinine Glomerular filtration	M 0.04–0.13 mmol/L F 0.04–0.10 mmol/L	Conditions of decreased filtration (hypovolaemia, hypotension), renal or postrenal obstruction	Low muscle mass, pregnancy < 0.06 → poor protein tissue bulk
Urea:creatinine ratio	70–90	> 90 → excess protein tissue breakdown	< 70 → dietary protein deprivation
Calcium Hypo- or hyperparathyroidism, malignancy*	2.10–2.60 mmol/L	Hyperparathyroidism, malignancy, sarcoidosis, vitamin A or D toxicity	Hypoparathyroidism, renal failure, osteomalacia, rickets, thyroid or parathyroid surgery Calcium < 2.3 + phosphate < 1.0 → calcium and phosphate deficiency
Phosphate Renal failure, hyper- or hypoparathyroidism, metabolic bone disease	0.90–1.35 mmol/L	Hypoparathyroidism, hypercalcaemia due to malignancy, renal failure	Hyperparathyroidism, use of magnesium or aluminium-containing antacids
Calcium:phosphate ratio	1.0–2.4	> 2.4 + phosphate < 1.0 → calcium deficiency	< 2.2 with phosphate > 1.0 → phosphate deficiency
Proteins			
Total protein Amount of albumin and immunoglobulins present in serum	60–80 g/L	Increased immunoglobulins, dehydration	Low albumin, reduced immunoglobulins
Albumin Hydration, nutritional status, liver disease, catabolic disorders	38–50 g/L	Dehydration, level may be overestimated in severe deficiency depending on analysis method	Acute phase response, impaired protein synthesis < 35 g/L → severe protein deprivation
Globulins Hypo- and hypergammaglobulinaemia	Consult pathologist	Chronic inflammation, infection, autoimmune disease	Catabolic enteropathy, humoral immunodeficiency
Liver function			
Bilirubin Hepatobiliary disease, haemolysis*	Total: < 20 μmol/L Direct: < 3 μmol/L	Gilbert's syndrome, hepatobiliary disease, megaloblastic anaemia, fasting or insulin resistance, lack of cofactors B3, B6, Mg, Fe or glutamine	
Alkaline phosphatase (ALP) Hepatobiliary or bone disease*	< 120 U/L	Paget's disease, liver damage, excess bone activity, tissue repair	Zinc deficiency, abnormal dentition and fragile bones

INVESTIGATION/APPLICATION	REFERENCE VALUE	POTENTIAL INCREASED LEVEL	POTENTIAL DECREASED LEVEL
Gamma glutamyltransferase (GGT) Liver disease*	F < 45 U/L M < 65 U/L	Liver dysfunction with cholestasis, diabetes, excess alcohol, pancreatitis, prostatitis, acute liver damage	Impaired protein synthesis, vitamin B6 deficiency
Alanine aminotransferase (ALT) Liver cell damage*	< 35 U/L	Hepatocellular damage	Vitamin B6, B1 or zinc deficiency
Aspartate aminotransferase (AST) Liver cell damage*	< 40 U/L	Hepatocellular damage, haemolysis during collection, muscle tissue breakdown, copper toxicosis	Vitamin B6, B1 or zinc deficiency
Lactate dehydrogenase (LD) Liver disease, malignancy, skeletal muscle damage	110–230 U/L	Myocardial infarction, liver disease, haemolysis, ineffective erythropoiesis, muscle disease and tissue damage, some malignancies	
Blood cells			
Red cell count (RCC)*	F 3.8–5.8 × 10^{12}/L M 4.5–6.5 × 10^{12}/L Reticulocytes: 0.5–2.0%	Polycythaemia, dehydration, in response to low oxygen levels (smoking, high altitude, chronic diseases)	Anaemia, haemorrhage, chronic infection or renal failure, pregnancy, overhydration, leukaemia, multiple myelomas
Haemoglobin Anaemia*	F 115–165 g/L M 130–180 g/L	Anaemia	
Mean cell volume (MCV) Macro or microcytic anaemia*	81–98 fL	Macrocytic anaemia, vitamin B12 or folate deficiency, hypothyroidism, chronic liver disease Drugs that affect B12 status (anticonvulsants, antimetabolics)	Microcytic anaemia, iron deficiency, malignancy, rheumatoid arthritis, haemoglobinopathies, radiation or lead poisoning
White cell count (WCC) Infection, inflammation, bone marrow failure*	4.0–11.0 × 10^9/L	Acute infection, tissue necrosis, leukaemias, collagen diseases, sickle cell anaemia, parasites, stress Drugs such as aspirin, heparin, digoxin, lithium	Viral infections, malaria, haematopoietic diseases, alcoholism, SLE, rheumatoid arthritis Drugs such as antibiotics, paracetamol, sulfanomides, diuretics, indomethacin, oral hypoglycaemic agents

(Continued)

INVESTIGATION/APPLICATION	REFERENCE VALUE	POTENTIAL INCREASED LEVEL	POTENTIAL DECREASED LEVEL
Neutrophils*	Band: 0.05 × 10^9/L Mature: 2.0–7.5 × 10^9/L	Acute bacterial infections, inflammation, tissue damage, solid tumours, excessive exercise, allergies, pregnancy and labour	Viral infections, overwhelming bacterial infection, aplastic anaemia, acute leukaemia, vitamin B12 or folate deficiency, malnutrition, SLE
Lymphocytes*	1.0–4.0 × 10^9/L	Stress, uraemia, neoplasia, infections, rickets, ulcerative colitis, Addison's disease	Aplastic and pernicious anaemia, burns, protein malnutrition, toxic chemical exposure, pneumonia, high dose adrenocorticosteroids
Eosinophils*	0.0–0.4 × 10^9/L	Parasitic worm infections, allergic diseases, Hodgkin's lymphoma	
Basophils*	0.01–0.1 × 10^9/L	Chronic myeloid leukaemia	
Monocytes*	0.2–0.8 × 10^9/L	Chronic bacterial infections, TB, subacute bacterial endocarditis, ulcerative colitis, cirrhosis, haemolytic anaemias, SLE	
Platelet count*	150–400 × 10^9/L	Acute illness, chronic inflammation, splenectomy, thrombocythaemia	Increased tendency to bleed and bruise
Cholesterol			
Total cholesterol*	< 5.5 mmol/L	Cardiovascular disease risk	
HDL	> 1.00 mmol/L		Cardiovascular disease risk
LDL	< 3.5 mmol/L	Cardiovascular disease risk	Acute illness
Triglycerides*	< 2.0 mmol/L	Secondary to nephrotic syndrome, hypothyroidism, pancreatitis, insulin resistance or diabetes, alcoholism, OCP or steroid medication	Chronic disease
Homocysteine	5–15 μmol/L	Lack of methylation cofactors vitamin B12, folate, methionine	
Thyroid function			
Thyroid stimulating hormone (TSH)*	0.3–5.0 mU/L	Hypothyroidism, elevated mercury levels	
T4	10.0–20.0 pmol/L	Hyperthyroidism	Hypothyroidism

INVESTIGATION/APPLICATION	REFERENCE VALUE	POTENTIAL INCREASED LEVEL	POTENTIAL DECREASED LEVEL
T3	3.3–8.2 pmol/L		With low T4 → low thyroxine activity secondary to nutrient deficiency such as iodine or autoimmune disease With normal T4 → impaired conversion due to nutrient deficiency such as selenium, hyperinsulinaemia
Thyroid antibodies	Consult pathologist	Hashimoto thyroiditis, other autoimmune thyroid dysfunctions, other tissue specific autoimmune disorders	
Food allergies—refer to Chapter 5 on food sensitivity			
IgA		Chronic infections, inflammatory bowel disease	Recurrent intestinal infection, dairy protein intolerance, other food sensitivities
IgE	Varies with age—consult pathologist	Allergic reactions	
IgG		Chronic infections, intestinal parasites, food sensitivities	Malnutrition
IgM		Viral infections, hepatobiliary disease, food sensitivities	Immune suppression, protein loss from bowel
Antigliadin antibodies		Gluten intolerance or coeliac disease	
Tumour markers			
PSA (prostate-specific antigen)	0–4.0 µg/L	Benign prostatic hypertrophy. Marked elevation is indicative of prostate cancer, but normal or slightly raised levels do not exclude it.	
CEA (carcinoembryonic antigen)	< 7.5 µg/L	Recurrence of colonic adenocarcinoma and breast carcinoma following resection	
AFP (alpha fetoprotein)	< 10 µg/mL	Detection and monitoring of hepatocellular carcinoma and germ cell tumours Assessment of risk for neural tube and other defects *in utero*, including Down syndrome (one of the components of the 'triple test').	
CA-125	< 35 U/mL	Marker for serous carcinoma, especially ovarian	

(Continued)

INVESTIGATION/APPLICATION	REFERENCE VALUE	POTENTIAL INCREASED LEVEL	POTENTIAL DECREASED LEVEL
Glucose			
Glucose (fasting)	3.5–6.0 mmol/L	Diabetes mellitus	Hypoglycaemia
Glucose (random)	3.5–9.0 mmol/L	Diabetes mellitus	Hypoglycaemia
HbA$_{1c}$	4.7–6.1%	Diabetes mellitus (indicative of levels over past 3 months)	
Other endocrine tests			
Cortisol 8 a.m.	130–700 nmol/L	Stress, OCP use, adrenal or ACTH-producing tumours, Cushing's syndrome	Addison's disease, hypopituitarism
Cortisol 4 p.m.	80–350 nmol/L	Stress, OCP use, adrenal or ACTH-producing tumours, Cushing's syndrome	Addison's disease, hypopituitarism
FSH adult	1.9 IU/L		
FSH ovulation	10–30 IU/L		
FSH post menopausal	4–200 IU/L		
Oestradiol menopausal	< 200 pmol/L		
Testosterone	F < 3.5 nmol/L M 10–35 nmol/L	Various interpretations—please see Chapter 31 on fertility	

Markers of inflammation: ESR and CRP

Comparison between ESR and CRP
- Both investigations are markers of inflammation and there tends to be a broad correlation between them.
- The CRP levels rise faster than the ESR.
- The levels are similar after 24 hours or so.
- CRP levels fall faster than the ESR.
- CRP levels (unlike ESR) are not affected by pregnancy.
- ESR may be very high with a normal CRP in giant cell arteritis/polymyalgia rheumatica.
- CRP costs more.

Relative values (mm/hour) of typical examples of erythrocyte sedimentation rate (ESR) readings

VERY HIGH (OVER 80 mm/hour)	HIGH (40–80 mm/hour)	MODERATE TO LOW ELEVATION (20–40 mm/hour)	LOW (< 1 mm/ hour)
Giant cell arteritis/ polymyalgia rheumatica/temporal arteritis Multiple myeloma Tuberculosis Deep abscess Bacterial endocarditis Acute osteomyelitis	Rheumatic fever Pyelonephritis Other bacterial infections Viral infections with cold agglutinins Collagen disorders (e.g. rheumatoid arthritis, SLE) Solid tumours, especially metastases Leukaemia/lymphomas Myocardial infarction Inflammation of healing	Most acute and chronic infections (e.g. recent viral) Severe other illness Anaemia Pregnancy Drugs, especially contraceptives Elevated serum cholesterol level Laboratory error (e.g. tilted tube) Idiopathic–normal	Idiopathic–normal Sickle-cell anaemia Polycythaemia NSAIDs Old specimen

There is a lag phase of 24–48 hours between the onset of inflammatory stimulation and the production of inflammatory proteins that increase in the ESR. There is also a delay in the fall of the ESR after resolution of the inflammation because the fibrinogen levels can remain elevated for 6 days or so after acute tissue damage—this can take 4–8 weeks to return to normal.

A normal value of < 20 mm/hour generally excludes inflammation. The OCP can push the level to 20–25 mm/hour.

Normal values of ESR—reference interval

Child	
	2–15 mm/hour
Adult male	
17–50 years	1–10 mm/hour
> 50 years	2–15 mm/hour
Adult female	
17–50 years	3–12 mm/hour
> 50 years	5–20 mm/hour

C-reactive protein levels (normal value < 10 mg/L)

MARKED ELEVATION > 40 mg/L	NORMAL TO MILD ELEVATION
Bacterial infection	Viral infection
Abscess	Ulcerative colitis
Crohn's disease	SLE
Active rheumatic disease:	Atherosclerosis
– rheumatic fever	Steroid/oestrogen therapy
Connective tissue disorders:	
– rheumatoid arthritis	
– vasculitis	
Malignant disease	
Trauma/tissue injury	

Interpretation of iron studies

CONDITION	SERUM Fe	TIBC	% TRANSFERRIN SATURATION	FERRITIN
Reference range	14–30 (μmol/L)	45–80 (μmol/L)	F 20–55% M 20–60% (Transferrin 2–3.5 g/L)	20–250 (μg/L)
Iron deficiency	↓	N or ↑	↓	↓↓
Thalassaemia	N or ↑	N	N or ↑	↑
Anaemia of chronic disease	↓	N or ↓	↓	N or ↑
Sideroblastic anaemia	N or ↑	N	N or ↑	↑
Haemochro-matosis	↑	↓	↑↑	↑↑

Appendix 5

Factors affecting nutritional status

Niikee Schoendorfer

ND, MHSc

A variety of factors other than dietary insufficiency may influence nutritional status and therefore should be taken into account if a particular deficiency is suspected or if a specific condition present. Some conditions may increase the need for a particular nutrient, while others may interfere with its absorption or excretion.

Vitamin A

- Levels are affected by preexisting conditions such as abetalipoproteinaemia, carcinoid syndrome, chronic infections, cystic fibrosis, disseminated tuberculosis, hypothyroidism,[1] liver disease or a systemic inflammatory response,[2] as well as diseases that cause fat malabsorption, including impaired pancreatic and/or biliary secretions such as Crohn's and coeliac disease, radiation enteritis, ileal resection or damage.[3]
- Zinc deficiency impairs the absorption, transport and metabolism of vitamin A.[4]
- Protein deficiency can markedly affect vitamin A nutriture and in turn vitamin A deficiency can also influence protein metabolism.[5]
- Preterm infants are generally considered to be at risk because their plasma retinol concentrations are usually low.[6]

Vitamin B1

- Levels are affected by chronic alcoholism, gastric bypass surgery and gastrointestinal disorders.[7]
- Thiaminases that degrade thiamine are present in raw fish, fish paste and betel nuts.[7]
- Antithiamine factors are also found in caffeic acid, tannic acid and salicylic acid, as well as blueberries, black currants, red cabbages, beetroots and brussels sprouts.[8]

Vitamin B2

- Levels are affected by alcoholism,[9] diabetes mellitus, thyroid and adrenal insufficiency, liver disease, and gastrointestinal or biliary obstruction.[10]
- Several metals form chelates or complexes that may affect their bioavailability, such as copper, zinc, iron, tryptophan and vitamins B3 and C, as well as caffeine and saccharin.[11]
- Protein–energy malnutrition leads to increased urinary losses.[12]
- Exercise increases requirements.[12]

Vitamin B3

- Alcoholism, Crohn's disease and anorexia[12]

Vitamin B6

- Levels are affected by alcoholism, asthma, carpal tunnel syndrome, gestational diabetes, lactation, malabsorption, malnutrition, neonatal seizures, normal pregnancies, occupational exposure to hydrazine compounds, pellagra, preeclamptic oedema, renal dialysis, uraemia,[1] liver disease, oestrogen therapy, rheumatoid arthritis and HIV.[13]

- Vitamin B6 antagonists exist in foods such as some varieties of mushrooms, flax-seed meal, jack beans and mimosa, possibly via a systemic effect rather than interfering with its absorption.[14]
- Levels are affected by vitamin B2 deficiency.[15]

Vitamin B12
- Inadequate peptic digestion and gastric acid,[16] pancreatic insufficiency[3] and alcoholism may result in deficiency due to inadequate ingestion and absorption, as well as enhanced utilisation and excretion.[17]
- Bacterial overgrowth,[18] tropical or non-tropical sprue, Crohn's disease and inflammatory bowel disease may cause decreased levels.[1]
- Absorption through receptor sites in the ileum occurs in alkaline pH in the presence of calcium.[10]
- Diabetes, leukocytosis, hepatitis, cirrhosis, obesity and protein–energy malnutrition may cause increased levels.[1]

Folate
- Hyperthyroidism, pregnancy, haemolytic anaemia, the need for intensive care or any other sustained metabolic drain may increase folate need up to six- to eightfold.[19]
- Malabsorption of folate occurs secondary to an infection with *Giardia lamblia* and bacterial overgrowth.[10]
- Achlorhydria, oral contraceptive agents,[14] oral oestrogen and antacids affect folate levels.[20]
- Conditions of increased cellular turnover such as cancer affect folate levels.[10]
- Vitamin B12 deficiency may induce a secondary folate deficiency by reducing the activity of the enzyme methionine synthase, which activates folate.[10]

Biotin
- Achlorhydria and alcoholism affect biotin levels.[21]
- Biotinases that degrade biotin are found in the protein avidin in raw egg white.[21]

Vitamin C
- Levels are affected by alcoholism, anaemia, cancer, haemodialysis, hyperthyroidism, malabsorption, rheumatoid disease[1] and oral contraceptive pills, while acute infection and stress may increase urinary excretion.[10]
- Deficiency can occur secondary to some disease states such as liver disease, cancer, gastrointestinal disorders, cigarette smoking and environmental exposure.[10]
- Aspirin usage affects levels.[22]
- Excess iron and copper affect levels.[14]
- Pregnancy also lowers serum levels due to haemodilution and active transfer to the fetus, especially during the last trimester.[10]

Vitamin E
- Fat malabsorption syndromes such as coeliac disease, cystic fibrosis and chronic cholestatic liver disease[23], chronic pancreatitis, pancreatic carcinoma, chronic cholestasis,[1] gastric surgery and alcoholism affect levels.[12]
- Levels are affected by abetalipoproteinaemia (which involves a defect in chylomicron synthesis), hyperthyroidism, cirrhosis of the liver, hereditary spherocytosis

and β-thalassaemia, as well as associated with conditions such as bronchopulmonary dysplasia and retrolental fibroplasia.[24]
- Those with protein energy malnutrition[25] and premature[26] and low birth weight infants[27] and children with cystic fibrosis are often found to have a vitamin E deficiency, which may also occur in children with chronic cholestasis.[28]
- Obstructive liver disease may increase levels.[1]

Vitamin D
- Nephrotic syndrome, advanced renal failure, chronic liver diseases, severe small-bowel disease, Fanconi's syndrome, vitamin D-dependent rickets type I, neonatal hypocalcaemia, osteomalacia, osteoporosis, renal osteodystrophy affect levels.[24]
- Bowel resection, coeliac disease, inflammatory bowel disease, malabsorption, pancreatic insufficiency and thyrotoxicosis affect levels.[1]
- Magnesium deficiency, which may be due to both the decrease in parathyroid (PTH) secretion and a renal resistance to PTH, affects levels.[29]
- Lack of exposure to UV light combined with a bad diet affects levels.[24]
- Increased levels occur in primary hyperparathyroidism associated with hypophosphataemia, vitamin D-dependent rickets type II or sarcoidosis.[24]

Vitamin K
- Chronic fat malabsorption, liver disease, primary biliary cirrhosis, cancer, surgery and chronic alcoholism,[6] Crohn's disease, ulcerative colitis, chronic gastrointestinal diseases or resection,[30] obstructive jaundice, pancreatic disease, diarrhoea in infants, haemorrhagic disease of the newborn and hypoprothrombinaemia affect levels.[1]
- Levels drop in subjects treated with antibiotics for extended periods, as approximately half of vitamin K intake is provided by bacterial synthesis in the jejunum and ileum.[6]
- Ingestion of supraphysiological doses of vitamins A and E[31] may be inhibited by competitive mechanisms.

Magnesium
- Levels are affected by cardiovascular disease, myocardial infarction, toxaemia of pregnancy, hypertension or postsurgical complications, excessive vomiting and/or diarrhoea, burns, protein malnutrition, malabsorption syndromes, endocrine disorders such as diabetes mellitus, parathyroid disease, hyperparathyroidism with hypercalcaemia, hyperthyroidism and hyperaldosteronism,[32,33] as well as alcoholism, chronic glomerulonephritis, haemodialysis, pancreatitis, severe loss of body fluids as in diarrhoea, sweating and laxative abuse.[1]
- Pregnancy and lactation affect levels.[1]
- High levels of carbohydrates and ethanol affect levels.[34]
- Diets high in caffeine, calcium, protein,[35] although intakes of protein < 30 g/day may reduce magnesium absorption.[10]
- High dietary fibre, phytate, oxalate and phosphate intakes reduce magnesium absorption by binding cations.[36]
- Potassium depletion[3] and hypophosphataemia stimulate magnesium excretion.[37]
- Magnesium also shares a common renal reabsorption pathway with sodium and increased sodium results in magnesuria.[32]
- Levels may be increased in Addison's disease, adrenocortical insufficiency, severe diabetic acidosis, multiple myeloma, overuse of antacids, renal insufficiency, systemic

lupus erythematosus, tissue trauma,[3], increased parathyroid hormone,[33] hypocalcaemia, fluid depletion and hypothyroidism inhibit magnesium excretion.[34]

Calcium

- Hypoparathyroidism,[6] hypomagnesaemia,[29] phosphate supplementation and impaired vitamin D synthesis are also associated with depression of serum calcium levels.[38]
- Malabsorption is associated with acute pancreatitis and gastrointestinal diseases such as Crohn's and coeliac diseases, intestinal resection or bypass, and patients with renal failure caused by the reduced synthesis of 1,25-dihydroxyvitamin D.[33]
- Calcium absorption may be decreased with age, diabetes, chronic renal failure, non-tropical sprue and primary biliary cirrhosis.[6] Low protein diets can also affect calcium absorption[39] and cause decreased in bone mineral density.[40]
- Diets high in protein increase the urinary excretion of calcium, which is not compensated by increased calcium absorption.[41] Caffeine and sodium also increase urinary losses, while high phosphorus intakes reduce urinary losses although increased faecal losses, which may negate any effects on calcium balance.[33]
- Calcium absorption in the intestine may be inhibited by the presence of oxalate, which is found in a variety of vegetables such as spinach, beets, celery, eggplant, greens, okra and squash, as well as fruits such as strawberries, blackberries, blueberries, gooseberries and currants, nuts such as pecans and peanuts, and beverages such as tea, Ovaltine and cocoa. Oxalate chelates calcium and increases faecal excretion of the complex.[33]
- Divalent cations such as magnesium and calcium compete for intestinal absorption whenever an excess of either is in the gastrointestinal tract, while diets high in phosphorus relative to calcium have also been shown to impair calcium balance.[33]
- Hyperparathyroidism is the most common cause of hypercalcaemia.[6]
- Elevated serum levels occur in association with hyperthyroidism, sarcoidosis and when large parts of the body are immobilised, as well as in vitamin D intoxication and in patients with kidney stones, usually due to excessive absorption.[10]

Zinc

- Malabsorption syndromes such as Crohn's disease, short bowel syndrome and cystic fibrosis affect levels.[42] Increased urinary losses occur in alcohol, cirrhosis, infections, diabetes mellitus, renal tubular diseases, anorexia, starvation, catabolism such as burns, dialysis, pregnancy, oral contraceptives and hypoalbuminaemia.[12]
- Disease processes such as infection, surgery, pancreatic insufficiency and alcoholism may sometimes alter zinc absorption in humans.[43]
- Gastric acid secretion inhibition, phytate such as in soy protein, fibre in wheat and corn flour, tea, coffee, cheeses and cow's milk, calcium supplements and pregnancy affect levels.[43]
- As albumin appears to be the main portal carrier for newly absorbed zinc. Changes in the systemic level of albumin, such as inflammation or protein deficiency, may also alter zinc balance,[43] while high levels of protein intake enhance urinary excretion.[41]
- Inorganic iron in pharmacological doses may increase zinc uptake, and other studies suggest haem iron has the same effect.[43]

Iron

- Lead poisoning may be associated with iron deficiency, as lead and iron share a common absorptive mechanism the activity of which is enhanced in iron deficiency.[44]
- Copper and vitamin A deficiencies can diminish iron status,[45] while intermediate to high levels of manganese interfere with iron metabolism as shown by decreased haemoglobin concentrations and reversal by dietary iron supplementation.[46]
- High levels of zinc also decrease iron bioavailability, but it is not entirely clear whether this is a direct effect or is mediated indirectly through the copper effect on iron metabolism.[46] A ratio of 3:1 iron to zinc is desirable to prevent competitive interference.[47]
- Ascorbic acid enhances the absorption of non-haem iron from foods consumed at the same meal, while absorption of haem iron is not affected by vitamin C intake.[45]

Selenium

- Catabolic states and deficiency over time may occur with increased oxidative stress and a concurrent inadequate dietary intake.[38]
- Premature infants are found to have lower plasma concentrations of selenium and glutathione peroxidase than full-term infants. To compound this problem, other commonly used supplements such as iron, calcium and phosphate may impair selenium absorption. These infants also have an increased need because of the high risk of oxidative diseases such as bronchopulmonary dysplasia and retinopathy.[48]
- Other groups prone to a low status include low birth-weight neonates, alcoholics, patients with Down syndrome or acquired immune deficiency disease, and those with malabsorption syndromes such as coeliac disease and cystic fibrosis.[10]
- Iron deficiency may affect selenium absorption or increasing selenium use in the body. Another possibility is that iron or an iron-containing protein may be needed for glutathione peroxidase activity.[33]

Iodine

- Secondary iodine deficiency may develop in the presence of a number of diseases of the thyroid gland, pituitary or hypothalamus.[10]
- Goitrogens that inhibit iodine activity occur naturally in foods such as cabbage, broccoli, turnips and cauliflower, as well as in soybeans and bacterial products of *Escherichia coli* in drinking water.[49]
- In populations with a high intake of cassava, the thiocyanate present may act as a goitrogen and impair the uptake of iodine by the thyroid gland.[6]
- Iodide in large doses has the potential to block the synthesis of thyroid hormone, usually temporarily, after which hormone synthesis resumes.[50]

EFAs

- Malabsorption, obesity-related bypass surgery, alcoholism, malignancy, biliary disease and multiple sclerosis affect levels, while surgery and trauma patients need increases up to fivefold.[12]

References

1. Van Leeuwen A, et L. Davis's comprehensive handbook of laboratory and diagnostic tests with nursing implications. 2nd edn. Philadelphia: FA Davis Company, 2006.
2. Fell G, Talwar D. Assessment of status [Review article]. Curr Opin Clin Nutr Metab Care 1998;1(6):491–497.
3. Heimburger D, et al. Clinical manifestations of nutrient deficiencies and toxicities: a resume. In: Shils ME, et al. Modern nutrition in health and disease. USA: Lippincott Williams & Wilkins, 2006.
4. Solomons NW, Russell RM. The interaction of vitamin A and zinc: implications for human nutrition. Am J Clin Nutr 1980;33(9):2031–2040.
5. Mejia L. Vitamin A–nutrient interrelationships. In: Bauernfeind JC, ed. Vitamin A deficiency and its control. Orlando: Academic Press, 1986.
6. Sauberlich HE. Laboratory tests for the assessment of nutritional status. 2nd edn. USA: CRC Press, 1999.
7. Butterworth RF. Maternal thiamine deficiency: still a problem in some world communities. Am J Clin Nutr 2001;74(6):712–713.
8. Hilker DM, Somogyi JC. Antithiamins of plant origin: their chemical nature and mode of action. Ann NY Acad Sci 1982;378:137–145.
9. Pinto J, et al. Mechanisms underlying the differential effects of ethanol on the bioavailability of riboflavin and flavin adenine dinucleotide. J Clin Invest 1987;79(5):1343–1348.
10. Gibson R. Principles of nutritional assessment. 2nd edn. USA: Oxford University Press, 2005.
11. Rivlin R. Riboflavin. In: Ziegler EE, Filer Jr LJ, eds. Present knowledge in nutrition. 7th edn Washington: ILSI Press, 1996:167–173.
12. Ryan AS, Goldsmith LA. Nutrition and the skin. Clin Dermatol 1996;14(4):389–406.
13. Rall L, Meydani SN. Vitamin B(6) and immune competence. Nutr Rev 1993;51(8):217–225.
14. Sauberlich HE. Bioavailability of vitamins. Prog Food Nutr Sci 1985;9:1–33.
15. Leklem J. Vitamin B6. In: Ziegler EE, Filer Jr LJ, eds. Present knowledge in nutrition. 7th edn ILSI Press: Washington, 1996:175–183.
16. Ralph C. Subtle and atypical cobalamin deficiency states. Am J Hematol 1990;34(2):108–114.
17. Kanazawa S, Herbert V. Total corrinoid, cobalamin and cobalamin analogue levels may be normal in serum despite cobalamin in liver depletion in patients with alcoholism. Lab Invest 1985;53:108–110.
18. Cooke W, et al. The clinical and metabolic significance of jujunal diverticula. Gut 1963;4(2):115–131.
19. Herbert V. Making sense of laboratory tests of folate status: folate requirements to sustain normality. Am J Hematol 1987;26(2):199–207.
20. Thongprasom K, et al. Folate and vitamin B12 levels in patients with oral lichen planus, stomatitis or glossitis. Southeast Asian J Trop Med and Public Health 2001;32(3):643–647.
21. Bonjour JP. Biotin in man's nutrition and therapy—a review. Internat. J Vit Nutr Res 1977;47:107–118.
22. Basu T. The influence of drugs with particular reference to asprin on the bioavailability of vitamin C. In: Counsell J, Hornig D, eds. Vitamin C. London: Applied Science Publishers, 1981:273–281.
23. Rader DJ, Brewer Jr HB. Abetalipoproteinemia: new insights into lipoprotein assembly and vitamin E. Metabolism from a rare genetic disease. JAMA 1993;270(7):865–869.
24. De Leenheer AP, et al. Chromatography of fat-soluble vitamins in clinical chemistry. J Chromatogr 1988;429:3–58.
25. Kalra V, et al. Vitamin E deficiency and associated neurological deficits in children with protein–energy malnutrition. J Trop Pediatr 1998;44(5):291–295.
26. Kelly FJ, et al. Time course of vitamin E repletion in the premature infant. Br J Nutr 1990;63(3):631–638.
27. Bieri JG, Evarts RP. Tocopherols and polyunsaturated fatty acids in human tissues. Am J Clin Nutr 1975;28(7):717–720.
28. Sokol RJ, et al. Vitamin E deficiency neuropathy in children with fat malabsorption studies in cystic fibrosis and chronic cholestasis. Ann N YAcad Sci 1989;570:156–169.
29. Fatemi S, et al. Effect of experimental human magnesium depletion on parathyroid hormone secretion and 1,25-dihydroxyvitamin D metabolism. J Clin Endocrinol Metab 1991;73(5):1067–1072.
30. Krasinski SD, et al. The prevalence of vitamin K deficiency in chronic gastrointestinal disorders. Am J Clin Nutr 1985;41(3):639–643.
31. Olson R. The function and metabolism of vitamin K. Ann Rev Nutr 1984;4:281–337.
32. Ryzen E. Magnesium homeostasis in critically ill patients. Magnesium 1989;8(3–4):201–212.
33. Groff J, Gropper S. Advanced nutrition and human metabolism. 3rd edn. USA: Wadsworth/Thompson Learning, 2000.
34. Whang R, et al. Magnesium homeostasis and clinical disorders of magnesium deficiency. Ann Pharmacother 1994;28(2):220–226.
35. Kesteloot H, Joossens JV. The relationship between dietary intake and urinary excretion of sodium, potassium, calcium and magnesium: Belgian Interuniversity Research on Nutrition and Health. J Hum Hypertens 1990;4:527–533.
36. Rude RK. Magnesium deficiency: a cause of heterogenous disease in humans. J Bone Mineral Res 1998;13(4):749–758.
37. Maclean AR, Renwick C. Audit of pre-operative starvation. Anaesthesia 1993;48(2):164–166.
38. Prelack K, Sheridan RL. Micronutrient supplementation in the critically ill patient: strategies for clinical practice. J Trauma 2001;51(3):601–620.
39. Kerstetter JE, et al. Dietary protein affects intestinal calcium absorption. Am J Clin Nutr 1998;68(4):859–865.
40. Hannan MT, et al. Effect of dietary protein on bone loss in elderly men and women: the Framingham Osteoporosis Study. J Bone Miner Res 2000;15(12):2504–2512.
41. Mahalko JR, et al. Effect of a moderate increase in dietary protein on the retention and excretion of Ca, Cu, Fe, Mg, P, and Zn by adult males. Am J Clin Nutr 1983;37(1):8–14.
42. Pironi L, et al. Urinary zinc excretion in Crohn's disease. Dig Dis Sci 1987;32(4):358–362.
43. Cousins RJ. Zinc. In: Ziegler EE, Filer LJ Jr, eds. Present knowledge in nutrition. 7th edn. ILSI Press: Washington, 1996:293–306.
44. Smith H. Diagnosis in paediatric haematology. New York: Churchill Livingstone, 1996:6–40.
45. Lynch SR. Interaction of iron with other nutrients. Nutr Rev 1997;55(4):102–110.
46. O'Dell B. Bioavailability of and interactions among trace elements. In: Chandra RK, ed. Trace elements in nutrition of children. Raven Press: New York, 1985:41–55.
47. Rushton DH. Nutritional factors and hair loss. Clin Exp Dermatol 2002;27(5):400–408.
48. Salmenpera L. Detecting subclinical deficiency of essential trace elements in children with special reference to zinc and selenium. Clin Biochem 1997;30(2):115–120.
49. Gaitan E. Goitrogens in food and water. Annu Rev Nutr 1990;10:21–39.
50. Wolff J, Chaikoff IL. Plasma inorganic iodide as a homeostatic regulator of thyroic function. J Biol Chem 1948;174(2):555–564.

Appendix 6

Taxonomic cross-reference of major herbs

BOTANICAL NAME	COMMON NAME
Achillea millefolium	Yarrow
Aesculus hippocastanum	Horse chestnut
Agathosma betulina	Buchu
Agropyron repens	Couchgrass
Albizzia lebbeck	Albizzia
Alchemillia vulgaris	Lady's mantle
Aloe spp.	Aloe vera
Althaea officinalis	Marshmallow
Andrographis paniculata	Andrographis
Anemone pulsatilla	Pasque flower, pulsatilla
Angelica sinensis	Dong quai
Apium graveolens	Celery seed
Arctium lappa	Burdock
Arctostaphylos uva-ursi	Uva ursi, bearberry
Arnica montana	Arnica
Artemisia absinthium	Wormwood
Asclepias tuberosa	Pleurisy root
Asparagus racemosus	Shatavari
Astragalus membranaceus	Astragalus
Avena sativa	Oats
Azadirachta indica	Neem
Bacopa monnieri	Bacopa, brahmi
Baptisia tinctoria	Baptisia
Berberis aquifolium	Oregon grape
Berberis aristata	Indian barberry
Berberis vulgaris	Barberry
Bupleurum falcatum	Bupleurum
Calendula officinalis	Calendula, marigold
Capsella bursa-pastoris	Shepherd's purse
Caulophyllum thalictroides	Blue cohosh
Centella asiatica	Gotu kola
Chamaelirium luteum	False unicorn root
Chelidonium majus	Greater celandine
Chionanthus virginicus	Fringe tree
Cimicifuga racemosa	Black cohosh
Cinnamomum zeylanicum	Cinnamon
Codonopsis pilosula	Codonopsis
Coleus forskohlii	Coleus

BOTANICAL NAME	COMMON NAME
Commiphora molmol	Myrrh
Crataegus monogyna	Hawthorn
Crataeva nurvala	Crataeva
Curcuma longa	Turmeric
Cynara scolymus	Globe artichoke
Dioscorea villosa	Wild Yam
Echinacea angustifolia Echinacea purpurea	Echinacea
Eleutherococcus senticosus	Siberian ginseng, eleutherococcus
Epilobium parviflorum	Willow herb
Equisetum arvense	Horsetail
Eschscholzia californica	Californian poppy
Euphorbia hirta	Euphorbia
Euphrasia officinalis	Eyebright
Filipendula ulmaria	Meadowsweet
Foeniculum vulgare	Fennel
Fucus vesicolus	Bladderwrack
Galega officinalis	Goat's rue
Galium aparine	Cleavers, clivers
Gentiana lutea	Gentian
Geranium maculatum	Cranesbill
Ginkgo biloba	Ginkgo
Glycyrrhiza glabra	Liquorice
Grindelia camporum	Grindelia
Gymnema sylvestre	Gymnema
Hamamelis vulgaris	Witch hazel
Harpagophytum procumbens	Devil's claw
Hemidesmus indicus	Hemisdesmus
Humulus lupulus	Hops
Hydrastis canadensis	Goldenseal
Hypericum perforatum	St John's wort
Hyssopus officinalis	Hyssop
Iberis amara	Bitter candytuft
Inula helenium	Elecampane
Iris versicolor	Blue flag
Lavandula spp.	Lavender
Leonurus cardiaca	Motherwort
Lycopus virginicus	Bugleweed
Marrubium vulgare	White horehound
Matricaria recutita	Chamomile
Melissa officinalis	Lemon balm

(Continued)

BOTANICAL NAME	COMMON NAME
Mentha piperita	Peppermint
Mentha spicata	Spearmint
Paeonia lactiflora	White peony, peony
Panax ginseng	Korean ginseng
Panax notoginseng	Tienchi ginseng
Passiflora incarnata	Passionflower
Peumus boldo	Boldo
Phytolacca decandra	Poke root
Piper methysticum	Kava
Piscidia erythrina	Jamaica dogwood
Plantago ovata	Psyllium
Prunus serotina	Wild cherry
Rehmannia glutinosa	Rehmannia
Rhamnus purshiana	Cascara
Rosmarinus officinalis	Rosemary
Rubus idaeus	Red raspberry leaf
Rumex crispus	Yellow dock
Ruscus aculeatus	Butcher's broom
Salvia officinalis	Sage
Sambucus nigra	Elder flower
Schisandra chinensis	Schisandra
Scutellaria baicalensis	Baical skullcap
Scutellaria lateriflora	Skullcap
Serenoa repens	Saw palmetto
Silybum marianum	Milk thistle, St Mary's thistle
Smilax ornata	Sarsaparilla
Solidago virgaurea	Goldenrod
Stellaria media	Chickweed
Symphytum officinale	Comfrey
Tabebuia avellanedae	Pau d'arco
Tanacetum parthenium	Feverfew
Taraxacum officinale	Dandelion
Thuja occidentalis	Thuja
Thymus vulgaris	Thyme
Tilia spp.	Linden, lime flowers
Trifolium pratense	Red clover
Trigonella foenum-graecum	Fenugreek
Turnera diffusa	Damiana
Tylophora indica	Tylophora
Ulmus fulva	Slippery elm
Uncaria tomentosa	Cat's claw

BOTANICAL NAME	COMMON NAME
Urtica dioica	Nettle, stinging nettle
Vaccinum prunifolium	Bilberry
Valeriana edulis	Mexican valerian
Valeriana officinalis	Valerian
Verbascum thapsus	Mullein
Verbena officinalis	Vervain
Viburnum opulus	Cramp bark
Viburnum prunifolium	Black haw
Viscum album	Mistletoe
Vitex agnus-castus	Chaste tree
Withania somnifera	Withania, ashwaganda
Zanthoxylum clava-herculis	Prickly ash
Zea mays	Cornsilk
Zingiber officinale	Ginger
Zizyphus spinosa	Spiny jujube

COMMON NAME	BOTANICAL NAME
Albizzia	*Albizzia lebbeck*
Aloe vera	*Aloe* spp.
Andrographis	*Andrographis paniculata*
Arnica	*Arnica montana*
Astragalus	*Astragalus membranaceus*
Bacopa, brahmi	*Bacopa monnieri*
Baical skullcap	*Scutellaria baicalensis*
Baptisia	*Baptisia tinctoria*
Barberry	*Berberis vulgaris*
Bearberry	*Arctostaphylus uva-ursi*
Bilberry	*Vaccinum prunifolium*
Bitter candytuft	*Iberis amara*
Black cohosh	*Cimicifuga racemosa*
Black haw	*Viburnum prunifolium*
Bladderwrack	*Fucus vesicolus*
Blue cohosh	*Caulophyllum thalictroides*
Blue flag	*Iris versicolor*
Boldo	*Peumus boldo*
Buchu	*Agathosma betulina*
Bugleweed	*Lycopus virginicus*
Bupleurum	*Bupleurum falcatum*
Burdock	*Arctium lappa*
Butcher's broom	*Ruscus aculeatus*
Calendula, marigold	*Calendula officinalis*

(Continued)

COMMON NAME	BOTANICAL NAME
Californian poppy	*Eschscholzia californica*
Cascara	*Rhamnus purshiana*
Cat's claw	*Uncaria tomentosa*
Celery seed	*Apium graveolens*
Chamomile	*Matricaria recutita*
Chaste tree	*Vitex agnus-castus*
Chickweed	*Stellaria media*
Cinnamon	*Cinnamomum zeylanicum*
Cleavers, clivers	*Galium aparine*
Codonopsis	*Codonopsis pilosula*
Coleus	*Coleus forskohlii*
Comfrey	*Symphytum officinale*
Cornsilk	*Zea mays*
Couchgrass	*Agropyron repens*
Cramp bark	*Viburnum opulus*
Cranesbill	*Geranium maculatum*
Crataeva	*Crataeva nurvala*
Damiana	*Turnera diffusa*
Dandelion	*Taraxacum officinale*
Devil's claw	*Harpagophytum procumbens*
Dong quai	*Angelica sinensis*
Echinacea	*Echinacea angustifolia* *Echinacea purpurea*
Elder flower	*Sambucus nigra*
Elecampane	*Inula helenium*
Euphorbia	*Euphorbia hirta*
Eyebright	*Euphrasia officinalis*
False unicorn root	*Chamaelirium luteum*
Fennel	*Foeniculum vulgare*
Fenugreek	*Trigonella foenum-graecum*
Feverfew	*Tanacetum parthenium*
Fringe tree	*Chionanthus virginicus*
Gentian	*Gentiana lutea*
Ginger	*Zingiber officinale*
Ginkgo	*Ginkgo biloba*
Globe artichoke	*Cynara scolymus*
Goat's rue	*Galega officinalis*
Goldenrod	*Solidago virgaurea*
Goldenseal	*Hydrastis canadensis*
Gotu kola	*Centella asiatica*
Greater celandine	*Chelidonium majus*
Grindelia	*Grindelia camporum*

COMMON NAME	BOTANICAL NAME
Gymnema	*Gymnema sylvestre*
Hawthorn	*Crataegus monogyna*
Hemisdesmus	*Hemidesmus indicus*
Hops	*Humulus lupulus*
Horse chestnut	*Aesculus hippocastanum*
Horsetail	*Equisetum arvense*
Hyssop	*Hyssopus officinalis*
Indian barberry	*Berberis aristata*
Jamaica dogwood	*Piscidia erythrina*
Kava	*Piper methysticum*
Korean ginseng	*Panax ginseng*
Lady's mantle	*Alchemillia vulgaris*
Lavender	*Lavandula officinalis*
Lemon balm	*Melissa officinalis*
Liquorice	*Glycyrrhiza glabra*
Linden, lime flowers	*Tilia* spp.
Marshmallow	*Althaea officinalis*
Meadowsweet	*Filipendula ulmaria*
Mexican valerian	*Valeriana edulis*
Milk thistle, St Mary's thistle	*Silybum marianum*
Mistletoe	*Viscum album*
Motherwort	*Leonurus cardiaca*
Mullein	*Verbascum thapsus*
Myrrh	*Commiphora molmol*
Neem	*Azadirachta indica*
Nettle, stinging nettle	*Urtica dioica*
Oats	*Avena sativa*
Oregon grape	*Berberis aquifolium*
Pasque flower, pulsatilla	*Anemone pulsatilla*
Passionflower	*Passiflora incarnata*
Pau d'arco	*Tabebuia avellanedae*
Peppermint	*Mentha piperita*
Pleurisy root	*Asclepias tuberosa*
Poke root	*Phytolacca decandra*
Prickly ash	*Zanthoxylum clava-herculis*
Psyllium	*Plantago ovata*
Red clover	*Trifolium pratense*
Red rasberry leaf	*Rubus idaeus*
Rehmannia	*Rehmannia glutinosa*
Rosemary	*Rosmarinus officinalis*
Sage	*Salvia officinalis*

(Continued)

COMMON NAME	BOTANICAL NAME
Sarsaparilla	*Smilax ornata*
Saw palmetto	*Serenoa repens*
Schisandra	*Schisandra chinensis*
Shatavari	*Asparagus racemosus*
Shepherd's purse	*Capsella bursa-pastoris*
Siberian ginseng, eleutherococcus	*Eleutherococcus senticosus*
Skullcap	*Scutellaria lateriflora*
Slippery elm	*Ulmus fulva*
Spearmint	*Mentha spicata*
Spiny jujube	*Zizyphus spinosa*
St John's wort	*Hypericum perforatum*
Thuja	*Thuja occidentalis*
Thyme	*Thymus vulgaris*
Tienchi ginseng	*Panax notoginseng*
Turmeric	*Curcuma longa*
Tylophora	*Tylophora indica*
Uva ursi	*Arctostaphylos uva-ursi*
Valerian	*Valeriana officinalis*
Vervain	*Verbena officinalis*
White horehound	*Marrubium vulgare*
White peony, peony	*Paeonia lactiflora*
Wild cherry	*Prunus serotina*
Wild yam	*Dioscorea villosa*
Willow herb	*Epilobium parviflorum*
Witch hazel	*Hamamelis vulgaris*
Withania, ashwaganda	*Withania somnifera*
Wormwood	*Artemisia absinthium*
Yarrow	*Achillea millefolium*
Yellow dock	*Rumex crispus*

Appendix 7

Traditional Chinese medicine: the six evils

Traditional Chinese medicine identifies six pernicious influences or environmental factors playing a role in disease. Combinations of these may also manifest. These may be adapted to contemporary naturopathic practice.[1,2]

EVIL	INDICATIONS	TONGUE	PULSE	TREATMENT
Heat	The body as a whole or in parts will feel or appear hot, such as red painful skin lesions, fevers, headaches and thirst, desire for cold or irritability.	Red tongue which may be long and/or yellow coating	Rapid	Cleansing and draining herbs
Cold	A person feels cold or has a pale appearance, with a corresponding aversion to cold, and seeks warmth. There are thin watery and clear fluid discharges, such as clear nasal discharge, pale urine or watery loose stools. The cold pathogen obstructs and contracts, leading to slow movement and underactivity, as well as blocking circulation and causing severe, sharp and cramping pain that is relieved by heat. There is a common saying: 'Retention of cold causes pain'.	White tongue coat and/or pale body	Slow	Stimulating and warming herbs such as sulfur or volatile, oil-rich species
Dry	Dry or cracked skin, scanty urination, dry lips and stools, which emphasise dehydration	Dry, cracked	Thin	Moistening herbs such as demulcent and soothing herbs. Increasing water intake and avoiding diuretics such as caffeine and alcohol would also be of benefit.
Damp	Wet, heavy and slow conditions that tend to linger and may present as a heavy dull pain as opposed to the sharp intense cold type of pain. Cloudy or sticky excretions may also present as heavy menstrual cycles, oozing skin eruptions or thickened mucus.[3] Damp can also obstruct Qi, leading to heavy, stiff limbs and aching joints, feelings of fullness in the chest or abdomen that may cause indigestion, loss of appetite, nausea or diarrhoea.	Sticky greasy tongue coat, white with cold or yellow with heat	Slippery	Drying herbs such as those with astringent and diuretic properties which may be rich in tannins or pungent. Heavy, rich, sweet and deep-fried foods should be avoided where a damp pathogen exists, particularly in the gastrointestinal tract.

(Continued)

EVIL	INDICATIONS	TONGUE	PULSE	TREATMENT
Wind	Wind in the body is similar of that in nature, where it produces rapid onset and changes in symptoms, while these move from place to place in the body. Related to movement, it is linked to pain, itching or skin eruptions that change location, tremors, twitching, dizziness, convulsions, sudden onset headaches, sneezing, coughs and an aversion to drafts.	Varies depending on whether associated with cold or heat	Floating	Diaphoretic or alternative herbal medicines
Summer heat	A purely external influence resulting from exposure to extreme heat; appears as a high fever with heavy sweating, which leads to exhaustion and depleted fluids.[3]	Red tip and sides	Rapid	Energetically 'cold' herbs, e.g. bitters, may be used to 'drain heat'.

References

1. Maciocia G. The foundations of Chinese Medicine. New York: Churchill Livingstone, 1996.

2. Ross J. Combining western herbs and Chinese medicine: principles, practice and materia medica. Seattle: Greenfields Press, 2006.

Appendix 8

Traditional Chinese medicine: tongue diagnosis

ATTRIBUTE[1]	DESCRIPTION[1]	CAUSE[1]
Colour	Pale	Deficiency of yang (tongue also wet) or Blood deficiency (dry tongue)
	Red	Heat
	Deep-Red	Severe heat
	Purple	Blood stasis
	Blue	Interior cold giving rise to Blood Stasis
Shape	Thin	Blood deficiency (pale) or yin deficiency (red)
	Swollen	Damp or damp heat (red)
	Stiff	Interior wind
	Flaccid	Yin deficiency
	Long	Heat (particularly heart heat)
	Short	Interior cold (if pale and wet) Yin deficiency (red and peeled)
	Cracked	Full heat or yin deficiency
	Quivering	Spleen Qi deficiency
	Teethmarks	Spleen Qi deficiency
Coating	White	Cold pattern
	Yellow	Full-heat pattern
	Grey/black	Extreme cold/heat (if wet/dry)

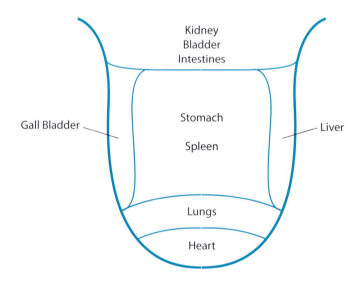

Reference

1. Maciocia G. The foundations of Chinese medicine. New York: Churchill Livingstone, 1996.

Appendix 9

Traditional Chinese medicine: pulse diagnosis

Aside from the aforementioned, the pulse may be felt on three levels: superficial, middle and deep, pertaining to the force of pressure applied to the wrist on palpation.[1]

PULSE DEPTH	ENERGY LEVEL	ORGANS
Superficial	Exterior	Heart and lungs
Middle	Stomach and spleen	Stomach and spleen
Deep	Interior	Kidneys and liver

A further differential diagnosis on a simple pulse technique is the pulse separated into three pulse positions—front, middle and rear—with the former position closest to the hand.[1]

PULSE POSITION	BODY POSITION	ORGANS
Front	Upper	Heart and lungs
Middle	Middle	Stomach and spleen
Rear	Lower	Kidneys and liver

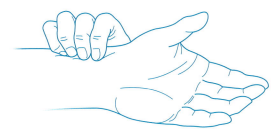

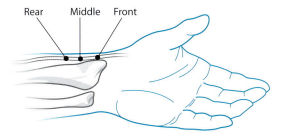

Reference

1. Maciocia G. The foundations of Chinese medicine. New York: Churchill Livingstone, 1996.

Appendix 10

Systematic review of herbal immunomodulators

From a systematic review of the literature, Spelman et al.[1] have identified a number of herbs as having their action through modulation of one or more cytokines. While some herbs were shown to stimulate pro-inflammatory cytokine secretion, other herbs had suppressive actions on these cytokines. Some herbs were shown to do both, depending on dosage, cell type and type of stimulus. It is important to know the context of the cells or animals used in order to know how results of in vitro, ex vivo (stimulation of cells to secrete cytokines after blood has been taken) and in vivo cytokine studies should be interpreted.

A case in point is that *Echinacea purpurea* was shown to stimulate pro-inflammatory cytokine production, in a manner comparable to lipopolysaccharides (*Echinacea* increased levels of IL-10, TNF-α, IL-1β and IL-6 ($p < 0.05$) more than culture medium alone).[2] While this may be desirable in the early stages of a respiratory tract infection in order to hasten the cell-mediated response to an infection, it may not be desirable in an individual with an overactive cell mediated response.

It would appear from this study that *Echinacea* may be contraindicated in chronic inflammation. However, based on this one study, this conclusion would be quite premature. The human macrophages used for this in vitro study came from one 50-year-old female. Details of possible confounds for cytokine production, such as preexisting health concerns, atopic status, stress or inflammatory status or medication intake, were not given. Further, oestrogen levels are usually fluctuating widely at this time of life, and the presence of oestrogen receptors on macrophages may influence cytokine production. For this reason, most studies of cytokines exclude perimenopausal women, and many exclude women altogether. This finding can hardly be considered representative.

While in vitro studies are interesting, they must not be taken as a 'gold standard' on how a herb may affect cytokine profiles. There are so many factors that influence cytokine production and, by taking cells out of context, in vitro and ex vivo studies risk overlooking factors that regulate cytokine production in the plasma. It is also difficult to extrapolate the in vivo equivalent concentrations from herb concentrations that have been effective in vitro. Some herbs have been found to be suppressive at low concentrations and stimulatory at high concentrations in vitro.[1] With these major methodological limitations in mind, those Western herbs included in the systematic review by Spelman et al.[1] that were shown to suppress or inhibit pro-inflammatory cytokine production have been summarised in the table below (see Table 6.4 in Chapter 6 for additional review).

Western herbs shown to suppress or inhibit pro-inflammatory cytokine production

INTERVENTION	METHODOLOGY	RESULT	COMMENT
Allium sativum (garlic, fresh crushed)[3]	In vitro study of stimulated whole blood and peripheral blood monocytes from healthy volunteers	↓ TNF-α, IL-1α, IL-6, IL-8, IFN-γ (all $p < 0.05$) ↑ IL-10 ($p < 0.05$)	Various concentrations of garlic were effective at down-regulating the pro-inflammatory cytokines and up-regulating the anti-inflammatory cytokine, IL-10

(Continued)

Western herbs shown to suppress or inhibit pro-inflammatory cytokine production *(Continued)*

INTERVENTION	METHODOLOGY	RESULT	COMMENT
Andrographolide from *Andrographis paniculata*[4]	In vitro study of human endothelial cells	↓ TNF-induced up-regulation of intercellular adhesion molecule-1 (ICAM-1) expression ↓ TNF-induced endothelial monocytes adhesion (dose-dependent)	The significance of the difference levels were not given in the study. However, andrographolide reduced adhesions comparable to the anti-ICAM-1 antibody, which significantly reduced adhesion ($p < 0.001$).
Astragalus membranaceus[5]	80 SLE patients randomly assigned into two groups. Both continued to receive conventional treatment (corticosteroids). One group were also given injection of radix astragali.	Both groups improved a range of immunological parameters (all $p < 0.05$) from baseline. *Astragalus* group improved significantly more than steroid treatment alone ($p < 0.05$)	Abstract only was available (article in Chinese) so unable to determine many factors such as how much *A. membranaceus* was used and for how long.
Astragalus membranaceus[6]	In vitro study of human amnion cells, stimulated with LPS	↓ IL-6 (dose-dependent) ($p < 0.05$) ↓ PGE_2 ($p < 0.01$) ↓ LTC_4 ($p < 0.01$) all compared with controls	*A. membranaceus* was anti-inflammatory by inhibiting IL-6 and both COX-2 and lipoxygenase (LO) pathways. Inhibition was substantial.
Hydrastis canadensis and *Astragalus membranaceus* extracts[7]	In vitro study with mouse macrophages	*H. canadensis*: ↓ TNF-α, ↓ IL-6, ↓ IL-12, ↓ IL-10 ($p < 0.05$). *A. membranaceus* not as effective but ↓ IL-6, ↓ IL-12, ↓ IL-10 at the highest doses ($p < 0.05$) but did not suppress TNF-α.	Herbs were commercially available, and two different brands of each herb were compared. One brand of *A. membranceus* suppressed cytokines at the highest dose (1:50 dilution). Both brands of golden seal were effective.
Panax quinquefolium[8]	Mice given oral doses of American ginseng 200 mg/kg or placebo before stress	↓ IL-6 and ↓ IL-2 in brain cortex and hippocampus induced by stress (both $p < 0.001$) compared with placebo	It was interesting to note that in this study, half the dosage of American ginseng (100 mg/kg) was not effective.
Smilacis glabrae radix[9]	Adjuvant-induced arthritis in rats, as an animal model for human rheumatoid arthritis	↓ IL-1 ↓ TNF-α ↓ NO products All compared with control ($p < 0.01$).	*S. glabrae* reduced inflammatory mediators almost to level of rats with no disease, much more so than the corticosteroid prednisolone.
Scutellaria baicalensis[10]	In vitro study of mouse microglial cells, stimulated with LPS	↓ TNF-α ↓ NO production ($p < 0.05$)	The compounds baicalein and wogonin were thought to exert the anti-inflammatory effects.
Withania somnifera[11]	Normal mice ($n = 3$ per group) were given one 20 mg dose *W. somnifera* and sacrificed 24 hours later, blood drawn from heart puncture.	↓ TNF-α ($p < 0.01$) ↑ IL-2 and ↑ IFN-γ (both $p < 0.001$)	When the anti-inflammatory drug cyclophosphamlde was administered, all three cytokines were reduced. *W. somnifera* increased IL-2 and IFN-γ to baseline.

Western herbs shown to suppress or inhibit pro-inflammatory cytokine production *(Continued)*

INTERVENTION	METHODOLOGY	RESULT	COMMENT
Echinacea spp. (Coneflower)	A range of in vitro and in vivo studies	Alkylamides bind to CB2 receptors invoking increased levels of IL-10, TNF-α, IL-1 β and IL-6[2,12]	In vitro studies using polysaccharides may not extrapolate to human effects due to low bioavailability

References

1. Spelman K, et al. Modulation of cytokine expression by traditional medicines: a review of herbal immunomodulators. Altern Med Rev 2006;11(2):128–150.
2. Burger RA, et al. Echinacea-induced cytokine production by human macrophages. Int J Immunopharmacol 1997;19(7):371–379.
3. Hodge G, et al. *Allium sativum* (garlic) suppresses leukocyte inflammatory cytokine production in vitro: potential therapeutic use in the treatment of inflammatory bowel disease. Cytometry 2002;48(4):209–215.
4. Habtemariam S. Andrographolide inhibits the tumour necrosis factor-α-induced upregulation of ICAM-1 expression and endothelial-monocyte adhesion. Phytother Res 1998;12(1):37–40.
5. Cai XY, et al. [Effects of radix *Astragali* injection on apoptosis of lymphocytes and immune function in patients with systemic lupus erythematosus]. Zhongguo Zhong Xi Yi Jie He Za Zhi 2006;26(5):443–445.
6 Shon YH, et al. Effect of Astragali radix extract on lipopolysaccharide-induced inflammation in human amnion. Biol Pharm Bull 2002;25(1):77–80.
7. Clement-Kruzel S, et al. Immune modulation of macrophage pro-inflammatory response by goldenseal and *Astragalus* extracts. J Med Food 2008;11(3):493–498.
8. Rasheed N, et al. Involvement of monoamines and pro-inflammatory cytokines in mediating the anti-stress effects of *Panax quinquefolium*. J Ethnopharmacol 2008;117(2):257–262.
9. Jiang J, Xu Q. Immunomodulatory activity of the aqueous extract from rhizome of *Smilax glabra* in the later phase of adjuvant-induced arthritis in rats. J Ethnopharmacol 2003;85(1):53–59.
10. Kim YO, et al. Cytoprotective effect of *Scutellaria baicalensis* in CA1 hippocampal neurons of rats after global cerebral ischemia. J Ethnopharmacol 2001;77(2–3):183–188.
11. Davis L, Kuttan G. Effect of *Withania somnifera* on cytokine production in normal and cyclophosphamide treated mice. Immunopharmacol Immunotoxicol 1999;21(4):695–703.
12. Gertsch J, et al. Echinacea alkylamides modulate TNF-alpha gene expression via cannabinoid receptor CB2 and multiple signal transduction pathways. FEBS Lett 2004;577(3):563–569.

INDEX